Fundamentals of Pediatric Surgery

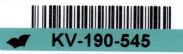

Fundamentals of Pediatric Surgery

Edited by

Peter Mattei, MD, FAAP, FACS

The Children's Hospital of Philadelphia, Philadelphia, PA, USA

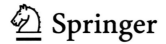 Springer

Editor
Peter Mattei, MD, FAAP, FACS
Assistant Professor of Surgery,
University of Pennsylvania School of Medicine,
Division of General, Thoracic and Fetal Surgery,
The Children's Hospital of Philadelphia,
Philadelphia, PA, USA

ISBN 978-1-4419-6642-1   e-ISBN 978-1-4419-6643-8
DOI 10.1007/978-1-4419-6643-8
Springer New York Dordrecht Heidelberg London

Printed on acid-free paper

Springer is part of Springer Science+Business Media (www.springer.com)

To my wife, partner, and best friend, Kim, for her support and encouragement every day, and To Kim, Gina, Peter, Joey, and Michael, for the inspiration and hope for the future I derive from watching them grow, learn and dream.

Preface

Fundamentals of Pediatric Surgery, like its predecessor *Surgical Directives: Pediatric Surgery*, provides practicing pediatric surgeons and adult general surgeons with authoritative discourses that were written by recognized experts and cover the fundamental principles of clinical pediatric surgery. The goal of the editor and the authors is simple: provide readers with a unique resource consisting of practical and clinically oriented chapters that reflect the real-world experience of expert pediatric surgeons. Given the pace of new advances in Pediatric Surgery, we felt the time was right for the book to be updated and improved. The result of these improvements and enhancements is *Fundamentals of Pediatric Surgery*.

Fundamentals of Pediatric Surgery is based on a simple but important philosophy: provide a practical and up-to-date resource for the practicing surgeon detailing the specific needs and special considerations surrounding the surgical care of children. We especially wanted to convey this information in an accessible and pleasing format. Written by an experienced surgeon or clinician, each chapter has been carefully edited to maintain continuity in style and format while preserving the unique voice of the experienced and knowledgeable contributing author. This new edition also includes highlighted textboxes that emphasize important points and critical concepts along with a list of suggested reading. Finally, every chapter is followed by the editor's comments, which are intended to provide more in-depth analysis, a distinct opinion, or simply additional useful information.

In addition to serving as a useful reference for pediatric surgeons and general surgeons in clinical practice, *Fundamentals of Pediatric Surgery* is also specifically designed to be used by general surgical residents rotating in pediatric surgery and chief residents who have chosen to obtain further specialized training in a Pediatric Surgery fellowship program. The American Board of Surgery and the Accreditation Council for Graduate Medical Education (ACGME) consider experience in the clinical aspects of pediatric surgery a necessary and important aspect of the education and training of the general surgeon and every General Surgery resident is expected to participate in a Pediatric Surgery rotation during their residency. These rotations are typically brief but can be quite hectic, with little time to read a comprehensive pediatric surgical textbook, especially when what one really needs is a practical guide to the everyday care of the pediatric surgical patient. The monographs provided by *Fundamentals of Pediatric Surgery* are concise and easy to read, filled with detailed and relevant information that can help you care for the patient in the clinic today or as a consultation on the Pediatrics service. The goal is not to describe every possible management strategy, but rather at least one reasonable and proven approach endorsed by an experienced surgeon in a context that includes a discussion of the underlying principles of care and essential issues to be considered when faced with a particular clinical entity.

The Pediatric Surgery fellow will find this book to be a rich and up-to-date source of pertinent information related to the actual day-to-day care of the child with a surgical disease process. Furthermore, it will provide the foundation for what will undoubtedly prove to be an exciting and life-long education in the complexities of the surgical care of children. Finally, it is intended to be a valuable resource and study guide for preparation for the written and oral American Board of Surgery certifying examinations in Pediatric Surgery.

It is our sincere hope that *Fundamentals of Pediatric Surgery*, designed with the more advanced practitioner in mind, will prove to be a useful and valuable complement to the many excellent pediatric surgical texts currently available.

Philadelphia, Pennsylvania   Peter Mattei, MD, FAAP, FACS
November 2010

Acknowledgments

This book is the result of a team effort that includes the support and encouragement of my Surgeon-in-Chief, N. Scott Adzick, the help and accommodations of my partners in the Division of General, Thoracic and Fetal Surgery, and the time and expertise of our administrative assistants. I was inspired to produce this book by my many excellent teachers and mentors when I was a resident and pediatric surgery fellow, and over the years I have been motivated to forge ahead by the experience of being a teacher and mentor to the many excellent pediatric surgery fellows and general surgery residents I have had the privilege to help train over the years. I must also acknowledge the hard work and dedication of the pediatric surgeons and other experts in the field who have contributed chapters for this text and, more importantly, their continued devotion to a career of working with children who need our help and who ultimately make it all worthwhile.

Contents

Part I   Perioperative Care

1 **Preoperative Assessment and Preparation** 3
Ari Y. Weintraub and Lynne G. Maxwell

2 **Prenatal Diagnosis and Genetic Counseling** 17
R. Douglas Wilson

3 **Epidural and Regional Anesthesia** 23
Arjunan Ganesh and John B. Rose

4 **Enteral Nutrition** 27
L. Grier Arthur and Shaheen J. Timmapuri

5 **Parenteral Nutrition** 33
Aaron P. Garrison and Michael A. Helmrath

6 **Fast-Track Protocols** 37
Peter Mattei

7 **Quality Improvement, Education, and Outcomes Research
in Pediatric Surgery** 41
Steven Teich and Marc P. Michalsky

Part II   Critical Care

8 **Shock** 49
John J. McCloskey

9 **Electrolyte Disorders** 57
Patrick J. Javid

10 **Vascular Access** 65
Stephen G. Murphy

11 **Acute Kidney Injury** 73
Peter A. Meaney and Kevin E.C. Meyers

12 **Respiratory Failure and Mechanical Ventilation** 83
Todd J. Kilbaugh

13 **Extracorporeal Membrane Oxygenation** 91
Edmund Y. Yang

Part III   Trauma

14   **Pediatric Trauma Resuscitation** 103
      Thane Blinman

15   **Head Trauma** 111
      Gregory G. Heuer and Phillip B. Storm

16   **Neck Injuries** 117
      Peter T. Masiakos and George C. Velmahos

17   **Burns** 123
      Gail E. Besner

18   **Abdominal Trauma** 135
      Michael L. Nance

19   **Thoracic Trauma** 145
      Martin S. Keller

20   **Spine Trauma** 151
      Robert W. Letton

21   **Vascular Injury** 157
      Barbara A. Gaines

22   **Pediatric Hand Injuries** 161
      Roger Cornwall

23   **Child Abuse** 169
      Richard A. Falcone, Jr. and Kathi Makoroff

Part IV   Head and Neck

24   **The Critical Airway** 177
      Karen B. Zur

25   **Bronchoscopy** 185
      Ian N. Jacobs

26   **Cystic Neck Masses** 195
      Oluyinka O. Olutoye

27   **Disorders of the Thyroid and Parathyroid** 203
      William T. Adamson

28   **Cervical Lymphadenopathy** 213
      Rajeev Prasad and L. Grier Arthur

Part V   Esophagus

29   **Esophageal Atresia and Tracheo-Esophageal Fistula** 223
      Jean-Martin Laberge

30   **Long-Gap Esophageal Atresia** 233
      Pietro Bagolan and Francesco Morini

31 **Esophageal Replacement** 247
Lewis Spitz

32 **Esophageal Injuries** 253
Kristin N. Fiorino and Petar Mamula

33 **Foregut Duplications** 267
Pablo Laje

34 **Achalasia** 273
J. Duncan Phillips

Part VI Thorax and Mediastinum

35 **Patent Ductus Arteriosus** 283
Stephanie Fuller and Peter J. Gruber

36 **Vascular Compression Syndromes** 289
Mark L. Wulkan

37 **Congenital Lung Lesions** 293
Bill Chiu and Alan W. Flake

38 **Thoracoscopic Biopsy and Lobectomy of the Lung** 299
Sanjeev Dutta and Craig T. Albanese

39 **Diseases of the Pleural Space** 305
Keith A. Kuenzler

40 **Pectus Deformities** 313
M. Ann Kuhn and Donald Nuss

41 **Mediastinal Masses** 323
Richard D. Glick

Part VII Stomach and Small Intestine

42 **Gastroesophageal Reflux Disease** 333
Thane Blinman

43 **Hypertrophic Pyloric Stenosis** 341
Marjorie J. Arca and Jill S. Whitehouse

44 **Surgical Enteral Access** 347
Tim Weiner and Melissa K. Dedmond

45 **Duodenal Atresia** 353
Keith A. Kuenzler and Steven S. Rothenberg

46 **Intestinal Atresias** 359
Peter F. Nichol and Ari Reichstein

47 **Abdominal Cysts and Duplications** 365
Patricia A. Lange

48 Anomalies of Intestinal Rotation 373
François I. Luks

49 Necrotizing Enterocolitis 381
Cynthia A. Gingalewski

50 Short Bowel Syndrome 387
Thomas Jaksic, Brian A. Jones, Melissa A. Hull, and Shimae C. Fitzgibbons

51 Meconium Ileus 395
Peter Mattei

52 Intussusception 401
John H.T. Waldhausen

53 Meckel's Diverticulum 409
Melvin S. Dassinger, III

54 Bariatric Surgery 415
Joy L. Collins

55 Chronic Abdominal Pain 425
Frazier W. Frantz

56 Crohn's Disease 437
Peter Mattei

57 Ileostomy and Colostomy 443
Oliver S. Soldes

Part VIII   Colon, Rectum, and Anus

58 Constipation 453
Linda Nicolette

59 Perianal Disease 461
Cynthia D. Downard

60 Pilonidal Cyst Disease 467
Daniel P. Doody

61 Hirschsprung Disease 475
Jacob C. Langer

62 Appendicitis 485
Shawn D. Safford

63 Ulcerative Colitis and Familial Polyposis 491
Stephen E. Dolgin

64 Anorectal Malformations 499
Marc A. Levitt and Alberto Peña

Part IX   Abdominal Wall, Peritoneum, and Diaphragm

65   **Gastroschisis**   515
      Aimen F. Shaaban

66   **Omphalocele**   523
      Kenneth W. Liechty

67   **Eventration of the Diaphragm**   531
      Samuel Z. Soffer

68   **Congenital Diaphragmatic Hernia**   535
      Peter Mattei

69   **Uncommon Hernias**   543
      Shaheen J. Timmapuri and Rajeev Prasad

70   **Umbilical Disorders and Anomalies**   547
      Adam J. Kaye and Daniel J. Ostlie

71   **Peritoneal Dialysis**   553
      Danny Little and Monford D. Custer

Part X   Liver, Biliary Tree, Pancreas, and Spleen

72   **Neonatal Hyperbilirubinemia**   561
      Clyde J. Wright and Michael A. Posencheg

73   **Biliary Atresia**   567
      Peter C. Minneci and Alan W. Flake

74   **Surgical Therapy of Disorders of Intrahepatic Cholestasis**   575
      Peter Mattei

75   **Cholecystitis**   579
      Andrè Hebra and Aaron Lesher

76   **Choledochal Cysts**   587
      Greg M. Tiao

77   **Hepatic Resection**   593
      Heung Bae Kim

78   **Portal Hypertension**   599
      Jaimie D. Nathan, Kathleen M. Campbell, Greg M. Tiao, Maria H. Alonso,
      and Frederick C. Ryckman

79   **Congenital Hyperinsulinism**   611
      N. Scott Adzick

80   **Disorders of the Pancreas**   617
      Marshall Z. Schwartz and Michael S. Katz

81   **Disorders of the Spleen**   625
      Melissa E. Danko and Henry E. Rice

Part XI   Genitourinary

82 Vesicoureteral Reflux 635
Pasquale Casale

83 Renal Abnormalities 641
Pierluigi Lelli-Chiesa and Gabriele Lisi

84 Penile Anomalies and Circumcision 651
Douglas A. Canning

85 Inguinal Hernia and Hydrocele 663
André Hebra and Joshua B. Glenn

86 Undescended Testis 673
Pasquale Casale and Sarah M. Lambert

87 The Diagnosis and Management of Scrotal Pain 679
Stephen A. Zderic

88 Cloacal Exstrophy 685
Michael C. Carr

89 Disorders of Sex Development 693
Thomas F. Kolon

90 Vagina: Diseases and Treatment 701
Edward J. Doolin

Part XII   Surgical Oncology

91 Neuroblastoma 709
Natasha E. Kelly and Michael P. La Quaglia

92 Wilms Tumor 715
Peter F. Ehrlich

93 Adrenal Tumors 725
Daniel von Allmen

94 Rhabdomyosarcoma 729
Ravi S. Radhakrishnan and Richard J. Andrassy

95 Sacrococcygeal Teratoma 735
Helene Flageole

96 Ovarian Tumors 741
Kirk W. Reichard

97 Pediatric Testicular Tumors 749
Ismael Zamilpa and Martin A. Koyle

98 Soft Tissue Tumors 755
Roman M. Sydorak and Harry Applebaum

99 Liver Tumors 761
Rebecka L. Meyers

100 Musculoskeletal Surgical Oncology 773
Jenny M. Frances and John P. Dormans

Part XIII Skin and Soft Tissues

101 Subcutaneous Endoscopy 785
Sanjeev Dutta

102 Benign Skin Lesions 795
Michael D. Rollins and Sheryll L. Vanderhooft

103 Atypical Nevi and Malignant Melanoma 805
Kenneth W. Gow

104 Necrotizing Soft Tissue Infections 815
Eric R. Scaife

105 Hemangiomas and Vascular Malformations 819
David W. Low

106 Disorders of the Breast 829
Mary L. Brandt

Part XIV Transplantation

107 Kidney Transplantation 839
Peter L. Abt and H. Jorge Baluarte

108 Liver Transplantation 847
Maria H. Alonso

109 Intestinal Transplantation 857
Thomas M. Fishbein

Part XV Miscellaneous

110 Gastrointestinal Bleeding 865
Katherine J. Deans

111 Fetal Surgery 871
Foong-Yen Lim and Timothy M. Crombleholme

112 Disorders of the Abdominal Aorta and Major Branches 881
Omaida C. Velazquez

113 Ventricular Shunts for Hydrocephalus 887
Gregory G. Heuer and Phillip B. Storm

114 Conjoined Twins 893
Gary E. Hartman

Index 901

Contributors

Peter L. Abt, MD
Department of Surgery, University of Pennsylvania, Children's Hospital of Philadelphia, Hospital of the University of Pennsylvania, Philadelphia, PA, USA

William T. Adamson, MD
Department of Surgery, University of North Carolina School of Medicine, North Carolina Children's Hospital, Chapel Hill, NC, USA

N. Scott Adzick, MD
Department of Surgery, Children's Hospital of Philadelphia, University of Pennsylvania School of Medicine, Philadelphia, PA, USA

Craig T. Albanese, MD, MBA
Department of Surgery, Stanford University, Lucile Packard Children's Hospital, Stanford, CA, USA

Maria H. Alonso, MD
Division of Pediatric and Thoracic Surgery, Cincinnati Children's Hospital Medical Center, Cincinnati, OH, USA

Richard J. Andrassy, MD
Department of Surgery, Memorial Hermann Hospital, MD Anderson Cancer Center, Houston, TX, USA

Harry Applebaum, MD
Division of Pediatric Surgery, David Geffen School of Medicine at UCLA, Kaiser Permanente Los Angeles Medical Center, Los Angeles, CA, USA

Marjorie J. Arca, MD
Department of Surgery, Medical College of Wisconsin, Children's Hospital of Wisconsin, Milwaukee, WI, USA

L. Grier Arthur, MD
Division of Pediatric General, Drexel University, Thoracic and Minimally Invasive Surgery, St. Christopher's Hospital for Children, Philadelphia, PA, USA

Pietro Bagolan, MD
Department of Medical and Surgical Neonatalology, Bambino GESU Children's Hospital, Piazza S. Onofrio, 4, Roma 00165, Italia

H. Jorge Baluarte, MD
Division of Pediatric Nephrology, Children's Hospital of Philadelphia, Philadelphia, PA, USA

Gail E. Besner, MD
Department of Surgery, Ohio State University College of Medicine, Nationwide Children's Hospital, Columbus, OH, USA

Thane Blinman, MD
General, Thoracic and Fetal Surgery, The Children's Hospital of Philadelphia,
34th and Civic Center Blvd., 5 Wood, Philadelphia, PA 19104, USA

Mary L. Brandt, MD
Department of Pediatric Surgery, Baylor College of Medicine, Texas Children's Hospital,
Houston, TX, USA

Kathleen M. Campbell, MD
Department of Gastroenterology, Cincinnati Children's Hospital
Medical Center, Hepatology and Nutrition, Cincinnati, OH, USA

Douglas A. Canning, MD
Department of Surgery, Division of Urology, University of Pennsylvania
School of Medicine, Children's Hospital of Philadelphia,
Philadelphia, PA, USA

Michael C. Carr, MD
Division of Urology, Children's Hospital of Philadelphia,
Philadelphia, PA, USA

Pasquale Casale, MD
Department of Urology, Children's Hospital of Philadelphia, Philadelphia, PA, USA

Bill Chiu, MD
Department of Surgery, Children's Hospital of Philadelphia, Philadelphia, PA, USA

Joy L. Collins, MD
Department of Pediatric General and Thoracic Surgery, University of Pennsylvania,
Children's Hospital of Philadelphia, Philadelphia, PA, USA

Roger Cornwall, MD
Division of Orthopedic Surgery, Cincinnati Children's Hospital Medical Center,
Cincinnati, OH, USA

Timothy M. Crombleholme, MD
Department of Pediatric Surgery, Cincinnati Children's Foundation,
University of Cincinnati College of Medicine, Cincinnati Children's
Hospital Medical Center, Cincinnati, OH, USA

Monford D. Custer, MD
Division of Pediatric Surgery, Children's Hospital at Scott and White,
Temple, TX, USA

Melissa E. Danko, MD
Department of Surgery, Duke University
Medical Center, Durham, NC, USA

Melvin S. Dassinger, III, MD
Division of Pediatric Surgery, University of Arkansas for Medical Sciences,
Arkansas Children's Hospital, Little Rock, AR, USA

Katherine J. Deans, MD, MHSc
Department of Surgery, Division of General Thoracic and Fetal Surgery,
University of Pennsylvania, Children's Hospital of Philadelphia,
Philadelphia, PA, USA

Melissa K. Dedmond, PA-C
Department of Pediatric Surgery, University of North Carolina,
UNC Hospitals, Chapel Hill, NC, USA

Stephen E. Dolgin, MD
Albert Einstein College of Medicine, Schneider Children's Hospital, 269-01 76 Ave 1,
New Hyde Park, NY 11040, USA

Daniel P. Doody, MD
Department of Pediatric Surgery, Massachusetts General Hospital, Harvard Medical School,
Boston, MA, USA

Edward J. Doolin, MD, BS Chemistry
Department of Pediatric General and Thoracic Surgery, Children's Hospital
of Philadelphia, Philadelphia, PA, USA

John P. Dormans, MD
Department of Orthopedics, Children's Hospital of Philadelphia,
Philadelphia, PA, USA

Cynthia D. Downard, MD, MMSc
Department of Surgery, University of Louisville, Kosair Children's Hospital,
Louisville, KY, USA

Sanjeev Dutta, MD, MA
Department of Surgery, Lucile Packard Children's Hospital, Stanford University,
780 Welch Road, Svite 206, Stanford, CA 94305, USA

Peter F. Ehrlich, MD, MSc
Department of Pediatric Surgery, University of Michigan,
CS Mott Children's Hospital, Ann Arbor, MI, USA

Richard A. Falcone, Jr., MD, MPH
Pediatric General and Thoracic Surgery, University of Cincinnati,
Cincinnati Children's Hospital Medical Center, Cincinnati, OH, USA

Kristin N. Fiorino, MD
Department of Pediatric Gastroenterology, Children's Hospital of Philadelphia,
Philadelphia, PA, USA

Thomas M. Fishbein, MD
Georgetown University Hospital, Transplant Institute, Washington, DC, USA

Shimae C. Fitzgibbons, MD
Department of Surgery, Harvard Medical School, Children's Hospital Boston,
Boston, MA, USA

Helene Flageole, MD, MSc, FRCSC, FACS
Department of Surgery, McMaster Children's Hospital, 1200 Main Street, Hamilton,
ON # L8N325, Canada

Alan W. Flake, MD
Department of Surgery, Children's Hospital of Philadelphia, Philadelphia, PA, USA

Jenny M. Frances, MD, MPH
Department of Orthopedic Surgery, New York University Hospital for Joint Diseases,
New York, NY, USA

Frazier W. Frantz, MD
Department of Pediatric Surgery, East Virginia Medical School,
Children's Hospital of The King's Daughters, Norfolk, VA, USA

Stephanie Fuller, MD
Department of Cardiothoracic Surgery, Children's Hospital of Philadelphia,
34th Street & Civic Center Boulevard, Ste. A2NWAD, Philadelphia, PA 19103, USA

Barbara A. Gaines, MD
Children's Hospital of Pittsburgh of UPMC, University of Pittsburgh,
Pittsburgh, PA, USA

Arjunan Ganesh, MBBS
Department of Anesthesiology, University of Pennsylvania,
Children's Hospital of Philadelphia, Philadelphia, PA, USA

Aaron P. Garrison, MD
Department of General Surgery, University of North Carolina at Chapel Hill,
Chapel Hill, NC, USA

Cynthia A. Gingalewski, MD
Department of General Surgery, George Washington University,
Children's National Medical Center, Washington, DC, USA

Joshua B. Glenn, MD
Department of Pediatric Surgery, Vanderbilt University Children's Hospital,
TN, USA

Richard D. Glick, MD
Department of Pediatric Surgery, Albert Einstein College of Medicine,
Schneider Children's Hospital, New Hyde Park, NY, USA

Kenneth W. Gow, MD, MSc, FRCSC, FAAP, FACS
Department of Surgery, Children's Hospital and Regional Medical Center, University of
Washington, 4800 Sand Point Way NE, MIS W-7729, PO Box 5371, Seattle, WA 98105, USA

Peter J. Gruber, MD, PhD
Department of Pediatric Surgery, Children's Hospital of Philadelphia,
Philadelphia, PA 19140, USA

Gary E. Hartman, MD, MBA
Department of Pediatric Surgery, Stanford University School of Medicine,
Lucile Packard Children's Hospital, Stanford, CA, USA

Andrè Hebra, MD
Department of Surgery, Medical University of South Carolina, Children's Hospital,
96 Jonathan Lucas Street, Charleston, SC 29425, USA

Michael A. Helmrath, MD
Department of Pediatric Surgery, University of North
Carolina at Chapel Hill, Chapel Hill, NC, USA

Gregory G. Heuer, MD, PhD
Department of Neurosurgery, University of Pennsylvania, The Children's
Hospital of Philadelphia, 877 N. 30th St. Philadelphia, PA 19130, USA

Melissa A. Hull, MD
Department of Surgery, Harvard Medical School, Children's
Hospital Boston, Boston, MA, USA

Ian N. Jacobs, MD
Department of Otolaryngology, University of Pennsylvania School of Medicine,
Children's Hospital of Philadelphia, Philadelphia, PA, USA

Thomas Jaksic, MD, PhD
Department of Pediatric Surgery, Children's Hospital Boston, Boston, MA, USA

Brian A. Jones, MD
Department of Surgery, Harvard Medical School,
Children's Hospital Boston, Boston, MA, USA

Patrick J. Javid, MD
Department of Surgery, Seattle Children's Hospital,
University of Washington, Seattle, WA, USA

Michael S. Katz, MD
Department of Pediatric Surgery, St. Christopher's
Hospital for Children, Philadelphia, PA, USA

Adam J. Kaye, MD
Department of Pediatric Surgery, Children's Mercy Hospital, 2401 Gillham Road,
Kansas City, MO 64108, USA

Martin S. Keller, MD
Department of Pediatric Surgery, Washington University,
St. Louis Children's Hospital, St. Louis, MO, USA

Natasha E. Kelly, MD
Department of Pediatric Surgery, Memorial Sloan Kettering Cancer Center,
New York, NY 10065, USA

Todd J. Kilbaugh, MD
Department of Anesthesiology and Critical Care, University of Pennsylvania,
Children's Hospital of Philadelphia, Philadelphia, PA, USA

Heung Bae Kim, MD
Department of Surgery, Pediatric Transplant Center, Harvard Medical Center,
Children's Hospital Boston, Boston, MA, USA

Thomas F. Kolon, MD
Department of Pediatric Urology, University of Pennsylvania
School of Medicine, Children's Hospital of Philadelphia, Philadelphia, PA, USA

Martin A. Koyle, MD, FACS, FAAP
Department of Pediatric Urology, University of Washington,
Seattle Children's Hospital, Seattle, WA, USA

Keith A. Kuenzler, MD
Minimally Invasive Pediatric Surgery, NYU Langone Medical Center, New York,
NY 10016, USA

M. Ann Kuhn, MD
Department of Pediatric Surgery, Eastern Virginia Medical School,
Children's Hospital of the King's Daughters, Norfolk, VA, USA

Michael P. La Quaglia, MD
Department of Surgery, Weill Cornell University Medical School,
Memorial Sloan-Kettering Cancer Center, New York, NY, USA

Jean-Martin Laberge, MD, FRCSC, FACS
Department of Pediatric General Surgery, McGill University, Montreal Children's Hospital
of the McGill Health Care Centre, Montreal, QC, Canada

Pablo Laje, MD
Department of General Pediatric and Thoracic Surgery, Children's
Hospital of Philadelphia, Aapt K-1103, Philadelphia, PA 19144, USA

Sarah M. Lambert, MD
Department of Urology, Children's Hospital of Philadelphia, Philadelphia, PA, USA

Patricia A. Lange, MD
Department of Surgery, University of North Carolina, Chapel Hill,
UNC Hospitals, Chapel Hill, NC, USA

Jacob C. Langer, MD, FRCSC
Hospital for Sick Children, Division of Thoracic and General Surgery, University of Toronto,
1526–555 University Avenue, Toronto, ON, M5GF 1X8, Canada

Pierluigi Lelli-Chiesa, MD
Department of Pediatric Surgery, Gabriele d'Annunzio
of Chieti-Pescara, Santo Spirito Hospital, Pescara, Italy

Aaron Lesher, MD
Department of Surgery, Medical University of South Carolina, Charleston SC, USA

Robert W. Letton, Jr., MD
Oklahoma University Health Sciences Center, Children's Hospital of Oklahoma,
Oklahoma City, OK, USA

Marc A. Levitt, MD
Colorectal Center for Children, Cincinnati Children's Hospital Medical Center, Pediatric
Surgery, 3333 Burnet Avenue, ML 2023, Cincinnati, OH 45229, USA

Kenneth W. Liechty, MD
Departments of General Thoracic and Fetal Surgery, University of Pennsylvania, Children's
Hospital of Philadelphia, Philadelphia, PA, USA

Foong-Yen Lim, MD
Department of Pediatric Surgery, Cincinnati Children's Hospital Medical Center,
3333 Burnet Avenue, MLC 11025, Cincinnati, OH 45229–3090, USA

Gabriele Lisi, MD, PhD
Department of Pediatric Surgery, Gabriele d'Annunzio of Chieti-Pescara, Santo Spirito
Hospital, Pescara, Italy

Danny Little, MD
Division of Pediatric Surgery, Scott and White Hospital, 615 West Garfield Avenue, Temple,
TX, USA and Department of Surgery, Texas A&M Health Science Center, Temple, TX, USA

David W. Low, MD
Department of Surgery, Division of Plastic Surgery, University of Pennsylvania
School of Medicine, Children's Hospital of Philadelphia, Philadelphia, PA, USA

François I. Luks, MD, PhD
Warren Halpert Medical School of Brown University, Providence, RI, USA,
Division of Pediatric Surgery, Hasbro Children's Hospital, 2, Dudley Street, Suite 180,
Providence, RI 02905, USA

Kathi Makoroff, MD
Department of Pediatrics, Cincinnati Children's Hospital Medical Center,
Cincinnati OH, USA

Petar Mamula, MD
Department of Endoscopy, University of Pennsylvania, Children's Hospital of Philadelphia,
Philadelphia PA, USA

Peter T. Masiakos, MS, MD, FACS, FAAP
Department Pediatric Surgery, Pediatric Trauma Unit, 55 Fruit Street, Warren 1155, Boston,
MA 02114, USA

Peter Mattei, MD, FAAP, FACS
Assistant Professor of Surgery, University of Pennsylvania School of Medicine,
Division of General, Thoracic and Fetal Surgery, Children's Hospital of Philadelphia,
Philadelphia, PA, USA

Lynne G. Maxwell, MD
Department of Anesthesiology, University of Pennsylvania, Children's
Hospital of Philadelphia, Philadelphia, PA, USA

John J. McCloskey, MD
Department of Anesthesiology and Critical Care Medicine, Children's
Hospital of Philadelphia, Philadelphia, PA, USA

Peter A. Meaney, MD, MPH
Department of Anesthesia and Critical Care, University of Pennsylvania,
Children's Hospital of Philadelphia, Philadelphia, PA, USA

Kevin E.C. Meyers, MB BCh
Department of Pediatrics and Nephrology, Children's Hospital of Philadelphia
and University of Pennsylvania, Philadelphia, PA, USA

Rebecka L. Meyers, MD
Primary Children's Medical Center, 100 North Medical Drive, Svite 2600, Salt Lake City,
UT 84113, USA

Marc P. Michalsky, MD
Department of Pediatric Surgery, Ohio State University, Nationwide
Children's Hospital, Columbus. OH, USA

Peter C. Minneci, MD
Department of Surgery, Children's Hospital of Philadelphia, 34th Street & Civic Center
Boulevard, Wood 5, Philadelphia, PA 19104, USA

Francesco Morini, MD
Department of Medical and Surgical Neonatology, Bambino Gesu Children's
Hospital – Research Institute, Rome, Italy

Stephen G. Murphy, MD
Department of Surgery, DuPont Hospital for Children, Wilmington, DE, USA

Michael L. Nance, MD
Department of Surgery, Children's Hospital of Philadelphia, Philadelphia, PA, USA

Jaimie D. Nathan, MD
Division of Transplantation, Division of Pediatric and Thoracic Surgery, University of
Cincinnati, Cincinnati Children's Hospitals Medical Center, Cincinnati, OH, USA

Peter F. Nichol, MD, PhD
Department of Surgery, University of Wisconsin School of Medicine
and Public Health, Madison, WI, USA

Linda Nicolette, MD
Department of Pediatric Surgery, Presbyterian Hospital, Albuquerque, NM, USA

Donald Nuss, MB, ChB
Department of Surgery, Eastern Virginia Medical School, Children's Hospital
of The King's Daughters, Norfolk, VA, USA

Oluyinka O. Olutoye, MD, PhD
Division of Pediatric Surgery, Michael E. DeBakey Department of Surgery,
Baylor College of Medicine, Texas Children's Hospital, Houston, TX, USA

Daniel J. Ostlie, MD
Department of Pediatric Surgery, University of Missouri Kansas City,
Children's Mercy Hospital and Clinics, Kansas City, MO, USA

Alberto Peña, MD
University of Cincinnati, Children's Hospital of Cincinnati, Cincinnati, OH, USA

J. Duncan Phillips, MD
Department of Surgery, University of North Carolina, Chapel Hill,
North Carolina Children's Hospital, Chapel Hill, NC, USA

Michael A. Posencheg, MD
Department of Neonatology, University of Pennsylvania School of Medicine,
Hospital of the University of Pennsylvania, Philadelphia, PA, USA

Rajeev Prasad, MD, FACS, FAAP
Department of Pediatric General Surgery, Drexel University College of Medicine,
St. Christopher's Hospital for Children, Philadelphia, PA, USA

Ravi S. Radhakrishnan, MD, MBA
Department of Surgery, MD Anderson Cancer Center, Memorial Hermann Hospital,
6431 Fannin Street, MSB 4200, Houston, TX 77030, USA

Kirk W. Reichard, MD
Thomas Jefferson School of Medicine, Alfred I. DuPont Hospital
for Children, Wilmington, DE, USA

Ari Reichstein, MD
Department of Surgery, University of Wisconsin School
of Medicine and Public Health, Madison, WI, USA

Henry E. Rice, MD
Division of Pediatric Surgery, Duke University,
Duke University Medical Center, Durham, NC, USA

Michael D. Rollins, MD
Department of Surgery, Division of Pediatric Surgery, Primary Children's Medical Center,
University of Utah School of Medicine, 100 North Mario Capecchi Drive, Suite 2600, Salt
Lake City, UT 84113–1100, USA

John B. Rose, MD
Department of Anesthesiology, University of Pennsylvania, Children's
Hospital of Philadelphia, Philadelphia, PA, USA

Steven S. Rothenberg, MD
Columbia University, Rocky Mountain Hospital for Children, Denver, CO, USA

Frederick C. Ryckman, MD
Division of Pediatric and Thoracic Surgery, Cincinnati Children's Hospital
Medical Center, Cincinnati, OH, USA

Shawn D. Safford, MD
Department of Surgery, National Naval Medical Center, Bethesda, MD, USA

Eric R. Scaife, MD
Department of Pediatric Surgery, University of Utah, 100 N. Mario Capecchi Drive, Street
2600, Salt Lake City, UT 84113–1103, USA

Marshall Z. Schwartz, MD
Department of Surgery, Drexel University College of Medicine,
St. Christopher's Hospital for Children, Philadelphia, PA, USA

Aimen F. Shaaban, MD
Department of Surgery, University of Iowa Carver College of Medicine,
University of Iowa Hospitals and Clinics, Iowa City, IA, USA

Samuel Z. Soffer, MD
Albert Einstein College of Medicine, Division of Pediatric Surgery, Schneider Children's
Hospital, 269–01 76th Avenue, New Hyde Park, NY 11598, USA

Oliver S. Soldes, MD
Department of Pediatric Surgery, Cleveland Clinic Foundation, Cleveland, OH, USA

Lewis Spitz, MB ChB, PhD, MD (Hon), FRCS, FRCPCH,
FAAP (Hon), FCS(SA) (Hon)
Department of Paediatric Surgery, Institute of Child Health,
University College, London, Great Ormond Street Hospital, London, UK

Phillip B. Storm, MD
Department of Neurosurgery, Children's Hospital of Philadelphia,
Philadelphia PA, USA

Roman M. Sydorak, MD, MPH
Department of Pediatric Surgery, Kaiser Permanente Los Angeles Medical Center,
4760 Sunset Boulevard, 3rd Floor, Los Angeles, CA 90027, USA

Steven Teich, MD
Department of Pediatric Surgery, Ohio State University,
Nationwide Children's Hospital, Columbus, OH, USA

Greg M. Tiao, MD
Department of Pediatric and Thoracic Surgery, Cincinnati Children's
Hospital Medical Center, Cincinnati, OH, USA

Shaheen J. Timmapuri, MD
Department of Pediatric Surgery, Drexel University, St. Christopher's
Hospital for Children, Philadelphia, PA, USA

Sheryll L. Vanderhooft, MD
Department of Pediatric Dermatology, University of Utah School of Medicine,
Primary Children's Medical Center, Salt Lake City UT, USA

Omaida C. Velazquez, MD, FACS
Jackson Memorial Medical Center, University of Miami Hospital 1611 NW 12th Avenue,
Holtz Building, Room 3016 (R-310), Miami, FL 33136, USA

George C. Velmahos, MD, PhD, MSEd
Department of Surgery, Harvard Medical School,
Massachusetts General Hospital, Boston MA, USA

Daniel von Allmen, MD
Department of Pediatric Surgery, University of North Carolina,
North Carolina Medical Hospital, Chapel Hill, NC, USA

John H.T. Waldhausen, MD
Department of Surgery, University of Washington, Children's
Hospital and Regional Medical Center, Seattle, WA, USA

Tim Weiner, MD
Department of Surgery, University of North Carolina, UNC Hospitals,
Chapel Hill, NC, USA

Ari Y. Weintraub, MD
Department of Anesthesiology, University of Pennsylvania, Children's Hospital
of Philadelphia, Philadelphia, PA, USA

Jill S. Whitehouse, MD
Department of Pediatric Surgery, Medical College of Wisconsin, Children's
Hospital of Wisconsin, Milwaukee, WI, USA

R. Douglas Wilson, MD, MSc
Department of Obstetrics and Gynecology, University of Calgary and Calgary
Health Region, Foothills Medical Center, Calgary, AB, Canada

Clyde J. Wright, MD
Department of Pediatrics, Children's Hospital of Philadelphia, 34th Street and Civic Center
Boulevard, Philadelphia, PA 19104, USA

Mark L. Wulkan, MD
Department of Surgery, Children's Healthcare of Atlanta at Egleston,
Emory Children's Center, Atlanta, GA, USA

Edmund Y. Yang, MD, PhD
Department of Pediatric General Surgery, Vanderbilt Children's Hospital,
Nashville, TN, USA

Ismael Zamilpa, MD
Department of Pediatric Urology, University of Washington,
Seattle Children's Hospital, Seattle, WA, USA

Stephen A. Zderic, MD
Department of Pediatric Urology, Children's Hospital of Philadelphia,
Philadelphia, PA, USA

Karen B. Zur, MD
Department of Otolaryngology, University of Pennsylvania
School of Medicine, Children's Hospital of Philadelphia, Philadelphia, PA, USA

Part I
Perioperative Care

Chapter 1
Preoperative Assessment and Preparation

Ari Y. Weintraub and Lynne G. Maxwell

All patients presenting for surgical procedures under anesthesia benefit greatly from a thorough preanesthetic/preoperative assessment and targeted preparation, which serve to optimize any coexisting medical conditions and minimize the potential for complications. An increasing number of procedures are being performed on an outpatient basis, and the preoperative assessment and preparation often occurs in the surgeon's office or even in the preoperative area on the day of surgery. In addition to identifying outstanding medical issues that may delay or lead to cancellation of their procedure on the scheduled date, the preoperative assessment is an excellent opportunity to prepare patients and families and to educate them about what to expect during and after administration of an anesthetic. For pediatric patients in particular, where the psychological needs of the patient differ depending on their age and the surgery and recovery involves and affects the entire family, the preoperative assessment has a crucial role in ensuring a smooth perioperative experience.

The goals of the preoperative evaluation are to identify any active medical issues and to ensure that the management of these conditions is optimized prior to anesthesia and surgery. Unresolved medical issues are often significant enough to warrant cancellation of procedures for further diagnostic workup or treatment. It is obviously in the best interest of all the involved parties to avoid this.

Risks of Anesthesia

The risk of dying from general anesthesia can only be extrapolated from large series and appears to be as low as 1 in 250,000 in healthy patients. To put this in perspective for parents, the risk of a motor vehicle collision on the way to the hospital or surgery center is greater than the risk of death

under anesthesia. Common minor adverse effects including discomfort from airway management and postoperative nausea and vomiting (PONV) should be discussed, along with assurances that everything will be done to prevent and treat these relatively common complaints.

The American Society of Anesthesiologists (ASA) physical status score is a means of communicating the physical condition of the patient. The physical status score was never intended to represent a measure of operative risk and serves primarily as a means of communication among care providers (Table 1.1). In addition, certain information is essential and should be included in the preoperative assessment of every patient: weight, blood pressure, oxygen saturation (SpO_2) by pulse oximetry in both room air (and with supplemental O_2, if applicable), allergies, medications, cardiac and murmur history, and previous subspecialty encounters.

Patients who have previously undergone general anesthesia should be asked specifically regarding a history of the adverse effects: emergence delirium, PONV, difficult intubation, and difficult intravenous access. Keep in mind that patients and parents are often very anxious about recurrence of these events. The family history should also be reviewed for pseudocholinesterase deficiency (prolonged paralysis after succinyl choline) or any first-degree relative who experienced malignant hyperthermia.

Airway/Respiratory System

Many congenital syndromes are associated with craniofacial abnormalities that may complicate or even preclude routine airway management techniques (Table 1.2). In addition to a detailed physical examination, a history of past intubations and details of the methods used to secure the airway are even more useful in planning an anesthetic. Some patients are given a "difficult airway letter" by an anesthesiologist and this information should be shared with the anesthesia care team in advance of the scheduled operation. In the absence of such information, prior anesthetic records should be obtained and reviewed to guide airway management.

A.Y. Weintraub (✉)
Department of Anesthesiology, University of Pennsylvania, Children's Hospital of Philadelphia, 34th Street and Civic Center Boulevard, Room 9329, Philadelphia, PA 19104, USA
e-mail: weintraub@email.chop.edu

P. Mattei (ed.), *Fundamentals of Pediatric Surgery*,
DOI 10.1007/978-1-4419-6643-8_1, © Springer Science+Business Media, LLC 2011

Table 1.1 American Society of Anesthesiology (ASA) physical status (PS) classifications

Classification	Definition	Example
PS 1	Normal healthy person	
PS 2	Mild systemic disease without functional limitations	Well-controlled asthma
PS 3	Severe systemic disease	Acute lymphocytic leukemia
PS 4	Severe systemic disease that is a constant threat to life	Extreme prematurity
PS 5	Moribund patient, unexpected to survive without the procedure	Congenital heart disease for initiation of ECMO
PS 6	Brain-dead patient for organ procurement	
E	Suffix added for emergent procedures	

Table 1.2 Syndromes and craniofacial abnormalities associated with difficult ventilation or intubation

Syndrome	Associated airway features
Apert	Craniosynostosis, midface hypoplasia
Beckwith–Wiedemann syndrome	Macroglossia
Crouzon	Craniosynostosis, midface hypoplasia
Freeman–Sheldon (whistling face) syndrome	Microstomia
Goldenhar syndrome	Hemifacial microsomia, mandibular hypoplasia (uni- or bilateral)
Klippel–Feil syndrome	Limited cervical mobility
Mucopolysaccharide storage disorders	Redundant facial, pharyngeal, and supraglottic soft tissue; neck immobility
Pierre-Robin sequence	Micrognathia, glossoptosis, cleft palate
Treacher-Collins syndrome	Maxillary/mandibular hypoplasia
Trisomy 21 (Down syndrome)	Macroglossia, subglottic stenosis, midface hypoplasia

Asthma (reactive airways disease) is one of the most common chronic diseases in children and many perioperative procedures can exacerbate the disease. These include induction and emergence from anesthesia and endotracheal intubation. As with all chronic conditions, asthma should be optimally medically managed prior to presenting for an operation or anesthesia. In addition to regular appropriate use of "controller medications" (inhaled corticosteroids, intermediate-acting bronchodilators, leukotriene modifiers), we recommend that patients with asthma use their bronchodilators every 6 h for 48 h prior to anesthesia to minimize perioperative bronchospasm. A history of a recent flare requiring oral corticosteroids suggests poorly controlled disease and might warrant delay of an elective procedure until better control is achieved. Some feel it is best to wait 4–6 weeks after an acute exacerbation for associated airway hyperreactivity to return to baseline. Patients with persistent poorly controlled reactive airways disease should be referred to their primary health care provider or pulmonologist for strategies to improve their status. These strategies sometimes include the administration of oral corticosteroids.

Children often have loose teeth as they transition from their primary to secondary dentition, or due to poor oral hygiene or an underlying disorder such as osteogenesis imperfecta or ectodermal dysplasia. There is a significant risk of aspirating a tooth that is accidentally displaced during orotracheal intubation, so loose teeth should be electively removed at induction. In some cases, it is best to recommend a preoperative visit to a dentist.

Obstructive sleep apnea is seen commonly in patients with adenotonsillar hypertrophy, obesity, and some syndromes. Symptoms (snoring, daytime somnolence), results of sleep studies, and the need for noninvasive ventilation (CPAP, BIPAP) should be included in the preoperative assessment as airway obstruction should be anticipated in the postoperative period, often making inpatient observation and monitoring necessary.

One of the most common questions confronting an anesthesiologist is whether to cancel a procedure because of an upper respiratory infection. This can be a vexing problem for all parties involved, and the decision is often a difficult one to make with confidence. The patient with current or recent URI undergoing general anesthesia is theoretically at increased risk of postoperative respiratory complications, including laryngospasm, bronchospasm, hypoxia, and apnea, with the patients under 2 years of age being at greatest risk. However, anesthetic management can also be tailored to reduce stimulation of a potentially hyperreactive airway. In addition, cancellation of a procedure can impose an emotional or economic burden on the patient, family, physician, and hospital or ambulatory surgical facility. Unless the patient is acutely ill, it is often acceptable to proceed with the anesthetic. Patients with high fever, wheezing, or productive cough may actually have a lower respiratory tract infection and surgery is more likely to be cancelled. Our approach is to discuss the urgency of the planned procedure with the surgeon and to review the risks and benefits of proceeding or rescheduling with the parents, including the possibility that the child may have another URI at the time of the rescheduled procedure. Allowing the parents to participate in the decision-making process when appropriate usually leads to mutual satisfaction among all parties involved.

The patient with a difficult airway might require advanced airway management techniques, which often necessitates additional OR time and, in some cases, a planned period of postoperative mechanical ventilation and an ICU stay.

The laryngeal mask airway is now being used routinely for general anesthesia. This technique allows the patient to breathe spontaneously, with or without pressure support from the anesthesia machine, and, in most cases, neuromuscular blocking agents are not used. Therefore, it is usually used for cases where skeletal muscle relaxation is not needed for safe conduct of the operation. Any requirement for muscle relaxation should be discussed with the anesthesiologist in advance.

Cardiovascular

At the time of the presurgical evaluation, up to 90% of children are found to have an innocent murmur, probably due to turbulent flow at the aortic or pulmonary roots or in the subclavian or pulmonary arteries. Most of these children do not require a cardiology consultation and can be safely observed. These murmurs are frequently episodic and are associated with a normally split second heart sound, normal exercise tolerance, and normal electrocardiogram. Concomitant medical problems such as anemia and fever augment audibility of innocent murmurs because they increase cardiac output.

Nevertheless, a thorough history and physical examination will occasionally reveal findings that raise greater concern in a child with a murmur: an infant with failure to thrive or diaphoresis or tachypnea during feedings, or the older child with dyspnea, tachypnea, exercise intolerance, or syncope. These findings warrant further evaluation, including an electrocardiogram, chest X-ray, consultation with a pediatric cardiologist, and, in some cases, an echocardiogram.

Children with congenital heart disease frequently undergo a general surgical procedure. Assessment of the child's current health status includes a full history and physical examination and recent evaluation by the child's cardiologist. This communication should include: a full description of the original lesion, documentation of any procedures performed for palliation or repair, residual abnormalities such as an intracardiac shunt or valve abnormality, current functional status, and results of the most recent echocardiogram.

Knowledge of the child's cardiac anatomy is essential to assess the risk of paradoxical emboli and endocarditis. Revised recommendations for antibiotic prophylaxis that are substantially different from those promulgated over the past 50 years were recently published by the American Heart Association. Specifically, genitourinary and gastrointestinal procedures have been eliminated from those requiring prophylaxis and prophylaxis for dental and respiratory tract procedures is restricted to patients with: (1) unrepaired cyanotic congenital heart disease, (2) congenital heart defect repaired with prosthetic material, (3) cardiac transplantation, or (4) a history of endocarditis. Endotracheal intubation itself is not an indication for antibiotic prophylaxis (Table 1.3). Patients with hemodynamically insignificant lesions such as bicuspid aortic valve or mitral valve prolapse no longer require prophylaxis for any procedure. Patients with congenital heart disease repaired with prosthetic material require prophylaxis only for the first 6 months after repair, after which time endothelialization will have occurred. This is true for VSD as well as ASD repairs as long as there is no residual defect. Patients with prosthetic valves or those palliated with shunts or conduits require prophylaxis. Some cardiologists differ with these new guidelines. It is therefore advisable to request a recommendation from the child's cardiologist based on the child's condition and planned procedure. Although antibiotic prophylaxis is frequently administered orally to adults, it is usually given intravenously in children. When indicated, our practice is to give the antibiotic intravenously at induction of anesthesia, because the surgical preparation time generally allows sufficient time to achieve adequate blood levels before the incision is made. Starting an intravenous catheter in an awake child solely to administer antibiotics for antibiotics is rarely, if ever, necessary.

Surgical patients with long QT syndrome (LQTS), in which ion channels involved in repolarization function

Table 1.3 Cardiac conditions for which prophylaxis with dental or respiratory tract procedures is recommended

Congenital heart disease (CHD)[a]
Unrepaired cyanotic CHD, including palliative shunts and conduits
Completely repaired congenital heart defect with prosthetic material or device, whether placed by surgery or by catheter intervention, during the first 6 months after the procedure[b]
Repaired CHD with residual defects at the site or adjacent to the site of a prosthetic patch or prosthetic device (which inhibit endothelialization)
Cardiac transplantation recipients who develop cardiac valvopathy
Prosthetic cardiac valves
Previous infective endocarditis

[a]Except for the conditions listed above, antibiotic prophylaxis is no longer recommended for any other form of CHD

[b]Prophylaxis is recommended because endothelialization of prosthetic material occurs within 6 months of the procedure

Source: data from: Wilson W, Taubert KA, Gewitz M et al. Prevention of infective endocarditis. Guidelines from the American Heart Association Rheumatic Fever, Endocarditis, and Kawasaki Disease Committee, Council on Cardiovascular Disease in the Young, and the Council on Clinical Cardiology, Council on Cardiovascular Surgery and Anesthesia, and Quality of Care and Outcomes Research Interdisciplinary Working Group. Circulation. Apr 2007; doi:10.1161/CIRCULATIONAHA. 106.183095

abnormally due either to a congenital defect or drug effect, are at risk for torsades de pointes, a potentially life-threatening ventricular tachycardia. Congenital LQTS occurs in 1:5,000 individuals and can present at any age with syncope, seizures or sudden cardiac death, usually after an increase in sympathetic activity such as exercise or emotional stress. Because volatile anesthetic agents and surgical stress increase the risk of developing ventricular tachycardia, a preoperative electrocardiogram should be obtained in patients who are symptomatic, have a family history of sudden death, or are taking drugs which predispose to the condition (www.azcert.org/medical-pros/drug-lists/drug-lists.cfm). A QTc of more than 470 ms in males and 480 ms in females is diagnostic of LQTS. Cardiology consultation should be obtained as preoperative medical treatment might be necessary.

Any patient with congenital heart disease, cardiomyopathy, arrhythmia, or unexplained syncope requires a thorough cardiology evaluation before undergoing an elective surgical procedure, especially one that requires a general anesthetic. In fact, anesthetists at most institutions will require that a letter of cardiology clearance be included in the medical record before the day of surgery. This letter is written by the consulting cardiologist and should include a detailed discussion of the anatomy of the defect, the current medical regimen, and specific recommendations regarding the peri-operative care of the patient.

Gastroesophageal Reflux Disease

The majority of infants and a significant number of children have some degree of gastroesophageal reflux and the diagnosis of gastroesophageal reflux disease is increasing. Symptoms of GERD in infants and children differ substantially from those seen in adults and are often primarily respiratory in nature: cough, wheezing, or pneumonitis. Yet, despite a theoretical increase in the risk of aspiration of gastric contents during the induction of anesthesia, children with a history of GERD do not have an increased incidence of pulmonary aspiration as long as fasting guidelines have been followed. Unless there is a history of aspiration when fasting, an intravenous rapid sequence induction is not usually indicated. Patient with GERD should be taking appropriate chemoprophylaxis H$_2$-blocker or proton pump inhibitor) as prescribed by their primary physician or gastroenterologist.

Obesity

Obesity is an increasing problem in children, with a recent estimated incidence of 15%. As in adults, obese children have an increased incidence of obstructive sleep apnea, which can be associated with adverse respiratory events in the perioperative period. Problems during induction include difficult mask ventilation. Preoperative evaluation of children with a body mass index of 30 or greater should include a careful history of snoring and daytime somnolence. Patients with suspected obstructive sleep apnea should be referred to a pulmonologist for a sleep study and considered for therapy with a positive-pressure breathing device. In addition to airway and respiratory complications, obese patients have been found to have an increased incidence of postoperative complications such as infection, wound complications, and deep venous thrombosis when compared to children of normal weight.

Diabetes

Approximately 1 in 500 people under age 20 has diabetes, however complications requiring surgical intervention, such as cardiovascular disease, are extremely rare in this age group. Nevertheless, patients with diabetes present for routine and emergent surgery with the same frequency as nondiabetic patients and their underlying diabetes must be addressed. As with any other chronic illness, the medical management of diabetes should be optimized before elective surgery and a plan for perioperative glucose and insulin management should be formulated by the endocrinologist and anesthesiologist in joint fashion. The stresses of surgery and its effects on a regular schedule can wreak havoc on normally well-controlled diabetes if not properly managed. The goal of perioperative management is no longer merely avoiding life-threatening hypoglycemia and severe hyperglycemia but to maintain euglycemia to the extent possible.

Regimens of multiple injections of long- and short-acting insulin are still common, but many patients with diabetes have insulin pumps that deliver a continuous subcutaneous infusion with on-demand boluses for carbohydrate intake or correction of hyperglycemia. Typical management includes the usual preoperative fast with clear liquids up until 2 h before the operation. Whenever possible, it is usually best to schedule the diabetic patient as the first case of the day. After consultation with the patient's endocrinologist, the insulin dosage regimen most often includes reduction of the long- or moderate-acting insulin dose with a reduced or skipped short-acting insulin dose on the morning of surgery. Insulin pump infusions may be continued up until the time of surgery. Blood sugar should be checked upon arrival. Hypoglycemia requires intervention but oral treatment might require delaying the procedure due to fasting guidelines. Hyperglycemia (>250 mg/dL) should be treated with subcutaneous insulin or a bolus via the insulin pump.

The presence of urine ketones will usually lead to cancellation or delay of an elective procedure.

Intra-operative management depends on the length of the procedure. Many institutions consider insulin pumps unauthorized medical devices and prohibit their use. For outpatient procedures that take <2 h, it is often sufficient to simply disconnect the insulin pump immediately before surgery and to monitor blood sugar by fingerstick regularly during the course of the anesthetic using subcutaneous or intravenous insulin to correct hyperglycemia, using a sliding scale agreed upon in advance with the child's endocrinologist, and intravenous dextrose as needed for hypoglycemia. Longer procedures, or those requiring postoperative admission, sometimes require continuous intravenous insulin infusion along with dextrose-containing fluids in order to maintain glucose homeostasis. This might require a longer preoperative preparation time for obtaining intravenous access and initiating the infusions.

Thyroid Disease

Thyroid disease is uncommon in childhood but is associated with certain pediatric conditions, including prematurity and trisomy-21. Hypothyroidism can lead to myocardial depression, arrhythmias, hypotension, hypothermia, and delayed gastric emptying, while hyperthyroidism can manifest as hyperthermia, tachycardia, hypertension, palpitations, and dysrhythmias. In addition, patients with large goiters sometimes require imaging to exclude airway involvement. Both hypo- and hyperthyroidism have anesthetic and cardiovascular implications, and, whenever possible, patients should be euthyroid prior to an elective procedure.

Corticosteroids

Although there is little evidence to support the practice, many textbooks and practitioners advocate steroid supplementation during the perioperative period for patients receiving steroid therapy. Theoretically, chronic corticosteroid administration might suppress the hypothalamic-pituitary-adrenal (HPA) axis to the degree that an adrenal crisis is precipitated by the physiologic stress of surgery and anesthesia. In practice, patients who receive a short "pulse" of steroids, for example for treatment of an acute asthma exacerbation, generally do not require supplementation. The administration of "stress-dose" steroids is sometimes recommended for patients who have received supra-physiologic doses, multiple short courses of steroids, or chronic steroids. Adrenal suppression diminishes with time from completion of steroid therapy. In addition, the need for

steroid supplementation and recommended doses and duration are also dependent on the degree of surgical stress. Patients exposed to minor surgical stress (hernia repair, extremity surgery) might require a single dose of hydrocortisone or methylprednisolone, whereas those who undergo a major operation (laparotomy with blood loss requiring transfusion) might need multiple doses during the 2–3 day period of maximal physiologic stress. Consultation with an endocrinologist should be sought in these situations.

Anemia

The normal hemoglobin level varies with age. Term infants have a hemoglobin level between 14 and 18 g/dL, which, due to rapid weight gain and expansion of blood volume in the face of relatively low levels of erythropoietin, normally decreases to physiologic nadir of 9 or 10 g/dL by the age of 2–3 months. Preterm infants start with a lower hemoglobin level and have an even lower nadir of between 7 and 9 g/dL.

Hemoglobin is the most commonly requested preoperative laboratory test. Because the incidence of previously undetected anemia in healthy children undergoing elective surgery is extremely low (approximately 0.3%), routine determination of hematocrit and hemoglobin is not necessary if the results of studies performed previously as part of well-child care have been normal. A selective hemoglobin determination should be performed in children with a chronic medical illness, those with acute blood loss (trauma, GI bleeding), and those about to undergo procedures with the potential for significant blood loss. Infants younger than 6 months should have hemoglobin measured because of the nadir. In addition, in premature infants, hemoglobin levels of less than 10 g/dL have been associated with an increased incidence of postoperative apnea. Children of African ethnicity who have not been screened for sickle cell disease and have not had a hemoglobin determination after 6 months of age should have such measurements performed before undergoing a major surgical procedure.

Anemia results in a decrease in oxygen-carrying capacity and an increase in cardiac output. Most children with chronic anemia are in a well-compensated state. However, intraoperative blood loss can lead to decompensation in the face of surgical stress and systemic vasodilation and myocardial depression caused by anesthetic agents. Obviously, the child with preoperative anemia is more likely to require a transfusion in the setting of moderate blood loss than children without anemia. Although the hemoglobin value at which individual anesthesiologists choose to transfuse varies greatly, most anesthesiologists allow a healthy child's hemoglobin to decline to the range of 7 or 8 g/dL before recommending a blood transfusion.

Sickle Cell Disease

Sickle cell anemia results from a single base mutation in the β-globin gene. Under conditions of hypoxia, acidosis, dehydration, hypothermia or the use of a tourniquet, HgbS can polymerize, causing sickling of red blood cells, resulting in microvascular occlusion, tissue ischemia, pain (crisis), and, when it occurs in the lung, impaired pulmonary function (acute chest syndrome). This is most common in children homozygous for the mutation, but can also occur with one HgbS gene combined with another abnormal gene such as $HgbO_{Arab}$ or HgbC. The optimum hemoglobin level in patients with sickle cell disease is unknown, but recent evidence indicates that simple transfusion to 10 g/dL is associated with morbidity no greater than that in patients treated with aggressive exchange transfusion to reduce the HgbS concentration to less than 30%, which was the standard recommendation for many years. That is not to say that the rate of morbidity is low; in fact, it is around 20–30% in both groups. These patients require: (1) pre- and postoperative hydration, (2) careful attention to maintenance of normothermia, (3) avoidance of tourniquets whenever possible, (4) supplemental oxygen to avoid hypoxemia, and (5) good analgesia. Patients with sickle cell trait (Hgb AS) have no apparent perioperative risk of sickling or acute chest syndrome, except rarely in conditions associated with extreme dehydration and electrolyte depletion (uncorrected GI losses from bowel obstruction).

Coagulation Disorders

Von Willebrand disease (vWD) is the most common the congenital bleeding disorder. Most patients with vWD have type I disease, which is a quantitative deficiency of Von Willebrand factor (vWF). Ninety percent of patients with type I vWD will respond to DDAVP with a two to threefold increase in vWF. The dose of DDAVP is administered intravenously, intranasally, or subcutaneously 30 min before the procedure. Because 10% of patients with type 1 vWD do not respond to DDAVP, advance determination of the quality of the response is fundamental to the preoperative evaluation of a patient with vWD. Type 1 non-responders, as well as patients with type 2 and type 3 vWD, require preoperative administration of plasma-derived factor VIII concentrate (Humate-P), which has a high concentration of vWF. All patients with vWD undergoing major surgical procedures require factor replacement preoperatively.

Hemophilia A, B and C are inherited deficiencies of factors VIII, IX and XI respectively. Perioperative management of these patients depends on the procedure planned. Patients undergoing major surgical procedures require factor VIII and factor IX levels that approximate 100% of normal from 30 min before the procedure through the first post-operative week. Factor administered to patients with hemophilia A can be plasma-derived or recombinant, and the regimen should be discussed with the child's hematologist ahead of time. Recombinant factor VIII products have become available, but are not necessarily associated with a lower rate of inhibitor or antibody formation. Patients undergoing minor procedures are usually fine with factor levels that are 50% of normal for the first two to three postoperative days. Some patients with mild hemophilia A have a sufficient response to DDAVP to provide adequate protection for minor procedures. The coagulopathy of patients with hemophilia C does not directly correlate with factor levels. The need for fresh-frozen plasma transfusion in these patients should be determined by a pediatric hematologist.

Malignancy

Children with cancer frequently receive medications that have the potential to cause profound perianesthetic complications. Many receive prolonged doses of corticosteroids as part of their chemotherapy, which places them at risk for adrenal suppression. The anthracycline drugs, doxorubicin and daunorubicin, can cause myocardial dysfunction, whereas mithramycin, carmustine (BCNU) and bleomycin can cause pulmonary fibrosis, especially when combined with radiation therapy. The fact that this pulmonary damage can be exacerbated by supplemental oxygen is of concern to the anesthesiologist. The effects of these drugs are not always apparent at the time of treatment and can present later in life or be unmasked by the additive effects of anesthetic agents (myocardial dysfunction) or oxygen exposure. As many protocols include serial echocardiographic evaluations, the most recent echocardiographic report should be included in the preoperative evaluation.

In addition to complications from chemotherapy and radiation, these children and their families frequently have psychological sequelae from prolonged treatment and the side effects associated with malignancy and bone marrow transplantation. They deserve careful evaluation and gentle treatment in the perioperative environment.

Anterior Mediastinal Mass

Patients presenting with an anterior mediastinal mass (especially lymphoma) are at particularly high risk of airway compromise and cardiovascular collapse with the induction of general anesthesia due to compression of the trachea or great vessels when intrinsic muscle tone is lost and spontaneous respiration ceases. Preoperative evaluation should begin with a careful history to elicit any respiratory symptoms, including dyspnea, orthopnea, stridor, or wheezing. A chest X-ray and complete echocardiogram must be performed, including evaluation of: the great vessels with respect to compression of inflow or outflow tracts, the pericardium for direct infiltration or effusion, and the atria and ventricles with attention to degree of filling and the presence of atrial diastolic collapse. If it can be done safely, computed tomography should be obtained to assess the degree of tracheal and bronchial compression. Pulmonary function studies do not predict outcome or help to guide management and are no longer considered necessary. When possible, percutaneous biopsy of the mass or surgical cervical lymph node biopsy using local anesthesia with minimal sedation is preferred over a procedure performed under general anesthesia because it poses the least risk to the patient. If general anesthesia is required and airway or vascular compression exists, having ECMO capability on standby is strongly recommended.

Cerebral Palsy

Cerebral palsy is a polymorphic set of motor disorders with a wide spectrum of severity. Children with CP frequently require surgery to treat GERD or orthopedic problems. Many have increased oral secretions, dysfunctional swallowing, and chronic pulmonary aspiration of both oral and gastric contents. These processes, together with an ineffective gag and inadequate cough, commonly result in the development of reactive airway disease and recurrent pneumonitis. Up to one third of patients with CP also have a seizure disorder. Patients are often taking several medications, including anticonvulsants, muscle relaxants, proton pump inhibitors or H_2 blockers, and drugs for reactive airways disease. Communication is important so that these essential medications are continued in the perioperative period. Confirmation of recent determination of adequate anticonvulsant blood level within the previous 6 months is helpful, although some patients have poorly controlled seizures and are expected to have seizures in the perioperative period despite adequate blood levels.

Preoperative assessment should include evaluation of room-air oxygen saturation and the degree of underlying reactive airway disease, as well as the presence of snoring and other obstructive symptoms suggestive of inadequate airway tone. In the most severely affected patients, scheduling elective procedures between episodic exacerbations of reactive airway disease and aspiration pneumonia is challenging. Since many of these children have ongoing increased airway reactivity, preoperative evaluation and preparation should be directed to ensuring that the child's pulmonary status is as good as it can be. Chest radiographs are helpful in the child who has had frequent pneumonitis.

Hypotonia

Children with generalized hypotonia often present for definitive diagnosis by muscle biopsy under general anesthesia and should be considered at risk for malignant hyperthermia. Malignant hyperthermia precautions are commonly taken, consisting of avoidance of succinyl choline and potent volatile anesthetics. Patients with muscular dystrophy or myotonia are also at risk for MH and MH-like events with exposure to triggering agents. Succinyl choline should always be avoided in patients with Duchenne muscular dystrophy due to the risk of rhabdomyolysis.

Developmental Disorders

An increasing number of children are receiving pharmacotherapy with stimulant medications for attention deficit disorder. Although the American Heart Association recommends that an electrocardiogram be performed prior to initiation of stimulant therapy to identify significant cardiac conditions (LQTS, hypertrophic cardiomyopathy, Wolff–Parkinson–White syndrome), the American Academy of Pediatrics does not agree with this recommendation. There is no evidence to suggest that patients with these diagnoses are at higher risk of sudden cardiac death with stimulant medications than the general population. Therefore, in the absence of a personal history, family history, or physical exam findings suggestive of cardiac disease, no additional testing or evaluation is required prior to anesthesia and surgery.

Children with pervasive developmental disorder or autism require special patience and care because of communication difficulty, emotional lability, possible aggressive behavior, and sensory hypersensitivity. Some of the medications used to treat the maladaptive behaviors in children with autism (atypical antipsychotic drugs) can cause LQTS, placing the patient at risk for torsade de pointes.

Prematurity

Infants born prematurely (<37 weeks gestation) may have sequelae such as bronchopulmonary dysplasia, GERD, intraventricular hemorrhage, hypoxic encephalopathy, laryngomalacia or tracheal stenosis from prolonged intubation and are at increased risk for postoperative apnea after exposure to anesthetic and analgesic agents. Preoperative assessment of ex-premies should therefore take these conditions into consideration.

Bronchopulmonary dysplasia is the most common form of chronic lung disease in infants and significantly complicates the perioperative management of infants born prematurely. The incidence of BPD has fallen as a result of the widespread use of surfactant over the past two decades. It is associated with airway hyperreactivity, bronchoconstriction, airway inflammation, pulmonary edema, and chronic lung injury. Corticosteroids are frequently used in an attempt to reduce inflammation and mitigate the extent of evolving BPD. Many infants with BPD also have pulmonary hypertension. Several effects of anesthesia, together or separately, may have life-threatening consequences. Pulmonary vasoconstriction after anesthetic induction can aggravate ventilation-perfusion mismatch and lead to profound hypoxemia. Anesthetic effects on myocardial contractility can result in impairment of right ventricular function, reduced cardiac output, and pulmonary blood flow, and profound cardiovascular compromise with hypoxemia, resembling acute cor pulmonale. Increased airway reactivity during anesthetic induction or emergence from anesthesia can result in severe bronchoconstriction, impairing ventilation and pulmonary blood flow. Increased oral and bronchial secretions induced by the anesthetic can further compromise airflow and lead to plugging of the airway or endotracheal tube, which, because of their diminished respiratory reserves, can quickly cause profound hypoxia and acute right-sided heart strain, arrhythmias or death.

The pulmonary status of these children must be evaluated and their condition optimized to minimize perioperative risks of bronchospasm, atelectasis, pneumonia, respiratory, and cardiac failure. Bronchodilators, antibiotics, diuretics, corticosteroid therapy and nutritional therapy should be considered in these children. Children with bronchospasm and pulmonary hypertension may benefit from preoperative treatment with elevated FiO_2 to decrease pulmonary vasoreactivity and improve cardiovascular function. The possibility of associated right-ventricular dysfunction should always be considered and, when indicated, evaluated with electrocardiography and echocardiography. Many children take diuretics such as furosemide and spironolactone on a long-term basis, which may cause electrolyte abnormalities that should be assessed preoperatively. Corticosteroids administered for 48–72 h might reduce the risk of perioperative bronchospasm. Infants with severe BPD require continuous postoperative monitoring and intensive pulmonary therapy for 24–48 h postoperatively. Risks of general anesthesia and intubation in these children can sometimes be avoided with the judicious use of either a laryngeal mask airway or a regional anesthetic.

If an infant was intubated for a prolonged period after birth, subglottic stenosis, granuloma or tracheomalacia may be associated with stridor but can be asymptomatic. A range of smaller uncuffed endotracheal tubes should be available at the time of surgery in the event that the initial size chosen is too large.

The risk of apnea is increased in premature infants because of immaturity of central and peripheral chemoreceptors with blunted responses to hypoxia and hypercapnia, even without the additional burden of drug-induced depression. In addition, anesthetic agents decrease muscle tone in the upper airway, chest wall, and diaphragm, thereby depressing the ventilatory response to hypoxia and hypercapnia further. Although postanesthetic apnea is often brief and frequently resolves spontaneously or with minor stimulation, even brief apnea in premature infants can result in significant hypoxia. Although most apneic episodes occur within the first 2 h after anesthesia, apnea can be seen up to 12 h postoperatively.

This increased risk of apnea affects the postanesthetic care of infants born prematurely, mandating that those at risk be admitted for cardiorespiratory monitoring, including ECG, plethysmography, and pulse oximetry. This increased risk persists until infants born at less than 37 weeks gestation reach 56–60 weeks postconceptual age. A hemoglobin concentration of less than 10 g/dL increases the risk above the mean for all premature infants. Infants undergoing surgery with regional (caudal or spinal) anesthesia alone are at less risk of postoperative apnea. Former premature infants who receive prophylactic caffeine intravenously also have a lower incidence of postoperative apnea and bradycardia, but the long half-life of caffeine may delay the appearance of apnea rather than prevent it. Regardless of the anesthetic technique used, our preference is to admit all prematures with a postconceptual age less than 60 weeks to a monitored, high-surveillance inpatient unit for 24 h after surgery. Similarly, because postanesthetic apnea has been reported in full-term infants up to 44 weeks postconceptual age, infants born at term must be at least 4 weeks of age to be candidates for outpatient surgery (Fig. 1.1).

Malignant Hyperthermia

Malignant hyperthermia is an inherited disorder of skeletal muscle calcium channels, triggered in affected individuals by exposure to inhalational anesthetic agents (isoflurane, desflurane, sevoflurane) or succinyl choline, resulting in an elevation of intracellular calcium. The incidence of MH in children is 1:15,000 general anesthetics but it is important to note that nearly half of patients who have an MH episode have undergone a prior general anesthetic without complication. The resulting MH crisis is characterized by hypermetabolism (fever, hypercarbia, acidosis), electrolyte

Fig. 1.1 Algorithm for eligibility for day surgery in young infants. (Reprinted from Galinkin JL, Kurth CD. Neonatal and pediatric apnea syndromes. Problems Anesth. 1998;10:444–54, with permission)

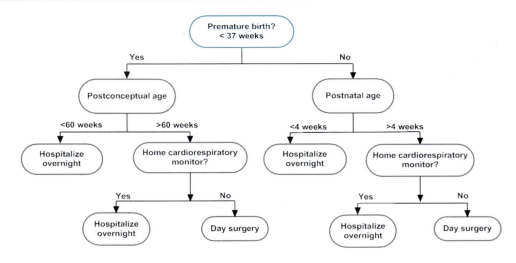

Table 1.4 Treatment of malignant hyperthermia (MH) crisis: "Some Hot Dude Better GIve Iced Fluids Fast"

Stop all triggering agents, administer 100% oxygen

Hyperventilate: treat **h**ypercarbia

Dantrolene (2.5 mg/kg) immediately

Bicarbonate: treat acidosis (1 mEq/kg)

Glucose and **i**nsulin: treat hyperkalemia with 0.5 g/kg glucose, 0.15 U/kg insulin

Iced intravenous fluids and cooling blanket

Fluid output: ensure adequate urine output: **f**urosemide and/or mannitol as needed

Fast heart rate: be prepared to treat ventricular tachycardia

Source: reprinted with permission from Zuckerberg AL. A hot mnemonic for the treatment of malignant hyperthermia. Anesth Analg. 1993;77:1077

Table 1.5 Conditions associated with MH-susceptibility

Previous episode of MH in patient or first-degree relative

Central core myopathy

King-Denborough syndrome

Other muscle diseases (e.g., Duchenne's muscular dystrophy, myotonic dystrophy) – associated with MH-like episodes

derangement (hyperkalemia), arrhythmias, and skeletal muscle damage (elevated CPK). This constellation of events can be lethal if unrecognized or untreated. Dantrolene reduces the release of calcium from muscle sarcoplasmic reticulum and when given early in the course of an MH crisis significantly improves patient outcomes. With early and appropriate treatment, the mortality is now less than 10%. Current suggested therapy can be remembered using the mnemonic "Some Hot Dude Better GIve Iced Fluids Fast" (Table 1.4). It should be noted that dantrolene must be prepared at the time of use by dissolving in sterile water. It is notoriously difficult to get into solution and the surgeon may be asked to help with this process.

Patients traditionally thought to be susceptible are patients with certain muscle diseases (Table 1.5), but many patients who develop MH have a normal history and physical examination but have a specific genetic susceptibility. In the past, patients with mitochondrial disorders have been thought to be at risk, but recent case series have concluded that anesthetic

gases are safe in this population, but it is still recommend that succinyl choline be avoided. An occasional patient will demonstrate signs of rhabdomyolysis (elevated CPK, hyperkalemia, myoglobinuria) without having true malignant hyperthermia.

Trisomy 21

Several common attributes of patients with Trisomy 21 have potential perianesthetic implications. Perioperative complications occur in 10% of patients who undergo non-cardiac surgery. Complications include severe bradycardia, airway obstruction, difficult intubation, post-intubation croup, and bronchospasm.

The risk of airway obstruction is increased by a large tongue and mid-face hypoplasia. The incidence of obstructive sleep apnea exceeds 50% in these patients and can worsen after anesthesia and surgery. Obstruction can persist even after adenotonsillectomy. Many patients with Trisomy 21 have a smaller caliber trachea than children of similar age and size, therefore a smaller endotracheal tube may be required.

Children with Trisomy 21 have a 40–50% incidence of congenital heart disease (ASD, VSD, AV canal) and should have a cardiology consultation and recent echocardiogram if congenital heart disease is present.

Patients with Trisomy 21 have laxity of the ligament that holds the odontoid process of C2 against the posterior arch of C1, resulting in atlanto-axial instability in 15%. Cervical spine instability can lead to spinal cord injury in the perianesthetic period. Preoperative X-ray screening for this condition is controversial but in the absence of an X-ray exam (sometimes performed as part of routine pediatric care or pre-participation sports physical examination) care should be taken perioperatively to keep the neck in as neutral a position possible, avoiding extreme flexion, extension or rotation. Any patient with Trisomy 21 who has neurologic symptoms such as sensory or motor changes, or loss of bladder or bowel control must have preoperative neurosurgical consultation to rule out cervical cord compression.

Allergies

Documentation of allergy status is an essential part of the preoperative evaluation. Prophylactic antibiotics are frequently administered prior to incision. Antibiotic allergy, especially penicillin, ampicillin, and cephalosporins are the most common medication allergies in children presenting for surgery. Although severe allergic reactions and anaphylaxis are rare in patients undergoing surgery, latex is still a common trigger. Such reactions can be life-threatening if not diagnosed and treated promptly. Children with spina bifida (myelomeningocele), bladder exstrophy, and those who have undergone multiple surgical procedures (ventriculoperitoneal shunts) are at greatest risk for such reactions. Although the etiology is unknown, these patients may be at higher risk because of repeated exposure to latex rubber products during repeated surgeries or other procedures, such as bladder catheterization. In 1991, the FDA recommended that all patients should be questioned about symptoms of latex allergy prior to surgery. The general consensus among the pediatric anesthesia community is that children in the high-risk groups noted above should never be exposed to latex-containing products. Since 1997, the FDA has mandated that all latex-containing medical products be labeled as such. Latex-free alternatives should be used instead. It has been well documented that prophylactic medications (steroids, histamine blockers) are ineffective in preventing anaphylaxis in susceptible patients. If anaphylaxis occurs (hypotension, urticaria or flushing, bronchospasm) the mainstays of treatment are: (1) stopping the latex exposure by aborting the operation, changing to non-latex gloves and removing any other sources of latex; and (2) resuscitation with fluids, intravenous epinephrine (bolus and infusion), corticosteroids, diphenhydramine, and ranitidine. If anaphylaxis is suspected, blood should be drawn within 4 h for measurement of tryptase levels, which can confirm whether anaphylaxis took place but does not identify the inciting agent. Patients should be referred to an allergist for definitive testing to identify the antigen.

Medications

Children are frequently taking medications for various illnesses, both chronic and acute. Dosing of some (anticonvulsants) are adjusted to ensure adequate therapeutic levels both by serum determination and clinical endpoint. Administration of most medications is continued at customary doses up to and including the day of surgery as long as excessive volume or co-ingestion of solid food is not involved. An increasing number of children are being treated for behavioral and depressive disorders with selective serotonin reuptake inhibitors (SSRI) such as fluoxetine (Prozac). Stopping these medications can cause withdrawal anxiety and agitation, therefore they should be continued. Most of these drugs have such long elimination half-times that unless prolonged fasting periods are contemplated, withdrawal is unlikely if only one dose is omitted. Anesthesiologists must be aware that patients are taking an SSRI because they are potent inhibitors of hepatic CYP 450 enzymes and such inhibition may result in prolonged or exaggerated effects of other drugs metabolized by the same enzyme system.

NSAIDs and Aspirin

Contrary to most other drugs, NSAIDS and aspirin should be stopped preoperatively because of their effects on platelets. Because of aspirin's irreversible binding, it should be stopped at least 10 days prior to surgery. Ibuprofen and naproxen are reversibly bound and can safely be continued until 2 days prior to surgery.

Herbal Medications

An increasing number of children are taking herbal or homeopathic medications, some of which can interact with anesthetic and analgesic drugs (St. John's Wort, kava kava, valerian) or increase the risk of bleeding (*Ginkgo*, ginseng). Many anesthesiologists advise stopping all herbal supplements for 2 weeks before a surgical procedure. Melatonin is often used to ameliorate sleep derangements associated with behavioral disorders and many practitioners will allow it to be continued throughout the perioperative period as there are no apparent interactions with anesthetic or analgesic drugs.

Preoperative Fasting

Aside from upper respiratory infections or other acute illnesses, violation of fasting guidelines is one of the most common causes for cancellation or delay of surgeries. Preoperative fasting is required to minimize the risk of vomiting and aspiration of particulate matter and acidic liquid during the induction of anesthesia. Research done at the authors' institution demonstrated that intake of clear liquids up until 2 h prior to the induction of anesthesia does not increase the volume or acidity of gastric contents. Our policy is to recommend clear liquids up until 2 h prior to the patient's scheduled arrival time. Breast milk is allowed up until 3 h before arrival, and infant formula is allowed until 4 h before arrival in infants less than 6 months old and until 6 h before arrival in babies between 6 months and 1 year old. All other liquids (including milk), solid food, candy, and gum are not allowed <8 h before induction of anesthesia. In order to minimize "NPO violations," we developed a color flyer with clear rules that is provided to families at their preanesthetic visit (Fig. 1.2).

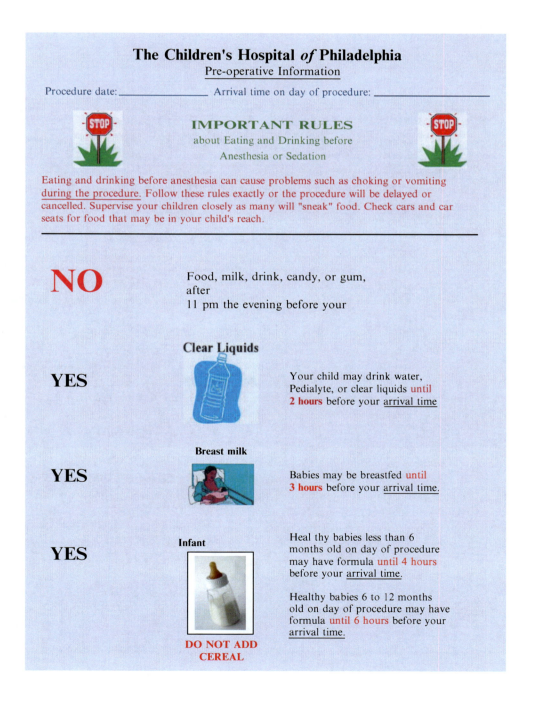

Fig. 1.2 Fasting instructions given to families at the preoperative visit

Laboratory Testing and Diagnostic Studies

For most procedures in healthy children, preoperative laboratory testing and/or diagnostic studies are not necessary. Patients with underlying diseases should have appropriate testing to ensure that they are in optimal health at the time of anesthesia:

Hemoglobin/hematocrit. At our institution, all neonates and infants less than 6 months of age must have their hemoglobin and hematocrit checked prior to surgery. For any procedure associated with the potential for significant blood loss and need for transfusion (tonsillectomy, craniotomy, spinal fusion), a complete blood count should be performed in the preoperative period.

Pregnancy testing. Routine screening for pregnancy in all females who have passed menarche is strongly recommended. An age-based guideline (any female 11 years of age or older) might be preferable. Although it is easiest to perform a point-of-care test for human chorionic gonadotropin in urine, if a patient cannot provide a urine sample, blood is drawn and sent to the laboratory for serum testing. Institutional policy may allow the attending anesthesiologist to waive pregnancy testing at their discretion.

Other studies. The nature of the planned surgical procedure may dictate additional studies. It is important to note that the results of any testing must be reviewed and interpreted before proceeding with surgery.

Summary Points

- For most children, general anesthesia is extremely safe, with a risk of dying at less than 1 in 250,000.
- The goals of the preoperative evaluation are to identify and optimize active medical issues prior to the scheduled date of an operation.
- ASA physical status score is a means of communication regarding a patient's physical condition but does not necessarily correlate with operative risk.
- The history should include a family history of serious anesthesia-related events and personal history of adverse reactions, such as difficult intubation, poor intravenous access, postoperative nausea/vomiting, or emergence delirium.
- Management of reactive airways disease should be optimized preoperatively with the help of the primary care providers and might include bronchodilator nebulizer treatments every 6 h for 48 h before the operation.
- Loose teeth should be sought for and preferably removed at induction before attempted intubation to avoid foreign body aspiration.
- Obese patients with sleep apnea can be difficult to intubate and often need to be monitored as an inpatient postoperatively.
- Patients with an upper respiratory infection but no signs of systemic illness and normal lung sounds on auscultation are generally safe to proceed with general anesthesia.
- "Innocent murmurs" are extremely common in children and in the absence of other symptoms do not require cardiology consultation or SBE prophylaxis.
- Antibiotic SBE prophylaxis guidelines have changed considerably in the past few years and it is now only recommended in certain specific situations.
- LQTS places the child at risk for torsades de pointes when exposed to certain medications.
- GERD is very common but does not appear to increase the risk of aspiration if NPO guidelines are adhered to.
- Management of blood sugar for patients with diabetes needs to be individualized and best coordinated with the patient's endocrinologist ahead of time.
- Most patients do not need "stress doses" of corticosteroids unless they have been on exogenous corticosteroids for a very long period of time or the planned operation is associated with significant physiologic stress.
- Only infants and children at risk for anemia or scheduled for operations associated with significant blood loss should have a complete blood count performed preoperatively.
- Premature infants and children with sickle cell disease should be transfused to a hemoglobin of 10 g/dL before an operation requiring a general anesthetic.

Editor's Comments

We are fortunate to live in an era in which general anesthesia, especially for healthy children, is extraordinarily safe. In fact, because it involves more secure control of the airway, it is probably associated with fewer serious complications than moderate sedation. Nevertheless, we should not be complacent, but instead should take every case involving general anesthesia very seriously. This means a meticulous and systematic approach to preoperative preparation based on evidence-based protocols and strict attention to detail. Many institutions utilize physician extenders to perform the preoperative assessment of every patient according to strict guidelines. Children at our institution are evaluated by surgery APNs, unless they have significant risk factors for an anesthetic or surgical complication, in which case they are seen in the Anesthesiology Department by specially trained APNs or an anesthesiologist.

Allergies are obviously important to document, but it is also clear that the majority of reported allergies are erroneous or exaggerated. This is partly due to overly anxious parents who are quick to label their children with an allergy and clinicians who are afraid of being held liable for inducing an allergic reaction. Falsely reported reactions prevent some patients from getting the medications they need or force clinicians to administer inferior alternatives. Moreover, the science of allergy immunology is clearly still inadequate to help us sort out these very important questions. Until better tests or preventive medications become available, we have no choice but to continue taking a careful history and using the current approach, albeit characterized by somewhat excessive caution.

Healthy children should not be subjected to phlebotomy or medical imaging unless absolutely necessary. It is useful to have very specific guidelines with clear triggers for various proposed tests. To avoid a delay or last-minute cancellation, consult with an anesthesiologist well in advance of the scheduled date of the operation.

Suggested Reading

American Academy of Pediatrics, Section on Anesthesiology. Evaluation and preparation of pediatric patients undergoing anesthesia. Pediatrics. 1996;98:502–8.

Cook-Sather SD, Litman RS. Modern fasting guidelines in children. Best Pract Res Clin Anaesthesiol. 2006;20(3):471–81.

Cote CJ, Zaslavsky A, Downes JJ, et al. Postoperative apnea in former preterm infants after inguinal herniorrhaphy. A combined analysis. Anesthesiology. 1995;82:809–22.

Harvey WP. Innocent vs. significant murmurs. Curr Probl Cardiol. 1976;1:1–51.

Kain ZN, Caldwell-Andrews AA. Preoperative psychological preparation of the child for surgery: an update. Anesthesiol Clin North Am. 2005;23:597–614.

Tait AR, Malviya S. Anesthesia for the child with an upper respiratory tract infection: still a dilemma? Anesth Analg. 2005;100: 59–65.

Williams RK, Adams DC, Aladjem EV, et al. The safety and efficacy of spinal anesthesia for surgery in infants: the Vermont infant spinal registry. Anesth Analg. 2006;102:54–71.

Wilson W, Taubert KA, Gewitz M, et al. Prevention of infective endocarditis. Circulation. 2007;116:1736–54.

Chapter 2
Prenatal Diagnosis and Genetic Counseling

R. Douglas Wilson

Birth defects are increasingly being identified prenatally, allowing the pediatric surgeon to become involved before presentation in the neonatal intensive care unit. Congenital malformations are the most frequent cause of mortality during the first year of life, accounting for approximately 20% of all infant deaths in the United States. The overall risk of birth defects for any couple undertaking a pregnancy is estimated at 3–5%, with 2–3% of those infants having major structural abnormalities identified prenatally and requiring evaluation and treatment as a newborn (Table 2.1). More functional birth defects and developmental changes, not recognizable as structural anomalies, can make up the additional 2–3% by the end of the first year of life. Minor birth defects are estimated at 8–10% but generally are not associated with significant morbidity.

The principal causes of birth anomalies are: (1) chromosome abnormalities, such as microdeletion and microduplication syndromes, (2) single gene disorders, (3) multifactorial disorders involving both genetic and environmental factors, (4) teratogenic exposure, and (5) idiopathic.

The most common prenatal diagnosis procedure is ultrasound, which is recommended as a routine evaluation for all pregnancies in the 18–22 week gestational age range. First trimester ultrasound is becoming more common for screening of pregnancies to identify early risks for aneuploidy and structural defects but this is not as frequently utilized as the second trimester ultrasound. The classification of fetal and birth defects has developed over the years with the Royal College of Obstetricians and Gynecologists in the United Kingdom looking at four specific subgroups: (1) lethal anomalies, (2) anomalies associated with possible survival and long-term morbidity, (3) anomalies that may be amenable to intrauterine therapy, and (4) anomalies associated with possible immediate or short-term morbidity.

R. Douglas Wilson (✉)
Department of Obstetrics and Gynecology, University of Calgary and Calgary Health Region, Foothills Medical Center, North Tower, 1403 29 Street NW, Calgary, AB T2N 2T9 Canada
e-mail: doug.wilson@calgaryhealthregion.ca

Genetic Inheritance Mechanisms and Other Birth Defect Etiologies

Autosomal recessive inheritance is common as all individuals are carriers for up five recessive genetic conditions. For common recessive conditions, the survival advantage conferred by being heterozygous is usually much more important than incidence of new mutations for maintaining the diseased gene at high frequency, the most obvious example being sickle cell disease, in which carriers are less susceptible to malaria. Heterozygotes do not usually manifest a phenotype or, if they do, it is a mild form of the disease. Affected siblings often follow a similar clinical course – more similar in fact than for many autosomal dominant disorders. Once a diagnosis of a recessive disorder is made, the parents are considered obligate carriers and the risk of another affected child is 25%. The healthy siblings of the affected individuals have a two-thirds risk of recessive carrier status.

Autosomal dominant diseases require a single mutant allele to be manifested and are characterized by significant clinical variability. Factors influencing this variability include penetrance, expressivity, somatic mosaicism, germline mosaicism, reproductive ability of the affected individual, new mutation rate, paternal age effect (new mutations occur with age greater than 50) and anticipation (worsening of the disease severity in successive generations). Carriers of autosomal dominant conditions have a 50% chance of passing the condition on to their offspring.

X-linked recessive disorders usually manifest in males who are hemizygous for the X chromosome but generally not in carrier females. The exception is the rare situation in which, rather than the usual 50–50 inactivation pattern, the inactivation of one X chromosome predominates, allowing an X-linked recessive condition to be clinically expressed. Mosaicism may also occur, as in Duchenne muscular dystrophy and androgen insensitivity syndrome. When a female X-linked recessive carrier has a pregnancy there are four possible outcomes that occur in equal proportion: normal daughter, carrier daughter, normal son, affected son. When an affected male initiates a

P. Mattei (ed.), *Fundamentals of Pediatric Surgery*,
DOI 10.1007/978-1-4419-6643-8_2, © Springer Science+Business Media, LLC 2011

Table 2.1 Congenital anomalies: classification and frequency

Classification	Frequency (per 1,000)	
	Isolated	Multiple
A Major malformations (mortality; severe morbidity)	30	7
B Deformations (mechanical; intrinsic or extrinsic)	14	6
C Minor malformations (limited or mild morbidity)	140	5

Source: Data from Connor and Ferguson-Smith 1993, p. 193

pregnancy, all of his daughters will be X-linked carriers and none of his sons will be affected.

X-linked dominant disorders affect males more severely and often lead to pregnancy loss or neonatal death. When a heterozygous affected female has offspring, there are four equally likely possibilities: normal daughter, affected daughter, normal son, severely affected son. When an affected male has a child, the daughters will inherit the mutation with some clinical features while none of the sons will be affected.

Multifactorial inheritance is the result of environmental interactions with genetic alleles at many loci and is the causes of a large number of common birth defects, such as cleft lip and palate, congenital dislocation of the hip, congenital heart disease and neural tube defects. The risk of the specific defect is greatest among close relatives and decreases with increasing distance of relationship. The risk is also higher when the proband is severely affected and if two or more close relatives demonstrate the defect. When there are several affected close relatives, the possibility of an autosomal dominant disorder with incomplete penetrance should be considered.

Genomic imprinting is when one allele is inactivated in utero by an epigenetic mechanism such as histone modification or DNA methylation. The imprint is maintained throughout the life of the organism. Imprints previously established are removed during the early development of male and female germ cells and thus reset prior to germ cell maturation. About 50 genes are known to be imprinted and these genes have important roles in growth and development as well as in tumor suppression. One additional aspect of imprinting is inheritance by uniparental disomy, in which one of the chromosome pairs has been inherited exclusively from one parent. If two identical homologs are inherited, this is called isodisomy; if nonidentical homologs are inherited, this is called heterodisomy. A trisomic zygote is then formed at fertilization and trisomic rescue with loss of the "paired" chromosome from the other parent. If uniparental disomy occurs in an imprinted region of the chromosome, this could determine a specific disease. Some diseases that are a result of an imprinting effect are: transient neonatal diabetes, Russell-Silver syndrome, Beckwith-Wiedemann syndrome, Prader-Willi syndrome, Angelman syndrome, and Albright hereditary osteodystrophy.

Chromosomal mosaicism is the presence of two or more cell populations derived from the same conceptus that are genetically disparate. Mosaicism can occur prenatally or postnatally, due to mitotic nondisjunction, trisomy rescue, or a new mutation. Prenatal chromosomal mosaicism is increasingly identified by invasive prenatal diagnostic studies and is found in 0.3% of amniocentesis specimens and approximately 2% of chorionic villi specimens. In chorionic villi, this is usually confined to the placenta with true fetal mosaicism occurring in less than 10% of cases. The morbidity from mosaicism is difficult to predict and may require analysis of more than one cell source from the fetus, such as amniocytes or fetal blood.

When evaluating a child with an anomaly, it is important that the appropriate terms be used so that a clear understanding of the etiology will be conveyed (Table 2.1). The causes of birth defects include: multifactorial inheritance in 25%, familial disorders in 15%, chromosomal defects in 10%, teratogens in 3%, single mutant genes in 3%, uterine factors in 2.5%, twinning in 0.4%, and unknown in 40%.

The four defined terms that should be used to describe birth anomalies are malformation, deformation, disruption, and dysplasia. The term *malformation* is used for intrinsic abnormalities caused by an abnormal completion of one or more of the embryonic processes. These anomalies are usually limited to a single anatomical region, involve an entire organ, or produce a syndrome affecting a number of different body systems. *Deformations* are secondary events that can be extrinsic or intrinsic to the fetus, such as mechanical forces that alter the shape or position of a normally formed body structure. Deformations usually occur during the fetal period. Intrinsic deformations are secondary to other malformations or neuromuscular disorders. *Disruption* is a structural defect of an organ, part of an organ, or larger region of the body that is caused by an interference with or an actual destruction of a previously normally developing organ or tissue. Disruptions result from mechanical forces as well as events such as ischemia, hemorrhage or adhesion of denuded tissues. Disruption anomalies are commonly involved with teratogen exposure. *Dysplasia* occurs when structural changes are caused by abnormal cellular organization or function within a specific tissue type throughout the body. Except for hamartomatous tumor development (hemangioma, nevi), this is usually caused by a primary defect caused by a major mutation.

Additional terms used in describing birth defects include syndrome, sequence, and association. A *syndrome* is a particular set of developmental anomalies occurring together in a recognizable and consistent pattern and known or assumed to be the result of a single etiology. A *sequence* is a pattern of developmental anomalies consistent with a primary defect but often with a heterogeneous etiology (oligohydramnios sequence). An *association* is a non-random collection of developmental anomalies not known to represent a sequence or syndrome that are seen together more frequently than would be expected by chance, such as the VACTERL association.

When evaluating a fetus or child, parents will want to know several things about the anomaly: the etiology, the genetics, the prognosis, the risk of recurrence in subsequent pregnancies, and what further studies might be available to better answer these questions. The history is very important and includes: the family history for at least three generations, pregnancy history and exposures, neonatal history and, if the child is older, developmental milestones and current school level. The physical examination will allow classification of the birth anomalies into the descriptive terms of malformation (multiple or isolated), deformation, and disruption. The pattern of the birth defects, both major and minor, will assist in syndrome identification as well as considering the possibilities of a sequence or an association pattern. This type of evaluation will assist in the investigations and directed diagnostic testing required (Table 2.2).

Table 2.2 Differential diagnosis of congenital anomalies based on results of screening studies

Neck
Cystic hygroma
  Isolated (sporadic)
  Trisomies 21 or 18
  45X
  Noonan's syndrome (AR)
Hemangioma
  Isolated (sporadic)
  Klippel-Trenauney-Weber
  Proteus syndrome (somatic mosaicism)
Teratoma
  Isolated (sporadic)

Chest
CCAM
  Isolated (sporadic)
  Genetic mutations reported for growth control
CPL
  AR associated with pleural effusions
CDH
  Isolated (60%)
  Trisomy 18, 21; tetrasomy 12p
  Chromosomal deletions (15q; 8p; 8q; 4p; 1q)
  Cornelia de Lange (AD, XL), craniofrontonasal dysplasia (XL)
  Donnai-Barrow (AR); Fryns (AR), Matthew-Wood (AR)
  Multiple vertebral segmentation defects (AR)
  Jarcho-Levin (AD), Simpson-Golabi-Behmel (XL)
  WT1 mutations
TEF/EA
  Trisomy 18, 21
  del22q11; 17qdel
  VATER/VACTERL (sporadic)

(continued)

Table 2.2 (continued)
  Goldenhar syndrome (sporadic)
  CHARGE sequence (sporadic)
  OEIS (sporadic)
  Feingold syndrome (AD)
  Opitz syndrome (XL,AD)
  AEG syndrome (SOX2 mutation)
  Martinez-Frias syndrome (AR)
  CHARGE sequence (sporadic)
  OEIS (sporadic)
  Feingold syndrome (AD)
  Opitz syndrome (XL,AD)
  AEG syndrome (SOX2 mutation)
  Martinez-Frias syndrome (AR)

Abdomen
Gastroschisis
  Isolated (sporadic)
Omphalocele
  Trisomy 13 or 18
  Beckwith-Wiedmann syndrome
  OEIS syndrome
Cloacal extrophy
  OEIS syndrome
Bowel obstruction
  Miller-Dieker syndrome (duodenal atresia) deletion 17p
  Short rib-polydactyly syndrome (Type I, III – AR)
  Trisomy 21 or 22
  Cystic fibrosis (AR)
  Fryns syndrome (AR)
  Feingold syndrome (AD)
  Martinez-Frias syndrome
Ascites
  Perlman syndrome (AR); Fraser syndrome (AR)
  Trisomy 21; 45X; alpha-thalassemia (AR)
  OEIS syndrome
  CHAOS syndrome
  Cystic fibrosis (AR)
  Infection (CMV, parvovirus, toxoplasmosis, syphilis)
Hyperechogenic bowel
  Intra-amniotic bleeding
  IUGR
  Trisomy 21
  Cystic fibrosis (AR)
  Alpha-thalassemia (AR)
  Infections (rubella, CMV, varicella)
Absent stomach
  CDH
  Trisomy 9 or 18
  Tetrasomy 12p
  Deletion 4p (Wolf-Hirschhorn syndrome)
  VATER/VACTERL sequence
  Tracheoesophageal fistula
Distended bladder
  Cloacal extrophy sequence
  Megacystitis-microcolon-intestinal hypoperistalsis syndrome (AR)
  PLUTO (posterior urethra valves, urethral hypoplasia/atresia)
  Bladder hypotonia

AR autosomal recessive; *AD* autosomal dominant; *XL* X-linked

Genetic Analysis and Techniques

Chromosome analysis is commonly performed for prenatal diagnosis when there is increased genetic risk due to screening risk, ethnicity, birth defects, multiple malformations, familial disorders, risk of neonatal mental retardation, infertility or a history of recurrent miscarriages (Table 2.3). Cytogenetic testing requires the cells that are replicating, including blood lymphocytes, bone marrow cells, skin fibroblasts, amniocytes, chorionic villus or solid tumors.

Most commonly the cell cycle is interrupted at metaphase so that chromosome analysis can be undertaken using light microscopy after staining. The most useful staining technique is G-banding, which combines the use of trypsin to denature associated proteins and a green dye. This produces the characteristic dark and light bands as seen on a standard karyotype. Q-banding uses fluorescent microscopy, while C-banding is used to enhance the centromeric regions and areas containing heterochromatin. Chromosome analysis can identify fetuses with trisomy 21 (1 in 800), trisomy 18 (1 in 5,000) and trisomy 13 (1 in 15,000), as well as sex chromosome abnormalities such as Klinefelter syndrome 46XXY (1 in 700 males), 47XYY syndrome (1 in 800 males), 47XXX syndrome (1 in 1,000 females) and Turner's syndrome 45X or mosaics (1 in 1,500 females).

Fluorescence in situ hybridization (FISH) is a sensitive and relatively rapid method for direct visualization of specific nucleotide sequences. Single stranded DNA is annealed with specific complementary probes that tagged with fluorescent markers. One of the major advantages of FISH over the standard cytogenetic techniques is the ability to recognize subtle chromosomal changes such as deletions or duplications. FISH probes are used to recognize specific microdeletions that may be suspected due to the pattern of congenital anomalies. An example of this is the 22q deletion sequence (DiGeorge sequence or velo-cardio-facial syndrome). Another advantage of FISH is that it can be applied to interphase nuclei of nondividing cells, thereby minimizing the need for cell culture. A disadvantage of FISH is that certain structural chromosome abnormalities cannot be detected with this technique.

The whole genome can be evaluated for copy number variants (CPN), indicating that there is too much or too little of a portion of a chromosome. This is known as array-based comparative genomic hybridization (array CGH) and is able to detect small changes in the amount of chromosomal

Table 2.3 Summary of prenatal diagnostic procedures: chorionic villus sampling (CVS) and cordocentesis

	Amniocentesis	CVS	Cordocentesis
Procedure	Amniotic fluid removed by needle and syringe	Chorionic villi removed by TC catheter or BF and syringe or TA needle insertion	Fetal blood from umbilical cord
Timing	15–37 weeks	TA 10–32 weeks TC 10^{+0}–11^{+6} weeks	18–37 weeks
Added risk of miscarriage due to procedure	0.5–1.0% (0.19–1.53%)	TA 1–2% TC 2–6%	1–2% 5% (IUGR)
Fetal malformation risks	–	1 in 3,000 vascular limb malformation if less than 10 weeks	–
Chance of successful sampling	Approximately 99%	Approximately 99%. If unsuccessful, can follow with amniocentesis	95%
Time required for cytogenetic diagnosis	1–2 weeks (FISH analysis 24 h)	1–2 weeks (rapid direct technique may be considered in specific situations)	3 days
Accuracy (chromosomes) for aneuploidy and major structural rearrangement	Highly accurate	Highly accurate	Highly accurate
Mosaicism	True fetal mosaicism – rare 0.3%	Confined placental – 1.0–2.0%	Rare
Open neural tube defects (NTDs)	AFP in amniotic fluid detects approximately 95% of NTDs	Maternal serum or ultrasound required for detection of NTDs	–
Molecular/DNA testing	Excellent	Excellent	Excellent
Twin risk	Reliable/safe 1.6%	Depending on placental location and chorionicity	Increased risk sampling
Rh negative prophylaxis	Anti-D immunoglobulin	Anti-D immunoglobulin	Anti-D immunoglobulin
Type of complication	PROM, infection, bleeding	Bleeding, placental abruption	Fetal bleeding

TC trans-cervical; *BF* biopsy forceps; *TA* trans-abdominal; *FISH* fluorescence in situ hybridization; *AFP* alpha-fetoprotein; *IUGR* intrauterine growth restriction; *PROM* premature rupture of membranes

material in the fetus but with the advantage of significant less analysis time than a standard karyotype. The limitations of array CGH are that it cannot detect defects in which the total amount of chromosome material is unchanged. Therefore, it cannot be used to identify balanced rearrangements such as reciprocal translocations, Robertsonian translocations or inversions. Array CGH cannot detect point mutations or small changes in the genes as it is designed to detect syndromes caused by duplications or deletions of large amounts of chromosome material. Chromosomal mosaicism may or may not be more identifiable depending on the level of the mosaicism. The level of the mosaicism needs to be higher than 15–30% of the cells. This type of array CGH analysis will also identify normal variants that are not associated with pathological changes. For this reason, when prenatal or neonatal array CGH testing is undertaken, parental bloods are used to compare for the presence of these "normal" variants.

In addition to FISH, other new molecular genetic methods for rapid aneuploidy detection include quantitative fluorescence polymerase change reaction (QF-PCR) and multiplex ligation-dependent probe amplification (MLPA), which might replace standard cytogenetics in the future due to their sensitivity, specificity, and cost saving compared to the full karyotype if aneuploidy (large chromosome defect) testing is the primary reason for the prenatal diagnosis.

An understanding of prenatal diagnosis techniques, genetic counseling issues, and birth defect terminology and etiologies will assist pediatric surgical specialists in their daily role of caring for fetuses, newborns, and children with birth defects.

Summary Points

- Birth defects are common – major malformations are detected at a frequency of 2–3% in utero and 1–2% postnatally.
- Terms to describe birth defects include *malformation, deformation, disruption,* and *dysplasia.*
- Types of genetic inheritance and mechanisms of genetic expression include *autosomal recessive, autosomal dominant, X-linked, sporadic, multifactorial, imprinting, uniparental disomy,* and *mosaicism.*
- Genetic invasive testing is done prenatally dependent on gestational age: chorionic villus sampling (CVS) 10–35 weeks, amniocentesis 15–38 weeks, and cordocentesis 18–37 weeks.
- Multiple anomaly terminology is described as *syndrome* (due to single etiology), *sequence* (primary defect but often heterogeneous etiology), and *association* (non-random collection of anomalies not known to represent a syndrome or sequence).
- Parental counseling is required to clarify and educate regarding the fetal or neonatal births regarding their possible etiology, diagnostic testing to evaluate, and surveillance or treatment (with morbidity and mortality risks) protocol to be considered.

Editor's Comment

Prenatal testing continues to evolve as newer and less invasive technologies are developed. Many women in the US undergo a quadruple screen (or "quad" screen, which has replaced the triple screen) in the second trimester, a test that measures serum levels of AFP, unconjugated estriol, hCG, and inhibin. It is more than 80% sensitive for neural tube defects and certain chromosomal abnormalities (trisomies 18 and 21), but has a 5% incidence of false positive results. A positive screen is usually followed by more detailed imaging or, in some cases, amniocentesis or CVS. Imaging modalities, including "3-D" ultrasound and fetal MRI, have also continued to improve significantly, allowing the prenatal characterization of complex structural anomalies such as heart defects and gastrointestinal abnormalities.

There are now a number of fetal diagnostic and therapeutic specialty centers where the care of the high-risk pregnant woman and fetuses with congenital anomalies can be coordinated and planned, sometimes allowing in utero intervention. What defines a pregnancy as high risk for birth defects is somewhat variable, but usually includes: women who are over 35 years of age; women who have a history of miscarriages or premature births or have given birth to a child with cardiac defects or genetic abnormalities; parents with an ethnic background associated with a high risk of certain genetic syndromes; multiple fetuses; and women with certain medical conditions (diabetes, systemic lupus erythematosus, seizure disorder). Regardless of the calculated risk of a birth defect, national groups like the American College of Obstetrics and Gynecology often recommend that all pregnant women be made aware of the prenatal screening tests that are available to them.

Suggested Reading

Benacerraf BR, editor. Ultrasound of fetal syndromes. 2nd ed. Philadelphia: Elsevier; 2008.

Bianchi DW, Crombleholme TM, D'Alton ME, editors. Fetology: diagnosis and management of the fetal patient. New York: McGraw-Hill; 2000.

Bui TH. Syndrome: an approach to fetal dysmorphology. In: Evans MI, Johnson MP, Yaron Y, Drugan A, editors. Prenatal diagnosis. New York: McGraw-Hill; 2006. p. 57–62.

Callen PW, editor. Ultrasonography in obstetrics and gynecology. 5th ed. Philadelphia: Elsevier; 2008.

Connor JM, Ferguson-Smith MA. Essential medical genetics. 4th ed. Oxford: Blackwell Scientific Publications; 1993.

Firth HV, Hurst JA, Hall JG, editors. Oxford desk reference clinical genetics. New York: Oxford University Press; 2005.

Gaudry P, Grange G, et al. Fetal loss after amniocentesis in a series of 5,780 procedures. Fetal Diagn Ther. 2008;23:217–21.

Jones KL, editor. Smith's recognizable patterns of human malformation. 6th ed. Philadelphia: Elsevier; 2006.

Sanders RC, Blackmon LR, Hogge WA, Spevak P, Wulfsberg EA, editors. Structural fetal abnormalities: the total picture. 2nd ed. St. Louis: Mosby; 2002.

Simpson JL, Elias S, editors. Genetics in obstetrics and gynecology. 3rd ed. Philadelphia: Saunders; 2003.

Wilson RD. Management of fetal tumors. Best Pract Res Clin Obstet Gynaecol. 2008;22(1):159–73.

Chapter 3
Epidural and Regional Anesthesia

Arjunan Ganesh and John B. Rose

Children undergoing surgical procedures benefit from many improvements in pain management that have occurred over the past few decades. These enhancements are the result of changes in the attitudes of physicians, nurses, hospital administrators, and patients and their families, coupled with increased pressure from external regulatory agencies mandating the adequate assessment and effective treatment of pain in children. It can no longer be debated that infants and children have the capacity to feel pain, or that the experience of pain by a child potentially results in negative short- and long-term consequences. In fact, the evidence continues to mount that inadequately treated pain in children can result in harmful physiological and behavioral consequences and delay recovery from surgical procedures as measured by time required to return to a regular diet, activity, and hospital discharge.

Systemic opiate therapy has long been the mainstay of treatment for postoperative pain management in children. However, one of the most important advances in pediatric pain management over the last few decades has been the recognition that the harmful side effects of systemic opiate therapy (nausea, vomiting, constipation, ileus, sedation, respiratory depression, pruritus) can be minimized by the judicious use of other analgesic agents and techniques that act at other targets in pain pathways. Furthermore, one of the most effective methods for reducing opiate consumption and opiate-related side effects is the use of an appropriate regional anesthetic technique.

Additional advantages of regional anesthesia include superior analgesia that is site-specific, lowering of the hormonal stress response, and improved patient and family satisfaction. The importance and advantages of providing adequate perioperative analgesia in infants and neonates have been well described. These include minimizing the endocrine and metabolic responses associated with surgical stress and decreasing the risk of neurobehavioral changes later in childhood.

Regional anesthetic techniques used in children undergoing general surgical procedures include epidural analgesia (single injection or continuous infusion), intrathecal (spinal) analgesia, penile block, ilioinguinal/iliohypogastric blocks, and rectus sheath blocks. Most techniques used in pediatric regional anesthesia are similar to the ones used in adults. However, drug dosages must be adjusted to body weight and pharmacokinetic differences, particularly in young infants. Also, unlike adults, most regional anesthetic techniques in children are performed under general anesthesia. Although regional anesthetic techniques performed under general anesthesia could potentially increase the risk of these procedures, large prospective observational studies have demonstrated that they can be safely performed by trained anesthesiologists. The recent use of ultrasound guidance to perform several of these procedures has increased the precision and success rate and lowered the volumes of local anesthetic used, potentially reducing the risk of local anesthetic toxicity.

Epidural Anesthesia

In neonates, the spinal cord usually extends to the level of L3 and the dural sac to the level of S3, but they gradually recede to the adult levels of L1 and S1 during the first year of life. It is therefore recommended that dural punctures for intrathecal (spinal) injections be performed below the level of L3 in infants. The epidural space is a potential space located outside the dura and consists of blood vessels, fat and lymphatics. In infants and young children, the epidural space can be accessed via the sacral hiatus, which is easily identified in this age group. This "caudal block" may be used for single-shot injections or for continuous infusions. The single-shot technique provides effective analgesia for surgical procedures below the level of the T10 dermatome.

The caudal approach to the epidural space is usually obtained with the patient in the lateral decubitus position.

A. Ganesh (✉)
Department of Anesthesiology, University of Pennsylvania, Children's Hospital of Philadelphia, 34th Street and Civic Center Boulevard, Philadelphia, PA 19104, USA
e-mail: ganesha@email.chop.edu

P. Mattei (ed.), *Fundamentals of Pediatric Surgery*,
DOI 10.1007/978-1-4419-6643-8_3, © Springer Science+Business Media, LLC 2011

After sterile preparation of the skin, the needle is advanced through the skin and the sacrococcygeal membrane until a loss of resistance is encountered. In the case of a single injection technique, aspiration is performed to rule out intravascular or intrathecal position of the needle tip and then a small test dose of local anesthetic combined with epinephrine (1:200,000) is injected while the patient's EKG is monitored continuously for changes in heart rate and the ST-T waveforms, which might indicate intravascular injection. Once proper epidural needle placement is confirmed in this fashion, a larger dose of long-acting local anesthetic such as ropivacaine or bupivacaine is administered in incremental doses to provide postoperative analgesia for over 4 h.

Continuous infusions of local anesthetics into the epidural space can be used to provide intra- and postoperative analgesia for a variety of surgical procedures performed below the T4 dermatome. Catheters may be placed in the epidural space via the caudal, lumbar or thoracic routes. Ideally, the tip of the epidural catheter is positioned in the center of the affected dermatomes. In infants, thoracic and lumbar dermatomal analgesia may be obtained by advancing a styletted epidural catheter to the thoracic and lumbar epidural level via the caudal approach. Although this technique might be safer than placing a catheter by the thoracic approach, incorrect dermatomal placement is occasionally the result. When a catheter is advanced via the caudal approach, a radiograph following injection of contrast through the catheter is used to document the location of the tip of the catheter.

When direct access to the lumbar or thoracic epidural space is desired, the epidural space is usually identified by a loss of resistance technique using saline as an epidural needle is advanced (usually in the midline). A catheter is then advanced into the epidural space up to 3–5 cm beyond the tip of the needle. After the catheter is placed in the epidural space, a test dose of a combination of local anesthetic and epinephrine is administered to rule out an intravascular injection as described above. Epidural infusions are typically started following a bolus injection in the operating room. The infusate may consist of a single agent (usually a local anesthetic) or a combination of local anesthetic plus an opioid and/or clonidine. At our institution, patients with continuous epidural infusions are followed on the floor by the pain management service, who are consulted soon after the epidural is placed. A full report of the patient's medical history, surgical procedure, location of the epidural insertion site, and medications administered via the epidural catheter needs to be communicated to the pain management service. Postoperative monitoring of these patients typically include continuous EKG monitoring, hourly respiratory rate, and recording of blood pressure, heart rate, mental status, and pain scores every 4 h. Also, these patients needed to be followed by a team of physicians and nurses with expertise in continuous epidural analgesia, in order to provide appropriate adjunctive analgesia as needed and to detect and respond appropriately to complications such as nausea and vomiting, pruritus, motor block, and infection. When opioids are administered epidurally, intravenous opioids are ideally avoided. However, additional intravenous opioids are sometimes be administered safely after consultation with the pain management service.

The most common problem noted with continuous epidural analgesia is inadequate analgesia due to incorrect dermatomal location and inappropriate infusion rate or solution. Mechanical problems include kinking and obstruction of the catheter, leakage, accidental displacement of catheter, and pump failure. Side effects related to opioids in the epidural infusion (nausea, vomiting, pruritus, over-sedation with respiratory depression) are managed with appropriate antidote medication (ondansetron, nalbuphine, naloxone). Another potentially serious but rare complication is local anesthetic toxicity related to systemic absorption or accidental placement or migration of the catheter into a blood vessel. Strict adherence to epidural analgesia dosing protocols is required to avoid excessive administration of local anesthetics. The pain management team should inspect all epidural infusions and infusion pumps regularly to confirm that the correct solutions and dosages are being administered. Neonates have a higher risk of developing local anesthetic toxicity by virtue of their immature hepatic and renal function and thus decreased metabolism and excretion of local anesthetics. A functioning intravenous line is required in patients with continuous epidural infusions. Also, a breathing circuit, oxygen source, and suction should be immediately available at the bedside in preparation for the rare respiratory complication.

Other complications related to epidural catheter placement include unintentional intrathecal injection resulting in a "high spinal" block, epidural hematoma, infection or epidural abscess, nerve injury, headache after inadvertent dural puncture, and chronic back pain. A high spinal block is managed by using supportive cardio-respiratory measures. Any suspicion of an epidural hematoma/abscess, usually manifested by back pain and neurological changes, should generate an immediate neurosurgical consult while concurrently performing a urgent spine MRI. Post-dural puncture headache is usually successfully treated using conservative measures that include rest, fluids, and caffeine. When conservative measures fail, an epidural blood patch is the usual definitive treatment.

Spinal Anesthesia/Analgesia

Although used sparingly, a spinal anesthetic technique may be valuable in children born prematurely and less than 60 weeks post conception, and those born full term but less that 44 weeks post conception, who are having surgery below the level of the T10 dermatome. In this population, it has been shown to decrease the incidence of post operative apnea when no additional opioids or sedative/hypnotics have been used. The infants do fairly well with this technique. However, this technique is limited by the duration of the block, which is usually in the range of 60–90 min. Spinal anesthesia is also a useful technique in children undergoing muscle biopsy, particularly in those at risk of malignant hyperthermia.

Spinal analgesia using intrathecal morphine can be used for operations performed on the lower extremities, abdomen, and thorax. A single injection of intrathecal morphine in the dose of 5 μg/kg can provide analgesia for 12–24 h. Although respiratory depression with this dose is rare, other side effects like pruritus and nausea/vomiting are more common. These side effects are dealt with in the same manner as those seen with epidural opioids.

Penile Block

A penile nerve block can be effective as the sole anesthetic technique for circumcision or for postoperative analgesia following hypospadias surgery. Several techniques have been employed. The simplest technique is to perform a ring block around the base of the penis while taking care to avoid the subcutaneous veins. The penile nerves can also be blocked in the subpubic area using the technique described by Dalens. Using a long-acting local anesthetic like bupivacaine or ropivacaine helps to prolong postoperative analgesia. Potential complications include hematoma formation and intravascular injection.

Ilioinguinal and Iliohypogastric Block

This block is commonly performed for inguinal hernia repair. The nerves lie between the internal oblique and the transversus abdominis muscle. Although the block is still performed using the "double-pop" technique (represents the popping of the needle through the external oblique aponeurosis and the internal oblique muscle), the use of ultrasound has increased the success of the block and lowered the quantity of local anesthetic needed. Complications include hematoma and intraperitoneal or intravascular injection.

Rectus Sheath Block

Effective intra- and postoperative analgesia following umbilical hernia repair and other midline abdominal procedures can be obtained by performing a rectus sheath block. The nerves supplying the 9th, 10th and 11th thoracic dermatomes are blocked bilaterally by infiltrating local anesthetic between the rectus abdominis muscle and the posterior rectus sheath. This technique is usually done using a short-bevel or a blunt-tipped needle and feeling the pop through the anterior rectus sheath and advancing the needle further until the resistance of the posterior rectus sheath is met. At this point local anesthetic is infiltrated. Ultrasound guidance is increasingly being used to precisely guide the needle to the target to ensure a higher level of success and also to accomplish the block with a smaller amount of local anesthetic.

Summary Points

- Inadequately treated pain in children who undergo surgical procedures can result in harmful physiological and behavioral sequelae can delays recovery from surgical procedures.
- The use of an appropriate regional analgesic technique can minimize opiate consumption and reduce the incidence of opiate-related side effects.
- Potential advantages of regional anesthesia/analgesia include superior site-specific analgesia, lowering of the stress response, reduced sedation, and improved patient and family satisfaction.
- In children, regional analgesia is almost always used as an adjunct to general anesthesia.
- In infants, the epidural space can be accessed via the sacral hiatus, which known as a "caudal block" and can be used to deliver a single dose of an analgesic or to place a catheter for infusion.
- The epidural catheter needs to be positioned properly such that the affected dermatome is adequately blocked.
- Complications of epidural analgesia include: inadequate analgesia due to incorrect positioning of the catheter, systemic effects of the narcotic or local anesthetic being administered, over-sedation, and, rarely, nerve root injury or epidural abscess.
- Spinal anesthesia can be used in premature infants who are having a brief (<45 min) surgical procedure below the T10 dermatome as an alternative to general anesthesia with endotracheal intubation.
- Regional blocks are used routinely for certain pediatric surgical procedures such as circumcision (penile block), inguinal hernia repair (ilio-inguinal block), and umbilical hernia repair (rectus sheath block) with good effect and excellent post-surgical analgesia.
- Ultrasound can be used to improve the accuracy and effectiveness of some regional analgesic techniques.

Editor's Comment

The vast majority of surgical procedures performed in children are performed under general anesthesia. Properly performed regional techniques, such as epidural analgesia and regional blocks, can very effective reduce the need for systemic narcotics, decrease the physiologic stress response, and provide lasting postoperative pain relief in these patients. The key ingredient, however, is accurate placement. This can be difficult to achieve, especially given that these procedures are technically demanding, therefore requiring a great deal of experience, and they are often placed when the child is already under general anesthesia, removing an element of feedback that is usually available when these are placed in adults. The use of ultrasound- and fluoroscopy-guidance seems to have greatly increased the accuracy of some of these procedures and certainly should be used more frequently.

When used as part of a post-operative fast-track protocol, epidural catheters used for postoperative pain relief after major bowel surgery have been shown to reduce the postoperative ileus and shorten hospital stay, but only when they are placed in the thoracic region and when local anesthetics are infused instead of opioids. Children with lumbar epidural catheters not only can have a prolonged ileus, but they require an indwelling Foley catheter for urinary retention, and they sometimes complain of lower extremity numbness or weakness, which delays ambulation. In addition, the failure rate of epidural analgesia can be as high as 40%. When it does occurs, it can be very painful for the child and extremely frustrating for the parents, unless there is an aggressive and rapidly instituted back-up plan, which usually includes systemic therapy with intravenous narcotics and, if necessary, adjuvant anxiolytics.

Suggested Reading

General

Fitzgerals M, Howard R. The neurobiologic basis of pediatric pain. In: Schechter NL, Berde CB, Yaster M, editors. Pain in infants, children, and adolescents. 2nd ed. Baltimore: Lippincott William & Wilkins; 2001. p. 19–42.

Lidow MS. Long-term effects of neonatal pain on nociceptive systems. Pain. 2002;99(3):377–83.

Taddio A, Katz J, Ilevsick AL, Koren G. Effect of neonatal circumcision on pain response during subsequent routine vaccination. Lancet. 1997;349:599–603.

Weisman SJ, Bernstein B, Schechter NL. Consequences of inadequate analgesia during painful procedures in children. Arch Pediatr Adolesc Med. 1998;152:147–9.

Epidural

Birmingham DK, Wheeler M, Suresh S, Dsida RM, Rae BR, Obrecht J, et al. Patient-controlled epidural analgesia in children: can they do it? Anesth Analg. 2003;96(3):686–91.

Krane EJ, Dalens BJ, Murat I, et al. The safety of epidurals placed during general anesthesia. Reg Anesth Pain Med. 1998;23:433–8.

Meunier JF, Goujard E, Dubuousset AM, Samii K, Mazoit JX. Pharmacokinetics of bupivacaine after continuous epidural infusions in infants with and without biliary atresia. Anesthesiology. 2001;95(1):87–95.

Tsui BC, Wagner A, Cave D, Kearney R. Thoracic and lumbar epidural analgesia via the caudal approach using electrical stimulation guidance in pediatric patients: a review of 289 patients. Anesthesiology. 2004;100(3):683–9.

Other Regional

Berde CB. Regional anesthesia in children: what have we learned? Anesth Analg. 1996;83(5):897–900.

Darbure C, Pirot P, Raux O, Troncin R, Rochette A, Ricard C, et al. Perioperative continuous peripheral nerve blocks with disposable infusion pump in children: a prospective descriptive study. Anesth Analg. 2003;97(3):687–90.

Hadzik A, Vloka J. Neurologic complications of peripheral nerve block. In: Hadzik A, Vloka J, editors. New York School of Regional Anesthesia: peripheral nerve blocks: principles and practice. New York: McGraw-Hill; 2004. p. 67–77.

Marhofer P, Greher M, Kapral S. Ultrasound guidance in regional anaesthesia. Br J Anaesth. 2005;94(1):7–17.

Chapter 4
Enteral Nutrition

L. Grier Arthur and Shaheen J. Timmapuri

Providing adequate nutrition is necessary for infants and children to grow and develop properly, especially following major surgery or trauma when catabolic demands are greater than normal. However, the need to provide additional nutritional support is sometimes overlooked as we focus on treating the primary disease and managing complications in the perioperative period.

While advances in parenteral nutrition have certainly had a dramatic impact on our ability to provide nutrition, especially in the perioperative period, enteral nutrition remains the mainstay of nutritional support in surgical patients. Enteral nutrition has numerous advantages including lower cost, ease of administration, fewer infectious complications, and a decreased incidence of cholestasis and liver dysfunction. These advantages probably derive from the fact that the enteral route is more physiologic and stimulates normal gastrointestinal and hepatic systems, and the fact that it does not require placement of an indwelling central venous line. With this in mind, in the child with a functioning gastrointestinal tract, enteral nutrition should always be the primary means of providing nutrition.

Growth requirements vary with age, the greatest requirement occurring during infancy. In addition, certain patients have specialized nutritional needs such as milk-protein allergy, lactase deficiency, short bowel syndrome, or chylothorax.

Nutritional Assessment

The first step in nutritional support is the assessment of overall nutritional status. Many physicians begin with a subjective global assessment (SGA) to identify patients with malnutrition. The SGA involves a history and physical examination focused on vomiting, weight loss, anorexia, diarrhea, feeding intolerance, and evidence of muscle wasting. A carefully conducted SGA can be as reliable as other nutritional assessment factors.

Age-matched anthropometric data, such as height, weight, and head circumference, are the next step in assessing a child's growth and development. These data can help to determine if the child is between the 5th and 95th percentiles. Daily weight gain can be a helpful marker when caring for neonates. Premature infants should gain 15–20 g/day and full term infants 30–35 g/day. Although daily weights as a nutritional parameter can be inaccurate because they can be influenced by fluid shifts and variations in scales, when followed on a weekly basis they can provide a useful marker for growth.

Biochemical markers can provide further information regarding the child's nutritional status. While the serum albumin level generally correlates with the nutritional state, because it has a half-life of 20 days it often lags behind true nutritional changes. Prealbumin (2- to 3-day half-life) and transferrin (9-day half-life) are more accurate measures of acute changes in nutritional status. However, all of these protein levels can be decreased during the acute phase response that typically occurs with the stress of surgery, trauma, infection or malignancy. It has therefore become our practice to measure C-reactive protein (CRP) as a marker for acute phase responses when checking nutritional parameters. When the CRP is elevated, the nutritional proteins are assumed to be artificially lowered due to an ongoing inflammatory response. When the CRP is normal, one can be more confident that low protein levels are indicative of poor nutrition.

Nutritional Requirements

Caloric requirements vary with age and, to some degree, on stage of development (Table 4.1). These recommendations are based on the concept of resting energy expenditure (REE), which should always be considered an estimation. Factors that increase metabolic demands, such as injury illness, should be considered but are difficult to predict or calculate with any degree of certainty. Patients need to be monitored

L.G. Arthur (✉)
Division of Pediatric General, Drexel University Thoracic and Minimally Invasive Surgery, St. Christopher's Hospital for Children, Erie Avenue at Front Street, Philadelphia 19134, PA, USA
e-mail: grier.arthur@tenethealth.com

Table 4.1 Approximate caloric requirements (kcal/kg) and protein needs (g/kg) in children based on age

Age	Caloric requirements (kcal/kg)	Protein (g/kg)
Premature	120	3.0–4.0
0–6 months	110	2.0–3.0
6–12 months	100	1.6
1–3 years	100	1.3
4–6 years	90	1.2
7–10 years	70	1.0

continuously to be sure they are receiving enough calories to heal, grow, and develop normally. Premature infants need approximately 120 kcal/kg/day. Because non-fortified infant formulas are 20 kcal/30 mL, this means that a premature infant needs approximately 180 mL of formula delivered enterally per day. Full-term infants need closer to 110 kcal/kg/day, which is approximately 165 mL of infant formula per day up to about 6 months of age. Between 6 months and about 3 years of age, the caloric needs are slightly less, usually estimated to be between 90 and 100 kcal/kg/day. At some point late in the first year, the child can usually switch to more concentrated formula that is by convention 30 kcal/30 mL. Caloric needs gradually decrease until between approximately 7 and 14 years of age, daily caloric intake decreases from around 75 to about 60 kcal/kg/day. In adolescents, caloric requirements are still slightly more than for adults being approximately 30–60 kcal/kg/day (of lean muscle mass, which is generally considered to be 50 kg for the average adult).

By convention, a well-balanced diet is composed of 15% protein, 35–45% fat, and 40–50% carbohydrates (Table 4.1). Because they continue to myelinate developing nerves, infants need a slightly higher fat component than older children. In addition, fat is higher in caloric density and serves as an important energy source in infants who have lower glycogen stores. While failure to provide the correct amount and proportion of any of the major dietary components can lead to inadequate nutrition and prevent normal growth and development, overfeeding of any or all of the components can lead to other undesirable consequences. Overfeeding carbohydrates can produce an osmotic diarrhea and can raise the respiratory quotient (more carbon dioxide is produced) thereby worsening the child's respiratory status and making it more difficult for to wean from mechanical ventilation. Elevated fat content can lead to steatorrhea and ketosis. Excess protein intake can cause azotemia.

Vitamins and trace minerals are also required for normal growth and development, but except for certain special clinical situations, supplementation does not vary widely from the accepted standard daily requirements. Because premature infants do not have the bone density of full term infants, premature infant formulas provide additional calcium, magnesium, and phosphorous. Without adequate supplementation, children with short bowel syndrome or fat malabsorption can become deficient in the fat-soluble vitamins A, D, E, and

K. Finally, without supplementation children with excessive diarrhea can develop zinc deficiency.

Feeding Access

The method and route of feeding a child is chosen based on several factors, depending on the child and the clinical situation. These include the child's age, the likely duration of need for enteral feeding access, the disease process itself, and the child's surgical history. Temporary feeding access can be obtained with the use of orogastric, nasogastric, or nasoduodenal feeding tubes. Long-term feeding access is usually provided by surgical or radiologically placed gastrostomy or gastrojejunostomy feeding tubes.

While there is no absolute algorithm for determining which type of feeding access to use, each route has advantages and disadvantages. Neonates will tolerate a tube in their nose, or even their mouth, for far longer than an older child and lack the ability to pull out the tube themselves. As a result, it might be possible to feed a neonate through a nasogastric feeding tube for weeks or even months, especially if the child is an inpatient. The type and nature of the disease process itself might also influence the decision. Certainly, a child in need of enteral feeds for less than 4–6 weeks would not be a good candidate for a surgically placed feeding tube. On the other hand, a child who is failing to thrive due to poor oral intake or a child whose oral intake drops significantly during chemotherapy is a better candidate for long-term feeding access.

The decision tree for temporary feeding access is fairly straightforward and usually involves a nasogastric feeding tube. These tubes can be placed in an awake patient and reasonably well tolerated. They allow bolus feedings and free the patient from a pump between feedings. The disadvantages of nasogastric feeding tubes are that they can irritate the nostril or induce sinusitis, they can be dislodged easily, and they can exacerbate reflux presumably by disrupting normal lower esophageal sphincter function. Orogastric feeding tubes are essentially identical to nasogastric tubes and are really only appropriate in small infants.

There has been some debate among clinicians as to the relative benefits of post-pyloric feeding tubes. Advocates of post-pyloric feeding tubes point to a lower risk of aspiration, while proponents worry about higher rates of intestinal perforation. A recent meta-analysis by McGuire *et al.* compared nasogastric and transpyloric feeding tubes and found no difference in nutritional outcomes or complication rates. In our practice, the large majority of children seem to be able to tolerate nasogastric feeding, but we use a transpyloric feeding tube in patients with slow gastric emptying or severe gastroesophageal reflux and those who are unable to protect their airway.

Children who require long-term feeding access are candidates for a surgical or radiologically placed gastrostomy tube. These can be placed using an open or laparoscopic surgical approach, or percutaneously with endoscopic (PEG) or radiologic guidance. The advantages of a G-tube include the ability to provide bolus feedings by gravity and to allow children to move freely between feedings. A decision as to which type of permanent G-tube to use is largely based on the clinical situation and clinician's preference. The PEG tube is generally safe, minimally invasive, and has a high success rate (up to 96%) even in small infants. The majority of complications that occur are minor and involve leakage and local wound irritation, but occasionally a more serious complication such as colocutaneous fistulas (1–2%) or liver injury can occur. Additionally, when compared to surgically placed tubes, PEG tubes have a higher rate of peritonitis when they become inadvertently dislodged.

We favor the laparoscopic approach, which allows the surgeon to directly visualize entry of the tube into the stomach. These can be inserted with two port sites, one in the umbilicus for the camera and one at the site of the intended G-tube. Radiologically placed G-tubes are a nice alternative: the stomach is distended with air by orogastric tube and confirmed to be aligned with the abdominal wall using fluoroscopy. The stomach is then accessed percutaneously and either a G-tube or gastro-jejunostomy (GJ) tube is placed. This procedure has the advantage of not requiring general anesthesia but does expose the child to ionizing radiation.

Jejunal tubes offer some benefits in patients who are prone to gastroesophageal reflux or delayed gastric emptying. Nevertheless, they are somewhat controversial among pediatric surgeons. Disadvantages include an inability to administer bolus feedings and thus the need for a pump to deliver feeds continuously. There are two basic types: the GJ-tube and the primary J-tube. A GJ-tube can be passed through a gastrostomy and into the jejunum during an open surgical procedure or, preferably, over a wire through a pre-existing gastrostomy by fluoroscopy. They can also be placed primarily by interventional radiology using fluoroscopy. All GJ-tubes have the potential of the jejunal port clogging or flipping back into the stomach, requiring repositioning by radiology. In our experience, GJ-tubes can be beneficial in the marginal operative candidate with gastroesophageal reflux disease who is felt to be a poor candidate for a Nissen fundoplication and having difficulty with gastric feedings.

Compared to the situation in adults, primary J-tubes are much more problematic in infants and small children because of the small caliber of the intestinal lumen. Standard Witzel J-tubes tend to narrow the lumen of the intestine in infants and small children causing a partial obstruction. Jejunostomies can also result in small bowel intussusception or segmental volvulus around the point of anterior abdominal wall fixation. In the rare child who cannot safely undergo a Nissen fundoplication and cannot tolerate GJ tubes, a roux-en-Y jejunostomy can be used; however these involve creation of an end-to-side jejunojejunostomy, which can leak or stricture and can also be the lead point for a segmental volvulus. As a result, it is in only rare circumstances that we would recommend this type of feeding access for a child requiring long-term enteral nutrition.

Formula Selection

There are now dozens of commercially available formulas for both infants and children. Formulas are selected based on age, disease process, nutrient requirements, and other patient and disease factors. Consultation with a nutritionist and the hospital formulary are recommended prior to selecting an appropriate formula.

For both premature and full term infants, the optimal enteral nutrition is human breast milk. Not only does breast milk provide sufficient macronutrients and electrolytes to allow for normal growth, it also supplies antibodies to help support the immature immune system. It has also been shown to decrease the incidence of necrotizing enterocolitis. It has been our practice to offer donor breast milk to those infants whose mothers cannot produce sufficient quantities of milk. Some preterm infants cannot grow adequately on breast milk alone. Human milk fortifiers can add an additional 4 kcal/ounce to increase caloric content. Alternatively, hind milk, which contains a higher proportion of fat content, can be used to increase the caloric intake in infants who are not growing adequately.

Standard infant formulas are cow's milk-based, are 20 kcal/ounce, and contain macronutrients in similar proportion to breast milk but higher levels of calcium, phosphorous, and iron. These formulas provide adequate nutrition for most full-term or large preterm infants (>1,800 g) with normal GI tracts and typical fluid requirements. Infants who are not gaining weight adequately on standard formulas can have their formulas supplemented with specialized powders to increase the caloric content. However, these additives increase the osmolarity of the formulas and can lead to increased stool volume or feeding intolerance. Alternatively, there are specialized pre-manufactured formulas that have higher caloric content. These formulas are not always significantly higher in osmolarity, but can be more expensive for long-term use.

Small preterm infants (<1,800 g) have different nutritional needs than term infants. Studies have shown that preterm infants fed standard infant formulas gain a higher proportion of fat than age-matched fetuses. Preterm formulas more closely approximate the growth and nutrition requirements of fetuses. These formulas provide more calcium and phosphorous because preterm infants are deficient in bone density when compared to term infants. Preterm formulas also contain less lactose and substitute lower osmolarity glucose polymers to achieve similar or higher caloric content without greatly elevating the formula osmolarity. These formulas are available in 20, 22, and 24 kcal/ounce preparations. The American Academy of Pediatrics does not recommend soy formulas for preterm infants because optimal macronutrient and mineral utilization is not well documented for these preparations. One consideration with preterm formulas that is not well studied is the timing for conversion to standard infant formulas. Our practice has been to continue the preterm formula until the child weans from formula to baby foods, but some clinicians convert preterm infants to standard formulas once they have begun to catch up with full term infants.

There are many specialized formulas available for specific disease processes and clinical situations. Soy formulas, which substitute corn syrup or sucrose for lactose, have several specific indications, such as lactase deficiency or galactosemia. Soy formulas can also be useful cow's milk protein allergy, but up to a third of patients with cow's milk allergy will also have a soy formula allergy. These patients sometimes benefit from the use of formulas that contain protein hydrosylates. Infants with malabsorption or short bowel syndrome need semi-elemental or elemental formulas. Semi-elemental formulas (Pregestimil, Alimentum) contain protein hydrosylates and medium chain triglycerides, which do not require bile salts and micelles for absorption but instead are absorbed directly across the intestinal mucosa. The protein in elemental formulas (Elecare, Neocate) is broken down even further into amino acids. These specialized formulas generally lack sufficient micronutrients for preterm infants, so vitamin and trace mineral supplementation is usually necessary.

Full-term infants have better renal function than prematures and therefore can tolerate a more concentrated formula. Standard formulas contain 1 kcal/mL or about 30 kcal per ounce. Soy and elemental formulas are also available for the pediatric age groups. Portagen is a specialized formula that contains 87% MCTs and is given to some children with fat malabsorption or chylothorax. There are also specialty formulas designed for specific disease states such as diabetes, renal failure, pulmonary disease, and inflammatory bowel disease.

Administration of Enteral Feeds

When compared to parenteral feeds, enteral feeds are less expensive, obviate the need for central venous access, and do not expose the patient to the risks of cholestasis or line sepsis. However, the use of enteral feeds requires a functioning gastrointestinal tract. Bowel obstruction, intestinal atresia, and inflammatory bowel disease flares are common contraindications to initiating enteral feeds. Following major gastrointestinal operations, most surgeons wait until resumption of bowel function before starting feeds. Most healthy children will tolerate the withholding of feeds for up to 1 week without significant impact on their nutritional status. However, preterm infants have far less energy stores and require nutritional supplementation almost immediately. Enteral feeds are also usually held in patients with extreme cardiovascular or pulmonary instability. These patients, especially preterm infants and those with cyanotic heart disease, may have relative gut hypoperfusion and enteral feeds under these circumstances place the infant at a higher risk of NEC.

Timing for initiation of feeds in a preterm infant can be controversial as there is no clear medical evidence to support the physician's decision. Several studies have found that earlier feeding correlates with a higher risk of NEC, but to date no study has been able to demonstrate which feeding strategy reduces the risk of NEC. The safety of starting with low-volume trophic feedings in an effort to reduce the risk of NEC has not been confirmed and, according to a meta-analysis by Tyson et al., these might actually increase the risk of NEC compared to withholding feedings. In the absence of clear guidelines, the general practice is to begin feedings within the first 5–7 days of life as long as the child is stable and has no contraindications to starting feeds. When breast milk is not available, a glucose-electrolyte solution or half-strength formula is used first. Advancement of feedings is generally no greater than 20 mL/kg/day. Full-term infants and older children can generally be started at 25% of their goal rate and advanced by 25% daily.

Tube feedings can be administered by intermittent bolus feedings or by continuous infusion. Bolus feedings are generally preferred since they are more physiologic and do not require the use of a pump. Continuous feedings can be beneficial in patients with severe gastro-esophageal reflux and it may allow better nutrient absorption in children with malabsorption or short bowel syndrome.

Another important consideration is to remember to encourage oral feedings even in children who rely on enteral feedings for the majority of their nutrition. Infants usually develop the ability feed orally by about 34 weeks corrected gestational age but can struggle to develop the skill later if they are not allowed to try early in life. We introduce oral suckling and allow the infant to develop this skill even while feeds are being advanced slowly. The services of an experienced speech therapist can be very valuable in these situations.

The simplest and perhaps the best measure of feeding tolerance is the presence of a normal stooling pattern and proper weight gain. Weight gain can be somewhat misleading in the peri-operative period, when large fluid shifts can occur. Excessive stool output is often the first indication that a child is not tolerating feeds due to malabsorption or rapid intestinal transit. In general, stool output greater than about 40 mL/kg/day is a sign of malabsorption and a significant loss of water and electrolytes. Other indicators include the presence of reducing substances (sugars) or fat in the stool. Infants with high stool output can also easily become may be sodium deficient. A urine sodium of less than 10 mEq/L is a reliable sign that sodium supplementation is necessary.

Many hospital units use abdominal girth and gastric residual volume after feedings to monitor feeding tolerance in infants. While both probably have some clinical value, inexperienced clinicians can frequently misinterpret their significance. In general, a good physical exam by an experienced surgeon is more accurate in the assessment of abdominal distention than serial measurements. Likewise, the presence of gastric residuals is frequently of concern to the caregivers of children who are being fed enterally. Though bile-tinged residuals can suggest the presence of an ileus or bowel obstruction, the significance of residuals that are a mixture of formula and gastric secretions is less clear. Certainly when the volume of the gastric residuals exceeds 50% of the administered volume, some concern should be raised about continuing feeds at that level because the stomach may not be emptying well and the patient may be at higher risk for aspiration. However, this is not an exact science and if a patient is otherwise showing all indications of tolerating feeds and has not vomited, a single high gastric residual should not be cause for concern.

Complications

Complications associated with enteral feeds can be gastrointestinal, metabolic or mechanical (tube-related). Malabsorption can be addressed by converting form bolus to continuous feeds or by changing formulas. Dumping can also be related to the high concentration of the formula and may be alleviated by dilution. Some children with dilated or dysfunctional bowel can develop bacterial overgrowth within a static intestinal loop. Bacterial overgrowth can lead to hyperosmolar diarrhea as well as fat malabsorption from conjugation of bile salts. Bacterial overgrowth can usually be treated with oral metronidazole. Dehydration and electrolyte abnormalities can occur in association with enteral feeds especially when the feedings are concentrated. Dehydration can be the result of a free water deficit or excessive stool output. Children on enteral feeds should be periodically monitored for electrolyte abnormalities, especially after feeds are initiated or altered significantly. Finally, aspiration pneumonia can be related to tube malposition but is more frequently related to gastroesophageal reflux or delayed gastric emptying. Treatment with H_2-blockers or proton pump inhibitors may be of some value, and when possible, feedings should occur with the patient in an upright position. We have used metaclopramide or erythromycin with some success in the treatment of delayed gastric emptying, though there is admittedly little definitive evidence of their efficacy in the literature.

Tube-related complications are common and can be very frustrating. Depending on which method was used, inadvertent tube dislodgment is potentially serious especially when it occurs within the first 2 weeks after placement of a feeding tube. The stomach or jejunum can fall away from the abdominal wall and leak into the peritoneum. Prevention of tube dislodgement begins at the time of surgery. The surgeon should ensure that the balloon on the selected tube is intact prior to its insertion. We also prefer to place button-type tubes because they are less likely to be inadvertently dislodged than standard long tubes and fix the new tube securely with skin sutures. When a tube is inadvertently removed, the tract can close within several hours if some type of tube is not re-inserted promptly. Some parents are comfortable performing this task themselves, but many will require a trip to the clinic or emergency department for tube replacement.

Another frequent problem is the buildup of granulation tissue around the tube. This tissue can bleed and contribute to tube leakage. Usually this is easily treated with silver nitrate application or 2- or 3-times daily 0.5% triamcinolone cream application for 10–14 days. Finally, probably the most frequent issue related to tube management is tube leakage. This ranges from a minor issue causing mild irritation around the tube site to a major issue in which so much leakage is occurring that feedings and medications are unable to be reliably delivered and significant irritation of the abdominal wall develops. Minor leakage can sometimes be treated with increasing the inflation of the balloon. When this does not work, short-term removal of the tube to allow the tract to narrow sometimes helps. Putting in a larger tube rarely ameliorates the problem and sometimes worsens it by enlarging the tract. When these maneuvers fail, revising or re-siting the tube may be necessary.

Summary Points

- The first step in nutritional support of pediatric patients is the assessment of the child's overall nutritional status.
- Energy requirements in the pediatric population vary by age and physiologic status with the greatest requirements for growth and development during the neonatal period.
- By consensus, a well-balanced diet is composed of 15% protein, 35–45% fat, and 40–50% carbohydrates.
- A determination of the method and route of feeding a child is based on several factors such as disease process, duration of need for enteral access, and previous surgical history.
- Formulas are selected based on age, disease process, and nutrient requirements.
- When compared to parenteral feeds, enteral feeds are less expensive, obviate the need for central venous access, do not expose the patient to the risks of biliary cholestasis or line sepsis, and require a functioning GI tract.

Editor's Comment

Any child who needs supplemental nutrition and has functional intestine should be given enteral feeds. This can be by nasogastric, nasoduodenal (post-pyloric) or nasojejunal tube, or by gastrostomy, gastrojejunostomy or jejunostomy tube. Each of these, even the more invasive ones, are preferable to parenteral feeds because of the lower risk of hepatic dysfunction, deep venous thrombosis, and line sepsis. However, surgically placed jejunostomy tubes, especially when done with a roux-en-Y technique, are dangerous due to the risk of volvulus, especially in patients who are neurologically impaired. Feeds are most conveniently given as gastric boluses, which are also said to be more "physiologic." Nevertheless, children seem to tolerate continuous feedings well and in some situations it clearly more practical. A regimen of bolus feedings during the day and continuous at night is often more convenient for parents and the night feeds allow more calories to be given. The disadvantages of continuous feedings include the need for a pump, the tethering effect of being attached to a tube, and the risk of contamination of the formula with microbes.

Some turn the simple procedure of advancing feeds into a complex art form with convoluted rules and restrictions that border on superstitious (gastric residuals). Enteral feeds are usually advanced very gradually in prematures because of the thought that rapid feeding advancement might precipitate bowel ischemia or NEC. Likewise, infants who have been treated for "medical" NEC are at risk for colonic strictures, which appear to be a risk factor for overwhelming sepsis when feeds are advanced quickly. For most other children, feeds should be advanced as quickly as tolerated – without pain, reflux or diarrhea. Which formula, how much, and by what route should be agreed upon and then feeds started at one quarter to one half of the goal rate. Some prefer to start with a glucose-electrolyte solution or diluted formula but as soon as it is clear that the patient is tolerating even a small amount of these solutions he or she should be switched to the appropriate full-strength formula. Advancing all the way to goal volume with anything other than formula makes little sense, except perhaps in the rare case of the child who is at risk for dehydration and has no intravenous access. (Recall that in infants, the goal rate for hydration is about two thirds of the goal rate for calories.) We usually start with one third volume feeds and then advance to two thirds and then full feeds every 8, 12, or 24 h, depending on how quickly the child is expected to tolerate it. About half of the total volume can usually be given at night as continuous feeds. The key is that the child must be assessed for reflux symptoms, discomfort, severe abdominal distension, and watery diarrhea at every step to be sure that they are tolerating the advancement. It is dangerous to put the schedule on auto-pilot. Gastric residuals and abdominal girths are generally not very accurate in assessing feeding tolerance. As always, it is important to keep the regimen as simple as possible.

Children with intestinal failure (short gut) are at risk for malabsorption and may not tolerate rapid feeding advancement. Similarly, infants with gastroschisis have bowel dysmotility and foreshortened intestine and are notoriously difficult to get up to full feeds except very slowly. It is useful to start with continuous feeds and then gradually consolidate the feeds into boluses after full volume is achieved. In these cases, we start with a very small amount (5 mL/h or less) and then advance by 1 mL/h/day, as long as stool output is less than 15 mL/kg/shift (45 mL/kg/day). More than this and fluid and electrolyte abnormalities become difficult to manage. If there is profuse diarrhea, feeds should be stopped for at least 8 h and then restarted at the last rate that was tolerated for a few days before trying to advance again. Children with proximal high-output stomas can be "re-fed" the effluent through a mucous fistula, in which case the only output that matters is the actual (more distal) stool output.

Parental Preparation

– Risks of enteral feedings include metabolic/gastrointestinal complications (diarrhea or dumping syndrome, aspiration pneumonia, dehydration) and tube-related/mechanical complications (inadvertent tube dislodgment, granulation tissue and/or leakage at tube site).

Suggested Reading

Axelrod D, Kazmerski K, Iyer K. Pediatric enteral nutrition. J Parenter Enteral Nutr. 2006;30(1):S21–6.

Chauhan M, Henderson G, McGuire W. Enteral feeding for very low birth weight infants: reducing the risk of necrotising enterocolitis. Arch Dis Child Fetal Neonatal Ed. 2008;93:F162–6.

Ching YA, Gura K, Modi B, et al. Pediatric intestinal failure: nutrition, pharmacologic, and surgical approaches. Nutr Clin Pract. 2007;22:653–63.

Coran A. Nutritional Support. In: Oneil JA, Grosfeld JL, Fonkalsrud EW, et al., editors. Principles of pediatric surgery. 2nd ed. St Louis: Mosby; 2004. p. 87–102.

Kleinman RE, editor. Pediatric nutrition handbook. 6th ed. Elk Grove Village: American Academy of Pediatrics; 2009. p. 61–104.

McGuire W, Bombell S. Slow advancement of enteral feed volumes to prevent necrotising enterocolitis in very low birth weight infants. Cochrane Database Syst Rev. 2008;(2):CD001241.

Tyson JE, Kennedy KA. Trophic feedings for parenterally fed infants. Cochrane Database Syst Rev. 2005;(3):CD000504.

Chapter 5
Parenteral Nutrition

Aaron P. Garrison and Michael A. Helmrath

Parenteral nutrition has advanced significantly since it was first developed by Shohl and colleagues in 1939. Numerous early problems included allergic reactions to heterogeneous protein hydrosylates, side effects from intravenous fat preparations, and sclerosing of peripheral veins due to hyperosmolar infusions. Over time, protein hydrosylates were replaced by amino acid preparations, the development of Intralipid allowed greater caloric density to be delivered isotonically, and the ability to deliver nutrients via central venous access proved to be invaluable. When used properly, parenteral nutrition can provide substantial benefit to pediatric surgical patients, but complications and comorbidities are still commonly encountered and need to be considered very carefully prior to instituting intravenous nutritional therapy.

Indications

We use parenteral nutrition only when the enteral route is not available or is unable to meet the patient's metabolic needs to sustain growth or fluid balance. This commonly occurs in neonates affected by conditions that preclude adequate early feeding, such as gastroschisis, intestinal atresia or necrotizing enterocolitis, and those who have undergone extensive intestinal resection or have developed complications such as an enterocutaneous fistula. The consideration to initiate parenteral nutrition is based on the patient's age and overall assessment of the anticipated duration of therapy. Newborn infants who cannot begin enteral feeds are generally started on parenteral nutrition on the second or third day of life, advancing up to the goal rate over 48–72 h. In older children, we use parenteral nutrition only if we anticipate not being able to provide enteral nutrition for more than 7 days. Although it might seem intuitive that early initiation of parenteral nutrition is beneficial, experience has shown the use of parenteral nutrition even for as little as 1–2 weeks actually significantly increases comorbidities of nosocomial infections, especially pneumonia and urinary tract infections. Therefore, we use intravenous fluids to resuscitate patients following a massive intestinal resection or trauma and delay the decision to initiate parenteral nutrition until the patient is stable and declares their clinical course. This can often take up to 5 days. Of course, the goal should always be to use enteral feeding whenever possible.

Most infants recover gastrointestinal function and are able to be transitioned back to enteral feeding, but the few patients who go on to develop chronic intestinal failure will require prolonged parenteral nutrition. Careful management of the type and amount of parenteral nutrition and enteral feeding provided to these high-risk patients is important to avoid life threatening complications. We feel that a significant number of these infants are given too many calories, leading to recurrent line infections and rapid progression of liver disease. A multidisciplinary approach to the management of these infants can avoid many of these complications.

Routes of Administration

We rarely utilize peripheral nutrition and almost always administer parenteral nutrition via central venous access. In newborn infants, umbilical venous lines provide ideal early central access. We never use umbilical artery catheters for parenteral nutrition as this has been associated with an increased risk of thrombosis. The widespread use of the peripherally inserted central catheter (PICC) has dramatically decreased the need for percutaneously or surgically placed central lines and are ideal for administration of parenteral nutrition. We always favor aggressive attempts at PICC placement. If long-term parenteral nutrition is indicated, we prefer to place a single-lumen tunneled Silastic catheter that is dedicated to parenteral nutrition use and preferably placed at a time remote from contaminated procedures. The use of

A.P. Garrison (✉)
Department of General Surgery, University of North Carolina at Chapel Hill, 1623 Providence Glen Drive, Chapel Hill, NC 27514, USA
e-mail: mahelmra@texaschildrenshospital.org

P. Mattei (ed.), *Fundamentals of Pediatric Surgery*,
DOI 10.1007/978-1-4419-6643-8_5, © Springer Science+Business Media, LLC 2011

subcutaneous venous access ports for parenteral nutrition is discouraged, unless the patient requires only intermiteent or supplemental administration.

In patients needing long-term nutritional therapy, venous access can be challenging. Formal venous imaging by duplex ultrasound or MRI should be performed in patients with a history of multiple central lines prior to surgical attempts at placement. In dire circumstances when patients with significant thombosis in central veins require placement of a new central line, interventional access can be obtained via an intercostal, inferior epigastric, or azygous vein, or the inferior vena cava. Parenteral nutrition can also be given through ECMO circuits, but we prefer to administer lipids intravenously as they can interrupt flow through the ECMO circuit.

Nutrient Requirements

Calories

The most widely used method to determine daily caloric needs involves estimating resting energy expenditure (REE). The formula for REE is based on the patient's age, height and weight and is supposed to reflect the basal metabolic rate. Indirect calorimetry provides the most accurate measurement of REE, but is of limited utility in neonates and intubated patients. The REE can be multiplied by a correction factor to increase total daily caloric needs during periods of mild stress (minor surgery, 1.3), sepsis or major surgery (1.5), or severe stress (1.7). Contrary to conventional teaching, due to decreased physical activity, premature infants probably do not have increased caloric needs in the face of external stress. Ultimately, weight gain is the most reliable measure of caloric delivery in infants and young children. Weight charts should be kept on all patients receiving parenteral nutrition and the total calories adjusted to avoid the common mistake of overfeeding based on miscalculated nutritional needs (Table 5.1).

Table 5.1 Intestinal failure associated liver disease (IFALD) – patient and parenteral nutrition factors

Prematurity
Low birth weight
Duration of PN
Lack of enteral nutrition
Recurrent septic episodes
Essential fatty acid deficiency
Taurine deficiency
Excess dextrose
Excess lipid emulsions

Protein

Administration of amino acids in neonates should begin at 1.0 g/kg/day and advanced to no higher than 3.0 g/kg/day. The usual range of amino acids administered to older children usually ranges from 1.0 to 2.0 g/kg/day. Current amino acid formulations consist of solutions of crystalline amino acids as opposed to the protein hydrosylates used in the past, but these were designed to provide the requirements of an adult fed enterally. Use of these solutions can lead to elevated levels of methionine, glycine and phyenylalanine, and low plasma concentrations of tyrosine and cysteine. TrophAmine was designed to normalize amino acid levels within a range found in a healthy 1 month old 2 h after breastfeeding and provides essential amino acids including taurine, tyrosine, and histidine. Arginine is an essential amino acid for children but not adults, meaning it cannot be synthesized de novo and therefore must be supplied in the diet. TrophAmine® might prevent the development of cholestasis by providing more physiologic levels of taurine, as taurine deficiency has been proposed as a possible cause of parenteral nutrition-associated cholestasis.

Carbohydrates

Glucose is the major source of nonprotein calories in parenteral nutrition and when provided in solution as D-glucose, its caloric yield is 3.4 kcal/g compared to the 4 kcal/g provided when glucose is taken enterally. Glucose also accounts for most of the osmolality in the solution and therefore limits the rate at which parenteral nutrition can be provided by peripheral vein. Stable infants should receive approximately 40–45% of their total caloric intake as carbohydrates. We usually begin with a glucose infusion rate (GIR) of approximately 6–8 mg of dextrose/kg/min, and can be increased up to 14 mg/kg/min as needed if delivered through a central catheter. Carbohydrates are initiated in a graded fashion to induce an appropriate endogenous insulin response and prevent glucosuria and a subsequent osmotic diuresis. In addition, excess glucose increases the production of carbon dioxide, which is associated with prolonged mechanical ventilation and infectious complications.

Fat

Intravenous lipid emulsions are a condensed source of calories and should provide between 30 and 50% of non-nitrogen caloric needs and the essential fatty acids, linoleic acid and linolenic acid. Twenty-percent lipid emulsions are better tolerated than 10% preparations because of the lower phospholipid-to-triglyceride ratio. The maximum intravenous fat dose provided should not exceed 3 g/kg/day. Patients who cannot be given large volumes of fluid or glucose can receive appropriate calories with additional intravenous fats, which are most appropriately administered continuously. Essential fatty acid deficiency is clinically important and manifest by decreased growth; dry, flaky skin; thrombocytopenia; and increased susceptibility to infection. Since biochemical evidence precedes clinical signs, a useful indicator of a deficiency is the triene: tetraene ratio. This is the ratio of 5,8-11-eicosatetraenoic to arachidonic acid, and a ratio >0.4 is indicative of EFA deficiency.

Electrolytes

Frequent monitoring of standard electrolytes is required. Preterm infants have much greater requirements for calcium, phosphorus, and zinc than term infants and older children. Zinc is a trace element that is lost in the stool and therefore should be monitored in some surgical patients.

Home Parenteral Nutrition

The ultimate goal for every patient receiving parenteral nutrition is to be able to receive 100% of nutritional requirements enterally. Most patients are able to be weaned off parenteral nutrition during their hospitalization. Documentation of daily oral intake can give an estimate of enteral calories, which are removed from parenteral nutrition in increments. When this cannot be achieved during the hospitalization, the transition can be done with home parenteral nutrition infusion. Though expensive, numerous studies have shown that home parenteral nutrition can improve quality of life for the families of patients with intestinal failure. Proper family and patient education is paramount so caregivers are aware of signs and symptoms of infection and can troubleshoot indwelling catheters for basic problems.

Complications

Complications related to nutritional therapy are common and careful patient selection is warranted. Mechanical complications such as pneumothorax and hemothorax can occur while obtaining central access. The risk of developing central venous thrombosis increases with time. Most importantly, catheter-related infections cause significant morbidity and even death in malnourished or physiologically stressed patients. Neonates and patients with short bowel syndrome have the greatest risk of catheter infection. These infections

can occur at the exit site or along the tunnel of the catheter, and may eventually lead to septicemia. Catheter infections are most commonly caused by flora endogenous to the skin (*Staphylococcus epidermis*) or a gastrointestinal source and therefore usually respond to empiric therapy with vancomycin, often used in combincation with a third-generation cephalosporin. Catheter removal is not always required for this type of infection unless the infection cannot be cleared with antibiotics, purulent drainage is identified at the exit site, or the infant's clinical condition is not improving with antibiotics. In contrast to bacterial infections, identification of yeast from catheter cultures requires the removal of the central line as medical therapy is generally not effective at clearing fungal infections. I try to avoid replacing the central line at the time of catheter removal, except in the rare situation that access cannot be obtained or central access is clinically needed. As the administration of parenteral nutrition is never a true emergency, the immediate placement of a new central line specifically for continuation of parenteral nutrition is not clinically indicated. Ideally, negative blood cultures and clinical resolution of the infection should be identified prior to replacing a new central line. We do not use prophylactic antibiotics in our patients with central lines as this does not appear to decrease the incidence of line sepsis and might increase the prevalence of antibiotic-resistant organisms.

Parenteral nutrition-induced cholestasis is a poorly understood condition that is currently an area of active research. Intestinal failure-associated liver disease (IFALD) is likely the result of a combination of patient factors and deleterious effects of parenteral nutrition (Table 5.2). Patient factors include immature bile secretory mechanism, bile stasis induced by fasting, and repeated septic episodes resulting in endotoxemia. Parenteral nutrition-associated factors include excessive glucose, which can cause fatty liver, excessive protein, which may result in reduced bile flow, and phytosterols present in intravenous lipid preparations, which might injure the liver directly. Preventive strategies include: decreasing GIRs, decreasing protein and parenteral lipid load. The most important factor that can prevent IFALD appears to be maximizing the percentage of calories provided by the enteral route. When this is not possible, we have had success with limiting intralipids to 1 mg/kg 1 day a week or eliminating their use altogether in patients with intestinal failure and parenteral nutrition-induced cholestatasis. If small amounts of enteral feeding are tolerated, administration of enteral fats via corn oil or safflower oil supplementation in the feeds can usually provide adequate essential fatty acids. When managing patients by reducing intralipids, we document that the triene-to-tetraene ratio is less than 0.4 every 1–2 weeks. Preliminary data on the intravenous administration of omega-3 fatty acid (fish oil) lipid solution may have a beneficial effect on IFALD in patients who cannot tolerate trophic feeds, but the use of this lipid formulation currently requires an Investigational New Drug application to the FDA to be used in the United States.

Table 5.2 Typical parenteral nutrition requirements by patient age

Age	Calories (kcal/kg/day)	Protein (g/kg/day) (15% of calories)	Carbohydrates (mg/kg/min) (45% of calories)	Fat (g/kg/day) (40% of calories)
Premature	100–120	2.5–3.0	6–8	0.5–1.0
Term infant	90–110	2.0–3.0	6–12	1.0
1–7 years	75–90	1.0–2.0	12	1.0
7–14 years	60–75	1.0–2.0	12	1.0
14–18 years	30–60	0.8–2.0	12	1.0

Summary Points

- Indications for initiating parenteral nutrition should consider both the age of the patient and anticipated duration of parenteral nutrition needs.
- In general, limited enteral nutrition for a short period of time (7–10 days) is preferred over a short course of parenteral nutrition due to fewer complications.
- PICC lines are ideal for parenteral nutrition.
- Patients requiring long-term treatment are best served by placing a single lumen tunneled catheter at a time remote from infection.
- Bacterial catheter infections can usually be treated with antibiotic therapy; fungal infections require removal of central lines.
- IFALD is more common in premature infants, and may be associated with overfeeding and recurrent infections.
- Limiting parenteral lipids to less than 1 mg/kg 1 day a week or providing all lipids enterally may slow the progression of liver disease, yet mandates checking essential fatty acid levels by monitoring the triene: tetraene ratio.
- A triene: tetraene ratio >0.4 indicates an essential fatty acid deficiency, which precedes clinical manifestations.
- Intestinal failure patients are best managed by a multidisciplinary approach.

Editor's Comment

There is no doubt that advances in the science of parenteral nutrition have saved countless lives; however until the mystery of parenteral nutrition-associated cholestasis is solved, it will continue to be simply a bridge to enteral nutrition. As a result, the goal for every patient receiving parenteral nutrition is to get off of it as soon as possible. Peripheral nutrition rarely provides enough nutrition to make a real difference and tends to require daily replacement of peripheral intravenous catheters, which can be torturous for the patient. It is incumbent on the surgeon or interventionalist who places central venous catheters in patients who will need long-term parenteral nutrition to do everything possible to preserve the central veins. This means placing only the smallest single-lumen catheter needed to meet the child's needs, having protocols and support staff available to help families avoid catheter dislodgement and line infections, and monitoring patients closely for catheter-associated vein thrombosis so that the catheter can be removed and treatment started early. Some of these patients will benefit from a work up for a hypercoagulable state.

Every year the literature is replete with reports of new breakthroughs in the understanding of parenteral nutrition-associated liver disease, but none have provided the definitive solution to the problem. The latest and perhaps most promising are taurine and omega-3 fatty acids, each of which, so far at least, appears to be protective against cholestasis.

The best preventative measure, of course, is to transition to enteral nutrition as soon as possible.

PICC lines have revolutionized the care of patients who need parenteral nutrition for up to several months at a time, but the risk of complications and catheter-associated blood stream infection remains relatively high. Perhaps the most significant advantage is that it has lowered the threshold for surgeons to begin (and patients to accept) the initiation of parenteral nutrition in borderline situations, especially in the postoperative period. While patients with prolonged ileus or multiple procedures in the past might have been reluctant to consider placement of a central venous catheter, they and their surgeons are now probably less inclined to fear placement of a PICC line at an earlier stage in their postoperative recovery, when it can make the difference between healing and the risk of multiple complications.

Suggested Reading

Chung DH, Ziegler MM. Central venous catheter access. Nutrition. 1998;14(1):119–23.

Kelly DA. Intestinal failure-associated liver disease: what do we know today? Gastroenterology. 2006;130(2 Suppl 1):S70–7.

Mascarenhas MR, Kerner Jr JA, Stallings VA. Parenteral and enteral nutrition. In: Walker WA, Durie PR, Hamilton JR, Walker-Smith JA, Watkins JB, editors. Pediatric gastrointestinal disease: pathophysiology, diagnosis, management. Hamilton: B.C. Decker; 2000. p. 1705–51.

Wessel JJ, Kocoshis SA. Nutritional management of infants with short bowel syndrome. Semin Perinatol. 2007;31(2):104–11.

Chapter 6
Fast-Track Protocols

Peter Mattei

It is increasingly clear that the application of systematic and evidence-based perioperative protocols can help make patients more comfortable and hasten their recovery. Many also believe that patient care should be straightforward and that patients should not be subjected to the discomfort and indignity of unnecessary procedures, worthless rituals, and therapies that are not supported by scientific evidence. Clinical pathways should address several aspects of postoperative care including: the return of bowel function, increasing activity levels, maximizing patient comfort, and eliminating superfluous maneuvers.

Postoperative Ileus

Traditional surgical teaching, passed on through generations of surgical residents, emphasized the idea that the postoperative ileus is a mandatory period of bowel inactivity that could not, and should not, be hastened or otherwise modified. This was especially true for patients who had undergone intra-abdominal procedures such as bowel surgery. Standard therapy mandated strict bowel rest and gastric decompression. Patients were typically forbidden to eat or drink until they had a bowel movement, which was supposed to signify the return of bowel function. An enlightened few would allow removal of the nasogastric tube and resumption of diet upon the passage of flatus or when the nasogastric tube drainage was no longer green. Regardless, the result of this strategy was that the typical length of time before resumption of regular diet could be anywhere from 3 to 14 days.

The postoperative period of paralytic ileus was considered not only mandatory but beneficial. The house officer foolhardy enough to remove a nasogastric tube prematurely, allow the patient to suck on ice chips or sip water, or induce

a bowel movement with a laxative or suppository was roundly castigated and accused of placing the patient at risk for such horrible complications as bowel obstruction, anastomotic dehiscence, and peritonitis with sepsis. Finally, a few intrepid pioneers in the late 1980s did the unthinkable and questioned this dogma by doing away with some of these firmly held beliefs. They found that not only did their patients survive but they got better faster, went home sooner, and were more comfortable throughout their postoperative course. Studies throughout the 1990s have confirmed that these "fast-track" protocols are safe and they have become standard at many forward-thinking surgical services around the world. Strangely, pediatric surgeons seemed initially reticent about adopting similar measures in the care of children.

Indications

Most likely to benefit from application of a fast-track postoperative program is the healthy child who has undergone an elective and uncomplicated intra-abdominal procedure and who is comfortable, neurologically intact, and spontaneously breathing. The absence of any of these components is not an absolute contraindication to applying the protocol, but the critically ill, comatose, mechanically ventilated patient with severe chemical peritonitis might not the best candidate. Although the patient who has undergone a minimally invasive procedure would naturally be expected to recover more quickly, children who have undergone an extensive operation through a more traditional open incision also appear to benefit from these measures.

Safe application of a fast-track protocol involves experience and good judgment. Relative contraindications include: age less than 6 months or weight less than 10 kg, or any infant whose respiratory status might be compromised by a distended abdomen; esophageal, gastric or duodenal procedures; inability to protect the airway in the event of emesis; positive-pressure ventilation, BiPAP, or CPAP; and conditions expected to cause a profound ileus such as high-grade bowel obstruction, fecal contamination of the peritoneum, or

P. Mattei (✉)
Department of Anesthesia and Critical Care, Children's Hospital of Philadelphia, 3400 Civic Center Boulevard, Philadelphia, PA 19146, USA
e-mail: mattei@email.chop.edu

massive ascites. On the other hand, we have safely utilized the protocol or a slightly modified version thereof in patients with perforated appendicitis, partial SBO, jejunal resection with primary anastomosis, hepatic resection, Meckel's diverticulitis, retroperitoneal tumor resection, nephrectomy, and many procedures that include creation of an ileostomy.

The Protocol

The basic tenets of a typical fast-track protocol include: no routine nasogastric tube, early diet advancement, minimization of narcotic analgesics, and early ambulation/physical rehabilitation (Table 6.1). Naturally, the protocol is modified according to the patient population, the procedure, preference of the surgeon, and, sometimes, the biases of the institution, but a common theme is that each component should be supported by the evidence.

Patient Expectations

The first step is to manage expectations by educating patients and their families that the discharge date is determined by

Table 6.1 Typical fast-track protocol in pediatric surgery

Patient education	Anticipate discharge to home by POD 2–3[a]
NO nasogastric tube	Except • After esophageal, gastric or duodenal surgery • Infants <6 months of age or <10 kg body weight • Placed postop as needed for comfort[b]
Diet	• Clear liquid diet immediately (sips at first) • Advanced to regular as tolerated[c]
Intravenous fluids	0.8 of calculated "maintenance" rate[d]
Pain management	• Minimize narcotics • Nalbuphine and/or ketorolac • If PCA, basal rate infusion should be *zero* • Thoracic epidural delivering local anesthetic[e]
Physical rehabilitation	Start to ambulate within first 12–24 h
Bisacodyl suppository	Start on POD 2 then BID until bowel movement

POD postoperative day; *PCA* patient-controlled analgesia; *BID* twice daily

[a]This is standard for an uncomplicated bowel resection but will vary depending on the procedure being performed
[b]Intractable emesis, extreme distension, gas bloat
[c]In the absence of symptoms (fullness, nausea, emesis) or abdominal distension
[d]Maximum rate: 84 mL/h (roughly 2 L/day)
[e]Lumbar epidural administration of narcotics are known to prolong postoperative ileus

how well the patient is doing and therefore inherently unpredictable. Some patients having the same operation will go home within a few days while others need more time, and still others will have setbacks that could delay discharge even more. However, families should be given some idea of what an average length of stay is expected to be. We have found it best to err on the side of too few days rather than too many, as parents who are told that their child will stay 5 days will feel like they are being rushed out the door or their care is being compromised if you declare on day 3 that they can are ready to go home. Because we have many patients who are ready for discharge on postoperative day 2 or 3 after laparoscopic-assisted ileocecectomy for ileal Crohn's disease, this is the length of stay we use for this procedure. Other operations have different anticipated lengths of stay. Do not underestimate the importance of the psychology of illness and wellness: in general, patients who think they should be sick for a certain number of days often feel ill for that many days while those who anticipate feeling better sooner often do.

Nasogastric Tubes

Nasogastric tubes were once thought to improve patient comfort by preventing postoperative emesis and to shorten the postoperative ileus by reducing bowel distension caused by intestinal secretions and swallowed air. However, most patients in fact do not experience severe postoperative bloating or emesis, and it appears that gastric decompression probably prolongs the postoperative ileus rather than shortens it. The reasons for this are unclear but one possibility is that postoperative emesis was much more common and more severe with older anesthetic drug regimens and before the development of modern antiemetics. Also, gastric decompression might prolong ileus by removing stimulants to downstream bowel motility that are normally secreted proximally. The tubes themselves are also known to increase the risk of infectious complications such as sinusitis and aspiration pneumonia.

Nasogastric tubes are therefore not routinely needed after most abdominal operations. But we still use them after operations in which gastric distension might disrupt a suture line or be otherwise disastrous, such as those involving the esophagus, stomach, or duodenum. Following small bowel or colorectal surgery, fewer than one in 20 patients will need to have a nasogastric tube placed, and this is usually for patient comfort: intractable emesis, severe distension, or symptomatic gastric gas bloat. We also still use them in small infants because even a moderate amount of gastric or abdominal distension can compromise their respiratory status.

Diet

There is rarely the need to strictly prohibit oral intake after uncomplicated abdominal or bowel surgery. With or without a nasogastric tube in place, taking sips of clear liquids in the immediate postoperative period is probably harmless as the volume is minuscule compared to the typical volume of saliva, gastric secretions, and pancreaticobiliary effluent that patients generate. Of course, excessive volume of intake or the gas from carbonated beverages can cause bloat, nausea, or vomiting early on, but, for the most part, limited early oral intake appears to stimulate the bowel in a way that is more beneficial than harmful. This makes sense from a physiologic standpoint given that promotility enterohormones are normally released in response to oral intake.

In the very early postoperative period, we let our patients take small amounts of clear liquids and then advance gradually to more substantive intake, as long as they are not feeling full or nauseated and if there is only minimal abdominal distension on physical examination. It is the rare patient who will not limit intake appropriately. Nevertheless, they need to be monitored closely for signs of significant ongoing dysmotility (abdominal distension, belching) at least 3 or 4 times in a 24-h period.

Intravenous Fluid

It has been suggested that bowel edema increases postoperative bowel dysfunction. This certainly appears to be the case when a patient has a bowel obstruction or chemical peritonitis, but whether the edema is a primary cause or simply a result of the injury is not clear. Some have suggested that excessive intravenous hydration during or after an operation prolongs the postoperative ileus and it has been posited that this could be due to third-space fluid entering the bowel wall, much as it does in a more visible way in the face and other soft tissues of the body. We therefore try to limit the amount of intravenous fluid, both in the operating room and in the postoperative period, to only that which is necessary to maintain adequate tissue perfusion and renal function. Though this is perhaps the part of the protocol with the weakest scientific support, there may be other benefits to avoiding excessive hydration intravenous fluids and certainly no reason why it would be advantageous. The traditional pediatric maintenance fluid formula is empirically based and was designed to err on the side of giving too much fluid. We therefore give 0.8 of the calculated maintenance rate and then, if a patient demonstrates a need for more fluid (low urine output, tachycardia), we provide a bolus of crystalloid solution (20 mL/kg). Increasing the maintenance rate

under these circumstances takes too long to have an effect and replaces third-space losses with mostly free water. Regardless of the calculated maintenance rate, we give no more than 84 mL/h since very few patients need more than 2 L of intravenous fluids in a 24-h period.

Pain Management

That narcotics have a detrimental effect on bowel motility is well documented. They also induce nausea and their sedative effects make it difficult for some patients to participate in a postoperative physical rehabilitation program. It is therefore preferable to minimize the administration of narcotics while still making sure the patient is comfortable. We prefer to use the combined agonist-antagonist narcotic drug nalbuphine (0.1 mg/kg IV every 3 h, as needed for pain), which has good analgesic properties and may have less of a detrimental effect on bowel motility than morphine or dilaudid. We also typically use ketorolac (0.5 mg/kg IV every 6 h, maximum dose 30 mg, around the clock), which has excellent analgesic properties and none of the adverse effects associated with opiates. Because of concerns regarding the use of an NSAID in this patient population, we routinely co-administer an intravenous H_2-blocker or proton pump inhibitor as prophylaxis against gastritis, and we limit the use of ketorolac to 72 h to minimize the risk of renal dysfunction. Patient-controlled analgesia is also an excellent option for postoperative pain relief but we have found it best to avoid a basal opiate infusion as it tends to make patients very sedated and appears to delay resolution of the ileus. Clinical trials are under way for use of an intravenous form of acetaminophen, but whether this will prove to be an effective alternative to opiates for postoperative pain relief is unclear. It is well known that narcotics administered through a lumbar epidural catheter prolong the postoperative ileus but that local anesthetics delivered by a thoracic epidural catheter have little such effect and provide excellent analgesia.

Ambulation

Contrary to traditional surgical teaching, patients cannot "walk off" their ileus. While being sedentary probably does prolong an ileus, making patients take more than two or three trips around the hospital ward per day is probably excessive, at least as far as the ileus is concerned. Nevertheless, early ambulation is beneficial for many reasons and we therefore encourage patients to walk early in the postoperative period, preferably the night of surgery for their first postoperative void, but certainly no later than the morning of the first postoperative day.

Constipation

Because the colon was thought to be the last segment of the intestine to recover from the postoperative ileus, the traditional recommendation was to maintain gastric decompression and nothing by mouth until the patient passed stool or flatus. In retrospect, it seems more likely that what was considered the final phase of the postoperative ileus was simply constipation. There are many factors that promote constipation in postoperative patients including general anesthetic agents, opiates, diminished activity, fluid shifts, and poor oral intake. In our experience, it is clear that inducing a bowel movement on the second or third day in patients who are otherwise recovering nicely from their operation makes them feel better, relieves abdominal distension, and improves their appetite.

Discharge Criteria

Barring a postoperative complication, patients are considered ready for discharge to home when they are afebrile, tolerating a regular diet, able to ambulate without assistance, and have good pain control with oral analgesics. It is also preferable that they have at least one bowel movement. We have found that it is very important that parents feel comfortable taking their child home, and this is where the preoperative education to anticipate an early discharge is vital.

The fast-track approach is not a one-size-fits-all regimen. The care of every patient must be individualized, which is only possible by getting to know each patient and following them closely in the postoperative period. Every patient should be examined at least 3–4 times daily to be sure that they are able to be advanced on their diet and that a complication has not developed. But the majority of patients will do well and advance appropriately.

Summary Points

- Patients and their families should be educated regarding the criteria for discharge and the fact that some patients are safely discharged in the early postoperative period.
- Routine nasogastric tube decompression prolongs the postoperative ileus, makes patients more uncomfortable, and ultimately extends the average length of hospital stay.
- Nasogastric tubes are used in patients who have had surgery on the esophagus, stomach, duodenum, or pancreas, and in infants for whom moderate gastric distension can compromise ventilation.
- Early postoperative oral intake appears to be safe and, in moderation, hastens recovery of bowel function.
- Administering excessive intravenous fluids might prolong the postoperative ileus by increasing bowel wall edema.
- Patients appear to benefit from having a bowel movement in the early postoperative period, which can safely be promoted by administering a rectal suppository.
- Patients who ambulate early and often recover more quickly, have fewer complications, and are discharged sooner.
- Narcotics, especially when delivered by lumbar epidural catheter or as a basal intravenous infusion, slow bowel motility and their use in the postoperative period should be limited to the minimum amount necessary to achieve adequate pain relief.
- Patients are considered ready for discharge to home when they are afebrile, ambulating, tolerating a regular diet, and have adequate pain relief with oral analgesics.

Suggested Reading

Delaney CP. Clinical perspective on postoperative ileus and the effect of opiates. Neurogastroenterol Motil. 2004;16 Suppl 2:61–6.

Delaney CP, Fazio VW, Senagore AJ, Robinson B, Halverson AL, Remzi FH. 'Fast track' postoperative management protocol for patients with high co-morbidity undergoing complex abdominal and pelvic colorectal surgery. Br J Surg. 2001;88(11):1533–8.

Holte K, Kehlet H. Postoperative ileus: a preventable event. Br J Surg. 2000;87(11):1480–93.

Kehlet H, Wilmore DW. Evidence-based surgical care and the evolution of fast-track surgery. Ann Surg. 2008;248(2):189–98.

Lobo DN, Bostock KA, Neal KR, Perkins AC, Rowlands BJ, Allison SP. Effect of salt and water balance on recovery of gastrointestinal function after elective colonic resection: a randomised controlled trial. Lancet. 2002;359(9320):1812–8.

Luckey A, Livingston E, Tache Y. Mechanisms and treatment of postoperative ileus. Arch Surg. 2003;138(2):206–14.

Nelson R, Edwards S, Tse B. Prophylactic nasogastric decompression after abdominal surgery. Cochrane Database Syst Rev. 2005;(1): CD004929.

Senagore AJ, Delaney CP, Mekhail N, Dugan A, Fazio VW. Randomized clinical trial comparing epidural anaesthesia and patient-controlled analgesia after laparoscopic segmental colectomy. Br J Surg. 2003;90(10):1195–9.

Waldhausen JH, Schirmer BD. The effect of ambulation on recovery from postoperative ileus. Ann Surg. 1990;212(6):671–7.

Chapter 7
Quality Improvement, Education, and Outcomes Research in Pediatric Surgery

Steven Teich and Marc P. Michalsky

Historically, there has been a great disparity in the advancement of pediatric clinical services and the development of pediatric quality and safety indicators. The development and expansion of pediatric care in the United States began with the opening of the Children's Hospital of Philadelphia in 1855. Despite this major advancement in the organization and administration of medical care for the pediatric population, a formalized mechanism to specifically address medical errors, quality of care, quality improvement, and longitudinal outcomes analysis did not take form until the middle of the twentieth century. In 1934 Ernest Codman, an orthopedic surgeon, advocated that every hospital should follow patients to determine if their treatment had been successful. Over the past half century, pediatric hospitals have become highly specialized facilities for delivering state-of-the-art medical care. The progression of medical specialization into pediatric subspecialties has led to a commitment to provide the best care possible for pediatric patients.

In this chapter we will discuss injuries among hospitalized children on a pediatric surgical service, with a focus on strategies to eliminate medical errors; the use of Morbidity and Mortality conference as a vehicle to discuss complications and how to use the conference as a teaching tool for surgical residents and medical students; and the state of surgical outcomes research and quality improvement in pediatric surgery.

Medical Injuries

Recent data suggest that patient safety events for hospitalized children occur at a comparable rate to hospitalized adults. This realization has led to increased scrutiny regarding the accurate assessment and prevention of pediatric medical errors. In 2003, Miller et al. analyzed 3.8 million pediatric discharge records from 22 states in the 1997 Healthcare Cost and Utilization Project State Inpatient Databases. They found that the Agency for Healthcare Research and Quality Patient Safety Indicator events were associated with a two to sixfold increase in length of stay and a 2- to 20-fold increase in total hospital charges. In a study of medical injuries among hospitalized children in Wisconsin, Meurer and colleagues documented that specific medical injuries had up to 56% excess adjusted mean LOS and $4465 excess mean adjusted hospital charges.

There are many safety issues that are unique to children's health care. These relate to the four Ds of childhood: developmental change, dependence on adults for accessing care, different disease epidemiology from adults, and demographic characteristics unique to childhood. The enhanced susceptibility of newborns to infections and the detection of life-threatening cardiac anomalies within the first few days of life are examples of developmental change. Children are dependent on adults for accessing medical care since they usually cannot be the primary historian for their medical complaints, they are not capable of questioning their medical care, and usually do not administer their own medications. Children also have unique illnesses, such as birth trauma and metabolic abnormalities that do not occur de novo in adults. Pediatric outcomes research is hampered by the low association between parental and child perspectives, the need for developmentally appropriate measures, low rates of medical conditions, long intervals necessary to detect treatment effects, and the need for case-mix adjustment.

Medication errors are the most common adverse events in hospitalized patients (nearly 20% of all events). One third of all adverse drug events are associated with medication errors and are therefore preventable. In adults, ADEs occur at a rate of 5 per 100 medication orders. Although a similar overall medication error rate occurs in the pediatric population, the nature of associated errors has several unique characteristics when compared to the adult population. Specifically, routine weight-based dosing in the pediatric population results in children being more likely to experience dosing errors as a result of simple mathematical errors. Such errors result in the inadvertent administration of medications at doses 10- or 100-fold higher than the prescribed amounts. Other unique

S. Teich (✉)
Department of Pediatric Surgery, Ohio State University, Nationwide Children's Hospital, Columbus, OH, USA
e-mail: steven.teich@nationwidechildrens.org

P. Mattei (ed.), *Fundamentals of Pediatric Surgery*,
DOI 10.1007/978-1-4419-6643-8_7, © Springer Science+Business Media, LLC 2011

factors to be considered include the errors associated with off-label drug usage and preparation. In addition, pediatric patients have a limited reserve to tolerate a dosing error and limited ability to communicate with health care personnel that an error has occurred or is about to occur. A prospective study of medication errors and adverse drug events at two academic pediatric hospitals demonstrated a medication error rate of 5.7%. Recent reports have concluded that 50–90% of ADEs are preventable, since medication errors occur frequently during drug order entry and may be corrected if the error is detected early in the ordering process.

Analysis of medication error causality on a pediatric surgical service concluded that the majority of medication errors are associated with the presence of rotating general surgery residents. Specifically, the authors suggest that general surgery residents, while often still in the process of familiarizing themselves with routine "adult" dosing guidelines are often less familiar with pediatric dosing and therefore, more likely to commit an error. In a study from Riley Hospital for Children, Engum and Breckler demonstrated that an incorrect dose of medication accounted for the largest number of errors, followed by dosage form, omission of information necessary to complete an order, and missed allergies. Most medication errors are identified by the pharmacy, go no further, and result in no harm to the patient. Medication orders should always include the milligram-per-kilogram dosing information, the patient's weight in kilograms, as well as the total dose requested. This allows the pharmacy to efficiently check medication orders. Computerized physician order entry (CPOE) is an important tool in this regard since it is designed to flag and refuse to accept a medication order without these critical parameters.

On the pediatric surgery service at Nationwide Children's Hospital, like most pediatric surgical services, the attendings and fellows are most experienced at writing pediatric medication orders, yet the majority of orders are written by inexperienced rotating general surgery house officers. Therefore, we have initiated standardized order sets for many pediatric surgical conditions including hypertrophic pyloric stenosis, acute appendicitis, and Nissen fundoplication. In addition to reducing the potential for medication error, we have demonstrated that the use of routine peri-operative order sets reduces overall hospital charges as well as length of stay.

Other strategies to decrease medication errors can also be useful. Pharmacy auditing and clinical pharmacist review are critical to identify medication errors involving drug interactions, incorrect drug doses, incorrect solutions, and inappropriate infusion rates. Adding a pharmacist to the ward team has been shown to decrease ADEs by 66% and has been widely adopted in both the pediatric and adult setting. Handheld PDAs with a drug prescribing reference can help reduce medication errors. However, not all commercially available drug dosing references have pediatric dosing information and many drugs are used off-label for pediatric patients.

Within our CPOE at Nationwide Children's Hospital, common dosages for prescribed drugs are listed to help guide physicians. In an effort to reduce errors on the pediatric surgery service, we also provide the house staff with a pediatric surgery pocket manual, which lists the common drugs used on the pediatric surgery service with the correct dosages. In addition, we highlight several specific services, such as pediatric burn surgery and trauma surgery, with supplemental pocket cards, which allow for immediate access to important drug dosing information in the acute care setting.

Morbidity and Mortality Conference

Surgical morbidity and mortality (M&M) conference has been the most important meeting for surgical education and quality assurance in the surgery department at teaching institutions ever since Ernest Codman developed his "End Results" system at the Massachusetts General Hospital in the early 1900s. The structure of M&M conference has remained essentially unchanged from Codman's description of a system which details the patient's history and outcome, along with adverse events and their causative errors.

Teaching at M&M conferences is based on the idea that analysis of our errors is a powerful educational tool. In a national survey, 80% of respondents stated that they would attend M&M conference even if it was not mandatory. This survey reflects the strong belief, among surgical residents and attendings, of the value of M&M conferences as an educational tool. M&M conferences are also an important tool for quality assurance since many surgeons demonstrate a willingness to change their clinical practice based on knowledge acquired at M&M conferences.

Over the past decade, surgical education has been strained by reduced resident work hours, the economic needs of the hospital, and further specialization within general surgery. In 2001, the Accreditation Council for Graduate Medical Education (ACGME) mandated U.S. residencies to implement a curriculum and evaluation process based on six general competencies: patient care, medical knowledge, practice-based learning and improvement, interpersonal and communication skills, professionalism, and system-based practice. In response to these challenges, surgical residencies have instituted a number of innovative changes including a Night Float System and a daily General Surgery Morning Report. However, a well run M&M conference remains the cornerstone to fulfilling many of the ACGME competencies, especially practice-based learning and improvement.

We have sought to increase the educational value of the surgical M&M conference through several proven techniques: direct questioning of the audience, more thorough explanation of cases, questions directed to attending surgeons, use of radiographic images, and teaching points specifically made for the medical students in attendance. Moreover, this weekly conference requires coordinated participation from an attending radiologist and pathologist, as well as other pediatric sub-specialists as dictated by the case under discussion. The result is a multidisciplinary discussion with maximal educational content.

Evidence-Based Practice in Pediatric Surgery

Evidence-based medicine (EBM) defines best practice based on the weight of best available evidence. It has been demonstrated in the adult medical literature that among different practice groups significant variations can exist in rates of hospitalization, medical therapy, and surgical procedures for the same medical conditions with no significant variation in quality or outcomes. Therefore, all specialties are seeking to define optimal care practices to reduce inappropriate utilization through the use of objective clinical data studies.

Evidence-based practice derives its data from the scientific literature. However, the pediatric surgery literature is replete with retrospective single-institutional series, often focusing on narrow surgical problems. There are many descriptions of surgical techniques, personal experiences, and unique cases. These observational studies do not provide strong support for defining best practices in pediatric surgery. Hardin et al. in a 1999 review of the core pediatric surgery literature, identified 9,373 pediatric surgery articles as of March 1998, with only 0.3% classified as prospective, randomized, controlled studies. Thus, the need for better outcomes research in pediatric surgery is obvious.

Several studies in children have suggested an association between hospital and surgeon volumes and outcome, yielding data similar to adult volume-outcome studies. A retrospective review of 11,000 infants with hypertrophic pyloric stenosis demonstrated that patients in low-volume hospitals were 1.6 times more likely to have complications than those operated at intermediate- or high-volume hospitals and patients operated on by low- and intermediate-volume surgeons were more likely to have complications. The same association between service delivery and outcomes has been demonstrated for biliary atresia. Stringer compared the centralized management of biliary atresia in the United Kingdom to the decentralized French system. Both systems improved outcomes for infants with biliary atresia but only the British centralized model improved the overall results for infants undergoing a Kasai porto-enterostomy. The clinical advantage of a centralized system is seamless transition from rapid evaluation of neonatal obstructive jaundice to prompt Kasai porto-enterostomy by an established, multi-disciplinary team at a single center.

The opportunity for evidence-based practice in minimal access pediatric surgery is evident. Pediatric surgeons were initially slow to embrace minimal access surgery until the 1990s when advances in technology allowed the creation of smaller instrumentation and camera systems suitable for children and infants. Orzech, Zamakhshary and Langer performed a systematic review of medical databases from 1995 to 2006. Only 1.5% of articles on minimal access pediatric surgery could be classified as level 1 randomized controlled studies or systematic reviews of randomized controlled studies while 71% were classified as level 4 case series. Any new surgical technique should be equal or superior to the conventional method that it is trying to replace but the quality of evidence for minimal access pediatric surgery remains extremely poor.

The non-operative management of blunt spleen and liver injuries in children serves as a model for the creation of evidence-based guidelines in pediatric surgery. In 1998, the American Pediatric Surgical Association (APSA) Trauma Committee devised evidence-based guidelines for resource utilization based on a retrospective review of 832 children with isolated liver or spleen injuries. Stylianos and the APSA Liver/Spleen Trauma Study Group then conducted a prospective study at sixteen centers to apply these evidence-based guidelines to children with isolated spleen or liver injuries. Compared with the patients in the retrospective study, the prospectively treated patients had a significant reduction in ICU stay, hospital stay, follow-up imaging, and interval of physical activity restriction within each grade of injury with no adverse sequelae. With validation, these guidelines have had direct economic impact while enhancing patient and family satisfaction.

Pediatric surgeons, like other health care providers, are being challenged to optimize utilization of resources while providing maximum patient safety. We now have the opportunity and need to apply evidence-based practice to define optimal care for our pediatric surgical patients on a prospective basis.

Surgical Outcomes Research in Pediatric Surgery

The assessment of surgical outcomes had its beginnings in the pioneering work of Ernest Codman at the Massachusetts General Hospital in the early 1900s. Among his many accomplishments were the development of the intra-operative anesthesia record, the first tumor registry, and the routine collection and reporting of individual surgeons' operative outcomes. His adverse operative outcome system is still in use today. The M&M conference and audits of physician performance were widely adopted by the surgical specialties but largely ignored by other branches of medicine. In the 1960s and 1970s, computer programs made it possible to audit large institutional surgical volumes as well as surgeon-specific outcomes. However, data collection was not uniform, there was no risk stratification, co-morbidities were not well assessed, and incomplete follow-up gave rise to inaccurate morbidity and mortality data.

In 1991, the National Surgical Quality Improvement Program (NSQIP) was initiated by the United States Department of Veteran's Affair and was subsequently adopted in a staged fashion by academic medical centers throughout the United States. Designed to measure the quality of adult surgical care within an institution utilizing prospective entry of patient risk and outcome data and the determination of risk-adjusted 30-day outcomes, initial NSQIP results from the VA system demonstrated a 47% reduction in overall 30-day post-operative mortality and a 43% reduction in overall 30-day post-operative morbidity.

Due to the great need for risk-adjusted and outcomes-driven quality improvement programs in pediatric surgery, the American College of Surgeons and the APSA are co-developing a Children's NSQIP. However, there are marked differences in children's surgery that do not allow for direct adaptation of the NSQIP model. Most complicated general pediatric procedures are performed infrequently and have a low peri-operative mortality rate. Also, because of age-related cognitive limitations, preoperative co-morbidities, postoperative outcomes, and quality of life assessments must be obtained through parents or caregivers for neonates, infants, and preschoolers.

The ACS/APSA committee has developed a three-phase system to implementation of the Children's NSQIP. Phase I is a 12-month pilot study of data collection in three hospitals to test and refine the data collection software. Phase II is a 2-year study in 10–15 hospitals to collect risk and outcomes data, on approximately 20,000–30,000 patients, to develop valid risk-adjustment models. Finally, Phase III will be national implementation.

Data will be recorded in three broad categories: neonatal, general, and trauma. The neonatal category will include all procedures performed on infants less than 30 days of age. The general category will include all procedures performed on patients from 31 days to 18 years of age. The trauma category will include all patients with the primary diagnosis of trauma undergoing a surgical procedure. Hundred and fifty eight variables will be divided into six groups: demographic patient information, surgical profile, patient-related preoperative risk factors, laboratory data, operative information, and postoperative data.

The philosophy of the children's NSQIP, like the adult version, is to provide pediatric surgeons with highly reliable data that they can use to make quality improvements. The aim is to not only provide a highly reliable data system to compare risk-adjusted outcomes among pediatric surgical programs and individual pediatric surgeons but also to provide robust data to permit intensive quality improvement efforts at the local hospital level.

Summary Points

- Patient safety events for hospitalized children occur at a comparable rate to hospitalized adults.
- There are many safety issues that are unique to children's health care, which are related to the four Ds of childhood: developmental change, dependence on adults, different disease epidemiology, and unique demographic characteristics.
- Medication errors are the most common adverse events in hospitalized patients.
- The majority of medication errors are associated with the presence of rotating general surgery residents.
- Standardized order sets for common pediatric surgical conditions the use of routine peri-operative order sets reduce the potential for medication error, overall hospital charges, and length of stay.
- Surgical morbidity and mortality (M&M) conference has been the most important meeting for surgical education and quality assurance in the surgery department at teaching institutions ever since Ernest Codman developed his "End Results" system at the Massachusetts General Hospital in the early 1900s.
- M&M conference remains the cornerstone to fulfilling many of the ACGME competencies, especially practice-based learning and improvement.
- The educational value of the surgical M&M conference can be improved by applying several techniques: direct questioning of the audience, more thorough explanation of cases, questions directed to attending surgeons, use of radiographic images, and teaching points specifically made for the medical students in attendance.
- The NSQIP, initiated by the United States Department of Veteran's Affair and adopted by academic medical centers throughout the United States, is designed to measure the quality of adult surgical care within an institution utilizing prospective entry of patient risk and outcome data and the determination of risk-adjusted 30-day outcomes.
- Efforts are under way to apply the NSQIP standards to the analysis of patient risk and outcome data at children's centers.

Editor's Comment

It is hard to believe that a focus on the issue of patient safety as it relates to the care of children has taken so long to take root in this country, especially when one considers the staggering statistics as it relates to the number of preventable injuries that occur every day. At many children's medical centers, the boards of trustees have taken ownership of the problem and this has helped to increase awareness and spark entire institutions to action. Every children's hospital should have a patient safety officer and deputies in every department. Meanwhile, the science of patient safety, though still in its early development, is being developed by pioneers who are applying many of the same techniques that have proved successful in other fields such as aviation and industry. A major advance is the concept that although some medical errors are due to human factors and the technological complexity of the medicine, the majority actually appear to be due to predictable and therefore preventable system failures. Analysis of errors and near-misses through root cause analyses and multi-disciplinary M&M conferences, without using traditional personal blame tactics, have helped to identify system modifications that should help to prevent similar errors. There are also efforts to make use of available technology such as computer-based medical entry to improve efficiency and minimize errors. Finally, it is clear that improving quality and patient safety follows naturally when medical care is evidence-based and standardized. Nevertheless, these are difficult to institute due to the traditional health-care culture that values physician autonomy, a rigid hierarchy with the physician as "captain of the ship," and learning by trial-and-error.

The M&M conference is a hallowed tradition in most surgery departments. Modifications in the traditional approach are long overdue and should result in vast improvements in the value of the conference without compromising its traditional usefulness. These modifications include: (1) making it a multi-disciplinary conference; (2) adopting a no-blame format; (3) distinguishing between known and expected complications from true patient safety issues, which should be forwarded to the department patient safety officer for systematic review; (4) discussing near-misses as well as complications; and (5) discussing cases in the context of the available scientific evidence. Finally, there should be a concerted effort to gather data prospectively rather than discuss each case individually and therefore out of context. Though much is to be learned by studying individual data points in depth, it is through the analysis of outcomes data and trends that improvements in the quality and safety of patient care can be realized more quickly and effectively.

Suggested Reading

Calkins C. Contemporary outcomes research: tools of the trade. Semin Pediatr Surg. 2008;17:69–78.

Christakis DA, Johnston BD, Connell FA. Methodologic issues in pediatric outcomes research. Ambul Pediatr. 2001;1:59–62.

Codman EA. The shoulder: rupture of the supraspinatus tendon and other lesions in or about the subacromial bursa. Boston: T. Todd Company; 1934.

Dillon P, Hammermeister K, Morrato E, et al. Developing a NSQIP module to measure outcomes in children's surgical care: opportunity and challenge. Semin Pediatr Surg. 2008;17:131–40.

Engum S, Breckler F. An evaluation of medication errors-the pediatric surgical service experience. J Pediatr Surg. 2008;43:348–52.

Forrest CB, Simpson L, Clancy C. Child health services research. Challenges and opportunities. JAMA. 1997;277:1787–93.

Forrest C, Shipman S, Dougherty D, et al. Outcomes research in pediatric settings: recent trends and future directions. Pediatrics. 2003;111:171–8.

Gore D. National survey of surgical morbidity and mortality conferences. Am J Surg. 2006;191:708–14.

Hardin W, Stylianos S, Lally K. Evidence-based practice in pediatric surgery. J Pediatr Surg. 1999;34:908–13.

Kaplan SH, Greenfield S, Connolly GA, et al. Methodologic issues in the conduct and interpretation of pediatric effectiveness research. Ambul Pediatr. 2001;1(1):163–70.

Kaushal R, Bates D, Landrigan C, et al. Medication errors are common in pediatric inpatient settings, and further efforts are needed to reduce them. JAMA. 2001;285:2114–20.

Khuri S, Henderson W, Barbour G, et al. The National Veterans Administration Surgical Risk Study: risk adjustment for the comparative assessment of the quality of surgical care. J Am Coll Surg. 1995;180:519–31.

Khuri S, Daley J, Henderson W, et al. The Department of Veterans Affairs NSQIP: the first national, validated, outcome-based, risk-adjusted, and peer-controlled program for the measurement and enhancement of the quality of surgical care. National VA Quality Improvement Program. Ann Surg. 1998;228:491–507.

Leape LL, Brennan TA, Laird NM, et al. The nature of adverse events in hospitalized patients: results from the Harvard Medical Practice Study II. N Engl J Med. 1991;324:377–84.

McGuire HH, Horsley JS, Salter DR, Sobel M. Measuring and managing quality of surgery. Statistical vs. incidental approaches. Arch Surg. 1992;127:733–7.

Meurer JR, Yang H, Guse CE, Scanlon MC, Layde PM, Wisconsin Medical Injury Prevention Program Research Group. Medical injuries among hospitalized children. Qual Saf Health Care. 2006;15:202–7.

Michalsky MP, Pratt D, Caniano DA, Teich S. Streamlining the care of patients with hypertrophic pyloric stenosis: application of a clinical pathway. J Pediatr Surg. 2002;37:1072–5.

Miller MR, Elixhauser A, Zhan C. Patient safety events during pediatric hospitalizations. Pediatrics. 2003;111:1358–66.

Morrato E, Dillon P, Ziegler M. Surgical outcomes research: a progression from performance audits, to assessment of administrative databases, to prospective risk-adjusted analysis-how far have we come? Curr Opin Pediatr. 2008;20:320–5.

Rosenfeld JC. Using the Morbidity and Mortality Conference to teach and assess the ACGME general competencies. Curr Surg. 2005;62:664–9.

Stiles B, Reece T, Hedrick T, et al. General surgery morning report: a competency-based conference that enhances patient care and resident education. Curr Surg. 2006;63:385–90.

Stylianos S, APSA Trauma Committee. Evidence-based guidelines for resource utilization in children with isolated spleen or liver injury. J Pediatr Surg. 2000;35:164–9.

Part II
Critical Care

Chapter 8
Shock

John J. McCloskey

Shock can be due to a variety of etiologies and is encountered frequently in the Emergency Department, Operating Room, and Pediatric Intensive Care Unit. Parameters of vital signs such as blood pressure, respiratory and heart rates, quality of perfusion, and mental status are frequently incorporated in descriptions of shock. However, the best unifying definition is an acute state of circulatory dysfunction that results in the inability to meet tissue metabolic demands. When dealing with a child in shock, this concept will help guide the evaluation, assessment, and treatment. Of equal importance in treating the patient with shock is time. A *rapid* evaluation, assessment, and treatment, especially when dealing with hypovolemic or septic shock, are paramount to a favorable outcome.

Types of Shock

Anaphylactic shock occurs when an allergen triggers degranulation of mast cells, releasing large amounts of inflammatory mediators that lead to systemic vasodilatation and hypotension, sometimes accompanied by laryngeal edema and bronchoconstriction. A typical presentation in the ED is the patient with a bee sting, while in the OR or PICU anaphylaxis is seen as a reaction to latex, drugs, or intravenous contrast material.

Neurogenic shock is encountered when a patient suffers a traumatic spinal cord injury above the T6 level. The hallmark of this type of shock is hypotension accompanied by bradycardia, caused by loss of sympathetic innervation and subsequent unopposed vagal innervation of the heart.

Cardiogenic shock can result from a variety of causes: failure after open heart surgery, myocardial contusion secondary to trauma, viral myocarditis, pericardial tamponade, congenital rhythm disturbances, and tension pneumothorax. Drug intoxication with tricyclic depressants or calcium- or sodium-channel blockers are also significant causes of cardiogenic shock. In neonates, patent ductus arteriosus-dependent cardiac lesions and inborn errors of metabolism can also produce cardiogenic shock.

Septic shock occurs in the setting of bacteremia and the initiation of a systemic inflammatory response. In the strictest sense, a positive blood culture is required to confirm the diagnosis, however there are many situations in which blood cultures remain negative. In surgical patients, septic shock might occur due to perforated viscus with peritonitis, wound infection, meningococcemia, necrotizing fasciitis, community- or hospital-acquired methicillin resistant *Staphylococcus aureus* (MRSA) infection, catheter-associated blood-stream infection, ventilator-associated pneumonia, or necrotizing enterocolitis.

Hypovolemic shock in the pediatric patient is usually due to either excessive fluid loss from the gastrointestinal tract or from hemorrhage. Examples of excessive fluid loss from the GI tract include the patient with pyloric stenosis, sequestration of fluid due to bowel obstruction, bacterial or viral gastroenteritis, or malabsorption syndromes. Hemorrhage can be due to resection of an intra-thoracic or intra-abdominal tumor, gastrointestinal bleeding, or trauma (Table 8.1).

Diagnosis

It cannot be overemphasized that there needs to be a rapid evaluation and assessment of the patient in shock. In the most severe forms, the child can rapidly progress to cardio-respiratory failure. Unlike adults, children can more easily tolerate circulatory dysfunction, but will decompensate more precipitously once unable to adequately meet their metabolic demands.

As always, the initial assessment should include the ABCs. Loss of a patent airway can be intrinsic (direct trauma to the airway or edema secondary to anaphylaxis) but usually in shock states the cause is extrinsic based on decreased

J.J. McCloskey (✉)
Department of Anesthesiology and Critical Care Medicine,
Children's Hospital of Philadelphia, 34th Street and
Civic Center Boulevard, Philadelphia, PA 10904, USA
e-mail: mccloskeyj@email.chop.edu

P. Mattei (ed.), *Fundamentals of Pediatric Surgery*,
DOI 10.1007/978-1-4419-6643-8_8, © Springer Science+Business Media, LLC 2011

Table 8.1 Types of shock

Type	Etiology	Pathophysiology	Treatment
Hypovolemic	Hemorrhage	Lack of preload	Fluid resuscitation
	Dehydration	Secondary vasoconstriction	Blood transfusion
Septic	Bacteremia	Peripheral vasodilation	Fluid resuscitation
		Afterload reduction	Pressors
			Antibiotics
Anaphylactic	Allergen	Peripheral vasodilation	Fluid resuscitation
	Histamine release	Afterload reduction	Pressors
			Histamine blockade
Cardiogenic	Multiple	Low cardiac output	Fluid resuscitation
	Cardiomyopathy	Decreased stroke volume	Pressors
	Valve dysfunction		Cardiac assist
Neurogenic	Spinal cord injury	Peripheral vasodilation	Fluid resuscitation
		Collapse of venous tone	Pressors
		Bradycardia	

perfusion to the brain. Establishment of a patent airway with spontaneous or assisted ventilation is crucial since hypoxia and hypercarbia will exacerbate the circulatory dysfunction seen with shock. If the airway is patent, then an assessment of respiratory effort can give clues to the severity of the shock state. In the early stages of shock, mild tachypnea will occur to help facilitate oxygen delivery. As the shock state worsens and oxygen delivery continues to deteriorate, the work of breathing will increase as manifested by a greater respiratory rate, retractions, and the use of accessory muscles of breathing. It will also increase as metabolic acidosis occurs secondary to decreased perfusion and there is a compensatory respiratory alkalosis. In the late stages, hypopnea, or decreased respiratory rate, is a harbinger of cardiovascular collapse. After securing the airway and ensuring adequate ventilation, circulation should be assessed.

Evaluation of circulation entails assessing the vital signs, heart rate and blood pressure, along with end organ perfusion, in particular the brain, skin, and kidneys. Like the respiratory rate, heart rate increases to compensate for a decrease in effective blood volume and the need to increase oxygen delivery. As the shock state worsens, the heart rate increases much like the respiratory rate. This harkens to what was learned in physiology – ventilation should match perfusion. Tachycardia is more robust in children as an initial compensatory mechanism for a decreased effective circulatory volume. Once hypotension occurs, the pediatric patient is at risk for impending cardiovascular failure.

An alteration in mental status is a sign of critical illness in the shock patient. The patient in shock who is confused, disoriented, lethargic, or difficult to arouse is not receiving adequate perfusion of the brain. This patient requires an immediate response in terms of assessment and therapy and close monitoring, preferably in a critical care setting.

Further assessment of circulation includes an evaluation of peripheral perfusion. This involves physical examination of pulses, extremities, and capillary refill. In hypovolemic and cardiogenic shock, pulses are usually diminished, the extremities are mottled and cool, and capillary refill is increased to greater than 2 s. This is due to a compensatory vasoconstriction that diverts blood flow from the skin and extremities to help preserve flow to vital organs such as the brain, heart, and kidneys. This constellation of signs is often referred to as "cold shock." In contrast, patients with "warm shock" have full and bounding pulses, warm extremities, and brisk capillary refill. This is due to peripheral vasodilatation from a loss of vasomotor tone and is typical of septic and anaphylactic shock. Aberrations in pulse pressure are also found in these shock states: narrow pulse pressure in "cold shock" and wide in "warm shock."

Physiologic Principles

Despite the myriad ways in which a patient can present with shock, therapy is essentially guided by improvement in clinical parameters along with correction of hemodynamic and oxygen utilization variables. Cardiac output is directly related to perfusion pressure and is inversely related to resistance. This is more clearly stated by the equation: $CO = (MAP - CVP)/SVR$. Perfusion pressure is the mean arterial pressure (MAP) minus the central venous pressure (CVP) and SVR is systemic vascular resistance. Furthermore, CO is the product of strove volume and heart rate: $CO = SV \times HR$; stroke volume is related to preload, afterload, and contractility.

Oxygen utilization is closely related to CO since it is oxygenated blood that is ejected from the heart and perfusing peripheral tissues. Oxygen delivery is defined by the equation: $OD = CO \times C_aO_2$; arterial oxygen content (C_aO_2) is defined by the equation: $C_aO_2 = (Hgb \times 1.34 \times S_aO_2) + (0.003 \times PaO_2)$. Hemoglobin (Hgb) is expressed as g/dL of blood,

1.34 is the constant that describes the amount of oxygen bound to hemoglobin (mL/g), S_aO_2 is oxygen saturation, 0.003 is the constant that describes the amount of oxygen dissolved in blood. After factoring out the units, the content is expressed as mL of O_2/dL blood. The first part of the C_aO_2 is the most important part of this equation since dissolved oxygen will contribute very little content unless the patient has profound anemia.

In reviewing these equations, it becomes obvious that one can increase oxygen delivery to peripheral tissues by increasing heart rate, preload, contractility, and hemoglobin and by decreasing afterload. These equations, however, do not take into account oxygen *extraction*. Normally, blood leaving the heart is 100% saturated and comes back 75% saturated – an extraction ratio of 25%. In periods of stress, such as exercise or shock, the body can compensate by increasing oxygen extraction. This effect, however, is short lived or limited by flow. Once the threshold for extraction is exceeded, anaerobic metabolism is initiated. This, in turn, leads to the development of lactic acidosis which is typically seen as shock progresses. Oxygen extraction also can be attenuated by cellular poisoning, such as with cyanide, or eventually, cell death.

Goal-Directed Guidelines

Despite some differences in presentation and therapy for specific forms of shock such as neurogenic shock secondary to spinal cord trauma, anaphylaxis, and hemorrhagic shock, the approach to therapy and principles guiding the therapy are similar for shock secondary to sepsis. The notable exception is in hemorrhagic shock secondary to trauma in which source control for active bleeding is paramount and the focus on resuscitation is on restoring intravascular volume with blood. The guidelines put forth by the Surviving Sepsis Campaign serve as a template for treating not only septic shock, but for any form of shock in pediatric patients.

The Surviving Sepsis Campaign was initiated by a number of international critical care groups to standardize the definition, diagnosis, and treatment of sepsis with the goal of improving overall mortality. The guidelines, one set for adults and another for pediatric patients, were developed by consensus groups of physicians after an exhaustive review of the medical literature. The reviewed studies were graded from weak to superior in terms of supporting evidence and incorporated into the guidelines. Since the initial publication in 2002, there have been studies on pediatric patients that have demonstrated improved outcomes with these "goal-directed" guidelines. In turn, these studies have lead to improvements that have been recently published.

First Hour of Resuscitation

Once the diagnosis of shock has been made – as evident by an altered mental status, tachycardia, diminished pulses, mottled skin, cool extremities, capillary refill >2 s, or, in the case of "warm" septic shock, bounding pulses, brisk capillary refill, and warm extremities – large bore intravenous access should be quickly established. If intravenous access is not established quickly, then one should consider an intraosseous approach. With establishment of vascular access, blood samples for a complete blood count, electrolyte panel, ionized calcium, glucose level, coagulation studies, and type and cross should be sent. If sepsis is suspected, blood cultures should also be sent. Once access is established, rapid infusions of normal saline or lactated Ringer's, should be given in 20 mL/kg boluses. Colloid, such as 5% albumin can also be used. A recent randomized, prospective study showed no difference in mortality when ICU patients were treated with crystalloid or colloid, except for head injured patients who demonstrated an increase in mortality when treated with colloid. If hemorrhage is occurring, resuscitation with packed red cells, fresh frozen plasma, and platelets in a 1:1:1 ration should be considered since recent literature on military casualty victims demonstrated improved mortality using this approach. O-negative blood can be used if needed immediately. O-positive blood can be considered in males but Rh incompatibility in future pregnancies is a potential problem for females.

The initial fluid resuscitation improves oxygen delivery by increasing preload, which leads to an increase in cardiac output. This is appropriate for all forms of shock, even cardiogenic, since the response to volume resuscitation should be guided by the improvement in clinical parameters or the development of rales or hepatomegaly. In patients with septic shock, this can take up to 200 mL/kg of fluid before there is significant improvement. Resuscitation with large amounts of fluid has not demonstrated an increased incidence of ARDS or cerebral edema.

During the fluid resuscitation, there should be an ongoing evaluation and assessment of clinical response. Heart rate should improve to within threshold limits; for neonates this is a rate >90 and <160, for older children >70 and <170. Capillary refill should return to <3 s, distal extremities should warm, pulses should become stronger, and most importantly, the patient's mental status should improve. If dealing with "warm" septic shock, the widened pulse pressure should decrease. If hypotension is present, there should be an improvement in blood pressure. (In deviating slightly from the guidelines, we use a dilute solution of epinephrine, 10 µg/mL, and give small boluses of 1–5 µg/kg to augment the blood pressure while the volume is being administered.) Other clinical parameters to monitor include urine output, as a measure of renal perfusion, and respiratory status.

Early in the shock state, patients are tachypneic and develop a respiratory alkalosis to compensate for an evolving metabolic acidosis. As the shock state worsens and mental status deteriorates, hypoxemia and loss of airway protective reflexes can lead to respiratory failure. Furthermore, work of breathing can increase dramatically due to changes in lung compliance secondary to fluid resuscitation. The increased work of breathing can significantly diminish cardiac output; changes in pleural pressure exerting increased pressure on the thoracic aorta, which can increase afterload. Typically, 8–10% of cardiac output is needed for normal respiratory effort, but with a severe increase in work of breathing this can lead to an increase of up to 40% of cardiac output. Securing the airway with endotracheal intubation and mechanical ventilation should be considered early if it appears the shock state is going to progress. Decreasing the work of breathing with mechanical support allows cardiac output to be diverted to other vital organs. Multiple agents can be used to sedate or induce anesthesia for placement of the endotracheal tube, but the sepsis guidelines recommend the use of ketamine (2 mg/kg) with atropine pretreatment and a benzodiazepine after intubation; the atropine reduces secretions and the benzodiazepine blocks the emergence phenomenon seen with ketamine. Ketamine is a good choice since it maintains blood pressure by the release of endogenous catecholamines. Caution should be taken, though, in using ketamine in patients with chronic heart failure. This subset of patients have a depletion of endogenous catecholamines and for them ketamine can be a myocardial depressant. Etomidate is no longer the drug of choice for intubation in patients with shock due to its effect on adrenal suppression, even with one dose. Epinephrine should be available during the intubation and initial mechanical ventilation due to their effects on cardiovascular function.

Antibiotics should also be considered in this first hour if the shock is thought to be due to infection. Empiric therapy should initially be broad. This typically requires a combination of agents. A third-generation cephalosporin, such as cefotaxime, and vancomycin provide excellent coverage for community-acquired pneumonia and meningitis. This combination will cover most Gram-positive and Gram-negative organisms; the vancomycin will cover resistant *Pneumococcus.* If there is concern for *Pseudomonas,* a fourth generation cephalosporin (cefipime) should replace cefotaxime. Ampicillin, gentamicin, and metranidazole are standard if perforation of an abdominal viscus is suspected. Strong consideration should also be given for an anti-fungal agent in the immunocompromised host, especially patients recently treated with antibiotics.

Typically, there should be some improvement in the shock state after 60 mL/kg of fluid. If not, the shock is described as being *fluid refractory*. At this point, a continuous infusion of a vasopressor should be started. Dopamine (5–10 µg/kg/min) is usually started. In this range, dopamine maintains blood pressure by indirectly stimulating the release of norepinephrine from sympathetic vesicles and by directly interacting with alpha-adrenergic receptors and increases cardiac output by its inotropic effect on the heart. Patient less than 6 months of age may not respond well to dopamine due to underdevelopment of the sympathetic nervous system. If the blood pressure and other clinical parameters are not responding to dopamine, epinephrine (0.05–0.3 µg/kg/min) should be used. For patients with septic shock, the dopamine should not be decreased to "renal" levels (3–5 µg/kg/min) as studies have shown it has no protective advantage in these patients. Norepinephrine (0.05–0.3 µg/kg/min) can be used instead of epinephrine for patients in "warm" shock. Dopamine at >10 µg/kg/min and epinephrine or norepinephrine at >0.3 µg/kg/min have predominantly alpha-adrenergic effects, which can cause marked vasoconstriction. Although it is recommended that these agents be given only through a central line, gaining central access in small children can take some time and studies have demonstrated that a delay in starting vasopressors is associated with increased mortality. Dilute solutions of dopamine and epinephrine should be given though a peripheral vein until central access is obtained.

If the blood pressure and other parameters are not responding appropriately to the vasopressors at this point, hydrocortisone 50 mg/m^2/day for patient at risk for absolute adrenal insufficiency (pituitary or adrenal abnormalities, chronic corticosteroid exposure, purpura fulminans) and Waterhouse–Friderichsen syndrome.

Laboratory values should be available at this point. Correction of ionized hypocalcemia is important since adequate intracellular stores of calcium are necessary for the effective use of inotropic agents. Calcium gluconate 50–100 mg/kg or calcium chloride 10–20 mg/kg can be given intravenously to correct the hypocalcemia. Calcium chloride should be reserved for central administration since extravasation into the subcutaneous tissues can cause necrosis. Metabolic acidosis decreases myocardial contractility; it should be corrected with sodium bicarbonate. The hemoglobin should be kept >10 g/dL and platelets >50,000/mm^3. If there is active bleeding, the platelet count should be maintained at >100,000. Coaugulation studies should be corrected with FFP 10 mL/kg and fibrinogen <100 mg/dL with cryoprecipitate 1–2 U/10 kg of body weight.

At this juncture, if the patient is not going to the operating room to control surgical bleeding or exploration for a source of infection, they should be transferred to an intensive care unit for closer and more invasive monitoring.

Beyond the First Hour: Advanced Care in the Intensive Care Unit

In the ICU, therapy is continued to achieve capillary refill <3 s, HR within range, normal pulses with no differential between peripheral and central pulses, warm extremities, urine output > mL/kg/h, and normal mental status. However, the goals of a mixed central venous saturation (SvO_2) >70%, a CVP of 8–12 mmHg, cardiac index >3.3 and <6.0 L/min/ m^2 with a normal perfusion pressure (MAP–CVP) for age, and lactate measurements are added. To facilitate the measurements of CVP, SvO_2, and possibly CI, central venous access must be obtained. If intubation has not occurred yet, this is an appropriate time to secure the airway since placement of a central line is more readily performed with sedation. An indwelling arterial line for direct measurement of blood pressure can also be placed while the patient is sedated.

Again, basic physiologic principles should be utilized for guiding therapy. Fluid is given to keep the CVP at 8–12 mmHg; this will aid CO by ensuring an adequate preload. SvO_2, obtained from samples drawn from the central line, will give an indirect measurement of cardiac output. If metabolic demands are not adequately met by effective cardiac output, then mixed venous saturations will be much less than 75%. Furthermore, the sepsis guidelines recommend the use of SvO_2 to determine the use of other vasoactive agents to improve oxygen delivery dependent on the particular shock state. At this point of the treatment algorithm, patients are classified as having cold shock with normal blood pressure, cold shock with low blood pressure, or warm shock with low blood pressure.

In both cold-shock states, epinephrine and fluids are already being administered to improve cardiac output and oxygen delivery. However, if the SvO_2 consistently stays <70% in the cold shock with normal blood pressure state, a vasodilator such as nitroprusside or nitroglycerin is indicated to decrease afterload and increase forward flow. Caution should be used with these agents since significant decreases in blood pressure can occur. Adequate volume status should be present and it is recommended to have volume readily available. Milrinone, a phosphodiesterase inhibitor, or dobutamine, a beta-adrenergic agent, are other choices; each has potent inotropic properties along with being a vasodilator. If SvO_2 remains <70% in the cold shock with low blood pressure state, norepinephrine should be added in conjunction with the epinephrine to improve the blood pressure. If SvO_2 continues to be low despite an improvement in blood pressure, milrinone or dobutamine should be added. In the warm shock with low blood pressure state, norepinephrine and fluids are already being administered. SvO_2 can be <70% based on maldistribution. A vasopressin infusion can be added to improve the blood pressure further. If SvO_2 remains below 70%, low-dose epinephrine can be added for its inotropic effects.

If the shock state continues to be resistant to vasoactive agents, other etiologies for shock should be investigated and corrected: ongoing blood loss, pericardial effusion, pneumothorax, increased intra-abdominal pressure, necrotic tissue, and occult infection. Although it is not utilized as often as it was in the past, a pulmonary artery catheter (PAC) can be placed to give a better picture of cardiac output. Improved outcome in pediatric patients has been shown when the CI was in the range of >3.3 and <6.0 L/min/m^2. Plus, many PACs offer the capability to measure SvO_2 continuously. Stress hormone replacement therapy can be administered, preferably after obtaining a baseline AM cortisol level. Thyroid replacement therapy, as an infusion, can be utilized if there is evidence of thyroid dysfunction. If the shock still continues, then as a last resort consider the use of veno-arterial ECMO.

If at any point along this algorithm the patient stabilizes, then this level of therapy should be continued as long as needed. With any shock state, an inflammatory cascade is triggered and can lead to multi-system organ failure. It is the goal of these therapies to continue adequate perfusion and oxygen delivery as the inflammatory state abates and the body is allowed to heal. As the patient's condition improves (normal blood pressure and heart rate, capillary refill <3 s, normal perfusion of extremities, improved mental status, resolving metabolic acidosis, decreasing serum lactate levels, improving coagulation profile), then supportive therapies can be slowly decreased. Some forms of shock (severe dehydration) can resolve in hours while septic shock can take days to weeks (Fig. 8.1).

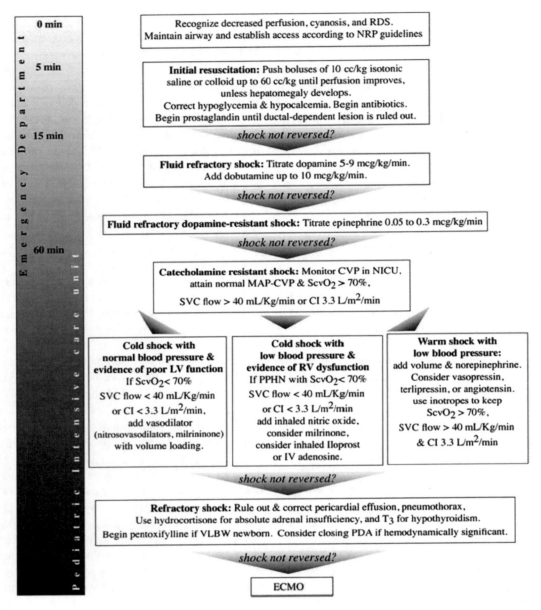

Fig. 8.1 Algorithm for the management of infants and children who require hemodynamic support. If shock persists, proceed to the next step. First-hour goals: heart rate within range, capillary refill ≤2 s, normal blood pressure, and appropriate oxygenation and ventilation. Subsequent goals (PICU): intervene, if necessary to restore and maintain normal perfusion pressure (mean arterial pressure [MAP]–ventral venous pressure [CVP]), oxygen saturation >70%, cardiac index (CI) >3.3, <6.0 L/min/m². *PICCO* pulse contour cardiac output; *CRRT* continuous renal replacement therapy. (Reprinted from Brierley et al. 2009, with permission.)

Summary Points

- Shock is defined as an acute state of circulatory dysfunction that results in the inability to meet tissue metabolic demands.
- *Rapid* evaluation, assessment and treatment, especially when dealing with hypovolemic or septic shock, are paramount to a favorable outcome.
- The initial assessment of a child in shock should include the ABCs.
- Unlike adults, children can more easily tolerate circulatory dysfunction, but will decompensate more precipitously once unable to meet their metabolic demands.
- In patients with "cold shock," pulses are diminished, extremities are mottled and cool, and capillary refill is increased to greater than 2 s due to compensatory peripheral vasoconstriction.
- Patients with "warm shock" have full and bounding pulses, warm extremities, and brisk capillary refill, due to peripheral vasodilatation from a loss of vasomotor tone.
- Management begins with securing an airway, maintaining ventilation, and establishing intravenous access.
- Treatment of the child in shock includes rapid fluid resuscitation with crystalloid and, if needed, pressors to support perfusion pressure.
- Besides clinical parameters such as heart rate and blood pressure, sensitive measures of tissue perfusion include: capillary refill, urine output, mixed venous oxygen saturation, and lactic acid levels.

Editor's Comment

A recurring theme in the care of the critically ill child is the need for a calm and systematic approach to the assessment and treatment of the patient in need. All accepted protocols (ACLS, ATLS, PALS) explicitly address the patient in shock. The ABCs should always be assessed first, although, in reality, multiple issues are addressed simultaneously. Most children in shock, unless they respond rapidly to the initial fluid boluses, should be intubated and maintained on mechanical ventilation. After securing the airway and establishing adequate ventilation, fluid resuscitation should always be initiated aggressively but judiciously to avoid fluid overload and pulmonary edema. If clinical parameters fail to improve despite seemingly adequate fluid resuscitation, pressors should be considered next; however one must always remember that the goal of therapy is to restore tissue perfusion – any intervention that increases central pressure at the expense of peripheral tissue perfusion will be counter-productive. This is why the use of drugs that induce intense peripheral vasoconstriction (norepinephrine) should be considered only as a last resort, if ever.

Given their characteristic clinical presentations, the common causes of shock (sepsis, hypovolemia, anaphylaxis) and even the less common causes (cardiogenic, neurogenic) are usually fairly easy to spot, especially when the history is known. However, there are rare causes of shock that should be considered when the presentation is not so clear-cut. Spontaneous pneumothorax, typically occurring in tall, lanky teenagers who smoke, can occasionally result in tension pneumothorax and shock. Careful physical examination and immediate thoracostomy can be life-saving (there is no time

for a chest X-ray). Pericardial tamponade is also quite rare but should be considered in the child who presents with what otherwise appears to be cardiogenic shock. Physical examination (muffled heart sounds, pulsus paradoxus) and ultrasound (FAST) should be used to confirm the diagnosis. Occult bleeding can cause hypovolemic shock after traumatic injury (scalp laceration, femur fracture, hemothorax), or in association with a GI source (esophageal varices) or massive hemolysis (toxins, rare infections). It is also easy to underestimate the ability of severe dehydration to cause shock in a child. Finally, children with severe respiratory compromise and hypoxia will eventually exhibit signs of cardiovascular collapse if not treated quickly and appropriately: yet another reminder that attention to the ABCs is vitally important in these cases.

Suggested Reading

Brierley J, Carcillo JA, Choong K, et al. Clinical practice parameters for hemodynamic support of pediatric and neonatal septic shock: 2007 update from the American College of Critical Care Medicine. Crit Care Med. 2009;37(2):666–88.

Ceneviva G, Paschall JA, Maffei F, Carcillo JA. Hemodynamic support in fluid-refractory pediatric septic shock. Pediatrics. 1998; 102(2):e19.

Dellinger RP, Levy MM, Carlet JM, et al. Surviving Sepsis Campaign: international guidelines for management of severe sepsis and septic shock: 2008. Intensive Care Med. 2008;34(1):17–60.

Han YY, Carcillo JA, Dragotta MA, et al. Early reversal of pediatric-neonatal septic shock by community physicians is associated with improved outcome. Pediatrics. 2003;112(4):793–9.

Perkin RM, Levin DL. Shock in the pediatric patient. Part I. J Pediatr. 1982;101(2):163–9.

Chapter 9
Electrolyte Disorders

Patrick J. Javid

The management of fluids and electrolytes is central to the care of the surgical patient and, given the unique aspects of fluid and electrolyte metabolism in infants and children, becomes even more important in pediatric surgery. Water is the largest constituent of the human body and the relative volume of water within the body changes with age: total body water is greatest in the fetus (85% of body mass at mid-gestation), less in the newborn (75% of body mass), and lowest when adult levels are reached followed puberty (55–60% of body mass). Body water is found in both the extracellular and intracellular spaces although the majority of water resides in the intracellular space. The cell membrane separates the intracellular and extracellular domains and plays an important role in fluid and electrolyte physiology. There are marked differences in solute concentration between the intracellular and extracellular fluid compartments. The key concept is that water is freely permeable through the cell membrane. Therefore, when a solute concentration changes in one fluid compartment, water moves across the cell membrane to correct the change in osmolality and to facilitate equilibrium between the two compartments.

It is important to remember the baseline electrolyte differences between intracellular and extracellular fluid. Potassium predominates in the intracellular space and sodium predominates in the extracellular space. The routine assessment of electrolyte levels is actually a measurement of the extracellular electrolyte concentration through sampling of the intravascular domain. The body's extracellular fluid volume and its sodium concentration are very tightly linked, and a discrepancy in one directly affects the other. The association between sodium and extracellular fluid has direct implications on the diagnosis and treatment of electrolyte imbalances.

Proper cellular function requires a narrow window of normal plasma osmolality, approximately 280–300 mOsm/kg. Plasma osmolality is estimated by the equation: plasma osmolality = (plasma sodium × 2) + (serum glucose/18) + (BUN/2.8). For the most common scenarios in pediatric surgery, the vital part of this equation is the doubling of the sodium concentration. In the absence of severe hyperglycemia or renal impartment, glucose concentration and BUN represent a small fraction of the overall plasma osmolality. In this way, total plasma osmolality is made up of the plasma sodium concentration plus the corresponding anions that serve to counteract the positive charge of sodium. Hence, doubling the sodium concentration is a reliable and consistent indicator of plasma osmolality. It follows that in the setting of hyponatremia, the plasma osmolality should be low and vice versa.

Urine osmolality, on the other hand, reflects the body's attempts to correct an electrolyte imbalance. To counteract the increased plasma osmolality that occurs with hypernatremia, the kidney is expected to retain free water and thus lower plasma osmolality. Hence, the urine should become more highly concentrated and urine osmolality increases. A finding of elevated plasma osmolality with normal or decreased urine osmolality reflects a severe fluid and electrolyte disturbance and is diagnostic of diabetes insipidus. In the setting of significant electrolyte disorders, urine osmolality should therefore be measured in conjunction with plasma osmolality to help make the correct diagnosis.

Hyponatremia

Hyponatremia refers to a plasma sodium concentration of less than 130 mEq/L. Recalling the relationship between extracellular water and plasma sodium, the diagnosis of hyponatremia simply means that there is a deficit of sodium relative to extracellular water. Symptoms of hyponatremia include lethargy, mental status changes, and seizures. Clinical severity is related to the rapidity of the sodium loss in addition to the absolute value of the sodium deficiency.

In general, hyponatremia is caused by either (a) the loss of sodium in excess of water, (b) a gain of water in excess of

P.J. Javid (✉)
Department of Surgery, Seattle Children's Hospital, University of Washington, 4800 Sand Point Way, NE. Mailstop W-7729, Seattle, WA 98105, USA
e-mail: patjavid@u.washington.edu

P. Mattei (ed.), *Fundamentals of Pediatric Surgery*,
DOI 10.1007/978-1-4419-6643-8_9, © Springer Science+Business Media, LLC 2011

Table 9.1 Etiology and treatment of hyponatremia

Hyponatremia with	Hypovolemia	Hypervolemia	Euvolemia
Causes	GI tract losses	CHF	SIADH
	High-output fistula	Cirrhosis	
	Burns	Nephrotic syndrome	
	Chronic diuretic use	Sepsis	
		Excessive fluid resuscitation	
Treatment	Fluid resuscitation (normal saline)	Treatment of underlying cause	Fluid restriction

sodium, or (c) a laboratory artifact related to volume shifts. Hyponatremia may be associated with hypovolemia, euvolemia, or hypervolemia (Table 9.1). The key to the diagnosis and treatment of hyponatremia is deciding whether the hyponatremia is associated with hypo- or hypervolemia.

Hyponatremia with Hypovolemia

In this condition, both water and sodium are lost, but the loss of sodium is greater. There is a deficit of total body water, which if severe enough can result in inadequate tissue perfusion. The most common cause of hyponatremia with hypovolemia in pediatric surgical patients is the loss of sodium-rich fluid from the gastrointestinal tract in the form of diarrhea or vomiting. This can be seen in small bowel obstruction, pyloric stenosis, gastroenteritis, and in massive stool losses in children with short bowel syndrome or intestinal malabsorption. Less commonly, it can be secondary to excessive output from an enterocutaneous fistula, severe burns, or chronic diuretic use.

This condition is relatively easy to diagnose after hyponatremia has been confirmed by laboratory measurement. An assessment of total body fluid volume will reveal evidence of clinical dehydration: dramatic weight loss in an infant, tachycardia, dry mucous membranes, sunken fontanelle, decreased skin turgor, elevated BUN, and hemoconcentration. The history is critical in making the diagnosis, as there is usually an associated symptom to explain the loss of sodium and water, such as diarrhea, vomiting, or chronic diurectic use. Urine specific gravity will be elevated, and the fractional excretion of sodium (FeNa) will be less than 10%. Fractional excretion of sodium (FeNa) = [(urine Na × plasma creat)/(plasma Na × urine creat)] × 100%.

The treatment of hyponatremia with hypovolemia consists of fluid resuscitation using an appropriate crystalloid solution. A bolus of 20 mL/kg of normal saline is given, and this should be repeated once or twice depending on the degree of dehydration. The crystalloid solution chosen for

resuscitation should ideally match the concentration of sodium in the fluid being lost. The most precise method is to measure the electrolyte concentration in a sample of the fluid. This is commonly performed when an enteric fistula is the source. In practical terms, the resuscitation fluid usually consists of either normal saline or ½-normal saline. One must carefully consider the time course for the full replacement of the sodium content as well as the amount of sodium to be replaced. Rapid correction (over a few hours) must be avoided given the risk of cerebral edema and central pontine myelinolysis. In general, correction to a normal sodium level should take place over the course of 24–48 h, at a rate of 0.5–1.0 mEq/L/h.

The rate and volume of the fluid replacement will depend on the sodium deficit and the fluid chosen for resuscitation. A simple equation to calculate the actual sodium deficit in a patient with hyponatremia is: sodium deficit (mEq) = (desired sodium level−actual sodium level) × 0.6 × body weight (kg), using 135 mEq/L as the desired plasma sodium level. A 10-kg toddler with a plasma sodium of 120 mEq/L after several days of diarrhea will appear hypovolemic on physical examination with tachycardia, dry mucous membranes, and poor skin turgor. The sodium deficit is 90 mEq. If we choose normal saline (154 mEq/L of sodium) as the replacement fluid, the patient would require 90 mEq/154 mEq/L = 0.58 L to replace this sodium deficit. Replacing this volume over 48 h would require a continuous infusion rate of 12 mL/h. This does not, however, take into account maintenance volume and sodium requirements, which for a 10 kg child is 40 mL/h of D5 ½NS with 20 mEq KCl/L. The simplest way to provide this is to infuse two separate crystalloid solutions to accomplish both replacement and maintenance fluid needs. This calculation also does not account for ongoing fluid and electrolyte loss, so additional replacement is sometimes necessary depending on the volume of ongoing losses.

In extreme or symptomatic cases of hyponatremia, hypertonic saline (3% saline contains 513 mEq/L of sodium) can be used as the replacement fluid. This will rapidly increase the plasma sodium concentration but must be used judiciously. In most cases, hypertonic saline is infused slowly over 4–6 h to rapidly increase the sodium concentration to a range in which symptoms, especially seizures, will be alleviated. In practice, attaining a plasma sodium level of 125 mEq/L over several hours should limit further hyponatremic seizure activity. The remaining correction of the sodium deficit is performed using normal saline over the course of 24–36 h.

For all methods of sodium correction, serial plasma electrolyte measurements must be performed. In the clinical setting, this translates into chemistry panels every 4–8 h depending on the degree of hyponatremia and the patient's symptoms.

Hyponatremia with Hypervolemia

This is characterized by a low plasma sodium concentration and an increase in total body water. In fact, patients with this condition have increased total body sodium as well, but the sodium is not located in the intravascular space but instead resides in the interstitial fluid compartment. It is commonly seen in patients with congestive heart failure, cirrhosis, nephrotic syndrome, sepsis, and other conditions associated with severe hypoproteinemia or low oncotic pressure. Normal oncotic pressure keeps fluid within the intravascular space. In each of these disease processes, there is a decrease in oncotic pressure, which allows fluid and electrolytes to leave the intravascular space and accumulate in the interstitial space. Thus, these patients present with peripheral edema, pulmonary edema. or ascites. The diminished circulating volume is sensed by the kidney and baroreceptors, which stimulate antidiuretic hormone (ADH) secretion and the renin-angiotensin cascade. Both increase resorption of water in the kidney and free water is retained to a greater degree than sodium. Thus, although total body water and sodium are increased, there is a dilutional hyponatremia within the intravascular space.

On the pediatric surgical services, the most common cause of hyponatremia with hypervolemia is excessive fluid resuscitation with hypotonic crystalloid solution. This is often seen in the early postoperative period when ¼ or 0.2 normal saline is administered at maintenance or higher infusion rates. Given the low sodium content of the fluid and the patient's propensity to "third-space" fluid into the interstitium during this phase of recovery, it is easy to see how a dilutional hyponatremia can develop.

Hyponatremia with hypervolemia is treated by addressing the cause of increased water retention rather than the sodium content per se. In postoperative patients, the hyponatremia resolves as the capillary leak diminishes and urine output increases, usually around postoperative day 2–3. The clinician can also decrease the infusion rate of the hypotonic fluid or switch to ½ normal saline or crystalloid solution. For other types of hyponatremia with hypervolemia, the condition is treated with sodium and fluid restriction, inotropes (in congestive heart failure), albumin supplementation (in cirrhosis), or aggressive antibiotic therapy (in sepsis).

Hyponatremia with Euvolemia

The main cause of hyponatremia in the setting of euvolemia is the syndrome of inappropriate antidiurectic hormone secretion (SIADH). Normally, ADH is secreted when plasma osmolality is elevated, thus increasing free water retention by the kidney. In SIADH, the hypothalamus secretes ADH at lower levels of plasma osmolality. This results in increased free water re-absorption, a decrease in plasma osmolality, and a dilutional hyponatremia. While hypervolemia can develop over time, the patient is initially euvolemic. Pediatric surgeons see SIADH in the setting of blunt head trauma, intracranial hemorrhage in the premature neonate, empyema, malignancy, or with certain medications. The diagnosis is made by comparing plasma and urine osmolality levels: the urine osmolality will be inappropriately high in the setting of a low plasma osmolality. The only appropriate treatment is fluid restriction, since any additional crystalloid fluid will only exacerbate water retention.

Pseudohyponatremia

Hyponatremia due to laboratory artifact is an example of hyponatremia with euvolemia. It occurs when hyponatremia is identified in the absence of a change in plasma volume or plasma osmolality. In this condition, plasma sodium levels are actually normal, and the discrepancy in the sodium measurement is due to an altered makeup of solutes within the extracellular space. The key point is that the plasma osmolality is normal. If there were an actual deficit in plasma sodium, one would expect a concomitant decrease in plasma osmolality since sodium is the most abundant solute in plasma and extracellular fluid in general.

Pseudohyponatremia can be seen in the setting of hyperlipidemia, hyperproteinemia (multiple myeloma), or hyperglycemia. In each of these instances, the abnormal increase in the solute concentration in plasma causes a decrease in plasma water and it is the plasma water that is used to measure the sodium concentration; hence, sodium concentration is normal, but because of the method in which sodium is measured, the level appears to be low. There is no treatment necessary since plasma sodium is normal and the challenge is making an accurate and timely diagnosis.

Hypernatremia

Hypernatremia is defined as a plasma sodium concentration greater than 150 mEq/L. There are two causes of hypernatremia in the pediatric patient (Table 9.2): loss of body water (hypernatremia with hypovolemia) and excessive intake of sodium (hypernatremia with hypervolemia). In children, the latter is rare, usually iatrogenic, and associated with hypervolemia, since this is the body's response to maintain a stable plasma osmolality. Like hyponatremia, hypernatremia also

Table 9.2 Etiology and treatment of hypernatremia

Hypernatremia with	Hypovolemia	Hypervolemia
Etiologies	Watery diarrhea	Incorrectly concentrated infant formula
	Excessive sweat loss	
	Insensible fluid loss	
	Diabetes insipidus	Saltwater ingestion
Treatment	Free water replacement	Correct error in formula
		Furosemide
		Hypotonic fluid infusion

leads to neurologic changes, including lethargy and a decreased threshold for seizure. These changes occur when the plasma sodium concentration is greater than 160 mEq/L.

Hypernatremia with Hypovolemia

In this condition, the patient has lost body water and sodium, but the loss of water is greater than the loss of sodium. Therefore, while total body sodium is low, the plasma sodium concentration is elevated in the remaining extracellular water. As expected, plasma osmolality is increased. Under normal conditions, in response to increased plasma osmolality, ADH is released by the hypothalamus and free water resorption is stimulated in the kidney. These mechanisms serve to increase total body water and decrease plasma osmolality to the normal range.

Hypernatremia with hypovolemia is commonly seen in gastroenteritis with watery diarrhea, excessive loss of sweat, and significant loss of insensible fluid. The latter is commonly seen in low birth weight premature infants who are placed under a radiant warmer and proceed to lose a large amount of hypotonic volume through the skin. Babies with short bowel syndrome who have excessive stool output most often present with hypernatremia with hypovolemia.

A unique cause of hypernatremia with hypovolemia is diabetes insipidus (DI), which is caused by ineffective function of ADH. Central DI occurs when ADH secretion from the pituitary gland is impaired and is seen in head-injured patients or premature babies with intracranial hemorrhage. Nephrogenic DI occurs when there is end-organ resistance to ADH at the level of the renal tubule. Nephrogenic DI can be congenital but is more often associated with certain medications, including lithium and demeclocycline. Diabetes insipidus is easy to diagnose if clinical suspicion is high. Under normal conditions, urine osmolarity should be elevated in the setting of hypernatremia and increased plasma osmolality, but in DI, the urine osmolality is inappropriately low because the kidney cannot resorb free water. Central DI is treated with exogenous vasopressin whereas nephrogenic DI is treated by cessation of the causative medication.

The treatment of hypernatremia with hypovolemia must include free water replacement. A bolus of isotonic fluid is initiated to help restore intravascular volume and organ perfusion. A 20-mL/kg volume of normal saline over 30–60 min is adequate and this is repeated depending on the degree of dehydration. Next, the actual free water deficit is calculated: free water deficit $(mL) = 0.6 \times body weight (kg) \times [(plasma sodium / 140) - 1]$. The free water deficit is then replaced over 24–48 h. The free water deficit in mL is divided by 48 h to determine an hourly rate and this volume is infused as 5% dextrose in water (D_5W). Alternatively, a portion of this volume replacement can be given enterally through a nasogastric feeding tube in the form of free water or by increasing the free water content of formula feeds. This can become complicated in patients with gastroenteritis and short bowel syndrome and is usually reserved for mild, asymptomatic cases of hypernatremia.

Hypernatremia with Hypervolemia

This constellation of findings is rare. It occurs when there is an increase in plasma sodium without evidence of dehydration. The patient will likely be volume overloaded, and peripheral edema and jugular venous distention might be noted on exam.

Hypernatremia with hypervolemia is caused by increased intake of sodium and is usually iatrogenic. An incorrectly concentrated infant formula can result in an increase in sodium intake. Other iatrogenic etiologies include resuscitation with an inappropriately hypertonic crystalloid solution, excessive use of hypertonic saline, or multiple doses of sodium bicarbonate in the intensive care unit. Rarely, the cause is ingestion of saltwater.

The patient becomes hypervolemic as a compensatory mechanism to the increased sodium concentration: water diffuses into the extracellular domain to counteract the imbalance in plasma osmolality, ADH is released to stimulate free water resorption from the kidney, and the neurologically intact patient will experience increased thirst. Ultimately, these mechanisms serve to normalize plasma osmolality at the expense of increasing total body water.

Treatment is usually limited and requires only correcting the error that led to increased sodium intake while at the same time providing maintenance intravenous fluid (D_5 ½ NS should suffice). In severe cases, diuresis with a loop diuretic along with partial fluid replacement with free water can be used.

Hypokalemia

Potassium is the major intracellular ion; in fact, 98% of total body potassium is stored inside the cell at any particular time. Therefore, the plasma measurement of potassium does

Table 9.3 Etiology of hypokalemia

Migration of potassium into the intracellular space
Increased non-renal losses
Increased renal losses
Insufficient potassium intake

not accurately reflect total body potassium. There is no precise and practical way to measure total body potassium. Keeping this in mind, disorders of plasma potassium must be analyzed carefully prior to the initiation of replacement therapies, and any therapy for potassium disorders must be coupled with frequent plasma laboratory surveillance.

Hypokalemia is defined as a plasma potassium concentration of less than 3.5 mEq/L. There are four potential sources for potassium loss: (1) migration of potassium into the intracellular space, (2) increased non-renal losses of potassium, (3) increased renal losses of potassium, and (4) decreased potassium intake (Table 9.3). This latter etiology is extremely rare given the kidney's remarkable capacity for potassium resorption and is seen only in settings of extreme starvation.

Movement of Potassium into Cells

Several systemic mechanisms serve to increase the movement of potassium against its concentration gradient and into the intracellular space. Alkalemia causes the transfer of protons out of the cell in exchange for potassium ions into the cell. This allows for the primary buffering of the extracellular space at the cost of hypokalemia. This is one of the reasons that dehydration and gastrointestinal losses, both prime etiologies for alkalosis, are often associated with hypokalemia (pyloric stenosis).

Other mediators of potassium transport into the cell include insulin, catecholamines, and paralysis. Insulin-induced hypokalemia is usually observed during treatment of diabetic ketoacidosis. Hypokalemia related to catecholamines is seen in the setting of shock, severe burns, and even temporarily following administration of β_2-agonist bronchodilators. It is important to note that in each of these scenarios total body potassium might not be altered but rather merely shifted to another body compartment. Hence, in general, these varieties of hypokalemia do not require aggressive potassium repletion but rather are alleviated by treating the primary cause.

Increased Non-Renal Losses of Potassium

Potassium can be lost from the intestine as well as the skin. Enterocytes preferentially absorb sodium chloride to aid extracellular volume expansion and secrete potassium bicarbonate in exchange. Thus, prolonged severe diarrhea can result in true hypokalemia. This is also one reason why children with bladder augmentation using intestinal segments often become hypokalemic and alkalotic. In patients with high-volume emesis, there can be some potassium lost in the gastric fluid. However, the main etiology for the severe hypokalemia associated with emesis is secondary to volume depletion and loss of potassium in exchange for sodium. Rarely, excess potassium can be lost from the skin in the form of severe sweating.

Increased Renal Losses of Potassium

The primary etiology of this process is hypovolemia-induced activation of the renin-angiotensin cascade, which ultimately stimulates aldosterone release. Aldosterone directly stimulates renal tubular excretion of potassium and protons as it works to increase the resorption of sodium. Patients who become dehydrated from prolonged emesis, as seen in both pyloric stenosis and gastroenteritis, sometimes present with classic hypokalemic metabolic alkalosis and paradoxical aciduria. This represents a true loss of total body potassium, although there is also some increase in movement of potassium into the intracellular space by the alkalemia alone. Diuretics, especially those of the loop variety, will also cause the kidney to lose excessive potassium. Patients given large boluses of furosemide must have careful electrolyte monitoring before and after the diuretic dose to follow plasma potassium levels. In patients prone to diuretic-induced hypokalemia, chronic oral potassium supplements should be administered. Rarely, especially in pediatrics, hypokalemia can be caused by inappropriate serum levels of aldosterone or renin in the setting of endocrine tumors or renal artery stenosis.

Treatment of Hypokalemia

Potassium needs to be replaced in the setting of severe hypokalemia. Low serum potassium levels can lead to cardiac arrhythmia, muscle weakness, lethargy, and delayed intestinal motility. Patients with critically low levels of potassium mandate continuous electrocardiographic monitoring and urgent electrolyte replacement. Potassium can be replaced by intravenous or oral routes and determination of the appropriate route of administration is based on the nature of the symptoms.

For intravenous replacement, potassium is administered as potassium chloride at a dose of 0.25–1.0 mEq/kg and at a rate of 0.25 mEq/kg/h, to minimize the effects of a rapid potassium bolus. The maximum dose in a child in a single administration is usually 10–20 mEq, and then plasma potassium concentration must be rechecked prior to additional dosing. The concentration of the potassium mixture must be diluted when a peripheral line is used for administration, which requires a greater volume for large potassium doses. Intravenous replacement should result in the immediate increase in plasma potassium.

In a less urgent clinical scenario, potassium can be gradually administered through a continuous crystalloid infusion with sodium chloride. In this way, maintenance fluids are usually administered as D_5 ½ NS with potassium as an additive to the solution. Potassium can be added in doses up to 80 mEq/L for peripheral access. While this is an effective mode for potassium replacement, the clinician must be careful to avoid over-dosing potassium in this fashion. Potassium must be checked at least twice daily when using high additive concentrations and, once serum potassium is normalized, remember to reduce the potassium concentration in the maintenance fluids.

For oral replacement, potassium is usually given as potassium chloride although potassium phosphate may also be used. Potassium chloride is dosed at 0.5–1.0 mEq/kg for the oral route, and this can be given 2–3 times/day with electrolyte monitoring once or twice each day.

Hyperkalemia

Hyperkalemia is defined as a plasma potassium level greater than 6.5 mEq/L and represents an urgent clinical scenario. Elevated serum potassium lead to alterations in the electrochemical gradient of the cell membrane and have a distinct effect on the action potential. This can result in depolarization of the myocyte and, hence, life-threatening cardiac arrythmias. Hyperkalemia needs to be confirmed quickly and treated aggressively.

Hyperkalemia has a variety of etiologies in the pediatric population. A common cause is impaired renal function. Potassium intake must therefore be restricted in patients with renal insufficiency. Other common causes of hyperkalemia in children include tumor lysis syndrome, hemolysis, rhabdomyolysis, and adrenal insufficiency. Serial potassium measurements are routine in patients at risk, including children with large tumors who are being given chemotherapy. Significant acidemia can cause hyperkalemia through the exchange of potassium into the extracellular domain for hydrogen ion into the cell. Certain medications, including spironolactone and angiotensin-converting enzyme (ACE) inhibitors, can cause a gradual increase in plasma potassium.

Finally, a common cause of apparent hyperkalemia in infants is a hemolyzed blood sample. This occurs when a small bore needle is used for a percutaneous blood sample; red blood cells are lysed as they pass through the needle and intracellular potassium is released into the specimen. Most often, the hospital laboratory will note the hemolyzed status

Table 9.4 Treatment of hyperkalemia

Temporizing
Sodium bicarbonate 1 mEq/kg IV bolus
Insulin 0.1 U/kg with D_{50} 1 mL/kg IV bolus
Definitive
Kayexylate 1 g/kg/dose q6 h PO or q2–4 h PR
Furosemide 0.5–1.0 mg/kg IV bolus
Hemodialysis

of the specimen in their results. In this setting, the plasma potassium should be re-measured if the patient is not symptomatic.

True hyperkalemia is treated aggressively with both temporizing and definitive techniques (Table 9.4). First, a thorough review of the patient's intravenous fluid regimen should be performed; any exogenous potassium must be eliminated, even if this means discontinuing the patient's parenteral nutrition in exchange for a potassium-free crystalloid solution. Calcium gluconate (10 mg/kg of 10% solution) is administered next in an attempt to stabilize the cardiac membrane.

Temporizing measures allow for the transfer of potassium into the intracellular space and will alleviate the potential for cardiac instability in the short term by decreasing the amount of potassium that the cardiac myocyte is exposed to. Sodium bicarbonate is administered as a 1-mEq/kg intravenous bolus to help exchange potassium for protons in the extracellular space. Insulin (with concomitant glucose) is an excellent agent for the temporary movement of potassium intracellularly. Insulin is given in a dose of 0.1 U/kg and to maintain euglycemia it is given just after a 1-mL/kg bolus of 50% dextrose solution (D_{50}). Both sodium bicarbonate and insulin/dextrose may be repeated as potassium levels increase again prior to definitive therapy.

Definitive therapy requires the loss of potassium from the body and this can be accomplished using sodium polystyrene (Kayexylate), administration of a loop diuretic, or hemodialysis. Kayexylate is a cation-exchange resin that binds potassium in the gastrointestinal tract and facilitates removal of the bound ion in the stool. It can be administered orally, through a nasogastric tube, or by enema. In most acute settings, either gastric or rectal administration is associated with the quickest effects on plasma potassium. The timing of kayexylate's effects is dependent on the patient's stool output, and therefore kayexylate might take hours to actually lower the plasma potassium level. Thus, kayexylate is most often used in conjunction with temporizing measures to lower the plasma potassium in the short-term. Furosemide 0.5–1.0 mg/kg given intravenously will also lower plasma potassium by promoting renal excretion. This can be repeated several times as long as plasma potassium and renal function are monitored carefully. Hemodialysis is reserved for the most severe, refractory, and symptomatic cases of hyperkalemia.

Summary Points

- Potassium predominates in the intracellular space, sodium in the extracellular space.
- Extracellular fluid volume and sodium concentration are tightly linked; a discrepancy in one directly affects the other.
- Symptoms of hyponatremia include lethargy, mental status changes, and seizures.
- The most common cause of hyponatremia with hypovolemia in pediatric surgical patients is the loss of sodium-rich fluid from the gastrointestinal tract in the form of diarrhea or vomiting.
- The treatment of hyponatremia with hypovolemia is fluid resuscitation using crystalloid solution.
- On the pediatric surgical services, the most common cause of hyponatremia with hypervolemia is excessive fluid resuscitation with hypotonic crystalloid solution
- The main cause of hyponatremia in the setting of euvolemia is the SIADH.
- Hypernatremia with hypovolemia is commonly seen in gastroenteritis with watery diarrhea, excessive loss of sweat, or significant loss of insensible fluid
- Hypernatremia with hypervolemia is caused by increased sodium intake and is usually iatrogenic.
- Low serum potassium levels can lead to cardiac arrhythmia, muscle weakness, lethargy, and delayed intestinal motility.
- Hyperkalemia can cause life-threatening cardiac arrythmias and needs to be treated aggressively.

Editor's Comment

Electrolyte disorders in surgical patients can be confusing but a simple algorithm for identification and treatment of the common problems should be part of the skill set of the pediatric surgeon. The most common imbalances seen in clinical practice involve sodium and potassium. Since most mild abnormalities are self-correcting, it is rarely necessary to even check electrolytes after an uncomplicated procedure in a healthy patient who resumes normal oral intake within 2–3 days of the operation. Patients who need regular routine monitoring of electrolytes include those who are NPO for several days, have high GI fluid losses, are being provided nutrition parenterally, or have another specific risk factor. Even these patients rarely need to have labs checked more than twice weekly unless there is a potentially dangerous value that is being actively corrected. It is still common to see daily or twice daily labs being drawn, especially in ICU patients, despite the values being minimally aberrant or entirely normal for days on end – this is a wasteful and potentially dangerous practice that should be abolished.

Mild hyponatremia is common in pediatric general practice due to a combination of factors: GI losses, over-resuscitation in the OR and postoperative period with hypotonic solutions, and a surgical stress-induced SIADH. Our current protocols for fluid resuscitation tend to err on the side of excess, which contributes to hyponatremia, dilutional anemia, and bowel edema/ ileus. Some fast-track protocols recommend a slightly lower calculation for "maintenance" fluids, a preference for crystalloid boluses as needed, and early reliance on oral intake and thirst to guide fluid management. It is also common for surgical residents to mistakenly use the fluid replacement strategy recommended for gastric fluid losses (½mL per mL of D5½NS + 20 mEq/L KCl) for other GI losses (ileostomy output, diarrhea, biliary drainage), which are all isotonic and have higher concentrations of potassium. Hypernatremia is less common and the cause is usually obvious, although insensible losses in infants can be more than expected. The most serious cases of hypernatremia (serum sodium >200) have occurred when parents are instructed to supplement their infant's formula with a pinch of salt. Regardless of the cause, correction of hypo- and hypernatremia should be gradual to prevent brain injury related to rapid fluid shifts.

Hyperkalemia can be dangerous but is very uncommon in the setting of normal renal function. It is much more commonly spurious, especially in infants, due to hemolysis of the specimen. Nevertheless, having to prove that it is normal is time-consuming (delays induction of anesthesia) and potentially dangerous in that potassium is withheld from an infant who more likely has hypokalemia (pyloric stenosis). Hypokalemia must be profound to have clinical effects but is dangerous because of the excitement it causes for nurses and physicians, who tend to overreact by giving large doses of potassium intravenously, which is hazardous, or orally, which induces vomiting and can make the problem worse. Calmly correcting acid-base imbalances, replacing potassium losses in GI fluids, and providing moderate concentrations of potassium in the maintenance fluids or parenteral nutrition solutions are usually all that is required.

Mild hypocalcemia is relatively common but is more often spuriously due to hypoalbuminemia. Patients who are risk (thyroidectomy) and symptomatic should be treated with oral calcium carbonate and calciferol. Rarely, intravenous calcium gluconate or calcium chloride is needed and should be administered according to institutional guidelines for rate and cardiac monitoring. Hypomagnesemia can be seen in patients with malnutrition or excessive GI fluid losses, often in conjunction with hypocalcemia. Oral magnesium supplements usually work best but intravenous replacement is occasionally necessary. Hypophosphatemia occurs commonly after massive hepatic resection and is due to a transient hyperphosphaturia rather than consumption by the regenerating liver. It typically peaks on postoperative day two and resolves by day 5. Supplementation is necessary to prevent life-threatening hypophosphatemia but will not prevent the underlying parathyroid hormone spike that is the likely cause.

Suggested Reading

Choong K, Kho ME, Menon K, Bohn D. Hypotonic versus isotonic saline in hospitalized children: a systematic review. Arch Dis Child. 2006;91:828–35.

Kim MS, Somers MJG. Fluid and electrolyte physiology and therapy. In: McMillan JA, Feigin RD, DeAngelis CD, Jones Jr MD, editors. Oski's pediatrics: principles and practice. 4th ed. Philadelphia: Lippincott Williams & Wilkins; 2006.

Roberts KB. Fluid and electrolytes: parenteral fluid therapy. Pediatr Rev. 2001;22(11):380–7.

Siegel NJ. Fluid, electrolytes, and acid-base. In: Rudolph CD, Rudolph AM, Hostetter MK, Lister G, Siegel NJ, editors. Rudolph's pediatrics. 21st ed. New York: McGraw-Hill; 2003.

Chapter 10
Vascular Access

Stephen G. Murphy

For the busy pediatric surgeon, vascular access issues arise frequently and often unexpectedly. One should be technically proficient and familiar with the various venous access options, indications, and complications.

Peripheral Intravenous Access

Expertise in establishing peripheral IV access is a useful skill. Pediatric surgeons are often requested to obtain access after other practitioners have had an opportunity. Most pediatric institutions have a pecking order of expertise from the IV team or pediatric house staff to the Anesthesiology/PICU and NICU staff. Ability to obtain peripheral IV access can convert a crisis into a more controlled situation and allow for administration of appropriate sedation. Neonates often have fragile, mobile or non-visible veins. Patients who are cold or hypotensive often develop peripheral vasospasm. The best place for a surgeon to maintain peripheral IV access skills is the OR. Anesthesia and surgical staff can work simultaneously to establish access in different extremities. The difficult IV access (DIVA) score predicts difficult IV access and takes into consideration four variables: prematurity (3 points), age (less than 1 year = 3 points, 1–2 years = 1 point), veins not palpable (2 points), and veins not visible (2 points). A score of 4 or more predicts difficult IV access.

Umbilical Vein

The umbilical vein access is a reliable route that can provide excellent venous access for up to 10 days. One should not overlook this easily accessible vein in the ill newborn: Check the cord for three vessels. Identify the lone umbilical vein. Dissect out a small segment of the vein. Pass a braided absorbable suture around it. The lumen is considerable. Thread the catheter cephalad. Complications include perforation of the liver capsule, infection, and thrombosis. The umbilical artery can also be cannulated for arterial access and moved to a site lateral to the umbilicus as described by Wolfson. Be wary of aortic thrombosis with this arterial site. It is best used for only a short time.

Peripherally Inserted Central Catheter

The PICC line, a centrally directed, peripherally accessed silicone catheter has several advantages: it is placed peripherally by the IV team, imaging specialists, NICU staff, or resident staff and avoids the need for general anesthesia. It is ideal for short-term, central venous access for antibiotics or parenteral nutrition. The principal disadvantage is the small caliber of the line (3.0 F or less), which limits the flow rate and makes it not suitable for blood draws. The antecubital route is the most common approach but access can also be achieved from the lower extremities. We advise an attempt at this route in the NICU patient needing long-term IV access before consideration of tunneled central venous access. Blindly inserted PICC lines need repositioning in up to 85% of cases, so insertion under fluoroscopic guidance is recommended. Catheter tip position is most influenced by arm movement. Complication rates vary but are generally very low. You may be called to remove the difficult or stuck PICC line. The catheters are flimsy so you need to be careful when pulling. (Avoid sudden yanking!) Involve Interventional Radiology if you feel the catheter is caught centrally.

S.G. Murphy (✉)
Department of Surgery, DuPont Hospital for Children,
Wilmington, DE 19899, USA
e-mail: smurphy@nemours.org

P. Mattei (ed.), *Fundamentals of Pediatric Surgery*,
DOI 10.1007/978-1-4419-6643-8_10, © Springer Science+Business Media, LLC 2011

Percutaneously Inserted Central Venous Catheter

The gold standard for insertion of percutaneous central lines has always been guidance by surface anatomy landmarks. The subclavian, internal jugular and femoral venous approaches account for the majority of central line insertions. The indications for this type of central access are cardiac arrest, need for central venous pressure monitoring or vasopressor therapy, ill patient requiring multiple lumen venous access for medications or fluids, and plasmaphoresis. This is generally a short-term (several days) central venous access route. Because the catheter lacks a cuff, it is more easily dislodged and the infection rate increases with time. If necessary, the catheter can also be changed over a guide wire using the Seldinger technique, although it is often preferable to replace it at another site.

Tunneled Central Venous Catheter

In some institutions the most commonly placed line is the cuffed tunneled central line. The indications for this catheter type include: long-term access for parenteral nutrition, chemotherapy for malignancy, long-term need for blood component therapy, plasmaphoresis, and the need for frequent blood sampling. Catheters with a polytetrafluoroethylene cuff have a lower infection rate than uncuffed central venous catheters. The cuff becomes densely adherent to the subcutaneous tissues and prevents inadvertent dislodgement. Medical staff should understand that with a cuffed catheter, there is no ability to adjust the position of the catheter tip or change the catheter over a wire once it is secured. The cuff is usually placed about 1.5 cm from the exit site and this is where it stays.

Despite the popularity of the PICC line, we are still frequently asked to place central lines in the NICU. Most NICUs are not set up to accommodate fluoroscopy, so central lines should be placed in the OR if tip location is considered vital. The will usually be an add-on case, waiting for an available room, OR, and anesthetist. Because performing the procedure in the NICU depends upon surgeon availability, there is greater flexibility. In this setting, I place a tunneled cuffed catheter. I can only verify that the catheter aspirates and flushes – the tip may be anywhere but it is still better IV access than the peripheral IV whether it is in the subclavian, innominate, jugular, SVC or IVC. Since the catheter is cuffed, manipulation of the catheter tip is not a practical option. Again, if catheter tip position is imperative, the catheter should be placed in the OR.

Upon arrival in the NICU for line placement, often the only light available is the room light and a nonfunctional isolette light, and the only instruments available are on an umbilical catheter tray. It is best not to proceed under these conditions. Rightly advocate for the fragile premature infant, a patient with no reserve who requires optimal conditions for success. Insist on the appropriate equipment. Have a good source of light. Use the bilirubin lights once the baby is covered. Bring magnification. Intubate, ventilate and paralyze the patient – they are not going home the next day. Bring the equipment with you. With an ophthalmic retractor, central venous catheter insertion is easy even if being done solo. Bring two small retractors, fine vascular forceps, #11 and #15 blades, several fine mosquito clamps, and a small right-angle clamp. Bring 4-0 braided absorbable suture and a non-absorbable suture to secure the catheter. I prefer the cervical approach as there are multiple veins available and practically no risk of pneumothorax. I incise at the midpoint between clavicle and ear lobe for 1 cm. If the external jugular vein is large enough, I dissect it out. Tunnel a 3- or 4-F single lumen catheter from an incision on the ipsilateral chest wall up to the neck. Create a small venotomy and pass the catheter or an introducer, then pass the catheter. When the catheter won't easily thread, change the angle of traction on the cephalic end of the vein. If won't go, tie it off and find the IJ vein. Control it proximally and distally and cannulate the vein through a small venotomy or venipuncture. Secure in place with an absorbable suture just tight enough to prevent back bleeding. Secure the catheter at the exit site. Since I am not worried about pneumothorax, if catheter aspirates and flushes and cuff is 1 cm from exit site, that is where I leave it. The catheter tip should be measured on the chest wall to reach the third interspace. I do not obtain CXR, avoiding both the radiation and the expense, unless a central location is imperative.

Implantable Central Venous Access

The subcutaneous venous access port is associated with high quality of life scores. When not accessed, the patient is free to swim, shower, and play sports. The infection rate is generally lower than for tunneled catheters, but once infected the infection is more difficult to clear. A disadvantage in the younger child is the need to pass a needle through the skin to access the silicone reservoir of the port. Apprehension results from visualizing the needle and anticipating pain. Topical local anesthetic cream can minimize the psychological distress. This access route is a good choice in the older patient. The Huber needle is a specially constructed large-bore needle that is slightly bent near the tip in such a way that the opening (the bevel) is at a right angle to the long axis of the needle. This prevents the creation of a hole in the silicone window with each access attempt.

Complications

Catheter thrombosis is a relatively frequent problem, especially with catheters of smaller caliber. Catheter thrombosis increases the risk of venous thrombosis and central-line associated blood stream infection. Catheters should be monitored and if they develop sluggish flow or inability to draw blood, the thrombosis is usually cleared easily with tissue plasminogen activator (tPA). A line that cannot be cleared should be replaced or removed.

Central-line associated blood stream infection (CLABSI) is a well-known complication of central venous access. Catheters can become infected due to contamination during insertion, by seeding from improper handling during use, or secondarily in the setting of bacteremia. Catheters can also become infected at the insertion site (tunnel infections). Prevention of CLABSI has become an important patient-safety issue. Measures that appear to minimize the risk include taking appropriate precautions during insertion (chlorhexidine antisepsis, strict aseptic technique), minimizing access to the lines, strict aseptic technique when the line accessed, and removing the line when no longer needed. Every institution should have protocols that address each of these factors.

During placement of a central venous line, it is common for ectopic heart beats (PACs, PVCs) to occur due to stimulation of the endocardium with the guide wire. In fact this is often a welcome sign that the wire has been directed centrally. Some patients are prone to tachyarrhythmias or ventricular tachycardia and this needs to be anticipated and treated appropriately. Persistent or intermittent sinus tachycardia can be due to a line that is positioned too deep in the atrium and needs to be pulled back or replaced. Pneumothorax can occur during line insertion, especially when the subclavian vein is being accessed, although this is much more common early on the learning curve of the practitioner placing the line. Catheters can break either externally or internally. External catheter breaks can usually be repaired with specialized catheter repair kits. Subclavian catheters that are inserted medial to the midclavicular line can be sheared off by the scissoring action of the first rib against the clavicle. This can result in a catheter embolus, which should be retrieved by an interventional radiologist.

Catheters whose tips are directed against the wall of a vein, the SVC or the right atrium can perforate, resulting in bleeding or instillation of fluid into the pleural cavity or pericardium. Prompt line removal usually results in spontaneous sealing of the perforation but patients need to be monitored closely or studied to rule out ongoing bleeding. The previous habit of cutting silastic catheters at a sharp angle increases the risk of perforation as well as inability to draw blood from the catheter due to a flap-valve effect against the wall of the vein. Central vein thrombosis is increasingly recognized and more likely to be treated with anticoagulation to prevent embolism and allow recanalization of the vein. Chylothorax can result from injury to the thoracic duct during left subclavian vein access or as a result of SVC thrombosis, which can also lead to SVC syndrome. The catheter should be removed and anticoagulation therapy started if indicated.

Ultrasound

There are some data to suggest that the use of real-time sonography can minimize complications with insertion of a central line. US certainly helps identify vascular structures, especially in adults. It seems logical that familiarity with this technology should minimize complications of insertion by identifying the vessels definitively rather than estimating vessel location by surface anatomy. There are some data in children demonstrating greater first pass success with use of sonography. Another utility of US is in patients who have had multiple prior central lines. US can demonstrate patency of subclavian or jugular vessels. However, one must bear in mind that previously thrombosed vessels may recanalize with smaller caliber pathways to the central circulation. A recanalized SVC thrombosis can still create difficulty in passing a venous catheter to a central position. US will likely make central venous catheter insertion safer and will become more prevalent.

Difficult Passage

With live fluoroscopy in OR, it is possible to direct the J-tip of the guide wire towards the right atrium. If the guide wire stops, one should check that it is not passing up into the jugular vein. If the guide wire is not passing as intended, one should instill contrast through a small catheter to verify anatomy. There are rare thoracic venous anomalies such as duplication of SVC in which the catheter will thread centrally but down the left side of the vertebral column.

Trauma

Central venous access is not an early priority in the resuscitation of the injured child. It is important to establish large-bore peripheral access for volume administration. The flow characteristics of a long central line make it less than ideal for rapid fluid administration. If peripheral IV access is not rapidly established, the next option should be an interosseous line. All fluids and medications can be administered through this route with rapid dissemination through the body. Interosseous access is rapidly, reliably, and simply obtained by use of commercially available devices. Contraindication is fracture in the same extremity. The infectious complication rate is low. Central venous access is reserved for later in resuscitation in the case of a patient remaining hypotensive in spite of volume resuscitation.

Removal of Central Lines

One should treat removal of central venous catheters seriously. Ports should be removed in a controlled OR setting. Be wary of the call to the NICU or floor to remove a central venous line before the patient is discharged. You might be provided with only a suture removal kit. Often the catheter is removed easily but one must be prepared for a difficult removal. It is important to optimize the conditions. With a central venous access, IV sedation may be administered. Dissect down to the cuff and separate it from the subcutaneous tissue. Never yank on the catheter! Rather, apply a steady pull. If the catheter is not coming out easily, stop! Consider bringing the patient to the OR. Place yourself in a situation in which the cuff can be dissected free. The catheter usually comes out easily when the cuff is free. I never dissect the cuff away from the catheter or leave the cuff behind. If the cuff is free and the catheter is still stuck, it is probably stuck at site of insertion. This occurs with an exit site on the chest wall and a hairpin turn in the catheter which is inserted into the jugular vein and secured by suture. The catheter could break and necessitate a call to interventional radiology. You should carefully dissect down to the site of catheter insertion on the vein and divide the suture. The catheter will then dislodge. This is a good reason to avoid the use of silk suture to secure the line. The catheter can be secured and back bleeding controlled with a small absorbable tie or manual pressure.

Removal of a central catheter in the NICU is a common scenario. I once accommodated a request to remove a central line in a NICU baby and was asked to replace the catheter later the same day. Avoid this situation. A good general rule is that a baby must tolerate full feeds for a time and be on no IV medications before considering removal of the central venous catheter. The NICU infection rate for CVCs is slightly higher than elsewhere so there is an argument for removal of the catheter when it is no longer in use. But intubating, sedating and incising a new route for IV access causes pain, leaves a scar and is not a benign intervention. It is best to know the CVC infection rate per 1,000 days in your ICU settings to help decide on the most prudent course.

I insert a central line through the internal jugular vein as I remove the venous cannula from a patient on ECMO. These babies remain critically ill and in need of venous access. The jugular vein is well-exposed and it can accommodate a large-caliber IV. Though there is a risk of thrombosis and infection, the alternative is a separate dissection elsewhere with attendant risks.

Pearls Gathered from the Recent Literature

- Routine use of CXR after fluoroscopic placement of a central line is not justified and is not cost-effective [1].
- Probability of vein wall penetration is increased if the catheter is bowed along its course and tapered at the point of contact [2].
- Ultrasound guided central venous catheterization has a high success rate (99% adults, 90% children), and a higher single wall puncture rate in adults (83%) compared to children 49% [3].
- Minocycline-rifampin coated central venous line vs. non-coated: no difference in rate of catheter site infection, but delayed onset of infection (5 days vs. 18) [4].
- Heparin-bonded venous catheters might reduce the incidence of catheter occlusion and catheter-related infections [5].
- Complications with removal of implantable venous access devices occur in 16%, all in catheters in place for 20 months or more [6].
- Arm position, rather than site or vein, is the significant variable influencing PICC movement [7].
- Incidence of venous thromboembolism was greater for femoral (32%) and subclavian (27%) sites than for jugular (8%), whereas catheter type and size did not influence the rate [8].
- The carina can be used as a radiographic landmark for the proper placement of central line tip (within 1.5 cm in 95% of cases) in pediatric patients [9].
- The cavo-atrial junction is the ideal location for the tip of a central venous catheter and it is reliably located two vertebral bodies below the carina [10].
- Age under 6 years and hematologic disease were risk factors in central line complications. Double lumen catheters had double the complication rate of single lumen catheters [11].
- Most PICC lines (85.8%) placed without fluoroscopy resulted in non-central initial position. With fluoroscopic guidance, final central position was achieved in 90.2% [12].
- When using the femoral approach, place the tip of the catheter at the level of L3 [13].
- Insertion of central venous catheters larger than 6 F in children less than 1 year old, less than 10 kg or less than 75 cm in height was associated with a higher complication rate [14].

- Use the right third intercostals space as an anatomic landmark to allow positioning of the catheter tip in the SVC near but not in the right atrium in children [15].
- Using US to determine ideal body position for optimal size of subclavian vein: head in neutral position, chin midline, no shoulder role all optimize size of the vein [16].
- Risk factors for PICC line infections include: weight <8 kg, cardiac failure, cancer, silicone catheter, obstructed catheter, >12 days dwell time [17].

- Removal of tunneled or implanted central lines should be considered if bacteremia persists or recurs 72 h after initiation of antibiotic treatment, also for *Staphylococcus aureus*, *Pseudomonas aeruginosa*, *Acinetobacter baumannii* or *Candida* species [18].
- Tunneled catheters were associated with a threefold higher rate of blood stream infections compared to implantable devices, and there was a shorter time to first infection (52 vs. 109 days) [19].

Summary Points

- Expertise in establishing peripheral IV access is a useful skill.
- The umbilical vein access is a reliable route that can provide excellent venous access for up to 10 days.
- The peripherally inserted central catheter (PICC) is ideal for short-term, central venous access for antibiotics or parenteral nutrition.
- The gold standard for insertion of percutaneous central lines has always been guidance by surface anatomy landmarks. The subclavian, internal jugular, and femoral venous approaches account for the majority of central line insertions.
- In some institutions the most commonly placed line is the cuffed tunneled central line.
- The subcutaneous venous access port is associated with high quality of life scores: the infection rate is generally lower than for tunneled catheters, but once infected the infection is more difficult to clear.

Editor's Comment

Pediatric surgeons have traditionally been considered the ultimate experts in securing all forms of vascular access in children, a role partially usurped of late by interventional radiologists and the nurse IV specialist. Nevertheless, the pediatric should strive to be the "go-to" person for difficult vascular access, including percutaneous, incisional, and rare surgical techniques. This comes with several important responsibilities: availability at all hours; a genuine willingness to accommodate the needs of the child and their caregivers; the technical proficiency to provide even difficult access safely and efficiently; and meticulous attention to every detail of the insertion technique, dressings, and postoperative use and care of the line. It is important to approach each line in every patient as a true life line and one that, if it becomes infected or stops working, can make for a miserable or dangerous situation.

Percutaneous access to central veins is a veritable art form that experienced surgeons are able to perform safely on the basis of anatomic landmarks alone; however, there are increasing calls from others, primarily regulatory outsiders, but also skeptical colleagues in Radiology and Anesthesiology, who assume that this "blind" approach is inherently unsafe and feel that every one of these procedures should be done with ultrasound guidance. The femoral approach is not nearly as straightforward in children as it is in adults. The femoral

vein lies close to and somewhat behind the artery, increasing the risk of arterial injury. Before a large cannula is placed, absolute confirmation that the guide wire is in the vein is essential – femoral artery injury can cause limb ischemia and not infrequently results in leg amputation. Femoral venous catheters are also associated with an increased risk of thromboembolic complications, infection, catheter malfunction, and activity restriction and should therefore be considered the access of last resort.

A cutdown approach to any vein is generally avoidable except in an emergency or when image guidance is unavailable. Most children have four good choices for percutaneous central venous access in the neck and chest: the internal jugular and subclavian veins. The entire anterior neck and chest should routinely be sterilely prepared when placing a central line so that all are available every time. The right internal jugular vein is the best choice in small children as the risk of subclavian thrombosis is relatively high and could become an issue in adulthood should the patient be at high risk for renal insufficiency and require a shunt. The safest approach is between the two heads of the sternocleidomastoid muscle: the vein is surprisingly superficial and can be entered with the needle at nearly a right angle to the skin. Carotid artery injury is rare, but in children the subclavian artery tends to arch up into the neck above the clavicle, placing it at risk of injury. The catheter should then be tunneled below the platysma and in such a way that all turns are smooth and without kinks. The catheter tip should ideally be at the cavo-atrial junction, which looks like the uppermost portion of the atrium on X-ray. This point is usually within two vertebral bodies below the carina and can be measured relative to the guide wire under fluoroscopy or on the basis of superficial landmarks (nipple, third intercostal space), which are notoriously inaccurate. Another option is to err on the long side and check length while the peel-away sheath is still in place. This way the catheter can be retrieved, trimmed, and placed back through the sheath. The neck incision is closed with a deep-dermal absorbable stitch and cyanoacrylate skin adhesive. The cuff of the catheter should be placed within 2 cm of the chest incision but it is better to pull it up higher and then bring it down to its proper location so that it is being held back by the fibrous septae in the subcutaneous fat. This helps to prevent accidental dislodgement before the cuff sets.

The subclavian vein is easily identified in most children but the window for safe access is relatively small: lateral to the intersection of the clavicle and first rib but medial to where the subclavian artery is at risk for injury. The best place is usually just lateral to the palpable first rib, with the needle aimed just above the sternal notch. No shoulder roll, or at most a very small one that only slightly exaggerates the normal anatomy, is best. In infants and small children, the arms can be pulled gently downward with hypoallergenic tape to the diaper or lower extremities. The anterior aspect of the shoulder should be left exposed, allowing the needle to travel in a plane parallel to the chest wall without the hub getting caught in the drapes. Pneumothorax should be rare if the tip of the needle passes close to the clavicle and the shaft of the needle is parallel to the chest. Catching the periostium of the clavicle is a well-known complication that should be avoided. Again, the catheter should be tunneled below the platysma (which extends down onto the upper chest) so that the catheter is not too close to the skin where it can be punctured with a suture needle or erode through the skin. Ports should be placed on the upper chest, medial for boys, slightly more lateral for girls, and always in the space between the Scarpa fascia and the pectoralis fascia – too superficial and skin erosion is a problem, too deep and the port is in the muscle.

As PICC lines become ever more popular, placement of the tunneled line in the premature newborn is a dying art. The procedure must often be completed without an assistant. Gather all instruments and disposables ahead of time and always use strict aseptic technique. The patient must be intubated, sedated, and immobilized. Percutaneous access to the subclavian vein is possible in infants more than 1,500 g but very difficult in smaller infants. The external jugular vein is unreliable due to its acute angle of insertion into the internal jugular in more than half of infants and is best avoided. The facial vein is ideal but not always easily identified. An incision placed in the uppermost skin crease just posterior and inferior to the angle of the mandible will usually reveal the vein, but if not present, the internal jugular is easily found a little deeper. Avoiding injury to the vagus nerve, control the IJV proximally and distally but do not ligate it. After tunneling a 2.7 F silastic catheter and cutting it to length with a sharp tapered point, create a venotomy with 19-gauge needle and the catheter should slide right in without back-bleeding. If fluoroscopy is not available, the catheters must be confirmed to be central by plain x-ray and then repositioned if not in the right position.

Differential Diagnosis

- Long-term access for parenteral nutrition
- Chemotherapy
- Ongoing need for blood component therapy
- Plasmaphoresis/hemodialysis
- Need for frequent blood sampling

Parental Preparation

- Complications of central venous access include infection, bleeding, arrhythmia, injury to adjacent structures (artery, nerve, thoracic duct), infection, thrombosis, pulmonary embolism, and pneumothorax.
- Life-threatening complications are rare but not unheard of.

References

1. Adwan H, Gordon H, Nicholls E. Are routine chest radiographs needed after fluoroscopically guided percutaneous insertion of central venous catheters in children? J Pediatr Surg. 2008;43(2): 341–3.
2. Towbin R. The bowed catheter sign: a risk for pericardial tamponade. Pediatr Radiol. 2008;38(3):331–5.
3. Tercan F, Oguzkurt L, Ozkan U, Eker HE. Comparison of ultrasonography-guided central venous catheterization between adult and pediatric populations. Cardiovasc Intervent Radiol. 2008;31(3): 575–80.
4. Chelliah A, Heydon KH, Zaoutis TE, et al. Observational trial of antibiotic-coated central venous catheters in critically ill pediatric patients. Pediatr Infect Dis J. 2007;26(9):816–20.
5. Shah PS, Shah N. Heparin-bonded catheters for prolonging the patency of central venous catheters in children. Cochrane Database Syst Rev. 2007;17(4):CD005983.
6. Dillon PA, Foglia RP. Complications associated with an implantable vascular access device. J Pediatr Surg. 2006;41(9):1582–7.
7. Connoly B, Amaral J, Walsh S, et al. Influence of arm movement on central tip location of peripherally inserted central catheters (PICCs). Pediatr Radiol. 2006;36(8):845–50.

8. Male C, Julian JA, Massicotte P, et al. Significant association with location of central venous line placement and risk of venous thrombosis in children. Thromb Haemost. 2005;94(3):516–21.

9. Yoon SZ, Shin JH, Hahn S, et al. Usefulness of the carina as a radiographic landmark for central venous catheter placement in paediatric patients. Br J Anaesth. 2005;95(4):514–7.

10. Baskin KM, Jimenez RM, Cahill AM, et al. Cavoatrial junction and central venous anatomy: implications for central venous access tip position. J Vasc Interv Radiol. 2008;19(3):359–65.

11. Fratino G, Molinari AC, Parodi S, et al. Central venous catheter-related complications in children with oncological/hematological diseases: an observational study of 418 devices. Ann Oncol. 2005;16(4):648–54.

12. Fricke BL, Racadio JM, Duckworth T, et al. Placement of peripherally inserted central catheters without fluoroscopy in children: initial catheter tip position. Radiology. 2005;234(3):887–92.

13. Shinohara Y, Arai T, Yamasita M. The optimal insertion length of central venous catheter via the femoral route for open-heart surgery in infants and children. Paediatr Anaesth. 2005;15(2):122–4.

14. Janik JE, Conlon SJ, Janik JS. Percutaneous central access in patients younger than 5 years: size does matter. J Pediatr Surg. 2004;39(8):1252–6.

15. Kim KO, Jo JO, Kim CS. Positioning internal jugular venous catheters using the right third intercostal space in children. Acta Anaesthesiol Scand. 2003;47(10):1284–6.

16. Lukish J, Valladares E, Rodriguez C, et al. Classical positioning decreases subclavian vein cross-sectional area in children. J Trauma. 2002;53(2):272–5.

17. García-Teresa MA, Casado-Flores J, et al. Infectious complications of percutaneous central venous catheterization in pediatric patients: a Spanish multicenter study. Intensive Care Med. 2007;33(3): 466–76.

18. Simon A, Bode U, Beutel K. Diagnosis and treatment of catheter-related infections in paediatric oncology: an update. Clin Microbiol Infect. 2006;12(7):606–20.

19. Adler A, Yaniv I, Steinberg R, et al. Infectious complications of implantable ports and Hickman catheters in paediatric haematology-oncology patients. J Hosp Infect. 2006;62(3):358–65.

Suggested Reading

Bagwell CE, Salzberg AM, Sonnino RE, Haynes JH. Potentially lethal complications of central venous catheter placement. J Pediatr Surg. 2000;35(5):709–13.

Barnacle A, Arthurs OJ, Roebuck D, Hiorns MP. Malfunctioning central venous catheters in children: a diagnostic approach. Pediatr Radiol. 2008;38(4):363–78.

Chung DH, Ziegler MM. Central venous catheter access. Nutrition. 1998;14(1):119–23.

Juno RJ, Knott AW, Racadio J, Warner BW. Reoperative venous access. Semin Pediatr Surg. 2003;12(2):132–9.

Radtke WA. Vascular access and management of its complications. Pediatr Cardiol. 2005;26(2):140–6.

Chapter 11
Acute Kidney Injury

Peter A. Meaney and Kevin E.C. Meyers

Acute kidney injury (AKI) is defined as a loss of renal function measured by a decline in glomerular filtration rate that develops over hours to days, and is the preferred term over acute renal failure. A decline in GFR results in impairment of nitrogenous waste product excretion and loss of water, electrolyte regulation and acid-base regulation.

One in twenty hospitalized adults develops AKI, which increases mortality fourfold and doubles the length of hospital stay. In children, AKI is due primarily to renal dysfunction in the setting of systemic illness. Approximately 20% of cases are due to renal ischemia, 15% to nephrotoxic medications, and 10% to sepsis. Primary renal disease accounts for less than 10% and hemolytic uremic syndrome (HUS) for less than 1%. Overall survival is 70% while survival for those requiring ICU admission or renal replacement therapy is 60%. Two-thirds of children with AKI eventually have full recovery of renal function.

The disease process underlying acute kidney injury typically affects one or more anatomic areas: the vascular supply, the glomeruli, the renal tubule, the urinary tract. Any process that interferes with the renal architecture or its functioning can compromise renal function. Although the etiology is best described by the renal anatomy affected by the disease process, it is often categorized functionally as pre-renal, renal, or post-renal (Table 11.1). In both pre-renal and post-renal AKI, kidney function is initially normal but compromise of renal perfusion or obstruction of urine flow leads to diminished renal function. If not corrected, this can progress to intrinsic acute kidney injury. Intrinsic AKI occurs when the kidneys are themselves primarily affected by a process that causes loss of renal function.

Progression of all types of renal failure results in acute tubular necrosis, characterized by a rapid decline in GFR and signs of tubular cell injury, including oliguria and electrolyte disorders. While the differential diagnosis for AKI is broad, most cases seen in the peri-operative setting are due to hypoperfusion (prerenal), either in isolation or in association with another nephrotoxic insult.

Acute tubular necrosis progresses through several phases: initiation, extension, maintenance, and recovery. Tubular damage by ischemia, nephrotoxins or both leads to decreased GFR by a combination of mechanisms (Fig. 11.1). The initiation phase is set in motion when reduction in blood flow further compromises the GFR and results in damage to the renal tubule epithelial cells. Vascular and inflammatory changes then account for the extension phase and contribute to a further decline in renal function. During the maintenance phase, cellular mechanisms are set in motion to permit repair. The GFR reaches its nadir at this time. Repair permits recovery of organ integrity and normalization of function with return of the GFR (Fig. 11.2).

There are clinical phases that parallel the cellular pathophysiology. During the initiation phase, oliguria is often the only sign. Although often subtle, it is important to recognize early because timely intervention might limit the degree of injury. Persistent oliguria and progressive azotemia signify the maintenance phase, in which pre- and post-renal forms of AKI transition to intrinsic renal injury. Renal function begins to improve during the recovery phase, which is often heralded by a brisk diuresis. This "polyuric phase" is due to an improvement in GFR at a time when the injured tubule cells still have poor reabsorptive and concentrating abilities. If unchecked, this can lead to fluid and electrolyte depletion and subsequent re-injury.

Diagnosis

The diagnosis of AKI is made by careful history, physical examination, and laboratory evaluation. Clinical history should include a search for exposures to potential nephrotoxic drugs, avenues of fluid loss and hypotension, potential sources of emboli, a history of umbilical lines in the neonatal period, and a family history of renal disease.

P.A. Meaney (✉)
Department of Anesthesia and Critical Care, University of Pennsylvania, Children's Hospital of Philadelphia, Philadelphia, PA, USA
e-mail: meaney@email.chop.edu

P. Mattei (ed.), *Fundamentals of Pediatric Surgery*,
DOI 10.1007/978-1-4419-6643-8_11, © Springer Science+Business Media, LLC 2011

Table 11.1 Categorization of acute kidney injury

Pre renal	Intrinsic renal	Post renal
Volume related	Glomerular	Urinary tract obstruction
Intravascular depletion	Hemolytic uremic syndrome	Posterior urethral valves
Ineffective circulation	Acute glomerulonephritis	Bilateral UPJ obstruction
Ischemic/thrombotic	Vasculitis	Bilateral nephrolithiasis
Abdominal compartment syndrome	Lupus nephritis	Neoplasm
Renovascular	Goodpasture syndrome	Retroperitoneal fibrosis
Renal vein thrombosis	Wegener's	Trauma
Renal artery stenosis	ANCA associated	
Neurohumoral signaling dysfunction	Vascular	
Hepato-renal syndrome	Hemolytic uremic syndrome	
Medications	Malignant hypertension	
Calcineurin	Tubular/interstitial	
Radio contrast agents	Uncorrected pre- or post-AKI	
ACEI and ARB	Asphyxia/hypoxia	
	Medications	
	Aminoglycosides/vancomycin	
	Amphotericin B	
	Amphotericin B	
	Poisons	
	Crystals (acyclovir and methotrexate)	
	Tumor lysis/urate nephropathy	
	Rhabdo/hemolysis: pigment nephropathy	

ACEI angiotensin converting enzyme inhibitors; *ARB* angiotensin receptor blockers; *ANCA* anti-neutrophil cytoplasmic antibodies; *UPJ* ureteropelvic junction obstruction

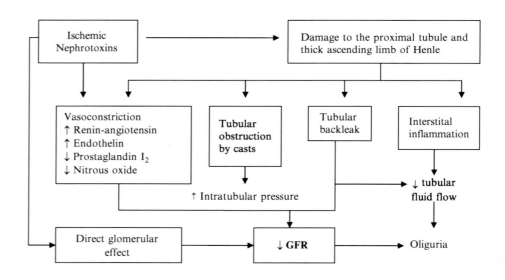

Fig. 11.1 Pathophysiology of acute kidney injury

The physical examination should focus on the patient's overall fluid status (weight gain, edema) and the current intravascular volume status (blood pressure, jugular venous distention, hepatomegaly, respiratory sounds). Abdominal examination might reveal a mass or palpable bladder.

The diagnosis of AKI is usually confirmed by elevations in BUN and creatinine levels, the normal values of which vary significantly by age (Table 11.2). An increase in creatinine concentration indicates a decrease in the GFR, even if the absolute level remains within the normal range. In the neonate, a doubling of the creatinine from 0.3 to 0.6 mg/dL corresponds to a decrease in GFR by 50%. In adults and older children with pre-renal disease, the BUN is often elevated out of proportion to the creatinine (BUN:Cr ratio >20:1) due to an increase in the passive reabsorption of urea that follows the enhanced proximal transport of sodium and water. This is not as useful in infants and smaller children as their serum creatinine levels are so much lower.

Fig. 11.2 Phases of acute tubular necrosis (Reprinted by permission from Macmillan Publishers, Ltd.: Sutton TA, Fisher CJ, Molitoris BA. Microvascular endothelial injury and dysfunction during ischemic acute renal failure. Kidney Int. 2002;62:1539–49.)

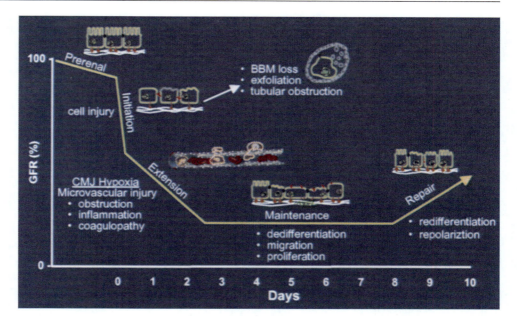

Table 11.2 Creatinine: normal values by age

Newborn	0.3–1.0 mg/dL (27–88 μmol/L)
Infant	0.2–0.5 mg/dL (18–35 μmol/L)
Child	0.3–0.7 mg/dL (27–62 μmol/L)
Adolescent	0.5–1.0 mg/dL (44–88 μmol/L)

Calculating the *fractional excretion of sodium* (FENa) is the most accurate way to determine if there is a significant pre-renal component in AKI:

$$FENa = \frac{U_{Na} \times P_{Cr}}{P_{Na} \times U_{Cr}} \times 100,$$

where U_{Na} = urine sodium, P_{Cr} = plasma creatinine, P_{Na} = plasma sodium, U_{Cr} = urine creatinine. It is a measure of the percent of filtered sodium that is excreted in the urine and is not affected by the rate of water reabsorption. A value of less than 1% signifies pre-renal disease, while a value >2% implies impairment of glomerular function. Because of the decreased ability to reabsorb sodium in newborns, pre-renal disease is associated with FENa values less than 2.5% while values greater than 2.5–3.5% usually suggest tubular dysfunction. A urine sodium concentration below 25 mEq/L is generally indicative of hypovolemia.

While a *urine osmolality* greater than 500 mOsm/kg usually indicates pre-renal disease, lower values are of little value in differentiating pre-renal from intrinsic renal disease. This is due to the fact that, regardless of the etiology, loss of concentrating ability is an early and almost universal finding in ATN.

Urinalysis is an important noninvasive test in the diagnostic evaluation of AKI. A normal or near-normal urinalysis, characterized by few cells with little or no casts or proteinuria, suggests pre-renal disease or urinary tract obstruction. Muddy brown granular casts and epithelial cell casts are suggestive of ATN, but their absence does not exclude the diagnosis. The presence of red cell casts and dysmorphic red cells is diagnostic of glomerulonephritis, while marked proteinuria suggests nephrotic syndrome. Granular casts with mild to moderate proteinuria, microscopic hematuria and sterile pyuria are suggestive of tubulo-interstitial disease.

The *urine specific gravity* is not very useful in the diagnosis of AKI as it is affected by the maturity of the kidney and by the presence of colloids including protein, glucose and mannitol.

Renal ultrasound with Doppler is utilized to document kidney size, shape, and consistency of the parenchyma, and to exclude urinary tract obstruction and vascular occlusion.

Kidney biopsy is most commonly obtained when noninvasive evaluation has been unable to establish the correct diagnosis, but it is rarely required prior to the institution of supportive therapy.

Proposed and developed by an expert panel, the RIFLE criteria stratifies renal injury into three levels based on the magnitude of the decrease in the GFR and duration and severity of the oliguria (Table 11.3).

Treatment

Initial management should be directed at mitigating the progression of AKI. For pre-renal disease, it is essential to improve kidney perfusion by intravascular volume resuscitation and weaning vasoconstrictive drugs. In the case of intrinsic renal disease, the underlying disease process should

Table 11.3 RIFLE criteria for the diagnosis of acute kidney injury

Level	Nomenclature	Increase in serum creatinine	Urine output
Level I	Risk of kidney injury	1.5× baseline	<0.5 mL/kg/h for >6 h
Level II	Kidney injury	2× baseline	<0.5 mL/kg/h for >12 h
Level III	Failure of kidney function	3× baseline or sCr >4 mg/dL with absolute increase of >0.5 mg/dL	<0.3 mL/kg/h for >24 h or anuria for >12 h
Loss of kidney function		Persistent renal failure for >4 weeks	
End-stage disease		Persistent renal failure for >3 months	

be treated and nephrotoxic agents eliminated. Acute management of post-renal AKI consists of decompressing the urinary tract with percutaneous drains or endoscopically placed stents. Despite preventative measures, progression to renal insufficiency can occur and is manifest by volume overload, hypertension, electrolyte abnormalities, acidosis, anemia, and impaired drug metabolism.

In the setting of reduced GFR, physiologic intake of sodium and water leads to plasma volume overload, which can lead to cardiac failure and pulmonary edema. Limiting intake and increasing intravascular fluid removal by judicious use of diuretics or dialysis are the keys to optimizing fluid management. Loop diuretics inhibit sodium, potassium and chloride ion transport mechanisms in the ascending loop of Henle, which is responsible for 20–30% of the total reabsorption of sodium and chloride in the renal medulla. Both furosemide and bumetanide inhibit the luminal chloride pump and therefore must be excreted into the urine in the proximal tubule to function properly. This favors a continuous mode of delivery and helps to avoid toxicity, which occurs at high peak serum concentrations. In adult ICU patients, continuous infusion combined with albumin supplementation can lead to significantly improved negative fluid balance. Loop diuretics also serve to increase venous capacitance, which can produce rapid relief of symptoms from congestive heart failure even before the diuretic effect is produced. These drugs can usually augment urine output in patients with mild to moderate AKI, but are often ineffective in severe cases.

Dopamine is synthesized in the kidney and participates in the regulation of renal blood flow, proximal tubular sodium reabsorption, and aldosterone-mediated distal tubular sodium reabsorption. Although laboratory research indicates that renal blood flow is increased by 20–40% with dopamine infusion rates of 0.5–2 µg/kg/min, clinical studies have been unable to demonstrate significant attenuation of AKI with its routine use. Likewise, fenoldopam mesylate, a selective dopamine receptor-1 agonist that increases renal blood flow in healthy adult volunteers, has not been shown to be clinically effective in the intensive care population.

Once euvolemia is achieved, strict fluid management is essential. Fluid administration should match insensible losses, which are approximately one third of calculated "maintenance" requirements. In patients who are mechanically ventilated, insensible loss is minimized by humidification of inspired gases; therefore fluid administration should be reduced to one quarter maintenance.

Hypertension in patients with AKI is the result of volume overload and activation of vasoconstrictor pathways including the renin-angiotensin-aldosterone system. Treatment strategies should therefore be directed at volume reduction and vasodilatation. In addition to loop diuretics, antihypertensive medications such as calcium channel antagonists are sometimes useful in the acute setting, while angiotensin receptor blockers and ACE inhibitors are useful for chronic therapy.

Patients with severe AKI commonly develop hyperkalemia, hyperphosphatemia, hypocalemia, and acidemia. Supplemental potassium and phosphorous should be eliminated in critically ill patients with a rising or elevated serum creatinine. Orally-administered binding resins, such sodium polystyrene sulfonate (Kayexalate) and sevelamer hydrochloride (Renagel) can be used to decrease intestinal absorption of potassium and phosphorus, respectively. Lowering serum phosphate will also tend to raise the serum calcium. Patients with hypocalcemia generally are not treated with intravenous calcium supplementation unless symptomatic. Electrocardiographic findings associated with life-threatening hyperkalemia consist of: peaking of T waves, followed by an increase in the PR interval, flattened P waves, widening of the QRS complex, bradycardia and, eventually, ventricular fibrillation. Metabolic acidosis should be corrected if the plasma bicarbonate concentration falls below 16 mEq/L or the arterial pH is less than 7.25, especially if the patient requires vasopressor therapy, as acidosis worsens myocardial dysfunction. Dialysis is indicated for refractory electrolyte disturbances and acidosis.

Renal injury suppresses production of erythropoietin, producing anemia. Patients with long-standing renal disease often benefit from recombinant erythropoietin and iron supplementation. Uremia also causes a coagulopathy, which, if clinically significant, is treated with administration of platelets, plasma, or desmopressin (DDAVP).

It is important to remember that impaired renal function decreases the clearance of medications commonly used in the peri-operative setting, such as antibiotics, anticonvulsants, paralytics, and H_2 blockers. Dose adjustments need to be made based on a patient's GFR and serum drug levels.

Despite meticulous management, some children with AKI progress to refractory volume overload or life threatening

Table 11.4 Factors associated with AKI in the peri-operative setting

Cardiac surgery
Medication associated
Hepatorenal syndrome
HUS/TTP
Abdominal compartment syndrome
Malignancy-associated
Radiocontrast effect
Rhabdomyolysis
HIV related nephropathy
Allergic interstitial nephritis

metabolic derangements necessitating renal replacement therapies (Table 11.4).

Specific Clinical Scenarios

Cardiac Surgery

AKI occurs in up to 30% of infants who undergo cardiac surgery and is associated with increased mortality. Patients at highest risk are those with low cardiac output, vasodilatory shock, or bleeding. There is no definitive evidence that the use of diuretics, vasodilators, dopamine or fenoldapam prevents or alters the course of AKI after cardiac surgery. Urodilatin (an atrial natriuretic peptide) is potentially useful but further prospective trials are underway.

Drug-Related AKI

Aminoglycosides, Amphotericin B, NSAIDs, and many chemotherapeutic agents have been implicated in pediatric medication-associated AKI (Table 11.5). Infants, children with chronic kidney disease, and children on multiple medications are at increased risk. The effect is usually mild and self-limited but only if recognized early and administration of the drug *and all other nephrotoxins* are stopped. The indications, alternatives, pharmacokinetics, and potential for drug interactions need to be considered for each potentially nephrotoxic medication administered in the peri-operative setting.

Hepatorenal Syndrome

AKI occurs in patients with cirrhosis for three reasons: prerenal azotemia, hepatorenal syndrome (HRS) and ATN, but clinical differentiation between these entities is not always

Table 11.5 Medication-associated AKI in the peri-operative setting

Antibiotics	Aminoglycosides
	Colistin
	Penicillins, cephalosporins
Antifungals	Amphotericin B
Nonsteroidal anti-inflammatory drugs	COX-1 inhibitors
	COX-2 inhibitors
Antivirals	Acyclovir, indinavir, foscarnet
	Adefovir, tenovir, cidofovir
Anti-epileptics	Dilantin
Diuretics	Furosemide
Sedatives	Propofol
Chemotherapeutics	Cisplatinum
Radiocontrast agents	
Antihypertensive agents	Angiotensin converting enzyme inhibitors and angiotensin receptor blockers
Immunosuppressives	Calcineurin inhibitors

Table 11.6 Differentiation of causes of AKI in children with advanced liver disease

AKI	Urine sodium (mEq/L)	FENa (%)	Urine sediment
Pre renal azotemia	<20	<1	Bland
HRS	<20	<1	Bland or bile-stained granular casts
ATN	>40	>2	Granular casts

Table 11.7 Criteria for the diagnosis of Hepatorenal syndrome

Liver disease with advanced hepatic failure and portal hypertension
Reduced GFR
Absence of shock, ongoing bacterial infection, volume depletion, or use of nephrotoxic drugs
Absence of sustained improvement in renal function after discontinuation of diuretics and expansion of plasma volume
Absence of proteinuria or obstructive uropathy or other renal disease

straightforward (Table 11.6). A form of functional renal failure, HRS is characterized by profound renal vasoconstriction (Table 11.7). The underlying pathogenesis is incompletely understood but is thought to be due to a cascade of events that begins with splanchnic vasodilatation, hyperdynamic circulation, and in effect arterial under-filling, which activates neuro-humoral vasoconstrictors and inhibition of local renal vasodilators. Two types are recognized, with type 1 being more fulminant and associated with a particularly poor prognosis. Successful treatment with octreotide, milrinone or vasopressin has been described anecdotally but none has been proved effective in clinical studies in children. Definitive therapy is liver transplantation. Renal replacement therapy should be used as a bridge to liver transplantation.

Hemolytic Uremic Syndromes and Thrombotic Thrombocytopenic Purpura

TTP and HUS are acute syndromes with multi organ system involvement. HUS is a thrombotic microangiopathy that is characterized by platelet aggregation and fibrin deposition within small vessels, leading to intravascular hemolysis, thrombocytopenia, and AKI. In many parts of the world, HUS is the most common cause of AKI in children Though sometimes associated with a urinary tract infection, HUS is usually seen in association with bloody diarrhea caused by shiga toxin-producing *Escherichia coli* 0157:H7. The course is severe in less than 10% of children but can be fatal due to neurological (seizures, coma), gastrointestinal (gangrenous colitis), or cardiorespiratory (congestive cardiac failure, respiratory distress syndrome) complications. HUS also infrequently occurs in association with pneumococcal infections, pregnancy or the use of drugs such as oral contraceptives or calcineurin inhibitors. Inherited causes of HUS are due to complement disorders (Factor H, Factor I, Membrane cofactor protein). Treatment is supportive, with plasma exchange indicated for Factor H-associated HUS and possibly when there are severe neurological manifestations of HUS.

TTP has many of the same clinical manifestations and comorbidities as HUS but is the term used when fever, hemolysis, thrombocytopenia, and neurologic symptoms predominate. AKI is much less commonly seen and is usually less severe in patients with TTP.

Abdominal Compartment Syndrome

Abdominal compartment syndrome (ACS) is caused by a sudden and severe increase in intra-abdominal pressure. Loss of kidney function in ACS appears to be primarily due to venous compression and indirectly to loss of cardiac output and sympathetic nervous system-mediated arterial vasoconstriction. The result is progressive loss of glomerular filtration and urine output. Oliguria is often seen at an intra-abdominal pressure of 15 mmHg and anuria at 30 mmHg, which can be measured using a commercially available pressure-sensor equipped Foley catheter. Treatment involves drainage of peritoneal fluid, if present, or urgent surgical decompression of the abdomen. Marked improvement in renal function is commonly observed within hours following decompression.

Malignancy

The etiologies of malignancy-associated AKI are varied and can be divided into pre-renal, intrinsic renal and post-renal causes (Table 11.8). Tumor lysis syndrome (TLS) results from massive lysis of tumor cells and causes AKI by decreasing GFR through pre-renal mechanisms and by increasing solute load, which impairs tubular function. Characterized by hyperkalemia, hyperphosphatemia, hyperuricemia, and metabolic acidosis, TLS is seen most commonly after initiation of therapy for lymphoreticular malignancies. In the setting of acidic urine, uric acid crystallizes in the tubules. A urine uric acid-to-creatinine ratio of greater than 1 is suggestive of uric acid nephropathy. The prevention of TLS centers on volume expansion and administration of urate oxidase (Rasburicase), an enzyme that converts uric acid to allantoin, which is five times more soluble in the urine than uric acid. Oliguric AKI due to TLS invariably requires institution of continuous renal replacement therapy (CRRT).

Rhabdomyolysis

Rhabdomyolysis is the result of fulminant destruction of skeletal muscle. Trauma and extensive operative dissection are the most common causes. Less common causes include extreme exertion, heat-related illness, status epilepticus, infections such as influenza, and malignant hyperthermia. A number of toxins have also been implicated (Table 11.9). Rhabdomyolysis

Table 11.8 Etiologies of malignancy associated AKI

Pre-renal	Intrinsic-renal	Post-renal
Extracellular fluid depletion	Acute tubular necrosis	Ureteral obstruction
Anorexia; vomiting; diarrhea	Medications; sepsis	Retroperitoneal tumors, lymphadenopathy, fibrosis
Hepatorenal syndrome	TTP/HUS	Bladder outlet obstruction
Hepatic veno-occlusive disease	Medications: Post BMT Parenchymal infiltration Leukemia; lymphoma Intratubular obstruction Methotrexate; acyclovir; tumor lysis syndrome	Rhabdomyosarcoma

Table 11.9 Medications and toxins associated with acute rhabdomyolysis

Antiretrovirals	Zidovudine
Antipsychotics	Haloperidol New atypical antipsychotics Phenothiazines
Lipid lowering agents	Statins Fibric acid derivatives
Vasoconstrictors	Cocaine Ephedrine plus vigorous exercise
Toxins	Multiple bee or wasp stings Snake-envenomation
Alcohols	Ethsanol

with AKI is usually seen in the context of intravascular volume depletion or concomitant exposure to additional nephrotoxins. It is characterized by an elevated serum creatine kinase (CK) concentration and myoglobinuria. Early vigorous fluid resuscitation with isotonic fluids reduces the incidence of oliguric kidney injury and the need for dialysis. Though not definitively proven to be effective, many advocate the use of mannitol as an osmotic agent and sodium bicarbonate to alkanize the urine when CK levels are greater than 10,000 U/L.

Radiocontrast Nephropathy

Radiocontrast nephropathy accounts for 10% of cases of hospital-acquired AKI in adults but is very uncommon in children. Risk factors for development of AKI include baseline renal insufficiency, congestive cardiac failure, diabetes mellitus, and exposure to a large dose of contrast material. The serum creatinine typically begins to increase 24–48 h after contrast administration, peaks within 3–5 days and returns to baseline within 7–10 days. Prior to contrast administration, medications including diuretics, NSAIDs and metformin should be withheld and volume depletion corrected. There is evidence that pre- and post-procedure volume expansion and the use of low osmolar contrast agents reduce the risk of AKI. The use of sodium bicarbonate, N-acetylcysteine or theophylline has not been proven to be of any value in preventing AKI.

HIV/AIDS

There are numerous etiologies of AKI in patients with HIV/AIDS. The most common is prerenal hypovolemia associated with opportunistic infections or drugs. Also seen with increased frequency in these patients are HUS/TTP, rhabdomyolysis, and acute interstitial nephritis. The protease inhibitor indinavir causes nephrolithiasis, crystal-induced AKI, and tubulo-interstitial nephritis. The nucleotide reverse transcriptase inhibitors tenofovir, adefovir and cidofovir cause AKI with proximal tubular injury and a Fanconi syndrome. Dose adjustments are required for most antiretroviral drugs in patients with renal impairment.

Acute Interstitial Nephritis

Acute interstitial nephritis (AIN) is classically represented by the triad of fever, rash and eosinophilia, although less than 10% of all cases have all three. Fifteen percent of cases of AIN are thought to be due to infectious causes, but the majority are drug-related. The most common drugs implicated are NSAIDs, penicillins and cephalosporins, rifampin, sulfonamides, and, much less often, diuretics, ciprofloxacin, and proton pump inhibitors. Additional causes include autoimmune disorders and a variety of infections, such as legionella, leptospirosis, cytomegalovirus and streptococcal organisms. Removal of offending agent or treatment of organism in combination with supportive therapy is all that is required as most cases improve after 3–5 days of appropriate treatment.

Prognosis

Acute kidney injury in children is associated with significant morbidity and mortality. In the peri-operative setting, the most important predictors of mortality are: hemodynamic instability, underlying systemic illness severity, and the degree of fluid overload at initiation of renal replacement therapy. Survival is better in children with primary renal disease, whereas mortality is greatest in the setting of multiple organ dysfunction, exceeding 50% in children requiring renal replacement therapy. In-hospital mortality is estimated to be between 30 and 50%. In a retrospective review of 254 AKI episodes in 248 children by Hui-Stickle et al., overall survival for the entire cohort was 70%, whereas 60% requiring ICU admission and 56% receiving renal replacement therapy survived. Two-thirds of children had full recovery of renal function, while 20% of hospital survivors died after discharge. Askenazi et al. estimated that about 20% develop stage 1 chronic kidney disease (CKD), 10% develop stage 2 chronic kidney disease, and almost a third of survivors progress to end-stage renal disease.

Future Directions

There is a considerable amount of ongoing research in the field of acute kidney injury, including studies of alternative markers of renal injury such as cystatin C, which may detect AKI 1–2 days earlier than serum creatinine concentration alone, potentially allowing clinicians to prevent the progression of renal injury. In addition, multiple therapeutic agents are under investigation, including atrial naturetic peptide, thyroid hormone, calcium channel blockers, oxyradical scavengers, and adenine nucleotides. It is likely that with earlier detection and newer treatment options, prevention and management of acute kidney injury in the pediatric population will continue to improve.

Summary Points

- Acute kidney injury (AKI) is defined as the loss of renal function measured by a decline in glomerular filtration rate (GFR) that develops over hours to days.
- In children, AKI is usually secondary to systemic illness.
- The etiology of AKI is best described by the renal anatomy most affected: pre-renal, renal, orpost-renal.
- Progression of renal failure results in acute tubular necrosis (ATN).
- A high BUN-Cr ratio is not as useful in infants and smaller children because their serum creatinine levels are so low.
- In newborns, because of their decreased ability to resorb sodium, pre-renal disease is associated with FENa values of less than 2.5% and ATN is associated with values greater than 2.5–3.5%.
- Initial management should be directed at halting the progression of AKI and minimizing complications.
- Electrocardiographic findings associated with life-threatening hyperkalemia consist of initial peaking of T waves, followed by an increase in the PR interval, flattened P waves, widening of the QRS complex, bradycardia, and ventricular fibrillation.
- There is no definitive evidence that the use of diuretics, vasodilators, dopamine or fenoldapam prevents or alters the course of AKI after cardiac surgery.
- Aminoglycosides, amphotericin B, NSAIDs, and chemotherapy are frequently implicated in pediatric medication-associated AKI.
- Hepato-renal syndrome is a form of functional renal failure that is characterized by severe vasoconstriction of the renal circulation.
- Rhabdomyolysis is caused by muscle injury or extensive surgery; vigorous fluid resuscitation with normal saline can lessen kidney injury.
- Radiocontrast nephropathy is very uncommon in children.
- Seventy percent of patients with AKI in hospital not requiring dialysis survive.
- Long-term results are excellent: over two-thirds of children with AKI go on to full recovery of renal function.

Editor's Comment

Acute kidney injury occasionally occurs in healthy children after major surgery, usually from exposure to a nephrotoxic drug like gentamicin. Transient renal dysfunction can also occur after exposure to ketorolac or in patients who are allowed to become extremely dehydrated. Renal injury due to intravenous contrast material appears to be exceedingly rare in children. Since frequent routine daily blood draws have (appropriately) become a thing of the past, the clinician needs to be vigilant for the subtle signs of renal dysfunction, including nausea, ileus, and a generalized malaise. Urine output is usually normal, or consistent with the usual fluctuations observed in the postoperative period, and is therefore not a reliable sign. Basically, any patient whose postoperative progress seems to have stalled or taken a step back for no apparent reason (sepsis, obstruction, and hemorrhage have been ruled out) should raise the question of AKI. Electrolytes with BUN and creatinine should be drawn, fluid status should be assessed, and a urinalysis with specific gravity and urine sodium and creatinine (for calculation of fractional excretion of sodium) should be ordered. If AKI is confirmed, all potential nephrotoxins should be discontinued, fluid intake should be decreased, and, if the patient is oliguric, potassium should

be removed from all intravenous solutions. The vast majority of these children will recover uneventfully without specific therapy or need for dialysis.

Infants and children with AKI will sometimes need to undergo dialysis or hemofiltration. The indication is usually either fluid overload, hyperkalemia, or, in the case of a prolonged recovery from ATN, azotemia. Options include peritoneal dialysis, standard hemodialysis, or continuous renal replacement therapy, usually in the form of continuous venovenous hemofiltration (CVVH). Peritoneal dialysis is more often used in infants due to their limited vascular access for hemodialysis. Peritoneal dialysis catheters need to be placed under general anesthesia but in most cases dialysis is well tolerated. Hemodialysis is sometimes considered in older children and requires placement of a large-bore double-lumen hemodialysis catheter in the jugular vein. These can be percutaneous or tunneled, depending on the length of time dialysis is likely to be needed. CVVH is generally used only in patients admitted to the ICU who are critically ill. Hemofiltration differs from hemodialysis in that water and solutes from the blood are forced through a semipermeable membrane by hydrostatic pressure generated by a pump (convection), rather than across a gradient generated by the presence of dialysate on the other side of the membrane (diffusion). It is slower than dialysis and requires daily sessions lasting 12–16 h. It has less of an effect on systemic blood pressure and may be better tolerated by patients who are hypotensive. Continuous arterio-venous hemofiltration, in which the patient's blood pressure provides the hydrostatic pressure needed to create the ultrafiltrate, is sometimes used in adults but is rarely an option for children. The pediatric surgeon is often asked to provide the vascular access required by these various therapies and must therefore be familiar with the equipment available and the flow rates needed. Subclavian vein catheters should be avoided in children at risk for chronic renal failure – in the event they need to have a graft or arterio-venous fistula created in the future, it would be best not to have created a subclavian vein stenosis.

Differential Diagnosis

Pre-Renal

- Volume related
- Intravascular depletion
- Ineffective circulation
- Ischemic/thrombotic
- Abdominal compartment syndrome
- Renovascular
- Renal vein thrombosis
- Renal artery stenosis
- Neurohumoral signaling dysfunction
- Hepato-renal syndrome
- Medications
- Calcineurin inhibitors
- Radio-contrast agents
- ACEI and ARB

Intrinsic Renal

Glomerular

- Hemolytic uremic syndrome
- Acute glomerulonephritis
- Vasculitis
- Lupus nephritis
- Goodpasture syndrome
- Wegener's
- ANCA-associated

Vascular

- Hemolytic uremic syndrome
- Malignant hypertension
- Tubular/interstitial
- Uncorrected pre or post AKI
- Asphyxia/hypoxia

Medications

- Aminoglycosides/vancomycin
- Amphotericin B
- Poisons
- Crystals (acyclovir and methotrexate)
- Tumor lysis/urate nephropathy
- Rhabdo/hemolysis: pigment nephropathy

Post-Renal

- Urinary tract obstruction
- Posterior urethral valves
- Bilateral UPJ obstruction
- Bilateral nephrolithiasis
- Neoplasm
- Retroperitoneal fibrosis
- Trauma

Diagnostic Studies

- FENa and urine sodium concentration
- Urinalysis
- Renal ultrasound

Parental Preparation

- Long-term results are excellent: over two-thirds of children with AKI go on to full recovery of renal function.

Technical Points

- Volume overload is treated with fluid restriction (1/3 maintenance + urine output), diuretics (furosemide 0.5–1 mg/kg dose), or dialysis.
- Hypertension is treated with diuretics (if volume overload) ± CCB (acute) or ACEI (chronic).
- Electrolyte abnormalities are treated by minimizing intake (especially potassium and phosphorous), kayexalate for potassium, and oral calcium carbonate and severamer for phosphorus.
- Metabolic acidosis should be corrected if the plasma bicarbonate concentration falls below 16 mEq/L or the arterial pH is less than 7.25, especially if the patient requires vasopressor therapy, as acidosis worsens myocardial dysfunction.

Suggested Reading

Andreoli SP. Acute kidney injury in children. Pediatr Nephrol. 2009; 24(2):253–63.

Askenazi DJ, Feig DI, Graham NM, Hui-Stickle S, Goldstein SL. 3-5 year longitudinal follow-up of pediatric patients after acute renal failure. Kidney Int. 2006;69(1):184–9.

Baker RJ, Pusey CD. The changing profile of acute tubulointerstitial nephritis. Nephrol Dial Transplant. 2004;19(1):8–11.

Bates CM, Lin F. Future strategies in the treatment of acute renal failure: growth factors, stem cells, and other novel therapies. Curr Opin Pediatr. 2005;17(2):215–20.

Bunchman TE, McBryde KD, Mottes TE, Gardner JJ, Maxvold NJ, Brophy PD. Pediatric acute renal failure: outcome by modality and disease. Pediatr Nephrol. 2001;16(12):1067–71.

Herget-Rosenthal S, Marggraf G, Hüsing J, Göring F, Pietruck F, Janssen O, et al. Early detection of acute renal failure by serum cystatin C. Kidney Int. 2004;66(3):1115–22.

Hui-Stickle S, Brewer ED, Goldstein SL. Pediatric ARF epidemiology at a tertiary care center from 1999 to 2001. Am J Kidney Dis. 2005; 45(1):96–101.

Skippen PW, Krahn GE. Acute renal failure in children undergoing cardiopulmonary bypass. Crit Care Resusc. 2005;7(4):286–91.

Sutton TA, Fisher CJ, Molitoris BA. Microvascular endothelial injury and dysfunction during ischemic acute renal failure. Kidney Int. 2002;62(5):1539–49.

Chapter 12
Respiratory Failure and Mechanical Ventilation

Todd J. Kilbaugh

Acute lung injury develops in response to a variety of pulmonary and extrapulmonary disease processes, ultimately resulting in widespread alveolar-capillary leak with extravasation of protein-rich, non-cardiogenic pulmonary edema. This acute phase leads to atelectasis, consolidation, surfactant degradation, and ultimately decreased lung compliance with progressive hypoxemia. Further progression of lung injury leads to a chronic stage, also known as the fibroproliferative stage, characterized by improvement in compliance despite continued poor lung function. Poor compliance at this stage is due to fibrosis and thickening of the lung interstitium. If the patient survives, the acute and fibroproliferative (chronic) stages, his or her lung function can vary from complete recovery to substantial long-lasting pulmonary functional deficits.

Clinical features of lung injury can vary from mild, self-limiting dyspnea to rapidly progressive and fatal respiratory failure. The clinical course of acute lung injury can be generalized into four phases; however, not every patient passes through all these phases and the condition can resolve at any stage (Table 12.1). Extensive research continues to develop predictive biomarkers and genomic arrays for severity and resolution of lung injury; however, to date there are no useful clinical biomarkers or genomic readouts for prediction or goal directed therapy.

Consensus clinical definitions have been constructed to define lung injury and give a common vernacular based on the pathophysiologic response to lung injury (Table 12.2). The definitions for acute lung injury (ALI) and acute respiratory distress syndrome (ARDS) are similar and include: a diffuse bilateral process, pulmonary edema due to capillary leak (as opposed to hydrostatic edema from cardiogenic failure), and hypoxemia. ALI and ARDS only differ by the degree of hypoxemia (measured by a decrease in PaO_2) and rising oxygen requirements (measured by an increase in

FiO_2). This ratio is numerically expressed as the PaO_2/FiO_2 ratio, which serves as a surrogate quantitative data point to define worsening lung injury. A patient has ALI if the P/F ratio is between 200 and 300, CXR reveals bilateral infiltrates, and the PCWP (usually estimated by echocardiogram) is less than 18 cm H_2O. A P/F ratio below 200 defines ARDS. But the P/F ratio can be misleading in a mechanically ventilated patient because it does not factor the level of mechanical support necessary for a patient to maintain an adequate PaO_2 for a given FiO_2. Therefore, physicians often discuss the degree of lung injury, progressive mechanical support, and optimization of oxygenation in terms of oxygenation index: $OI = (MAP \times FiO_2)/PaO_2$.

If lung injury can result from a varied group of disease processes, how can we use a broad set of definitions to define/ and discuss lung injury? In response to this question, authors have proposed that patients with ALI/ARDS be considered as two separate groups. Pulmonary lung injury results from clinical conditions that cause direct lung injury, such as pneumonia, whereas extrapulmonary lung injury follows an indirect mechanism of injury mediate by systemic mediators of inflammation such as sepsis (Table 12.3). In fact, despite meeting the same criteria for ARDS, the two subgroups of lung injury differ with respect to pathologic mechanisms, appearance on CT, respiratory mechanics, and response to ventilatory strategies. However, despite diverse etiologies, the ultimate histological appearance of lung injury is remarkably consistent. This consistent histologic appearance, despite varied direct or indirect injury, allows ARDS to be considered a discrete clinical entity and this definition of ARDS has been used to study incidence and mortality.

Ventilator-Associated Lung Injury

Many factors contribute to lung injury in patients who are mechanically ventilated, or ventilator-associated lung injury (VALI): excessive airway pressure (barotrauma); excessive alveolar volume (volutrauma); oxygen toxicity; tissue damage due to release of cytokines and inflammatory mediators

T.J. Kilbaugh (✉)
Department of Anesthesiology and Critical Care,
University of Pennsylvania, Children's Hospital of Philadelphia,
Philadelphia, PA, USA
e-mail: kilbaugh@email.chop.edu

P. Mattei (ed.), *Fundamentals of Pediatric Surgery*,
DOI 10.1007/978-1-4419-6643-8_12, © Springer Science+Business Media, LLC 2011

Table 12.1 Phases in the clinical development of lung injury

Phase	Clinical picture	CXR findings	Duration
1	Dyspnea Tachypnea	None	Variable
2	Hypoxemia Normal or subnormal PaCO$_2$	Minor abnormalities	24–48 h
3	Diagnostic criteria of ALI Severe hypoxemia Decreased pulmonary compliance	Bilateral diffuse infiltrates	Variable
4	Massive bilateral consolidation Unremitting hypoxemia Increased dead space Rising PaCO$_2$	Dense bilateral infiltrates	Often terminal

Table 12.2 Criteria for definition of acute lung injury (ALI) and acute respiratory distress syndrome (ARDS)

	ALI	ARDS
Hypoxemia	√	√
Bilateral infiltrates on CXR	√	√
PCWP <18 cm H$_2$O	√	√
P/F ratio >200 and <300	√	
P/F ratio <200		√

CXR chest X-ray; *PCWP* pulmonary capillary wedge pressure; *PaO$_2$* arterial partial pressure of oxygen; *FiO$_2$* fraction of inspired oxygen; *P/F ratio* P$_a$O$_2$/FiO$_2$ ratio

Table 12.3 Causes of direct and indirect lung injury classified by relative prevalence

	Direct lung injury	Indirect lung injury
Common	Pneumonia	Sepsis
	Aspiration	Severe non-thoracic trauma
	Pulmonary embolism	Transfusion-associated acute lung injury (TRALI)
Less common	Pulmonary contusion	Acute pancreatitis
	Near drowning	Cardiopulmonary bypass
	Inhalational injury	Burns
	Fat/amniotic fluid embolism	
	Reperfusion edema	

(biotrauma); and the effects of recurrent alveolar collapse and expansion (atelectrauma).

As lung injury progresses in response to pulmonary or extrapulmonary injury, the lungs can be divided into three hypothetical regions: (1) Areas with severe collapse and alveolar flooding – dependent areas; (2) recruitable areas with alveolar atelectasis – intermediate areas; and (3) "normal lung – non-dependent areas" (Fig. 12.1). The goal of mechanical ventilation is to recruit intermediate areas, which improves gas exchange, spares normal areas of lung from ventilator

associated lung injury (VALI), gives dependent collapsed regions of lung with alveolar flooding time to recover, and, it is hoped, inhibits further injury while the primary process resolves. Lung recruitment of intermediate areas and prevention of VALI is accomplished by using positive end-expiratory pressure (PEEP) and limiting tidal volume and plateau pressures. As alveolar airway pressure increases there is an opening pressure (P_{flex}) required to overcome airway resistance and alveolar compliance (Compliance=$\Delta V/\Delta P$). Pressures below P_{flex} lead to alveolar collapse (atelectasis). If airway pressure cycles above and below P_{flex}, alveoli continually open and collapse, leading to wall shear stress and eventual damage: atelectrauma. Following the pressure-volume curve to the upper extent of the inspiratory limb, as pressure increases, there comes a point (P_{max}) whereby the alveoli start to become over-distended. Above P_{max}, shear stress again leads to alveolar damage (volutrauma). Therefore, in theory, we attempt to keep tidal volumes on the most compliant part of the volume-pressure curve, above P_{flex} and below P_{max}, leading to the concept of "open lung ventilation." Triggered by the ARDSnet initial study, the use of low tidal volumes (6–8 mL/kg) with the addition of PEEP (open lung strategy), might reduce morbidity and mortality in patients with ARDS. However, as lung injury to the normal and intermediate areas of the lungs progresses, the volume-pressure curve moves to the right as the compliance of the lungs decreases, leaving a smaller therapeutic window, requiring an increase in PEEP and resulting in higher mean airway pressure (MAP) to maintain recruitment of areas of normal and recruitable lung. Lung protective strategy attempts to decrease VALI by limiting volutrauma, barotrauma, atelectrauma, oxygen toxicity, and biotrauma.

Low Tidal Volume

Despite the lack of usual control groups in the ARDSnet original study, the low tidal volume approach (6–8 mL/kg) has become standard of care to prevent alveolar over-distension, stretch, and volutrauma. There is increasing animal data that hyperinflation induces pulmonary edema by both permeability and filtration mechanisms. In addition, alveolar over-distension leads to alteration in surfactant function. These deleterious effects are sometimes greater in patients with pre-existing lung injury.

PEEP

The advantages of PEEP as a distending pressure include: increase in FRC, improvement of respiratory compliance, improvement of ventilation/perfusion (V/Q) mismatch, and

Fig. 12.1 Typical inspiratory volume-pressure curve in a ventilated patient. Three zones are represented in this idealized representation. The *green triangle* represents the optimal balance of alveolar filling that avoids both over-distension (*red triangle* to the *right*) and subsequent barotrauma and volutrauma, and under-filling of the alveoli (*red triangle* to the *left*), which results in alveolar collapse and subsequent atelectrauma. Compliance is defined as $\Delta V/\Delta P$

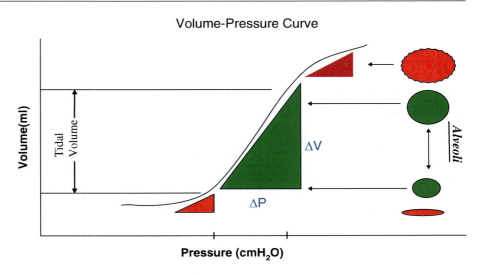

redistribution of lung water (edema). Thus, PEEP ultimately improves arterial oxygenation. The use of low tidal volumes has been consistent across multiple recent trials, but the selection of PEEP in these trials has been highly variable. Animal models have shown that setting PEEP just above P_{flex}, 1–2 cm H_2O, minimizes lung injury and inflammation, suggesting that perhaps an "open-lung" strategy does limit atelectrauma. Clinically, it can be difficult to determine the critical opening pressure of alveoli in children, especially in those with severe, heterogeneous disease such as ARDS. Therefore, most clinicians initially use a minimal distension strategy by setting PEEP between 5 and 9 cm H_2O, then, as lung injury progresses and hypoxemia worsens, by increasing PEEP to increase mean plateau pressures (<30–35 cm H_2O), and thus recruiting intermediate areas of lung. These strategies have yet to show a decrease in mortality but have shown improvement in secondary outcomes.

Other methods to determine optimal PEEP in a patient with ARDS include titration with dynamic compliance or static pressure-volume curve. It is important to remember that as PEEP is increased and lung is recruited, intrathoracic pressure is also increased and can inhibit cardiac output by reducing venous return. Therefore, despite an improvement in oxygenation, oxygen delivery to vital organs might be compromised.

Limiting Plateau Airway Pressures

Sustained plateau airway pressures >35 cm H_2O can lead to barotrauma: pneumothorax, pneumomediastinum, subcutaneous emphysema. In an attempt to limit barotrauma, $PaCO_2$ is allowed to increase (permissive hypercapnea).

Avoiding Oxygen Toxicity

While exposure to brief periods of 100% oxygen appears to be safe, long-term exposure leads to cellular damage, especially in the lung, due to the formation of superoxide radicals. Although the safe level of inspired oxygen in patients with ARDS is unknown, a reasonable goal seems to be an $FiO_2 < 0.6$, weaned to tolerate oxygen saturation as measured by pulse oximetry (S_pO_2) greater than 88–90%.

Partial Ventilatory Support

By avoiding neuromuscular blockade, spontaneous ventilation can occur during mechanical ventilation. Partial ventilatory support can lead to improve alveolar recruitment, V/Q mismatch, venous return, and weaning from mechanical ventilation. Avoidance of neuromuscular blockade can also lead to decreased needs for sedation, and possibly a decreased risk for post-traumatic stress disorder following critical illness.

Recruitment Maneuvers

Recruitment maneuvers, or sigh breaths, employ sufficient pressure to overcome critical opening pressures in areas of collapsed lung. The degree of pressure and timing is controversial but it appears that it is only helpful in early phases of acute injury, not in the fibroproliferative stage. Further research in pediatric patients is needed.

Basic Modes of Mechanical Ventilation

The most basic mode of mechanical ventilation is controlled mandatory ventilation (CMV), which delivers a set tidal volume at a set respiratory rate, thereby ensuring a constant minute-ventilation (minute ventilation = tidal volume × respiratory rate). CMV delivers a preset tidal volume at a preset rate regardless of the patient's effort. Unlike CMV, intermittent mandatory ventilation (IMV) allows the patient to breath spontaneously between mandatory ventilator breaths. The most common type of IMV is synchronized intermittent mandatory ventilation (SIMV), whereby mandatory ventilator breaths are synchronized with spontaneous breaths. SIMV has a time-assist window, a period of time measured in seconds that is dependent on the set mandatory breaths. During the assist window, if the ventilator does not sense a spontaneous breath from the patient, the ventilator will deliver a mandatory breath

SIMV is commonly combined with pressure support (PS): SIMV + PS, in which case the ventilator senses the initiation of a breath and a preset positive pressure is delivered during the patient's breath in an attempt to support an adequate minute ventilation. Pressure support is often set between 5 and 20 cm H_2O. SIMV + PS is advantageous because it allows for partial ventilatory support, which improves cardiopulmonary mechanics and improves the patient's ability to wean from mechanical support. The disadvantage of SIMV + PS is that it does not assure minute ventilation as the mechanical breaths are decreased and the patient becomes less dependent on mandatory breaths to maintain minute ventilation. If the patient is not ready for decreased support, work of breathing can increase and ventilation will be impaired.

Regardless of the mode of ventilation, the clinician must determine the type of ventilator breath to be delivered, generally classified as either pressure-controlled or volume-controlled. Pressure-controlled (PC) ventilation delivers a pressure-limited breath at a preset respiratory rate and inspiratory time. Tidal volume is a dependent variable during PC ventilation, and is determined by the preset pressure limit and the compliance of the respiratory system. If compliance decreases (or airway resistance increases), the preset pressure limit might not be adequate to maintain a tidal volume necessary to support minute ventilation. During PC ventilation the flow waveform is a decelerating pattern that follows a pressure gradient between the pressure delivered and alveolar pressure. Therefore, gas flows into airways along this pressure gradient: as alveolar volume increases and the pressure gradient between delivered breath and alveolar pressure narrows, gas flow slows. When the clinician sets the inspiratory time (Ti), gas flow maintains a decelerating pattern and, even after the gas flow has stopped, mean airway pressure is maintained for the length of the set Ti. This combination of a high initial flow with a decelerating flow pattern and consistent

airway pressure over the set Ti might improve aeration by recruiting stiff, non-compliant sections of lung. PC might also be useful in patients with an air leak (broncho-pleural fistula or around the endotracheal tube) by maintaining gas flow until the set pressure and tidal volume are achieved.

Volume-controlled ventilation (VC) delivers a preset tidal volume during a preset inspiratory time and at a preset respiratory rate. Gas flow is constant during Ti. This prevents alveolar over-distension, thus limiting volutrauma. During VC ventilation, airway and alveolar pressures are dependent variables, and as lung injury worsens, mandatory tidal volumes are maintained despite a rising PIP (although high PIPs can lead to barotrauma). VC may also be advantageous in patients with changing airway compliance, such as during chest or abdominal surgery.

Advanced Modes of Mechanical Ventilation

Conventional mechanical ventilation fails due to inadequate CO_2 clearance (despite permissible hypercapnea, usually with persistent acidosis), poor oxygen delivery, exacerbation of lung injury beyond limits of protective ventilation, and inhibition of cardiovascular function due to increasing intra-thoracic pressure. Traditionally, high frequency oscillatory ventilation (HFOV) and airway pressure release ventilation (APRV) have evolved as alternatives to failed conventional ventilation; however, APRV and HFOV are sometimes used as a primary mode of ventilation in certain situations: air leak syndrome and after pneumonectomy. Both modes have the advantage of ventilating patients at full lung volumes on the expiratory limb of the pressure-volume curve while attempting to avoid phasic changes.

HFOV has become the mainstay of mechanical ventilation in pediatric patients with evolving ALI that is unresponsive to conventional modes of ventilation. In fact, some authors have suggested that early institution of HFOV during ALI improves survival by providing open lung ventilation and limiting VALI. HFOV allows for optimal alveolar recruitment with lower airway pressures while minimizing phasic alveolar opening and closing. A piston/diaphragm creates gas flow through bulk axial flow, interregional gas mixing (Pendelluft), and molecular diffusion. Tidal volumes are dependent on compliance, endotracheal tube size, device frequency, and device amplitude. Tidal volume is inversely related to cyclic frequency: $VCO_2 = frequency \times VT^2$. Transitioning from conventional modes of ventilation to HFOV, the initial power setting (ΔP/amplitude) is adjusted to visible chest "wiggle" spanning from the clavicles to the abdomen or pelvis. Mean airway pressure (MAP) is initially set at approximately 5 cm H_2O greater than the last MAP on conventional ventilation. Traditionally, tidal volumes in HFOV are considered to be just above FRC; however, it is difficult to measure actual tidal

Table 12.4 Initial frequency settings for high-frequency oscillatory ventilation (HFOV) based on dry body weight

Patient weight (kg)	Initial frequency setting (Hz)
<2	15
2–15	10
16–20	8
21–30	7
31–50	6
>50	5

Table 12.5 APRV formulas

$$MAP = (P_{high} \times T_{high}) + (P_{low} \times T_{low})/T_{high} + T_{low}$$

$$\text{Number of cycles (respiratory rate)} = 60 \text{ s}/T_{high} + T_{low}$$

volumes and provide precise optimal lung volumes strategy. Clinically, MAP is titrated upward by 1–2 cm H_2O until oxygenation improves and FiO_2 can be weaned to less than 0.60. While titrating MAP, it is important to assess for overdistension by following chest radiographs: flattened hemidiaphragms or greater than nine posterior ribs visible. Initial frequency settings (in Hz) are based on body weight (Table 12.4) and then titrated accordingly.

HFOV is the only mode of ventilation with active expiration. If hypercarbia leads to profound respiratory acidosis and patient instability, minute ventilation can be increased by several means. First, inline suction is used to ensure adequate airway and endotracheal tube patency – this overcomes one of the drawbacks of HFOV, namely the lack of spontaneous ventilation and airway clearance. Second, ΔP can be increased to maximize lung recruitment and effectively increase minute ventilation. Third, frequency can be slowly decreased to enhance lung recruitment and increase minute ventilation. Finally, the endotracheal tube cuff should be deflated to allow additional escape of CO_2 around the endotracheal tube.

Disadvantages of HFOV include the inability to provide partial ventilatory support leading to increased requirements for sedation and paralysis, cardiopulmonary interactions due to higher MAP and decreased venous return, and loss of alveolar recruitment if circuit detached for suctioning or manual ventilation.

Airway pressure-release ventilation (APRV) is essentially CPAP with brief intermittent release coupled with spontaneous ventilation. The high CPAP level (P_{high}) maintains alveolar recruitment and aids in oxygenation over a period of time (T_{high}), and the timed release to a low pressure (P_{low}) minimizes resistance to expiratory flow and carbon dioxide removal. In addition, the patient is able to breathe spontaneously during all phases potentially allowing for improved pulmonary mechanics and gas exchange. APRV differs from other modes of ventilation because it relies on an intermittent decrease in airway pressure instead of an increase in airway pressure to maintain an open lung strategy for ventilation. Therefore, the release time (T_{low}) should be set long enough to allow for an adequate tidal volume (6–8 mL/kg) but short enough to avoid alveolar collapse and atelectrauma.

The operator-controlled parameters in APRV are: P_{high}, T_{high}, P_{low}, T_{low}, and FiO_2. Guidelines for implementing APRV

in children are extrapolated from adult recommendations. P_{low} is initially set at zero. P_{high} can be set by several methods such plateau pressures or 75% of peak inspiratory pressure; however, when transitioning from conventional modes of ventilation P_{high} is often based on MAP (Table 12.5) where the MAP is set 2–3 cm H_2O above conventional MAP. To determine T_{high} and T_{low}, first determine the total cycle time according to a normal respiratory rate range for the patient's age: a respiratory rate of 20 yields a total cycle time of 3 s. T_{high} will be the total cycle time minus a T_{low} of 0.2–0.6 s, initially starting at 0.4 s.

Transitioning to APRV, like transitioning to HFOV, will take time for optimal lung recruitment. After several hours, if the patient continues to have severe hypoxemia, T_{high} or P_{high}, can be increased to aid in oxygenation. Once established, P_{low} and T_{low} usually do not require further changes; however as lung compliance improves P_{high} can be decreased and T_{high} increased to wean a patient toward a target of continual CPAP of 5–6 cm H_2O in preparation for extubation. APRV has the potential benefit of allowing the patient to breathe spontaneously throughout the ventilatory cycle, improving respiratory mechanics and reducing the need for sedation and neuromuscular blockade. However, some authors are concerned that there might be a higher incidence of cyclic alveolar collapse during the airway release phase (atelectrauma).

Non-invasive Mechanical Ventilation

Non-invasive positive pressure mechanical ventilation (NIPPV) relies on a patient interface (nasal prongs, nasal mask, face mask) to deliver ventilator support without placement of an endotracheal tube or tracheostomy. Although there have been no randomized, controlled trials to determine the efficacy of NIPPV in patients with mild to moderate respiratory failure, multiple case series have demonstrated utility in acute respiratory distress (bronchiolitis, asthma, pneumonia), chronic respiratory distress (neuromuscular disease), and acute on chronic respiratory distress (chronic lung disease with acute viral bronchiolitis). A trial of NIPPV may be initiated in early respiratory distress; however, the need for tracheal intubation should be constantly questioned. Contraindications to NIPPV include loss of protective upper airway reflexes, change in mental status due to hypercarbia or hypoxemia, and recent gastrointestinal surgery, in which case swallowed air can be a problem.

Adjuvant Therapies for ARDS

Prone Positioning

Prone positioning can improve oxygenation in patients with ARDS and has been safely applied in children. Prone positioning improves lung recruitment in certain patients but selection criteria and optimal duration are unclear. It is likely that a subgroup of patients respond to prone positioning early after lung injury and immediate responders might benefit from prolonged prone positioning. While prone positioning improves oxygenation, this improvement has not been shown to improve mortality; however, future studies will emphasize functional outcomes.

Surfactant Therapy

Exogenous surfactant therapy is standard of care in neonates suffering from respiratory distress syndrome (RDS); however, the utility of surfactant therapy in the treatment of older children with ALI and ARDS is uncertain. Recent studies have shown immediate improvement in oxygenation and a trend toward improved survival with exogenous surfactant therapy with calfactant. Research is ongoing to determine patient selection, timing, and effectiveness with other therapies.

Nitric Oxide

Inhaled nitric oxide (iNO) acts as a selective pulmonary vasodilator to improve V/Q mismatch (intrapulmonary shunting), decrease pulmonary hypertension, and reduce right ventricular cardiac work. NO upregulates cGMP, ultimately resulting in smooth muscle relaxation and pulmonary arteriolar vasodilatation. It is delivered directly to ventilated lung units and improves perfusion in these areas of lung without significant effects on the rest of the pulmonary vascular bed, thereby improving V/Q mismatch and oxygenation in patients with ARDS. Toxic side effects of iNO are methemoglobinemia and formation of nitrogen dioxide. However, these are rare when iNO is delivered within recommended dose range of 5–20 ppm. Much like prone positioning and surfactant therapy, iNO can result in transient improvements in oxygenation but further research is needed to prove that NO therapy leads to a decrease in mortality or improved functional outcomes in children with ARDS.

Permissive Hypercapnea

Permissive hypercapnea appears to be well tolerated in infants and children with ALI and ARDS. It is designed to limit tidal volume and alveolar over-distension and thus decrease VALI. Multiple studies with animal models of ALI/ARDS have suggested a possible protective role for hypercarbia. Clinically, a mild respiratory acidosis (pH of approximately 7.25) is considered acceptable, as long as the patient is able to compensate and remains clinically stable. Hypercapnea and the resulting respiratory acidosis can lead to increased pulmonary vascular resistance, increased intracranial pressure (due to increased cerebral blood flow), and cardiovascular dysfunction. If arterial pH falls below 7.25 or the patient demonstrates cardiopulmonary instability, minute ventilation can be increased or an intravenous base, such as sodium bicarbonate or THAM, is administered.

Permissive Hypoxemia

Tolerating S_pO_2 between 88 and 90%, to avoid prolonged high FiO_2 levels and subsequent lung toxicity, has become a tenet of lung protective strategies in children with ALI/ARDS. Whether permissive hypoxemia improves mortality or functional outcome is unclear at this time; however multiple animal studies show that hyperoxia is a directly toxic to the lung parenchyma due to formation of superoxide radicals that inhibit cellular signal transduction and ultimately lead to cell death.

Summary Points

- The definitions for acute lung injury (ALI) and acute respiratory distress syndrome (ARDS) are similar and include: a diffuse bilateral process, non-cardiogenic pulmonary edema, and hypoxemia.
- ALI is defined by a PaO_2/FiO_2 ratio between 200 and 300 and ARDS by a PaO_2/FiO_2 ratio below 200.
- Factors that contribute to ventilator-associated lung injury (VALI) include: barotrauma, volutrauma, oxygen toxicity, biotrauma, and atelectrauma.
- As lung injury progresses, the lungs can be divided into three regions: dependent areas (severe collapse and alveolar flooding), non-dependent areas (normal lung), and intermediate areas (atelectatic but recruitable).
- The low tidal volume approach (6–8 mL/kg) has become standard of care to prevent alveolar overdistension, stretch, and volutrauma.
- The advantages of PEEP include: increase in FRC, respiratory compliance, and V/Q mismatch, redistribution of lung edema, and protection from atelectrauma.
- In an attempt to limit barotrauma, $PaCO_2$ is allowed to increase (permissive hypercapnea).
- High frequency oscillatory ventilation (HFOV) allows for optimal alveolar recruitment with lower airway pressures while minimizing phasic alveolar opening and closing.
- Airway pressure-release ventilation (APRV) is essentially CPAP with brief intermittent release, coupled with spontaneous ventilation.
- Non-invasive positive pressure mechanical ventilation (NIPPV) relies on a patient interface (nasal prongs, nasal mask, face mask) to deliver ventilator support without placement of an endotracheal tube or tracheostomy.
- Prone positioning, exogenous surfactant, inhaled nitric oxide, and permissive hypoxemia are being investigated as potentially beneficial adjuncts in children with acute lung injury.

Editor's Comment

For most of us, mastering the art of ventilator management is one of the most gratifying rites of passage during residency. Check the $PaCO_2$, make a subtle adjustment in the ventilatory rate or the PIP, and the patient weans – you have the power and the skill and your patients are the better for it. Nevertheless, what we have been slow to realize is that, at least for our sickest patients, the treatment can be as detrimental as the disease. Ventilator-associated lung injury is a concept that has been around for a long time but is just now being accepted by the clinicians on the front lines of critical care medicine, including surgeons. This elegant concept posits that barotrauma, volutrauma, atelectrauma, oxygen toxicity, and biotrauma all contribute to lung injury and that minimizing the effects of these factors helps our patients recover more quickly and with fewer sequelae. It is tempting as surgical fellows and attendings, who learned about ventilator management several years before, to be openly critical of the young critical care physician who has instituted a strange new ventilator strategy in the care of our patient. Although obviously it is important to avoid the use of

untested or investigative techniques outside of a clinical trial, it is also important for us to attempt to understand the basis for any novel or counterintuitive approach – there might very well be compelling scientific evidence behind it that you were not aware of.

When both conventional and advanced modes of ventilation fail, the next step for otherwise viable patients with reversible lung injury (influenza, aspiration pneumonitis) might be ECMO. There is now considerable experience with the use of ECMO in adolescents and even adults and it appears to be a viable option in select cases. Every tertiary care children's center should have established criteria and a practical algorithm for patients with severe respiratory failure so that this potentially life-saving technology can be made available in a timely fashion. One of the most common issues related to the application of ECMO is waiting too long to consider it. The patient with multiple pneumothoraces and chest tubes has probably already had irreversible lung injury due to barotrauma for ECMO to be of any practical value. The same can be said of patients who have ventilator-associated pneumonia, severe pulmonary edema, or multiple areas of refractory and severe atelectasis.

Suggested Reading

Brower RG, Lanken PN, MacIntyre N, Matthay MA, Morris A, Ancukiewicz M, et al. Higher versus lower positive end-expiratory pressures in patients with the acute respiratory distress syndrome; National Heart, Lung, and Blood Institute ARDS Clinical Trials Network. N Engl J Med. 2004;351(4):327–36.

Hanson JH, Flori H. Application of the acute respiratory distress syndrome network low-tidal volume strategy to pediatric acute lung injury. Respir Care Clin N Am. 2006;12(3):349–57.

Mols G, Priebe HJ, Guttmann J. Alveolar recruitment in acute lung injury. Br J Anaesth. 2006;96(2):156–66.

Priebe GP, Arnold JH. High-frequency oscillatory ventilation in pediatric patients. Respir Care Clin N Am. 2001;7(4):633–45.

Slutsky AS. Ventilator-induced lung injury: from barotrauma to biotrauma. Respir Care. 2005;50(5):646–59.

The Acute Respiratory Distress Syndrome Network. Ventilation with lower tidal volumes as compared with traditional tidal volumes for acute lung injury and the acute respiratory distress syndrome. N Engl J Med. 2000;342(18):1301–8.

Chapter 13
Extracorporeal Membrane Oxygenation

Edmund Y. Yang

Extracorporeal membrane oxygenation (ECMO) is a life saving measure, but like all treatments, the technique has limitations. The basic concept is that an oxygenator will perform all gas exchange similar to the native lung via extracorporeal blood circulation. A pump must drive the blood through the oxygenator back to the body. In venovenous ECMO, the oxygenated blood is returned to the right side of the heart where it is mixed with native blood. It passes through the lungs and then back out to the body. In venoarterial ECMO, the blood bypasses the heart and returns to the arterial side under pressure where it mixes with the native circulation. In contrast to VV-ECMO, VA-ECMO provides support for low cardiac output and blood pressure. It also provides slightly higher systemic oxygen delivery.

The basic ECMO circuit can be broken down into a pump, an oxygenator, a warmer, the tubing, and the cannulas. Most North American ECMO programs use a roller pump, but centrifugal pumps are gaining in popularity. There is much more diversity in oxygenator use. The standard is the silicone membrane oxygenator (Medtronic, Minneapolis, Minnesota). However, many programs have changed to hollow fiber oxygenators (Minimax Plus, Medtronic, Minneapolis, Minnesota; Quadrox, Maquet, San Jose, California). The hollow fiber oxygenators are highly efficient gas exchangers and set up quickly.

Cannula selection is more important. For babies between 2 and 2.5 kg, VV-ECMO will be more difficult to perform simply because the smallest effective double-lumen VV cannula is 12 Fr (Origen, Austin, TX) and the internal jugular vein in babies this size is quite small. Usually, an 8 or 10 Fr arterial cannula is used and a 10 or 12 Fr venous cannula is used to initiate VA-ECMO. In larger babies, one has the choice of VV- or VA-ECMO and the corresponding double or single lumen cannulas. This decision should be based on the patient condition and desired clinical course.

For pediatric or adolescent patients, VV-ECMO is more commonly used than VA and cannulation can be performed percutaneously with the Seldinger technique. For larger patients, two venous cannulas are often necessary to provide adequate venous drainage. One venous cannula is usually placed in the right IJ vein and another in a femoral vein. Since the femoral cannula is in the intra-abdominal IVC, I usually initiate flow of oxygenated blood to return to the SVC, but one sometimes needs to switch the flow around because of recirculation between the two cannulas.

Indications

ECMO should be considered when standard medical management fails to correct a severe cardiopulmonary derangement (Table 13.1). It should only be considered when the derangement is potentially reversible, but this is not always predictable. Certainly, patients with fatal genetic anomalies, intracerebral hemorrhages, and congenital heart defects are not good candidates for ECMO, but often in the absence of a clear diagnosis, ECMO is used to allow more time for diagnostic procedures. A good example is the patient with alveolar capillary dysplasia, in which case ECMO can provide time for lung biopsy and pathologic diagnosis.

Guidelines for ECMO initiation have been established to help promote appropriate use. In reality, each institution must gauge their expertise and appropriate clinical indications for initiating ECMO.

Hypoxia

Respiratory failure is the most common indication for ECMO. If the hypoxia is worse than a PaO_2 of 40 mmHg for more than 2–4 h on 100% O_2 despite measures such as inhaled nitric oxide (iNO), high-frequency jet ventilation (HFJV), and high-frequency oscillatory ventilation (HFOV), then ECMO might be indicated. Many use additional indices

E.Y. Yang (✉)
Department of Pediatric General Surgery, Vanderbilt Children's Hospital, 2200 Children's Way, Suite 4150 Doctor's Office Tower, Nashville, TN 37232, USA
e-mail: edmund.yang@vanderbilt.edu

P. Mattei (ed.), *Fundamentals of Pediatric Surgery*,
DOI 10.1007/978-1-4419-6643-8_13, © Springer Science+Business Media, LLC 2011

Table 13.1 Diagnoses and utility of ECMO

Problem	Goal while on ECMO
Primary lung disease	
Pneumonia/ARDS	Optimize pulmonary function
PPHN	Optimize pulmonary function
ACD	Time for diagnosis
Surfactant deficiency	Time for diagnosis
Pulmonary hypoplasia	Optimize pulmonary function
MAS	Optimize pulmonary function
Airway problems	
CHAOS (tracheal atresia/web)	Create/repair airway
Bronchogenic cyst	Remove obstruction
Massive cystic hygroma	Remove obstruction, obtain airway
Massive cervical teratoma	Remove obstruction, obtain airway
Primary cardiac problems	
HLHS with intact atrial septum	Perform atrial septostomy
Cardiomyopathy	Optimize cardiac function or transplant
Infectious	
Sepsis	Control infection
Trauma	
Drowning with hypothermia	Warm patient, assess CNS
Post-traumatic ARDS	Optimize pulmonary function

ARDS acute respiratory distress syndrome; *PPHN* persistent pulmonary hypertension of the newborn; *ACD* alveolar capillary dysplasia; *MAS* meconium aspiration syndrome; *CHAOS* congenital high airway obstruction syndrome; *HLHS* hypoplastic left heart syndrome; *CNS* central nervous system

of worsening pulmonary function such as an (A-a) $DO_2 > 400$ mmHg or an oxygenation index $(OI = F_iO_2 *$ Mean Airway Pressure$)/P_aO_2)$ of >45 to guide initiation. Maximal ventilatory support should also be differentially limited depending on the clinical pathology. For neonates with pulmonary hypoplasia, such as with CDH, an OI of 25 is a better cut off to prevent barotrauma and all blood gas measurements should be taken from a preductal arterial line. For patients with previously normal lungs, and especially for older patients, the limits of barotrauma are less clear. When ventilatory pressures rise to the point that the patient is at risk for pneumothorax or if barotrauma is evident, then iatrogenic pulmonary injury could be worsening the chances of recovery and ECMO should be strongly considered.

Hypercarbia

Severe acute hypoventilation that cannot be managed with increased mechanical ventilatory support is also an indication for ECMO. The usual scenario involves a neonate with pulmonary hypoplasia (CDH). Pediatric and adult patients will usually have ARDS such as from trauma or severe pneumonia.

Hypoxia is almost always coincident with hypoventilation so the same principles for initiating ECMO apply. When maximal ventilatory support and medical therapy has failed, then ECMO should be considered. Again, ECMO should be initiated before iatrogenic lung injury is evident.

Cardiac Failure

Primary cardiac failure such as from cardiomyopathy is rare. In neonates, congenital heart disease should be ruled out with an echocardiogram. Usually one is treating secondary cardiac failure with ECMO, such as from hypoxia, sepsis, or metabolic derangement. If primary, then one should consider VA-ECMO since VV-ECMO is dependent on intact cardiac function. If the cardiac failure is secondary, then VV-ECMO will usually suffice. When the heart receives improved oxygen supply and there is correction of acidosis, function usually improves and vasopressor support can be weaned.

Metabolic Acidosis

This is a rare indication for ECMO and usually involves a patient with an inborn error of metabolism. Usually the acidosis is secondary to another problem such as cardiac failure. If an exhaustive search for the cause of the acidosis is not revealing, ECMO can be used to provide more time for diagnosis through metabolic correction.

Preoperative Preparation

Head ultrasound is essential in neonates to document the absence of intracerebral hemorrhage prior to initiating ECMO. If more than a grade I hemorrhage is evident, ECMO is not advised since the patient will need to be fully anticoagulated and the hemorrhage is likely to worsen. In older patients, clinical instability usually precludes our ability to obtain neuroimaging. One can rely on prior neurologic examination and if neurologic function is in question, it can be studied after ECMO by bedside examination and neuroimaging when the patient is clinically stable.

Echocardiogram is a critical step in the workup of a patient for ECMO. In the neonate it is most important to exclude congenital heart disease that is not survivable even with ECMO. Echocardiogram also provides excellent information about cardiac function. In nearly all patients, pulmonary hypertension is an issue. If this has not been treated, iNO can be initiated, cardiac function can be optimized, and one can reassess the need for ECMO. The echocardiogram can also reveal abnormalities of venous and arterial anatomy. Patients with duplicated SVC usually have a dominant right SVC draining into the right atrium, but rarely the left SVC is the larger of the two and should therefore be used for cannulation.

Exclusion criteria are relative, based on outcomes, technical limitations and risks of complications. Certainly patients with a fatal anatomic anomaly or genetic anomaly that precludes a reasonably good quality of life should be excluded. In patients with ongoing bleeding or coagulopathy, efforts should be made to control these problems before considering ECMO.

Small neonatal size poses a technical limitation for cannulation but it is not the best predictor of poor outcome. When the baby weighs less than 2 kg, cannulation becomes very difficult. No double-lumen cannula is available for such small vessels, so VA-ECMO is required. The smallest cannula available is 6 Fr. In the Extracorporeal Life Support Organization (ELSO) database more than 600 neonates with birth weight <2 kg have been put on ECMO. Thus, cannulation is certainly technically feasible. Although the overall survival rate for this population was significantly lower than that for babies who weigh more than 2 kg (53 vs. 77%), gestational age was found to be a better predictor of survival and ICH outcome. For reference, regression analysis revealed that a birth weight of 1.6 kg was associated with a survival of 40%, so this weight is perhaps a better cut off than the old standard of 2 kg for initiating ECMO.

Exclusionary issues regarding gestational age have more to do with the risk of intracranial bleeding. The largest data series reveals that the risk of ICH and subsequent death rises below 32 weeks gestation. More recent data, which takes into account postnatal age, reveals that postconceptual age (PCA) is the single greatest factor that correlates with risk of ICH, not the gestational age at birth. At 38 weeks PCA the incidence of ICH on ECMO is about 5%. The incidence rises to about 25% at 32 weeks. Since the relationship is approximately linear, there is no single PCA below which ICH increases dramatically. A reasonable guideline is that the risk of ICH increases to above 15% below 35 weeks PCA.

The issue of disease reversibility is a much harder exclusion to define. A limit of 10–14 days of mechanical ventilation is generally defined as a point of irreversibility. Although there is little modern data to define a temporal exclusionary limit, the period of healing time that ECMO provides cannot reverse end-stage respiratory disease. ECMO is a tool that temporizes and it should be conceptualized as such, rather than as a rescue or last-ditch therapy. The important difference in this approach is that one must consider the optimum time of ECMO initiation when it is conceptualized as a tool. Initiating ECMO too late, when end-organ damage has already occurred, leads to irreversibility. The more severe the

pathologic processes, such as 10–14 days of mechanical ventilation for pneumonia, the more time it takes to heal and correct the problems. Theoretically then, less severe cardiopulmonary derangements should be easier and quicker to correct, and earlier ECMO should achieve better results.

VV vs. VA-ECMO

VA-ECMO has been declining in use. VV-ECMO is technically easier, safer (fewer embolic events), and equally effective in most patients for providing gas exchange and oxygen delivery. There are two situations in which I prefer VA-ECMO: the patient with primary cardiac dysfunction (cardiomyopathy), in whom cardiac function will not improve simply with improved oxygen delivery, and the newborn patient with an element of fixed pulmonary hypertension due to pulmonary hypoplasia (severe CDH), in which case the pulmonary hypertension will not resolve quickly with improved oxygen delivery. The pulmonary hypertension while on VV-ECMO will likely still be severe and could cause ongoing cardiac dysfunction and systemic hypotension. This in turn limits diuretic effects and improvements in lung compliance. In this situation, VA-ECMO decompresses the heart and optimizes blood pressure and lung compliance, providing the best chance of survival.

Neonatal ECMO Cannulation

I usually give the patient 100 units/kg of heparin just before starting the operation. The patient is placed in the supine position with the head turned to the left and the neck extended to expose the full length of the neck. The right neck, shoulder, sternum, and chest are sterilely prepared and draped. Preparing the shoulder and sternum allows for the rare exposure of the more proximal vessels in case difficulty is encountered with neck cannulation. A transverse incision is made about one third of the way up the right sternocleidomastoid. Blunt dissection is carried down to expose the left internal jugular vein. The size of these vessels should be noted so that appropriately sized cannulas can be chosen. The IJ should be exposed for a length of at least 2 cm and controlled with proximal and distal ties. The same should be done for the common carotid artery if the patient is to be placed on VA-ECMO. If the patient is to be placed on VV-ECMO, sometimes it is useful to place a small vessel loop around the carotid artery to identify it in case one has to convert to VA-ECMO in the future. The vessel loop can be used to facilitate dissection of the carotid in an inflamed field, and it can be removed at decannulation.

The IJ is cannulated first. For VV-ECMO, a 12 Fr double lumen cannula is used. It is designed for use in the right IJ so that the re-infusion is directed back into the right atrium. I usually insert it about 7 or 8 cm for a term neonate, secure it with heavy silk ties, usually tied over small pieces of a silastic vessel loop ("bumpers") and flush it with heparinized saline, removing any air bubbles. For VA-ECMO, the neonatal IJ will usually accept a 12 Fr cannula, but if possible a 14 Fr cannula should be used for better venous return. For the carotid artery, usually an 8 Fr arterial cannula is used. I insert it to 2.5–3.0 cm for a term neonate, secure, and flush it. After the cannulas are connected to the ECMO circuit, flow is initiated and advanced to about 100 mL/kg/min over several minutes. If there are problems with flow, usually it is one of venous return and you can feel chatter in the circuit tubing. Volume should be given, and I gently manipulate the position of the venous cannula to see if one position or another improves flow. The chest radiograph and an echocardiogram can also be used to examine the venous cannula position. For the double-lumen cannula it is critical that the catheter be secured in a straight line to the heart because the outer wall of the cannula is thin and easily crimped over time.

Pediatric and Adult ECMO Cannulation

In this population, ECMO is almost always performed for respiratory failure. Pneumonia is usually the issue in pediatric patients whereas in adults, ARDS is the more common problem. In all of these patients VV-ECMO is commonly sufficient treatment. When the heart starts to receive oxygenated blood, function improves and pressors can usually be weaned within the first day of ECMO.

VV cannulation is via a femoral vein and right IJ approach. In the adolescent or large child, percutaneous access is easily achieved using the Seldinger technique and commercially available percutaneous insertion kits. In younger children, a cut-down operation might be required.

If VA-ECMO is required in a young child or adolescent, I prefer a cut-down to cannulate the vessels. The common femoral artery is used for arterial cannulation and the ipsilateral IJ or contralateral femoral vein is used for venous cannulation. For distal arterial flow, I like to place a 7 Fr central line or similar small bore catheter into the distal artery through the same arteriotomy and divert some oxygenated blood to the distal limb. Although this common femoral artery inflow set up is good for maintaining blood pressure, the downside is that it does not provide highly oxygenated blood to the brain. Just as in the neonate, I advocate right carotid artery cannulation for the rare pediatric VA-ECMO patient.

Initial Management on ECMO

After initiating ECMO, initial concerns are focused on volume requirements and coagulation issues. Just after cannulation, volume requirements are usually significant, probably because patient blood-to-circuit surface contact causes immediate vasodilatation, capillary leak, and third spacing. The patient can be raised higher to facilitate siphoning, however if circuit flow begins to cut out then volume must be given to improve venous return.

The other concern after initiating ECMO is preventing coagulopathy. General goals for coagulation are to maintain platelets >100,000/mm^3, INR <1.4, and fibrinogen >200 g/L. After initiating ECMO, these values usually plummet and almost all blood components require replacement. The activated clotting time (ACT) is also monitored. Initially, this rises dramatically to hundreds of seconds due to the heparin bolus from cannulation and the heparin used to prime the circuit. When it begins to decline, a heparin drip is started and titrated to target an ACT of between 180 and 200 s.

Goals on ECMO

The primary goals on ECMO are to provide tissue perfusion and oxygenation. End points should be a normal blood pressure, normal lactate, adequate mixed SvO_2 (75%), and adequate gas exchange. On VV-ECMO, mixed SvO_2 is not as reliable because of recirculation.

Peripheral O_2 delivery can be maintained by maximizing O_2-carrying capacity with a hematocrit in the high 1930s and by maintaining adequate cardiac output. On VV-ECMO, there is always a maximum arterial O_2 saturation because of mixing of desaturated blood. A peripheral O_2 saturation of 80–90% is acceptable, but O_2 delivery may need compensation by increasing cardiac output. On VA-ECMO, peripheral O_2 saturations of 90% or greater are feasible, except in the larger pediatric and adult population where cardiac output may exceed circuit flow. Blood pressure should be maintained in the normal range. While limiting volume, vasopressors, and inotropes are often necessary to maintain the blood pressure. Urine output can also be used as a measure of tissue perfusion. Usually it correlates well with blood pressure.

Since ECMO is usually performed for respiratory failure, pulmonary management is of critical importance. What ECMO provides is a period of pulmonary and cardiac rest, and during this time the physiologic problems that are preventing survival must be reversed. In neonates with a pulmonary indication, that problem is almost always a combination of hypoventilation and pulmonary hypertension. Whether the patient has CDH or meconium aspiration, the major problem is one of pulmonary compliance. In meconium aspiration, poor compliance is due to inflammation. In CDH, the poor compliance is due to pulmonary hypoplasia, often with superimposed inflammation secondary to barotrauma. In the pediatric patient, the compliance is poor due to infection and inflammation. Ultimately, the infection must be controlled in order for compliance to improve.

Once ECMO has been initiated and O_2 saturations start to improve, the ventilator is put into "rest" mode. For a neonate we use a pressure-control mode with a rate of 10, PEEP of 10 cm H_2O and PIP of 20 cm H_2O. Probably the only important setting is the PEEP. Increased PEEP has been shown to decrease the length of time on ECMO. When pulmonary inflammation resolves and compliance improves, the increased PEEP helps recruit alveoli. In older children and adults the optimal rest settings are less clear. A PEEP of 10–15 cm H_2O with a PIP of 30 cm H_2O is reasonable. For all patients, the clear objective is not to add to pulmonary inflammation or even slow the process of healing. This objective is especially relevant on VV-ECMO. If one cannot provide adequate ventilation, oxygenation, and cardiac output on VV-ECMO without lung rest, then one should consider conversion to VA-ECMO.

We usually repeat the head ultrasound every day for the first 3 days in neonates to rule out bleeding. In older children, we perform a head CT if there is a change in neurologic examination after going on ECMO. Daily CXRs while on ECMO are also useful to show changes in atelectasis or fluid collections which could affect weaning.

Weaning from ECMO

The process of weaning from ECMO begins within a few days of cannulation. The ECMO run is of limited duration, so each day matters immensely in preparing the patient for weaning. First, the third spacing associated with ECMO must begin to resolve. This is evident by decreased fluid requirements. We promote loss of extra body fluid to decrease pulmonary interstitial fluid and optimize pulmonary compliance. Although I prefer medical diuresis (furosemide 1–2 mg/kg/dose, BID or TID) to achieve this goal, ultrafiltration can also be used effectively.

One must also assess whether adequate pulmonary healing has occurred. This assessment will guide you as to when to initiate ventilation. The healing time is variable depending on the degree of inflammation and injury. The patient with severe barotrauma and pneumothoraces may need 4–7 days to adequately seal a leak. If rest ventilator settings cause continued air leak, then the ventilator pressures should be turned even lower to promote healing of the bronchopleural fistula. A patient with meconium aspiration usually takes 3–4 days

for the inflammation to resolve. Forcing ventilation into lungs with significant ongoing inflammation and healing will only add to the inflammatory process and probably diminish survival.

A good guide to patient readiness and the resolution of pulmonary inflammation is improvement in atelectasis on chest X-ray. With diuresis and increased PEEP, the lung commonly opens up on its own. At this point, one can decrease the PEEP to 5 cm H_2O, set the PIP to 25–30 cm H_2O and measure the tidal volume and compliance. With more aggressive diuresis, one should start to see increased tidal volume and improvements in the chest X-ray. Low level vasopressors (dopamine at <5 μg/kg/min) can be used to promote diuresis and maintain adequate blood pressure in the face of relative hypovolemia.

Finally, pulmonary hypertension must be addressed. Diuresis and good lung expansion are the initial primary treatments. Once both of these goals have been achieved and pulmonary compliance has been maximized, an echocardiogram should be obtained. On VA-ECMO there is a significant diversion of blood flow around the pulmonary system which will mask pulmonary hypertension. In the neonate, even 50–100 mL/min will change the echocardiographic findings. So, on VA-ECMO, we usually begin by ventilating the patient in a pressure-control mode at a rate of 40 breaths/min, PIP of 25 cm H_2O (higher in older children), PEEP of 5 cm H_2O, and 60% FiO_2. The flow is weaned over 2–3 h and blood gases are checked periodically. Commonly in the neonate with CDH, we see an increased O_2 requirement, postductal right to left shunting, and hypotension. Since the weaning has failed, an echocardiogram will confirm suprasystemic pulmonary hypertension. Inhaled nitric oxide, inotropes (milrinone), and even further diuresis can be initiated prior to another ECMO weaning trial. If the weaning blood gases are acceptable, then the VA circuit is clamped for 30 min and an echocardiogram is obtained. Systemic or suprasystemic pulmonary pressures do not portend survival after ECMO, so it is advisable to go back on full flow and further optimize the physiology.

On VV-ECMO, there is no diversion of blood around the right heart and lungs, so pulmonary hypertensive issues should be more apparent on full ECMO flows. Ventilation should be achieved and an echocardiogram should be obtained. If the pulmonary pressures are systemic or higher, then the pulmonary hypertension should be treated prior to decannulation.

Metabolic preparation is also important for the patient with hypoventilation, such as in CDH. I try to achieve a metabolic alkalosis with aggressive diuresis and with parenteral nutrition. In the patient with severe CDH physiology, it is useful to have the HCO_3^- in the high 1930s, so that a respiratory acidosis can be compensated. Nutritional supplementation has unknown benefit during ECMO, but we know that all ECMO patients are profoundly catabolic. In the neonate, we try to deliver at least 120 kCal/kg/day in small volumes. If the patient is on less than 5 µg/kg/min of vasopressors, then enteral nutrition can be given as well. In the pediatric patient, similar principles are applied.

Standard criteria for decannulation should be established at each institution. Optimally, the goals are to come off ECMO with: (1) subsystemic pulmonary artery pressures, (2) ventilator settings which are non-injurious and provide adequate gas exchange, and (3) moderate or less vasopressor requirements (<10 µg/kg/min).

Ideal ventilator settings for decannulation of the neonate are: pressure control mode, rate of 40 breaths/min, PIP of 25 cm H_2O, PEEP of 5 cm H_2O, and 60% FiO_2. After multiple optimization attempts, often one has to use higher ventilator settings, such as a higher rate, PIP, or vasopressor level. About 24 h after decannulation, usually one sees a slight worsening in gas exchange or cardiac function. Conservative decannulation settings are designed to allow for this short term decline.

Surgery on ECMO

The risk of bleeding due to surgery on ECMO is significant, probably on the order of 10–25%. If bleeding ensues, it is usually microvascular and difficult to control. If surgery is necessary while on ECMO, one should ensure that coagulation factors are normalized. One can use 6-aminocaproic acid (Amicar) prophylactically, and give activated factor VII to control postoperative bleeding. Often however, the only guaranteed way to stop hemorrhage is to stop the heparin or come off ECMO. For these reasons surgery should be optimally delayed until the child can be taken off ECMO, unless the surgical problem will prevent further progress or there is proven benefit to immediate surgery. A good example is the neonate with respiratory failure in which one suspects alveolar capillary dysplasia. The lung biopsy on ECMO is necessary to determine the diagnosis and make decisions about further medical care.

For the patient with CDH on ECMO, there is no convincing evidence that the timing of CDH repair relative to the ECMO run has any relationship to survival. There are published institutional series in which repair early in the ECMO run and late in the run achieve excellent results. However, there is also contradictory evidence that repair on ECMO has significant bleeding risk and may worsen survival. The optimal strategy would be to decannulate all patients and repair the CDH after decannulation. However, for many tenuous CDH patients there is a fear that the surgical insult of a CDH repair could push the patient back to barotrauma-inducing ventilatory settings. Furthermore, many suspect that for patients with severe CDH, optimal lung expansion and compliance can only be achieved if the CDH has been repaired and there is no external pressure on the lungs such as from the liver and intestine. To compromise, many institutions repair the CDH when the patient is nearly ready for decannulation. This strategy provides physiologic stability post-operatively and, if bleeding ensues, the patient can come off ECMO relatively safely.

If surgery must be performed while on ECMO, I feel that a strategy of preventing bleeding is far more effective than stopping bleeding after it has started. Acceptable strategies to prevent bleeding are to decrease the heparin infusion to achieve an ACT 20–40 s lower than normal (160–180 s) and to infuse Amicar for 72 h. I actually prefer to stop the heparin infusion for at least 6–12 h while giving Amicar. This strategy yields normal surgical field hemostasis during the operation and it allows for microvascular clot formation prior to re-initiation of heparin. The Amicar should prevent further thrombolysis of the surgical clot while on heparin. Short-term heparin-free ECMO can be performed safely with both Trillium-coated and Carmeda-coated circuits. We usually see significant fibrin stranding the next day, so it is beneficial to start the heparin-free period with a new circuit.

Decannulation

For decannulation of patients with percutaneously inserted venous cannulas, simple removal and manual pressure is adequate for control of bleeding. Patients who have had cut down insertion of cannulas require surgical removal. For the neonate, we re-open the neck wound, gain proximal and distal control of all the vessels and remove the cannulas. The vessels are ligated. The common carotid artery can be reconstructed and long term patency can be achieved, however this maneuver has never been shown to be beneficial in terms of neurodevelopmental outcome. A tunneled central line can also be placed in the same venous cannulation site without increased risk of infection. For adolescents who have had cut down cannula insertion, I usually reconstruct both the artery and vein, recognizing that the vein has little chance of long term patency.

Complications

The major complications from ECMO involve hemorrhage. Recent data from the ELSO database demonstrate that in neonates there is an incidence of any kind of bleeding of 25–35%. In pediatric patients, the incidence was 35–50%. These data include cannula and surgical site bleeding as well as pulmonary, gastrointestinal and brain bleeding. Gastrointestinal bleeding is much less common than other sites of bleeding. The other sites experience hemorrhage in about 5–7% of neonatal patients and 9% of pediatric patients. Of note, in older pediatric patients, cannula site bleeding is seen in about 20% of patients, likely due to the predominance of percutaneous access in these patients.

Once post-operative bleeding is evident, the strategies discussed in preventing bleeding should be implemented. For the cannulation site, local measures such as direct pressure or wrapping of the cannulas with thrombotic agents can assist in control. I suggest that in any patient with uncontrolled bleeding who is not ready for decannulation, one should aggressively normalize coagulation factors, lower the ACT and start Amicar. If these measures do not work, then one should try activated factor VII (aFVII) or a heparin-free trial with Amicar infusion. If all else fails, then decannulation is the only answer.

Blood stream infection occurs in 4–7% of neonatal ECMO patients and 17–23% of pediatric patients. Although the predominant organisms involved are coagulase negative *staphylococcus* organisms, usually appropriate antibiotics can control the infection. The infection may originate from other access points in the patient and not in the circuit itself. The use of prophylactic antibiotics in ECMO is somewhat controversial. I think it wise to cover for *Staphylococcus*, especially in pediatric patients.

Results and Expectations

Overall survival to discharge for neonatal and pediatric ECMO patients is about 70 and 50%, respectively. However for individual diagnoses, the survival rate can vary considerably (Table 13.2). The reversible neonatal respiratory diseases such as meconium aspiration, respiratory distress syndrome, and persistent pulmonary hypertension of the newborn, all have very high survival rates. These data should be in mind not only in discussion with parents, but also in deciding criteria for ECMO. When medical and ventilator

Table 13.2 Survival outcomes for ECMO based on diagnosis

Diagnosis	% Survived
Neonatal	
MAS	94%
RDS	84%
PPHN	79%
Sepsis	75%
CDH	53%
Pediatric	
Aspiration pneumonia	65%
Viral pneumonia	62%
Bacterial pneumonia	54%
ARDS, not postop/trauma	52%
Acute respiratory failure, non-ARDS	47%

MAS meconium aspiration syndrome; *RDS* respiratory distress syndrome; *PPHN* persistent pulmonary hypertension of the newborn; *CDH* congenital diaphragmatic hernia; *ARDS* acute respiratory distress syndrome

management escalates to a point where survival becomes less than that with ECMO, then obviously ECMO is indicated.

It is important to understand our own long-term outcomes for invasive therapies like ECMO. After a patient has been successfully decannulated, neuroimaging is obtained prior to discharge. The study of choice is a brain MRI to look for infarcts, bleeds, atrophy or hydrocephalus. If an MRI cannot be done, then a head CT would be second choice.

It should be emphasized to parents of neonatal and infant patients that regular neurodevelopmental follow up should be arranged to allow for early intervention should it become necessary. Findings are translated into early intervention program therapy, hearing aids, and vision aids. In general, about 20–30% of ECMO patients have long-term neurodevelopmental outcome deficits, but there is evidence from limited randomized controlled trials that ECMO patients may fare better than patients managed with conventional medical therapy. The primary diagnosis seems to have the strongest effect on long-term outcome since ECMO patients with CDH have the worst outcomes.

Summary Points

- ECMO is a life-saving tool but it must be used before end-organ damage has occurred.
- If lung rest and adequate cardiopulmonary support cannot be achieved on VV-ECMO, then change to VA-ECMO.
- The process of weaning from ECMO requires incremental daily optimization.
- Uncorrectable suprasystemic pulmonary artery pressures portend a poor outcome.

Editor's Comment

ECMO should be considered for any patient with severe respiratory compromise that fails to respond to all other available therapeutic measures and is potentially reversible.

For patients at the extremes of age and size, technical issues might preclude a successful application of the technology, but it is difficult to define absolute limits of applicability as they continue to change. For larger patients, arterial access is limited due to the adverse effects of ligating the vessel that is cannulated and venous return can be a significant issue, requiring sometimes two or three venous cannulas to support flow. A distal internal jugular cannula ("brain drain") can provide substantial additional flow even in neonates.

Veno-venous ECMO has become the preferred approach except when there is significant primary cardiac disease and in most babies with CDH, who often have poor venous drainage due to cardiac hypoplasia and severe mediastinal displacement. Especially in older patients, percutaneous VV cannulation has also become available and should be used whenever possible. A significant problem with VV-ECMO has been the development of transient cardiac dysfunction ("stun"), presumably due to cytokine release or electrolyte abnormalities, which sometimes leads to early emergent conversion to VA-ECMO. This has been effectively avoided at The Children's Hospital of Philadelphia since the introduction several years ago of a protocol that includes: low initial flow through the circuit (10 mL/kg/min) for 8 min, calcium gluconate 100 mg/kg (50 mg/kg in pediatric patients) given as an intravenous bolus during this initial period, and a very slow increase in flow (10 mL/kg/min every 2–3 min) up to the goal of 100–120 mL/kg/min.

Cannulation can be harrowing in neonates and should not be taken lightly. The internal jugular vein tears easily, sometimes requiring ligation and a second or third attempt. One should always use the smallest cannula expected to provide sufficient flow as a large cannula is more likely to injure the vein and can be surprising difficult to place even when the vein appears to be huge. In extremely rare cases, a portion of the clavicle can be resected to expose the vein in the chest or a sternotomy with direct placement of a cannula in the atrium is required. Unfortunately, the right jugular vein is essentially the only vein available in the neonate for safe cannulation and it should therefore be carefully protected. A common problem is for the cannula to pass for a short distance and then for there to be resistance to passage of the last few centimeters into the atrium. Firm pressure might be all that is required but perforation of the SVC or right atrium is a significant concern. It is useful in these situations to: gently spin the cannula as it is being advanced, lift the baby's thorax off the bed for a short distance, and change the degree of traction applied to the vein in an attempt to straighten it (more traction) or prevent the natural narrowing that occurs when a tubular structure is stretched (less traction). Rather than forcing it and risking a catastrophe, it is usually best to remove the cannula, regroup, and try again with a smaller cannula. Sterile water-soluble lubricant is also useful.

Cannulation of the artery is usually much more straight-forward, but there is a risk of placing the cannula in a subintimal plane, which is potentially disastrous. One should be very careful to place the tip of the cannula within the true lumen. If an intimal flap has occurred, it might be prudent to tack it down with fine polypropylene stitches prior to attempting cannulation. Probably the most common mistake in arterial cannulation is in the positioning of the tip of the cannula too far into the aortic arch, which can limit flow into the right arm and coronary arteries. The tip should be advanced no more than about 2.5–3 cm, just enough for it to be secured in the carotid artery. It does not need to be placed within the aorta proper.

When called about a patient who needs to be considered for ECMO, there are certain very specific steps that should be taken: assessment of the patient's candidacy in the context of available institutional resources; activation of the "ECMO team"; STAT echocardiography and head ultrasound; type and crossmatch for blood needed to prime the ECMO circuit; and informed consent obtained from the parents after a frank discussion of the indications, alternatives, anticipated benefits (ECMO is a bridge, not a therapy in and of itself), and potential risks of the procedure (especially bleeding and intracranial hemorrhage). For every patient, a limit should be agreed upon regarding what length of time is reasonable before considering ECMO a failure.

Ultimately, the goal for any patient on ECMO is to get them off ECMO as soon as possible, and every maneuver every day should be with that goal in mind. It is important to avoid the situation in which the focus is on the minutia of everyday care while the bigger picture is being neglected: avoid fluid overload and start a forced diuresis early; gently increase ventilator settings to recruit native lung function as early as is practical; wean pressors and unnecessary medications; provide adequate intravenous nutrition throughout the ECMO run; and have frequent discussions with the family to review progress and discuss limitations. Finally, when the infant is not responding to therapeutic measures as expected, repeat the echocardiogram a second or third time as some congenital heart lesions can be very difficult to identify early on.

Diagnostic Studies

- Pre-ECMO
- CXR
- Head ultrasound
- Echocardiogram
- On ECMO
- Daily head ultrasound for 3 days
- Daily chest X-ray
- Weaning
- Echocardiogram
- Post-ECMO
- Brain MRI

Parental Preparation

– ECMO provides time and clinical stability but does not correct underlying pathophysiology
– Significant bleeding risk which is life threatening
– Survival is variable depending on the diagnosis
– Significant risk of developmental delay

Preoperative Preparation

☐ Understand venous and arterial anatomy
☐ 100 μ/kg heparin iv bolus just prior to cannulation
☐ Assortment of appropriately sized cannulas in hand

Technical Points

• Transverse incision over vessels for cut down insertion.
• In neonate, tip of venous cannula in right atrium (7–8 cm) and tip of arterial cannula at aortic arch (2.5–3 cm).
• In older child, large bore venous cannulas in SVC and IVC (VV-ECMO).
• Avoid crimping the double lumen VV-ECMO cannula.
• Tunneled central line can be placed in vein at decannulation.
• Carotid reconstruction in neonate has long term patency, but no clear benefit.

Suggested Reading

Hardart GE, Hardart MK, Arnold JH. Intracranial hemorrhage in premature neonates treated with extracorporeal membrane oxygenation correlates with conceptional age. J Pediatr. 2004;145(2): 184–9.

Hirschl RB, Schumacher RE, Snedecor SN, Bui KC, Bartlett RH. The efficacy of extracorporeal life support in premature and low birth weight newborns. J Pediatr Surg. 1993;28(10):1336–40; discussion 41.

McNally H, Bennett CC, Elbourne D, Field DJ. United Kingdom collaborative randomized trial of neonatal extracorporeal membrane oxygenation: follow-up to age 7 years. Pediatrics. 2006;117(5): e845–54.

Rozmiarek AJ, Qureshi FG, Cassidy L, et al. How low can you go? Effectiveness and safety of extracorporeal membrane oxygenation in low-birth-weight neonates. J Pediatr Surg. 2004;39(6): 845–7.

Sigalet DL, Tierney A, Adolph V, et al. Timing of repair of congenital diaphragmatic hernia requiring extracorporeal membrane oxygenation support. J Pediatr Surg. 1994;30(8):1183–7.

Van Meurs K, Lally KP, et al., editors. ECMO extracorporeal cardiopulmonary support in critical care. Ann Arbor: Extracorporeal Life Support Organization; 2005.

Vazquez WD, Cheu HW. Hemorrhagic complications and repair of congenital diaphragmatic hernias: does timing of the repair make a difference? Data from the Extracorporeal Life Support Organization. J Pediatr Surg. 1994;29(8):1002–5; discussion 1005–6.

Part III
Trauma

Chapter 14
Pediatric Trauma Resuscitation

Thane Blinman

Care of the injured child differs in important ways from that of the injured adult. The pediatric trauma surgeon must account for these differences when crafting a plan of care. Pediatric patients differ from adults in measurable, distinct biomechanical ways: less mineralization of bone means that the skeleton offers less protection to structures in the CNS, thorax, and abdomen; decreased muscle strength per unit volume means not only diminished protection of the cervical spine and abdomen, but decreased Starling effect in the heart; increased surface area relative to body mass means dramatically increased vulnerability to radiative and evaporative loss of heat and fluid; and scaling of energetics means that babies require three times the energy per kilogram of body mass than adults and have far less reserve.

Not only are the patterns of injury different than in adults (pulmonary contusion even in the absence of rib fracture) but the physiologic responses to hemorrhage and resuscitative interventions differ substantially from those exhibited by adults (increased heart rate is more important than preload-recruitable stroke work for driving cardiac output). Failure to consider these differences can lead to treatment that is incorrect, either in terms of therapeutic choice (early splenectomy for spleen laceration) or of degree (over- or under-resuscitation of the child with shock or traumatic brain injury). In addition, the largely nonoperative nature of pediatric trauma has lulled some into believing that injured children do not need surgical consultation, a baseless myth easily dispelled by the case logs of any major children's trauma center. In any case, only a surgeon can judge when *not* to operate.

As with adults, the objectives of the trauma resuscitation are simple: (1) effectively deliver oxygen (ABCs); (2) systematically discover injuries; (3) make a treatment plan; (4) rapidly reach the destination (OR, ICU, CT scanner) where assessment and management of injuries can continue; and (5) do no harm. The slower pace of pediatric care generally allows clinicians to neglect the *Plan* and *Destination* portions of the resuscitation, and babies frequently end up stalled in the trauma bay, but it is the surgeon's job to remember these goals…and to keep an eye on the clock.

Pre-Hospital Care

In general, the evidence shows that paramedics deliver good pre-hospital care to children. Although properly-sized equipment is often absent on a standard rescue ambulance, paramedics improvise and adapt existing equipment well to protect the injured child. Response times and extrication methods are independent of patient age, but heavy use of helicopter evacuation and transport (in patients who tend to have less severe injuries) is perhaps evidence that, especially when treating children, EMS providers prefer to err on the side of caution.

Nevertheless, pre-hospital providers struggle with some important aspects of pediatric care, especially the pediatric airway, intravenous access, and c-spine immobilization. Recent evidence indicates that airway management short of endotracheal intubation (in particular, oral airway and bag-valve-mask ventilation) is superior to unsuccessful attempts at field intubation, especially in a child with traumatic brain injury. Meanwhile, complications are seen in as many as half of pre-hospital intubation attempts, with unrecognized esophageal intubations alarmingly common. As a result, current recommendations are to avoid attempts at endotracheal intubation in the field and to transport using an oral airway and bag valve mask ventilation with chin-lift/jaw-thrust, unless these maneuvers are demonstrably inadequate. An exception might be the pediatric patient requiring prolonged transport who requires a stable airway. EMS staff who must intubate a child should clearly understand the anatomic differences of the pediatric airway. Moreover, the chaotic pre-hospital environment means that the clinician receiving the patient in the trauma bay must *prove* that the endotracheal tube actually dwells properly in the trachea: In addition to visualization, auscultation and end-tidal carbon dioxide detection, a *chest X-ray* should be obtained as soon as the patient is moved from

T. Blinman (✉)
General, Thoracic and Fetal Surgery, The Children's Hospital of Philadelphia, 34th and Civic Center Blvd., 5 Wood, Philadelphia, PA 19104, USA
e-mail: blinman@email.chop.edu

P. Mattei (ed.), *Fundamentals of Pediatric Surgery*,
DOI 10.1007/978-1-4419-6643-8_14, © Springer Science+Business Media, LLC 2011

the ambulance gurney to the bed. This initial chest X-ray is an important part of the *Airway* section of the primary survey.

The child's small veins and surfeit of subcutaneous fat may foil attempts to gain intravenous access. A high percentage of pediatric trauma patients arrive in the ED with *no* IV access. Intra-osseus catheters seem under-used, despite their demonstrated effectiveness in children. While Gulf War traumatologists have learned that the sternum is a viable IO site in injured soldiers, the thin sternum of a child makes this location contraindicated; practitioners should use the proximal tibia. The risk of infection remains and in the hospital setting definitive IV access should be established as soon as feasible.

Cervical-spine precautions are often misapplied or not employed. Pediatric patients whose c-spines are immobilized often suffer from one of three errors: an incorrectly sized collar (almost always so large that it slips over the chin, simultaneously obstructing the airway and providing no c-spine protection); an absent collar (usually with the possibly effective but inadequately tested work-around of a rolled towel and tape); or inadequate padding beneath the thoracic spine to compensate for the prominent occiput of the child (which produces flexion at the neck instead of neutral positioning). These errors should be recognized during the primary survey and corrected.

Initial hospital care of the pediatric trauma patient parallels standard ATLS protocols, and, the usual rubric of Primary Survey (ABCDE), Secondary Survey (Plan and Destination), and Tertiary Survey (double check everything) allows a systematic (or "automatic") method for managing the injured child in a way that reduces the chance of doing too much, doing too little, or missing an injury.

Primary Survey

Airway

Safe control of the airway is paramount in pediatric trauma resuscitation. Success here prevents secondary injury from hypoxia, but depends on a clear understanding of the indications for intubation, an organized clinical approach, and facility with airway anatomy. All trauma centers should have an established protocol for pediatric intubation, a pediatric intubation cart stocked with appropriate sizes of tubes and laryngoscopes, and a guide (such as a Broselow tape) that facilitates choice of tubes and dosing of key medications.

Rapid sequence intubation aims to quickly secure a stable airway while minimizing the risk of aspiration of stomach contents. While every institution should maintain its own rapid sequence intubation protocol (Fig. 14.1), virtually all RSI methods employ some combination of paralytic, sedative, cricoid pressure (Sellick maneuver), and a shorter period of preoxygenation than would be used for induction of general anesthesia. Any unstable child should be intubated by the

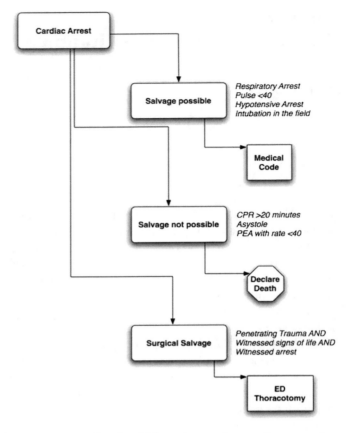

Fig. 14.1 Algorithm for children who sustain a cardiac arrest after traumatic injury

most experienced person present; unstable trauma patients cannot tolerate multiple unskilled attempts.

The pediatric airway differs from the adult in (at least) seven particular ways: (1) shorter trachea (even relative to body size); (2) anteriorly displaced epiglottis; (3) prominent occiput; (4) high larynx; (5) proportionately larger tongue and smaller mouth; (6) an airway that is narrowest at the cricoid cartilage; and (7) greater vulnerability to airway restriction from debris or edema because of the greater relative sensitivity to flow resistance at smaller airway radius.

These differences mean that a different strategy for intubation of the child is required. The short trachea demands extra caution to avoid a mainstem intubation. One strategy is to carefully observe the double lines on the ETT: when these have just passed the cords, the tube is likely in good position. Careful auscultation in the axilla and observation of the chest can reveal poor tube position. The anterior epiglottis can be compensated for by less aggressive head tilt (to be avoided if the c-spine is not cleared), opting instead for a gentle "sniffing" position.

A common error is to use too much hyperextension, a maneuver that tends to cantilever the larynx anteriorly, then when visualization is difficult, the clinician tries to compensate with more extension, which pulls the larynx even farther from view, and so on. Break this cycle by placing gentle padding behind the shoulders (not the neck) to overcome the prominent occiput and using little or no neck extension. Meanwhile, an assistant can direct the epiglottis into a more favorable position with cricoid pressure, even maneuvering the larynx slightly to the left or right as needed.

The small mouth and large tongue are handled by having reliable suction at the ready, using a correctly sized laryngoscope (especially the narrower Miller blade), and having the assistant apply gentle traction at the side of the mouth to give a better view. Finally, the narrowing at the level of the cricoid cartilage has traditionally translated into the use of uncuffed tubes for children in order to avoid subglottic stenosis from balloon pressure injury. While some have recently questioned this practice in the ICU setting, it remains true that a correctly-sized uncuffed tube is easier to place (the classic heuristic is to choose a tube with the same external diameter as the pinky finger). A small amount of water-soluble lubricant on the gently-curved stylet makes tube dislodgement in the short trachea less likely when the stylet is removed. Finally, all of these anatomic differences mean that esophageal intubation is common but easily-detected and corrected with the use of now widely available end-tidal CO_2 devices.

Indications for intubation include: (1) inability to spontaneously protect the airway (GCS ≤ 8, overdose, drugs, facial trauma); (2) inability to ventilate (flail chest); and (3) inability to oxygenate (pulmonary contusion, smoke inhalation, cardiac instability).

Breathing

Several factors not seen in adults can inhibit breathing in infants and children. Infants are obligate nose-breathers, so tubes, debris and blood in the nose can impede air movement. As in adults, auscultation and inspection are essential for proper evaluation of breathing. A tension pneumothorax should never be diagnosed by X-ray, but by recognition of tracheal deviation away from the pneumothorax, hyper-resonant sounds, and dyspnea. The first maneuver should be a "dart" to the anterior chest, followed by tube thoracostomy, since in the child this procedure always takes far longer and is more difficult than anticipated. Dyspnea is manifested by grunting, nasal flaring, belly-breathing, and engagement of the sternocleidomastoid and other accessory muscles with each breath. Stridor is evidence of critical narrowing and, especially in a burn patient, is an indication not for bronchoscopy but for intubation.

Calculations for minute ventilation are different in that children require higher respiratory rates and lower tidal volumes, especially during bag-valve-mask ventilation, and bradypnea/respiratory arrest is the most common of cardiac arrest in babies. The clinician should give rapid breaths (30–40/min) using a pressure valve, taking care to not exceed peak inspiratory pressures of 25–30 mmHg. Higher pressures are unlikely to improve tidal volume and are more likely to inflict barotrauma/volutrauma. Moreover, since gastric distension is one of the chief causes of respiratory embarrassment in the younger pediatric trauma patient, the overflow ventilation at higher pressures actually can *diminish* tidal volumes. Early recognition and tube decompression of a distended stomach in a crying, injured child can prevent unnecessary ventilation failure.

Circulation

The total circulating blood volume of the child can be surprisingly small. For young children, blood volume is approximately 80 mL/kg, thus a 5 kg baby has just 400 mL of total blood volume, and has sustained a 40% hemorrhage (class IV shock) with a loss of only 160 mL. Similarly, a 25 kg child with a total blood volume of 2,000 mL can quickly and quietly lose 25% of his blood volume from a scalp wound that bleeds just 8 mL/min or 500 mL in an hour. The small starting volumes can fool the complacent clinician who ignores these seemingly small but persistent sources of blood loss in the resuscitation suite.

Pediatric patients have a remarkable ability to compensate for blood loss. In the child, the initial response to hypovolemia is not hypotension, but tachycardia. Nevertheless, in the excitement of a trauma resuscitation, it is unsurprising to see tachycardia in a frightened, injured child. Distinguishing the source of the tachycardia can be challenging. Often, the pediatric patient will maintain a normal blood pressure until 40% or more of the estimated blood volume has been lost. It is this tendency to compensate and then abruptly and catastrophically decompensate that makes hypotension especially alarming.

For this reason, the C in ABC really means access to the circulation. According to ATLS protocol, two attempts should be made to place large bore IV cannulas in the upper extremities, but in children clinicians should not forget other relatively large veins such as the saphenous at the medial malleolus and the cephalic vein over the lateral distal radius (the "intern's vein"). If adequate IV access cannot be quickly obtained, an IO line can be placed in the tibia, which allows infusion of a large volume of fluid as well as blood products and IV medications. However, they should be regarded as temporary, unstable, and prone to infection; rarely should a child leave the trauma bay with an IO catheter in place.

In general, a central venous catheter should not be the first line access in the trauma bay. They take too long to insert and usually have much higher resistance to flow than a large-bore IV. On the other hand, in larger patients in shock, a Cordis catheter sheath can be used to deliver large volumes quickly. In any case, if a central line is the best option, it should be regarded as having been placed under dirty conditions and good practice is to remove and replace them with another form of access as soon as the patient is stabilized, usually within 48 h of admission.

The elements governing oxygen delivery (DO_2) in children are the same as in adults. However the relative contribution of each of these to oxygen delivery differs importantly in children. Oxygen delivery depends on blood oxygen content multiplied by cardiac output, which in turn is governed by two simultaneous equations: $CO = HR \times (EF \times EDV)$ and $CO = (MAP - CVP)/SVR$, where the five important elements are: heart rate, end-diastolic volume (preload), ejection fraction (contractility), mean arterial pressure, and systemic vascular resistance (afterload). We neglect central venous pressure since it is typically a very small value, and is really not a good "lever" for manipulation of cardiac output, especially compared to mean arterial pressure. Any intervention one employs to optimize cardiac output must work through at least one of these elements. The mainstay of resuscitation in adult trauma patients has been to maintain circulating volume and to optimize oxygen delivery by taking advantage of preload-recruitable increases in cardiac output. In other words, aggressive volume resuscitation in an otherwise healthy adult will boost cardiac output and oxygen delivery as far as EDV can be pushed upward by volume infusion. While enthusiasm for "supraphysiologic" DO_2 (appropriately) has waned, it is largely true that large volumes can be administered to healthy adults with little negative effect.

The same is not true for babies and children. Starling's law does not function over nearly the same range of preload and children rely more on an increased heart rate to increase cardiac output. Rather than responding to increased stretch with increased stroke work, the pediatric heart will more quickly yield to edema (which increases wall stiffness) and begin to fail. Consequently, clinicians must use caution to avoid over-resuscitation. Frequently, children in shock require earlier use of pharmacologic agents to alter SVR/afterload or EF/contractility rather than the aggressive fluid volume resuscitation that succeeds in adults and teens.

This has implications for choice of resuscitation fluid. Recommendations for the sick pediatric trauma patient include limiting crystalloid volume resuscitation to just two boluses of 20 mL/kg, then switching to type-O⁻ blood (usually in aliquots of 10 mL/kg) for ongoing hemodynamic instability. In this way, circulating volume is more likely to approach "euvolemia" while also preserving oxygen carrying capacity, thus maximizing DO_2.

This need for optimal resuscitation reveals measurement of preload as the single largest information gap in pediatric critical care: only measurement of end-diastolic volume is a true preload measure, but this is rarely done. Other commonly employed lines of evidence (CVP, X-ray, physical examination) provide only indirect, and often misleading, evidence. Remember that peripheral edema is a reflection of interstitial fluid, not intravascular volume, a misconception that leads to the abuse of diuretics in many pediatric intensive care units. (Lasix does not carry oxygen!) In practice, the best way to achieve "just right" is to tie specific treatments to explicit clinical endpoints: normalization of HR, improved skin color and extremity warmth, clearing sensorium, increasing mean arterial pressure, production of urine (2 mL/kg/h in infants, 1 mL/kg/h in adolescents), resolution of acidosis, and normal mixed venous oxygen saturation (SvO_2 60–80%).

Disability

A modified Glasgow coma scale has been validated in children (Table 14.1). As in adults, a GCS of 8 or less is an indication for intubation. Importantly, a low GCS is also an independent risk factor for other major injury. Though children are more likely to have seizures and transient altered mental status from post-ictal somnolence, the routine use of prophylactic anti-seizure medication has not been shown to be helpful: a second seizure in a well-resuscitated child is rare. (The same is *not* true later in definitive care of specific intracranial injuries.) Children seem to suffer more mental status degradation from shock, and therefore exhibit better recovery from resuscitation.

Children are more prone to severe traumatic brain injury. The head makes up a larger fraction of body mass than in adults and is less well supported by the neck. Because the larger relative head mass shifts their center of gravity upward, falling or ejected children tend to lead with the head, yet the brain is less protected by the bony skull. More importantly, children suffer disproportionately more from transient deficiencies in cerebral oxygen delivery: hypoxia, hypotension, or even hypoglycemia. Episodes of hypoxia or hypotension measurably increase the risk of death and disability in severe TBI. Timely and adequate resuscitation, quick diagnosis and repair of operative intracranial injury, and aggressive treatment of elevated intracranial pressure preserve function whereas even short delays allow its destruction: time is brain.

Table 14.1 Glasgow Coma Scale revised for use in pediatric population

Best response	Pediatric GCS	Score
Eye	No eye opening	1
	Eye opening to pain	2
	Eye opening to speech	3
	Eyes open spontaneously	4
Verbal	No vocal response	1
	Inconsolable, agitated	2
	Inconsistently consolable, moaning	3
	Cries, but is consolable, inappropriate interactions	4
	Smiles, oriented to sounds, follows objects, interacts	5
Motor	No motor response	1
	Extension to pain	2
	Flexion to pain	3
	Withdrawal from pain	4
	Localizing to pain	5
	Obeys commands	6

While most resuscitation efforts focus on oxygen, remember that oxygen is nothing more than an ash-can for spent electrons during aerobic metabolism. Babies have far less hepatic glycogen reserve relative to their metabolic needs and diminished ability to rapidly shift to ketogenesis to provide a backup substrate to the brain. They are more prone to hypoglycemia, and less able to compensate for it. Substrate (glucose) is equally crucial for cell survival. Not only should any child with any head injury or altered level of consciousness have oxygen and fluid resuscitation, but serum glucose (d-stick) should be measured often (every 30 min) during resuscitation. Critical hypoglycemia (glucose <50 mg/dL) may produce overt signs such as altered mental status and seizure or no signs at all. A quick check can protect brain cells from damage that can be as severe, and as preventable, as hypoxia. Treat critical hypoglycemia in a child or infant with a bolus of 0.25 g/kg of dextrose by pushing 2.5 mL/kg of D_{10} solution intravenously, followed by $D_{10}LR$ or $D_{10}NS$ at maintenance rates and a repeat sugar check at 20 min.

Exposure

Exposure in the pediatric trauma patient should be understood to mean unobstructed visualization and palpation of the entire body, determination of exposure to toxins (carbon monoxide, acid, petroleum distillates), and protection from hypothermia.

While complete exposure and examination of the injured child is crucial, so then is protecting the child from hypothermia. Babies expend energy at around 5 W/kg, but have more trouble containing that energy to maintain temperature. To overcome the cooling from just 10 mL evaporative loss over an hour from a 5-kg baby requires an additional 25% of metabolic power. Radiative losses add even more energy cost and since babies cannot mount this kind of reserve power, hypothermia manifests quickly. After the traditional "strip and flip," covering the child with warm blankets greatly protects against iatrogenic heat loss. Covering or bundling can also decrease anxiety (and tachycardia) in the awake child. Meanwhile, a warm ambient temperature in the trauma bay, overhead warming lights, underbody warmers and warm fluids should be employed to prevent hypothermia. Efforts should also be made to remove all trauma patients, even those with known spinal injury, from hard spine boards, which provide added protection only during transport and can cause skin injury in less than an hour.

Secondary Survey

The purpose of the secondary survey is to complete a detailed head-to-toe examination while the resuscitation team applies other monitors or interventions. More advanced diagnostic procedures are also considered and anticipated during this phase. Once again, the standard approach that is applied to every adult trauma patient is tempered and adjusted for the child, including routine ECG monitoring, BP cuff, and pulse oximetry.

Chest X-ray

The ordinary AP CXR is a rich source of information and is fast. It is a good practice to have a plate positioned on the table before the child arrives and to shoot the film during the primary survey. Often, problems with airway or breathing (mainstem intubation, pneumothorax, gastric distension) are identified or confirmed by this film.

Foley Catheter

Placement of a bladder catheter is only necessary in the critically injured child and should not be routine, especially given the high incidence of urethral injury and subsequent stricture that can result. If on gentle physical examination of the perineum and urethral meatus show no evidence of injury, a size-appropriate bladder catheter can be placed – a rectal examination or pelvic tilt maneuver to rule out a pelvic fracture is rarely necessary or advisable. Resistance or blood indicates the need for urethrogram, especially in the setting of pelvic fracture demonstrated by X-ray.

Nasogastric Tube

The NG tube is useful to decrease the risk of aspiration of gastric contents, to administer oral contrast, and to diminish abdominal respiratory compromise from gastric distention. Gastric distension can be profound in the child who is crying or being ventilated by bag-valve-mask. In this case, the ventilatory compromise can produce hypoventilation severe enough to lead to cardiac arrest. NG tubes are contraindicated in cases of basilar skull fracture or midface instability; an OG tube can be substituted in this case. Common sense indicates that gastric tubes are not to be inflicted on every patient arriving in the trauma bay.

Lab Studies

Recent literature indicates that *few* laboratory studies (LFTs, metabolic panel) are useful for directing care. Little effort should be made at attempting blood draws in injured children, except for CBC and a type & crossmatch. An arterial blood gas might add some information in the critically injured child since the admission base deficit reflects injury severity and predicts mortality. Mortality markedly increases in children with a base deficit less than −8 mEq/L, and is strong evidence of potentially lethal injuries or uncompensated shock. In patients with significant head injury, thrombin and partial thromboplastin times should be drawn to help determine the need for correction of coagulation abnormalities.

Digital Rectal Exam

The digital rectal exam is mentioned largely to be condemned. It is plain that in the pediatric trauma patient the DRE yields scant information. While a perineal examination is important, especially to search for entrance and exit wounds in penetrating trauma, the DRE is generally useless in the pediatric blunt trauma patient. Blood on the glove is more likely to have been caused by the exam than revealed by it, detecting masses is not the object in a blunt trauma context, and "rectal tone" is a poor indicator of neurologic deficits, which are always demonstrated more plainly other ways. "Tubes and fingers in every orifice" may be good practice in adults, but a selective approach is plainly indicated in the small patient.

Re-Evaluation

Resuscitation is a dynamic process. The practitioner must frequently reassess the physiologic response to resuscitation to ensure goals have been achieved. At the same time, the trauma team leader should anticipate a plan and destination for the child (CT scanner, PICU, operating room, transfer to a higher level of care). It is the trauma team leader's principal responsibility to drive the patient toward efficient implementation of a treatment plan.

Diagnostic Procedures

Unstable patients with penetrating trauma to the peritoneal cavity or an obvious source of ongoing hemorrhage need to go directly to the operating room. In this circumstance, the primary decision to be made once ABCs are secured is operative approach and incision. But these obvious occasions are uncommon in the pediatric patient and the surgeon usually requires more information to answer the question: Operate or not? Even when the answer is "no operation," imaging is still required to determine the hospital plan. Several diagnostic tools are available to help with this diagnostic process. However, imaging must be selected with awareness of the relatively increased sensitivity to ionizing radiation that the children have. "Scan them all" is a poor approach.

Plain radiographs are useful screening tools, but are probably less helpful overall than in adults because of the variable sizes and extent of ossification of bony structures. The anterior-posterior chest film, ideally taken immediately on patient arrival, is probably the most helpful and might reveal pneumothorax, hemothorax, pneumoperitoneum, foreign objects, widened mediastinum, or misplaced tubes (especially endotracheal tubes).

Other films are not as useful. Pelvic X-rays are both less sensitive and less specific for fractures in children. Cervical spine films should be considered screening tools only: positive findings always require further definition (CT or MRI) but even negative results should be viewed with suspicion in a child with a suggestive mechanism of injury or tenderness on physical exam. Injuries to the spinal cord without bony injury are much more common in children.

Most centers report that ultrasound (FAST) is reliable in discerning the presence or absence of fluid in the abdominal cavity, the thorax, and the pericardium, where it is the test of choice for tamponade. It does not, however, demonstrate the actual source of fluid. In experienced hands, FAST is reported to be useful to exclude the abdomen as a source of bleeding in the unstable child. However, it is critical to validate physician-performed diagnostic accuracy before employing FAST as a basis for operative decisions.

CT scanning has become the workhorse of trauma diagnostic information. While there are reports of measurable, albeit very small, lifetime increases in cancer risk from CT radiation, these worries should be tempered in the face of immediate injury. Rather, scanning protocols that employ weight-specific radiation dosing should be utilized. The rapid scan acquisition and processing made possible by multi-slice scanners and modern software mean few children need to be restrained or sedated in the scanner.

Intravenous contrast is contraindicated in initial head scans. For abdominal CT scans, intravenous contrast is required to optimally visualize the solid organs and in particular to determine active extravasation. For most injuries, CT angiography has supplanted more invasive methods of detecting injury to thoracic and carotid vessels, and can even exclude some extremity vascular injuries. Meanwhile, oral contrast is often omitted during initial abdominal CT scans since administration of contrast takes time, typically elicits vomiting, and usually does not have time to travel to the distal bowel. Oral contrast may, however, help identify proximal injuries such as duodenal hematomas, and certainly may be used in "second look" CT scans in patients with new or worsening symptoms after a blunt injury.

CT scanning reliably detects bony injuries, but children can sustain severe injuries to brain, spinal cord, lung, and GU tract without fractures because of the decreased mineralization and stiffness of the bony structures protecting these organs. In particular, CT is poor at detecting spinal cord injuries without radiologic abnormality (SCIWORA); MRI is the modality of choice here, but only in the stabilized patient. Currently, MRI has no role in the acute setting.

Diagnostic peritoneal lavage is rarely used in children now as the information it provides is similar (fluid or no fluid) to that gleaned from other sources. It can give some information about the source of fluid but is more difficult to perform, takes more time, and has greater associated risk. Nevertheless, it is still conceivable that DPL could be useful in detecting hemorrhage in a trauma patient when FAST or CT is unavailable. DPL is performed similarly to adults, with a few differences: (1) decompress the bladder and stomach (Foley and NG tube); (2) use a *supra-umbilical* incision to avoid the high-riding pediatric bladder and use the open or Seldinger technique to direct a catheter toward the pelvis; (3) gross blood is a positive result. If no blood is seen, instill 10 mL/kg (up to 1 L) of warmed Ringer's lactate solution and allow to drain. As in adults, with microscopic analysis, a positive test is given by: >100,000 RBC/mm^3, >500 WBC/mm^3, bile, urine, or food material.

ED Thoracotomy

Emergency Department thoracotomy has a poor track record in all trauma patients, but in children it has been particularly unhelpful. As early as 1987, it was apparent that in pediatric blunt trauma, ED thoracotomy had no influence on survival. Later, it was demonstrated that if pediatric patients had no signs of life in the field, they *never* survived, even with ED thoracotomy. Worse, there have been no *neurologically intact* survivors among pediatric blunt trauma patients who presented to the trauma bay without signs of life. Even those with limited signs of life on presentation had a survival of only 25% with the risk of fatality after CPR increased for children with a systolic blood pressure below 60 mmHg on arrival. While children with penetrating injury had better survival, for all survivors of traumatic arrest, nearly two thirds had at least one impairment in the functional activities of daily living. These findings and other data have consistently demonstrated that, contrary to the popular perception of extraordinary resilience in the pediatric patient, the potential for survival in pediatric trauma arrest is quite poor. Emergency thoracotomy may have value only in cases where arrest occurs in the trauma bay, regardless of mechanism (Fig. 14.1).

Tertiary Survey

Around one in 20 pediatric patients have some injury missed during the primary and secondary survey. Most of these are orthopedic injuries, missed either because the small child cannot complain, the initial films were not sensitive enough for the relatively demineralized bone, or there were other priorities (such as control of hemorrhage). However, there may be operative intra-abdominal injuries such as small bowel perforations, that are both hard to detect and slow to cause symptoms. Meanwhile, neurologic injuries can continue to progress over days. Injuries attributed to "accidents" may be discovered to stem from abuse. For these reasons, pediatric traumatologists routinely add a "tertiary survey" to the classic primary and secondary surveys. In the tertiary survey, when there is calm, a reliable historian and more time, a proper history and a more thorough head-to-toe exam can be done. This is often the best time to clear the c-spine (avoiding an expensive MRI), and to coordinate multiple consulting services.

Summary Points

- The patterns of injury in children are different those commonly seen in adults.
- Children are more likely to develop spinal cord injury without radiographic abnormality (SCIWORA), internal injuries without bone fractures, and airway compromise with minimal change in the diameter due to edema or compression.
- The physiologic response of children to injury is different than that of adults.
- Children increase cardiac output in response to hypovolemia by increasing heart rate. Any degree of hypotension suggests massive hypovolemia and impending shock.
- The role of the pediatric trauma surgeon is to protect the child by keeping the trauma bay focused on the plan and destination, preventing iatrogenic injury, and managing surgical injuries (either operatively of non-operatively).
- All procedures performed in the field or during transport (endotracheal intubation, intravenous access, cervical spine immobilization) should be confirmed to be appropriate in the trauma bay – never assume they were done properly.
- Digital rectal examination is rarely useful and should be performed only when absolutely necessary.
- Except for a single AP CXR, routine radiographic imaging of the pelvis, abdomen or spine is usually unnecessary.
- Most children can have their cervical spine cleared on the basis of physical examination and a single lateral cervical spine X-ray.

Editor's Comment

The standardization of trauma care for adults and children with incorporation of science-based protocols is one of the most significant advances in medical science of the twentieth century. Modern pediatric trauma systems are examples of the benefits of teamwork and the practical application of evidence-based diagnostic and therapeutic concepts. The trauma bay should have one recognized leader who nevertheless welcomes input from any member of the team. The leader should use a gentle but firm voice without shouting or bullying. Every finding and intervention should be carefully recorded on paper and videotaped for later review and as part of a formal quality assurance program. Parents should be allowed to be present and every aspect explained to them by an experienced observer at their side. The child should be kept warm and comfortable, with narcotics and anxiolytics if necessary, and everything should be explained in an age-appropriate manner. All procedures should be done by experienced personnel or residents in training, but never by a "first-timer" – the stakes are too high and the teaching value overrated.

In pediatric trauma, there is a tendency for exaggerated personal emotional reaction and heavy-handedness in the delivery of care: over-hydration, over-exposure to cold and radiation, over-protection (incomplete physical examination, tubes and catheters that are too small), superfluous laboratory studies, excessive concern about medical liability, and failing to use the proper size implements. In every aspect of the injured child's care, one should strive for a "just-right" approach based on scientific evidence and experience.

Diagnostic Studies

- Thorough primary, secondary, and tertiary physical examinations.
- Anterior-posterior chest radiograph on admission.
- Cervical spine X-rays (lateral ± AP ± odontoid) when there is any sign of injury to the head or neck.
- FAST/abdominal US (indications in children still unknown).
- Diagnostic peritoneal lavage (used only in very unusual circumstances).
- Flexion-extension cervical X-rays.
- Plain X-rays at all sites that are clearly injured or tender.
- Computed tomography of the head, neck, chest, or abdomen when indicated.
- Head and/or spine MRI when diffuse axonal injury of brain or SCIWORA is suspected.
- CT-angiography when major vascular injury is suspected.
- CT-cystogram if bladder injury is suspected.

Parenteral Preparation

- Your child is being treated according to well-established and scientifically-based protocols and by experienced and caring individuals.
- We need to be thorough but we will be gentle and thoughtful at every step.

Technical Points

- Intravenous access can be difficult in young children, making the intra-osseous catheter an excellent option in many cases.
- In children, endotracheal intubation can be challenging and dangerous. In the emergency setting children should be intubated by the most experienced clinician using appropriate rapid induction techniques.
- Gastric distension can compromise ventilation and sometimes causes bradycardia and hypotension – consider placing a naso- or orogastric tube to decompress the stomach.
- Foley catheters are not routinely placed except in critically injured children, in which case an appropriate size catheter should be placed with gentle technique to prevent urethral injury and subsequent stricture.

Suggested Reading

Adelson PD, Bratton SL, Carney NA, et al. Guidelines for the acute medical management of severe traumatic brain injury in infants, children, and adolescents. Chapter 3. Pre-hospital airway management. Pediatr Crit Care Med. 2003;4:S9–11.

Blinman T, Maggard M. Rational manipulation of oxygen delivery. J Surg Res. 2000;92:120–41.

Chung CY, Chen CL, Cheng PT, See LC, Tang SF, Wong AM. Critical score of Glasgow Coma Scale for pediatric traumatic brain injury. Pediatr Neurol. 2006;34:379–87.

Edil BH, Tuggle DW, Jones S, Albrecht R, Kuhn A, Mantor PC, Puffinbarger NK. Pediatric major resuscitation – respiratory compromise as a criterion for mandatory surgeon presence. J Pediatr Surg 2005;40:926–8; discussion 928.

Nance ML, Stafford PW. Pediatric trauma is a surgical disease. Ann Emerg Med 2003;41:423–4; author reply 424–5.

Stafford PW, Blinman TA, Nance ML. Practical points in evaluation and resuscitation of the injured child. Surg Clin North Am. 2002;82: 273–301.

Chapter 15
Head Trauma

Gregory G. Heuer and Phillip B. Storm

Trauma is the leading cause of death in the pediatric population, and brain injury is the most significant cause of trauma-related mortality. The best "treatment" is prevention through the use of car seats, seat belts, and bike helmets. Even with effective preventative measures, a large number of patients with head injuries still present every day to emergency rooms and trauma centers and their outcome is greatly affected by prompt and effective neurosurgical care.

Diagnosis

Head-injured patients are initially evaluated in the emergency room or trauma bay. As part of the secondary survey, a detailed neurologic exam is performed whenever possible. A specific note should be made of the admission Glasgow Coma Scale score, which includes assessment of eye opening, language, and motor activity (Table 15.1). The GCS is useful as it correlates with the degree of injury and is a simple and reproducible test that can be used to follow patients after admission. A GCS of 13–15 suggests a minor traumatic brain injury, 9–12 a moderate TBI, and 3–8 a severe TBI.

The initial management of the head-injured child is supportive and requires efficient management of airway, breathing, and circulation by the coordinated efforts of first responders, trauma surgeons, and neurosurgeons. Trauma patients often present with other injuries that can lead to cardiopulmonary compromise. It is important to treat hypoxia and hypotension as these can lead to secondary neurologic injury. Hypotension in particular has been shown to be associated with poor prognosis. A primary goal is to maintain cerebral perfusion pressure (CPP) by maintaining blood pressure and avoiding hypoxia. Hypotension is defined as a systolic blood pressure less than the fifth percentile for age or the presence of clinical shock.

Although the initial assessment and management of the child with traumatic brain injury (TBI) is the same as for any other trauma patient, it is important to move through the protocol quickly and efficiently so as to avoid any delay in the diagnosis and treatment of the head injury. Ideally, the logistics and individual resources of the particular institution not withstanding, the patient should get the necessary imaging studies within 15–30 min of arrival to the trauma bay. In addition, every patient with a head injury should be presumed to have a spine injury until proven otherwise, which means that cervical spinal immobilization and transportation on a rigid backboard are essential.

Once the patient is hemodynamically stable, a quick but thorough neurologic exam is performed as the patient is prepared for non-contrast computed tomography of the brain, which is usually the only imaging necessary to assess brain injury. Imaging should be considered in patients who have a history of having lost consciousness, a depressed or declining GCS, a fixed neurologic deficit, or an injury that is judged to place the patient at risk for brain injury. Magnetic resonance imaging is rarely indicated in the acute management of head trauma as the head CT and serial neurologic examinations determine the medical and surgical management of the patient.

The presence of an epidural or subdural hemorrhage is usually a neurosurgical emergency and requires immediate evacuation to lower intracranial pressure (ICP). Intraparenchymal hemorrhages and skull fractures are usually managed non-surgically unless they are extensive. Patients with non-surgical lesions should be closely monitored and aggressively managed in the intensive care unit.

Patients with severe head trauma who do not have a reliable exam often require placement of an ICP monitor. The usual criteria for placement of an ICP monitor include the presence of a non-surgical injury in a patient who is not localizing on exam or has a GCS of 8 or less. There are several options: a simple ICP monitor, a dual monitor that records ICP and brain tissue oxygen, or a ventriculostomy.

G.G. Heuer (✉)
Department of Neurosurgery, University of Pennsylvania, Children's Hospital of Philadelphia, 3400 Civic Center Blvd, Philadelphia, PA 19104, USA
e-mail: gregory.heuer@uphs.upenn.edu

P. Mattei (ed.), *Fundamentals of Pediatric Surgery*,
DOI 10.1007/978-1-4419-6643-8_15, © Springer Science+Business Media, LLC 2011

Table 15.1 Glasgow Coma Scale, modified for children

Score	Eyes open	Verbal	Motor
6	–	–	Spontaneous
5	–	Age appropriate	Localizes
4	Spontaneous	Cries/consolable	Withdraws
3	To voice	Irritable	Flexion posture
2	To pain	Restless	Extension posture
1	None	None	None

(see also table 14.1)

The ventriculostomy has the advantage of being diagnostic and therapeutic. It is our practice to place a ventriculosotomy if the lateral ventricles are accessible (based on the head CT). If not, we favor placement of a dual monitor that measures ICP and brain-oxygenation (Licox monitor, Integra LifeSciences, Plainsboro, NJ). The goal of therapy is an ICP under 20 mmHg, CPP (mean arterial pressure minus the ICP) greater than 50 mmHg, and brain tissue oxygenation greater than 20 mmHg. Additionally, it is important to prevent spikes in ICP or brain oxygen desaturations, both of which have been associated with poor outcome.

If a ventriculostomy is present, ICP is lowered by draining cerebrospinal fluid. Medical therapy includes: elevating the head of the bed to greater than 30°, preserving normothermia, avoiding hyponatremia, maintaining adequate analgesia and sedation, and using nondepolarizing paralytic agents. Patients with acute spikes in ICP and the absence of a mass lesion are also treated medically with hyperventilation, mannitol, or hypertonic saline. After a bony decompression, the ICP monitor waveform and values are not representative, but brain tissue oxygenation values will still give accurate readings that can be used to guide therapy.

Skull Fractures

Skull fractures are found in more than 20% of children hospitalized with head injury and the rate is higher in young children. As many as 40–60% of children under 1 year of age hospitalized with head injury are found to have a skull fracture. Fractures are classified as linear, depressed, or basilar.

Linear skull fractures are the most common type. In the absence of any significant underlying hemorrhage, patients with this type of fracture rarely need surgical intervention. Depressed skull fractures vary in significance depending on the age of the child. This is because skull anatomy and structure is different in infants compared with older children. Prior to 4 years of age, the skull is thin and pliable. As a result, young children often present with fractures in which the skull is depressed inward without a fracture line, similar to the way a dent forms in a ping-pong ball. This type of fracture rarely needs surgery and patients are usually followed clinically. We reevaluate in 4–6 weeks, after all of the post-traumatic swelling has resolved. With time, this type of

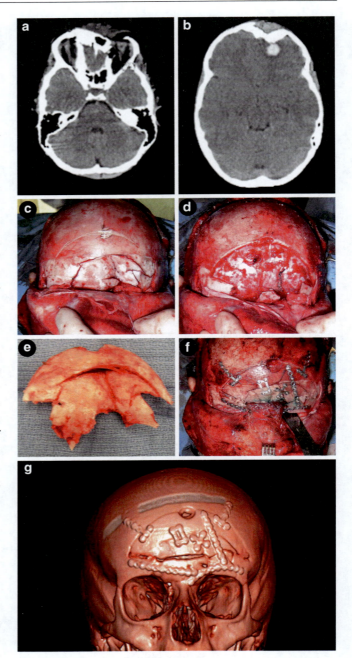

Fig. 15.1 A child who suffered a skull fracture after a blow to the head with a baseball. (**a–b**) Representative CT images demonstrating a skull fracture involving the orbit and an underlying contusion. (**c–d**) Intraoperative images demonstrating the skull fracture and the dura after elevation of the fracture and repair of the dural tear. (**e**) Elevated fracture. (**f**) Intraoperative image after plating of the fracture. (**g**) Postoperative CT reconstruction

fracture will spontaneously resolve as the bone remodels under the pressure of the growing brain.

True depressed skull fractures most often are diagnosed by CT (Fig. 15.1). These lesions are often associated with clinically significant underlying brain injury and often require surgical intervention. The indications for operation are: a large or otherwise clinically significant underlying hematoma, a neurologic deficit that is directly related to the depressed fracture, the presence of a break in the overlying skin with gross contamination of the wound, CSF leaking through the wound, and location of a fracture in a site that will result to a poor cosmetic outcome.

There are several goals of surgical intervention. First, the fractured segment must be elevated (Fig. 15.1). In ping-pong ball fractures that need treatment, a burr hole can be placed next to the depressed segment and the area can be flexed-out using an elevator. In some instances, fractures in older children can be similarly elevated directly with a Penfield dissector or other tool. In some instances where the bone is fragmented, a craniotomy is performed around the fracture, and then the fracture can be elevated along with the craniotomy. After the segment is elevated, a clinically significant underlying hematoma should be evacuated and hemostasis obtained. Dural tear should be repaired either primarily with suture or with a duroplasty. In cases where the fracture extends into the frontal or other sinuses, the sinus needs to be cranialized, the mucosal exenterated, and the remaining sinuses separated from the intra-cranial compartment with a vascularized pericranial graft. The last step in repairing a skull fracture is molding the bone back to a normal shape (Fig. 15. 1). In rare instances, it is necessary to perform a cranioplasty by reattaching the bone to the skull with mini-plates.

A unique complication of skull fractures in children, occurring is less than 1% of cases, is the growing skull fracture with leptomeningeal cyst. This lesion presents as an enlarging scalp lesion in a patient with a prior skull fracture. A growing skull fracture occurs in young children (usually less than three but not more than 6 years of age) and is associated with a torn dura and CSF leak. The CSF leak occurs within the fracture line and arachnoid tissue is caught within the fracture. As a result, the fracture line cannot heal and instead widens with time. A growing skull fracture presents as a pulsatile mass at the site of previous trauma and can result in seizures or focal neurologic deficit. These lesions are effectively treated by performing a craniotomy around the previous fracture, dissected the dura from the bone edges, and repairing the dura in a water-tight fashion.

Basilar skull fractures involve the bones of the skull base. It is imperative to identify these fractures due to their frequent association with other injuries. They can extend into the auditory canals, leading to sensorineural hearing loss. They can also extend into the sinuses or produce a CSF leak, which often requires surgical repair to prevent a persistent leak or infection. Finally, a fracture into the petrous bone can cause a facial nerve injury or carotid artery dissection. An angiogram is sometimes necessary to evaluate for a dissection, which is treated with antiplatelet therapy, anticoagulation or, rarely, endovascular stenting or surgery.

Hematoma

Epidural hematoma (EDH) normally results from birth trauma in neonates or, in older children, from a localized blow to the head. Trauma associated with an epidural bleed can lead to a classic pattern of neurologic decline. A patient may have an initial loss of consciousness, a subsequent period of apparent recovery (the lucid interval), and finally, as the EDH enlarges, distinct clinical deterioration. Epidural hematomas are caused by a tear in a meningeal artery or large vein, which leads to the accumulation of blood in the space between the skull and the dura. Most are confirmed by head CT, which reveals a classic biconvex (lentiform) hematoma that does not cross suture lines (Fig. 15.2). The suspicion for these lesions should be high in any patient with a skull fracture. The classic EDH occurs after a fracture in the squamous temporal bone in which the middle

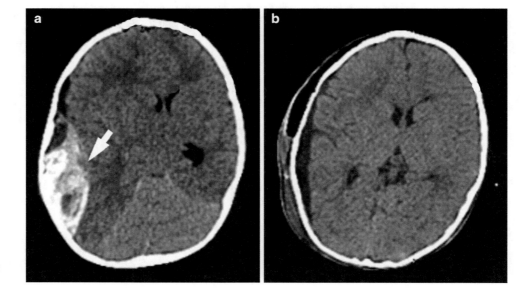

Fig. 15.2 Representative CT image of an epidural hematoma (EDH). (**a**) CT demonstrating a right temporal-parietal EDH. (**b**) Post-operative CT demonstrating evacuation of the EDH

meningeal artery is torn, however in children they more commonly result from bleeding from the fractured bone itself rather than an arterial injury.

Even if the head CT fails to demonstrate a fracture, one is always identified intra-operatively. Management of EDH depends on the clinical picture and the size and location of the lesion. A patient with a decreased level of consciousness and a several-centimeter EDH is considered a neurosurgical emergency. Controversy arises when the patient has a GCS of 15 and is neurologically intact. Some neurosurgeons advocate conservative management for all intact patients regardless of the size and location of the hematoma. Our practice is to intervene surgically on intact patients if the lesion is expanding on serial imaging, or if the patient is complaining of severe or worsening headaches. We also have a much lower threshold to operate if the lesion is in the middle fossa and pushing on the temporal lobe.

The surgical treatment of an epidural hematoma begins with a craniotomy over the lesion (Fig. 15. 2). The craniotomy needs to be large enough to evacuate the hematoma and to localize and coagulate the bleeding blood vessels. Bone wax should be applied to the bone edges and dural tack-up sutures should be placed to re-approximate the dura to the bone, eliminating any dead-space. This reduces the risk of re-accumulation of the hematoma.

Subdural hematoma (SDH) occurs when blood collects between the dura and the brain. On head CT, these lesions typically have a concave appearance and, unlike epidural hematomas, they do cross suture lines (Fig. 15.3). They are much more common than EDH and seldom require surgical intervention. If a patient with a reliable neurologic exam has no history of coagulopathy or a bleeding disorder and the SDH is causing minimal brain compression, he or she can be observed closely in the intensive care unit. Indications for surgical intervention include significant mass effect and enlargement documented by serial imaging. Decompressive hemicraniectomy may be indicated for small SDH that are associated with significant cerebral edema. When studied systematically with all variables controlled for, outcomes for patients with SDH are much worse than for those with EDH. Subdural hematoma portends a worse outcome because the blood accumulates as a result of injury to the brain itself, rather than the skull or dura. EDH can occur in the absence of any brain injury at the time of the initial insult.

Cerebral contusion and intraparenchymal hematoma (IPH) are common findings after head trauma (Fig. 15. 4). These injuries commonly result from acceleration–deceleration injuries in which the brain impacts the inside of the skull. It is important to note that in head-injured patients, IPH can enlarge with time, particularly during the first 24–48 h after admission. This enlargement ("blossoming") needs to be followed closely as it can lead to significant cerebral edema and increased ICP.

Intraparenchymal hemorrhages are managed using a strategy similar to that used for patients with SDH. In the absence of mass effect or cerebral edema, no surgical intervention is required. If medically intractable ICP develops, the goal of surgical intervention is decompression but not complete evacuation. It is also important to establish a complete history of the trauma and assure that the cerebral contusion is consistent with the trauma history. In those patients in whom there is an unexplained IPH, a non-traumatic cause, such as a vascular malformation, infarct or tumor, should be considered.

Traumatic brain injury is a serious and potentially fatal condition in the pediatric population. The effective treatment of these patients requires the prompt identification of the pathology and the institution of the correct therapeutic intervention. The coordinated efforts of a multimodality team can result in a good outcome in the majority of patients.

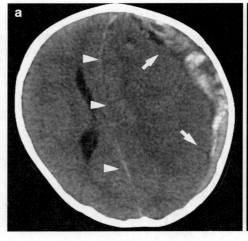
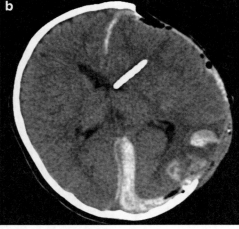
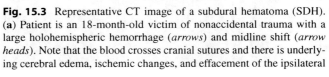

Fig. 15.3 Representative CT image of a subdural hematoma (SDH). (**a**) Patient is an 18-month-old victim of nonaccidental trauma with a large holohemispheric hemorrhage (*arrows*) and midline shift (*arrow heads*). Note that the blood crosses cranial sutures and there is underlying cerebral edema, ischemic changes, and effacement of the ipsilateral ventricle. (**b**) Postoperative head CT after the patient was managed with a decompressive craniotomy, clot evacuation, and placement of a venticulostomy. The ipsilateral ventricle is now visible, and the midline shift is much improved. There remains interhemispheric and intraparenchymal blood

Fig. 15.4 Head CT of an intraparehchmal hemorrhage. Patient is a 14-year-old girl who was riding her bike without a helmet and was struck by an SUV. There is an intraparenchymal clot in the anterior temporal lobe (*arrows*) and uncal herniation (*arrowhead*). She was managed with an ICP monitor and medical therapy

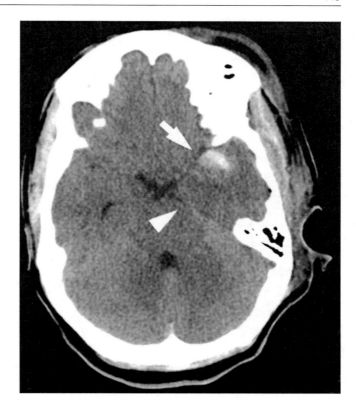

Summary Points

- Trauma is the leading cause of death in children, and brain injury is the leading cause of trauma-related mortality.
- The best "treatment" is prevention: car seats, seat belts, and bike helmets.
- The initial management of the head-injured child is supportive and requires efficient management of airway, breathing, and circulation.
- Hypoxia and hypotension can lead to secondary neurologic injury.
- Ideally, the head-injured child should get necessary imaging studies within 30 min of arrival to the trauma bay.

Editor's Comment

The child with a potential head injury should be managed according to standard ATLS protocols, with initial assessment of airway, breathing, and circulation, and rapid but thorough primary and secondary surveys. Time is of the essence and the patient needs to have a CT scan of the head as soon as possible; but sending an unstable patient to the CT scanner defeats the purpose. Temperature should be regulated to avoid both hyperthermia and hypothermia. Despite its potential benefit in the case of spinal cord injury, at this time corticosteroids have no role in the management of traumatic brain injury. The comatose patient (GCS≤8) should be intubated prior to leaving the trauma bay, with careful in-line traction of the neck and minimal extension of the neck. An orogastric tube should be used to decompress the stomach; nasogastric tubes are avoided due to the possibility of a cribiform plate fracture and subsequent intracranial penetration. During the primary survey the scalp should be carefully inspected and palpated. Scalp lacerations can bleed extensively and in a small child this can lead rapidly to exsanguination. Puncture wounds of the scalp or forehead in an infant can be a sign of a penetrating head injury. To avoid dangerous intracranial pressure elevation, seizures should be treated aggressively with rapid IV administration of fosphenytoin. Finally, it should be kept in mind that brain injury can result in significant coagulopathy due to release of brain tissue thromboplastins, which can have significant systemic consequences.

Nowadays, there appears to be a very low threshold to recommend head CT in children with a potential head injury. Although regional and institutional protocols vary, for the most part any child with evidence of injury above the clavicles, a suggestive mechanism, or a history of loss of consciousness or even the slightest mental status change or neurologic deficit will get a scan. Although a period of observation with serial neurologic assessment is probably just as safe and avoids unnecessary exposure of the developing brain to ionizing radiation, there seems to be a widespread belief that frequent scanning is the best way to avoid a missed injury (and a lawsuit). MRI is also being used with increasing frequency to assess the degree of diffuse axonal damage and previously under-appreciated cervical ligamentous injuries. Whether this is of any clinical significance in most cases is unclear. Nevertheless, head CT remains the initial study of choice in the assessment of acute brain injury.

Differential Diagnosis

- Diffuse axonal injury
- Intraparenchymal hemorrhage
- Epidural hematoma
- Subdural hematoma
- Linear skull fracture
- Depressed skull fracture
- Growing skull fracture with leptomeningeal cyst

Parental Preparation

- The goal for treatment after a head injury is to prevent secondary brain injury from hypoxia, hypotension, and increased intracranial pressure.
- Fractures and hematomas are not dangerous in and of themselves, but only to the extent that they cause underlying brain injury.
- Even after the initial management of the injury, there is often a long period of physical rehabilitation required to achieve maximal recovery.

Preoperative Preparation

- ☐ Airway, Breathing, Circulation
- ☐ Intravenous access
- ☐ Fluid resuscitation
- ☐ Arterial cannula
- ☐ Prophylactic antibiotics
- ☐ ICP monitoring
- ☐ Detailed imaging

Diagnostic Studies

- CT scan
- Arterial blood gas
- Serum sodium level
- Intracranial pressure measurement

Technical Points

- Every patient with a head injury should be presumed to have a spine injury until proven otherwise: cervical spinal immobilization and transportation on a rigid backboard.
- The presence of an epidural or subdural hemorrhage is often a neurosurgical emergency requiring immediate evacuation to lower intracranial pressure.
- Patients with severe head trauma who do not have a reliable exam should undergo placement of an ICP monitor.
- Hyperventilation ($PaCO_2$ 30–34 mmHg) is used only transiently until other medical therapies are instituted.
- The patient with persistent ICP elevation can be treated with hypertonic saline to maintain a sodium level of 155 mmol/L.
- Patients with refractory ICP elevation can be treated by pentobarbital-induced coma.
- If medical management of increased ICP is inadequate, move to surgical decompression (hemi- or bifrontal craniectomy).
- With a depressed skull fracture, indications for operation are: large underlying hematoma, neurologic deficit, break in the skin with gross contamination of wound, CSF leak, and location that will result to poor cosmetic outcome.

Suggested Reading

Choux M. Incidence, diagnosis, and management of skull fractures. In: Raimondi AJ, Choux M, editors. Head injuries in the newborn and infant. New York: Springer; 1986. p. 163–82.

Figaji A, Fieggen A, Argent A, LeRoux P, Peter J. Does adherence to treatment targets in children with severe traumatic brain injury avoid brain hypoxia? A brain tissue oxygenation study. Neurosurgery. 2008;63:83–92.

Hahn YS, Chyung C, Barthel MJ, Bailes J, Flannery AM, McLone DG. Head injuries in children under 36 months of age. Demography and outcome. Childs Nerv Sys. 1988;4:34–40.

Harwood-Nash DC, Hendrick EB, Hudson AR. The significance of skull fractures in children. A study of 1, 187 patients. Radiology. 1971;101:151–6.

Jagannathan J, Okonkwo D, Yeoh H, Dumont A, Saulle D, Haizlip J, et al. Long-term outcomes and prognostic factors in pediatric patients with severe traumatic brain injury and elevated intracranial pressure. J Neurosurg. 2008;2:240–9.

Reilly PL, Simpson DA, Sprod R, Thomas L. Assessing the conscious level in infants and young children: a paediatric version of the Glasgow Coma Scale. Child's Nervous System. 1988;4:30–3.

Stiefel MF, Udoetuk JD, Storm PB, Sutton LN, Kim H, Dominguez TE, et al. Brain tissue oxygen monitoring in pediatric patients with severe traumatic brain injury. J Neurosurg. 2006;105:281–6.

Stiver S, Manley G. Prehospital management of traumatic brain injury. Neurosurgical Focus. 1008;25:E5.

Chapter 16
Neck Injuries

Peter T. Masiakos and George C. Velmahos

Pediatric traumatic neck injuries are uncommon, occurring in less than 5% of trauma cases involving children. Despite their low frequency, they are associated with mortality rates approaching 10%. The management of such injuries can be challenging and continues to be debated. Injuries to the neck can be blunt or penetrating. Despite improvements in imaging technology and surgical care, neck injuries of either type continue to pose diagnostic and therapeutic challenges because a missed injury can result in significant morbidity and mortality. Unless the patient is hemodynamically unstable or an emergent surgical airway is required, blunt injuries to the neck are traditionally investigated using a variety of imaging modalities. Furthermore, the traditional and somewhat dogmatic *a priori* surgical exploration of penetrating neck injuries that violate the platysma has been challenged by many who advocate clinical paradigms that support a selective but methodical non-operative approach. No matter the paradigm, management of these injuries requires a systematic approach to assess for potential injury to the aerodigestive, nervous and vascular systems.

Blunt trauma to the neck typically results from forceful impact injuries. The most common causes in children are motor vehicle crashes and sports-related injuries. The mechanism is a direct blow to the neck either by a stationary object (steering wheel, seatbelt, dashboard) or a moving object in the form of fists, hands, feet, arms or sports equipment (sticks, bats, balls, pucks). Blunt forces applied to the anterior neck are likely to cause injuries to the larynx or trachea, however forces that severely hyperextend or rotate the neck can cause complete disruption of major blood vessels or, more commonly, an injury to the vascular intima leading to thrombosis. Neck injuries can also be broadly classified based on the nature of the weapon that was used to create them: *low velocity* or *high velocity* injuries. Each has a distinctive associated pattern of injury: injuries caused by stabbing mechanisms deliver significantly lower kinetic energy and tend to damage tissue in proximity to the injury, while injuries caused by a missile are defined by the velocity and mass of the object, which can cause injury to tissue remote to their trajectory. Location of the injury and knowledge of the structures that are proximate to the injury site and trajectory is of paramount importance in dealing with penetrating injuries.

Anatomy

The neck is invested by two major fascial layers: the superficial fascia (the platysma and its investing fascia) and the deep fascia, which invests the deeper muscles, the thoracic duct, blood vessels, nerves, glands, trachea and esophagus. For decades, clinical dogma has mandated the surgical exploration of any neck wound that has violated the platysma. Penetrating injuries that violated the deep fascia were approached differently depending on which anatomic zone was involved (Fig. 16.1, Table 16.1). Although a through knowledge of the location of major structures within these zones is important and should be used to direct the diagnostic approach to an injury, the blind approach of treating the patient simply according to which zone is involved has, for the most part, been abandoned. A more appropriate approach is to consider the trajectory of the missile in relation to the anatomy within the three zones. This individualized approach becomes important when considering the important "next steps" in the diagnostic paradigm and whether a patient should be taken directly to the operating room.

Diagnosis and Initial Management

As in other types of trauma, trauma to the neck should be managed according to Advanced Trauma Life Support (ATLS) standards. In most cases, a history and focused examination of the neck is enough to establish the diagnosis. For example, a history of significant hemorrhage at the scene

P.T. Masiakos (✉)
Department Pediatric Surgery, Pediatric Trauma Unit, 55 Fruit Street, Warren 1155, Boston, MA 02114, USA
e-mail: pmasiakos@partners.org

Fig. 16.1 Anatomic zones of the neck. (Modified with permission from Bee TK, Fabian TC. Penetrating neck trauma. In: Cameron JL, editor. Current Surgical Therapy, 7th ed. St Louis, Mosby, 2001.)

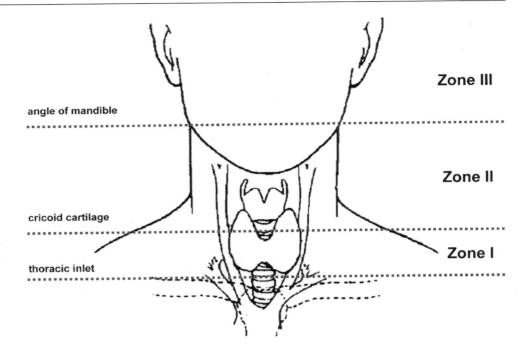

Table 16.1 The three zones of the neck, their anatomic borders and contents

Zone I: clavicle to inferior cricoid – includes the structures of the thoracic inlet contents

Vascular	Aerodigestive tract	Nerves
Proximal carotid artery	Esophagus	Brachial plexus
Subclavian artery	Trachea	Spinal cord
Vertebral artery		

Zone II: inferior cricoid to angle of mandible – most commonly injured (60–80%)

Vascular	Aerodigestive tract	Nerves
Carotid artery	Esophagus	Spinal cord
Vertebral artery	Larynx	Vagus nerve
Jugular vein	Trachea	Rec. Laryngeal nerve

Zone III: angle of mandible to base of skull

Vascular	Aerodigestive tract	Nerves
Distal internal carotid artery	Pharynx	Spinal cord
Vertebral artery	Parotid gland	

mandates a more thorough investigation of the vessels in a hemodynamically stable patient who has no hard signs of vascular injury. Finally, the mechanism of injury should be ascertained since identification of a blunt or penetrating mechanism would raise suspicion for certain injury patterns and may dictate the next steps in the diagnostic work up or surgery if the patient is unstable at any time.

First and foremost, the airway should be assessed and, if the patient is awake and alert, care should be taken to maintain a patent airway. If the patient is neurologically or hemodynamically unstable or unable to ventilate or oxygenate adequately, the airway should be secured by endotracheal

intubation or, if necessary, a cricothyroidotomy. The fiberoptic approach is ideal for intubation, although it might not be tolerated by a restless patient. In extreme circumstances, an endotracheal tube can be carefully placed through an open tracheal wound; however care must be taken not to completely disrupt the trachea, which can retract into the mediastinum. Large-bore intravenous access should be obtained. If the patient is exhibiting signs of a tension pneumothorax in the context of laryngeal of tracheal injuries, immediate decompression of the affected hemithorax must be performed. If active hemorrhage is identified, external compression should be applied and emergent but controlled surgical exploration of the neck should be undertaken.

If the patient is hemodynamically stable, a systematic review of the patient should be performed, otherwise operative exploration of the neck is mandated. The secondary survey should focus on associated and distracting injuries including closed head injuries. Chest and cervical spine radiographs might demonstrate a pneumothorax, pneumomediastinum, or subcutaneous air, which would be suggestive of an aerodigestive injury.

If a cervical collar is in place, it should be gently removed in order to allow evaluation of the neck (Table 16.2). The neck should be visualized and the cervical spine should be evaluated in the usual fashion. All bruises and wounds should be noted. Care should be taken to look for signs of potential vascular injuries, such as a pulsatile masses or expanding hematoma. Stridor, hoarseness, difficulty with phonation, and crepitance are each suggestive of a laryngotracheal injury. Hemoptysis is a sign of tracheal injury, whereas hematemesis is a sign of esophageal injury, although in an uncooperative patient with a mouth full of blood this distinction can be

Table 16.2 Signs of injury that call for immediate surgical exploration in most cases include

Signs of laryngeotracheal injury
 Voice alteration/hoarseness
 Drooling
 Hemoptysis
 Stridor
 Respiratory distress, dyspnea, tachypnea
 Decreased breath sounds/pneumothorax
 Sucking, hissing, or air frothing or bubbling through the neck wound
 Subcutaneous emphysema and/or crepitus
 Continuous air leak persisting after chest tube insertion
 Tracheal shift
Signs of heart or great vessel injury
 Hemorrhage
 Hemothorax
 Cervical or supraclavicular hematoma
 Bleeding from the entrance wound
 Cervical bruit/thrill
 Hypotension
 Pericardial tamponade
 Weak or absent carotid or brachial pulse
 Paradoxical pulse
 Upper extremity ischemia
 Contralateral hemiparesis
 Respiratory distress secondary to tracheal compression
 Decreased level of consciousness or coma
Signs of pharyngeoesophageal injury
 Dysphagia
 Bloody saliva, bloody nasogastric aspirate
 Sucking neck wound
 Pain and tenderness in the neck
 Resistance of neck with passive motion testing
 Crepitus

difficult to make. The most commonly encountered neurological injuries include unilateral upper extremity deficits (brachial plexus), hoarseness (recurrent laryngeal nerve), Horner's syndrome (stellate ganglion), elevated hemidiaphragm (phrenic nerve), or paralysis (spinal cord). It is important to document such injuries before any intervention is undertaken to prevent an allegation that nerve damage was iatrogenic.

Operative Technique

It is critical for the surgeon to know when a patient with a neck injury needs to have an emergency operation. This includes any patient who is hemodynamically unstable, and the hemodynamically stable patient with "hard signs" of injury: (a) active bleeding, large or expanding hematoma, or evolving stroke, which are indicative of a major vascular injury; (b) sucking neck wound, which suggests an injury to the pharynx or esoph-

agus; or (c) bubbling of air through the wound or subcutaneous emphysema, which are signs of a laryngotracheal injury.

Vascular Injuries

Not every vascular injury in the neck needs surgical repair. Jugular venous injuries usually result in significant bleeding but will sometimes tamponade on their own. If it is not actively bleeding, there is little reason to uncover such an injury. However, when bleeding persists despite gentle pressure, direct suturing of the venous defect is the preferred method of repair. Although ligation of one jugular vein is usually well tolerated, simultaneous ligation of both is potentially catastrophic and should be avoided.

Penetrating carotid artery injuries usually require surgical repair, but not all are accessible. Primary repair or placement of a graft can be performed either with or without the use of a stent, according to individual conditions. The management of blunt carotid injuries, on the other hand, is a matter of some debate. Surgical exploration is often difficult for several reasons: (a) they usually involve the internal carotid artery above the bifurcation, (b) the distal extent of the injury is unknown and might be intracranial, and (c) there is sometimes significant associated brain injury or fixed neurologic deficits at the time of diagnosis. In adults, repair of surgically accessible injuries that have not produced neurologic deficits is recommended. Percutaneous placement of a stent is an alternative but there are no long-term data. In children, the administration of anticoagulation or antiplatelet agents has been shown to decrease embolic events by 60% and is recommended as long as there is no other risk factor for bleeding. Finally, there are patients who have blunt carotid injuries that are surgically inaccessible (high carotid injuries) or who have significant injuries that preclude anticoagulation and are simply observed.

Penetrating injuries of the vertebral artery are very difficult to manage when they are bleeding freely, which happens uncommonly. Operations that include opening of the vertebral canal and direct ligation of the artery have been described but are rarely performed. In such circumstances the best course of action is usually to perform a damage-control operation (insertion of a foley balloon into the hole, packing of the neck, leaving the wound open) and take the patient urgently to the Interventional Radiology suite for embolization.

Blunt vertebral artery injuries are the subject of some debate as well. Most defects are managed by anticoagulation or antiplatelet therapy, or, if these are contraindicated, careful observation. Surgical embolization of an injured vertebral artery is an option if contralateral blood supply and a complete circle of Willis are confirmed angiographically and if there is a defect that is considered a potential nidus for an embolic event. Surgical repair of blunt vertebral arteries is almost never appropriate.

Pharyngo-Esophageal Injuries

Pharyngeal injuries can usually be managed nonoperatively. The dense layer of overlapping muscles at the pharyngeal level creates an optimal environment for fast healing. If a leak occurs, this is usually contained in the neck and can easily be drained percutaneously or by open incision.

Injuries below the level of the sixth cervical vertebrae can involve the esophagus. The soft tissue planes around the esophagus are more delicate and a leak can easily result in mediastinitis and life-threatening sepsis. We recommend surgical exploration for all esophageal injuries. Primary repair of the injury is adequate in almost all cases. Esophageal exclusion or a directed fistula by placing of a foley catheter inside the wound are surgical options reserved only for very extensive wounds or cases with delayed presentation. Unfortunately, delayed presentation is not uncommon, particularly in the developing world. This is because an esophageal injury can be very subtle at first, often associated with minor signs and symptoms, such as a very small quantity of extraluminal air on the plain film or mild odynophagia. The result of a missed diagnosis is neck abscess, esophago-cutaneous fistula or, in the worst cases, mediastinitis and sepsis.

Standard surgical practices (drainage and wound management) can be applied when treating a patient with a localized infectious process. Patients with an uncontrolled leak or frank sepsis require more aggressive attempts to control the soilage, including diversion or complex drainage procedures designed to create a controlled fistula.

Laryngotracheal Injuries

These injuries are rarely subtle. Active bubbling of the wound and major subcutaneous emphysema, often accompanied by hemoptysis, are the hallmarks of injury. Although small wounds have been managed non-operatively, most tracheal injuries mandate immediate intervention. Exploration can be performed through a lateral incision along the anterior border of the sternocleidomastoid muscle or a collar incision, if a through-and-through injury is suspected. There are no universal guidelines for the routine use of tracheostomy to protect a primary repair of a tracheal injury. As a general rule, small injuries can be repaired primarily without an additional procedure, while large injuries and those associated with extensive local tissue damage are usually more safely managed by performing a tracheostomy in addition to the primary repair. In the presence of difficult injuries, for example those involving the membranous portion of the trachea, we have performed tracheostomy only, without attempting a repair. The cuff is inflated below the level of injury and in all cases healing of the injury was uneventful.

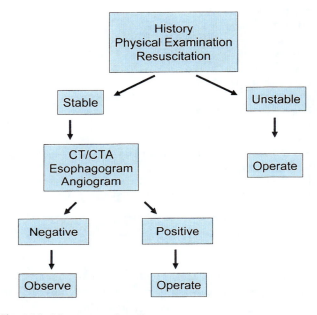

Fig. 16.2 Management flow diagram

Summary Points

- Pediatric traumatic neck injuries are uncommon but are associated with mortality rates approaching 10%.
- Unstable patients with hard signs of vascular or aerodigestive injury should be managed operatively.
- Stable patients with possible injuries should be further evaluated (Fig. 16.2).
- Esophageal injuries are rare and often present in a completely asymptomatic patient, going unnoticed for days.
- Esophageal injuries should be excluded by standard imaging practices in the context of a penetrating injury to the neck.
- The blind approach of treating the patient simply according to which zone is involved has for the most part been abandoned.
- A systematic diagnostic approach that considers the possibility of injury to major blood vessels, the esophagus, and the airway is the preferred approach

Editor's Comment

Neck injuries have been traditionally associated with a significant concern over missed injuries and aggressive attempts to exclude injuries with invasive diagnostic procedures and the frequent use of surgical exploration. Recent advances in medical imaging have helped to minimize both missed injuries as well as iatrogenic trauma. Based on the mechanism and a thorough physical assessment for soft signs of injury to the vascular and aerodigestive structures of the neck, one can now use Doppler US, CT, CT angiography, or MRI to produce accurate and detailed images of the complex anatomy of the neck.

It is becoming increasingly common to detect intimal injuries of the carotid artery after blunt trauma or deceleration injuries of the neck. Most are minor (slight irregularity, small thrombus) and can be managed safely with anticoagulation and follow-up angiography. More serious injuries (transections, pseudo-aneurysms, significant occlusive thrombus) should be treated surgically. If the vessel is inaccessible or completely occluded by thrombus, the patient is probably best treated with anticoagulation. Consultation with an experienced interventional radiologist is critical as endovascular techniques such as stenting or embolization of smaller vessels might be available options.

The surgical approach in children is usually best done through a transverse incision in one of the skin creases, though occasionally a traditional oblique carotid incision is necessary. The exposure should be generous and all structures should be dissected carefully to avoid iatrogenic nerve injury. The thigh should be sterilely prepared in case saphenous vein graft is needed. If the patient is stable, a brief rigid bronchoscopy and esophagoscopy before intubation can be very useful and should be part of the standard surgical approach in most cases. Vocal cord position and movement should be documented before exploration is undertaken. Vascular injuries are treated using standard principles such as proximal and distal control and direct suture repair. Patch repairs should be done with autologous vein. The external jugular vein can be used but needs to be doubled (by eversion) to prevent aneurysm in the long term. Postoperative anticoagulation or aspirin therapy should be considered for complex repairs.

Most pharyngeal or cervical esophageal injuries can be treated nonoperatively or with simple drainage, though associated airway injury needs to be excluded. Airway injuries can usually be treated with simple direct repair, but intra-operative control of the airway can be treacherous and requires coordination with the anesthesiologist and a carefully planned approach, including consideration of fall-back positions in the event of an airway catastrophe. A multi-disciplinary approach that includes a vascular surgeon who specializes in adults, otolaryngologist, neurosurgeon or oral surgeon should also be considered.

Diagnostic Studies

- Vascular injuries
- CT arteriogram
- Arteriography
- Pharyngeoesophageal injuries
- CT esophagogram
- Contrast esophagogram
- Laryngotracheal injuries
- Plain radiographs of the neck and chest
- CT scan of the neck and chest
- Bronchoscopy

Suggested Reading

Bee TK, Fabian TC. Penetrating neck trauma. In: Cameron JL, editor. Current surgical therapy. 7th ed. St Louis: Mosby; 2001. p. 1170–4.

Thal ER. Injury to the neck. In: Feliciano DV, Moore EE, Mattox KL, editors. Trauma. 3rd ed. Connecticut: Appleton and Lange; 1996. p. 329–44.

Gonzalez RP et al. Penetrating zone II neck injuries: does dynamic computed tomographic scan contribute to the diagnostic sensitivity of physical examination for surgically significant injury? A Prospective Blinded Study. J Trauma. 2003;54(1):61–5.

Demetriades D et al. Complex problems in penetrating neck trauma. Surg Clin Am. 1996;76(4):661–83.

Demetriades D et al. Penetrating injuries of the neck. In: Shoemaker WC, Ayers SM, Grenvik A, Holbrook PR, editors. Textbook of critical care. Philadelphia: WB Saunders Company; 1999.

Chapter 17
Burns

Gail E. Besner

Thermal injuries are a cause of significant morbidity and mortality in the pediatric population. Each year, approximately 440,000 children receive medical treatment for burns in the United States, among whom over 75,000 require hospitalization, 10,000 suffer severe permanent disability, and 2,500 eventually die. Recent advances in the care of the critically burned patient and the use of an aggressive multidisciplinary approach have led to significantly improved outcomes.

The etiology of pediatric thermal injury includes scald burns, flame burns, burns from contact with a hot object, electrical burns, and chemical burns. Scald burns due to household accidents or child abuse account for two-thirds of pediatric burns and are the most common type of burns seen in children under the age of 3. In older children and teenagers, flame burns become more common. Since 10–20% of child abuse cases present as burns, abuse must always be excluded. Clues to child abuse include evidence of other injuries, a history that is inconsistent with observed injuries, a conflicting story from parents and child, a history of prior injuries or abuse, a delay in medical attention, and the presence of bilateral, symmetrical burns (stocking-glove distribution).

Diagnosis

Diagnostic dilemmas in burn care mainly relate to the ability to determine the severity of the burn. The severity of a burn is directly related to its depth and the percent of total body surface area (%TBSA) involved. Burn depth is generally classified as partial-thickness or full-thickness. Partial-thickness burns are further divided into superficial partial-thickness burns and deep partial-thickness burns (Table 17.1). Determination of burn depth is important since it directly impacts the likelihood of the need for skin grafting. It is important to note that

children less than 2 years of age have especially thin skin, which means burns that initially appear partial-thickness might actually turn out to be full-thickness.

There are three ways to calculate the %TBSA burned in children: (1) The pediatric rule of nines (Fig. 17.1) provides a quick estimate of the area involved. This is an adaptation of the adult rule of nines, but takes into consideration the fact that the head is relatively larger in children (18% in young children compared to 9% in adults) and the lower extremities are relatively smaller (14% in young children compared to 18% in adults). (2) Lund and Browder charts (Fig. 17.2) are the most accurate method of determining area burned. These charts more precisely detail the %TBSA represented by each area of the body according to the age of the patient. (3) Estimation using the size of the patient's palm (approximately ½ %TBSA) is useful for multiple small, scattered burns.

Upon initial examination, it is important to determine whether the patient needs to be hospitalized or can be treated as an outpatient. Admission criteria generally include: partial-thickness burns greater than 10% TBSA; full-thickness burns greater than 2% TBSA; concomitant inhalation injury; significant burns of face, hands, genitalia, perineum, or feet; circumferential burns; burns over major joints; most electrical burns; chemical burns; all burns caused by child abuse; burns in patients with pre-existing medical disorders that could complicate management, prolong recovery or affect mortality; and cases in which it is determined that it is in the best interest to admit the child (parental inability to care for the burn). In children with major burns, consideration should be made for transferring the patient to a pediatric burn center with special expertise in the complex management of these critically ill patients.

Treatment

As with any trauma patient at initial presentation, rapid assessment and treatment of immediately life-threatening conditions are carried out: an airway is established, breathing is maintained, circulation is assessed and supported.

G.E. Besner (✉)
Department of Surgery, Ohio State University College of Medicine,
Nationwide Children's Hospital, 700 Children's Drive, Columbus,
OH 433205, USA
e-mail: besnerg@chi.osu.edu

P. Mattei (ed.), *Fundamentals of Pediatric Surgery*,
DOI 10.1007/978-1-4419-6643-8_17, © Springer Science+Business Media, LLC 2011

Table 17.1 Burn depth characteristics

Partial vs. full-thickness	Degree	Appearance of injury	Result
Partial thickness – very superficial Injury to epidermis only	First degree	Wounds are dry but extremely erythematous, painful	Heals spontaneously within a week without scarring
Partial thickness – superficial Injury to epidermis and superficial dermis	Second degree	Ruptured weeping blisters, erythematous, painful	Heals spontaneously within 2–3 weeks, usually without scarring
Partial thickness – deep Injury to epidermis and deeper dermis, but some viable dermis remains	Second degree	Wound appears whiter and less erythematous as depth into dermis increases. May be hard to distinguish from full-thickness burns initially	Heals spontaneously but often after 3–4 weeks. Degree of hypertrophic scarring related to length of time needed for re-epithelialization
Full thickness Injury to epidermis and entire dermis	Third degree	White, brown or black, leathery, insensate eschar	Will not heal (except for very small wounds that heal by contraction)

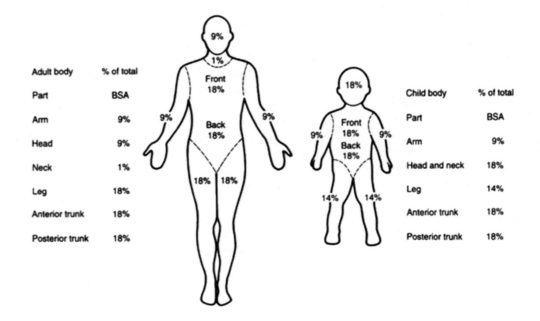

Fig. 17.1 Pediatric rule of nines (From Herndon DN, ed. Total burn care. London: WB Saunders; 1996, p. 35, with permission from Elsevier)

Endotracheal intubation is indicated in children with respiratory distress or airway compromise due to airway edema. The smaller diameter of the pediatric airway predisposes it to obstruction, so a low threshold for intubation should be maintained. Children with burns affecting more than 10% TBSA should receive intravenous fluid resuscitation. Attention must be paid to keeping the pediatric burn patient warm, since thermoregulation is made difficult by their greater body surface area and smaller muscle mass, and the inability of infants less than 6 months of age to shiver. During the secondary survey, a detailed history and physical exam should be performed. The burn wounds themselves initially need to be covered only with dry sterile sheets. Wet sheets or cooling packs should be avoided because this contributes to hypothermia. Tetanus immunization should be administered as needed.

Airway

Inhalation injury causes the majority of deaths in burn patients. Signs of potential inhalation injury include increased respiratory rate, hoarseness, a history of being burned in an enclosed space, altered mental status, head and neck burns, singed nasal hairs, inflamed oral mucosa, and carbonaceous sputum. Inhalation injury mandates endotracheal intubation, as does evidence of compromised upper airway patency, the need for ventilatory support as manifested by poor gas exchange or increased work of breathing, and compromised mental status. If in doubt, it is generally safer to intubate than to defer intubation, which can result in life-threatening occlusion of the small pediatric airway. In addition, since airway edema might not peak for 48 h, any suspicion of inhalation

Fig. 17.2 Lund and Browder chart (From Herndon DN, ed. Total Burn Care. London: WB Saunders; 1996, p. 36, with permission from Elsevier)

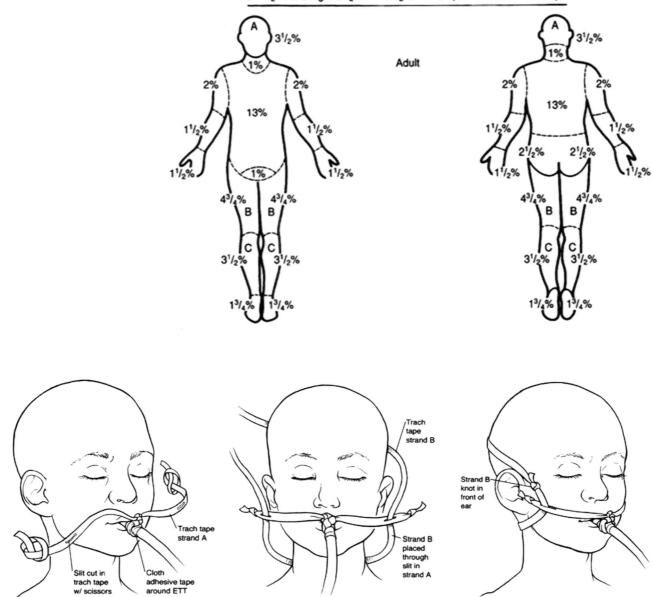

Age	0–1	1–4	5–9	10–14	15
A – ½ of head	9½%	8½%	6½%	5½%	4½%
B – ½ of one thigh	2¾%	3¼%	4%	4¼%	4½%
C – ½ of one leg	2½%	2½%	2¾%	3%	3¼%

Fig. 17.3 Endotracheal tube immobilization in children. The figure demonstrates a method using umbilical tape to secure a pediatric endotracheal tube in patients with facial burns. (Copyright 2003 A.S. Baker)

injury mandates, at minimum, admission for close observation. Regarding the pediatric airway, it is important to remember that in children the larynx is more cephalad and thus the glottis is more acute angulated, children with upper airway edema and alveolar-capillary block deteriorate faster than adults, and repeated intubation attempts cause edema and obstruction. Therefore, it is important to have experience in pediatric intubation and to avoid accidental dislodgement, especially in patients with facial burns, by securing the airway extremely well (Fig. 17.3).

Breathing

Exposure to carbon monoxide and cyanide is potentially fatal in patients with inhalation injury. CO has 250 times the affinity for Hgb as O_2, thereby shifting the Hgb–O_2 disassociation curve to left and impairing O_2 unloading at the tissue level. This causes a switch to anaerobic metabolism and severe metabolic acidosis. CO toxicity should be suspected when a metabolic acidosis persists despite adequate volume resuscitation. Remember that PaO_2 and O_2 saturation will be normal in the presence of CO toxicity. All patients with inhalation injury should therefore be treated with 100% inspired O_2, which reduces the half-life of CO from 4 to 1 h. Hyperbaric oxygen therapy (3 atm) leads to rapid displacement of CO in 20 min and should be considered for patients with CO levels greater than 50%, severe neurological compromise, and failure to respond to 100% O_2. The burning of natural materials such as wool, silk, cotton, and paper or synthetic products such as polyurethane, plastic, nylon, and acrylic produces hydrocyanide gas. Cyanide binds to the cytochrome oxidase system, inhibiting cellular metabolism and ATP production. It causes a shift to anaerobic metabolism, profound metabolic acidosis, and obtundation. Treatment includes the administration of sodium thiosulfate (8 g i.v. if <12 year, 12.5 g i.v. if >12 year), which converts cyanide to non-toxic, water-soluble, excretable thiocyanate. Therapy should not be delayed while awaiting the return of cyanide levels, which can take a long time to be reported.

Smoke inhalation can also induce airway inflammation, leading to microbial colonization, pneumonia and the need for ventilatory support. In severe cases, oscillator ventilation or even extracorporeal membrane oxygenation (ECMO) may be required.

Circulation

Thermal injury results in vasodilation and local edema. Patients with >30% TBSA burn also develop systemic edema. Children have nearly three times the body surface area-to-body mass ratio that adults have and fluid losses are proportionately higher. Consequently, children have relatively more evaporative water loss and greater fluid resuscitation requirements.

Fluid resuscitation begins with calculation of fluid needs. These formulas serve only to estimate fluid needs. Resuscitation should be continually revised based on the patient's response. Intravenous access may be obtained percutaneously or by cutdown, either peripherally or centrally. Peripheral access in an unburned area is preferred. Intra-osseous infusion is sometimes necessary and can be lifesaving in the severely burned patient (Fig. 17.4).

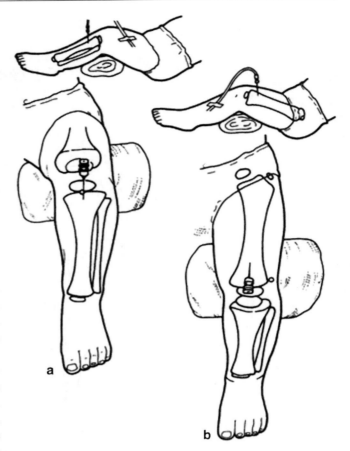

Fig. 17.4 Intraosseous line placement in the proximal tibia (**a**) and distal femur (**b**) (From Herndon DN, ed. Total Burn Care. London: WB Saunders; 1996, p. 354, with permission from Elsevier)

There are several burn resuscitation formulas that can be used in pediatric burn care, including the Parkland formula, which is modified for small children (Table 17.2). In children who weigh more than 20 kg, the Parkland formula can be used without modification to calculate resuscitation fluids. In children who weigh less than 20 kg, the formula is modified to include the addition of maintenance fluids to take into account the larger body surface-to-mass ratio and larger fluid losses. One half of the calculated fluid needs are administered in the first 8 h after injury, and the remaining half is administered over the next 16 h. The resuscitation fluid commonly used is Ringer's lactate solution. Since young children are susceptible to hypoglycemia due to their smaller liver glycogen reserves, maintenance fluids should be administered as Ringer's Lactate solution with 5% dextrose. The administration of pre-hospital fluids must be taken into account. If pre-hospital fluid resuscitation is inadequate, the fluid deficit must be added to the fluid rate calculated for the first 8 h of resuscitation. Note that these calculations should be based on the %TBSA of second and third degree burns only. Most importantly, rates of fluid administration are altered according to the patient's response.

Table 17.2 Pediatric fluid resuscitation guidelines

Weight <20 kg	Weight ≥20 kg
Modified Parkland formula (Parkland formula plus maintenance fluids):	Parkland formula:
Resuscitation fluids: 3–4 mL RL × weight (kg) × %TBSA burned (2 and 3 degree) 1/2 in first 8 h (from time of injury)[a] remaining 1/2 in next 16 h	*Resuscitation fluids*: 3–4 mL RL × weight (kg) × %TBSA burned (2 and 3 degree) 1/2 in first 8 h (from time of injury)[a] remaining 1/2 in next 16 h
Maintenance fluids: D5 RL: 4 mL/kg/h for 0–10 kg + 2 mL/kg/h for 10–20 kg + 1 mL/kg/h for each kg > 20 kg	

[a]Pre-hospital fluids must be taken into account. If pre-hospital fluid resuscitation is inadequate, the fluid deficit must be added to the fluid rate calculated for the first 8 h of resuscitation

RL Ringer's lactate solution; *D5 RL* Ringer's lactate solution with 5% dextrose

The response to fluid administration in the pediatric burn patient is best assessed by measurement of urine output via an indwelling urinary catheter, which should always be placed in patients with burns >15% TBSA. For major burns, fluid resuscitation needs to be reassessed at least hourly. In children weighing less than 30 kg, urine output should be 1 mL/kg/h. In children weighing greater than 30 kg, a urine output of 30–50 mL/h should be maintained. Adequacy of resuscitation is also assessed by monitoring mental status, blood pH, and peripheral perfusion.

Temperature Regulation

Children younger than 2 years have thin layers of skin and insulating subcutaneous tissue. As a result, they lose more heat and water, and they lose these more rapidly. In very young children, temperature regulation is partially based on nonshivering thermogenesis, which further increases metabolic rate, oxygen consumption, and lactate production. Hypothermia in the pediatric burn patients should be avoided by paying careful attention to increasing the room temperature, minimizing exposure time, and using radiant warmers and fluid warmers.

Systemic Antibiotics

Prophylactic systemic antibiotics are not used in the treatment of burn patients since this increases the risk of infection with resistant organisms. Instead, systemic antibiotics should be used to treat specific infections and administered at the first sign of clinical infection. Antibiotic regimens are then modified as culture results and antimicrobial sensitivity results become available. Burn wound cellulitis refers to infection spreading in dermal lymphatics in the non-burned skin surrounding a burn, usually occurring in the first few days after burn injury. Burn cellulitis is commonly caused by *Streptococcus pyogenes*. Invasive burn wound sepsis leads to systemic toxicity with high fever, bacteremia, and a hyperdynamic circulatory state with hypotension and cardiovascular collapse. Diagnosis can be made by either clinical examination, or by quantitative burn wound cultures or burn wound histology. Clinical signs include a change in the appearance of the burn in the patient with signs of toxicity. The burn may demonstrate punctuate hemorrhages, new drainage, changes in color, or wound liquefaction. Treatment should be based on clinical diagnosis so as not to delay therapy while cultures or histology are pending. Treatment includes parenteral antibiotics, aggressive resuscitation, and burn wound excision with temporary allografting.

Laboratory Studies

Monitoring of electrolytes and blood counts is often helpful, especially with large burns requiring aggressive fluid resuscitation. Carboxyhemoglobin levels are important in patients with inhalation injury, especially those burned in an enclosed space. Pre-albumin levels should be monitored weekly in patients with >20% TBSA burns. Pediatric burn patients typically spike fevers until the burn is healed. Fever workups with each temperature spike would be excessive, however one or two complete fever workups (including CBC with differential, urinalysis, CXR, and cultures of blood, urine, and sputum) should be obtained. Burn wound swab cultures may be obtained but do not definitively diagnose burn wound sepsis. Most burn wounds will become colonized with bacteria within a few days of hospitalization though the burns are not truly infected. If invasive burn wound sepsis is suspected (clinical deterioration, change in the appearance of the burn, odor to the burn) the diagnosis can be confirmed by performing quantitative burn wound cultures, in which a small piece of the burn tissue is excised at the bedside (at least 1 g of tissue is required) and the microbiology laboratory is alerted that quantitative wound cultures are required. Invasive burn wound sepsis is defined as more than 10^5 organisms/g of tissue. An alternative method is burn wound biopsy with histologic examination showing viable tissue being invaded by bacteria.

Wound Care

Devitalized skin and ruptured blisters should be debrided. Topical antibiotic therapy should be used to delay bacterial colonization. Silver sulfadiazine cream (Silvadene) is a commonly used broad-spectrum topical antimicrobial cream. It is applied as a thin layer with gauze dressings twice daily. It can cause transient neutropenia, which resolves even with continued use of the agent. If burn wound sepsis occurs or is suspected, mafenide cream (Sulfamylon) should be used instead due to its more active penetrating ability. Facial burns are usually treated with an antimicrobial ointment, or an immunomodulating cream such as beta-Glucan (a cream containing complex carbohydrate isolated from the cell wall of oats). Use of silver sulfadiazine cream on the central face is avoided because it can cause severe ocular irritation. Ear burns should be treated with the more potent Sulfamylon cream because the thin subcutaneous tissue in the ears predisposes to the development of chondritis.

Hydrotherapy provides wound and body cleansing with gentle removal of loose eschar and topical ointments, but should be limited to 15-min daily sessions to decrease promotion of infection. Topical enzyme preparations that contain papain and urea (Accuzyme) or collagenase (Santyl) can accelerate debridement of devitalized tissue without injury to viable tissue, allowing for earlier assessment of a clean wound bed and more rapid re-epithelialization.

To avoid the need for painful dressing changes, artificial skin substitutes, such as Aquacel Ag, may be used for the treatment of partial-thickness burns. Aquacel Ag is a hydrofiber dressing in which antibacterial silver (Ag⁺) ions are incorporated into the dressing and released in a sustained-release fashion for continuous topical antimicrobial effects. The fibers in the dressing hydrate upon contact with the burn surface creating a viscous gel that prevents fluid loss and traps bacteria. Aquacel Ag usually becomes adherent to the burn surface within 24–48 h and can be left in place for up to 2 weeks, during which time epithelialization is usually complete (Fig. 17.5). If epithelialization is not complete by that time, the Aquacel Ag can be reapplied. Its use eliminates the painful twice daily dressing changes associated with standard dressings, and, once it adheres to the burn, pain is virtually eliminated. Other temporary biological skin substitutes, such as EZ-Derm (porcine xenograft), can be used in a similar fashion to treat partial-thickness burns.

Escharotomy

Escharotomy is sometimes needed to relieve vascular compromise (extremity escharotomy) or ventilatory impairment (chest wall escharotomy). Vascular compromise to an extremity is the result of circumferential burns that create an inelastic eschar. Although vascular compromise usually occurs in extremities affected by full-thickness burns, it can occur in areas of partial-thickness burns, or occasionally in non-burned extremities. If left untreated, underlying tissue edema results in impaired venous outflow, followed by impaired tissue perfusion, and eventually diminished arterial

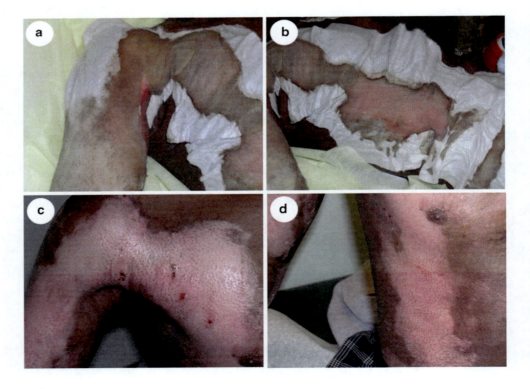

Fig. 17.5 Aquacel® Ag use in partial thickness burn. (**a, b**) Appearance of Aquacel® Ag adherent to the burn on post-burn day 3; (**c, d**) Healed burn on post-burn day 10. The Aquacel® Ag has separated from the burn which is totally re-epithelialized

inflow. All extremity burns at risk should be monitored with at minimum hourly vascular checks of palpable or audible Doppler pulses. Decreased pulses, direct measurement of compartment pressures with pressures >40 mmHg, or clinical symptoms (severe pain, paresthesias, decreased motor function) necessitate extremity escharotomy. One should not wait for loss of pulses to immediately treat this condition, for by that time neurovascular damage is already occurring.

The chest wall and lungs are more compliant in the child compared to the adult. The child may therefore become rapidly exhausted by the edema and restriction of a circumferential chest wall burn. Impaired ventilation, with progressive increase in ventilatory requirements, signal the need for chest wall escharotomy.

Escharotomy is typically performed in areas of full-thickness injury and therefore analgesics are not needed. The procedure can be performed at the bedside or in the operating room. Incisions can be made with a scalpel, but, if available, the electrocautery device is preferable. Extremity escharotomy is begun with a longitudinal incision medially or laterally in the extremity, beginning above the burned area and extending below the inferior aspect of the burn (Fig. 17.6). The incision is carried down to the subcutaneous fat, which bulges into the wound once an adequate incision is made. Medial and lateral incisions in the extremity are typically required. Adequate escharotomy should produce return of arterial pulses. Chest wall escharotomy is performed with incisions along the anterior axillary lines bilaterally, extending onto the abdomen, with transverse bridging incisions across the chest (Fig. 17.6). Adequate chest wall escharotomy should result in immediate improvement of lung compliance and ventilation.

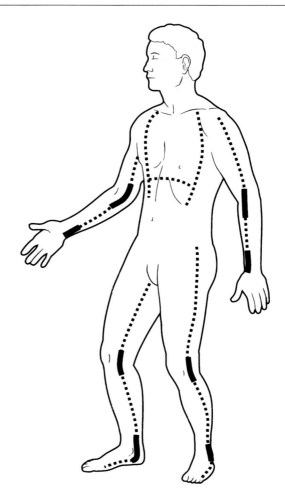

Fig. 17.6 Location of escharotomy sites. The *dotted lines* show the preferred incision sites. The *solid lines* emphasize the importance of extending the incisions across the joints (From Carrougher GJ, ed. Burn Care and Therapy. St. Louis: Mosby; 1998, p. 234, with permission from Elsevier)

Nutrition

Maximizing caloric intake is extremely important to ensure optimal burn wound healing. Adequate nutrition blunts the typical injury-induced hypermetabolic response and hypercatabolism, and prevents loss of muscle mass and depletion of fat stores. Protein and energy are important for new collagen synthesis and to help maintain visceral protein stores for optimal immune function. Nutritional support should be started as soon as possible, preferably within the first 24 h of admission. Enteral feeds are usually best. A high-calorie, high-protein formula is used and may include commercial supplemental beverages as needed. Vitamin and mineral supplementation, including especially vitamin C and zinc, is also important. If oral intake does not meet nutritional demands, a nasogastric or nasojejunal feeding tube should be placed. Calorie counts should be recorded by a dietitian, and daily weights obtained. If the enteral route is not feasible or unable to provide an adequate number of calories, then total or supplemental parenteral nutrition should be instituted.

Chemical Burns, Electrical Burns and Frostbite

Chemical burns in children are treated as in adults. Contaminated clothing is removed, powdered chemicals are brushed off the skin, and the contaminated area should be irrigated with copious amounts of water for at least 20 min and until the patient experiences a decrease in pain in the wound. Chemical injuries to the eye are treated by forcing the eyelid open and flushing the eye with water or saline. With gasoline injuries, the petroleum products may cause severe full-thickness cutaneous tissue damage, and absorption of the hydrocarbon may cause pulmonary, hepatic or renal failure.

Electrical burns in children include low voltage injuries (<1,000 V) and high voltage injuries (>1,000 V). Examples of low voltage injuries include injuries that result from biting an electrical cord, placing an object into a wall socket, and contacting a live wire or appliance indoors. High voltage injuries are usually due to contact with a live wire outdoors or being struck by lightning. Children who have sustained high voltage electrical injury need admission to the ICU, with cardiac monitoring, serial electrocardiograms and determination of CPK, urinalysis and urine myoglobin levels. Myoglobinuria or hemoglobinuria should be treated with aggressive hydration, osmotic diuretics and alkalinization of the urine to avoid renal failure. Extremities need to be monitored carefully for the development of compartment syndromes, and fasciotomy carried out as needed. Many patients who have sustained low voltage injury can be treated as an out-patient if: (1) there is absence of cardiac dysfunction, loss of consciousness or a history of tetany or wet skin during the accident, (2) the patient remains asymptomatic after 4 h of observation, (3) the cutaneous wounds can be managed appropriately, and (4) the patient can return for a wound check the following day. Parents of patients with oral commissure burns need to be instructed in the application of pressure to the lip in the event that the burn erodes into the labial artery, a complication that can develop several days after the injury.

Frostbite usually involves the ears, nose, hands, or feet, and results from prolonged exposure to severe cold. Ice crystal formation in the tissues results in cellular dehydration. Venous dilation and arterial vasoconstriction result in peripheral blood pooling and tissue necrosis. Signs and symptoms include red, blue or pale skin, a prickling sensation with superficial frostbite, painless rigid skin with deep frostbite, and functional impairment. Treatment involves placing the patient in a warm environment, removing articles of clothing from the affected region, and rewarming the area by immersion in water at 100–105°F, for up to 45 min. Dry heat and massage should be avoided.

Preoperative Preparation

Successful burn wound management in children demands conversion of open wounds to closed wounds as soon as possible. The concept of early removal of burn eschar and immediate wound closure to decrease the incidence of invasive burn wound sepsis has gained widespread acceptance. Evidence suggests that early eschar removal is effective in decreasing morbidity and improving survival. With the exception of very small injuries that are allowed to heal by contraction, full-thickness burns should be grafted. The goal

is to excise the wound within 7 days of the injury. Additionally, deep partial-thickness burns that take more than 3 weeks to heal usually benefit from grafting, with less hypertrophic scarring and a better cosmetic result.

Preoperative patients must be hemodynamically stable and have optimal acid–base, fluid and electrolyte balance. Adequate blood must be available for transfusion prior to excision and grafting. A prophylactic dose of a first-generation cephalosporin antibiotic is generally administered in the operating room. Attention to maintenance of body temperature is extremely important.

Surgical Technique

Burn excision involves serial tangential removal of thin layers of devitalized tissue until profuse pinpoint bleeding from a healthy, well-vascularized wound bed is observed, usually in the subcutaneous fat. Meticulous hemostasis is then obtained using epinephrine-soaked (1:100,000) sponges, topical spray thrombin, and electrocautery, followed by immediate grafting with thin sheets of autograft. Skin grafting involves harvesting partial-thickness autografts from donor sites on unburned areas using a dermatome. The thickness of the harvested skin commonly is 0.008–0.012 in., depending on the age and skin thickness of the patient. Meshed autografts are harvested from the donor sites and then passed through a meshing machine that cuts a series of parallel offset slits in the grafts at various expansion ratios (1:1, 2:1, 3:1, 4:1, etc.). This technique allows expansion of the graft to cover a larger surface area. In addition, the interstices in the graft allow for drainage of fluids under the graft so that the grafts do not lift off their beds. Unfortunately, the meshed patterns of the graft persist after healing and often lead to suboptimal cosmetic results. Non-meshed, or sheet grafts, are harvested from the donor sites in the same way, but are not passed through a meshing machine. The use of sheet grafts leads to a better cosmetic result, however, since the grafts cannot be expanded, it is difficult to cover large areas of injury with sheet grafts alone. Nonetheless, sheet grafts should be used in highly visible and functional areas, such as the face, neck, hands, and over joints. Though meticulous attention to hemostasis should be utilized in all grafting procedures, it is particularly important with sheet grafts. The harvested grafts are then applied to the wound bed and secured in place. This usually involves stapling the grafts, but small grafts can be secured by suturing with absorbable sutures. Bulky dressing with the addition of splints if grafts cross joints are critical to ensure immobilization of the grafts in the early post-operative period.

Autografts are always preferred but for very large burns sufficient donor skin may not be available. In these cases, burns can be excised and temporarily covered with one of several commercially available biological dressings (allografts, xenografts) or skin substitutes. As autograft donor sites become available, the temporary wound coverings are removed and the wounds regrafted. Growth hormone (0.15–0.2 mg/kg/day) administered intramuscularly appears to speed donor site healing, allowing more rapid reharvesting of healed donor sites.

Postoperative Care

Sheet grafts should be inspected after approximately 48 h so that any underlying fluid can be aspirated to avoid loss of the graft. For meshed grafts, dressings can be left in place for up to 5 days if desired, as long as the suspicion for infection is low. Dressings are usually changed daily thereafter.

Complications

Complications in the immediate post-operative period include bleeding, infection and graft loss. If infection is suspected, dressings should be changed to include broad-spectrum aqueous Sulfamylon solution. Invasive infection and bacteremia should be treated with appropriate systemic antibiotics. Bleeding from freshly excised wounds or under grafts can be prevented by maintaining meticulous hemostasis in the operating room and avoiding coagulopathy with good nutrition and, if necessary, supplementation with exogenous clotting factors.

Long-term complications mainly involve scar hypertrophy and contracture formation. As these can be quite challenging to deal with once they are established, it is advisable to initiate preventive measures early in the course of therapy.

For burns that are grafted or take longer than 3 weeks to heal, hypertrophic scarring can be minimized with the use of compression therapy. Custom-made garments that apply 25–30 mmHg pressure to all wounds usually work best. Gel pads can be used underneath or sewn into the garments, to apply extra compression. Compression therapy is continued throughout the wound healing process (12–18 months). Application of emollients with massage therapy helps to keep grafted areas soft and supple.

Contractures are scars that impair joint function or range of motion. Aggressive occupational and physical therapy is necessary to ensure optimal results. Active and passive range of motion exercises are instituted early and splints are worn at night and between exercise periods. Burn patients at risk for contractures are followed for years to monitor for the development of these complications.

Burn injuries can lead to significant psychological sequelae and the assistance of a trained psychologist or psychiatrist is an important addition to the overall care of these patients.

Recent Advances

There is a great deal of ongoing clinical and basic science research in the areas of burn physiology and treatment. One such area of interest is the hypermetabolic response to severe burns and the observation that patients have significantly increased energy expenditure and muscle-protein catabolism despite appropriate nutritional support. These studies are promising because attenuation of muscle-protein losses may improve strength and accelerate recovery.

A recent prospective, randomized, controlled trial of recombinant human growth hormone (rHGH) in combination with the beta-blocker propranolol demonstrated attenuated hypermetabolism and inflammatory and acute phase responses after severe burn injury. Human growth hormone improves post-traumatic hypermetabolism, but its use alone is associated with hyperglycemia, increased free fatty acids, and triglycerides. Concomitant administration of propranolol improves fat metabolism and insulin sensitivity and avoids the adverse effects of rHGH alone.

Another active area of research is in the development of cultured skin to treat very large burns. At present, cultured epidermal autografts, which are grown from the patient's own uninjured epidermis, are commonly used. However, these grafts are very thin and fragile. In the future, cultured bilayered skin (epidermis and dermis) should lead to better functional and cosmetic results.

Prognosis

Survival rates after burn injury have improved significantly, even in very young children. Improved survival can be attributed to refinements in resuscitation, intensive care, multidisciplinary management, and surgical techniques. In the past decade, the size of a survivable injury has increased from 70 to >95% BSA in children under 15 years of age. In the absence of severe inhalation injury, even children who are very young or who have large burns are expected to survive.

Summary Points

- Inhalation injury is the leading cause of death in pediatric burn patients.
- Child abuse comprises up to 10–20% of pediatric thermal injuries and must be ruled out.
- Due to the larger body surface area to mass ratio of children compared to adults, the modified Parkland formula, which adds maintenance fluids to resuscitation fluids, is used in the resuscitation of smaller children.
- Fluid resuscitation should be guided by the patient's response (urine output).
- Extremity escharotomy may be needed to prevent compartment syndrome, and chest escharotomy may be needed to prevent respiratory compromise.
- Recent developments of silver-impregnated sustained release dressings (e.g., Aquacel® Ag) have allowed for the treatment of partial-thickness burns in a nearly painless fashion.
- Recent advances in the care of the critically burned patient with use of an aggressive multidisciplinary approach have led to significantly improved outcomes in children.
- A multidisciplinary approach to burn care including participation of surgeons, nurses, occupational therapists, physical therapists, dieticians, play therapists, social workers, psychologists, and discharge planners, leads to the best outcome.

Editor's Comment

In addition to management of the physical injury and the ABCs of trauma care, care of the burned child demands careful consideration of many simultaneous and sometimes competing issues: social and legal concerns, the psychological and emotional care of the child, alleviating pain and anxiety, and, of course, ruling out other injuries. Making matters more difficult is the fact that for severely injured children, the care provided in our trauma bay is likely to be transitional as they need to be accepted from the first responders and safely prepared for transfer to a pediatric burn center. Transfers of care increase the risk of medical errors, increasing the importance that we maintain attention to detail and anticipate potential snags. One should never assume that the care provided at another institution or in the field was adequate: always check endotracheal tube position by auscultation and a chest X-ray, be sure that the cervical spine is properly immobilized, and perform a careful physical assessment yourself. Likewise, if the patient is being transferred, it is important to think ahead as to what will be needed on the receiving end: rather than applying cream or ointment, cover the burns with dry sterile dressings that can be easily removed for a proper assessment of the depth and extent of the injury; secure adequate intravenous access and hydrate the patient well; avoid long-acting muscle relaxants to allow an accurate assessment of neurologic status after transfer; be sure that copies of all films and medical records accompany the patient; and so on.

Silvadene has been the therapy of choice for many years, though many prefer to use patrolatum-based antibiotic ointments, which are transparent, keep the wounds moist, and do not need to be removed or washed off before every application. The antibiotic concentration in most topical antibiotic preparations is too high for use in the eye, so in little children, it is best to use ophthalmic-strength ointment for burns on the face or hands.

Diagnostic Studies

- Chest X-ray if inhalation injury is suspected
- Carboxyhemoglobin levels for suspected inhalation injury
- CBC, chemistry studies if significant fluid resuscitation required
- Fever workup (CBC; U/A; blood, urine, sputum, wound cultures) as clinically indicated
- Quantitative wound cultures or wound histology for suspected invasive burn wound sepsis

Parental Preparation

- Explanation of grafting procedure, location of donor sites, expected cosmetic result
- Possibility of complications including graft failure, infection, progression of partial-thickness burns to full-thickness burns
- Possibility of psychological sequelae related to scarring and post-traumatic stress

Preoperative Preparation

- ☐ Fluid resuscitation
- ☐ Prophylactic antibiotics
- ☐ Type and crossmatch
- ☐ Informed consent

Technical Points

- Always have sufficient blood available for intra-operative transfusion.
- Pay careful attention to preserving body temperature and avoiding hypothermia.
- Utilize measures to minimize blood loss (tourniquets, epinephrine solution, topical thrombin)
- Use sheet graphs when possible, especially on cosmetically and functionally sensitive areas such as the face, hands, and over joints.
- Pay careful attention to securing of grafts, preventing sheer stress on grafts, and avoiding build up of fluid or blood under grafts.

Suggested Reading

Jeschke MG, Finnerty CC, Kulp GA, Przkora R, Micak RP, Herndon DN. Combination of recombinant human growth hormone and propanolol decreases hypermetabolism and inflammation in severely burned children. Pediatr Crit Care Med. 2008;9:209–16.

Paddock H, Fabia R, Giles S, Hayes J, Lowell W, Besner G. A silver-impregnated antimicrobial dressing reduces hospital length of stay for pediatric burn patients. J Burn Care Res. 2007;28:409–11.

Sheridan RL. Sepsis in pediatric burn patients. Pediatr Crit Care Med. 2005;6:S112–9.

Sheridan RL, Schnitzer JJ. Management of the high-risk pediatric burn patient. J Pediatr Surg. 2001;36:1308–12.

Sheridan RL, Remensnyder JP, Schnitzer JJ, Schulz JT, Ryan CM, Tompkins RG. Current expectations for survival in pediatric burns. Arch Pediatr Adolesc Med. 2000;154:245–9.

Chapter 18
Abdominal Trauma

Michael L. Nance

Trauma is the leading cause of death and disability in the pediatric population. While head injuries are the most likely to be lethal, the abdomen is the most common sight of occult injury that results in death. The management of abdominal injuries has evolved in recent decades as non-operative strategies have been met with increasing success.

The initial approach to a child with trauma should begin with the standard American Trauma Life Support teachings, namely assessing airway, breathing and circulation. It is during the secondary survey that the abdomen is evaluated. Concern for an intra-abdominal injury might arise as a result of the clinical history, as part of the physical examination performed during the secondary survey, or both. Hemodynamically unstable patients with concern for an intra-abdominal source for hemorrhage are best managed in the operating room, however this represents a small proportion of the abdominal trauma population. The physiologic condition of most children undergoing evaluation allows for a thoughtful, but timely, evaluation.

There are anatomic differences between children and adults that make intra-abdominal injuries more likely. The intra-abdominal organs, especially the liver and spleen, are protected in the adult by the thoracic cage, but are proportionately larger in the child and can extend beyond the costal margin, exposing them to traumatic external forces. Because of increased compliance of the ribs, more energy is transmitted to the underlying structures and less diffused by fracture. Also, in the younger children, the abdominal wall musculature is less well developed and thus affords relatively little protection to the underlying internal organs.

There are several physical findings that should increase your index of suspicion for an abdominal injury. Notably, bruising of the abdomen (classic seatbelt sign or more subtle bruising of the abdominal wall) greatly increases the risk of intra-abdominal injury in the setting of a motor vehicle crash-related injury. As such, advanced imaging should be considered for these patients. Periumbilical ecchymosis (Cullen's sign) or flank ecchymosis (Grey-Turner's sign) should raise concern for intra-abdominal or retroperitoneal injury and the need for advanced imaging. Likewise, fractures of the lower ribs are indicative of significant force and should also raise concern for intra-abdominal injury.

After completion of the primary and secondary survey, a plan of care should be formulated for both global concerns as well as the abdomen. The need for laboratory and imaging studies should be considered. The routine use of laboratory studies in the evaluation of the patient with abdominal trauma remains controversial. Most studies have demonstrated limited utility to the use of laboratory studies such as liver function studies or amylase and lipase for routine screening. As a screening tool, they may better be reserved for selected cases, such as possible child abuse, in which the mechanism is uncertain and thus the level of suspicion for intra-abdominal injury less clear. In patients with real concerns for intra-abdominal injury, a CBC (a normal hemoglobin level may be falsely reassuring in the acute setting but important to follow over time) and serum electrolytes should be obtained. Urinalysis (or dip stick assessment for blood) should be performed as well. A specimen for type and crossmatch should also be strongly considered as guided by the clinical scenario. Other laboratory studies, (PT/PTT, Ca, PO_4) are utilized selectively but infrequently.

Intravenous access can be challenging in the pediatric patient but is of utmost importance. Ideally, two age-appropriate large-bore intravenous catheters should be placed in any patient with concerns for abdominal trauma. At least one of these catheters should be placed above the level of the diaphragm in case a major venous injury exists in the abdomen. In the unstable patient, limited attempts should be made at peripheral catheters before central venous access is obtained. Intraosseus lines should also be considered in young children (up to age 6 years, perhaps older) as a reliable initial access site. These lines can be used for volume and blood infusions as well as for medication administration. However, these lines are unstable and should be replaced with more durable sites as soon as feasible.

M.L. Nance (✉)
Department of Surgery, Children's Hospital of Philadelphia,
34th and Civic Center Boulevard, Philadelphia, PA 19104, USA
e-mail: nance@email.chop.edu

P. Mattei (ed.), *Fundamentals of Pediatric Surgery*,
DOI 10.1007/978-1-4419-6643-8_18, © Springer Science+Business Media, LLC 2011

Diagnosis

Imaging studies are commonly employed in the evaluation of the child with a suspected intra-abdominal injury. Plain films of the abdomen are typically of limited value but might demonstrate free air if a bowel perforation has occurred. Pelvic films may be useful in patients with a possible fracture, however, most such patients should be considered for computed tomography of the abdomen and pelvis, in which case the plain films are superfluous. The mainstay of evaluation of the pediatric abdomen for trauma is the CT scan, however the need for CT should always be questioned and the study obtained only if clinically indicated. The CT scan should include the abdomen and pelvis and should be performed with intravenous contrast enhancement. The ability to characterize solid organ injuries is greatly diminished without IV contrast. The utility of oral contrast in the trauma setting is still of some debate. We prefer to use oral contrast when safe (if a nasogastric tube is in place or if the subject is willing and able to drink) as it provides greater detail in evaluating the proximal bowel. Forcing oral contrast or placing an NG tube for the sole purpose of contrast administration should be discouraged. In the adult trauma population, ultrasound of the abdomen (FAST exam) has been widely embraced and utilized. The utility of FAST in the pediatric population is less clear. As most of our treatment algorithms are predicated on the grade of organ injury (rather than the presence or absence of free-fluid in the abdomen), FAST has been used only sparingly. However, FAST might be of value in determining if there is an evolving intra-abdominal process in hemodynamically unstable inpatients or in patients for whom transport to a CT scanner is deemed hazardous. Clinical deterioration of a trauma patient already in the operating room for other procedures (craniotomy) might also be an indication for FAST. In today's armamentarium of noninvasive studies, diagnostic peritoneal lavage is currently of limited value. DPL can be an alternative in selected clinical scenarios if FAST is unavailable.

Penetrating Injuries

Penetrating injuries account for 5–10% of trauma admissions in most major pediatric centers. In most cases, penetrating injuries to the abdomen generally warrant laparotomy after full completion of the ATLS-based evaluation and resuscitation. Determination of the trajectory is key in management of this population. Many patients with intra-abdominal injuries will have remote entrance wounds (thigh, buttock, or chest), and it is important to remember that 15% of children with an intra-abdominal injury will also have injuries to other body regions. Diagnostic imaging plays a vital role in trajectory determination and is also important in accounting for all projectiles: what appear to be entrance and exit wounds could in fact represent two entrance wounds.

Physical examination is, of course, necessary and, in conjunction with imaging, one can estimate the likelihood of internal injuries. Hemodynamic instability or clear evidence of peritonitis mandates urgent laparotomy, typically through a midline abdominal incision. In selected patients, a nonoperative strategy might be reasonable. Such an approach should only be considered in the hemodynamically stable patient with a trajectory that does not suggest major vascular injury or hollow visceral injury. The patient with a simple solid organ injury from a low-energy missile (stab wound) that is not actively bleeding can potentially be observed, but those having sustained a high-energy mechanism (gunshot wound) or in whom the trajectory is not clear need to be promptly explored. Though CT has been advocated for determining trajectory, clinical deterioration or evidence of peritonitis is an absolute indication for surgical exploration.

Laparoscopy can be used in patients whose extent of injury is unclear, such as when local wound exploration suggests minimal violation of the fascia or when CT findings suggests that the missile's trajectory was in proximity to vital structures. Indications for repair of penetrating organ injuries and conversion to laparotomy are the same in children as in adults. It is generally prudent to sterilely prepare the patient widely to include the chest and both lower extremities in case the laparotomy incision needs to be extended to include a thoracotomy or if autologous vein graft material is needed for vascular reconstruction. Available surgical techniques include: suture repair or partial resection of injured structures, control of active bleeding, judicious placement of closed suction drains, and, in the rare case of severe devitalizing injuries of the bowel or rectum with extensive peritoneal soilage, creation of a protective ileostomy or colostomy. In the stable patient, partial splenectomy is preferred over total splenectomy and drainage of a penetrating pancreatic injury is usually adequate and avoids prolonged and complicated repairs. In the unstable child with uncontrolled hemorrhage, salvage procedures that include packing the abdomen, temporary fascial closure, a period of resuscitation in the ICU and return to the operating room in 12–24 h for definitive repair are also acceptable and certainly preferred over heroic measures that ultimately fail.

Solid Organ Injuries

Over the last several decades, the management of solid organ injuries has evolved to a largely non-operative approach. Guided by early studies demonstrating the safety and efficacy of this approach for the management of splenic injuries, this strategy has subsequently been successfully applied to liver and kidney injuries as well. Contemporary studies have demonstrated success rates in excess of 90% for non-operative management of solid organ injuries, even for severe injuries. Solid organ injuries are graded using the Organ Injury Scaling system devised by the American Association for the Surgery of Trauma (Table 18.1). We use the injury severity score to guide our treatment protocols but not as an indication for surgical intervention.

Although the patterns for peak time to operative intervention vary for the specific organs injured and injury severity, most children with a solid organ injury requiring surgery will need operative intervention within 24 h of admission. Children who fail a non-operative strategy due to ongoing hemorrhage, do so in predictable patterns. The "non-responder" does not improve with the initial infusion of intravenous fluid (two 20 mL/kg boluses of warmed normal saline or lactated ringer's solution), needs early consideration for transfusion of blood products, and will frequently require operative intervention. "Transient responders" improve with initial fluid challenges but later require additional fluid or blood due to a physiologic deterioration and should be considered candidates for angioembolization for control of ongoing hemorrhage. The majority of children are "responders." That is, initial volume resuscitation, when

Table 18.1 Organ injury scale for spleen, liver, and kidney

Organ, grade[a]	Injury type	Description of injury	AIS
Spleen			
I	Hematoma	Subcapsular, <10% surface area	2
	Laceration	Capsular tear, <1 cm parenchymal depth	2
II	Hematoma	Subcapsular, 10–50% surface area; intraparenchymal, <5 cm in diameter	2
	Laceration	Capsular tear, 1–3 cm parenchymal depth that does not involve a trabecular vessel	2
III	Hematoma	Subcapsular, >50% surface area or expanding; ruptured subcapsular or parenchymal hematoma; intraparenchymal hematoma ≥5 cm or expanding	3
	Laceration	>3 cm parenchymal depth or involving trabecular vessels	3
IV	Laceration	Laceration involving segmental or hilar vessels producing major devascularization (>25% of spleen)	4
V	Hematoma	Completely shattered spleen	5
	Laceration	Hilar vascular injury devascularizes spleen	5
Liver			
I	Hematoma	Subcapsular, <10% surface area	2
	Laceration	Capsular tear, <1 cm parenchymal depth	2
II	Hematoma	Subcapsular, 10–50% surface area: intraparenchymal <10 cm in diameter	2
	Laceration	Capsular tear 1–3 cm parenchymal depth, <10 cm in length	2
III	Hematoma	Subcapsular, >50% surface area of ruptured subcapsular or parenchymal hematoma; intraparenchymal hematoma >10 cm or expanding	3
	Laceration	>3 cm parenchymal depth	3
IV	Laceration	Parenchymal disruption involving 25–75% hepatic lobe or 1–3 Couinaud's segments	4
V	Laceration	Parenchymal disruption involving >75% of hepatic lobe or >3 Couinaud's segments within a single lobe	5
	Vascular	Juxtahepatic venous injuries, i.e., retrohepatic vena cava/central major hepatic veins	5
VI	Vascular	Hepatic avulsion	6
Kidney			
I	Contusion	Microscopic or gross hematuria, urologic studies normal	2
	Hematoma	Subcapsular, nonexpanding without parenchymal laceration	2
II	Hematoma	Nonexpanding perirenal hematoma confirmed to renal retroperitoneum	2
	Laceration	<1.0 cm parenchymal depth of renal cortex without urinary extravasation	2
III	Laceration	>1.0 cm parenchymal depth of renal cortex without collecting system rupture or urinary extravagation	3
IV	Laceration	Parenchymal laceration extending through renal cortex, medulla, and collecting system	4
	Vascular	Main renal artery or vein injury with contained hemorrhage	4
V	Laceration	Completely shattered kidney	5
	Vascular	Avulsion of renal hilum that devascularizes kidney	5

AIS abbreviated injury scale

[a]Advance one grade for bilateral injuries up to grade III

Source: Tinkoff G, Esposito GJ, Reed J, et al. American Association for the Surgery of Trauma Organ Injury Scale I: spleen, liver, and kidney, validation based on the National Trauma Databank. J Am Coll Surg. 2008;207:646–55, reprinted with permission from Elsevier

necessary, adequately restores any existing physiologic abnormalities and maintenance fluid administration alone is utilized subsequently.

Children who fail non-operative management typically do so secondary to ongoing hemorrhage or peritonitis. Failure due to hemorrhage is apparent based on physiologic deterioration or ongoing transfusion requirements. Those who fail due to the evolution of an intra-abdominal process such as hollow organ injury with perforation can be more difficult to detect. These patients require constant vigilance and frequent re-examination of the abdomen. Blood in the abdomen or contusion of the abdominal wall will cause tenderness to exam but are not necessarily indicative of the need for an operation. This must be distinguished from a progressive worsening of pain or tenderness suggesting peritonitis and a need for laparotomy.

Missed injury is the nemesis of the trauma surgeon. In the patient with a solid organ injury, there should also be concern for an associated hollow viscus injury. Fortunately, such associated injuries are uncommon and correlate more with the multiplicity of injuries (spleen and liver, kidney, spleen) rather than the severity of the individual organ injury. And, when a hollow viscus injury does occur and is missed on initial work-up, morbidity and mortality are not significantly increased by delay in diagnosis or treatment.

Controversy continues regarding the optimal transfusion threshold for failure of non-operative management in this patient population. It is generally accepted that if the transfusion requirement exceed 40 mL/kg, intervention is indicated. However, this criterion must be considered in context. The patient who requires 40 mL/kg of blood in the first several hours of care is quite different than one who requires the same volume transfused over several days. For patients requiring transfusion, we generally target a post-transfusion hemoglobin of 10 g/dL.

Accepted algorithms, most based on the American Pediatric Surgical Association's guidelines, are employed in the management of this patient population (Table 18.2). These algorithms base the care of the patient on the anatomic grade of injury (as demonstrated by CT) and include specific recommendations regarding the need for ICU monitoring, bed

Table 18.2 Treatment algorithm for abdominal solid organ injuries

Clinical parameter	CT grade of injury			
	I	II	III	IV or V
ICU stay (day)	None	None	None	1
Hospital stay (day)	2	3	4	5
Predischarge imaging	None	None	None	None
Postdischarge imaging	None	None	None	None
Activity restriction (weeks)	3	4	5	6

Source: Modified from Stylianos S. Evidence-based guidelines for resource utilization in children with isolated spleen or liver injury. The APSA Trauma Committee. J Pediatr Surg. 2000;35(2):164–7

rest, fluid resuscitation, repeat imaging, and time to discharge. Generally, lower grade injuries (1–3) can be managed on the ward with initial bed rest followed by a scheduled escalation of activity. Higher grade injuries (4 or 5) are managed in the ICU for close physiologic monitoring and hemoglobin checks. The management algorithms also address activity restrictions following hospital discharge. Lower grade injuries typically have a period of limited activity ("house arrest") of 2–3 weeks, followed by a period of limitation in contact sports of 2–3 months. Activity restrictions for higher grade injuries are typically 3 weeks of house arrest and 3 months of only non-contact sports. Routine follow-up imaging (ultrasound or CT) has not been shown to be of benefit and is therefore not recommended. However, a change in clinical condition (worsening pain, pallor, other symptoms) necessitates additional imaging. These algorithms are frameworks for care and well validated in the pediatric population. However, not all children will fit or adhere to a pathway and individualization (repeat CT scan for pain or prolonged bed rest) might be indicated. While the plan of care is based on the grade of injury, the need for intervention should be based on the physiologic response of the patient to the injury.

Spleen

The spleen is the most commonly injured intra-abdominal organ. Splenic trauma is suspected in any blunt trauma to the lower chest or upper abdomen. Patients often demonstrate pain and tenderness in the left upper quadrant, abdominal distension, tachycardia, and pain referred to the left shoulder. Lower rib fractures should raise suspicion for underlying injury as they suggest that a significant transfer of energy has occurred.

Most children with splenic injuries can be safely treated without operation or transfusion. Although associated with higher grades of injury, a contrast blush on the CT scan does not mandate embolization nor does it predict the need for surgical intervention in children with blunt splenic trauma. Severe splenic injuries with a blush on the initial CT scan can be successfully treated nonoperatively as guided by the stability of the patient. However, patients with evidence of ongoing hemorrhage should be considered for angioembolization (Fig. 18.1). Selective embolization of arterial branches can preserve functioning spleen, but evaluation of splenic function is difficult and these patients might require vaccination even if they avoid splenectomy. Embolization is associated with an increase in the need for blood transfusion, but this appears to be due to the severity of the injury, not the intervention itself.

For patients with ongoing hemorrhage or physiologic deterioration, laparotomy is indicated. Depending on the

Fig. 18.1 Algorithm for management of solid organ injury in children that incorporates angioembolization as an alternative to surgery in stable patients who have evidence of ongoing bleeding. Note hemodynamically unstable patients should undergo urgent laparotomy rather than attempts at embolization

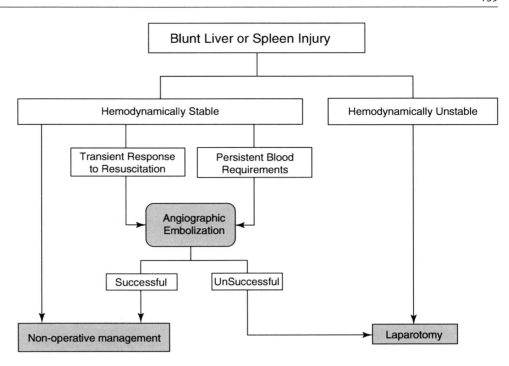

condition of the patient, attempts at splenic preservation should be pursued. Many techniques for splenic salvage have been described, including the use of an absorbable mesh to wrap the damaged organ and arrest bleeding through a tamponade effect. Hemostatic agents (thrombin, oxidized cellulose, hemostatic matrix gel) are also sometimes useful. If splenectomy is necessary, patients should receive vaccinations (against encapsulated organisms, *Streptococcus pneumoniae*, *Hemophilus influenzae*, and *Neisseiria meningitides*) to reduce the risk of overwhelming post-splenectomy infection (OPSI). Although OPSI is estimated to be rare (0.23–0.42% per year), it can be lethal. The risk for OPSI has been reported to be higher in children than in adults. In addition to vaccination, most recommend maintenance of daily oral penicillin until the age of 18 years. Complications of non-operative management include abscess, delayed hemorrhage, or chronic pain but are acceptably uncommon.

Liver

Liver laceration after blunt trauma is the second most common abdominal injury in pediatric trauma, but the most likely intra-abdominal injury to result in death. Non-operative management strategies, while typically successful, are not always free of complication. Delayed hemorrhage, biloma, and hemobilia have all been reported in patients managed non-operatively. A small proportion (5–10%) of children will require laparotomy. Liver injuries necessitating operation

are typically higher grade and can be quite challenging to the surgeon.

Experience in adults has demonstrated the utility of damage-control techniques, which have been useful in the pediatric population as well. This management approach involves an initial abbreviated laparotomy with the goal of hemorrhage control and limitation of soilage rather than definitive repair of injuries. The abdomen is packed with laparotomy pads to tamponade bleeding and the abdomen closed temporarily. Patients are then taken to the ICU for rewarming, correction of coagulopathy, and ongoing resuscitation. Following a period of stability, typically 12–24 h, the patient returns to the operating room for definitive repair of injuries. Angioembolization may also be of use for the control for persistent bleeding.

Kidney

The kidney is the third most commonly injured solid organ in blunt trauma. As with liver and spleen injuries, the majority of kidney injuries are amenable to a non-operative strategy. Because of the potential for injury to the collecting system, renal injuries pose unique challenges. With higher grade injuries (3–5), there is a risk of delayed extravasation of urine. For such injuries, follow-up CT scan at 48–72 h post-injury is recommended. Even in the face of significant extravasation, patients are likely to respond to closed techniques (ureteral stenting, percutaneous nephrostomy) obviating the need for laparotomy and minimizing possible renal loss. Selective embolization can also play a role in control of hemorrhage and organ preservation. Interventional techniques might also be of use in non-hemorrhagic vascular injuries to the kidney. If laparotomy is necessary, attempts at salvage should be pursued if feasible.

Pancreas

Pancreatic injuries are comparatively rare, but present challenging management issues. The pancreas might be injured when a child sustains a focused blow to the mid-abdomen (fist, handlebar), which crushes the body of the pancreas against the vertebral column. A child who presents immediately after injury is often deceptively asymptomatic and well-appearing until the destructive effects of pancreatic enzymes result in local tissue injury. As such, many pancreatic injuries are missed initially due to a paucity of symptoms. At times, assessment of the abdomen happens so efficiently, that edema planes resulting from an enzyme leak have not yet occurred and even the CT scan will be falsely reassuring. Persistent symptoms and clinical concerns warrant follow-up imaging (CT or ultrasound). Computed tomography (with IV contrast timed to highlight the pancreas) will reveal the injury.

Treatment of pancreatic injuries depends on the severity of injury and the timing of presentation. Minor injuries without evidence of major duct disruption will typically respond well to non-operative management. More significant injuries involving the main pancreatic duct respond variably to non-operative management. The rate of complications (pseudocyst formation, pancreatic necrosis, abscess) is much greater when the duct has been disrupted. If uncertainty exists regarding the integrity of the main pancreatic duct, ERCP allows definitive delineation of the duct anatomy and allows stent placement even in young children. Non-operative management typically includes a period of bowel rest to minimize pancreatic stimulation. The diet is then gradually liberalized and pancreatic enzymes followed to detect pancreatitis.

In general, complete or near-complete pancreatic transection in stable patients is managed with spleen-preserving distal pancreatectomy. Long-term functional results of distal pancreatectomy are generally excellent. Pancreatic exocrine insufficiency is rare and there are no reported cases of diabetes or other endocrine dysfunction.

Bladder

Most bladder injuries result from blunt trauma. Children are at greater risk of bladder injury because the bladder resides out of the pelvis and is thus less well protected. Any lower abdominal blunt trauma (such as a lap belt injury) can lead to rupture of the bladder.

Injury to the bladder is suggested by the injury mechanism, the presence of blood from the urethra or gross hematuria, abdominal pain, and presence of intraperitoneal fluid on imaging studies. The diagnosis is confirmed by conventional cystogram but CT cystogram with delayed and postvoid images might be more accurate.

Isolated extraperitoneal bladder perforation can be managed with Foley catheter drainage for 7 days, antibiotics, and pain control. Intraperitoneal bladder injury is managed by laparotomy and primary repair. A layered method using absorbable suture is most commonly used. Female urethral and bladder neck injury can occur with pelvic fracture, presents with gross hematuria or blood at the introitus, and requires operative repair for avulsions and longitudinal lacerations. These patients are at risk for significant sexual and lower urinary tract dysfunction and require careful follow up by an experienced pediatric urologist.

Duodenum and Small Intestine

Intestinal injuries comprise up to 15% of intra-abdominal injuries in children. While the duodenum is most commonly injured after blunt trauma in children, small bowel injuries, such as mesenteric avulsion, enterotomy, and even transections, are also well described. Overall, intestinal injuries in children are rare, but still carry a high mortality risk (>25%) likely due to the high energy transfer required to produce these injuries. Like pancreatic injuries, bowel injuries can easily be missed on initial assessment due to a paucity of clinical findings. Serial physical exams and a high index of suspicion are necessary to make the diagnosis when not apparent on initial evaluation.

Duodenal injuries result from a similar mechanism (epigastric blow from a handlebar or fist) and are frequently associated with pancreatic injuries. Diagnosis is confirmed by CT (or UGI) demonstrating intramural hematoma and proximal dilation. These injuries are typically managed with nasogastric decompression, bowel rest, and parenteral nutrition. A nasojejunal feeding tube can be threaded beyond the relative obstruction caused by the hematoma to allow enteral feedings. Most duodenal hematomas will resolve without late sequelae within 1–2 weeks. Patience is rewarded in the management of these injuries, with well over 90% able to be managed non-operatively. In cases where repair is required (perforation, failure of conservative treatment), primary repair by simple hematoma evacuation or primary closure is usually possible. More severe injuries sometimes require pyloric exclusion or gastrojejunostomy.

In contrast, small bowel perforations and transections must be repaired. Any blunt trauma to the abdomen can result in injury to the small intestine but diagnosis is difficult since free air is frequently absent and even CT has low sensitivity for these injuries. The diagnosis should be considered in all patients with a suspicious mechanism (seat-belt sign, handlebar injury, forceful direct blow to the epigastrium), focal tenderness, or intra-abdominal fluid without solid organ injury on CT scan. Limited perforations may be managed with simple repair. More extensive injuries or tissue devitalization from mesenteric injuries should be resected. Stable mesenteric hematomas should not be disturbed if the adjacent bowel is clearly viable. Most small bowel injuries can be managed without diversion.

Colon and Rectum

Injuries to the colon and rectum are relatively uncommon, but like small bowel injuries, operative management is typically necessary. Focal injuries without tissue devitalization can in most cases be managed with simple repair. More extensive injuries however will likely need resection and anastomosis. Criteria outlining those wounds needing fecal diversion are not well established in pediatric trauma, however most will do well with repair alone. Fecal diversion should be considered in the setting of hemodynamic instability, large-volume blood loss, extensive contamination, or when damage-control laparotomy is necessary.

Isolated Abdominal Free Fluid

Free fluid on CT scan in the absence of a solid organ injury raises the possibility of a hollow visceral injury. However, most studies have concluded that laparotomy is not mandated in these situations and that watchful waiting is a safe alternative. If symptoms worsen or the clinical picture is unclear, such patients are candidates, assuming they are hemodynamically stable, for diagnostic laparoscopy to exclude a bowel injury.

Child Abuse

One of the unfortunate aspects of pediatric trauma care is the prevalence of non-accidental injury. Many abused children suffer abdominal injuries. Given the often erroneous history in this setting, a high index of suspicion is necessary to make the diagnosis. It is not uncommon that a young child will present *in extremis* only to have evidence subsequently of an intra-abdominal injury from non-accidental trauma as the cause.

Impalements

Impalements involving the abdomen pose unique challenges to the healthcare team. Like other penetrating injuries, determination of trajectory and assessment of possible organ injuries is of paramount importance. Diagnostic imaging (beyond plain films) might not be practical if the foreign body remains in situ. Removal of the impaling object however should only occur in the controlled setting of the operating room. The operative team should be prepared to manage major vascular injury and have blood available. Specific management is based on injuries identified at the time of removal.

Summary Points

- Most blunt solid organ injuries can be managed non-operatively with a regimen of close observation, adequate fluid resuscitation, and gradual return to normal activities.
- In a patient with a solid organ injury, the indications for intervention include hemodynamic instability unresponsive to fluid resuscitation and ongoing hemorrhage.
- In the stable patient, many solid organ injuries with ongoing hemorrhage can be managed with selective angiography and embolization.
- Liver injuries that require surgery are associated with a significant mortality.
- Small bowel injuries can present in a delayed fashion and patients at risk (handlebar injury, epigastric blow) should be monitored carefully for signs of peritonitis.

Editor's Comment

The only indication for surgical intervention in the child with blunt solid organ injury is bleeding. Contrary to the protocols still used in many adult trauma centers, the child with free intraperitoneal blood, a blush on CT scan, the need for blood transfusion, or persistent abdominal pain does not require laparotomy unless there is also evidence of ongoing bleeding or hemodynamic instability. In the stable patient, embolization is also an excellent alternative to laparotomy. Though some children have significant discomfort after embolization, in experienced hands it appears to be safe and effective. At laparotomy in the stable patient, partial splenectomy should always be considered and pediatric trauma surgeons should be acquainted with the various techniques that have been described. Liver injuries that require laparotomy are always life-threatening and there should be a low threshold to resort to a damage-control approach if the patient becomes unstable in the OR. Retrohepatic caval injuries are the most serious and, whenever possible, one should consider enlisting the help of an experienced transplant surgeon, who might be able to apply the portal venous bypass techniques commonly used during transplant hepatectomy to allow repair or reconstruction of the vena cava.

Renal injuries that require surgical repair commonly lead to kidney loss, justifying sometimes seemingly extreme efforts to treat non-operatively. Injuries to the head of the pancreas should be treated non-operatively whenever possible. Transections of the neck or body of the pancreas that involve the main pancreatic duct can be treated non-operatively (drains, ERCP with stenting, parenteral nutrition) but the subsequent clinical course can be extremely long and complicated. On the other hand, distal pancreatectomy or, if the transection is at the neck of the pancreas, a Roux-en-Y pancreaticojejunostomy is well tolerated and usually results in a much shorter time to full recovery. The operation can be performed within 72 h of the injury, but clearly an operation performed within 24 h is best. The proximal duct needs to be oversewn but, especially in small children, it is often impossible to visualize. In this case, it is preferable to oversew the entire cut surface or use a gastrointestinal stapling device across the parenchyma. Regardless, it is prudent to leave a closed-suction drain in case of a leak.

Frank small bowel perforation can develop up to 72 h after an injury to the abdomen, most commonly associated with a handlebar or seatbelt sign. These patients do not necessarily need to be hospitalized during the entire observation period but parents need to understand that a delayed presentation is not uncommon and what signs to look for. Laparoscopy is an excellent way to diagnose and treat isolated small bowel injuries, which can usually be simply oversewn. Mesenteric defects should be repaired and hematomas left undisturbed. Ileostomy or colostomy should rarely, if ever, be necessary except possibly as part of a damage-control operation in a patient who has multiple bowel injuries.

Differential Diagnosis

Solid organ injury

- Spleen
- Liver
- Kidney
- Pancreas

Hollow viscus injury

- Duodenum
- Small intestine
- Colon
- Bladder

Parental Preparation

- Most solid organ injuries produced by blunt trauma can be managed without surgery but this involves a strict adherence to activity restrictions, usually for several weeks.
- When we operate for ongoing bleeding, there is a possibility that we will need to take extreme measures such as removing part of the organ involved or multiple operations.
- In most cases, once the injury has healed, we expect that the child will have normal organ function throughout life.

Diagnostic Studies

- Computed tomography
- Ultrasound
- CT cystogram

Technical Points

- Splenic injuries that require surgery should be managed with partial splenectomy if possible.
- Simple duodenal injuries can be repaired without diversion or extensive drainage.
- Distal pancreatic transection can be managed by spleen-preserving distal pancreatectomy and oversewing the proximal pancreatic duct.
- Patients with massive hemorrhage should be considered for damage control or salvage surgery in which the abdominal cavity is packed and partially closed and the patient is brought back to the ICU for resuscitation until a second operation 24–48 h later.
- Small and large bowel injuries can usually be safely repaired primarily.
- Colostomy or ileostomy should rarely be necessary and only when there is no other safe option.

Suggested Reading

Blinman TA, Nance ML. Special considerations in trauma in children (Chap. 53). In: Schwab CW, Trunkey D, Flint L, Meredith W, Taheri P, editors. Trauma: contemporary principles and therapy. Philadelphia: Lippincott Williams & Wilkins; 2007. p. 575–94.

Holmes IV JH, Tataria M, Mattix KD, Wiebe DW, Groner JI, Mooney DP, et al. The failure of non-operative management in solid organ injury: a multi-institutional pediatric trauma center experience. J Trauma. 2005;59:1309–13.

Moore EE, Shackford SR, Pachter HL, et al. Organ injury scaling: spleen, liver and kidney. J Trauma. 1989;29:1664–6.

Nance ML, Cooper AR. The visceral manifestations of child physical abuse. In: Christian C, Reece RM, editors. Child abuse: a medical reference. 4th ed. New York: Churchill Livingstone; 2008. p. 167–88.

Nance ML, Holmes IV JH, Wiebe DJ. Timeline to operative intervention for solid organ injuries in children. J Trauma. 2006;61(6):1389–92.

Stylianos S, Pearl R, Babyn P. Abdominal trauma in children. In: Wesson D, editor. Pediatric trauma. New York: Taylor & Francis; 2006. p. 267–302.

Chapter 19
Thoracic Trauma

Martin S. Keller

Clinically significant thoracic trauma occurs in 4–6% of injured children. Although the frequency of penetrating injuries continues to increase in both urban and rural centers, injuries due to blunt trauma, primarily from motor vehicle crashes and pedestrian trauma, predominate, accounting for more than 85% of cases. Isolated thoracic injuries are rare in children, and instead occur much more commonly in association with multi-system trauma. When present, they are a marker for severe, life threatening injuries. In fact, regardless of the mechanism, an associated thoracic injury more than triples the risk of death. Data from the National Pediatric Trauma Registry reports an overall mortality of 15% for children with blunt thoracic injury.

Children are at greater risk for thoracic trauma for several reasons. Incomplete rib ossification results in increased chest wall compliance and more efficient transmission of mechanical energy to internal organs without skeletal injuries or obvious external findings. When injury to the thoracic cage is present, it implies that significant blunt force energy was involved. The increased mobility of mediastinal structures places children at greater risk for the development of a tension pneumothorax, and significant physiologic compromise or cardiovascular collapse after simple pneumothorax. In addition, because of a relatively small size to body surface area, children are at higher risk for injuries to multiple organ after blunt trauma.

The initial management of a child with suspected thoracic injury should follow standard Advanced Trauma Life Support (ATLS) protocols. A positive physical exam (stridor, chest pain, tracheal deviation, distended neck veins, abnormal or diminished breath sounds, crepitus or dullness to percussion) in the appropriate clinical setting is highly suggestive of thoracic injury, but is neither sensitive nor specific. Before trying to completely define the injury, the priority should be to secure the airway, to make sure the patient is breathing, and to stabilize the circulation. Many thoracic injuries will require definitive treatment during the primary survey. All penetrating wounds should be identified as the patient is exposed during resuscitation to help determine trajectory and, in turn, potential organ injuries. In general, radiographic imaging is required to confirm diagnosis in children sustaining thoracic trauma.

Diagnosis

The diagnostic workup of a child with suspected thoracic trauma begins with a supine antero-posterior chest radiograph. Most thoracic injuries can be identified and managed on the basis of this standard plain film. Although the issue has been raised in several small series of blunt trauma patients, there is no consensus as to whether a thorough physical examination can safely obviate the mandatory screening chest radiograph in children. The treating physician must be cognizant of the normal anatomic variants of childhood, such as the relatively large thymic silhouette, which can make interpretation of the radiograph much more difficult. Nevertheless, such diagnostic difficulties often make it necessary to proceed with more advanced imaging studies in the evaluation of children with suspected thoracic trauma in order to guide appropriate management.

Helical CT and CT angiography of the chest can better delineate injuries identified on plain radiographs. These imaging modalities, however, are not necessary in the majority of children with blunt thoracic trauma and should not be used for screening purposes. In hemodynamically stable children with penetrating injuries, CT can often better define injuries and ballistic trajectory to guide management decisions. A modified focused abdominal ultrasound for trauma (FAST) of the thorax has reported utility for the immediate diagnosis of life threatening injuries such as pericardial effusion, pneumothorax, and hemothorax in the unstable adult trauma patient. Due to limited availability and poor sensitivity for abdominal injuries, its use as a screening test in children has not yet been as enthusiastically received by pediatric trauma surgeons. Two-dimensional transthoracic or transesophageal

M.S. Keller (✉)
Department of Pediatric Surgery, Washington University, St. Louis Children's Hospital, St. Louis, MO 63110, USA
e-mail: kellerm@wustl.edu

P. Mattei (ed.), *Fundamentals of Pediatric Surgery*,
DOI 10.1007/978-1-4419-6643-8_19, © Springer Science+Business Media, LLC 2011

echocardiography can assist with the diagnosis of pericardial effusion and tamponade as well as the detection of heart wall motion abnormalities in children with myocardial contusions. A water-soluble contrast esophagram is sometimes necessary in cases of suspected esophageal perforation.

Treatment

Injury to the lungs and pleural space are the most common thoracic injuries in children. Pneumothorax occurs frequently after both blunt and penetrating injury and can typically be managed by standard tube thoracostomy. Aggressive management is warranted due to the increased risk of tension pneumothorax physiology. Needle decompression of a tension pneumothorax may be required prior to definitive management with tube thoracostomy. Open pneumothorax (sucking chest wound) should be initially managed with a semi-occlusive dressing prior to tube thoracostomy. Occasionally, an asymptomatic pneumothorax will be identified incidentally on the lower chest images obtained during an abdominal CT scan. Although these "occult" pneumothoraces rarely become clinically significant and thus infrequently require tube thoracostomy, the patient should be monitored with serial examinations and follow-up chest X-rays, especially if positive pressure ventilation is required.

Pulmonary contusions are commonly identified by chest X-ray and confirmed by CT (Fig. 19.1). Due to the lack of comorbidities and excellent pulmonary reserve, these injuries are seldom of clinical significance. Extensive or multilobar injuries, however, can lead to respiratory compromise requiring aggressive support with mechanical ventilation.

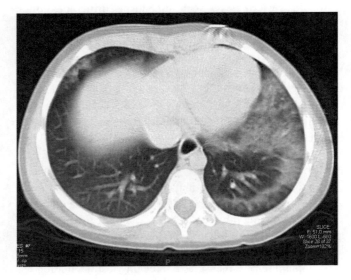

Fig. 19.1 Patchy bilateral infiltrates of lung bases representing pulmonary contusion in patient with blunt chest injury

Progression to respiratory distress syndrome has also been observed. Children with minimal symptoms but significant X-ray findings should therefore be monitored closely. Excessive intravenous fluid resuscitation can worsen pulmonary function in these patients. Late complications also occur, including pneumatoceles, which are due to air accumulation within an associated pulmonary laceration. These complications are rarely of clinical consequence but take weeks or months to completely resolve radiographically.

Cardiac contusions likely occur with a greater frequency after blunt trauma than is clinically appreciated. The excellent cardiac reserve of children masks the typical signs and symptoms of this injury seen in adults. An electrocardiogram should be obtained in all children to identify abnormalities in conduction, rhythm, and rate. Hemodynamically stable children in normal sinus rhythm may be monitored without further work-up, as complications from this injury are typically evident immediately. Serum creatine phosphokinase-MB (CPK-MB) and cardiac troponin levels (T and I) will demonstrate enzyme leak from injured myocardium but have limited clinical utility in routine patient management. Two-dimensional transthoracic echocardiography or TEE will demonstrate heart wall motion abnormalities, pericardial effusions, pericardial tamponade and valvular dysfunction in symptomatic children, and can guide pharmacologic support and, rarely, surgical intervention. Finally, central venous cannulation can be helpful in the resuscitation of children with functional compromise.

Tracheal and major bronchial injuries are rare in children and are typically the result of blunt chest trauma with a closed glottis. Laceration of the membranous portion of the trachea is the most common injury. Numerous reports have described successful "conservative" management of lacerations of the membranous trachea by endotracheal intubation (stenting) and broad-spectrum antibiotic coverage. However, unstable patients with significant air leak and respiratory compromise require operative intervention for repair. Bronchial injuries are characterized by persistent pneumothorax and often massive air leak following tube thoracostomy. The "fallen lung sign" on chest radiographs after tube thoracostomy is suggestive of this injury. These injuries uniformly require operative repair and often necessitate pulmonary resection. Bronchoscopy, in a controlled setting, can help to localize the site of injury. Extracorporeal life support has been used for stabilization and salvage in patients who are *in extremis*. Long-term follow up with serial bronchoscopy is required in all patients with tracheo-bronchial injuries to identify subsequent airway stenosis. Traumatic asphyxia may also result from compressive chest trauma applied against a closed glottis. Patients typically present with mental status changes and respiratory distress. The diagnosis is confirmed by the presence of edema and cyanosis with petechiae of the upper chest, neck and face. Subconjunctival and retinal hemorrhages may also be seen.

Treatment is supportive but must include a thorough assessment to exclude other injuries. Despite the dramatic clinical presentation, traumatic asphyxia is rarely life threatening. However, an occasional patient will require ventilatory support with positive end-expiratory pressure (PEEP) for significant pulmonary contusions or other associated injuries.

Esophageal perforation is rare following blunt thoracic trauma and is more likely the result of penetrating mechanisms. Diagnosis is best made with water-soluble contrast esophagram. Esophagoscopy is a complementary study and may increase the diagnostic yield. Thoracotomy and primary repair is recommended for injuries diagnosed early with minimal contamination. Pleural and mediastinal drainage is required. Esophageal perforation diagnosed late (more than 24 h after injury) may require esophageal diversion with a cervical esophagostomy to allow for healing.

Injury to the thoracic duct may occur anywhere along its intrathoracic course. Non-bloody pleural fluid, high in triglyceride levels and lymphocyte counts should raise suspicion. Although extremely rare, both blunt and penetrating mechanisms have been reported. Child abuse should be suspected in a child with associated rib fractures or an inconsistent history. Management typically requires tube thoracostomy to allow the lung to reexpand. Dietary modification with restrictions to medium chain triglycerides or a period of gut rest and total parenteral nutrition may facilitate closure of the leaking duct. Successful closure with octreotide, to limit chyle production, has been reported. Operative intervention should be reserved for children with persistent leakage over multiple weeks who fail conservative managements. Thoracic exploration via thoracoscopy or thoracotomy with pre- and intraoperative administration of cream into the gastrointestinal tract should demonstrate the site of injury and allow for ligation. Mechanical pleurodesis may also be required to obliterate the pleural space in children who fail other managements.

Injury to the ribs and thoracic cage in children is a rare consequence of blunt trauma. A child's skeletal immaturity results in increased chest wall compliance and typically allows for transmission of impact energy through the chest wall to be absorbed by internal structures. Rib fractures represent a sign that significant mechanical force was delivered and, as such, are a marker of potentially severe internal injuries. Rib fracture location is important to note during the work-up. Fractures to the lower ribs are associated with upper abdominal solid organ injuries and are an indication for further workup with an abdominal CT. First rib fracture and sternal fractures have been associated with injuries to the mediastinum, particularly the aortic arch, and should be followed up with a chest CT. Posterior rib fractures are associated with non-accidental trauma. These injuries are often found in various stages of healing during skeletal surveys obtained in the evaluation of non-accidental trauma. Most rib

and sternal fractures require only supportive management and pain control. Rarely, a displaced sternal fracture will require open reduction and internal fixation.

Flail rib segments result from ribs injuries with two or more points of fracture and represent the most severe injury to the thoracic cage. Respiratory embarrassment can result from paradoxic chest wall motion and ineffective respiration, but is more commonly due, in these injuries, to the underlying pulmonary contusion. Supportive management with aggressive analgesia, including thoracic epidural anesthesia, and positive pressure ventilation, may be necessary. Operative rib fixation is rarely needed.

Injury to the diaphragm occurs most frequently from severe blunt abdominal and penetrating thoraco-abdominal trauma. Recent series document that both hemidiaphragms are equally at risk. Most diaphragmatic injuries can be diagnosed by standard anteroposterior radiographs demonstrating an elevated hemidiaphragm, herniated bowel loops or a nasogastric tube tip within the chest. Computed tomography with coronal and sagittal reconstructions may assist with diagnosis in questionable cases. Although thoracoscopic repair has been described, laparotomy is favored due to the high (greater than 50%) likelihood of associated hollow viscus injury.

As in adults, blunt injury to the aorta and great vessels occurs most often following rapid deceleration. Diagnosis, in children with a concerning mechanism, should be suspected with widening and abnormal contour of the mediastinum on anteroposterior chest radiograph. The normal thymus gland in young children often makes interpretation of these X-rays difficult for the inexperienced. Helical CT and TEE are accurate in diagnosing this injury, and have replaced traditional angiography as a screening tool. Operative management with and without left heart bypass as well as endovascular stenting has reported success in case reports.

Unfortunately, penetrating thoracic trauma has increased in frequency in the pediatric population across all ages. Overall, 50% of children sustaining penetrating injury to the thorax will require surgery. The need for surgical intervention increases to over 90% in children presenting with unstable vital signs. After either blunt and penetrating mechanisms, children with a significant hemothorax and thoracostomy tube drainage greater than 15–20 or 2–3 mL/kg over 3 or more hours, require thoracotomy for hemorrhage control. Children who are hemodynamically stable should undergo radiographic imaging to identify injuries.

The radiographic work-up of a child with penetrating thoracic trauma typically begins with standard anterior-posterior plain radiographs. Use of radio-opaque markers over or adjacent to the wounds and additional views can assist with the determination of ballistic trajectory which may, in turn, help define injuries. Intravenous contrast-enhanced helical CT scanning is also effective in evaluating transthoracic gunshot

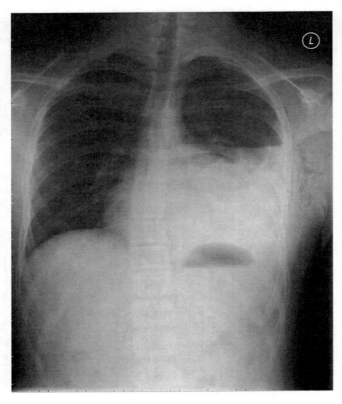

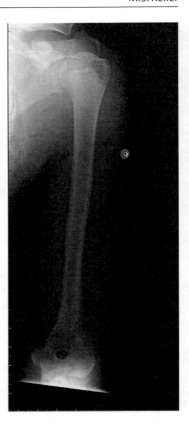

Fig. 19.3 Plain roentgenogram of humerus with wound marker in same patient in Fig. 19.2

Fig. 19.2 Massive hemopneumothorax in hemodynamically stable patient with stab wound to left shoulder

wounds. Positive results may warrant immediate operative intervention or further radiographic work-up with a water soluble contrast esophagram, arteriogram, bronchoscopy or echocardiography. Children with negative scans can be safely observed in a monitored setting without further evaluation. The shoulders and upper arms should be included with wounds of the torso and are considered at marker for potential associated intrathoracic injuries (Figs. 19.2 and 19.3). Hemodynamically unstable patients with penetrating thoracic injuries require immediate operative exploration, which should not be delayed by radiographic imaging.

Simple pneumothorax and hemothorax are the most common injuries due to penetrating thoracic trauma. The majority of these may be managed with tube thoracostomy alone. Cessation of air-leak and bleeding, along with full re-expansion of the lung and complete evacuation of the pleural space are all encouraging signs to guide therapy. Failure to improve with pleural space decompression warrants repeat thoracostomy or operative intervention. Thoracoscopy and thoracotomy both have utility in the management of selected cases. Pulmonary debridement, wedge resection, tractotomy, lobectomy and pneumonectomy may be necessary depending upon the operative findings.

Penetrating injury to the anterior thorax between the nipple lines and between horizontal lines drawn through the

manubrium and inferior costal margin ("the box") requires evaluation for potential cardiac and mediastinal injury. Hemodynamically stable children may be evaluated with CT-angiography and echocardiography. Many children will require a formal subxiphoid or transdiaphragmatic pericardial window. A positive pericardial window mandates sternotomy, pericardotomy and exploration of the pericardial sac for pericardial or cardiac injury.

When managing a child with a penetrating thoracic injury, the potential for injury outside of the thorax must also be recognized. The dome shape of the diaphragm allows for extension of the peritoneal cavity within the lower thoracic cage. Penetrating chest injuries below the level of the nipples or the tip of the scapula suggest the possibility of sub-diaphragmatic injuries. Thoracic and abdominal CT may suggest intraperitoneal injury with the demonstration of blood or free air in the abdomen but does not always define the injury, especially if a hollow viscus is involved. The hemodynamically stable child with a penetrating injury to the liver in which the trajectory of the missile or knife is defined may be safely observed, while significant hemoperitoneum or a CT evidence of extravasation is often an indication for operative intervention. Diagnostic laparoscopy or thoracoscopy is of utility in hemodynamically stable patients in whom diaphragmatic injury and concomitant intraperitoneal injury cannot be excluded by other imaging modalities. Exploratory thoracotomy and/or laparotomy are required in the hemodynamically unstable patient.

The role for emergency department thoracotomy in children remains undefined. Despite improved survival in children sustaining non-traumatic cardiac arrest, the outcome following emergency department thoracotomy for traumatic arrest continues to be no different from that in adults. Given this poor outcome, emergency department thoracotomy should be reserved for those children sustaining penetrating trauma who present with signs of life and develop a loss of vital signs in the trauma bay during resuscitation. Emergency department thoracotomy is futile for children who present with an absence of vital signs of longer duration and those who arrest from blunt mechanisms.

Summary Points

- Because most injuries are the result of blunt mechanisms, associated injuries are common and impact outcome.
- Immaturity of the bony thoracic cage allows for significant internal injury to occur without external signs.
- Most pneumothoraces and hemothoraces can be managed by tube thoracostomy.
- Rib fractures and thoracic duct injury, in the absence of a defined mechanism, should raise concerns for child abuse.
- Most pulmonary and cardiac contusions can be managed supportively.
- Determination of ballistic trajectory helps identify organ injury.

Editor's Comment

The life-threatening injuries that we commonly see in adults after a blunt thoracic trauma mechanism are rarely seen or significantly less morbid in children: aortic dissection, myocardial contusion, pericardial tamponade, pulmonary contusion, sternal fracture, and flail chest physiology. Children appear to less vulnerable to these types of injuries perhaps due to superior tissue resiliency and durability, more favorable dissipation of kinetic energy due to size/volume differences, and, in the case of a head-on automobile collision, the absence of steering wheel-induced injuries. Nevertheless, these injuries are occasionally seen in children and a proper diagnostic algorithm should be followed whenever the mechanism is suggestive.

After blunt trauma, a CT scan of the chest will sometimes reveal a small amount of mediastinal air or a tiny pneumothorax. In the absence of other signs of significant organ injury, these findings can generally be regarded as incidental. Nevertheless, these patients warrant a meticulous evaluation and careful observation.

Penetrating injuries in the form of stabbings and gun shot wounds are becoming more common in children and require a thoughtful and scrupulous diagnostic approach in order to identify latent injuries. Trajectories based on the location of entry and exit wounds are notoriously inaccurate for several reasons: the victim might have been in a contorted position at the moment of impact, missiles can follow tissue planes and therefore fail to travel in a straight line, and bullets can ricochet within the bony cage of the thorax. Not every patient with a gunshot wound or knife injury to the chest will require an operation, perhaps because most patients with potentially operative injuries never make it to the hospital, but a trauma surgeon needs to be involved with every aspect of the care of these children. The most important diagnostic and therapeutic maneuver in a child with a gunshot wound to the chest is the placement of a chest tube. The stable child with a stab wound should have a chest radiograph and could potentially avoid a chest tube if there is no evidence of a pneumo- or hemothorax. Placing a chest tube in a child should be done with a delicate technique, under sterile conditions, and after sedation and injection of a local anesthetic. In young children, a small incision that passes through the chest wall obliquely is all that is necessary (not big enough to insert your finger) but it is surprisingly easy to inadvertently place the tube into the subcutaneous tissues and for it to erroneously appear to be in perfect position on a chest film.

The primary indication for operative intervention in the child with a thoracic injury is bleeding. There is no absolute amount of bloody chest tube effluent that can be used to decide if an operation is needed; this must be based on good judgment. Lung injuries can be oversewn or repaired with stapling device using a vascular cartridge. Esophageal injuries can almost always be repaired primarily provided there is little devitalized tissue and good drainage can be maintained. The same is true for most tracheal injuries, but when there are injuries to both the airway and the esophagus, viable tissue should be placed between the two suture lines to prevent the formation of a tracheo-esophageal fistula. The vagus and phrenic nerves should be carefully identified and protected throughout the procedure. Major vascular injuries should be repaired using standard vascular techniques, including the principle of proximal and distal control of the vessels and the use of side-biting clamps whenever feasible.

Diagnostic Studies

- Anterior-posterior plain radiograph
- Helical computed tomography
- Computed tomography angiography
- Transthoracic echocardiogram
- Transesophageal echocardiogram
- Contrast esophagram
- 12-lead electrocardiogram

Parental Preparation

- Possible major operation, large incision, long recovery
- High rates of morbidity and mortality
- Delayed operations may be necessary

Preoperative Preparation

- ☐ Type and cross
- ☐ Informed consent

Technical Points

- Tube thoracostomy is by same technique employed for adults
- Pulmonary injury may require debridement, wedge resection, tractotomy, lobectomy or pneumonectomy
- Enteral administration of cream may facilitate identification of thoracic duct injury
- A positive pericardial window (blood) mandates sternotomy and formal pericardial and cardiac exploration
- Esophageal perforations identified early may be managed with primary repair and drainage, late injuries (greater than 24 h) may require esophageal diversion

Suggested Reading

Barsness KA, Cha E-S, Bensard DD, et al. The positive predictive value of rib fractures as an indicator of nonaccidental trauma in children. J Trauma. 2003;54:1107–10.

Bliss D, Silen M. Pediatric thoracic trauma. Crit Care Med. 2002;30: S409–15.

Dowd DM, Krug S. Pediatric blunt cardiac injury: epidemiology, clinical features, and diagnosis. J Trauma. 1996;40:61–7.

Nance ML, Sing RF, Reilly PM, et al. Thoracic gunshot wounds in children under 17 years of age. J Pediatr Surg. 1996;31:931–5.

Stassen NA, Lukan JK, Spain DA, et al. Reevaluation of diagnostic procedures for transmediastinal gunshot wounds. J Trauma. 2002;53: 635–8.

Vane DW, Keller MS, Sartorelli KH, Miceli AP. Pediatric trauma: current concepts and treatments. J Int Care Med. 2002;17:230–49.

Chapter 20
Spine Trauma

Robert W. Letton

The pediatric spine is more flexible than the adult spine, making it more resilient and therefore less susceptible to traumatic injury. The incidence of spinal column injury in children is low with rates varying from 1 to 5%. However, this increased flexibility contributes to the differing injury patterns seen in pediatric trauma when compared to the adult. In addition, due to physical and psychological immaturity, the clinical assessment and diagnosis can be extremely difficult. Significant head injury is a risk factor for cervical spine injury and any child with a suspected spinal injury should be immobilized in a hard cervical collar on a pediatric spine board. Since significant force is required to injure the spine, other regions may also be injured, with almost half of children having concomitant injuries.

The common signs of spinal cord injury include absence or asymmetry of the deep tendon reflexes, paralysis, and clonus, but these are sometimes delayed in presentation. There may be a transient (24- to 72-h) period of "spinal shock" defined by paralysis, areflexia, and hypotonia, which is usually followed by return of reflexes and progressive spasticity. Although corticosteroids have been recommended in adult spinal cord injury in the past, to date no study has evaluated their efficacy in pediatric spinal cord injury, and the eighth edition of the advanced trauma life support (ATLS) course states there is insufficient evidence to support the routine use of steroids in children with spinal cord injury.

The spinal column undergoes significant anatomic and biomechanical changes during the first 15 years of life. Ossification centers enlarge and the spinal articulations fuse and slowly increase the stiffness of the child's spine. The paraspinal musculature and ligamentous structures are underdeveloped and in young children the spine lengthens to a much greater degree than the spinal cord, allowing cord injuries to occur without vertebral column injury. The facets of the upper cervical spine are more horizontal, allowing for greater motion, and may present on radiographs as pseudosubluxation of the upper cervical spine. These features of the immature spine result in a much higher prevalence of injury above C4 in children who are younger than 8 years of age.

The incidence of spinal injuries has two peaks: one around 5 years of age and the other in those older than 10 years. Spinal Cord Injury WithOut Radiological Abnormality (SCIWORA) usually occurs in children less than 8 years of age. SCIWORA describes an acute spinal cord injury that can result in some degree of sensory and/or motor deficit without radiographic evidence of vertebral fracture or alignment abnormalities. The concept of SCIWORA was proposed in 1907, but the acronym was coined in 1982. The incidence in children with a spinal cord injury varies but in some series it is as high as 60%. The cause is unknown but it is likely a result of a combination of factors: a relatively inelastic spinal cord housed within a fairly elastic spine, transient intervertebral disc herniation, or cord infarction. It most commonly occurs in the cervical spine, followed by the thoracic spine. Plain radiographs and CT scan are usually normal, but MRI will often reveal signs of trauma, such as a signal change within the cord. Children with SCIWORA can develop paraplegia up to 4 days after the injury.

The cervical spine is more commonly involved probably because of the excessive spinal movement of the upper cervical spine in children younger than 3 years. Upper cervical SCIWORA appears to have more severe neurologic consequences than lower cervical SCIWORA. Thoracic SCIWORA is less common because the splinting effect of the rib cage prevents the thoracic spine from forced flexion or extension. The lumbar spine is very rarely affected, probably because the spinal cord normally ends at L2 and because severe lumbar spinal injuries are more frequently associated with lethal injuries such as aorta rupture.

If at any time the neurologic examination of a child with a history of trauma is abnormal, the child should be assumed to have a spinal cord injury and should be immobilized appropriately. If plain radiographs and CT scans show no evidence of fracture or malalignment, magnetic resonance scans should be obtained. Likewise, if a child is unconscious after injury, rigid

R.W. Letton (✉)
Department of Pediatric Surgery, The Children's Hospital of
Oklahoma, 1200 Everett Drive, Suite 2320, Oklahoma City,
OK 73104, USA
e-mail: robert-letton@ouhsc.edu

P. Mattei (ed.), *Fundamentals of Pediatric Surgery*,
DOI 10.1007/978-1-4419-6643-8_20, © Springer Science+Business Media, LLC 2011

immobilization should be maintained while plain radiographs and CT scans are obtained. If these studies are normal, MRI should be considered if the child remains unconscious.

Diagnosis

Spinal cord injuries are easily recognized in conscious patients with neurologic dysfunction below the level of the injury. In children with multiple injuries, the diagnosis of a spinal injury can be more difficult. Cord injuries may cause significant neurogenic shock, characterized by hypotension, bradycardia, hypothermia, and peripheral vasodilation. Other signs of spinal cord injury include paradoxic breathing, priapism, and Horner's syndrome. Severe cord injury results in symmetric flaccid paralysis and sensory loss. Lesser injuries can result in transient dysfunction of the limbs, bowel or bladder. Any history of transient neurologic dysfunction regardless of duration must be recognized and evaluated further.

A child who is alert (and not intoxicated) and has no history of transient neurologic dysfunction, midline spine tenderness, or a distracting injury can be cleared clinically without radiographs. All other children should have their spine immobilized with an appropriately fitted cervical collar until they can be cleared clinically and radiographically. Due to the size of the occiput relative to the rest of the body, a pediatric spine board should have adjustable padding that allows the torso to be elevated with respect to the head, thus keeping the cervical spine in a neutral position and preventing excessive anterior cervical flexion.

There are a number of normal anatomic variants and radiographic anomalies associated with the pediatric spine that can confuse the diagnosis. Pseudosubluxation is commonly noted in children less than 8 years of age, the atlanto-dens interval may be larger in children, and children have a relative kyphosis across the mid-portion of the cervical spine, which would be considered abnormal in an adult. Interpretation of soft tissue anatomy can also be more difficult in children as the posterior pharyngeal soft tissues appear thickened in the child who is crying and uncooperative during the examination. The size variability in children requires that the soft tissues be judged in reference to vertebral body size, with normal prevertebral soft tissues being two-thirds or less of the length of the adjacent vertebral body.

Despite the increasing use of MRI, a set of carefully performed flexion-extension radiographs remains an important tool in the assessment of pediatric cervical injuries. Specifically, patients in a very young age group who are incapable of participating in a meaningful evaluation because of cognitive impairment or emotional distress benefit from early fluoroscopy using traction and flexion-extension evaluation by an experienced examiner to assess for ligamentous instability.

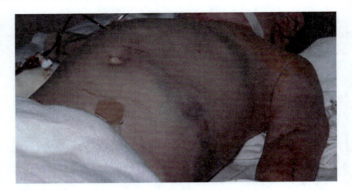

Fig. 20.1 A helical CT scan reconstruction of C2 "Hangman's" fracture in a "1-year-old"

Helical CT scans with digital reconstruction provide excellent delineation of osseous injury patterns (Fig. 20.1). Routine three-dimensional studies and sagittal and coronal reconstructions provide the physician with a detailed understanding of the injury. MRI scanning often requires general anesthesia and occasionally results in diagnostic ambiguity with regards to ligamentous signal abnormalities. Nevertheless, MRI plays an increasingly important role in the evaluation of pediatric spinal trauma as it allows superior soft-tissue and neural element visualization, providing specific advantages in the pediatric population. Protocols involving MRI have been shown to be cost effective, especially in the head-injured patient in the ICU setting whose spine cannot be cleared clinically. The inherent instability of the pediatric spine, a higher prevalence of SCIWORA, and a significant incidence of late instability makes clearance of the cervical spine in the uncooperative, multiply injured or head-injured child quite challenging.

The ability to quickly rule out problems in the cervical spine greatly facilitates the care of patients in the ICU. Delays in obtaining this information can interfere with bedside care, patient positioning, initiation of therapy, airway management, extubation, and operative procedures. Magnetic resonance imaging protocols have been clearly demonstrated to be useful in detecting injuries that were not appreciated on plain radiography, ruling out the presence of injuries suspected on the basis of plain radiographs, predicting cervical stability and allowing for collar removal, and evaluating the potential for recovery in patients with spinal cord injuries.

Preoperative Preparation

The most common operative scenario involves the child who requires urgent surgery and there is not enough time to completely clear the cervical spine prior to induction of general anesthesia. This is particularly worrisome in the child with a traumatic brain injury who needs urgent operative decompression. The great majority already have a secure airway, but positioning for the craniotomy can be of concern. In the conscious child with a distracting injury such as a long bone fracture or possible intra-abdominal injury requiring general anesthesia, it is likely that obvious fracture will be able to be excluded; however, SCIWORA or other types of occult injury will not have been ruled out. Since by definition these children have a distracting injury, the surgeon and anesthesiologist must assume that the child has a spine injury until proven otherwise by clinical criteria or with MRI, and therefore full spine precautions must be followed at all times. Once the distracting injury is treated, the child's spine can often be cleared the next day. In the event of severe head injury, MRI may be necessary depending on the anticipated length of disability. Any child who is hypotensive and in shock needs to have any question of hemorrhagic shock addressed before it can be attributed to neurogenic shock and treated with pressors.

Treatment

Prevention of secondary spinal cord injury is the principal treatment objective just as preventing secondary brain injury is in children with traumatic brain injury. Resuscitation with effective support of oxygen delivery is vitally important. Small children tend to have injury to the upper cervical spine more often than adults; therefore impairment of ventilatory function tends to occur early and require elective endotracheal intubation and mechanical ventilation. A nasogastric tube should be placed for associated delayed gastric emptying and a Foley catheter inserted to monitor urine output. Hypotension should be assumed to be secondary to hemorrhagic shock and is treated with ATLS resuscitation protocols until hypovolemia is ruled out. Once blood loss is excluded, neurogenic shock should be treated with euvolemic fluid resuscitation and pressors to minimize excessive fluid administration.

Specific Injuries

Atlanto-occipital injuries are associated with high energy transfer and are frequently fatal. Children appear to be at increased risk for this injury, especially when they are a front-seat passenger and an air bag is deployed. The injury is frequently associated with severe cord and brainstem injury, causing respiratory arrest. The early diagnosis of this problem can be challenging because the initial displacement is reduced with cervical immobilization. In addition, anatomic variation, adjacent level trauma, and poor visualization make

radiographs difficult to interpret. Frequently, the instability can be appreciated only if traction is applied for a radiographic study or when a large rigid cervical collar imparts a distractive force across the atlanto-occipital junction.

Treatment of atlanto-occipital injuries is challenging because the patients are usually intubated, are multiply injured, and have a major brain injury. Determining the extent of brain and spinal cord injury can be very difficult. Associated cranial nerve injuries can further confuse the issue as the patient might be conscious but unable to communicate. Communicating with family members is extremely important when making decisions for these patients.

In adolescents, *ondontoid fractures* are similar to those seen in adults. In young children, on the other hand, they can occur after relatively minor trauma and may not be detected at the time of the initial evaluation because the injury typically represents a fracture through the synchondrosis at the base of the ondontoid. Radiographic interpretation is challenging due a poorly unossified transverse line that is normally present at the base of the ondontoid. Although relatively uncommon, the injury can be associated with neurologic injury. Ondontoid abnormalities are easily missed and can lead to future instability and the risk of delayed neurologic injury. In questionable cases, careful clinical and radiographic assessment should prompt examination by CT with sagittal reconstruction.

Ondontoid injuries usually heal well with adequate immobilization. If displacement is evident on initial presentation, then closed reduction and halo immobilization should be undertaken. Closed reduction under sedation may safely allow neurologic assessment of the child. Nondisplaced injuries can be managed with halo-jacket immobilization in cooperative patients.

Injuries of the subaxial cervical spine are uncommon in children younger than 9 years. In adolescents, the injury patterns are similar to those in adults. Injury types include fracture-dislocations, burst fractures, simple compression fractures, facet dislocation, and posterior ligamentous injuries. These injuries usually involve major trauma and are most frequently related to motor-vehicle collisions.

Instrumentation and fusion in children is less commonly performed because of concerns about subsequent growth. Pediatric fracture-dislocations and burst injuries should be managed by realigning the canal and immobilizing the spine, usually with a halo-vest. Stable *compression fractures* require collar immobilization for 4–6 weeks. Unilateral and bilateral *facet dislocations* require reduction under sedation, which allows for a controlled reduction in a cooperative patient. Three months of halo immobilization followed by evaluation by dynamic flexion-extension radiography should be sufficient for most of these injuries. *Facet fracture-dislocation* is an unstable injury for which conservative management is more likely to fail. Primary posterior instrumentation and fusion is usually required to provide long-term stability in these patients. Young children can present with a *growth plate separation*, which is frequently associated with neurologic injury and should be considered very unstable. They are difficult to visualize radiographically and are often only appreciated by MRI. After being properly reduced and stabilized, these injuries usually heal rapidly.

Injuries to the thoracic and lumbar spine are rare in the pediatric population though the literature suggests that spinal injuries in children are relatively balanced between the cervical and thoracolumbar spine. Young children sustain thoracolumbar spine injuries as a result of abuse or motor-vehicle collision, whereas older children are likely to sustain them during sports activities such as snowboarding and mountain-biking. Most such injuries are centered around the thoracolumbar junction and are often related to a seat-belt injury while being improperly restrained. Patients who present with fractures in this region often have multisystem injuries. Initial physical examination might demonstrate features that are indicative of major spinal trauma, including abdominal bruising and evidence of a posterior distraction injury. Neurologic injury is not uncommon in these patients and can be partial or complete.

The mechanism of injury in the thoracic and lumbar spine determines the fracture pattern that is seen and is reflected in fracture classification and spinal stability. Moderate flexion moments can lead to compression fractures and a greater axial load leads to a burst pattern. The Chance fracture is created with a posterior distractive force and a violent flexion moment and is commonly referred to as a flexion-distraction injury. The anterior column can fail as a result of compression in these injuries or it may remain intact. Fracture-dislocations are rare in children and are characterized by severe instability, translational displacement, and a high prevalence of neurologic injury.

Spinal injuries in children have a greater potential for remodeling, especially if the injury is reduced and the end-plate growth has been preserved. Pediatric spinal instrumentation systems have increased in sophistication, allowing stable instrumentation to be established across fewer spinal segments, thus minimizing long-term effects on spinal health.

Compression injuries most commonly occur at the thoracolumbar junction. They are characterized by failure of the anterior column in the absence of either clinical or radiographic evidence of posterior element injury. The superior end plate fails more commonly than the inferior end plate. These injuries can occur over multiple levels and with a relatively low-energy injury in a growing patient. Most can be managed conservatively, either with activity restriction or orthotics. Long-term kyphosis is rare since anterior growth is preserved and often leads to correction. Injuries with more than 50% compression of the anterior column should be evaluated for evidence of posterior injury and closely followed over time. Instrumentation is sometimes required to control kyphosis.

Flexion-distraction injuries due to seat-belt injuries in children have been well recognized by clinicians since the original description by Chance in 1948. Almost all injuries are the result of a motor-vehicle collision and inappropriate lap belt restraint (Fig. 20.2). While in older children and adolescents the injury typically involves L1, in younger children the injury is likely to be more caudal and tends to occur at L3. It is important to consider the possibility of a major vascular injury, including aortic dissection, and major abdominal injuries, which occur in almost half of these children (Fig. 20.3). Jejunal transection and small-bowel perforation is also a common finding in these patients. These intra-abdominal injuries may present up to 3 days after injury, possibly placing the patient at greater risk of complications.

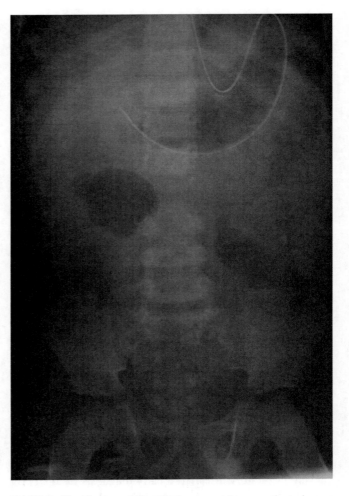

Fig. 20.2 Significant seatbelt stripe in a young trauma patient who was improperly restrained with a lap belt

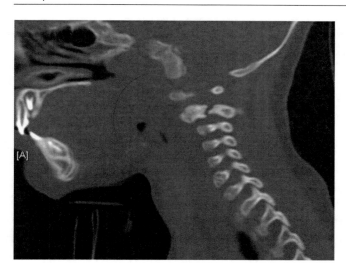

Fig. 20.3 A flexion-distraction, or Chance fracture, of the lumbar spine in the patient shown in Fig. 20.1. Notice the significant distance between the L2 and L3 vertebral bodies. This patient succumbed from an associated abdominal aortic transection

Optimal management of flexion-distraction injuries in children has not been well defined. Injuries that have a major osseous component but remain well aligned should heal well with immobilization alone and are usually associated with good long-term stability. Indications for operative manage-

ment include the presence of multisystem injuries and severe or progressive kyphosis.

Complications

There are numerous potential complications from spinal cord injury. Children with high cervical lesions often have serious associated injuries, such as vascular transection and brain injury, which are often lethal. Chance fractures are associated with major vascular and intestinal injury. And, of course, paralysis or disability may result from an associated spinal cord injury. In addition, these children are at risk for nosocomial and iatrogenic complications, such as ventilator-acquired pneumonia and central line, blood stream, and urinary tract infections. Pressure sores from prolonged immobilization are known risks in patients with a documented spine fracture, but even patients without spine fracture who are immobilized on a backboard or in a hard cervical collar for a long period of time are at risk for decubitus ulcers. Perhaps the most tragic complication is conversion of a partial or fully functional spinal injury into a complete cord injury by not realizing that a patient is at risk for spinal injury and subsequently subjecting them to improper immobilization, inappropriate work up and delay in diagnosis.

Summary Points

- Immaturity of the pediatric spine makes it susceptible to different injury pattern than in adults.
- Children are especially susceptible to spinal cord injury without radiographic abnormality (SCIWORA).
- Children less than 8 years of age have a higher incidence of injury above the level of C4.
- There is currently insufficient evidence to support the routine use of steroids in spinal cord injury in children.
- Children who are cooperative, without altered level of consciousness, have no distracting injuries, no history of neurologic impairment, and who have no spine tenderness can be safely cleared clinically without extensive radiographic work-up.
- The great majority of patients that cannot be cleared with physical exam alone can be cleared with a combination of plain radiographs or helical CT scanning with digital reconstruction. MRI should be reserved for those with negative imaging and a history of neurologic deficit or coma.
- Shock should be treated empirically as hemorrhagic shock with appropriate fluid resuscitation. Only after hemorrhagic shock is ruled out should pressors be added to treat neurogenic shock.
- CT angiography should be performed in upper cervical spine fractures to rule out vertebral artery injury or thrombosis.
- The flexion-distraction fracture (Chance fracture) is often the result of inappropriate restraining of a child in a motor vehicle and is associated with intra-abdominal visceral and major vascular injuries.

Editor's Comment

Spinal cord injuries are among the most devastating injuries that can occur in children. Because of anatomic, physiologic and emotional differences, all aspects of care in children,

including especially identification of an injury and treatment of a known injury, are more challenging than the corresponding issue in adults. Ruling out a spine injury can be exceptionally difficult. Though CT and MRI are known to be more sensitive than clinical examination and plain radiographs, they are also associated with some risk and higher costs. Developing effective and efficient protocols that incorporate these modalities in everyday clinical practice is proving to be difficult. Trauma protocols that unambiguous guidelines in place help to avoid both over-use and under-use of these useful tools.

Though there is as yet no specific recommendation to administer intravenous corticosteroids in children with spinal injuries as there is in adults, I suspect most trauma centers that deal with children are doing it, based on a simple calculus that weighs the relatively small risks and the potential reward of the therapy. Nevertheless, until more data become available, it is not a recommended practice. It is much more important to avoid progression of the injury by proper immobilization (properly fitting hard collar, taking into consideration the relatively large size of the child's occiput) and fastidiously addressing airway, breathing and circulation.

Differential Diagnosis

Shock

- Neurogenic
- Hemorrhagic

Neurologic Deficit

- Spinal "shock"
- Permanent disability

Diagnostic Studies

- Plain radiographs
- Helical CT with reconstruction
- CT angiography
- Flexion-extension radiographs
- MRI

Parental Preparation

- Permanent disability
- Rehabilitation
- Preventive strategies with front seat air-bags and age appropriate restraints

Preoperative Preparation

- □ Rule out source of hemorrhagic shock
- □ Clear cervical spine if possible
- □ Informed consent

Technical Points

- Get patient off of spine board as soon as possible to avoid pressure sores.
- One must elevate the torso on pads to keep spine in neutral position.
- When deciding between stabilization with internal fixation and external bracing, consider the effects on growth.

Suggested Reading

D'Amato C. Pediatric spinal trauma: injuries in very young children. Clin Orthop Relat Res. 2005;432:34–40.

Launay F, Leet AI, Sponseller PD. Pediatric spinal cord injury without radiographic abnormality: a meta-analysis. Clin Orthop Relat Res. 2005;433:166–70.

Platzer P, Jaindl M, Thalhammer G, et al. Cervical spine injuries in pediatric patients. J Trauma. 2007;62:389–96.

Reddy SP, Junewick JJ, Backstrom JW. Distribution of spinal fractures in children: does age, mechanism of injury, or gender play a significant role? Pediatr Radiol. 2003;33:776–81.

Sanchez B, Waxman K, Jones T, et al. Cervical spine clearance in blunt trauma: evaluation of a computed tomography-based protocol. J Trauma. 2005;59:179–83.

Viccellio P, Simon H, Pressman BD, et al. A prospective multicenter study of cervical spine injury in children. Pediatrics. 2001;108(2):E20.

Chapter 21
Vascular Injury

Barbara A. Gaines

While trauma is the leading cause of morbidity and mortality in the pediatric population, most pediatric trauma is the result of blunt force, with a predominance of head and truncal injuries. Vascular injuries are quite uncommon and therefore management is less well defined. Even in busy pediatric trauma centers, vascular injuries account for fewer than 1% of total hospital admissions, and therefore individual experience with these injuries is limited, largely abstracted from the adult literature, and often multi-disciplinary.

Two large, recently published studies have defined the demographics of the pediatric trauma victim with a vascular injury. Patients are predominantly male, around 10 years of age, and the victims of penetrating trauma. The association of penetrating mechanism with vascular injury in children is striking: whereas only 6% of one center's total admissions were the result of a penetrating mechanism, 55% of vascular injuries occurred by this type of mechanism. The types of penetrating injuries range from gunshot and stab wounds to dog bites and lawn mower injuries. One mechanism deserves to be highlighted, since it is somewhat unique to the pediatric population: wounds from glass account for a significant number of injuries (the majority in one large series of peripheral vascular injuries). Blunt mechanisms include motor vehicle and all-terrain vehicle (ATV) crashes, falls, and child abuse.

The most frequently injured vessels are those of the upper extremity. Radial and ulnar arteries are often injured by glass, the classic case of the child thrusting his arm through a window. Brachial artery injuries are strongly associated with supracondylar humerus fractures and with falls, especially in younger children. Injuries to the superficial femoral artery are associated with femur fractures, although these injures are generally the result of a penetrating mechanism. Lawnmowers are a unique mechanism for arterial injuries below the level of the popliteal, frequently presenting as a "mangled extremity" with significant bony and soft tissue injury, and a high rate of ultimate limb loss.

Blunt injury to the cerebral vasculature is a problem of significant interest in the adult trauma population. While these injuries are infrequently described in children, the true incidence is possibly underestimated, and anechdotal reports suggest that high energy blunt trauma to the neck can result in significant injury to the carotid or vertebral vessels. Penetrating trauma to the head or neck can also result in vascular injury. One unusual mechanism for an internal carotid injury is the penetrating palate injury. In this scenario, the palate is punctured by a sharp object (such as a pencil), which then damages the internal carotid artery at the skull base.

Finally, vascular injury to the torso is frequently the result of violent, penetrating mechanisms, although blunt force, such as that encountered with motor vehicle crashes, can also result in damage to visceral vessels. Traumatic injury to the thoracic aorta, a well-described deceleration injury in adults, is rare in children. When it does occur, motor vehicle crashes are primarily responsible, although other high velocity mechanisms, such as ATVs and motorcycle crashes have also been implicated.

Diagnosis

Physical examination and arteriography remain the mainstays of the diagnosis of arterial injuries in children, although CT and CT angiography are important in the evaluation of abdominal and cerebrovascular arterial injuries. In the unusual case of suspected injury to the thoracic aorta, helicial CT scan is frequently definitive. If necessary, confirmatory studies include aortography or transesophogeal echocardiography.

Absence of palpable pulses or other hard signs of vascular injury mandate operative intervention in penetrating injury, and further evaluation in the case of blunt mechanisms. An ankle–brachial index of less than 0.9 is also highly suggestive of an injury. Conversely, proximity of a wound to a major vessel alone, in the absence of physical signs, does not warrant invasive diagnostic evaluation. Reduction of an associated fracture (often in the operating room) usually results in restoration of blood flow and pulses. If this does not occur, arteriography is recommended. If the patient is already in the

B.A. Gaines (✉)
University of Pittsburgh Children's Hospital of Pittsburgh of UPMC,
3705 5th Avenue, 4A489, Pittsburgh, PA 15213, USA
e-mail: barbara.gaines@chp.edu

P. Mattei (ed.), *Fundamentals of Pediatric Surgery*,
DOI 10.1007/978-1-4419-6643-8_21, © Springer Science+Business Media, LLC 2011

operating room, the surgeon should consider performing an on-table arteriogram. It is important to note that, in contradistinction to vascular problems in adults, there is a high rate of vasospasm in children, especially those under 10 years of age. In one series, over a quarter of children initially evaluated for peripheral vascular insufficiency were ultimately diagnosed with vasospasm and managed conservatively.

Injury to the cerebral vascular vessels should be strongly considered in children with evidence of significant blunt or shearing force to the neck. Other injuries associated with blunt injury to the carotid artery include basilar skull fractures and combined head and chest trauma. CT angiography with an appropriately timed contrast bolus can definitively identify such lesions. In the setting of multiple injuries, consultation with radiology is important in order to maximize diagnostic information and minimize radiation and intravenous contrast exposure.

Arteriography can be performed safely in children and the role of the interventional radiologist in pediatric vascular trauma is increasing. Angiograms provide important diagnostic information, and can also be therapeutic. Most therapeutic procedures in children involve embolization of bleeding vessels or pseudoaneurysms, although there are scattered reports of balloon angioplasty and endovascular stent placement in the literature. One difficulty with endovascular techniques in children is the lack of devices small enough for pediatric vessels, and issues related to long term vessel growth. New techniques and devices available to pediatric interventional cardiologists may help bridge this gap, although any such use would certainly be investigational in the peripheral or cerebral vascular setting.

Treatment

Management of vascular injuries in children is often multidisciplinary, with involvement of pediatric surgeons, plastic surgeons, neurosurgeons, adult vascular surgeons, orthopedic surgeons, cardiothoracic surgeons, and interventional radiologists. Accurate diagnosis of the cause of vascular insufficiency must be determined. In the patient with no pulses after penetrating trauma to an extremity, exploration without any further diagnostic testing is justified. In other cases, some type of imaging is recommended, either arteriography or CT. CT angiography is utilized frequently for truncal and cerebrovascular injuries, whereas arteriography remains the gold standard for evaluation of peripheral vascular lesions. Arteriography also has the advantage of being potentially therapeutic, although in a more limited fashion than in adults.

Vasospasm may be simply observed and should resolve without intervention. Intimal flaps with no evidence of occlusion (particularly those involving the cerebral vessels) are most often treated by anticoagulation. Large pseudoaneueyerisms or bleeding from a visceral or pelvic vessel may be treated with angioembolization. Operative repair ranges from ligation of small distal arteries with good perfusion to primary repair and repair with grafts. Debridement of the injured vessel with end-to-end reconstruction is frequently employed, if the technique can be performed without undue tension to the repair. In cases in which an interposition graft is required, autologous reversed saphenous vein is the preferred conduit. Rarely, bypass grafts are required.

Axillo-femoral, innominate-axillary, and femoral-popliteal bypasses have been described for the management of unusual injuries or in the face massive tissue destruction. Again, an autologus tissue graft is preferred. Because saphaneous vein is the preferred conduit, any case in which the potential for vascular injury exists requires full sterile preparation and draping of both lower extremities for possible vein harvest. In addition, it is recommended that in the case of lower extremity injury, vein from the contralateral leg be harvested in order to prevent potential complications arising from combined arterial and venous insufficiency. Arterial injury in a young child often requires a team approach, with pediatric or vascular surgeons obtaining access to the field and a surgeon with microvascular expertise performing the actual vascular repair.

Injuries to the major abdominal vessels are frequently associated with other injuries, including those to the intestine, pancreato-biliary system, and solid organs. If the patient is not *in extremis*, a thorough exploration for these types of injuries is necessary. Successful application of damage control vascular surgical techniques such as the placement of temporary shunts has been reported in the military literature. There is little experience with these procedures in children but in cases of physiologic collapse, it would seem reasonable to attempt some sort of temporizing measure.

Outcomes

Outcome after vascular injury in pediatric patients often depend on associated injuries and the mechanism. The high rate of lower extremity amputation secondary to lawnmower injuries is due in part to the fact that the vascular injury is frequently associated with significant bony and soft tissues deficits. While information on specific long-term vascular outcome is lacking in most studies, repair of peripheral vascular injuries in children appears to be well tolerated and associated with a viable and functional extremity. In the future, data regarding vessel and/or graft patency will hopefully be collected and reported.

Blunt injury to the cerebral vascular vessels is associated with significant morbidity and risk for stroke. There are reports of fatal cerebral infarction in a child with a blunt carotid injury and a cerebellar stroke from a vertebral injury. Anticoagulation is the treatment of choice in these situations, but the optimal management of these lesions in the multiply injured child with a contraindication to anticoagulation has yet to be determined.

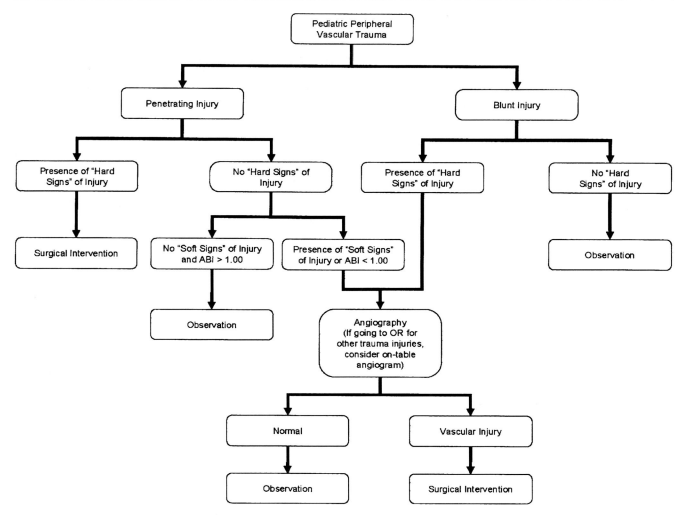

Fig. 21.1 Proposed algorithm for the management of peripheral vascular trauma in children. Hard signs of injury include: distal ischemia, absent pulses, active hemorrhage, expanding or pulsatile hematoma, and the presence of a bruit or thrill. Soft signs of injury include: a history of pulsatile bleeding, stable hematoma, or proximity to a known vessels (Adapted with permission from Shah et al. (2009))

There is minimal experience with the use of endovascular techniques for the treatment of such lesions in children.

Although the data are limited, injury to the thoracic aorta in children, as in adults, is associated with significant morbidity. Management of uncomplicated intimal flap injuries with anti-hypertensive medications appears to be well tolerated with few long-term complications. Injuries requiring interposition grafting, on the other hand, are associated with serious complications including paraplegia, renal failure, sepsis, and recurrent laryngeal nerve injury.

Abdominal vascular injuries are often associated with significant hemorrhage, and the outcome is dependent upon rapid control of the bleeding vessels, as well as repair of other visceral damage (Fig. 21.1).

Summary Points

- Vascular injury is unusual in pediatric trauma patients.
- Penetrating mechanisms result in a disproportionate number of pediatric vascular injuries.
- Management of these injuries often involves a multi-disciplinary team including specialists from general pediatric surgery, vascular surgery, neurosurgery, plastic and microvascular surgery, cardiothoracic surgery, neurosurgery, and interventional radiology.
- Vasospasm resulting in transient vascular insufficiency is more common in children than in adults.
- Blunt cerebral vascular injury may result in serious sequelae including stroke and death.
- Outcome after peripheral vascular injury in children is generally associated with a viable and functional limb, except in cases of the "mangled extremity" such as those seen as a result of lawnmower injuries.

- An abnormal vascular exam mandates further investigation.
- In the case of penetrating trauma, an abnormal exam is all that is necessary for surgical exploration.
- For peripheral vascular injuries, arteriography provides diagnostic information and in some cases may be therapeutic.
- CT angiography is extremely useful for the evaluation of cerebral vascular injuries.
- In the patient with normal hemodynamics, multi-detector helical CT scanning of the chest and/or abdomen can identify significant vascular abnormalities.

Editor's Comment

Vascular injuries in children are approached using the same basic techniques commonly applied in adults, but with special attention paid to using microvascular techniques when needed, avoiding artificial graft material whenever possible, and accounting for the need of children to grow both in length and tissue mass over time. Proximal and distal control of the vessel with proper flushing of heparin solution is critical but it is important to remember that excessive heparin flushes can cause systemic anticoagulation in a small child. Primary repair should be employed whenever possible, if the arterial ends can be debrided and the repair done without tension. Circumferential repairs should be done at least partly with interrupted sutures or with a "growth stitch" to allow for radial growth of the vessel as the child grows. Reversed saphenous vein is the best conduit or patch graft material but other veins can be used as an alternative. In the neck, the external jugular vein can be used but, because it is thin and prone to aneurysm, some have described everting it in order to effectively double the thickness of its wall. The same is true for the gonadal vein in the abdomen and other expendable but thin-walled veins in other body compartments. When reversed saphenous vein graft is used for bypass of major abdominal vessels in children, the graft can be reinforced with a sleeve of artificial graft material to prevent subsequent aneurysm formation.

Although ligation of some large arteries with good collateral blood supply such as the external iliac artery are compatible with limb salvage, subsequent claudication and limb-length disparity due to insufficient blood supply is a common result. Bypass grafting procedures are effective in reversing these symptoms and can allow significant catch-up growth of the affected extremity if done before the age of skeletal maturity.

Finally, extremities that have been ischemic for any length of time are at risk for compartment syndrome when perfusion is restored. Fasciotomy should be performed empirically in children who are at risk for this potentially devastating complication.

Diagnostic Studies

- Computed tomography
- CT angiography
- Ultrasound with Doppler
- Arteriography
- Helical CT (for aortic deceleration injuries)

Preoperative Preparation

- ☐ Intravenous access/fluid resuscitation
- ☐ Sterile preparation of both thighs for possible saphenous vein graft harvest
- ☐ Consultation with appropriate specialists

Technical Points

- Most cases of vasospasm may be treated conservatively with observation.
- Intimal flaps, especially in surgically inaccessible locations, are treated with anticoagulation.
- Angioembolization may be useful for the control of pelvic or visceral arterial bleeding.
- Endovascular techniques are in their infancy for the management of pediatric vascular problems.
- Open surgical techniques include primary repair of the injured vessel, end-to-end reapproximation of the injury, interposition grafting (most often with saphenous vein), and bypass grafts.

Suggested Reading

Anderson SA, Day M, Chen MK, et al. Traumatic aortic injuries in the pediatric population. J Pediatr Surg. 2008;43:1077–81.

Hamner CE, Groner JI, Caniano DA, et al. Blunt intraabdominal injury in pediatric trauma patients: injury distribution and markers of outcome. J Pediatr Surg. 2008;43:916–23.

Klinkner DB, Arca MJ, Lewis BD, et al. Pediatric vascular injuries: patterns of injury, morbidity, and mortality. J Pediatr Surg. 2007;42:178–83.

Puapong D, Brown CVR, Katz M, et al. Angiography and the pediatric trauma patient: a 10 year review. J Pediatr Surg. 2006;41:1859–63.

Shah SR, Wearden PD, Gaines BA. Pediatric peripheral vascular injuries: a review of our experience. J Surg Res. 2009;153(1):162–6.

Chapter 22
Pediatric Hand Injuries

Roger Cornwall

The hand is the most frequently injured part of the child's body. Household injuries dominate in the younger child and sports-related injuries account for the majority of hand injuries in older children and adolescents. The child's hand is important for exploration, socialization, and development, and its function in these realms can be affected by serious injuries.

In keeping with the trend toward increasingly specialized surgical disciplines, the majority of pediatric hand injuries will be treated by surgeons with orthopedic, plastics, or hand surgery training. Nonetheless, the general surgeon must be aware of the principles of evaluation and management of pediatric hand injuries, as they often occur in the setting of concomitant general surgical problems. Hand injuries can occur in the setting of major skeletal and visceral injuries, and must not be underappreciated by the general trauma surgeon directing the care of the pediatric polytrauma patient. Likewise, the general surgeon must be aware of potential complications of diagnostic and therapeutic procedures that can occur in the hand and require emergent specialized treatment.

While most fractures in the child's hand will heal uneventfully following closed treatment, several fractures and injuries require prompt diagnosis and specific treatment to avoid long-term problems such as deformity, dysfunction, or infection.

Diagnosis

Examining the injured hand can be challenging, especially in the young or multi-injured child. For this reason, the evaluation of the child's hand relies heavily on observation and passive tests. Observe the resting posture of the hand. Tendon injuries can be detected by simply observing the cascade of the fingers without needing the patient to actively flex a finger (Fig. 22.1). Similarly, since the extrinsic finger flexor and extensor tendons cross the wrist joint, the examiner can use wrist tenodesis to flex or extend a finger in an attempt to detect tendon incompetence or rotational deformities of the digits (Fig. 22.2). Wrinkling of digital skin in water ("pruning") requires intact sensory nerve function and its absence can be used to detect digital nerve injuries in children who are too young to cooperate with a formal sensory examination. Simple observation of the child's use of the hand may also provide valuable information regarding the location, nature, or severity of an injury.

Radiographs of the injured hand must be specific for the parts of the hand that are injured. The leading cause of poor outcome in pediatric finger fractures is failure to appreciate the fracture displacement due to inadequate initial lateral radiographs. A lateral radiograph of the hand with the fingers overlapping is insufficient for the evaluation of a finger fracture (Fig. 22.3). Similarly, forearm radiographs are not sufficient for evaluating fractures in the wrist, hand and digits due to the parallax distortion of structures at the edges of a radiograph. Computed tomography and MRI are rarely necessary in pediatric hand trauma, but can be very useful for evaluation of complex or occult carpal injury.

Specific Hand Fractures and Dislocations

Phalangeal Neck and Condyle Fractures

Phalangeal neck fractures account for 13% of pediatric hand fractures and in the majority of cases are displaced. Sagittal displacement impairs adjacent interphalangeal joint motion given the periarticular location of the fracture (Fig. 22.4). Coronal and rotational displacement can lead to permanent deformity given the lack of remodeling in these planes. The fracture is also inherently unstable and not amenable to splint or cast immobilization following reduction given the high rate of redisplacement. For these reasons, anatomic reduction and

R. Cornwall (✉)
Division of Orthopedic Surgery, Cincinnati Children's Hospital
Medical Center, Cincinnati, OH, USA
e-mail: roger.cornwall@cchmc.org

P. Mattei (ed.), *Fundamentals of Pediatric Surgery*,
DOI 10.1007/978-1-4419-6643-8_22, © Springer Science+Business Media, LLC 2011

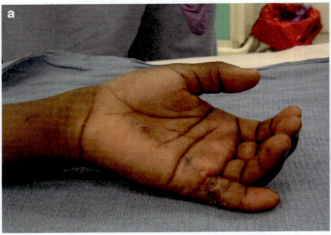

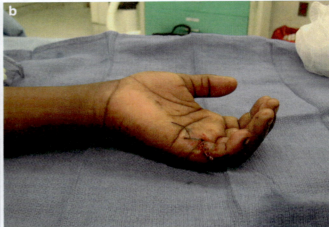

Fig. 22.1 (**a**) Altered cascade (resting posture) of the small finger from a laceration of the flexor tendons. (**b**) Note the restored flexion cascade following tendon repairs (Cornwall R, Waters PM. Pediatric trauma and infections. In: Trumble TE, Budoff JE, eds. Hand surgery update IV. American Society for Surgery of the Hand, 2007)

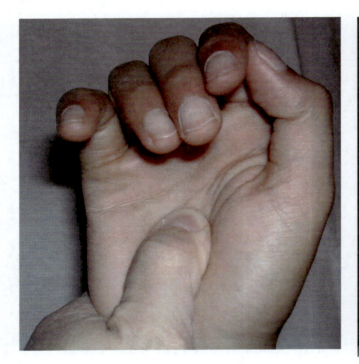

Fig. 22.2 Passive wrist extension creates enough tenodesis flexion of the fingers to detect a rotational deformity, such as in this proximal phalanx fracture of the small finger (Cornwall R, Waters PM. Pediatric hand trauma. In: Core knowledge in orthopaedics: hand, elbow, shoulder. Elsevier, p. 406)

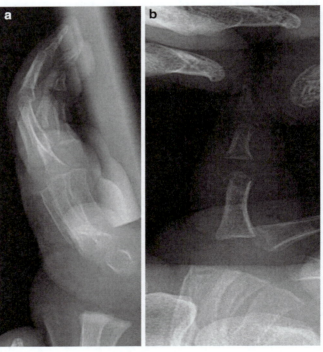

Fig. 22.3 (**a**) Lateral radiograph of the hand with the fingers overlapping is insufficient for evaluation of finger fractures. (**b**) Isolated lateral radiograph of the injured finger demonstrates a displaced proximal phalanx neck fracture in the same patient (Cornwall R. Pediatric hand fractures. In: Budoff JE, ed. Fractures of the upper extremity: a master skills publication. American Society for Surgery of the Hand, 2008)

pin fixation are required. Complicating the care of these fractures is the often subtle clinical picture and rapid healing that can lead to a malunion within 2–3 weeks. Such an incipient malunion cannot be easily corrected due to the risk of avascular necrosis of the fracture fragment from attempts at late open reduction. Therefore, the fracture must be identified and radiographically evaluated quickly to allow prompt treatment.

Phalangeal condyle fractures are intra-articular fractures of the distal end of the proximal or middle phalanx. Similar to phalangeal neck fractures, they cause significant deformity and dysfunction if displaced and require prompt reduction and fixation. The window of opportunity of fixation of these fractures is similarly short due to the rapid healing and the risks of attempted reduction once healing has begun.

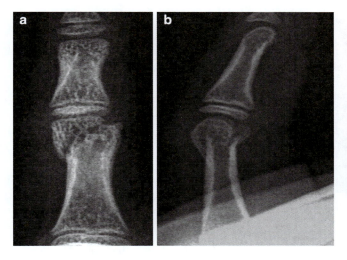

Fig. 22.4 (**a**) Anteroposterior (Cornwall R. Pediatric hand fractures. In: Fractures of the upper extremity: a master skills publication. American Society for Surgery of the Hand, p. 108) and (**b**) lateral radiographs of a displaced phalangeal neck fracture

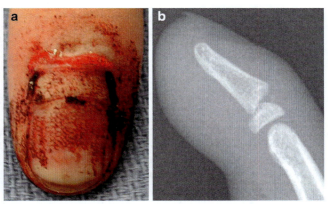

Fig. 22.5 (**a**) Clinical photograph (Cornwall R, Waters PM. Pediatric hand trauma. In: Core knowledge in orthopaedics: Hand, elbow, shoulder. Elsevier, p. 417) and (**b**) lateral radiograph of a Seymour fracture. Note the avulsed proximal end of the nail and the dorsally widened physis (Cornwall R. Pediatric hand fractures. In: Fractures of the upper extremity: a master skills publication. American Society for Surgery of the Hand, p. 113)

Seymour Fracture

A fracture of the distal phalanx physis with tearing of the proximal nailbed has been termed the Seymour fracture (Fig. 22.5). The torn nailbed and avulsion of the proximal end of the nail from the eponychial fold make this injury an open fracture that is prone to deep infection unless urgently irrigated and debrided. Furthermore, the torn nailbed often becomes entrapped in the fracture site, preventing proper reduction of the fracture. Any proximal nail avulsion or flexion deformity of the tip of the finger with bleeding at the cuticle should prompt immediate dedicated radiographs of the distal phalanx to rule out a Seymour fracture. If such a fracture is identified, the nail plate should be removed to allow irrigation, debridement, and reduction of the fracture. Care must be taken during irrigation and debridement to avoid further injury to the physis and nailbed, and this procedure is best done with appropriate magnification, lighting, and training. Osteomyelitis, growth arrest, and nail deformity can result if the diagnosis is delayed for even 1 day.

Scaphoid Fracture

As it is in the adult, the scaphoid is the most commonly fractured carpal bone in the skeletally immature. The precarious blood supply to the proximal pole of the scaphoid makes nonunion likely unless the fracture is immobilized properly during healing. Because of the intricate anatomy and kinematics of the carpus, malunion or nonunion of a scaphoid fracture can cause severe post-traumatic wrist arthrosis. Scaphoid fractures must therefore be identified, evaluated, and treated promptly. However, they often cause minimal swelling and can be difficult to identify on initial radiographs, even with dedicated scaphoid views. As many as two thirds of scaphoid fractures in adolescents present as nonunions, due largely to the initially underwhelming physical findings. Snuffbox tenderness in the setting of wrist trauma should raise suspicion for occult scaphoid fracture and prompt evaluation with either MRI or repeated plain radiographs after 1–2 weeks of immobilization. Displaced fractures are typically easily identified on plain radiographs, although the degree of displacement is best evaluated by a dedicated wrist CT scan. Displaced fractures require reduction and fixation by a qualified surgeon.

Metacarpophalangeal Dislocation

Metacarpophalangeal dislocations are more common than interphalangeal dislocations in children, and they are more common in children than in adults. Metacarpophalangeal (MCP) dislocations are irreducible in up to 50% of cases, usually because of entrapment of a torn volar plate, a plate of fibrocartilage on the palmar side of the joint that resists hyperextension. A reducible (simple) dislocation can be iatrogenically converted to an irreducible (complex) dislocation by inappropriate use of longitudinal traction during reduction attempts. Longitudinal traction applied to a dislocated MCP joint will create a vacuum within the joint that can pull the torn volar plate into the joint, creating a block to reduction. Instead, the proximal phalanx should be held in hyperextension and guided palmarly around the metacarpal head without longitudinal traction. If closed reduction attempts fail, open reduction should be performed urgently.

Soft Tissue and Combined Injuries

Flexor Tendon Injuries

Flexor tendon lacerations are not as common in children as they are in adults, but they may be more difficult to diagnose as the child will often refuse to try to flex an injured finger. Any alteration of the normal cascade or resting posture of the fingers should raise suspicion, especially in the setting of penetrating or crushing trauma to the palmar side of the fingers, hand, or forearm. Flexor tendon repair must be performed promptly, as scarring and retraction of the proximal stump and loss of flexor sheath patency will preclude successful primary repair beyond 2–3 weeks. Later reconstructive options are available, but with inferior results. Of particular concern is laceration of multiple tendons and at least one nerve or artery in the wrist ("spaghetti wrist") or forearm. Emergent exploration and repair is indicated in the setting of poor distal perfusion or difficulty obtaining hemostasis, but otherwise, the wound may be closed primarily for later repair of nerves and tendons within 7–10 days. Significant scarring and stiffness can result, but outcomes are surprisingly good overall.

Nerve Injuries

Nerve injuries of the hand are uncommon in children. Digital nerves can be lacerated in penetrating trauma or crushing injuries to the finger. Lacerations to the wrist may include laceration of the median, palmar cutaneous, ulnar, dorsal ulnar sensory, and radial sensory nerves, all of which cross the wrist crease. The function of each nerve underlying any laceration to the hand or wrist should be individually examined. Young children cannot participate in a typical sensory examination, but finger tip wrinkling in water can be used to assess sensory nerve function. Motor examination requires patience, and is often aided by bandaging the wound so that the child cannot see the laceration. When a nerve injury cannot be ruled out, surgical exploration is indicated, although this can be delayed for 7–10 days, if necessary, due to concomitant injuries.

Nerve injuries in the setting of a displaced fracture are usually neuropraxias and resolve spontaneously over the course of weeks or months. Formal surgical exploration is warranted in cases of incomplete recovery or worsening neurologic deficit. Knowledge of specific innervation within the hand and forearm is critically important for the diagnosis and follow up of nerve injuries, as electromyography can be highly variable and unpleasant in children.

Vascular Injuries

Vascular injuries to the hand typically occur in the setting of penetrating trauma. Pulsatile bleeding from the hand and wrist should be controlled with local pressure, not with a tourniquet, which can cause ischemia to the entire distal limb. If hemostasis can be obtained with local pressure alone and perfusion remains adequate, the wound need not be formally explored. Close follow up should be provided following wound closure, however, given the possibility of developing a pseuodoaneurysm from partial arterial injury. If hemostasis cannot be obtained, which is often the case with longitudinal arterial or major venous laceration, emergent exploration is indicated. Actively bleeding vessels in the hand and wrist should not be tied off in the emergency department, given the intimate proximity of important nerves. Arteriography is rarely helpful and will delay necessary surgical exploration.

Ischemia in the setting of a displaced fracture is often a result of tenting or compression of nearby arteries, such as the brachial artery in the setting of a displaced distal humerus fracture. Fracture reduction usually restores arterial flow, although emergent exploration and arterial repair is necessary if the limb remains ischemic following reduction. Ischemia in the setting of penetrating trauma warrants emergent surgical exploration.

Amputations

Fingertip amputations and partial amputations are common in young children, as toddlers have an uncanny interest in inserting their fingers into the hinge side of closing doors. Most such injuries involve fractures of the distal aspect of the distal phalanx and degloving of soft tissue and nail bed. Absorbable sutures should be used to repair all fingertip injuries in children, as later suture removal is both difficult and traumatic for the child and provider. If the part is completely detached and composed of only soft tissue, it can be sutured in place as a composite graft. The part may survive following such a repair in infants, but rarely in older children. Nonetheless, the part serves as a biological dressing following necrosis, under which the tip can heal by secondary intention. If the amputated part is unavailable, healing by secondary intention can work remarkably well in young children, although wet-to-dry dressing changes can be tedious for the child and parents. Formal graft or flap coverage is rarely indicated in the fingertip in children.

Microvascular replantation is generally reserved for amputations at or proximal to the level of the distal interphalangeal joint. Single digit replantation, while generally contraindicated in adults, is indicated in children given the possibility of a good functional result if the part survives. However, given the smaller size of the vessels, the salvage rate for distal replantation in children is slightly less than that for adults. Furthermore, successful venous reanastomosis is difficult in distal pediatric replantations, often requiring the use of leeches to treat postoperative venous congestion until the skin heals and new venules form.

Hand Compartment Syndrome

Compartment syndrome can occur in any of the ten compartments of the hand. While no series of pediatric hand compartment syndrome has been reported in the literature to date, it is my experience that hand compartment syndrome is generally seen after severe crush injuries with multiple metacarpal fractures or in the setting of severe intravenous line infiltration in the sedated or obtunded patient.

The most sensitive indicator of impending compartment syndrome in a child is increasing analgesic requirements. Other clinical signs include pain out of proportion to the injury and severe swelling with loss of the normal concavity of the palm (Fig. 22.6). Perfusion of the digits remains normal and brisk capillary refill should never be used to rule out a compartment syndrome in the hand.

Formal evaluation of a possible compartment syndrome in the hand is more difficult than in the forearm. The muscles affected by hand compartment syndrome are the intrinsic muscles, not the extrinsic finger flexors typically affected by volar forearm compartment syndrome. Therefore, in order to assess pain on passive stretch of the involved muscles, the intrinsic muscles must be stretched by either abduction of the fingers or combined metacarpophalangeal joint hyperextension and proximal interphalangeal joint flexion. Such maneuvers can be difficult and painful in the injured hand. Further complicating the diagnosis of compartment syndrome in the hand is the small size of the compartments and the difficulty in accurately measuring pressures using invasive techniques.

The compartments most reliably accessed with a pressure monitoring needle are the thenar and hypothenar compartments, but access to these compartments is through the very sensitive palmar skin, making invasive pressure measurement very painful for the awake child.

For these reasons, if a compartment syndrome is clinically suspected, the child should be taken emergently to the operating room for fasciotomy with or without pressure measurement under general anesthesia. In young children and infants, mean arterial pressure may be very low, and pressure values considered diagnostic of compartment syndrome in adults may not apply. Very often, therefore, faciotomies are performed based entirely on clinical grounds. The ten compartments can be approached through four incisions, one each for the thenar and hypothenar compartments, and two longitudinal incisions over the index and ring metacarpals for the interosseus compartments. Following fasciotomies, wounds can be left open for staged closure once the swelling subsides 2–3 days later. Skin grafting is rarely required.

Blast Injuries

Blast injuries to the hand are not uncommon where explosive devices such as fireworks are available. Contrary to popular belief, the incidence of blast injuries in children does not cluster around holidays typically associated with fireworks. Most injuries occur when the child finds an old device stored at home, which might be months to years old and not functioning properly. The age range is generally from 7 to 14 years, but children of any age can be affected. The hand is typically injured while the device is still in the hand, with the epicenter of the blast in the first webspace. As a result, the thumb is often the most severely injured digit. The amount of damage depends on the size of the device, and can range from superficial burns to partial or complete amputation of the hand (Fig. 22.7).

Any child with a blast injury to the hand should be emergently evaluated for percussive trauma to the chest and abdomen, as well as burns to the face and eyes. The hand must then be urgently irrigated and debrided. In general, parts amputated by the blast are too severely injured to be replanted, and much of the remaining tissue is nonviable and must be removed. Significant scarring and deformity can occur in the salvaged parts, leading to greatly compromised function.

Prevention is the best means of addressing blast injuries to the hand in children. Explosive devices should not be stored in a location accessible to children, and the handling of explosive devices should be left to properly trained individuals.

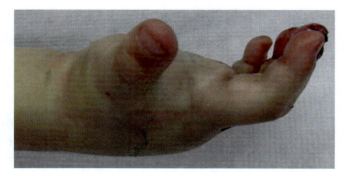

Fig. 22.6 Clinical photograph of a child with compartment syndrome of the hand following crush injury. Note the loss of palmar concavity

Fig. 22.7 (**a**) Severe blast injury to the hand of a 7-year-old boy from commercially available fireworks. (**b**) Same hand following skeletal reconstruction and coverage with a groin flap

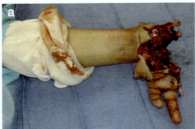 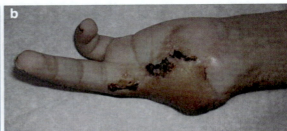

Summary Points

- The frequency of hand injuries in children and the wide variety of injury type and severity together pose challenges for the general surgeon treating the injured child.
- Thorough examination, though difficult, is crucial for determining the severity of injury. Always check for rotational deformity in injured digits.
- Dedicated radiographs of the injured digit are essential for evaluation of finger fractures. Similarly, forearm radiographs are not adequate for assessment of carpal fractures.
- Because of the rapid healing of fractures in the child's hand, permanent malunions may develop quickly unless definitive fracture treatment is provided within the first 1–2 weeks.
- Severe swelling in the hand with increasing analgesic requirements should raise suspicion for hand compartment syndrome.
- Major soft tissue injuries in the child's hand demand prompt and specialized care, but the rapid and reliable soft tissue healing in children usually allow rewarding results.

Editor's Comment

Definitive care of hand injuries requires a great deal of expertise and experience, preferably by a dedicated hand surgeon, but the initial assessment and treatment are important aspects of the care of the injured child. General and pediatric surgeons therefore need to be prepared to deal with these situations and should not be intimidated when they occur. In general, a minimalist approach is best: observe and gently examine the hand without excessive manipulation, try to assess distal neurovascular function, obtain appropriate dedicated radiographs, and discuss the case personally with a pediatric hand surgeon as soon as possible. If there is bleeding, one should apply direct pressure by hand, never with a "pressure" dressing or weights. Apply only the minimum pressure necessary to stop the bleeding; excessive pressure occludes the artery and causes distal ischemia. Severe ischemia or pulsatile bleeding should always prompt emergent surgical exploration, not additional diagnostic studies. Always assume that a subungual hematoma could be the result of an underlying distal phalangeal fracture and perform a dedicated radiograph to rule this out. To preserve amputated parts for possible reimplantation, it is probably best to wrap the tissue in saline-soaked gauze, place it in a specimen cup, and place this into a specimen bag containing ice and water.

Finally, remember to document every aspect of the physical examination and any therapeutic maneuvers in great detail in the medical record as this will help the hand surgeon during subsequent follow up and could help reduce medical liability if the functional outcome is less than optimal.

Differential Diagnosis

- Bony fracture
- Soft tissue injury
- Dislocation
- Tendon injury
- Nerve injury
- Vascular injury
- Hand compartment syndrome

Diagnostic Studies

- Dedicated radiographs with multiple views
- Computed tomography
- Magnetic resonance imaging
- Measurement of compartment pressures

Preoperative Preparation

- ☐ Prophylactic antibiotics, if appropriate
- ☐ Tetanus prophylaxis, if appropriate
- ☐ Meticulous physical examination and imaging studies

Parental Preparation

- The primary goal is the best long-term functional result possible.
- Some injuries require immediate or emergent treatment while others are best managed in a delayed fashion.
- Reimplantation of an amputated digit is not always indicated or possible and, when they are attempted, because of the small size of the blood vessels in children, the ultimate outcome is somewhat unpredictable.
- As with all trauma, prevention is best.

Technical Points

- Always carefully examine the hands of children who present with severe or multi-system injuries.
- Examination of the child's hand requires patience, careful observation, and passive tests as they are often frightened and in pain and therefore rarely cooperative.
- Control pulsatile or severe bleeding with direct pressure, not with a tourniquet.
- Never try to clamp or ligate a bleeding vessel without proper instruments, lighting, magnification, and experience, as nerve injuries are frequently the result.
- Do not attempt to reduce metacarpophalangeal dislocations by applying longitudinal traction, as this creates a vacuum that can draw in the volar plate or other soft tissue and prevent proper healing. If the dislocation cannot be reduced by gentle manipulation, it should be performed in the operation room.

Suggested Reading

Al-Qattan MM. Extra-articular transverse fractures of the base of the distal phalanx (Seymour's fracture) in children and adults. J Hand Surg [Br]. 2001a;26(3):201–6.

Al-Qattan MM. Phalangeal neck fractures in children: classification and outcome in 66 cases. J Hand Surg [Br]. 2001b;26(2):112–21.

Bae DS, Kadiyala RK, Waters PM. Acute compartment syndrome in children: contemporary diagnosis, treatment, and outcome. J Pediatr Orthop. 2001;21(5):680–8.

Cornwall R, Waters PM. Pediatric hand trauma. In: Trumble TE, Budoff JE, Cornwall R, editors. Core knowledge in orthopaedics: hand, elbow, shoulder. Philadelphia: Elsevier; 2006. p. 406–21.

Hastings H, Simmons BP. Hand fractures in children. A statistical analysis. Clin Orthop. 1984;188:120–30.

Light TR. Carpal injuries in children. Hand Clin. 2000;16(4):513–22.

Vadivelu R et al. Hand injuries in children: a prospective study. J Pediatr Orthop. 2006;26(1):29–35.

Chapter 23
Child Abuse

Richard A. Falcone, Jr. and Kathi Makoroff

Child abuse is a significant problem in the United States, with 905,000 children determined to be victims of abuse or neglect in 2006. More than 15% of these children were victims of physical abuse and almost 10% suffered sexual abuse. The consequence of missed cases of abuse is significant, with 25% of these children suffering more severe subsequent injuries before an appropriate diagnosis is made. In 2006 there were more than 1,500 deaths resulting from child abuse, making it the leading cause of death for children between 6 and 12 months of age. It is crucial that all health care providers properly identify and evaluate cases of child abuse. In addition, it is mandated by law that physicians report all suspected cases of suspected child abuse.

Eighty percent of the victims of child abuse, or non-accidental trauma (NAT) are less than 5 years old and 40% are less than a year of age. Children who are born prematurely or with disabilities are at increased risk of being physically abused. In more than 75% of cases, the abuser is a parent, related caretaker, or an acquaintance of the family. A male acquaintance of a single mother is a common perpetrator. In another 15–20% the abuser is an unrelated babysitter. It is important to recognize that parents who have been involved with other forms of domestic violence, alcohol or substance abuse are more likely to inflict harm on their children. Also, parents who have been physically or emotionally abused and those who are socially isolated or have high life stresses are more likely to abuse a child.

Diagnosis

Unusual patterns of injuries or a discrepancy between the history of the injury and the extent of injuries should prompt further evaluation for possible NAT. Early recognition and reporting of physical abuse can prevent the predictable progression to more serious injuries or death. Treatment of injuries should follow standard trauma care principles.

Head Injuries

It is estimated that 95% of serious intracranial injuries in children under a year of age are a consequence of NAT. In addition, more than 80% of deaths from head trauma in children younger than 2 years of age are the result of non-accidental injury. The principal mechanical forces that produce closed head injuries are translational (secondary to impact) and rotational (sudden acceleration-deceleration: shaking). Although most minor head injuries in children are accidental, skull fractures or intracranial injuries in children less than 1 year of age that occur without a witnessed or reliable mechanism should prompt further evaluation for possible non-accidental injury.

Subdural hematomas (SDH) occur secondary to disruption of bridging veins between the brain and the dura, and occur uncommonly from simple household falls or minor head trauma. SDH in an infant with no plausible explanation strongly suggest a non-accidental injury. The presence of concurrent skeletal or cutaneous injuries should prompt a presumption of non-accidental injury. Infants and children with non-accidental head injury ("shaken-baby syndrome") may initially present without any history of trauma and present only with lethargy and decreased responsiveness. The progressive neurologic deterioration is generally related to increased intracranial pressure secondary to cerebral edema and delay in treatment. It is important to remember that children with non-accidental head injury often have no significant external findings or associated skull fracture. Retinal hemorrhages, which can be bilateral or unilateral, are often present, but up to 20% of children with non-accidental head injury do not have retinal hemorrhages.

R.A. Falcone (✉)
Pediatric General and Thoracic Surgery, University of Cincinnati,
Cincinnati Children's Hospital Medical Center, Cincinnati, OH, USA
e-mail: richard.falcone@cchmc.org

P. Mattei (ed.), *Fundamentals of Pediatric Surgery*,
DOI 10.1007/978-1-4419-6643-8_23, © Springer Science+Business Media, LLC 2011

Abdominal Injuries

Although abdominal injuries following NAT are uncommon, these injuries are associated with a mortality rate of nearly 50% and are the second most common cause of death resulting from physical abuse. These children tend to be slightly older than those with head injuries with a mean age of around 2 years old.

Patterns of abdominal injury secondary to NAT are variable. The mid-abdomen is especially vulnerable to direct blows that result in compression injuries to the viscera. Blunt abdominal injuries that should always be considered suspicious include: gastric rupture, duodenal hematoma, or duodenal perforation. Likewise, intestinal shearing injuries that result in mesenteric hematoma, intestinal hematoma or bowel perforation most commonly result from non-accidental injury (Fig. 23.1). The most common site of intestinal shearing is at the duodenal-jejunal junction. Pancreatic contusion or transection following a blow to the abdomen should also raise suspicion. Additionally, solid organ injury, especially liver injury, is a common cause of hemorrhagic shock and death.

Infants and children with non-accidental abdominal injury usually do not have bruising over the abdomen, so evaluation for intra-abdominal injury should be performed even if the child has no cutaneous findings. Certainly if the child presents with abdominal bruising, further evaluation is warranted.

These children will often present late for care secondary to a failure to recognize the severity of the injury or an attempt to conceal the injury. Often a story inconsistent with the injury is provided, such as the child fell from a couch or bed, fell onto another piece of furniture, or was hit by a sibling. Again, there should be a high level of suspicion when

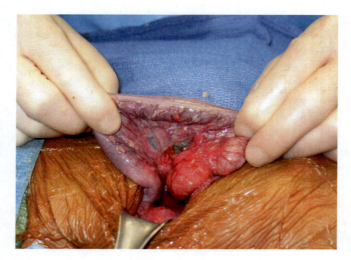

Fig. 23.1 Bowel injury secondary to non-accidental trauma

the identified injuries do not fit the provided mechanism or there has been a prolonged delay in seeking care.

Fractures

Fractures are present in approximately 25% of physically abused children. Long-bone fractures are the most common and skull fractures are second most common. Inflicted fractures can be transverse, comminuted, buckle, oblique, spiral or greenstick fractures. The age and developmental capabilities of the child can be helpful in determining the appropriate level of suspicion. In the absence of a significant accidental injury, certain fractures should be considered highly concerning for physical abuse: metaphyseal corner fractures, posterior rib fractures, scapular fractures, sternal fractures, and spinous process fractures. In addition, fractures in a non-ambulating child, untreated healing fractures, and subperiosteal hematomas due to pulling or twisting the child's limb should be considered highly suspicious for physical abuse.

Rib fractures have been reported in up to 25% of abused children. The presumed mechanism for posterior rib fractures in infants is violent anteroposterior compression of the chest. Accidental falls or chest compressions from cardiopulmonary resuscitation in infants and young children rarely cause rib fractures. As a consequence, in the absence of clear major trauma or preexisting disease, rib fractures in infants must be considered very concerning for non-accidental injury.

Conditions that cause bone fragility must be considered when unexpected fractures are discovered, even though such cases are quite rare. The most frequently discussed bone fragility disorder is osteogenesis imperfecta, a rare inherited connective tissue disorder. Associated features seen in some children include blue sclerae, wormian bones (seen on skull X-ray), and osteopenia. A family history of bone fragility, hearing loss, dental problems, miscarriages, and short stature is often present. When the etiology of a fracture is uncertain, a pediatric radiologist should carefully review the images and, when needed, a pediatric geneticist should be involved.

Burns

Approximately 10–20% of abuse cases involve burns. Most victims are younger than 2 years of age. Inflicted burns range from brandings with hot objects or cigarettes to life-threatening immersion burns. Scalding by hot water is the most common type of inflicted burn. Any scald burn with a sharp border, especially of the hands, feet or buttocks is suspicious

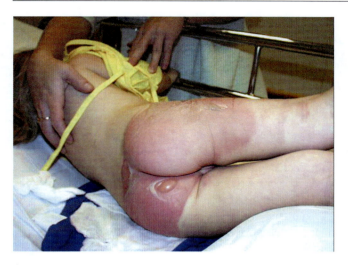

Fig. 23.2 Immersion burn of the buttock

Accidental or straddle injuries more commonly injure the external genitalia and perineum, and are usually unilateral. However, a penetrating straddle injury can injure the hymen, vagina and ano-rectal structures. In these cases, there is usually a history that supports the findings.

Inflicted Bruises and Bites

Bruises are the most common manifestation of physical child abuse. Child abuse should be suspected whenever bruises are over soft body areas such as the thighs, buttocks, cheeks, abdomen, or genitalia; when they are more numerous then expected; they are multiple and of different ages; they are in the shape of objects such as belts, cords or hands; they are

for child abuse (Fig. 23.2). A child who has had a hand placed in hot water and held there will often reflexively close the fingers leading to sparing of the palm and finger tips. Additionally, children who are "dipped" into a bath of hot water often show sparing of the feet or buttocks because they are held firmly against the tub's relatively cooler porcelain bottom. Burns from a solid source often have identifiable characteristics. Children held against a clothing or curling iron, hot plate or heating grate often have wounds with uniform depth and pathognomonic shapes. Cigarette burns typically appear as circular, punched-out ulcers of similar size that are often found on the palms of the hands or the soles of the feet. Any suspicious burns should prompt further evaluation for signs of abuse or other injuries.

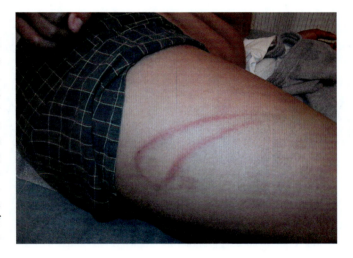

Fig. 23.3 Bruising in the pattern of a belt loop

Ano-Genital Injuries

Sexual abuse should be considered in all patients with genital or anal injuries unless there is a history of a significant accidental trauma. Penetrating injury can result in penetration of the peritoneal cavity and visceral injury. Blunt objects inserted into the rectum or vagina can cause laceration or perforation. The majority of genital and ano-rectal injuries from sexual abuse, however, do not require surgical repair.

If sexual abuse is suspected, testing for sexually transmitted infections should be done. If acute sexual abuse is suspected (within 72 h), evidence collection should be performed before surgical repair if possible. Photographs of the injury before repair should also be obtained.

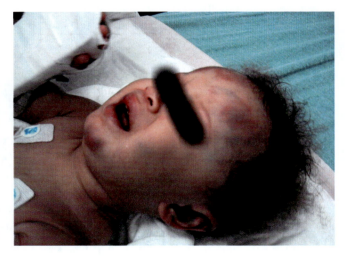

Fig. 23.4 Bruising of the face in a non-ambulating child

noted in young non-ambulating children (Fig. 23.3). Frequently bruising is an incidental finding, unrelated to the reason the child presented for medical care. In infants and young children, bruises to the head (except the forehead), neck, ears, and torso, rarely result from accidental injury mechanisms. Non-ambulating children who have bruising to the head and/or face should be evaluated for occult non-accidental head injury (Fig. 23.4).

Using the color of a bruise to determine dating of the injury is imprecise. Emergency medicine physicians, pediatricians and other physicians have been found to be unable to consistently and correctly determine when the injury happened using the color of the bruise. When an infant or child presents with multiple bruises, even patterned bruises, the presence of bleeding disorders and coagulopathies should be excluded.

Any lesion that is circular or oval could be a human bite, even if individual teeth marks are not discernible. It is important to differentiate between a child's bite and an adult's bite. A general rule-of-thumb is that adults have an inner-canine distance of more than 30 mm. Any suspected bite should be photographed and swabbed for potential DNA evidence. If available, a forensic dentist should be consulted.

Evaluation

Any child with findings suspicious for the possibility of physical abuse should be completely evaluated. This evaluation should occur regardless of the family's race, insurance status, education level or social standing as abuse occurs across all segments of society. Reporting cases of suspected physical or sexual abuse is mandatory and clinicians should be familiar with the appropriate agencies for reporting in their region. Substantiation of inflicted injury is critical to successful prosecution in child abuse cases, and documentation must be complete and accurate including photographs when needed. Digital photography is recommended and all lesions should be photographed with and without a measuring device.

A complete skeletal survey should be performed in all children under 2 years of age with suspicion of abuse. An older child, especially a child for whom it is difficult to assess pain or disability, can have a skeletal survey performed if physical abuse is suspected. The skeletal survey should include a minimum of 19 radiographs including anteroposterior and lateral views of the axial skeleton and tightly collimated anteroposterior views of the appendicular skeleton. Ideally, all studies should be read by a pediatric radiologist. Because acute rib fractures are often not visible on radiographs, a radionucleotide bone scan at the time of the initial evaluation or a follow-up skeletal survey within 10–14 days of the initial survey should also be obtained.

Suspicion of abdominal trauma or elevated liver enzymes should prompt evaluation of the abdomen by computed tomography. Careful evaluation of the abdomen should occur in all children with severe brain injury, in which case the clinical examination of the abdomen is usually limited.

Bruising on the head or face of a non-ambulating child, any fracture in an infant less than 6 months of age, or any concerns of non-accidental injury in a child less than 12 months of age should prompt evaluation of occult head injury with a head CT.

Until child abuse can be eradicated by prevention, it is the responsibility of all of us who care for children to be vigilant in the early and appropriate recognition of potential child abuse. Immediate recognition and intervention may prevent subsequent further injury or death. A high level of suspicion and comprehensive radiologic evaluation will assure prompt recognition and management with the best chance for a favorable outcome.

Summary Points

- Non-accidental trauma is still a leading cause of injury and death for children.
- Health care professionals are ethically and legally obligated to notify the proper authorities whenever there is a suspicion of non-accidental injury of a child.
- There are specific patterns of injury that suggest the likelihood of a non-accidental injury and pediatricians, emergency room physicians, and pediatric surgeons should be aware of the more common signs.

Editor's Comments

It is sometimes difficult to maintain equanimity when faced with the responsibility of caring for a child who has been intentionally harmed, especially for those of us who care for children on a daily basis. It is an unfortunate fact of life, and our emotions cannot interfere with our duty to help the child.

In most tertiary-care pediatric centers, there are experienced social workers and dedicated teams of health care professionals whose job it is to deal with the myriad social and legal issues involved in these cases. For physicians, it is important to meticulously document every aspect of the child's care and not to compound the injuries with a diagnostic or therapeutic misstep.

The perpetrator is very often an adult guardian (it is astonishing how often a single mother's boyfriend is the culprit) but it seems increasingly common to see older siblings, cousins, and peers involved. What might have been ascribed an accident or horse play could very well have been a deliberate act perpetrated by a bully. It is important to identify these patterns because it is disturbingly common to see a child returned home to a dangerous environment only to come back later with a more serious injury.

Diagnostic Studies

- Chest X-ray
- Skeletal survey
- Bone scan
- Computed tomography (brain, abdomen, and/or chest)
- Ophthalmologic examination for retinal hemorrhages

Suggested Reading

Jenny C, Hymel KP, Ritzen A, et al. Analysis of missed cases of abusive head trauma. JAMA. 1999;81:621–6.

Kaczor K, Pierce MC, Makoroff K, Corey TS. Bruising and physical child abuse. Clin Pediatr Emerg Med. 2006;7:153–60.

Lane WG, Rubin DM, Monteith R, Christian CW. Racial differences in the evaluation of pediatric fractures for child abuse. JAMA. 2002;288:1603–9.

Leventhal JM, Thomas SA, Rosenfield NS, et al. Fractures in young children, distinguishing child abuse from unintentional injuries. Am J Dis Child. 1993;147:87–92.

Makoroff K. Fifty very useful child abuse articles for pediatric emergency medicine physicians. Clin Pediatr Emerg Med. 2006;7:204–11.

Sugar NF, Taylor JA, Feldman KW. Bruises in infants and toddlers: those who don't cruise rarely bruise. Arch Pediatr Adolesc Med. 1999;153:399–403.

Chapter 24
The Critical Airway

Karen B. Zur

Imagine you are asked to evaluate the airway of a 4 months old with noisy breathing. Surrounded by anxious parents and helpless staff, you find an emaciated infant with biphasic stridor and suprasternal and subcostal retractions. He has been feeding poorly and intermittently cyanotic for several days. The first thing you must remember *not* to do is panic. The critical airway can be safely and effectively managed when a composed surgeon follows a sensible thought process and conducts a directed work up as part of a multidisciplinary care team.

It is important to have a clear understanding of what stridor is and how to distinguish it from other sources of noise in a child. Stridor is noisy breathing that can be a manifestation of any number of congenital or acquired lesions. It is the result of an obstruction of the upper airway, which includes the supraglottic structures (epiglottis, arytenoids), glottis (vocal folds), subglottis or trachea. It can be inspiratory, expiratory or biphasic, a distinction that helps localize the pathology to a certain level of the airway. In general, inspiratory stridor is the result of glottic or supraglotitc pathology, expiratory stridor arises from the trachea, and biphasic stridor represents a fixed extrathoracic, subglottic obstruction. Stridor may sound like a gentle wheeze over the neck or a loud high-pitched or low-pitched sound. The higher frequency sounds represent a more proximal pathology, whereas the deeper, grunting noises are more suggestive of distal airway pathology.

In contrast to stridor, other upper airway noises that are commonly heard in children include nasal sounds such as snoring (stertor), which is a more palatal or nasopharyngeal noise that resembles a snorting sound. Stertor can be a result of nasal secretions, adenoid hypertrophy, pharyngomalacia (floppy throat) or pathology of the base of the tongue. Because some children can have obstruction at multiple levels, one should develop a keen ear for the quality of sounds through exposure to these children.

The critical airway is not limited to the child with stridor, but should also be suspected in the child who fails multiple attempts at extubation or a child with a chronic tracheostomy who is unable to be decannulated.

Diagnosis

The first step is to assess the urgency of the situation. Alar retraction, suprasternal or subcostal retractions, cyanosis, palor, agonal breathing, or sudden loss of stridor all indicate that the child is struggling and that an urgent intervention might be necessary. A pulse oximeter will demonstrate normal oxygenation if the child is in the early stages of airway obstruction, but it is important to consider measuring end-tidal CO_2, an elevation of which could suggest imminent respiratory failure.

The remainder of the work up varies depending on the clinical findings. Though tailored to the individual child and the circumstances, my approach always begins with a thorough history and physical examination. The history should include perinatal issues such as gestational age, history of intubation and maternal complications, in addition to the onset and duration of symptoms. It is important to know if there are associated signs such as retraction, cyanosis, nasal flaring or dysphagia. To assess the severity of the symptoms, I want to know if the child has been thriving, whether there are any episodes of apnea or cyanosis, and whether there are is ever any choking or gagging with feeds. A detailed surgical and medical history should be elicited, with a focus on GI, pulmonary, central nervous system, and cardiac issues. These are especially important due to the important influence of gastroesophageal reflux or laryngopharyngeal reflux on airway edema, CNS function on muscle tone, pulmonary disease on paO_2, and vascular anomalies on airway compression. Patients who have undergone cardiothoracic surgery are at risk for recurrent laryngeal nerve injury and vocal cord paralysis, weak cry, and dysphonia. An allergy history should also be sought, as food allergies can manifest as airway inflammation (eosinophilic esophagitis).

K.B. Zur (✉)
Department of Otolaryngology, University of Pennsylvania School of Medicine, Children's Hospital of Philadelphia, 34th Street and Civic Center Boulevard, 1 Wood ENT, Philadelphia, PA 19104, USA
e-mail: zur@email.chop.edu

P. Mattei (ed.), *Fundamentals of Pediatric Surgery*,
DOI 10.1007/978-1-4419-6643-8_24, © Springer Science+Business Media, LLC 2011

On physical examination, it is important to note the overall appearance and status of the child. At this point, the most crucial aspect of the evaluation is to assess whether the patient is *in extremis* or has an impending airway compromise. Noisy breathing that is associated with adequate oxygentation *and* ventilation – a normal oxygen level does not rule out CO_2 retention – with no agonal breathing, provides an opportunity to do a thorough evaluation including diagnostic studies rather than an emergent intubation or surgical airway. The child should be thoroughly evaluated for evidence of maxillofacial skeletal abnormalities, which can contribute to airway compromise, and genetic abnormalities such as CHARGE, VACTERL, Down syndrome, or Pfeiffer syndrome, all of which are associated with significant airway pathology.

If the patient is stable, I might start with *flexible laryngoscopy* at the bedside to evaluate the upper airway for supraglottic sources of obstruction: adenoid hypertrophy, choanal atresia, nasopharyngeal mass, base of tongue collapse (glossoptosis), base of tongue mass, laryngomalacia, vocal fold paralysis, glottic stenosis, or evidence of laryngopharyngeal reflux, epiglottitis or tonsillar hypertrophy. If the upper airway appears normal or if the stridor is more severe than could be explained by the findings at laryngoscopy (mild laryngomalacia), I would obtain plain radiographs of the neck in anterior–posterior and lateral projections or an airway fluoroscopic study to rule out the possibly of a clinically significant synchronous lesion. My preference is the plain film in patients with laryngomalacia for whom my level of suspicion for a synchronous lesion is low, and airway fluoroscopy with barium esophagram in children who have a more complex stridor, such as the deeper and harsher sounds characteristic of a tracheal abnormality. In patients with tracheomalacia, for example, the barium esophagram can help to exclude a vascular ring. If the level of suspicion for a distal pathology is still high despite normal radiography, the gold standard of diagnosis of an airway abnormality is formal microlaryngoscopy and bronchoscopy (MLB) under general anesthesia.

I would suggest that surgeons who manage and evaluate children with airway disorders think of the child as a whole and work to assemble a multi-disciplinary team for the care of these patients. In elective or semi-elective situations, I will often ask my GI colleagues to join me in the operating room when performing an airway evaluation if I am concerned about the possibility of clinically significant GERD or EE, or have a pulmonologist present during bronchoscopy if the patient has a history of recurrent pneumonia, hypoxia or asthma.

The critical airway does not always present acutely. I see many patients with tracheostomy tubes who have a very high grade stenosis that is considered a critical airway, but who otherwise have a stable airway and are undergoing diagnostic

procedures to help in planning future reconstruction. These patients should have a multidisciplinary evaluation, especially from GI and pulmonary, to assess to what degree other active processes are involved. In addition, due to the proximity of the trachea and esophagus and the dynamics associated with respiration and swallowing, ct of the evaluation, dysphagia and aspiration are very common in the airway patient. I therefore spend a considerable amount of time discussing voice and swallowing issues with the family. Many of my patients need a gastrostomy tube or fundoplication and I need to explore what their oral feeding is like. Because the risk of aspiration is high, we work with the speech pathologist to perform either office-based evaluation of swallowing (functional endoscopic evaluation of swallowing, FEES) or a video swallow study. Though clearly not appropriate in the acute setting, these more thorough evaluations should be done at some point during the work up.

Airway Assessment in the Operating Room

The operative airway evaluation needs to be a well orchestrated procedure, with a clear understanding of the plan for the evaluation. The anesthesiologist, the airway surgeon and the nurses in the room all need to have a working knowledge of the equipment needed prior to the child's arrival to the operating room and a proposed plan of airway management needs to be in place. I always survey the bronchoscopy table ahead of time, making sure that the equipment is available and functional (Fig. 24.1). Our standard setup includes: (1) ventilating

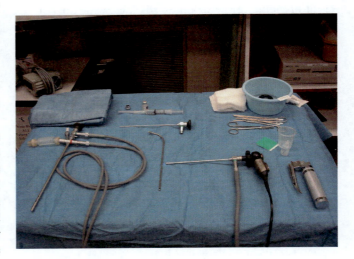

Fig. 24.1 Standard bronchoscopy table set up for evaluation of the critical airway: rigid bronchoscopes of various sizes, including a ventilating bronchoscope, suction cannula, laryngoscope, lidocaine solution, saline, mouth guard (in the basin of saline), cotton-tipped applicators, 4×4 gauze sponges, scissors, and anti-fog solution are all available and placed in the same place every time the table is set up. A tracheostomy tray is available on a separate table

bronchoscopy setup with a goose-neck connector, (2) suction, (3) 1 mL syringe containing 1 mL of 2% topical lidocaine, (4) tooth guard, (5) Philips laryngoscope (#1 for children <5 years of age, #2 for children >5 years of age), and (6) Hopkins rod lens connected to a camera head. In case of emergency, a tracheostomy tray is available nearby. Cuffless endotracheal tubes of expected sizes are available on the bronchoscopy table. The digital video recording system needs to be functional and ready to allow video recording of the airway during the case. The camera needs to be focused and white-balanced to ensure proper color visualization.

Even in the controlled setting of the operating room, evaluation of the airway is not always straightforward, especially when the child is *in extremis* and the airway has yet to be visualized or secured. In these situations, one should adhere to the same principles that apply during a trauma resuscitation. As time is of the essence, one should be thoroughly prepared ahead of time. Our approach is to set up the bronchoscopy table as planned for an elective procedure. If feasible, I like to start with a ventilating rigid bronchoscope and oxygen adapter. An age-appropriate setup is proper unless the child is unstable, in which case I select a relatively small bronchoscope. If the child desaturates during the bronchoscopy, I will try to intubate with a small endotracheal tube fitted with a stylet, which adds rigidity to the tube and might allow me to gently bypass an area of narrowing. Sometimes, especially in young infants, a gentle twisting of the endotracheal tube is needed to achieve an appropriate angle for intubation. During an emergency, transoral access of intubation is always preferable to the transnasal route. If the endotracheal tube cannot be inserted beyond the stenotic segment, it might be necessary to use the bronchoscope to establish a temporary airway. This must be done with extreme caution so as not to perforate the trachea.

In the presence an upper airway obstruction, such as base of the tongue pathology, or when transoral access is difficult due to trismus, a flexible bronchoscope prepared with an endotracheal tube over it should be prepared ahead of time. This will allow the anesthesiologist or surgeon to attempt fiberoptic transnasal bronchoscopy and intubation. If the child is stable and an airway cannot be secured with the bronchoscope or the endotracheal tube, consider placing a laryngeal mask anesthesia (LMA) tube, which can allow oxygen delivery while a surgical airway is created.

Whenever possible, I prefer to perform airway bronchoscopy with the patient spontaneously breathing, which allows me to evaluate the dynamics of the airway and the child to breathe on her own in case of emergency. This mode of anesthesia with no muscle relaxation is tenuous and requires the anesthetist to be comfortable with relinquishing control of the airway. I turn up the pulse oximeter volume so I can hear the heart rate and pitch. I use a Philips laryngoscope blade to expose the glottis and, to prevent laryngospasm, I spray the vocal folds with 2% topical lidocaine. The tip of the blade is routinely inserted into the vallecula. In most instances, this allows a nice exposure of the epiglottis, arytenoids, and vocal folds. I use a camera head that is connected to an appropriately sized Hopkins rod lens to perform the MLB. Four views are routinely captured: (1) hypopharynx, (2) vocal folds, (3) immediate sublottis, and (4) carina and mainstem bronchi. If pathology is identified in other portions of the airway I promptly photodocument these lesions, which is indispensable for communication with other providers and to allow a prospective follow-up.

The final portion of the airway evaluation is sizing of the airway: cannulate the airway with an endotracheal tube and calculate the expected vs. actual endotracheal tube size that fits the airway to estimate the degree of stenosis. The estimated endotracheal tube size can be estimated by: age/4 + 4.

Published in 1994, the Cotton–Myer grading system helps surgeons document and communicate the degree of subglottic stenosis: Grade I is a 0–50% obstruction of the lumen, Grade II is a 51–70% luminal obstruction, Grade III is a 71–99%, and Grade IV is complete obstruction.

Tracheostomy

Tracheostomy is most commonly performed in a child who is intubated and stable. The neck is extended with a shoulder role and a small amount of 1% lidocaine with 1:100,000 epinephrine is infiltrated at the level of the cricoid. It is important to recognize the anatomical landmarks (hyoid, thyroid cartilage, cricoid cartilage and trachea) prior to skin incision. In an infant, these cartilaginous structures are very close to one another and it is important to not only secure the airway, but also to avoid injury to the larynx and surrounding structures. A horizontal skin incision is made at the level of the cricoid and blunt dissection is used to separate the strap muscles in the midline raphe. I usually use Senn retractors and a fine mosquito to get from the subcutaneous skin to the anterior laryngotracheal complex. It is important to avoid violating the cartilaginous structures and to avoid stripping the perichondrium. Once the cricoid is identified, the overlying soft tissue is cleared with blunt dissection and if the thyroid gland is located relatively high in the neck overlying the desired site of incision in the trachea (third to fourth tracheal rings), then the thyroid gland is split in the midline with either suture ligature or electrocautery. Two retention 3-0 polypropylene sutures are placed alongside the vertical length of the trachea, spanning the second to fourth tracheal rings. These sutures will be used to apply gentle retraction during the operation and are left in place postoperatively in case of accidental decannulation. A beaver blade is used to incise the third or fourth tracheal ring in the midline. It is important to let inform the anesthesiologist that an air leak will be created and that they should be prepared to remove the endotracheal tube. Under direct visualization of the airway, and after ensuring that the age-appropriate tracheostomy tube is in hand, the anesthesiologist is asked to slowly remove the endotracheal tube and hold it immediately above the tracheotomy. Once the tracheostomy tube is inserted and its position in the airway and above the carina is confirmed by flexible tracheobronchoscopy, the tracheostomy tube is connected to the ventilator circuit, the tracheostomy ties are secured, and the endotracheal tube is removed. The retention sutures are labeled "right" and "left" using stickers and the suture is rolled up and secured to the anterior chest wall using small transparent plastic dressings.

Immediate surgical complications are unusual but it is extremely important to identify the landmarks and to keep the dissection in the midline. Inadvertent lateral tracheotomy can lead to esophageal perforation or vascular injury. To exclude the presence of a high-riding innominate artery, it is vital to palpate the distal tracheal deep to the strap musculature prior to incision of the trachea. Injury to the innominate artery can also occur postoperatively from erosion of the tracheostomy tube into the blood vessel, which produces catastrophic bleeding. Repair of an innominate artery injury can involve sternotomy or a trap-door incision and sometimes requires ligation of the vessel. Esophageal injuries can usually be repaired primarily with absorbable sutures and adequate drainage. Tracheo-esophageal fistula can result from aggressive insertion of a tracheostomy tube during the procedure and can require a complex reconstructive procedure. It is clearly preferable to avoid these potentially devastating complications with careful preparation and meticulous technique.

Definitive Treatment

Definitive therapy for an airway lesion is sometimes possible at the time of an urgent intra-operative airway evaluation. This depends on the nature of the lesion and whether associated pathology such active pulmonary disease or severe craniofacial abnormalities might place the child at increased risk for failing anything more than an intubation or a tracheostomy. Once the airway is secured an immediate plan can be executed.

When the child is unstable or if I suspect a glottic obstruction (glottic atresia), then I have a tracheostomy tray open and set up in the operating room. I always ask the scrub nurse where the knife is in case an emergent tracheostomy ("slash trach") is required. Pediatric tracheostomies should be performed by trained surgeons. The airway is much smaller than in the adult and must be respected as such. Cricothyroidotomies are not recommended in children less than 10 years of age as complication rates as high as 40% have been reported. More

recent innovations such as needle cricothyrotomy with transtracheal jet ventilation have been discussed in the pediatric emergency literature for management of airway compromise outside the operating room. In such a situation, a 14-gauge angiocatheter connected to a 5-mL syringe filled with 3 mL saline is used. The non-dominant hand stabilizes the trachea and the needle is angled caudad and inserted through the cricothyroid membrane. Aspiration of the syringe will show air bubbles in the saline when the airway is entered and, with care not to puncture the posterior tracheal wall, the catheter is slipped in and the needle is connected to an oxygen source. This can provide oxygenation for up to 60 min, allowing for more definitive surgical airway stabilization under controlled conditions in the operating room.

Some lesions can be managed endoscopically in the same setting as the diagnostic evaluation. These include base of tongue lesions, laryngeal cysts of varying types, subglottic cysts, pedunculated lesions, and granulation tissue.

When I consent the family for a diagnostic MLB, I usually mention that if I find a lesion that can be properly managed at the same time, I would secure the airway and then speak to them regarding a treatment plan. Since the airway is often tenuous and the diagnosis not known going in, it may not be possible to fully consent the family for additional procedures. I tell them that in cases of impending airway obstruction with no clearly resectable lesion, especially in a child with significant neurologic impairment or an active inflammatory process, a period of intubation or a temporary tracheostomy may be needed to allow for airway stabilization, clinical improvement, and further work up.

Children being considered for laryngotracheal reconstruction need to be evaluated thoroughly. Active disease processes that contribute to airway inflammation, such as GERD or eosinophilic esophagitis, can place a child with a low grade stenosis at risk of a worse outcome. Therefore, I feel that every effort should be made to protect the airway before attempting reconstruction, even if this means performing a temporary tracheostomy, at least until the associated conditions are under better control. However, it is important to remember that performing a tracheostomy in a child is not trivial and carries significant risks, such as tube obstruction or dislodgement, pneumothorax, and tracheo-innominate fistula, to name a few. It is also important to evaluate the psychosocial dynamics of the family. Our social workers are involved in this evaluation and, if deemed appropriate, our airway nurse practitioners begin family teaching. The child is discharged only after the family demonstrates proficiency in tracheostomy care and CPR.

The spectrum of airway pathologies leading to obstruction is varied and the management can vary from observation with supportive measures such as humidification, heliox, racemic epinephrine, corticosteroids, reflux management, and nebulizers to surgical approaches like endoscopic procedures or open reconstruction.

Laryngotracheal reconstruction generally refers to procedures in which a cartilaginous graft is used to augment the airway. Tracheal or cricotracheal resections (CTR) refer to procedures in which the stenotic or diseased segment of the subglottis or trachea is removed and an end-to-end anastomosis is performed. The standard laryngotracheal procedures are augmentative and involve placement of a "spreader graft" between the cut edges of the anterior cricoid, posterior cricoid or both. The cartilage graft can be taken from a rib, the thyroid ala, or the conchal cartilage of the auricle but other sources of autograft have been described.

Preoperative Preparation

Following a thorough airway evaluation and once concomitant active inflammatory conditions have been controlled, the child can be scheduled for a reconstruction. The initial decision is whether an augmentation procedure or resection is most appropriate. In general, if the lesion is more than about a few millimeters below the vocal folds and relatively discrete, measuring less than half of the length of the trachea, then a resection should be feasible. The best candidates for resection are those with concentric stenotic lesions that involve a few tracheal rings and begin several millimeters below the glottis. Since the decision can only be made after entering the airway, the approach should almost always be a vertical cricoid split. If the anterior cricoid is opened horizontally and excised as for a standard cricothyroid resection, this might preclude an augmentative procedure if is then felt to be more appropriate.

The second decision is whether a single-staged or a double-staged procedure should be used. A single-staged reconstruction means that the child will no longer have a tracheostomy tube, whereas after a double-staged reconstruction the tracheostomy remains. The best candidates for a single-staged reconstruction are neurologically intact and have a tracheostomy stoma that is close to the diseased segment. On the other hand, a double-staged reconstruction is a better option for patients whose pulmonary status is marginal, those with multiple associated anomalies whose ability to recover quickly and follow simple commands is limited, and children who are felt to be difficult to lightly sedate while a nasotracheal tube is in place. In addition, a double-staged reconstruction is advisable for patients whose tracheal stoma is located more distal to the diseased segment and have no significant stomal pathology. The double-staged procedure avoids a prolonged period of nasotracheal intubation and sedation with or without muscle relaxation, which can lead to withdrawal symptoms, a difficult recovery, and the constant threat of reintubation. A disadvantage of the double-staged procedure is that the tracheostomy tube can worsen stoma irritation and granulation formation at the site

of reconstruction. In general, the more difficult cases are done as double-staged procedures – although they are not as satisfying at the onset, the outcomes are good.

Preoperatively, I review all of the surgical options for management of suglottic stenosis and inform the family that some decisions can only be made in the operating room. I explain that palpation of the trachea during the full exposure of the laryngotracheal complex allows me to determine whether a graft will be well supported by the remaining tracheal rings and cricoid cartilage. As part of the informed consent, aside from the generic surgical risks, I discuss the risks of pneumothorax, mediastinitis, re-stenosis, need for postoperative dilatation, granulation tissue in the airway, need for future reconstruction or tracheostomy, pain (mostly related to rib graft harvest), scarring, dysphonia, vocal fold injury, dysphagia, and aspiration. I review the differences in recovery and postoperative sedation requirements between a single- and a double-staged reconstruction, especially in younger patients who need more sedation and for whom the risks of withdrawal symptoms are higher. I routinely recommend a weaning protocol to help avoid withdrawal. I remind the parents that after a double-staged procedure, the child will have a tracheostomy tube. This can be disconcerting to some parents who place their child at risk of surgery with the explicit goal of removing the tracheostomy. For that reason, the process of stent removal, follow-up bronchoscopies, possible dilatations, and the decannulation process are reviewed in detail.

To rule out colonization with methicillin-resistant *Staphylococcus aureus* (MRSA) or *Pseudomonas aeruginosa*, children with a tracheostomy should have a tracheal aspirate sent for culture 10–14 days before planned reconstruction. These two pathogens have been associated with significant postoperative morbidity related to graft infection and laryngotracheal separation. If the cultures are positive, I prescribe a 3-day course of trimethoprim/sulfamethoxyzole for MRSA or ciprofloxacin for pseudomonas. In addition, antibiotics directed at these strains are administered perioperatively.

I do not routinely obtain a preoperative chest X-ray unless the child has had a recent increase in oxygen requirement, in which case the procedure might need to be postponed. Close communication with the child's pulmonologist, cardiologist, and other subspecialists is important to be sure that decannulation is considered a safe option. My bias is also to hold off on reconstruction until any other planned elective operations (fundoplication) have been completed.

Laryngotracheal Reconstruction

In patients who have a tracheostomy, I replace the indwelling tracheostomy tube with a flexible, reinforced anode tube secured to the anterior chest wall using 2-0 silk sutures.

Patients without a tracheostomy are intubated and a trache-otomy is performed. This allows an unobstructed view of the diseased segment. The cervical skin incision is made at the level of the cricoid or around an existing tracheostomy tube and superior and inferior skin flaps are elevated and secured. The strap muscles are separated in the midline and retracted laterally, allowing exposure of the anterior laryngotracheal complex. This can be difficult in patients who have previ-ously had an airway reconstruction, and the use of very sharp scissors or a jeweler's bipolar forceps cautery can facilitate delicate dissection through scar. Once the laryngotracheal complex is identified, the cricoid plate is incised in the mid-line using a Beaver blade, taking care to avoid cutting through the anterior commissure of the vocal folds.

When a laryngofissure is needed for posterior cricoid exposure, I have the first assistant perform microlaryngos-copy while I use a 12-blade to carefully cut through the ante-rior commissure and thyroid cartilage, thus separating the vocal folds in the midline and allowing for better posterior subglottic and glottic exposure. I then decide how far distally the trachea needs to be incised to properly augment the air-way. If significant submucosal cricoid scarring is seen, I use very sharp scissors to remove the scar in a submucosal plane. The mucosal flap can then be sutured to the lateral cricoid plate with fast-absorbing 5-0 suture. The next step is to decide whether a posterior cricoid plate split would help properly augment the airway. This decision should be made with some caution, since the posterior split can lead to prolonged post-operative dysphagia or arytenoid prolapse and dysphonia.

To prevent scarring after a laryngofissure had been created, it is imperative to reapproximate the vocal folds at the same level vertically and in an anterior–posterior dimension. I use 4-0 polypropylene suture to meticulously perform this step. The sutures are tied down after the posterior graft is in place.

A rib cartilage graft is harvested and fashioned to the dimensions of the anterior and posterior cricoid split. To re-size the new airway, I place an appropriately sized endotra-cheal tube within the airway through the operative site to ensure that full closure and proper augmentation can be accomplished without an airleak. The posterior graft is inserted within the cut posterior cricoid plate in a sutureless fashion and the anterior graft is sutured such that the per-ichondrium is intraluminal. Mattress sutures are placed such that the graft is secured at an equal depth around its circum-ference. The knots and suture are placed extraluminally to prevent the formation of granulation tissue.

Cricotracheal Resection

The preoperative preparation and initial intraoperative approach is the same for CTR. I like to have appropriately sized bougie in the esophagus to allow for its intraoperative identification. I make two antero-lateral incisions alongside the cricoid carti-lage, thus removing the anterior cricoid plate. I almost never use a horizontal incision as this would preclude an augmenta-tion, if one becomes necessary. Once the cricoid plate is removed anteriorly, I inject the posterior trachealis and cricoid plate with a small amount of lidocaine/epinephrine solution, to help with hydro-dissection, and then use sharp scissors to ele-vate the trachealis off the esophagus in the common party wall. This dissection begins somewhat below the arytenoids, incis-ing the posterior cricoid mucosa horizontally, exposing the cricoid plate, avoiding injury to the arytenoids. This is impor-tant to provide a mucosal edge for anastomosis and to avoid placement of sutures too close to the glottis. Extreme care is taken to avoid esophageal perforation and that the dissection around the trachea is not carried too laterally, where the recur-rent laryngeal nerve can be injured in the tracheo-esophageal groove. Carefully hugging the trachea in a subperichondreal plane helps to avoid this potentially devastating complication.

Once the trachea is dissected far enough distally to allow for adequate upward mobilization, I resect the diseased tra-cheal rings, leaving a trachealis flap to help suture the tra-chea to the posterior cricoid mucosa. The remaining cricoid plate is inspected, and if scarred, is either drilled or shaven down with a Beaver blade, to maintain structural integrity of the cricoid while removing the disease. I then place 5-0 Monocryl or PDS sutures are placed to approximate the tra-chealis flap to the cricoid mucosa posteriorly. It is important to avoid "bunching" of the posterior mucosa to avoid obstruc-tion in the area, and care must be taken to prevent suturing of the vocal folds. Two relaxing sutures are placed alongside the lateral thyroid cartilage and lateral distal trachea to help appose these segments with no tension. If tension-free clo-sure is not possible, then either the distal trachea is mobilized further or other maneuvers such as a supra- or infra-hyoid release may be needed. To complete the anastomosis, 4-0 prolene sutures are placed extraluminally in the anterior tra-cheal and thyroid cartilages. It is important to avoid wide placement of the sutures or else buckling of the tracheal rings may result. In the single-staged procedure, the patient is nasotracheally intubated prior to tying down the knots. For the double-staged procedure, a stent is inserted. Sizing the airway is straightforward: cut a cuffless endotracheal tube of appropriate estimated size (based on the formula age/4 + 4), and match a Montgomery T-tube (cut or uncut) of equal size. With the stent in place, the sutures are carefully placed and tied down. The wound is irrigated, Tisseal is applied and a penrose drain is inserted. Following either CTR or tracheal resection, chin-to-chest (Grillo) sutures are placed to prevent excessive upward movement of the head, minimizing the risk of laryngotracheal separation. I usually leave these safety sutures for 7–10 days, depending on the duration of intuba-tion or stent placement.

Postoperative Care

For both resection and augmentation procedures, a similar postoperative course is advised. The patient is placed in a monitored setting (pediatric ICU for single-staged procedures, step-down unit for the double-staged procedures). A chest X-ray is obtained to rule out pneumothorax. Intravenous antibiotics are administered for 48–72 h. My bias is to keep the patients on IV antibiotics for as long as the neck drain is in place. I ask the speech therapist to see the patients on the first or second postoperative day to evaluate for feeding, with a focus on the risk of aspiration. The use of narcotics and muscle relaxants should be minimized, especially after a single-staged procedure. The day prior to planned extubation, I like to perform a bronchoscopy in the operating room to evaluate the reconstruction and confirm that the graft or suture line is covered with healthy mucosa. I also try not to keep a suprastomal stent for more than 2 weeks; for more complex reconstructions that require prolonged stenting, I prefer to use a T-tube instead. T-tubes are risky in young patients because of the possibility of plugging and loss of the airway, so unless the child is old enough to tolerate it (4 years or older) and allow an 8-mm T-tube to be placed, I use a cut T-tube and suture it to the trachea. Cut stents are not ideal, however, because they can generate more granulation tissue at the proximal and distal ends. Less traumatic stents are being devised but are not yet commercially available.

In general, a follow-up bronchoscopy is performed about 1 week after the stent is removed or the child is extubated. If the area has healed nicely and the child is doing well, surveillance bronchoscopy is performed to rule out the presence of granulation tissue, collapse or re-stenosis at 1, 3, 6 and 12 months after reconstruction.

Summary Points

Technical Points

- In a child with noisy breathing, one must consider: the acuity of the child's airway and to establish whether the noise is stridor vs. stertor.
- A bedside flexible laryngoscopy can help establish the status of the nasopharynx, base of tongue, supraglottis and vocal fold mobility or pathology. More distal lesions cannot be reliably seen during this type of endoscopy in a young child.
- Plain films and airway fluoroscopy can give clues, but are not diagnostic for airway pathology.
- A swallowing study may be used in conjunction with an airway fluoroscopy to rule out a vascular ring or sling.
- MLB are the gold standard for evaluation of stridor.
- Always communicate the plan with the anesthesiologist, establish the airway, and do not remove the anterior cricoid cartilage unless it is clear that a CTR is to be performed. Avoid a laryngofissure unless absolutely necessary for posterior exposure. Avoid vocal fold injury.
- Avoid a T-tube in young patients <4 years old and in patients with airways that would not accommodate an 8 mm T-tube.
- Preoperative cultures to rule-out MRSA and pseudomonas in the airway.
- Patients should undergo a multi-disciplinary evaluation: otolaryngology, pulmonology, gastroenterology, speech pathology. When indicated: genetics, general surgery and critical care.

Editor's Comment

Few situations are as terrifying as the child with acute compromise of the airway. As always, a calm and systematic approach is best. Mask ventilation should be attempted first while preparations are made for endotracheal intubation, temporary airway, and tracheostomy, usually in that order. In the trauma setting, neutral position of the neck must be maintained. Needle cricothyroidotomy with jet insufflation is an excellent option but care should be exercised in that excessive pressure, especially in an infant, can cause pneumothorax and life-threatening decompensation. Even in the setting of oral injury or bleeding, one brief attempt at orotracheal intubation – by the person with the most experience – is usually reasonable.

Emergency tracheostomy is rarely indicated in a child. It is truly a very delicate operation. The lack of adipose tissue and the presence of clean planes of dissection in some ways make it easier; but the small caliber of the trachea greatly increases the risk of iatrogenic injury. As always, meticulous technique, good lighting, and proper instrumentation are critical. All maneuvers should be deliberate and never forced. A trap-door tracheal incision, popular in adults, should not be used in children and, of course, it is important to avoid injury to the cricoid cartilage. If a tracheostomy tube is not available, an appropriate size cuffed or uncuffed endotracheal tube works just as well. In elective cases, some prefer to create a true fistula by suturing the edge of the tracheotomy to the skin.

Costal cartilage harvest is a straightforward procedure that involves removing a portion of one of the lower rib cartilages. Ribs seven through nine are often fused near the sternum, providing a wider graft, if needed. Although a graft can be taken from the costal margin, this can cause discomfort and a noticeable cosmetic defect. It is important to know exactly what size graft the airway surgeon needs for that particular patient. Most ask for a piece that has perichondrium on one side, allowing preservation of the posterior perichondrium; however, some request that there be perichondrium on both sides. This almost always results in violation of the pleura and pneumothorax, which should be evacuated with a soft rubber catheter under water seal or displaced with saline. Rarely is a chest tube required. Typically, the surgeon will sterilely prepare the neck and the chest as a unit and begin the airway portion of the operation. After determination of the size of the graft that is needed, a second surgeon is sometimes called on to harvest the graft. A small transverse incision is made over the lower rib cartilages, the pectoralis muscle fibers are separated, (not divided), and the site for the graft is marked with cautery. The cartilage can be incised with a scalpel and peeled off the posterior perichondrium. If both perichondrial surfaces are needed, the pleura can be attempted to be peeled off the perichondrium, but this is rarely completely possible. Injury to the intercostal vessels or internal mammary artery can result in significant bleeding. Inadvertent lung injury is rare but necessitates placement of a chest tube.

Differential Diagnosis

- Laryngomalacia
- Vocal fold paralysis
- Subglottic stenosis
- Subglottic cyst
- Tracheal stenosis
- Tracheomalacia
- Bronchomalacia
- Nasal obstruction

Diagnostic Studies

- MLB is gold standard
- Plain radiograph
- Airway fluoroscopy
- Barium swallow
- Modified barium swallow
- Functional endoscopic evaluation of swallowing (FEES)

Parental Preparation

- It might not be possible to take away the tracheostomy at this stage of the repair.
- Decision regarding laryngotracheal reconstruction vs. CTR might need to be made intra-operatively.
- Harvest of rib artilage graft might be necessary.
- There is a risk of postoperative dysphagia and aspiration.

Preoperative Preparation

- ☐ Communication with anesthesiologist and critical care team
- ☐ Bronchoscopy table set up, camera checked and white-balanced
- ☐ Informed consent
- ☐ Rule out tracheal pathogens (MRSA, *Pseudomonas*) in child with a tracheostomy tube

Technical Points

- Have the same approach to the bronchoscopy; know how to manipulate the camera and bronchoscope while performing the procedure.
- Vertical incision for tracheostomy.
- Horizontal cervical skin incision at level of cricoid for reconstruction.
- Avoid horizontal tracheal incision and removal of cricoid plate unless the need for a CTR is confirmed.
- Avoid CTR if the stenosis involves the vocal folds.
- Have a bougie in the esophagus for resections.
- Tension-free anastomosis is critical to the success of a resection.

Suggested Reading

Boardman SJ, Albert DM. Single-stage and multistage pediatric laryngotracheal reconstruction. Otolaryngol Clin North Am. 2008;41(5): 947–58.

Koempel JA, Cotton RT. History of pediatric laryngotracheal reconstruction. Otolaryngol Clin North Am. 2008;41(5):825–35.

Myer III CM, O'Connor DM, Cotton RT. Proposed grading system for subglottic stenosis based on endotracheal tube sizes. Ann Otol Rhinol Laryngol. 1994;103(4 Pt 1):319–23.

White DR, Cotton RT, Bean JA, Rutter MJ. Pediatric cricotracheal resection: surgical outcomes and risk factor analysis. Arch Otolaryngol Head Neck Surg. 2005;131(10):896–9.

Wrightson F, Soma M, Smith JH. Anesthetic experience of 100 pediatric tracheostomies. Paediatr Anaesth. 2009;19(7):659–66.

Chapter 25
Bronchoscopy

Ian N. Jacobs

Bronchoscopy is the detailed endoscopic examination of the trachea and bronchi with a telescopic lens, rigid open-tube bronchoscope, flexible fiberoptic scope, or a combination of these optical devices. The decision to perform rigid or flexible largely depends on the clinical situation. Both offer a detailed direct examination of the lower airway and each has its advantages and disadvantages. Bronchoscopy is often done in combination with direct laryngoscopy or microlaryngoscopy, which allows for exposure and examination of the larynx prior to performing bronchoscopy. In children, bronchoscopy is often performed under general anesthesia, but can also be performed in an endoscopy suite under moderate sedation.

A detailed examination of the tracheal anatomy offers significant advantages over radiologic examination and allows interventional procedures such as therapeutic lavage and culture, dilatation, removal of a foreign body, excision of recurrent respiratory papillomas or biopsy of a suspected neoplasm. The open-tube bronchoscope airway also permits simultaneous ventilation of the patient and passage of instruments.

Indications for Bronchoscopy

In most situations, bronchoscopy is elective and can therefore be planned ahead. The indications vary by age. In premature or small for gestational age infants, one of the most common indications for bronchoscopy is the failure to extubate. When an infant has had difficulty after extubation, it is important to determine if the cause is an upper airway obstruction. Premature infants who have endured long-term ventilation can develop subglottic stenosis and often require urgent intervention, such as a tracheotomy. Other possibilities include an

I.N. Jacobs (✉)
Department of Otolaryngology, University of Pennsylvania School of Medicine, The Children's Hospital of Philadelphia, Philadelphia, PA, USA
e-mail: jacobsi@email.chop.edu

obstructing subglottic cyst, which can be excised, or a soft subglottic stenosis, which can be gently dilated. An infant might also be difficult to extubate because of distal tracheal or lower airway problems such as vascular compression of the trachea, tracheomalacia or bronchopulmonary dysplasia. Direct endoscopic exam will be best to diagnose these problems as soon as it is feasible to proceed.

The infant is nearly always examined in the operating room under general anesthesia. The anesthesiologist will extubate the patient while the endoscopist slides a ventilating bronchoscope into the airway. This sometimes discloses fixed obstructive lesions of the larynx, trachea or bronchi, but fails to determine more dynamic obstructive problems such as laryngomalacia or tracheomalacia. These problems require a dynamic examination of the airway while the baby is extubated and breathing spontaneously. A normal airway finding might also indicate that the lungs are the cause of the extubation failure (bronchopulmonary dysplasia).

In the extubated infant with stridor, cyanotic spells or feeding difficulties, the work up of other congenital problems such as tracheoesophageal fistula, vascular compression or primary tracheobronchomalacia is necessary. The initial workup might include radiologic screening (barium swallow), but definitive diagnosis is made by rigid bronchoscopy. Bronchoscopy, along with MR angiography, aids in the diagnosis of vascular compression and tracheal compression.

In the toddler, the most common indications for bronchoscopy are recurrent croup, chronic stridor, and suspicion of foreign body aspiration. In the case of recurrent croup (laryngotracheobronchitis), it is important to rule out an airway problem as a cause: subglottic stenosis, subglottic cyst, hemangioma, or tracheal stenosis. These lesions tend to narrow the subglottic airway and predispose to croup and chronic stridor.

Tracheal and bronchial foreign bodies are a common indication for bronchoscopy in the toddler. A history of choking often occurs before the onset of wheezing and respiratory distress. Chest radiographs sometimes show a radiopaque object, air trapping, or post-obstructive atelectasis. Occasionally the radiographs are normal despite a history strongly suspicious for FB aspiration. Ultimately, bronchoscopy is needed to exclude a FB with certainty or to allow its extraction if confirmed. In fact, when films are equivocal and there is strong enough suspicion, bronchoscopy should be the next step.

Bronchoscopy is useful for evaluation of the child with chronic stridor. In this situation, after history, physical examination, and appropriate radiologic evaluation helps narrow the differential diagnosis, the child is taken to the OR to determine the cause of the noisy breathing. Potential causes of chronic stridor include laryngomalacia, tracheomalacia, subglottic stenosis, TEF, and vocal cord paralysis. Full dynamic and structural examinations during spontaneous ventilation is useful for determining the cause.

Microlaryngoscopy and bronchoscopy (MLB) are important in the preoperative planning for laryngotracheal reconstruction (LTR) for laryngotracheal stenosis. It can also be used to assess the airway during healing and help to determine the need for additional interventions (balloon dilation). MLB is useful in determining when a child's airway is suitable for decannulation. Appropriate interventions such as excision of suprastomal granulation or recurrent respiratory papillomatosis.

Contraindications and Special Airway Precautions

The few absolute contraindications to bronchoscopy include severe cardiovascular compromise and some cardiac arrhythmias. Severely compromised pulmonary status with hypoxemia that could worsen during bronchoscopy and lead to cardiopulmonary arrest is a relative contraindication since the airway problem could be contributing to the respiratory difficulty. Potentially useful interventions in this situation include lavage of distal mucoid secretions. An anterior mediastinal mass (lymphoma, teratoma) can lead to severe cardiopulmonary compromise during the induction of anesthesia and is also a relative contraindication. Finally, in any clinical situation, a poorly prepared or inexperienced bronchoscopy team or lack of ancillary support can make bronchoscopy more hazardous. If the patient is stable, he or she should be transferred to an environment where there is more support.

Distal tracheal airway obstruction (long-segment tracheal stenosis) requires special preparation as complete obstruction can occur beyond the ventilation bronchoscope and lead to rapid respiratory compromise. Conditions such as tracheal stenosis, bacterial tracheitis or tracheal/bronchial neoplasms might worsen after edema or bleeding starts and could quickly lead to complete airway compromise. In extreme situations, a back-up plan (ECMO, cardiopulmonary bypass) should be in place and all scenarios should be considered before starting.

There are a number of special hazardous airway situations that should be considered. One is the difficult exposure from oromandibular abnormalities such as severe mandibular ankylosis, microstomia, or scarring from trauma or burns. In such cases, exposure and intubation with a rigid laryngoscope can be difficult or impossible and only the flexible scope will visualize the airway. The endotracheal tube can be passed over the flexible scope after it is situated beyond the cords.

Another challenging situation is the infant with severe glossoptosis and Pierre Robin sequence, in which the tongue base prolapses against the epiglottis and the epiglottis is posteriorly displaced. The larynx is difficult to expose with conventional laryngoscopes. Significant cricoid pressure is required to lift up the epiglottis and occasionally an anterior commissure laryngoscope is needed to expose the larynx. The endotracheal tube can be passed directly through the scope. An alligator forceps is used to grasp the ETT and the scope is removed as the tube is secured distally.

Preoperative Evaluation

The history and physical examination will usually help to localize the site of airway obstruction and determine the urgency. Subsequent imaging and endoscopy will confirm the diagnosis. It is essential to know about the chronicity of stridor including its onset and any associated signs or symptoms such as croupy cough. A history of prematurity, intubation or meconium aspiration is important. Problems with voice quality would indicate a glottic (vocal cord) obstruction. Cyanosis with feeds can be caused by vascular obstruction or TEF. Worsening of stridor while in the supine position suggests the possibility of laryngomalacia.

The degree of respiratory distress and the past history dictate the urgency of the situation. If the child is in marked respiratory distress, emergent intervention and endoscopy is required. The examination is directed toward the general appearance of the child – the presence of retractions, tachypnea, and cyanosis all indicate an urgent situation. In most cases, stridor is subacute and a systematic workup is appropriate. The history should address birth history, intubation, ventilation, and presence of scalp hemangiomas. In toddlers and pre-school age children it is important to ask about possible foreign body aspiration or choking event.

The examination should determine three important characteristics of stridor: intensity, pitch, and phase of respiration. Intensity of the stridor correlates to some degree with the severity of the obstruction. The higher the intensity, the more urgent the situation. Pitch might suggest the location of the obstruction: high-pitched related to larynx or trachea, low-pitched sonorous obstruction from the nasopharynx.

The most important sign is the phase of respiration. Stridor that is inspiratory is usually due to a supraglottic cause of airway, such as laryngomalacia. Stridor that is biphasic will usually be related to upper tracheal causes such as subglottic stenosis. Expiratory stridor is most often related to lower tracheal causes as tracheomalacia.

Radiographic Evaluation

Imaging is essential in supporting the endoscopic approach and useful in preparing for the operating room. During the workup of stridor or recurrent croup, plain magnified neck radiographs might reveal evidence of a subglottic mass, suggesting the possibility of a cyst (usually the result of a previous intubation) or hemangioma. In cases of acute laryngotracheobronchitis, the films sometimes demonstrate a classic steeple sign (Fig. 25.1). Plain films are also important to confirm a normal trachea and rule out distal airway problems (long-segment tracheal stenosis), which might require special preparation in the OR.

Airway fluoroscopy and barium swallow are useful in the workup of vascular rings and tracheomalacia (Fig. 25.2). More advanced imaging with MRI will define the vascular anatomy and help determine the approach. Bronchoscopy is sometimes useful for visualizing the compressive vascular lesion and aid in the surgical repair. After surgical intervention, bronchoscopy helps confirm the improvement in the tracheal compression.

When FB aspiration is suspected, plain inspiratory and expiratory chest films are useful for determining the location of the FB. Air-trapping or mediastinal shift indicates a bronchial FB with airway obstruction due to a ball-valve mechanism. In less cooperative toddlers and infants, lateral decubitus views are useful: a lack of shift downward with air-trapping

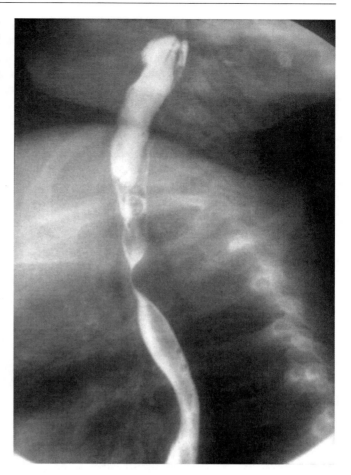

Fig. 25.2 Barium swallow showing complete vascular ring

suggests FB impaction of the main stem bronchus. Complete bronchial obstruction causes segmental or lobar atelectasis.

Review of Endoscopic Anatomy

The bronchoscopist should be familiar with both normal and abnormal anatomy of the tracheobronchial tree in infants and children as well as the expected age-related changes. The trachea begins at the base of the cricoid cartilage and ends at the carina. The length of the trachea varies with age. In a newborn the trachea is approximately 3 cm in length, in toddlers it is 5–7 cm, and in adults it is 9–15 cm. The transverse diameter averages approximately 6.5 mm in infants, 8 mm in toddlers, 14 mm in adult females, and 16.5 mm in adult males.

The endoscopist must understand the normal airway anatomy in different positions during the course of endoscopy and be able to appreciate abnormal pathology. In exposing the larynx, the endoscopist will encounter several important landmarks including the base of tongue and tip of epiglottis. Placing the rigid laryngoscope blade against the base of the

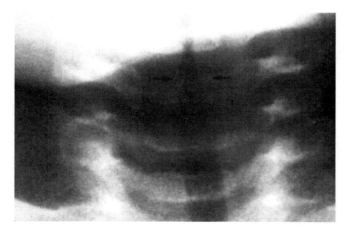

Fig. 25.1 Plain AP neck radiograph showing tapered subglottic airway (Steeple sign)

tongue exposes the epiglottic frenulum and the vallecula. The vallecula is formed by the medial and the two lateral glossoepiglottic ligaments which run from the tongue base to the epiglottis. Lateral to the lateral glossoepiglottic folds are the pyriform recesses of the pharynx (Fig. 25.3). A cantilever maneuver exposes the aryepiglottic folds (Fig. 25.4). Further anterior angulation exposes the arytenoids, glottic opening, and the anterior commissure. This is the ideal exposure for placing the rigid bronchoscope into the endolarynx.

Next, the cricoid cartilage is visualized as a complete cartilaginous ring of approximately 1.5–2 cm length starting just below the vocal folds (Fig. 25.5). The trachea has well defined c-shaped anterior rings and a flat posterior aspect comprised of the trachealis muscle (Fig. 25.6). The number of rings varies from 16 to 20. In most children, the soft posterior wall is subject to changes during the phases of the respiratory cycle while the anterior rings provide rigidity. The trachea is ovoid-shaped with the anterior tracheal wall form-

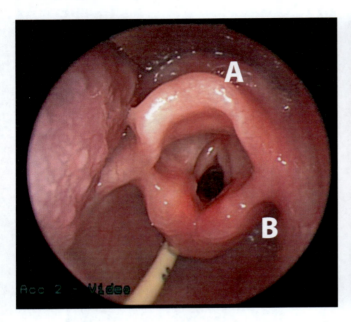

Fig. 25.3 Endoscopic exposure of the epiglottis and vallecula including the glossoepiglottic ligaments (*A*) and the pyriform sinuses (*B*)

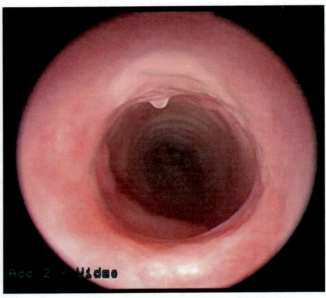

Fig. 25.5 Exposure of the subglottis showing a complete cartilaginous ring (the cricoid cartilage)

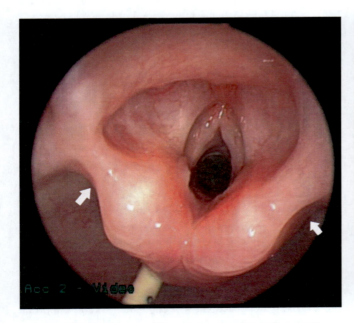

Fig. 25.4 Endoscopic exposure putting the aryepiglottic folds on stretch (*arrow*). The vocal cords are clearly visible

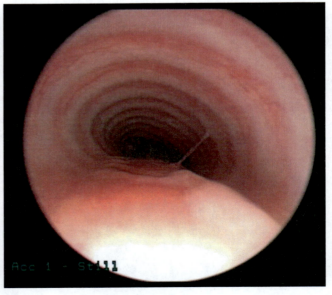

Fig. 25.6 Exposure of the main trachea showing 16–20 tracheal rings that form an arch and soft posterior trachealis muscle (membranous portion of the trachea)

ing an arch and the posterior wall being relatively flat. There is normally a 3:1 ratio of the circumference of the tracheal rings to the posterior wall. In cases of tracheobronchomalacia or major airway collapse, the ratio can be 2:1 or less due to loss of cartilaginous support. The carina is a sharp keel-shaped structure in the adult and a blunt ovoid in the infant.

The right main stem bronchus is approximately 1.5 cm in length in the adult and 6–8 mm in the infant. The right upper lobe bronchus is first seen at approximately 100° and sometimes comes off the distal trachea at the same angle. The main bronchus continues on as the bronchus intermedius. The left bronchus comes off at a more obtuse angle and ends in the left lower lobe and the upper lobe bronchus. Foreign bodies are more likely to become lodged in the right bronchus because of the diminished angle.

Preparation for Bronchoscopy

It is essential to select, assemble, and check all essential equipment prior to the patient's entering the room. The patient's age, size, airway conditions, and clinical situation determine the type of equipment to prepare. This needs to be communicated to the nursing staff early.

There are a variety of flexible bronchoscopes with and without suction. The smallest ultra-thin scopes, which easily fit through smallest endotracheal tubes, generally do not have suction, while the 3.5 mm diameter flexible bronchoscope is equipped with side port suction. Laryngoscopes are sized according to age and will help with examination of the larynx and introduction of the ventilation bronchoscope. Most kits will have sizes for infants, toddlers, and older children. We prefer the Benjamin laryngoscope because of its open side and ease of suspension. For cases involving the laser, we prefer the closed and protected Lindholme laryngoscope. Its enclosure protects the surrounding tissue from laser energy.

Age-specific rigid ventilating bronchoscopes are also useful. The size of the ventilating bronchoscope is also determined by age and modified for degree of airway stenosis. We prefer to do most diagnostic bronchoscopies with a no-touch technique using only the telescope. We use the 4 or 2.7-mm, zero-degree Storz-Hopkins rod telescope. However, there are situations that demand a rigid ventilating or open-tube bronchoscope for therapeutic intervention, such the removal of an aspirated airway foreign body. The size of the ventilating bronchoscope is dictated by the patient's age and the diameter of the airway. It is also sometimes useful to have a suspension apparatus available to free up one's hands.

When necessary, equipment necessary for foreign body removal should be set up with the nature of the FB in mind. This includes both optical and non-optical equipment that is specialized for the type of FB suspected. These instruments have a standard design for common foreign bodies such as peanuts, vegetable matter, and coins. For more challenging situations, there are also a range of non-optical forceps, some dating back to the days of bronchoscopy pioneer Chevalier Jackson. Some were designed specifically for certain FBs, such as nails, screws, beads, and even the open safety pin. One should be familiar with the various FB forceps and not rely exclusively on optical instruments for all objects. All the equipment should be neatly set up on an endoscopy table and positioned on the right side of patient for the right-handed surgeon. A monitor must be visible to all staff including nursing, anesthesia, and technicians.

Anesthetic Coordination and Induction

Most compromised airways and almost all rigid bronchoscopes require general anesthesia. Flexible bronchoscopy can be performed in select patients under moderate sedation. Regardless, close communication with the anesthesiology team is essential for the smooth performance of safe endoscopy. It is important to discuss the anesthetic plan before the patient enters the room. There are a number of important issues for the endoscopy and anesthesia teams to reconcile, including the overall surgical plan and goals, the technique of anesthesia, and the mode of ventilation: spontaneous ventilation, insufflation, complete paralysis, or jet ventilation. It is important to decide this ahead of time and all equipment, supplies, and medications should be in the room prior to the start of the procedure. In addition, the team must communicate clearly during the case and adjust to challenges. There must be a poised calm in the room and a quiet, undistracted atmosphere.

Flexible Bronchoscopy

The competent endoscopist is skilled with both flexible and rigid endoscopy. There are advantages to each approach and they will complement each other in the OR. The flexible scope is useful for dynamic evaluation of the airway and conditions such as epiglottic collapse, laryngomalacia, vocal cord paralysis, tracheomalacia, and vascular compression. In addition, the flexible scope can be used to examine the entire tracheobronchial tree.

Flexible scopes come in a variety of sizes ranging from ultra-thin fiberoptic scopes (1.9 mm) to larger bronchoscopes that are over 3.5 mm and have side ports for suction and biopsy. The ultra-thin scope in useful in small endotracheal or tracheotomy tubes to help visualize the distal airway, but does not have suction. In the older child, a 3.5 mm scope with suction can be used through the nose to examine the entire airway.

To help pass the flexible fiberoptic scope, oxymetalozine is sprayed in the nares to open the nasal passages. A mask with a PEEP valve is used to ventilate the patient during the endoscopy. The scope is introduced into the nasal cavity and passed along the floor of the nose and then inferiorly through the choanae into the nasopharynx. At this point, one can visualize the Eustachian tube, soft palate, and adenoid pad. The epiglottis is visualized as is the relative position of the epiglottis to the posterior larynx. The epiglottis might appear in the normal upright position or collapsed against the posterior pharyngeal wall. In addition, the structure and position of the aryepiglottic folds and arytenoids should be noted. The degree of arytenoid abduction and prolapse are noted.

Lidocaine spray can be used for topical anesthesia to reduce laryngospasm and to decrease reactivity of the vocal folds. After a light plane of anesthesia is established, vocal cord mobility is assessed. The presence of active abduction is confirmed and correlated with inspiration. Once this is seen and anesthesia alerted, the scope is passed below the vocal cords through the cricoid and into the trachea. One can examine for subglottic stenosis and tracheomalacia while observing the dynamic motion of the tracheal walls. Tracheobronchomalacia is confirmed when there is a less than 3:1 ratio of the anterior trachea to the posterior wall. The flexible scope is then passed down to the carina and then into each bronchus and terminal bronchial passage. The bronchi are examined for the presence of granulation tissue, foreign bodies or purulent fluid. A bronchial alveolar lavage can be performed to test for bacteria or lipid-laden macrophage, which correlates with aspiration.

Rigid Bronchoscopy

Rigid microlaryngoscopy and bronchoscopy (MLB) is best performed in a systematic fashion. It is essential to have all the necessary equipment organized and ready for immediate use. There needs to be a discussion about the anesthetic plan before starting. All staff including nurses, technicians, house staff and anesthesiologists need to be aware of the plan. In addition, all alternative or backup plans should be discussed and ready to go prior to start of the procedure. Close communication and frequent feedback is needed throughout the case. A tracheotomy set needs to be in the room and opened in case of a critical airway deterioration.

The patient is mask ventilated as the OR table is turned to a comfortable position for endoscopy. The patient is turned with the head toward the endoscopist and away from the anesthesia team. The neck in the neutral position or slightly hyperextended on a shoulder roll depending on operator preference. The hyperextended position provides more direct assess to the endolarynx, while the neutral position is the most physiologic and yields a more natural configuration of airway structures.

Once the patient is at the optimal depth of anesthesia, the endoscopist should insert a mouth guard to protect the teeth. The scrub nurse, who sits to the right of the surgeon, passes the laryngoscope and suction. An age-appropriate rigid laryngoscope such as the Benjamin or Parsons is inserted into the pharynx with the left-hand. The blade of the scope is used to "toe in" on the tongue base. Additional torque exposes the endolarynx. Two percent lidocaine spray is administered by atomizer to anesthetize the larynx in order to prevent laryngospasm. The right hand is used to suction secretions in the endolarynx and then the 4-mm Hopkins rod telescope or rigid ventilating bronchoscope is inserted into the endolarynx. Anti-fog solution is used to prevent fogging on the lens.

It is best to enter the midline of the oral cavity and lift up on the central tongue and tongue base. Pressure at the vallecula will lift up the epiglottis to expose the endolarynx allowing immediate visualization of the vocal cords. The telescope provides an excellent view of the endolarynx and avoids contact with the airway mucosa. The telescope is easily passed into the subglottis and down the entire trachea in infants and small children; however one might be limited by the 20-cm length of the Storz-Hopkins zero-degree telescope in older children. When the entire trachea and bronchi need to be examined in an older patient a longer telescope should be used.

In cases in which an open-tube bronchoscope is needed, the scope is inserted with the dominant hand into the endolarynx with the blade (blunt tip) end of the bronchoscope oriented anterior and then rotated as the scope is inserted. It is best to have the height of bed at a level such that the endoscopist is at eye level with the airway. The surgeon should not have to bend to view the airway.

Once the bronchoscope is placed in the trachea, the laryngoscope is passed off and the non-dominant fingers are used to grasp the shaft of the bronchoscope like a pool cue stick. The endoscopist then passes the telescope or bronchoscope down to the carina and directs the scope into each bronchus. The bronchus intermedius is at an acute angle to the right and the endoscopist may pass the scope directly down to visualize the right middle and lower lobe bronchus. This is often the site of an aspirated foreign bodies. The endoscopist needs to turn his or her body in order to direct the scope at 90° to the right to examine the right upper lobe bronchus. In some individuals the right upper lobe takeoff comes off the trachea at a more proximal position in the airway (Fig. 25.7). This so-called pig's bronchus makes it difficult to get the entire bronchoscope into the right upper lobe, but an entry level view might be enough.

The left main bronchus and lobular segments can be examined by angling at 20–30° to the left. While holding the bronchoscope with the left hand, specific surgical manipulations can be performed with the dominant hand such as foreign

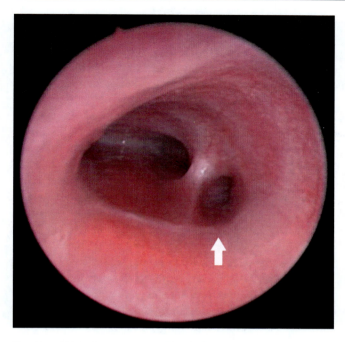

Fig. 25.7 High right upper lobe takeoff (tracheal or "pig's" bronchus, *arrow*). The carina and right and left mainstem bronchi are visible to the *left*

body removal, suctioning, or balloon dilation. The telescope can be removed to allow passage of a FB forceps down the shaft of the bronchoscope. Familiarity with all the parts and function of the bronchoscope are important.

Complications

Complications are related to anesthesia, ventilation, equipment use, or surgical intervention. Anesthetic complications increase with clinical complexity, the severity of the airway problem, and the overall status of the patient. Anesthetic complications are usually due to airway manipulations and include laryngospasm and bronchospasm. These can be related to certain techniques of anesthesia such as spontaneous ventilation or jet ventilation. Irritants such as blood and secretions also increase the risk. Topical anesthesia might reduce the risk of laryngospasm and should be applied before instrumenting the airway. Jet ventilation, which allows for clear laryngeal exposure, can lead to barotrauma (pneumothorax, pneumomediastinum). Other anesthetic complications include aspiration, cardiac arrhythmias, and malignant hypertension. Careful preparation, communication, and flexibility are vital.

Mechanical or equipment-related complications include injury from the laryngoscope to the teeth or soft tissues. A mouth guard should always be used when placing a laryngoscope. Loose teeth should be identified preoperatively and removed after induction of anesthesia. Instrumentation,

especially with the rigid ventilation scope, can cause laryngeal edema. This is best avoided by utilizing a no-touch technique and corticosteroids. Flexible fiberoptic bronchoscopes can cause epistaxis, which is best avoided by the use of oxymetalozine spray.

Ventilation complications include airway obstruction: laryngeal edema, mucosal tears and irritation, or loss of the airway leading to hypoxic events. Avoidance is best by planning for such mishaps ahead of time and having alternative pathways. Flexibility and close communication are essential. In high-risk airway cases such as distal tracheal obstruction, alternative modes of ventilation and resuscitation (ECMO) need to be planned.

Parental Considerations

Parent participation is an important consideration when performing endoscopy in infants and children. The indications and all possible alternatives need to be fully discussed. The major complications and possible outcomes should also need to be discussed and included in the consent. The person giving informed consent should discuss the risk of not performing the endoscopy. In addition, the family should be prepared for a possible emergency procedure such as tracheotomy.

Immediately after the endoscopy, color prints are very helpful in explaining the findings and future management plans with the parents. A copy can be given to the family for their own records.

Foreign Body Removal

One of the most challenging clinical situations is the removal of a foreign body from the pediatric airway. The presentation varies dramatically from a sudden fatal asphyxia to a more subtle problem of recurrent pneumonias or croup. It is incumbent upon the endoscopist to suspect the possibility of FB aspiration in any child who has a sudden change in respiratory status, focal respiratory findings (right lower lobe infiltrate), or a witnessed choking episode. The diagnosis is often supported by radiographic findings. Radiopaque foreign bodies are easily seen, but more often foreign bodies are non-radiopaque, in which case, indirect effects such as air-trapping or mediastinal shift may be the only radiologic sign from a partial or complete blockage of the bronchus. Inspiratory/expiratory phase images and decubitus films are sometimes helpful in the uncooperative child. On the other hand, a normal radiograph does not rule out the possibility of a FB. When clinical suspicion is high, endoscopy should be undertaken regardless of the negative physical and radiographic findings. Failure to identify an airway FB is associated with potentially serious or fatal seque-lae, justifying a 10–15% negative exploration rate.

The timing of airway endoscopy to remove a foreign body depends on the acuity of the presentation and the degree of respiratory distress. Other factors include the availability of optimal personnel, risk of sudden shift of the FB to another bronchus, and stability of the patient for general anesthesia. Laryngeal or tracheal foreign bodies, which present in a rather dramatic manner, should be extracted as soon as possible.

The patient with a laryngeal foreign body is induced by the anesthesiologist and all instruments should be available at the start. An open laryngoscope such as a Parsons or Benjamin is used and forceps can be used to quickly extract the object upon induction, after which the airway is secured. In rare cases, a sharp, large or deeply embedded FB will need to be removed through an open approach (tracheotomy).

Tracheal and bronchial foreign bodies, are not usually as acute or dramatic. Bronchoscopy can be planned on a semi-urgent basis when optimal equipment and staff can be assembled. Equipment should include appropriate-sized lar-yngoscopes, open-tube bronchoscopes, optical telescopes, and at least two non-optical forceps. One of these should be double-action fenestrated forceps and the other an alligator type. The experienced endoscopist will select and practice with the instruments on the suspected FB and have alterna-tive instruments available.

The technique of FB removal starts and ends with close communication with the anesthesiologist. The endoscopic approach often involves a rapid-sequence mask induction and tracheal intubation with an open-tube bronchoscope. Once the appropriate depth of anesthesia is achieved, a mouth guard is placed and the non-dominant hand places the laryn-goscope to expose the endolarynx. The dominant hand places the ventilating bronchoscope. Once the scope is in the air-way, the laryngoscope is removed and handed off to the scrub nurse. The optical lens inside the ventilating bronchoscope is then used to examine the trachea and bronchi until the FB is seen. The first order of business is to identify the FB as well as its position in the airway. Long suction cannulas are needed to clear secretions and aid in the identification of the FB. It is important to recognize the FB as free or embedded in the soft tissues because additional equipment such as en endoscopic cautery might be required. The position and presenting side of the FB will influence the strategy of removal.

Once the identity, shape, and position of the FB are estab-lished, a decision is made about which forceps to use. The eye piece is taken off and the optical lens removed. The forceps, either optical or non-optical, are used to engage the FB. The for-ceps should be carefully opened and closed over the object and it should be pulled close to the scope to avoid accidental strip-ping of the item. If the FB is larger than the diameter of the bronchoscope, the FB and scope are removed as a unit. A smaller FB can be drawn into the scope. The bronchoscope is immediately reinserted to examine for additional FBs. There are a variety of non-optical forceps that are designed for spe-cific foreign bodies: forward grasping, side curved, spherical grasping, basket or the Clerf-Arrowsmith safety pin closer.

Very distal fragments of nut and other matter in segmental bronchi can be removed with flexible single-action forceps introduced down the suction port of the rigid bronchoscope. This requires a thinner telescope. Special flexible endoscopic suctions can be passed down the side arm as well. Other situ-ations of difficult to remove FBs warrant the use of Fogarty balloons catheters, urologic baskets, or Busby cautery, if granulation is present. The patient with severe inflammation might benefit from treatment with corticosteroids, broncho-dilators, or antibiotics.

Bronchoscopic Surgery

Laser ablation or biopsy of papillomas, granulation tissue, or tumors can also be performed through an open-tube ventilat-ing bronchoscope. In these cases, the laryngoscope is placed into position and attached to a rigid suspension system as surgical interventions are best performed when both hands are free. A right-angle suspension device attached to the side rail of the OR table provides a stable set-up. It also allows the use of a microscope and microlaryngeal instruments.

Summary Points

- In the small child, the most common indications for bronchoscopy are recurrent croup, chronic stridor, and suspi-cion of foreign body aspiration.
- Bronchoscopy is often done in combination with direct laryngoscopy or microlaryngoscopy, which allows for expo-sure and examination of the larynx prior to performing bronchoscopy.
- Distal tracheal airway obstruction requires special preparation as complete obstruction can occur beyond the ventila-tion bronchoscope and lead to rapid respiratory compromise.
- One of the most challenging clinical situations is the removal of a foreign body from the pediatric airway.
- When a foreign body is aspirated, chest radiograph might show a radiopaque FB, air trapping, or post-obstructive atelectasis.
- The airway assessment should be recorded in video format and reviewed with the family.

Editor's Comment

Bronchoscopy, flexible and rigid, should part of the armamentarium of the pediatric general surgeon. Even if otorhinolarygologists do most of the primary airway surgery and foreign body removal at one's institution, it is a skill that can be invaluable in certain situations in the ICU, OR or even the ED. In general pediatric surgery, probably the most common indication for rigid bronchoscopy is as an adjunct prior to repairing esophageal atresia with TEF. These are usually straightforward procedures but they are important for confirming the diagnosis prior to thoracotomy and for ruling out the presence of a second more proximal fistula. It is a procedure with which one should be facile and effective. The infant should oriented transversely on the OR table and positioned properly with the neck slightly extended and bumps placed under the shoulder and, if necessary, the occiput. The surgeon should personally inspect and put together the equipment and make sure there is proper suctioning equipment readily available. Some prefer to use a ventilating scope, although using just the telescope for a brief assessment makes things less complicated and avoids insufflation of air through the fistula into the stomach. Some also prefer to have the patient breathing spontaneously so as to be able to identify moving vocal cords and assess the degree of tracheomalacia, although this information is rarely useful in the actual care of the patient. The surgeon should mask ventilate the child and then place a mouth guard or moistened gauze sponge against the upper gums. After visualization of the cords with a standard laryngoscope, the scope should be passed gently, without forcing or torquing, so that it enters the trachea without traumatizing the delicate structures of the airway. The surgeon should immediately be able to orient the view properly by identifying the membranous (posterior) portion of the trachea. The scope can be passed directly to the carina and then more slowly withdrawn to look for the primary fistula (sometimes located in one of the mainstem bronchi) and the rare second fistula. The scope should be withdrawn gracefully and the child should be immediately intubated in preparation for the operation. The entire procedure should take no more than 5 min.

Extraction of a foreign body from the airway is an art that is honed with experience. Most foreign bodies can be easily removed with rigid bronchoscopy and specialized graspers suited to the particular object. While extracting a foreign body from the bronchus, the object can become lodged in the trachea, converting a partial airway obstruction to a complete airway obstruction. If the object cannot be calmly and easily removed with a brief second attempt, it should be pushed back into the right mainstem bronchus temporarily while the patient is oxygenated, the staff take a deep breath, and a plan is formulated. It is important to not panic and to have a backup strategy. Another significant problem is the long-standing foreign body that is now embedded in the wall of the trachea or bronchus and cannot be dislodged. Endobronchial surgical techniques can be attempted (debridement of granulation tissue, balloon catheters), but bleeding is a significant concern. Although exceedingly rare, tracheotomy (or thoracotomy) is a last resort.

Flexible bronchoscopy is most useful in intubated patients who have severe lobar collapse and concern for mucous plugging of the distal airway. Again, the surgeon should be familiar with the equipment and be able to perform such a procedure at the bedside with confidence, competence, and skill. If opportunities for practice are rarely encountered, one should take the opportunity participate in airway courses or simulation labs at least once a year, or spend an afternoon with an ENT colleague observing and assisting in several airway cases. Regardless of one's experience, when preparing to do a detailed evaluation of the distal airways for hemoptysis, foreign body, or suspected tumor, it is a good idea to review the normal bronchial anatomy in a good surgical atlas and, if possible, to have a large diagrammatic illustration posted visibly in the OR during the procedure.

Differential Diagnosis

- Foreign body aspiration
- Tracheal stenosis
- Complete tracheal ring
- Subglottic stenosis
- Vocal cord paralysis
- Subglottic cyst
- Hemangioma
- Tracheomalacia/laryngeal malacia
- Tracheo-esophageal fistula
- Papillomatosis
- Granulation tissue

Diagnostic Studies

- Plain radiographs of the neck
- Chest X-ray (inspiration/expiration, ±decubitus views)
- Chest CT scan (for anterior mediastinal mass)
- MRI (for vascular rings)

Preoperative Preparation

- ☐ Prepare and test all equipment
- ☐ Discuss anesthetic plan with Anesthesiology team
- ☐ Review airway and bronchial anatomy
- ☐ Prepare for all possible scenarios, including emergency tracheostomy
- ☐ Prophylactic antibiotics

Parental Preparation

- Discuss risks of need for intubation and mechanical ventilation, tracheostomy, or ECMO.

Technical Points

- The endoscopist should assemble and check all equipment ahead of time.
- Lidocaine spray can be used topically to reduce laryngospasm and reactivity of the vocal folds.
- All airway procedures begin and end with close communication with the anesthesiologist.
- Nurses, technicians, house staff, and anesthesiologists need to be aware of the plan and be able to see the monitors throughout the case.
- Remain flexible and adjust plans if the situation changes.

Suggested Reading

Cortese DA, Prakash UBS. Anatomy for the bronchoscopist, Chapter 2. Bronchoscopy. New York: Raven; 1994.

De Wever W, Vandecaveye V, Lanciotti S, Verschakelen JA. Multidetector CT-generated virtual bronchoscopy: an illustrated reviews of the potential clinical applications. Eur Respir J. 2004;23(5):776–82.

Grillo HC. Anatomy of the trachea, Chapter 1. Surgery of the trachea and bronchi. New York: BC Decker; 2004.

Griscom NT, Wohl ME. Dimensions of the growing trachea related to body height. Length, anteroposterior and transverse diameters, cross-sectional area, and volume in subjects younger than 20 years of age. Am Rev Resp Dis. 1985;131(6):840–4.

Handler SD. Craniofacial surgery: otolaryngological concerns. Int Anesthesiol Clin. 1988;26(1):61–3.

Marsh BR, Kelly SM. Airway foreign bodies. Chest Surg Clin N Am. 1996;6(2):253–76.

Mairs EA, Parsons DS. Pediatric tracheobronchomalacia and major airway collapse. Ann Otol Rhinol Laryngol. 1992;101(4):300–9.

Rahbar R, Ferrari LR, Borer JG, Peters CA. Robotic surgery in the pediatric airway: application and safety. Arch Otolaryngol Head Neck Surg. 2007;133(1):46–50.

Rosen CA, Bryson PC. Indole-3-carbinol for recurrent respiratory pcxapillomatosis: long-term results. J Voice. 2004;18(2):248–53.

Chapter 26
Cystic Neck Masses

Oluyinka O. Olutoye

Head and neck masses in children are common and virtually always benign. The location of the mass is often an excellent clue to the differential diagnosis of the mass (Table 26.1). The age, history, and physical examination will also provide significant clues to aid in the diagnosis. Determining whether the lesion is cystic or solid helps to narrow the differential diagnosis. The vast majority of cystic cervical lesions are embryologic in origin; thus a proper understanding of the relevant embryology is important.

By the fourth week of embryonic development, bulges develop in the proximal foregut caudal to the stomodeum or future mouth. These bulges are due to paired branchial arches that form from specialized tissue. There are initially six paired branchial arches lined on the inner surface by endodermal derivatives and on the outer surface by ectodermal derivatives. Each arch contains a blood vessel, cartilage, and cranial nerve. The structures derived from each pharyngeal or branchial arch are supplied by the respective artery and cranial nerve. The inner indentations lined by endoderm form the branchial pouches, while the outer indentations lined by ectoderm form the branchial clefts. In lower vertebrates, these indentations communicate and the branchial arches form gills. In humans, only the first pharyngeal pouch and cleft meet to form the structures of the middle ear and external auditory canal, respectively. The fifth pharyngeal arch resolves without a trace.

Each of the pharyngeal clefts and pouches contributes to the major soft tissue, bony, and neural structures of the head and neck. The first cleft becomes the external auditory meatus while the second, third, and fourth cleft coalesce to form a common opening, the cervical sinus of His, which invariably obliterates. Persistence of this structure leads to the formation of a branchial cleft sinus or cyst. The persistent cervical sinus of His can either connect with the second, third, and possibly fourth pharyngeal pouches, creating an internal sinus or, if the skin opening remains patent, a fistula. The location of the internal opening is determined by the branchial cleft of origin. The second branchial fistula or sinus tracts drains internally at the tonsillar fossa. The third branchial pouch gives rise to the inferior parathyroid glands and thymus. These structures descend into the lower neck after detaching from the pharynx. Third branchial sinus or fistula tracts open at the pyriform sinus. The fourth and sixth aortic arches undergo asymmetric involution. This asymmetric involution results in the different paths of the right and left recurrent laryngeal nerves (derived from the fourth pharyngeal arch). Likewise, one would predict that the paths of a fourth branchial cleft sinus (between the fourth and sixth pharyngeal arches) would vary between both sides, but this is a theoretical consideration as these anomalies have not been described.

The embryologic development of the aortic arches and cranial nerves also helps clarify the anatomy of the second and third branchial cleft anomalies. The third aortic arch becomes the internal carotid artery. Second cleft anomalies course between the internal and external carotid arteries to drain into the supratonsillar bed. In contrast, third cleft anomalies pass behind the internal carotid artery, traverse the thyrohyoid membrane, and drain into the pyriform sinus. First branchial cleft anomalies are close to the origin of the facial nerve. The glossopharyngeal nerve innervates the second branchial arch and is at risk during dissection of second branchial cleft lesions. Dissection of third cleft anomalies place the superior laryngeal nerve at risk during dissection. In addition, there is risk of injury to the glossopharyngeal and hypoglossal nerves as the fistula courses behind the internal carotid artery.

The thyroid gland is derived from the endoderm as a ventral diverticulum and caudal migration from the cranial end of the endodermal tube. It originates from the junction of the anterior two-thirds and posterior one-third of the tongue (foramen cecum). The path of descent of the developing thyroid is through the body of the developing hyoid bone as it comes to rest in its final location with the isthmus anterior to

O.O. Olutoye (✉)
Division of Pediatric Surgery, Michael E. DeBakey Department of
Surgery, Baylor College of Medicine, Texas Children's Hospital,
Houston, TX, USA
e-mail: oolutoye@bcm.tmc.edu

P. Mattei (ed.), *Fundamentals of Pediatric Surgery*,
DOI 10.1007/978-1-4419-6643-8_26, © Springer Science+Business Media, LLC 2011

Table 26.1 Differential diagnosis of pediatric neck masses by location

Anterior midline	Thyroglossal duct cysts
	Dermoid cyst
	Epidermoid cyst
Anterior Lateral	Branchial cleft cyst
	Torticollis
	Carotid body paraganglioma
	Primitive myxoid mesenchymal tumor of infancy
Anterior (both midline and lateral possible)	Thyroid nodule
	Reactive adenopathy
	Ectopic thymus
	Neuroblastoma
	Ganglioneuroma
	Rhabdomyosarcoma
	Teratoma
Posterior	Dermoid cyst
	Lymphadenopathy
	Mononucleosis
	Tuberculosis
Any location	Pilomatrixoma
	Bronchogenic cyst

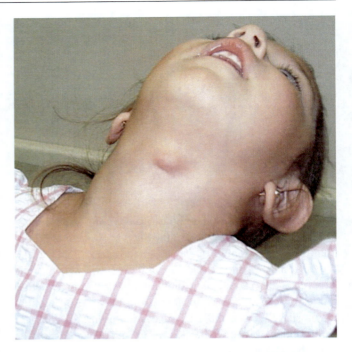

Fig. 26.1 External appearance of a typical thyroglossal duct cyst. Though classically in the midline, they can tend to fall to either side of the midline

the third to fifth tracheal cartilages. The thyroglossal duct then obliterates. Incomplete obliteration of the thyroglossal duct results in a thyroglossal duct cyst. Thus the cyst can be found anywhere along the path of the thyroglossal duct, from the thyroid isthmus to the base of the tongue at the foramen cecum.

Thyroglossal Duct Cyst

Thyroglossal duct cysts (TGDC) comprise one third to one half of all cervical lesions in children. The majority are located close to the hyoid bone or, less commonly, between the hyoid bone and the base of the tongue. They are less frequently located in the lower neck. A thyroglossal duct cyst typically presents as a smooth, firm or cystic swelling in the anterior neck, usually in or close to the midline, which has been present for weeks to months (Fig. 26.1). A gradual increase in size of a non-tender mass over time is sometimes reported, particularly in patients with an upper respiratory tract infection.

Patients also occasionally present with an acute infection of a thyroglossal duct cyst. Although the infection can be from oral flora through a patent sinus tract or duct, the most commonly identified bacteria are *Haemophilus influenzae* and *Staphylococcus aureus*. A history of a sour, foul taste in the mouth suggests decompression of an infected cyst through a patent foramen cecum. Some lesions present as a draining sinus. Sinuses form from spontaneous drainage or following incision and drainage of an inflamed cyst. Multiple sinus tracts have also been described. Thyroglossal duct cysts

are rarely located far from the midline, but when they drain, the sinus openings can appear to be lateral. Intra-thyroid thyroglossal duct cysts have also been reported.

Thyroglossal duct cysts can almost always be identified based on the history and physical examination. Although extremely rare, two synchronous cysts have been reported, one at the level of the hyoid, and the other in the thyroid. Because of the path of the thyroglossal duct through the central portion of body of the hyoid bone, the lesion will often move with tongue protrusion or rise with deglutition, however these clinical signs are not 100% reliable. Although thyroglossal duct cysts are cystic, they sometimes appear solid on physical examination.

It is important to differentiate a thyroglossal duct cyst from an ectopic thyroid gland. There is a 1–2% incidence of ectopic thyroid misdiagnosed as a TGDC. In this condition, the descent of the thyroid was arrested and the patient presents with a mass very similar in appearance to a TGDC. If not recognized and properly treated, accidental removal of a lingual thyroid will result in hypothyroidism. If recognized at surgery, the gland may be re-implanted in the strap muscles or forearm. Postoperative hypothyroidism necessitates life-long thyroid supplementation.

Palpation of the normal thyroid gland is difficult in young children. An ultrasound study of the neck will identify the normal thyroid gland while also confirming the cystic nature of the lesion. Radioisotope scanning has no additional value except when a normal thyroid gland is not identified by ultrasound.

In such a case, radioisotope scanning will confirm the lesion to be a lingual thyroid.

An infected cyst should be initially treated with a course of antibiotics. If not adequately controlled with antibiotics, cyst aspiration or incision and drainage is required. Initial efforts should be made to avoid incising an infected TGDC as this can result in a persistent draining sinus and increase the risk of recurrence following definitive excision. Surgical removal of an infected TGDC should be delayed until the infection and associated inflammation have subsided. The risk of recurrence is markedly increased if any excision is attempted while there is active inflammation. Recurrent cyst infection will sometimes occur while waiting.

The treatment of a thyroglossal duct cyst is surgical excision. The procedure (Sistrunk operation) involves resection of the cyst and the entire tract, including the central portion of the hyoid bone (through which the thyroglossal duct courses) to the base of the tongue.

The operation is performed under general anesthesia and can be performed as an outpatient procedure. A discussion with the anesthesiologist about the optimal method of airway control is prudent. While these cases can be accomplished with laryngeal mask anesthesia, occasionally it is necessary to have the anesthesiologist push on the tongue or pharynx. This makes the LMA less suitable, especially in younger children. Prophylactic antibiotics should be given, especially if there is a history of an infected cyst.

The patient is positioned supine with a shoulder roll across the back and the neck gently hyperextended. The head is supported on a donut gel pad and may even be taped to the bed. The preparation is similar to that for a thyroid resection. A small skin crease incision is made over the cyst and platysmal flaps elevated superiorly and inferiorly. Careful evaluation for other cysts is made once the platysma is elevated. A patent thyroglossal duct will connect to the cranial portion of the cyst and this part is dissected last. Whether or not a duct is clearly defined, the fibrotic tissue in the cranial portion of the cyst is preserved and dissected cephalad. Multiple ducts or sinus tracts sometimes exist, thus skeletonizing the duct is not advisable. The fibrous tissue is dissected up to the hyoid bone, which is then resected between the two lesser horns with bone cutters. In younger children, a heavy Mayo scissors is equally effective and easier to maneuver into the small space. The dissection should not extend lateral to the lesser horn of the hyoid to avoid injury to the hypoglossal nerves. The dissection is then continued cephalad to the base of the tongue. The anesthesiologist is instructed to push down on the posterior one-third of the tongue to facilitate this aspect of the dissection. Alternatively, the surgeon or assistant can place a double-gloved finger in the mouth for the same purpose. A ligature is placed on the stump at the base of the tongue with fine absorbable sutures and the duct is divided. Following the resection, the specimen is inspected

on the back table to identify any visible duct. Such findings should be stated in the operative report. The specimen is then oriented and submitted to pathology. All efforts are made to excise the cyst without rupture and keep the cyst, hyoid bone, and thyroglossal duct remnant intact. Rupture of the cyst, failure to remove the central portion of the hyoid bone or failure to remove a core of tissue up to the base of the tongue are all risk factors for recurrence. A clean and dry operative field is verified and the incision is closed in layers. The cut edges of the hyoid bone are not approximated but the strap muscles are brought together in the midline. A drain is typically not required after an uncomplicated procedure. Subcuticular skin closure with fine absorbable sutures is performed after infiltrating the wound with long-acting local anesthetic. Fluffed gauze dressing is applied. A patient who demonstrates no breathing or swallowing difficulties in the recovery room can be discharged home to a reliable family.

Excellent surgical technique will reduce the incidence of bleeding and infection. Simple excision of a TGDC carries a higher risk of recurrence (38–70%) compared to a formal Sistrunk operation (2.6–5%). Risk factors for recurrence include skin involvement, multiple or lobulated cysts, previous infection, history of surgical drainage or aspiration, and young patient age. Recurrent thyroglossal duct cysts require a more extensive excision. The pyramidal lobe of the thyroid gland, wider re-excision of the central portion of the hyoid bone and even removal of the central portion of the strap muscles down to the pretracheal fascia is indicated. The extensive aborization that is sometimes present with some TGDC necessitate this wide excision.

Carcinoma can develop within a thyroglossal duct remnant, presumably the result of chronic inflammation. In less than 1% of TGDC pathologic specimens, malignancy can be diagnosed incidentally. These are typically well-differentiated thyroid malignancies. Most are papillary carcinomas but other thyroid tumors have been described (with the exception of medullary carcinoma). In these cases, need for further management would be based on tumor biology and stage.

Branchial Cleft Cysts

Branchial anomalies comprise up to one third of cystic cervical lesions in children. The location of the cysts and paths of the sinus tracts and fistulae depend on their embryologic origin. The vast majority of branchial cleft anomalies are derived from the second branchial cleft. Much less common are derivatives from the first branchial cleft. Third branchial cleft anomalies are rare, and fourth branchial cleft anomalies are practically unheard of (and might not exist at all).

Branchial cleft anomalies present as cysts, sinuses or fistulae. Branchial cysts are remnants of the cervical sinus that are filled with fluid and have no communication with the skin or pharynx. The cysts tend to be lined by squamous epithelium. Branchial sinuses are cysts that maintain a connection to either the skin or the pharynx. These are typically lined by ciliated or non-ciliated columnar epithelium. Persistence of the pharyngeal and dermal communications results in a fistula.

Initial treatment with antibiotics is recommended for infected cysts. Needle aspiration is indicated if antibiotics fail to resolve the infection. If possible, incision and drainage should be avoided to facilitate complete excision once the infection is cleared.

The treatment of branchial cleft anomalies is surgical excision. Surgery is delayed until the acute infection subsides. The timing of surgery in younger children is controversial. Some recommend waiting until the child is older, but many of these lesions can become infected while waiting, leading to scarring that makes definitive surgery more challenging. The standard approach has been a skin crease incision made over the lesion. The more cosmetically appealing retroauricular hairline incisions should be considered for selected cases.

First branchial cleft remnants usually present due to infection and are located just anterior to the tragus of the ear, always cephalad to a horizontal line drawn through the hyoid. They can be difficult to confirm. The average delay to diagnosis and treatment is 4 years. A high index of suspicion of a superficial infection in the preauricular or parotid region would guide the astute physician. The external canal should be examined by otoscopy. Computed tomography is occasionally necessary to determine the relationship of a sinus tract to the middle ear and facial nerve.

Excision of a first branchial cleft remnant requires a careful understanding of facial nerve anatomy. Reviewing preoperative imaging studies is important before attempting to excise a deep-seated lesion. An important step in the operation is the identification of the facial nerve trunk and tracing its branches peripherally. Superficial lesions, lateral to the facial nerve, are easily excised. A superficial parotidectomy is sometimes required. If the tract courses deep to the facial nerve, a total parotidectomy is required. The tract should be followed to the ear canal and the adjacent cartilage and skin lining of the ear canal removed to reduce the risk of recurrence.

Second branchial cleft remnants typically present when the family describes a tiny punctuate opening that intermittently drains a small amount of clear fluid. Gentle downward stroking of the sternocleidomastoid sometimes allows expression of saliva. Branchial cysts and sinuses present as soft tissue swellings along the mid to upper third of the anterior border of the sternocleidomastoid muscle. The cysts are sometimes deep to the muscle and difficult to palpate. These lesions are non-tender unless they are infected. A gradual increase or fluctuation in size is sometimes noted. Some of these lesions present for the first time as a painful mass of an acutely infected cyst. Deep-seated lesions can enlarge enough to cause stridor, odynophagia or sore throat. Compression of the hypoglossal nerve manifests as ipsilateral hypoglossal nerve palsy.

History and physical examination usually suffice to make the diagnosis of a second branchial cleft fistula. Lesions with an atypical presentation benefit from further investigation with panendoscopy, or imaging with ultrasound, CT or MRI.

The treatment of a second branchial cleft sinus is surgical excision. If a cyst is present, a skin crease incision is made centered over the cyst. The cyst is carefully dissected out and any communication to the pharynx identified. When an external opening is present, an elliptical incision is made incorporating the external orifice. The tract can be probed with a lacrimal probe or 0 polypropylene suture. Injection of methylene blue into the tract can be helpful, provided there is no spillage. Staying close to the tract avoids injury to adjacent nerves (Fig. 26.2). Unlike thyroglossal duct cysts, multiple tracts are not typically present so one can safely stay close to the defined tract. The pliable skin of a young child allows for the incision skin to be retracted, permitting dissection from the skin of the lower neck up to the pharynx. In older children or adults, stepladder incisions are sometimes necessary. Special care is taken to avoid injury to the internal carotid artery, glossopharyngeal, superior laryngeal, and hypoglossal nerves.

Third and fourth branchial cleft anomalies (pyriform sinus fistula) are more common on the left side and present as a neck mass, recurrent superior neck abscess, or recurrent acute thyroiditis (particularly left sided). A fistula to the apex of the pyriform sinus is more likely to be of fourth cleft origin.

Unusual presentation of third and fourth branchial cleft anomalies frequently requires additional imaging modalities.

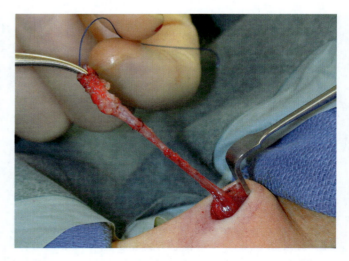

Fig. 26.2 Branchial sinus tract dissection. The entire dissection can usually be performed through a single incision but occasionally a counter-incision or step-ladder incisions will be required

Ultrasound is the initial modality of choice. If ultrasound is non-conclusive, CT can be helpful. A gas pocket seen in relation to the upper left pole of the thyroid is pathognomonic. CT is superior to MRI in visualizing gas in the soft tissues. Barium esophagram might define the tract. In suspected third or fourth cleft lesions, endoscopy and visualization of an opening in the pyriform sinus can aid in pre-operative planning.

Third and fourth branchial sinuses extend from the pyriform sinus to the thyroid, or the perithyroid tissue. Excision of superior pole of thyroid (or hemithyroidectomy if necessary) and high ligation of the tract decreases the risk of recurrence. It is important to perform laryngoscopy for cauterization of the pyriform sinus tract, either at the time of excision or 4–6 weeks later.

Bronchogenic Cysts

Bronchogenic cysts are rare anomalies of the foregut that most commonly present in the mediastinum. Occasionally, however, they can present in the inferior midline, lateral or posterior neck. In one large series, bronchogenic cysts represented fewer than 1% of cystic neck masses seen in children. Patients usually present with a palpable, fluctuant, non-tender mass. These cysts cannot be distinguished pre-operatively from other cysts and, depending on their location might be thought to be thyroglossal duct cysts, branchial cleft cysts, dermoid cysts, or vascular lesions. Diagnosis is made on pathological examination, with the presence of respiratory epithelium, mucinous glands and, sometimes, hyaline cartilage. The treatment is resection. Although malignancy has not been reported in children, malignant degeneration in adulthood has been reported.

Epidermoid and Dermoid Cysts

Epidermoid and dermoid cysts are closely related. Epidermoid cysts have only epidermis present in the cyst lining. Dermoid cysts have adnexal structures in addition to the epidermis. Embryologically then, epidermoid are derived from one germ cell layer (ectoderm) while dermoid cysts are derived from two (ectoderm and mesoderm). Epidermoid cysts can be either congenital or acquired but presentation and histology are the same regardless. Premalignant and malignant degeneration has been reported in adults. The majority of dermoid cysts in children present with a mass, most commonly (601%) in the periorbital region. The next most common site is the neck, often in the submental or suprasternal location. Epidermoid cysts in the neck can be easily confused with other cystic neck lesions. When located in the anterior neck, a thyroglossal duct cyst must also be considered.

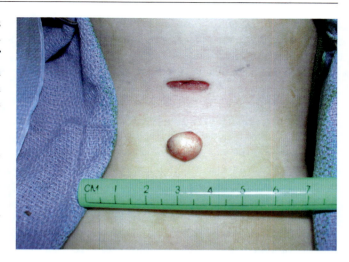

Fig. 26.3 Well circumscribed dermoid cyst clearly containing sebum (keratin)

Treatment is complete surgical excision. These cysts tend to be well circumscribed and filled with keratin (Fig. 26.3). A simple excision will usually suffice. However, if the location suggests the possibility of a thyroglossal duct cyst, a Sistrunk procedure is recommended.

Cervical Lesions of the Thymus

Descent of the thymus starts with elongation of the thymic buds from the third pharyngeal pouch to create the thymopharyngeal duct. This then separates cranially, and they "descend" (as a result of elongation of the embryo), fusing in the midline in the mediastinum. Thus, remnants can be found from the angle of the mandible to the mediastinum. Thirty percent of pediatric autopsies reveal thymic rests in the neck. Thymic lesions in the neck can present as ectopic thymus, thymic cyst and thymoma. Ectopic thymus and thymoma tend to be solid compared to thymic cysts.

Cervical thymic cysts are rare with about 150 cases reported in the literature in children between the ages of 2 and 11 years. The most common location is anterior to the left sternocleidomastoid muscle but can occur anywhere on the path of the descent. Most patients are diagnosed pre-operatively with branchial cleft remnant or lymphangioma. The treatment is complete excision.

Lymphatic Malformations

Abnormal development of the cervical lymph sacs in the embryo results in cervical lymphatic malformations. These are static (non-proliferative) vascular anomalies incorrectly termed lymphangioma or cystic hygroma. Most are diagnosed at birth and 90% are evident before age two. They are often located in the posterior neck.

Lymphatic malformations present as a soft, fluctuant, non-tender mass that sometimes increase in size with associated upper respiratory infections. Ultrasound imaging may be used to determine if the lesion is macrocystic or microcystic. MRI is helpful to determine the extent of the lesion, as they can extend into the axilla or chest. Large lesions can cause airway distortion or compression. Prenatal diagnosis of these lesions is increasingly common. Controlled delivery with ex-utero intrapartum treatment (EXIT procedure) avoids perinatal asphyxia.

Treatment can be operative, non-operative or a combination of both. Small lesions can be simply observed. Surgical therapy has traditionally been the primary modality used for treatment. It is currently best used for lesions that are completely resectable, however there is a high risk of recurrence and complications. In one series, complete resection was only possible in 60% of patients. Unlike solid lesions, lymphatic malformations do not merely displace structures but wrap around the structures along tissue planes. Careful knowledge of the anatomy is necessary to avoid serious complications.

Sclerotherapy is particularly effective in the treatment of macrocystic lesions, which are also the lesions easily treated by surgery. It is the preferred mode of treatment for lesions that infiltrate vital structures and when complete resection is not be feasible (floor of the mouth, tongue, pharynx). Multiple injections are sometimes needed depending on the extent of the lesion. Treatment of large lesions is limited by the toxicity of the agents.

The agents used vary by institutional and operator preference. Doxycyline is considered by many to be the preferred agent for sclerotherapy. It is less toxic than ethanol and is a nonspecific metalloproteinase inhibitor that might affect the angiogenesis of the lesion. Macrocystic lesions respond better (90%) than do microcystic lesions (60%). An average of two injections are needed. Hypoglycemia has been reported in some patients following treatment. This agent should be used with caution in pre-pubertal children.

Commonly used in Asia and Europe, OK-432 is a lyophilized mixture of low-virulence group A *Streptococcus* containing penicillin G potassium. In a report of 55 patients (adults and pediatric) followed for an average of 63 months (range 30–144), there was an initial response in 84% and long-term response in 76%.

Other agents used for sclerotherapy include 95% ethanol and bleomycin. Both are highly effective but therapy can be painful and extravasation can cause extensive local tissue injury.

Spontaneous resolution has been reported in up to 12.5% of patients with cervicofacial lymphatic malformations. The time to regression was about 2–7 months. The characteristics of patients with spontaneous resolution were those with macrocystic lesions, fewer than five septae, and limited extent (one location, usually posterior in the neck). The mechanism of regression is unknown but two hypotheses have been proposed: new collaterals develop that drain the lesion or inflammation/hemorrhage leads to spontaneous sclerosis.

Summary Points

- Most common cervical cysts in children are thyroglossal duct cysts and branchial cleft anomalies.
- Second branchial cleft anomalies are more common than those from other branchial clefts.
- Most cervical cysts can be identified by history and physical examination.
- In the case of anterior lesions, establish location of a normal thyroid gland prior to surgery.
- Avoid surgery in the presence of infection.
- For infected cysts, antibiotics and needle decompression are preferable to incision and drainage.
- CT scan is helpful for complex or deep-seated lateral neck lesions.

Editor's Comment

Sistrunk's operation for the excision of thyroglossal duct cysts is an elegant and relatively straightforward procedure with a high success rate and relatively low complication rate. Done well, it can be very satisfying. Carelessly performed, it can result in serious complications, including injury to the airway, hypoglossal nerve injury, and recurrence. The head must be positioned anteriorly (sniffing position) to lift the hyoid bone off of the tracheolaryngeal complex. Letting the head fall back compresses the hyoid bone against the airway, inviting injury. To avoid injury to the hypoglossal nerves, only the central 1-cm segment of the hyoid bone should be excised. And the tract must be followed nearly all the way to the foramen cecum. Postoperative wound infection almost always portends a recurrence, but it is more likely that the recurrence caused the infection, not vice versa. Recurrent thyroglossal duct cyst excisions can be frustratingly difficult, often resulting in a second recurrence and a great deal of misery for the patient and surgeon. A wide excision of all previously disrupted tissue, being sure to stay in the midline, is the most appropriate strategy.

Excision of branchial cleft cysts and sinuses is also usually straightforward, although it takes patience to dissect the entire tract all the way to its origin in the pharynx. Injection of blue dye is rarely helpful and more often leads to extensive tissue staining and a messy operative field. Not all branchial cleft sinuses will track all the way to the pharynx; some instead end somewhat abruptly in a thin-walled cystic structure with multiple tentacle-like projections that simply peter out in the soft tissues of the neck. This always raises concerns about recurrence, which occurs in a minority of cases.

Lymphatic malformations (cystic hygromas) are increasingly being managed by injection sclerotherapy. Surgical excision is very difficult, is associated with high complication and recurrence rates, and frequently results in an unacceptable cosmetic appearance. The cysts tend to interdigitate between and around vital structures, including the individual fibers of nerves such as the spinal accessory and the recurrent laryngeal nerves, which can easily be severed despite meticulous technique. Unfortunately, the cysts that most easily excised are also the most likely to respond to sclerotherapy.

Before undertaking excision of any cervical mass, it is important to review the vascular and neural anatomy very carefully and to recall that distortion of normal anatomic relationships is to be expected. One should also be prepared for the occasional unexpected vascular malformation, metastatic focus of papillary thyroid carcinoma, or carotid body tumor, each of which can be extremely vascular.

Differential Diagnosis

- Thyroglossal duct cyst
- Branchial cleft cysts
- Cervical bronchogenic cyst
- Cervical thymic cysts
- Lymphatic malformation
- Dermoid or epidermoid cysts
- Ectopic thyroid

Technical Points

- If unsure about diagnosis of a midline neck lesion, perform a Sistrunk operation.
- Stay close to the branchial cleft sinus tract but perform wide excision of thyroglossal duct tract.
- Complete excision is paramount to avoid recurrence.

Diagnostic Studies

- Ultrasound
- CT
- Panendoscopy for suspected low branchial cleft fistulas

Parental Preparation

- Outpatient procedure
- High risk of recurrence
- Risk of nerve injury

Suggested Reading

Acierno SP, Waldhausen JH. Congenital cervical cysts, sinuses and fistulae. Otolaryngol Clin North Am. 2007;40:161–76.

Dasgupta R, Adams D, Elluru R, et al. Noninterventional treatment of selected head and neck lymphatic malformations. J Pediatr Surg. 2008;43:869–73.

De Caluwé D, Ahmed M, Puri P. Cervical thymic cysts. Pediatr Surg Int. 2002;18:477–9.

Poldervaart MT, Breugem CC, Speleman L, Pasmans S. Treatment of lymphatic malformations with OK-432 (Picibanil): review of the literature. J Craniofac Surg. 2009;20(4):1159–62.

Roh JL, Yoon YH. Removal of pediatric branchial cleft cyst using a retroauricular hairline incision (RAHI) approach. Int J Pediatr Otorhinolaryngol. 2008;72:1503–7.

Teissier N, Elmaleh-Bergès M, Ferkdadji L, et al. Cervical bronchogenic cysts: usual and unusual clinical presentations. Arch Otolaryngol Head Neck Surg. 2008;134:1165–9.

Chapter 27
Disorders of the Thyroid and Parathyroid

William T. Adamson

Thyroid Disorders

Both functional and neoplastic thyroid disorders frequently challenge the pediatric surgeon. Symptoms of hyperthyroidism are the most common abnormality. Surgical treatment is occasionally indicated in hyperthyroid autoimmune conditions such as Graves' disease or Hashimoto's thyroiditis. Thyroid cancer is rare, with an overall incidence of 1/2,500 children. Presentation with a nodule or mass in the anterior neck demands a workup for thyroid malignancy. Both differentiated and medullary thyroid carcinoma are best treated with total thyroidectomy and appropriate lymph node dissection. Identification of non-malignant conditions requiring surgery and prompt diagnosis and treatment of a thyroid carcinoma are crucial elements of successful surgical management.

The thyroid gland develops from the base of the tongue ventral to the hyoid bone. Ectopic or accessory thyroid tissue may develop anywhere along the thyroglossal duct from the base of the tongue to the midline anterior neck. The thyroid gland consists of two lobes on either side of the midline connected by an isthmus of thyroid tissue. At the cellular level, follicular cells surround a reservoir of colloid thyroglobulin. Thyroglobulin is iodinated to produce thyroid hormone at the interface between colloid and follicular cells. Thyroid hormone circulates in plasma as free T4 (tetraiodothyronine) or protein-bound T3 (3,5,5 triiodothyronine) or T4. Thyroid hormone binds to a number of tissues, generally stimulating metabolic activity by increasing cellular oxygen consumption and protein synthesis. Other cells within the thyroid gland are parafollicular C cells, which derive from ultimobranchial bodies and are dispersed throughout the gland.

W.T. Adamson (✉)
Department of Surgery, University of North Carolina School of Medicine, North Carolina Children's Hospital, Chapel Hill, NC, USA
e-mail: william_adamson@med.unc.edu

Functional Thyroid Disorders

Simple enlargement of the thyroid gland, or goiter, is the most common thyroid abnormality in children. Autoimmune disorders, which can be associated with either hyper- or hypothyroidism, are next most common. Workup must begin with determining whether the patient is euthyroid or not. Abnormal thyroid function can result from a defect in hormone production and/or from inflammatory causes.

The first step is to obtain serum levels of circulating thyroid hormone. Free T4, which circulates unbound in the plasma, is not affected by levels of protein binding globulin and is most reliable. Plasma T3 and T4 measurements must be interpreted in the context of levels of thyroid binding globulin (TBG). Thyroid stimulating hormone (TSH) is produced by the anterior pituitary and stimulates production of thyroid hormone. TSH is increased in response to low levels of circulating thyroid hormone and suppressed in hyperthyroid conditions.

Imaging studies can be extremely useful in evaluating the thyroid. Ultrasound can identify the presence of a midline neck mass and its relationship to the thyroid. Ultrasound can differentiate between cystic and solid thyroid masses and determine if nodules are solid or multiple. Ectopic thyroid tissue and abnormal lymph nodes can also be identified by ultrasound. Work up frequently also includes a thyroid scan. Both ^{123}I and ^{131}I scintigraphy are effective in identifying functioning thyroid tissue. Less commonly employed scans such as technetium-99m pertechnetate can offer more precise imaging of thyroid gland nodules or masses.

Goiter, or diffuse enlargement of the thyroid gland, results from overstimulation of the gland. Increased size of the thyroid gland can be an appropriate response to a defect in hormone production or synthesis. Over 80% of goiters are simple adolescent goiter in a euthyroid patient. Decreased dietary iodine can result in low circulating levels of thyroid hormone, resulting in a TSH-stimulated increase in the size of the thyroid. Certain medications or foods, such as soy and cruciferous foods including broccoli, Brussels sprouts and cauliflower are goitrogens, which can stimulate the thyroid

P. Mattei (ed.), *Fundamentals of Pediatric Surgery*,
DOI 10.1007/978-1-4419-6643-8_27, © Springer Science+Business Media, LLC 2011

leading to goiter. Congenital hypothyroid goiter results from transplacental exposure of the fetus to maternal antithyroid drugs or iodides. Hormone or receptor defects at the pituitary or thyroid level can also result in stimulation of the thyroid gland with overproduction of thyroid hormone.

Adolescents with goiter are rarely helped by resection of the goiter. Over 60% of adolescents with goiter will have a normal size thyroid gland later in life. Thyroidectomy is reserved for those patients in whom the size of the gland produces airway compromise or swallowing difficulty.

Autoimmune Thyroid Disorders

Autoimmune inflammatory thyroid disorders are relatively common conditions that can result in both hypothyroid and hyperthyroid states. Inflammation can be mediated by lymphocytic, immunoglobulin, viral, or even bacterial causes. Most common are Graves' disease (antibody-mediated thyroiditis) and Hashimoto's (lymphocytic) thyroiditis.

Hashimoto's thyroiditis, or chronic lymphocytic thyroiditis, results from stimulation of CD4 T cells. These T cells are activated against thyroid antigens and recruit cytotoxic CD8 cells, which attack the follicular cells. While some adolescents with this condition are hyperthyroid initially, most are euthyroid and gradually progress to a hypothyroid state. Hashimoto's thyroiditis is much more common in girls than in boys. A feature of Hashimoto's that helps distinguish it from Graves' is that the thyroid is sometimes tender. Autoantibodies are detected in 95% of patients, and most have low T3 and free T4 levels. TSH is increased in 70% of patients.

Infectious causes of thyroiditis are rare. DeQuervain's thyroiditis is thought to be virally mediated. Treatment is supportive and many of these patients respond to non-steroidal anti-inflammatory medications or steroids. Rarely, suppurative inflammation of the thyroid is seen. Drainage, with or without ultrasound guidance, and antibiotics are usually effective. These patients are usually euthyroid.

Graves' disease, or autoimmune thyroiditis, results from an IgG-mediated autoimmune reaction against elements of the thyroid follicular plasma membrane, probably including the TSH-receptor. Infection may play a role in eliciting an antibody response. Graves' disease presents five times more commonly females than in males, typically in adolescence. Patients present with exopthalmos, myxedema and decreased performance in school. As the condition progresses, heat intolerance, sweating, palpitations, tremor, weight loss, and malaise become obvious. Diagnosis is confirmed by the presence of increased T3 and free T4 levels. TSH is usually suppressed and TSH receptor antibodies are present in 95% of patients. Scintigraphy shows rapid, diffuse uptake.

Initial treatment for Graves' disease is non-operative. Most patients will respond to antithyroid medications. Thionamides, such as propylthiouracil and methimazole, are the mainstays of treatment. These medications inhibit organification of iodide by the follicular cells. Iodotyrosines are blocked from coupling to thyroglobulin at the membrane, thus limiting thyroid hormone production. Response to these medications generally takes about 8 weeks and is successful in approximately two-thirds of patients. Beta-blockers such as propranolol can be effective in controlling symptoms of hyperthyroidism while thionamide medication takes effect. Remission of Graves' is seen in 25% of patients at 2 years, with an additional 25% remission every 2 years.

In addition to limiting production of T4 and T3 at the follicular membrane level, propylthiouracil limits conversion of T4 to active T3 in circulation. Thus, propylthiouracil may work faster than methimazole. Methimazole, however, has become the mainstay of antithyroid treatment for Graves' disease because of increased potency and longer half-life than propylthiouracil, characteristics which may correlate with better compliance. Side effects of these medicines such as nausea, rash, and pruritis are usually well tolerated, but some patients develop granulocytopenia, thrombocytopenia, or even hepatic dysfunction.

The treatment of choice for Graves' disease in adults and older adolescents has been thyroid ablation with ^{131}I therapy. Delivery of this medication effectively ablates the thyroid, rendering most patients hypothyroid in the process. All patients who have received ^{131}I therapy require long-term thyroxine supplementation. Fear of increased cancer risk and effects on fertility have limited the use of this option in younger children. Treatment with ^{131}I may also disrupt parathyroid function.

Surgery in Graves' disease is reserved for the rare patient who does not respond to medical treatment or whose condition warrants more rapid or permanent therapy. Thyroidectomy effectively reverses symptoms of Graves' disease. Most patients will require long-term thyroid replacement medication. Preoperative considerations prior to thyroidectomy for autoimmune thyroiditis include a course of antithyroid medications for 2–8 weeks. Once the gland is suppressed, waiting an additional 1–2 months can facilitate resection. Beta-blockade can help if symptoms demand surgery prior to this pretreatment period. Most surgeons suppress the vascularity of the thyroid gland with Lugol's solution (5–10 drops 1–3 times daily) for 5–10 days before the surgery.

It remains controversial whether subtotal or total thyroidectomy is the best surgical solution for Graves' disease. Subtotal thyroidectomy may offer a better chance of avoiding surgical complications such as recurrent laryngeal nerve injury or hypoparathyroidism. In subtotal thyroidectomy for Graves' disease, a rim of tissue, no more than 1 g per side, can be left to protect the parathyroid glands. Nevertheless, subtotal thyroidectomy carries a risk of hypoparathyroidism of up to 54%. Graves' symptoms recur in as many as 14% of patients who have undergone subtotal thyroidectomy.

Most surgeons feel that total thyroidectomy can be safely accomplished for cure in patients with Graves' disease. Elimination of thyroid tissue effectively cures the condition. If the parathyroid glands are compromised in the procedure, autotransplantation to the sternocleidomastoid muscle or non-dominant forearm can successfully prevent hypoparathyroidism. Both subtotal and total thyroidectomy pose significant risks to the recurrent laryngeal nerve and to the parathyroid glands. Meticulous approach and high surgeon volume correlate with better outcomes. Thyroid "storm" can result from manipulation of the inflamed gland. Thyroid storm is characterized by fever, cardiovascular compromise (tachycardia, dysrhythmias, congestive failure), neurologic abnormalities (irritability, agitation, tremor, coma, psychosis), and gastrointestinal upset (nausea, vomiting, diarrhea, jaundice). Appropriate preoperative treatment can avoid this condition. Treatment includes propranolol, antithyroid medications, potassium iodide, and steroids.

Thyroid Carcinoma

Thyroid cancer represents 3% of childhood malignancies. It is twice as common in females than in males, with a peak incidence between 10 and 18 years. Thyroid cancer in children is divided into differentiated (follicular and papillary) and medullary histologic types. Controversies persist regarding extent of surgical treatment for both types. Survival for papillary and follicular carcinoma is greater than 95%, despite high recurrence rates for these tumors.

Differentiated thyroid cancer, which includes papillary, follicular and mixed histologic subtypes, is the most common endocrine malignancy in children. Children typically present with advanced stage disease and a higher frequency of metastatic disease, but have a lower overall mortality. Eighty percent of pediatric thyroid cancer is papillary, 17% follicular, and 2% medullary. Anaplastic tumors are rare and uniformly fatal. Risk factors for differentiated thyroid cancer include exposure to radiation. Radiation for benign conditions has decreased over the last few decades with a corresponding decrease in the incidence of differentiated thyroid carcinoma. It is well documented that nuclear accidents, such as the Chernobyl disaster, have resulted in a marked increase in thyroid cancer in the surrounding pediatric population. Understanding of the molecular biology of papillary cancer has increased greatly in recent years. Genetic rearrangements (as opposed to point mutations) at the RET/PTC locus of the RET proto-oncogene have been seen in 35% of papillary cancers in children.

Second malignancies following chemotherapy for childhood cancer are commonly located in the thyroid gland. Thyroid cancer is the most common second malignancy occurring after treatment of both Hodgkins and non-Hodgkins

lymphoma and third most common following treatment for leukemia. Those patients treated with alkylating agents are most likely to develop thyroid malignancy.

Papillary and follicular thyroid carcinoma usually present as a thyroid mass. Lymph node involvement is present in 60–80% at presentation, 10–20% of patients have metastatic disease at presentation, primarily in the form of pulmonary nodules. During resection, FNA or frozen section may confirm presence of cancer in adjacent nodes, a finding which would direct further dissection.

Medullary carcinoma of the thyroid derives from parafollicular C cells. Calcitonin is frequently elevated in medullary thyroid cancer. Medullary thyroid cancer (MTC) accounts for 5% of pediatric thyroid cancers. MTC occurs in families as an autosomal dominant mutation. If not identified by genetic analysis of kindreds of known patients, MTC is usually metastatic with poor outcome at the time of presentation. Mutations of specific loci within the RET protooncogene on chromosome 10 are markers for the development of MTC. Families have been grouped into MEN 2A, MEN 2B, and familial MTC based on associated phenotypes and genotypes. Patients with MEN 2A develop pheochromocytoma (50%) and parathyroid hyperplasia (30%). These patients develop MTC after age 5. Eighty percent of MEN 2A patients identified at 10.5 years or older already have MTC. Patients with MEN 2B also develop pheochromocytoma (50%), but typically have a marfanoid body habitus and can develop mucosal neuromas and do not have parathyroid disease. Some patients with MEN 2B have been known to develop MTC at less than 2 years of age. Another familial subgroup of MTC patients (FMTC) develops medullary thyroid carcinoma alone.

Within the MEN 2 syndromes, medullary thyroid carcinoma typically presents before other associated malignancies and is responsible for the mortality in MEN 2 patients. For these patients, thyroidectomy before MTC develops offers the best chance for cure. Molecular biologic differentiation of specific subcategories of mutations within the RET protooncogene allows prediction of timing of development of MTC. Appropriate age selection for thyroidectomy is based on the earliest known presentation of MTC for the specific subtype. Current recommendations include thyroidectomy for MEN 2A patients before age five and for MEN 2B patients before age 1.

Surgical Therapy

Surgery for thyroid carcinoma is based on presentation, extent of disease and histologic subtype. Because of the overall excellent prognosis despite variations in operative therapies and extent of metastatic disease, controversy persists regarding the surgical management of differentiated thyroid cancer in children. Medullary thyroid cancer, however, is managed with total thyroidectomy and central lymph node dissection in all patients at an age determined by mutational subgroup.

Most papillary and follicular thyroid cancers present as a solitary nodule. Twenty percent of all solitary thyroid nodules are cancer. Work up for a solitary thyroid nodule should be expedient and focused on confirming or excluding the diagnosis of cancer while minimizing morbidity. An algorithm for management of the solitary thyroid nodule is described in Fig. 27.1. A thorough history should elicit signs of hyper- or hypothyroidism, risk factors such as radiation exposure, and a family history of head and neck cancer. Physical exam should assess for associated lymph node involvement and adherence to surrounding tissues. Laboratory tests should include serum T3, free T4, TSH, calcium, and calcitonin levels. ^{131}I scintigraphy can determine uptake of iodine in a functioning thyroid gland. A functioning (hot) nodule that takes up the radiotracer might represent a hyperthyroid mass and require preoperative suppression prior to biopsy or resection. Nonfunctioning (cold) nodules within the thyroid are more frequently malignant and demand biopsy. Scintigraphy is also helpful to identify ectopic thyroid tissue, such as a lingual thyroid gland.

A chest X-ray should be performed to assess for pulmonary metastases, which are identified preoperatively in up to 6% of patients with thyroid cancer.

Ultrasound of the neck and thyroid can be extremely helpful and should be performed in all patients with a midline neck mass or nodule. Ultrasound can determine if the mass is solid or cystic, characterize the relationship of the mass to the surrounding thyroid gland, identify abnormal lymph nodes, and help define the role of fine needle aspiration (FNA) or other biopsy. Solid masses should undergo FNA or biopsy. Cystic masses should be aspirated, and if they completely disappear may be observed. Any residual solid component of a cyst should be biopsied.

Routinely performed in adults and older adolescents with a midline neck nodule, FNA can identify benign nodules that are inflammatory or cystic. Though usually benign, hot nodules can also be thyroid cancer, so FNA might even be useful in these situations. The diagnosis of papillary carcinoma, the most common type of thyroid carcinoma, can frequently be confirmed by FNA, but it does not always allow differentiation of follicular carcinoma from normal thyroid tissue. Thus, FNA of a solid mass can confirm the diagnosis of cancer and preclude additional biopsy, but an equivocal result may yet

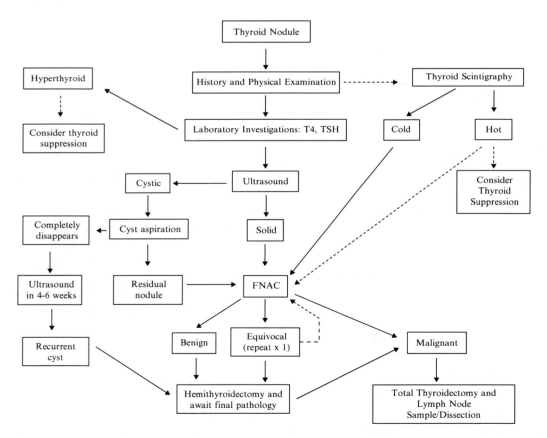

Fig. 27.1 Algorithm for the evaluation of pediatric thyroid nodules. The *dotted lines* indicate an optional pathway of the algorithm that may be deemed appropriate for individual cases (From The Canadian Pediatric Thyroid Nodule Study Group. The Canadian Pediatric Thyroid Nodule Study: an evaluation of current management practices. J Pediatr Surg. 2008;43:826–30. Reprinted with permission from Elsevier.)

demand more thorough operative biopsy. Hemithyroidectomy (lobectomy with isthmusectomy) for biopsy is recommended if the FNA is indeterminate. If malignancy is determined by FNA or biopsy, thyroidectomy is indicated.

Fine needle aspiration is recommended in children who are greater than 13 years of age. These patients are more cooperative and the likelihood that a nodule is malignant is decreased. Only 11% of midline neck nodules in teenagers will be malignant; this number is significantly higher in smaller children. For children less than 13 years of age, excision of the nodule, usually requiring thyroid hemithyroidectomy, is indicated.

Surgical Technique

As with thyroidectomy for benign disease, controversy exists regarding the extent of thyroidectomy for carcinoma. Morbidity following thyroidectomy is primarily related to the extent of dissection. Permanent injury to the recurrent laryngeal nerve is infrequent, but devastating. Transient abnormalities in calcium metabolism are common. Permanent hypoparathyroidism resulting from devascularization or resection of all parathyroid glands is as high as 25% in some series.

Subtotal thyroidectomy involves leaving thyroid tissue around the recurrent laryngeal nerve and/or around the parathyroid glands to preserve perfusion of these glands. It is presumed by those advocating subtotal resection that recurrent laryngeal nerve or parathyroid complications will be decreased. Advocates of subtotal resection note that there is the same overall mortality for patients whether subtotal or total thyroidectomy is performed.

Total thyroidectomy involves removing all thyroid tissue, if possible. This approach minimizes local recurrence. If the recurrent laryngeal nerve or other functional structures are involved, these tissues should be spared. No more than 1 g of thyroid tissue should be left on each side. Postoperative ablative ^{131}I treatment, recommended for patients with differentiated thyroid carcinoma, will eliminate the remaining thyroid tissue. Removing as much thyroid tissue as possible increases the sensitivity of postoperative ^{131}I scans. Complete removal of the primary also allows more of the ^{131}I to localize and treat distant metastases. Reported complications of total thyroidectomy are reduced in more recent studies; many surgeons feel that the parathyroid and recurrent laryngeal nerve areas can be safely navigated. Devascularized parathyroid glands can be autotransplanted into the sternocleidomastoid muscle or forearm.

Some authors recommend initial resection limited to lobectomy and isthmusectomy for confirmed papillary thyroid carcinoma if disease is limited to one lobe and there is no radiographic evidence of metastasis. A selective dissection of involved lymph nodes with curative intent is recommended in these patients as well. Comparable overall mortality is seen in these series. However, the high incidence of bilaterality (two thirds) and multicentricity for differentiated thyroid cancer persuades most authors to recommend total or near-total thyroidectomy. Papillary carcinoma may be bilateral in up to 85% of reported cases. Tumors are multifocal in more than 80%. Residual or multifocal disease can be found in the other lobe in as many as 16% of specimens. Furthermore, sensitivity of postoperative ^{131}I scans and effectiveness of ^{131}I treatment are limited by absorption of the tracer by the remaining lobe.

Regardless of the extent of thyroid gland resection, thyroidectomy for papillary or follicular thyroid cancer should be accompanied by central lymph node dissection as well as resection of any enlarged adjacent lymph nodes. A functional, rather than radical, neck dissection is advocated. This dissection includes nodes in the central compartment as bordered by the jugular veins laterally, the thyroid notch or hyoid superiorly, and the superior mediastinum inferiorly. Involved nodes adjacent to the central compartment should also be removed, with sparing of motor and sensory nerves, sternocleidomastoid muscle and the jugular vein. Thirty to 80% of patients will have positive nodes at dissection.

Total or near-total thyroidectomy with central node dissection for differentiated thyroid carcinoma is recommended by most authors. This approach minimizes local recurrence and affords the best opportunity for control of distant metastases with ^{131}I ablation and can be accomplished with acceptable morbidity, although it might be associated with more complications than a lesser resection. Removal of the thyroid gland also makes it possible to screen for recurrence by measuring thyroglobulin levels. Another putative benefit of total thyroidectomy is the elimination of the possibility of dedifferentiation of tumor left behind in the remaining thyroid gland. All patients with and at risk for medullary thyroid carcinoma should also undergo total thyroidectomy with central nodal dissection at the appropriate age.

Incision for thyroidectomy is a curvilinear low anterior cervical incision along skin lines. The platysma is divided and strap muscle retracted laterally. Meticulous hemostasis can prevent the need for drain placement in many cases. Resection of all thyroid tissue, including the posterior capsule, is advocated. Involvement of nodes beyond the central compartment may be assessed clinically or with intraoperative FNA or frozen section to help direct the extent of resection. If parathyroid tissue is compromised, autotransplantation is indicated.

Postoperatively, all patients with differentiated thyroid carcinoma should undergo ^{131}I scanning. If residual disease is detected, a therapeutic dose of ^{131}I can be given. Radioablative therapy decreases the risk of local recurrence and improves sensitivity of future scans. All patients who undergo thyroidectomy and ablation will require replacement therapy with exogenous thyroglobulin, L-thyroxine, to suppress TSH-mediated stimulation of thyroid tissue.

Surveillance following thyroidectomy for carcinoma includes serum thyroglobulin levels. Chest X-ray can identify pulmonary metastases. Computed tomography and CT/PET are probably more effective than chest radiography for identifying distant metastases. Radioiodide scans reveal metastases with high sensitivity following total thyroidectomy and ablation. Serum calcitonin levels should be monitored in medullary carcinoma patients. Finally, ultrasound of the neck may identify recurrence in the thyroid bed or adjacent lymph nodes.

Overall outcomes for differentiated thyroid cancer are excellent, with long-term survival reported to be 95–98%. Carcinoma recurs in 10–35% of patients. Local recurrence is common in the lateral neck and thyroid bed, while most metastases recur in the lungs. Follicular and follicular-variant of papillary carcinoma have higher rates of recurrence. Mortality is poorest in children less than 10 years old, in those with pulmonary metastases involving trachea or larynx, and in those with medullary carcinoma.

Parathyroid Disorders

Overproduction of parathyroid hormone by one or more of the four parathyroid glands can disrupt calcium homeostasis and lead to symptoms of hyperparathyroidism. The parathyroid glands in the neck, usually four in number, produce parathyroid hormone, an important regulator of bone growth and remodeling. Parathyroid hormone (PTH) mobilizes calcium from bone in a vitamin D-dependent process. Hyperparathyroidism produces pathologic increases in serum calcium. Patients with hyperparathyroidism may commonly present with fatigue, lethargy, nausea, abdominal pain, vomiting, and polydipsia. Nephrolithiasis, as well as diarrhea, depression, and joint pain are not uncommon. Treatment for hyperparathyroidism is primarily surgical.

Understanding the embryology of the parathyroid glands is paramount in localizing glands at surgery. The inferior glands derive from the third branchial pouch and migrate inferiorly with the thymus until they stop on the dorsal surface of the inferior thyroid gland. The superior glands derive from the fourth branchial pouch and descend to a point superior and lateral to the thyroid gland. Interruption of the downward migration can result in ectopic position of any of the four glands.

Primary Hyperparathyroidism

Primary hyperparathyroidism is rare, occurring with an incidence of less than 5/100,000 individuals. Symptoms result from hypercalcemia. Many patients with hyperparathyroidism may already have end-organ damage at presentation, including nephrocalcinosis, bone involvement, nephrolithiasis or acute pancreatitis. In children, there is a slight female preponderance, but it is not as pronounced as it is in adults.

Almost all children with primary hyperparathyroidism have hypercalcemia with an inappropriately elevated plasma PTH. In younger children, a single adenoma producing excess PTH can be seen in as many as two-thirds of patients. Solitary adenomas are rarer in older adolescents. Diffuse overproduction of PTH results from hyperplasia of all four glands in as many as one-fourth of children with hyperparathyroidism. While solitary adenomas are generally sporadic in children, four-gland hyperplasia is frequently associated with a familial syndrome. These include MEN 1 and 2A. More than half of children with primary hyperparathyroidism due to four-gland hyperplasia have MEN 1.

Primary hyperparathyroidism in infancy is rare but severe, often resulting in death. An infant with primary hyperparathyroidism may present with hypotonicity, respiratory distress, failure to thrive, lethargy and polyuria. All have elevated PTH resulting from diffuse four-gland hyperplasia and require emergent resection. This syndrome is familial in half of patients.

The differential diagnosis for hypercalcemia in children that is not related to hyperparathyroidism is listed in Table 27.1. None of these have hypercalcemia with elevations in PTH. Two of these conditions deserve special mention. Hypocalciuric hypercalcemia is an autosomal dominant condition that results from a defect in the calcium-sensing receptor gene. These patients have low PTH and low urinary excretion of calcium. Most patients who are heterozygous for this condition do not benefit from surgery. If both parents are carriers, infants may present with severe hypercalcemia in the neonatal period. This can be associated with four-gland hyperplasia requiring surgery.

Neoplasia commonly results in hypercalcemia in adults due to production of a parathyroid hormone-related polypeptide. While much less commonly a source of elevated calcium in children, childhood cancers in children can produce peptides that lead to elevated serum calcium. (Table 27.1).

Secondary and Tertiary Hyperparathyroidism

Secondary hyperparathyroidism results from renal insufficiency or calcium malabsorption. Decreased circulating calcium levels stimulate parathyroid production of PTH in these conditions. Medical therapy to decrease gastrointestinal phosphate absorption can help reestablish calcium homeostasis. In some cases, persistently elevated PTH production precipitates renal osteodystrophy, characterized by fractures and metastatic calcifications. In these cases, total parathyroidectomy with autotransplantation is indicated.

Table 27.1 Differential diagnosis of hypercalcemia in children with normal parathyroid hormone levels

Familial hypocalciuric hypercalcemia
Cancer (producing PTH-like peptide)
Neuroblastoma
Lymphoma
Malignant rhabdoid tumor
Mesoblastic nephroma
Rhabdomyosarcoma
Small cell carcinoma of the ovary
Hypervitaminosis A and D
Hypophosphatemia
Parenteral nutrition (iatrogenic)
Sarcoidosis
Subcutaneous fat necrosis
Prolonged immobilization
Thiazide diuretics
Thyrotoxicosis
Williams syndrome

Tertiary hyperparathyroidism occurs when elevated PTH production persists even after the hypocalcemic stimulus to the parathyroid is corrected. Following successful renal transplantation, for example, some patients have persistent elevations in PTH with resulting osteodystrophy. Presumably, chronically stimulated parathyroid tissue produces PTH autonomously, irrespective of calcium homeostasis. Total parathyroidectomy with heterogeneous autotransplantation is indicated.

Surgical Technique

Classically, treatment for hyperparathyroidism has been to proceed directly to surgery after a diagnosis of hypercalcemia with elevated PTH has been made. Routine preoperative imaging studies have not traditionally been recommended. This approach, certainly in cases of four-gland hyperplasia, has been proven effective and safe. More recently, there has been increasing support in the literature for preoperative imaging studies in children, especially in cases where four-gland hyperplasia is not suspected. Hyperparathyroid patients who are infants, who have familial hyperparathyroid syndromes, such as MEN 1 and MEN 2A patients, or who have renal causes of hyperparathyroidism, are likely to have four-gland hyperplasia and should be explored without routinely pursuing further imaging studies.

Regarding the initial operation for hyperparathyroidism, a debate continues between those favoring total resection vs. those favoring subtotal resection. The surgical approach involves exploration of the neck through a low cervical incision. All four parathyroid glands must be identified. Biopsy of each gland confirms the tissue as parathyroid. Most authors recommend removal of all four glands with heterotopic autotransplantation of part of one gland into skeletal muscle of

the forearm. Parathyroid tissue can also be transplanted into the adjacent sternocleidomastoid muscle. Some authors favor removal of 3½ glands, leaving ½ of one gland in place, marked with non-absorbable suture or clip.

Total parathyroidectomy with heterotopic autotransplantation of minced pieces of one gland into skeletal muscle offers specific advantages over the 3½-gland approach. If hyperparathyroidism persists postoperatively, repeat neck exploration to remove more tissue is avoided. The forearm site, for example, can be reexplored and some of the parathyroid tissue removed. This method has been shown to be safe in children, even infants. In fact, improved survival rates are reported in infants with severe hypercalcemia who undergo total parathyroidectomy with autotransplantation when compared with subtotal resection.

If all four glands cannot be located, the missing gland is most likely located along its path of embryologic descent. A missing parathyroid may be found along the tracheoesophageal groove, within the thymus, lateral to the thyroid in the carotid sheath, or within the thyroid gland itself. If a gland cannot be found, cervical thymectomy or thyroid lobectomy on the side of the missing gland should be considered. Because if a small but significant percentage of the population that ectopic or supernumerary parathyroid glands located in the upper mediastinum, many authors recommend routine cervical thymectomy in cases of secondary or tertiary hyperparathyroidism.

If a solitary adenoma and three normal glands are found, the adenoma alone can be resected. The other three parathyroid glands are biopsied, marked and left in place. This more limited resection is particularly successful when preoperative imaging identifies a solitary functioning adenoma.

Recurrent hyperparathyroidism after surgery almost always indicates that an adenoma was missed or that too much tissue was left behind following subtotal resection. Several imaging techniques can identify residual or ectopic parathyroid tissue. Sestamibi scintigraphy is highly sensitive and specific for parathyroid tissue in the neck or mediastinum. High-resolution ultrasound or CT scan can also identify an ectopic adenoma. One or more of these techniques should be employed prior to reoperation.

Imaging prior to initial surgery may be helpful in selected cases. Sestamibi scintigraphy and high-resolution ultrasound are extremely effective when combined with intraoperative rapid PTH assays for identification of parathyroid tissue. This technology has made image-guided minimally invasive exploration possible. In cases in which a solitary adenoma is suspected, sestamibi- or US-directed resection of a solitary adenoma without exploration of the other three glands may be an attractive option. This approach should be reserved for those cases in which four-gland hyperplasia is unlikely. Proponents of preoperative imaging cite a higher incidence of solitary adenomas in children and a higher incidence (9–13%) of ectopic glands as reasons to obtain ultrasound or sestamibi scans prior to surgical exploration. Others cite a 20% rate of failed primary operations for hyperparathyroidism in children when compared with adults as a reason to pursue preoperative imaging.

Minimally invasive image-guided resection of a single parathyroid gland should not be considered in cases of MEN 1, MEN 2A, familial hyperparathyroidism, or cases of hyperparathyroidism secondary to renal disease. All four glands must be identified and inspected in these cases.

Postoperative Care

Surgical complications from neck exploration for hyperparathyroidism include bleeding and damage to adjacent structures. Recurrent laryngeal nerve injury, usually temporary, is seen in approximately 4% of patients.

The most common problems following parathyroidectomy involve abnormalities of serum calcium levels. Hypercalcemia following parathyroidectomy for primary hyperparathyroidism suggests that an inadequate subtotal resection was performed or an adenoma was missed. Short-term hypocalcemia is common following parathyroid surgery, likely due to transiently decreased PTH production by the autotransplanted or remnant parathyroid tissue. Symptoms of hypocalcemia include paresthesias, Chvostek's sign and Trousseau's sign. Central nervous system symptoms are also common, including headache, slurred speech, tetany and arthralgias. In most cases, prophylactic calcium supplementation in the immediate postoperative period can avoid these problems.

Hyperparathyroidism in children is a rare problem that is successfully addressed with surgical resection. Familial hyperparathyroid syndromes, such as MEN 1 and MEN 2A, must be considered and suspected. In most cases, total parathyroidectomy with heterotopic autotransplantation is curative. Identification of all four parathyroid glands ensures a successful surgical technique. Sestamibi scintigraphy and high-resolution ultrasound are invaluable tools in reoperative parathyroid surgery and, in selected cases, prior to initial resection.

Summary Points

Thyroid

- Presence of a thyroid mass demands workup to determine if it is cystic or solid and if it is functional or non-functional.
- Goiter, a common cause of thyroid enlargement in children, does not usually require surgery.
- Graves' disease, a type of autoimmune thyroiditis, is usually managed with propylthiouracil or methimazole in children.
- Older adolescents with Graves' disease may be candidates for ^{131}I ablative therapy.
- Thyroidectomy for severe cases of Graves' disease is effective but may result in thyroid storm.
- Differentiated thyroid cancer, papillary and follicular, is the most common endocrine malignancy in children and is responsible for 3% of childhood malignancies.
- Differentiated thyroid cancer has a high recurrence after surgery, but overall survival is greater than 95%.
- Medullary thyroid cancer occurs in families as an autosomal dominant mutation associated with MEN 2A and 2B syndromes.
- Medullary thyroid cancer demands total thyroidectomy at an appropriate early age to avoid ultimately fatal metastases.
- Twenty percent of solitary thyroid nodules in children are cancer; all demand workup including biopsy if solid.
- FNA of a solid nodule can be helpful in older children; younger children may require hemithyroidectomy for diagnosis.
- Most thyroid cancers in children should be treated with total thyroidectomy and appropriate lymph node dissection.
- [131]I ablative therapy is effective for treatment of residual or metastatic thyroid cancer tissue in patients with differentiated thyroid carcinoma.

Parathyroid

- Hyperparathyroidism presents with fatigue, lethargy, nausea, abdominal pain, vomiting, and polydipsia.
- Primary hyperparathyroidism in children is more likely to result from a single adenoma than in adolescent and adult patients who often have four-gland hyperplasia.

- Four-gland parathyroid hyperplasia in children is frequently associated with MEN 1 and MEN 2A syndromes.
- Secondary and tertiary hyperparathyroidism result from prolonged systemic hypocalcemic stimulation of PTH, such as in renal disease.
- Total parathyroidectomy with reimplantation of minced parathyroid tissue into skeletal muscle is effective and safe in children with four-gland hyperplasia.
- Parathyroidectomy for a solitary nodule in a child may be limited to identification and resection of the enlarged nodule alone.
- Preoperative imaging prior to parathyroidectomy is not usually indicated, but is indispensible if a solitary nodule is suspected and limited resection of that nodule is planned.
- All four glands should be identified at surgery for hyperplasia; missing glands can be found along predicted paths of embryologic descent.
- Recurrent or persistent hyperparathyroidism after surgery demands multiple imaging techniques to identify residual or ectopic parathyroid tissue.

Editor's Comment

Thyroid nodules occur rarely in children but frequently raise the possibility of carcinoma. Because of the higher risk for malignancy, there tends to be a more aggressive approach towards biopsy and resection. Hot nodules are usually benign but not always, and FNA can be difficult or impossible in some children. Therefore, there is a very low threshold for recommending biopsy in the form of thyroid lobectomy. Although no imaging study is 100% accurate, ultrasound has become invaluable in the assessment of the thyroid gland and the lymph nodes of the neck, with some experienced ultra-sonographers able to distinguish benign nodules and lymph nodes from malignant ones. In rare cases, a needle-core biopsy can be done for palpable lesions or with ultrasound guidance under general anesthesia. Bleeding is a risk but gentle pressure along the biopsy tract is an effective tamponade.

If the nodule is proven to represent malignancy, total thyroidectomy is usually recommended, even for small papillary carcinomas. This protects the patient from bilateral disease, allows more effective treatment of metastases with ^{131}I ablative therapy, permits the use of thyroglobulin as a marker for recurrence, and increases the sensitivity of postoperative scans. In experienced hands, the risk of recurrent laryngeal nerve injury or hypoparathyroidism after total thyroidectomy should be quite low. In the end, regarding the question of total vs. subtotal thyroidectomy, the surgeon must make the decision that is safest for the child in the context of the resources available at their institution, the preferences of the endocrinologists who will be following the child after the operation, and his or her own experience and skill set. In some situations, this should prompt the family to be referred to a tertiary care center or other institution with more experience and a safe track record.

The surgical technique for thyroidectomy is essentially the same as it is in adults. The cleaner planes of the child's neck allow the surgeon to maintain a plane of dissection essentially right on the capsule of the thyroid throughout the operation. The recurrent laryngeal nerve is usually easily identified and is frequently much larger than expected given the size of the child. Recurrent laryngeal nerve monitoring should be considered standard of care for reoperative surgery, for children with pre-existing unilateral vocal cord paralysis, and when the tumor is infiltrative or invasive; however, for primary operations in healthy children with nonaggressive tumors it is optional. The parathyroid glands can be difficult to identify in children but every attempt should be made to do so. A tiny piece of any questionable tissue should be sent for biopsy and, if it appears to be ischemic, should be placed on ice until the frozen-section diagnosis is returned. If confirmed to be parathyroid tissue, it should be implanted into the sternocleidomastoid muscle. It is also extremely important to perform a proper lymph node dissection when dealing with any carcinoma, but especially medullary cancer. The surgeon should be familiar with all the anatomic zones of the neck including their borders and their contents and the details of the operation should be recorded with precision for staging purposes. For metastatic papillary carcinoma, removing all clinically positive nodes is usually sufficient and second or third operations to remove newly positive nodes is not unheard of. Even in the presence of metastases, papillary thyroid carcinoma is associated with an extremely good prognosis.

Parathyroid adenomas are rare but there should be an earnest attempt to localize it preoperatively with ultrasound, sestamibi scan or even MRI of the neck. Surgical treatment of four-gland hyperplasia is somewhat controversial, but given the dynamic nature of a child's metabolism and unpredictable changes in endocrine status with growth and development, it seems prudent to remove all glands and place a portion in the muscle of the forearm while preserving some extra tissue properly frozen in the event more is needed in the future. To have to return to the neck for a second operation seems unnecessarily risky.

Differential Diagnosis

Thyroid

- Thyroiditis: autoimmune (Hashimoto's, Graves'), inflammatory.
- Mass: goiter, thyroiditis, differentiated (papillary or follicular) carcinoma, medullary thyroid cancer.

Parathyroid

- See Table 27.1

Diagnostic Studies

Thyroid

- Ultrasound
- Serum T3, free T4, thyroid binding globulin, TSH
- Serum calcitonin and genetic studies
- ^{131}I scintigraphy
- Chest X-ray

Parathyroid

- Serum calcium, PTH
- Urinary calcium excretion
- Ultrasound, sestamibi scintigraphy, CT scan

Parental Preparation

Thyroid

- Potential complications: hemorrhage, recurrent laryngeal nerve injury, hypoparathyroidism
- Need for life-long thyroid replacement therapy

Parathyroid

- Risk of RLN injury
- High incidence of short-term hypocalcemia following parathyroidectomy
- Higher rate of failed primary operation in children than in adults

Preoperative Preparation

Thyroid

- For Graves' disease, antithyroid medication, beta-blockade, Lugol's solution
- Ultrasound can assess nodal involvement and direct dissection
- Informed consent

Parathyroid

- Suspicion of solitary adenoma should direct need for preoperative imaging
- Informed consent

Technical Points

Thyroid

- Curvilinear low anterior cervical incision
- Identification and avoidance of RLN and parathyroids
- Assess and remove all involved nodes; central lymph node dissection for MTC

Parathyroid

- Low anterior cervical dissection with identification and biopsy of each gland
- Missing glands can be found along tracheo-esophageal groove, within thymus or thyroid, lateral to thyroid in carotid sheath
- Cervical thymectomy or thyroid lobectomy considered for missing gland
- Intraoperative US and PTH assay can help localize adenoma or difficult to find glands

Suggested Reading

Dinauer CA, Breuer C, Rivkees SA. Differentiated thyroid cancer in children: diagnosis and management. Curr Opin Oncol. 2008; 20:59–65.

Gingalewski CA, Newman KD. Seminars: controversies in the management of pediatric thyroid malignancy. J Surg Oncol. 2006;94:748–52.

Kollars J, Zarroug AE, van Heerden J, et al. Primary hyperparathyroidism in pediatric patients. Pediatrics. 2005;115:974–80.

Massimino M, Collini P, Fagundes Leite S, et al. Conservative surgical approach for thyroid and lymph-node involvement in papillary thyroid carcinoma of childhood and adolescence. Pediatr Blood Cancer. 2006;46:307–13.

Schlosser K, Schmitt CP, Bartholomaeus JE, et al. Parathyroidectomy for renal hyperparathyroidism in children and adults. World J Surg. 2008;32:801–6.

Skinner MA, Moley JA, Dilley WG, et al. Prophylactic thyroidectomy in multiple endocrine neoplasia type 2A. N Engl J Med. 2005;353: 1105–13.

Skinner MA, Safford SD. Endocrine disorders and tumors. In: Ashcraft KW, Holcomb III GW, Murphy GW, editors. Pediatric surgery. 4th ed. Philadelphia: Elsevier Saunders; 2005. p. 1088–104.

Sosa JA, Udelsman R. Total thyroidectomy for differentiated thyroid cancer. J Surg Oncol. 2006;94:701–7.

The Canadian Pediatric Thyroid Nodule Study Group. The Canadian Pediatric Thyroid Nodule Study: an evaluation of current management practices. J Pediatr Surg. 2008;43:826–30.

Chapter 28
Cervical Lymphadenopathy

Rajeev Prasad and L. Grier Arthur

Cervical lymphadenopathy is common in children. The condition frequently results in a child's referral to a pediatric surgeon for further evaluation, and surgical intervention is often required. The majority of these masses represent benign disease, but the possibility of a malignancy exists. Parents often experience a significant amount of anxiety, and so it is important that pediatric surgeons are comfortable with the evaluation and management of these common lesions.

In general, neck masses in children can be congenital, neoplastic or inflammatory. Not all of these lesions cause cervical lymphadenopathy. Congenital lesions, including thyroglossal duct cysts, branchial cleft cysts, dermoid cysts, hemangiomas and lymphangiomas, are a part of the differential diagnosis of a neck mass in a child. Neoplastic causes of neck masses include relatively uncommon primary tumors such as neuroblastoma and rhabdomyosarcoma. Neoplasia that results in cervical lymphadenopathy is much more common and includes lymphoma and metastatic disease (most commonly thyroid cancer).

Inflammatory lesions are the most common etiology of cervical lymphadenopathy. Acute lymphadenitis, either viral or bacterial, is most often seen. Pediatric surgeons, however, will also encounter cases of subacute or chronic lymphadenitis, and the management of these can differ significantly. Some of the causes of these more indolent infections include atypical mycobacteria, tuberculosis, *Bartonella henselae* (cat scratch disease), and rarer fungal, parasitic or opportunistic infections. Finally, there are several miscellaneous conditions that can cause cervical lymphadenopathy in children as well.

R. Prasad (✉)
Department of Pediatric General Surgery, Drexel University College of Medicine, St. Christopher's Hospital for Children, Erie Avenue at Front Street, Philadelphia, PA 19134, USA
e-mail: rajeev.prasad@tenethealth.com

Acute Cervical Lymphadenitis

Acute cervical lymphadenitis in children is most commonly associated with a viral respiratory tract infection. The lymph nodes generally undergo reactive hyperplasia due to the viral infection and are usually bilateral, multiple, and small. Erythema is uncommon, and suppuration rarely occurs. Viral agents frequently associated with a respiratory tract illness include adenovirus, coronavirus, influenza virus, parainfluenza virus, reovirus, respiratory syncytial virus, and rhinovirus. Other common viruses that cause cervical lymphadenitis include Ebstein-Barr virus and cytomegalovirus. Less common causes include measles, mumps, rubella, and varicella. When bilateral enlarged lymph nodes appear in conjunction with typical upper respiratory tract infection symptoms, further work-up is not immediately necessary. The lymph node enlargement generally subsides spontaneously within 2–3 weeks. Enlarged nodes that persist beyond this time or continue to enlarge will likely require further investigation.

Acute bacterial lymphadenitis in children usually occurs due to an infection by *Staphylococcus aureus* or *Streptococcus pyogenes*. In infants less than 1 year of age, Group B *Streptococcus*, *Haemophilus influenza* type B, and anaerobes (*Bacteroides*, *Peptococcus*, *Peptostreptococcus* species) are possible causative agents. The lymph node groups that are affected, in decreasing order of frequency, include the submandibular, upper cervical, submental, occipital, and lower cervical nodes. The adenopathy is occasionally bilateral but more often unilateral. The involved node is usually solitary, large, and tender. Erythema and suppuration are common. Other associated findings include fever, pharyngitis, malaise, otitis, tonsillitis, dental caries, or periodontal disease.

Initial treatment is with antibiotics unless there is obvious suppuration requiring incision and drainage. Antibiotic therapy should be directed at the most likely organism. In general, an antibiotic with broad spectrum coverage, particularly against beta-lactamase producing organisms, is instituted first. However, coverage against methicillin-resistant *S. aureus* might be necessary given the increasing prevalence of this organism in the community. In about 25% of cases, one finds that an initially firm and tender lymph node, initially associated with mild overlying erythema, will suppurate after the institution of antibiotics. Incision and drainage or aspiration may then be required.

Subacute and Chronic Cervical Lymphadenitis

Lymphadenitis that persists beyond approximately 2 weeks is considered to be subacute or chronic. These localized infections can be caused by a variety of organisms. Atypical mycobacteria, specifically *Mycobacterium avium intracellulare* and *M. scrofulaceum*, are the most common cause of subacute lymphadenitis. Other less common strains include *M. kansasii, M. fortuitum,* and *M. hemophilum.* Patients with atypical mycobacterial lymphadenitis commonly present with a rapid onset of unilateral lymph node enlargement near the angle of the mandible. Typically, the nodes are only mildly tender and gradually increase in size over the course of 2–3 weeks. Erythema, induration, and fluctuance are often present. The skin overlying the nodes often becomes dry and flaky, and can develop a pink or purple hue. Patients rarely have other symptomatology, and a tuberculin skin test is at most mildly reactive. Antibiotic therapy is generally ineffective, and excision of the involved nodes is indicated. Simple drainage can sometimes lead to formation of a chronic draining fistula or simply a recurrence and therefore should be avoided.

Chronic lymphadenitis due to *M. tuberculosis* has a similar appearance to the other atypical infections. However patients may have constitutional symptoms. There is usually systemic disease as evidenced by an abnormal chest radiograph. A tuberculin skin test is positive, and there is a history of contact with an infected individual. Multi-agent antituberculous antibiotic therapy for 12–18 months is indicated.

Cat scratch disease is a lymphocutaneous disorder in which regional lymphadenitis occurs after infection with the bacterium *B. henselae*. There is usually a skin lesion in the area of inoculation. Over the course of days to weeks after inoculation, regional adenopathy occurs. The neck is the second most commonly affected area after the axilla. Patients sometimes have mild constitutional symptoms. Typically, there is a single enlarged lymph node in the chain that drains the area of inoculation. The lymph node is usually tender and firm, and suppuration can occur. If cat scratch disease is suspected, the diagnosis can be confirmed by serologic testing. The infection usually is self-limited, but antibiotic therapy with a macrolide antibiotic is often helpful in facilitating resolution of the adenopathy. Once the diagnosis has been confirmed, surgical intervention is not necessary unless purulence develops, in which case incision and drainage may be necessary.

Fungal infections is occasionally the cause of cervical lymphadenopathy in children. Histoplasmosis, blastomycosis, and coccidiomycosis are examples of these infections and are caused by *Histoplasma capsulatum, Blastomyces dermatitidis* and *Coccidioides immitis*, respectively. These organisms, which are endemic to certain regions of the country, usually cause a pulmonary infection that subsequently leads to involvement of cervical lymph nodes. Most cases are self-limited, but severe infections require systemic anti-fungal therapy.

Toxoplasmosis is caused by the consumption of tainted meat or milk products. The intracellular protozoan *Toxoplasma gondii* is the causative organism. Lymphadenopathy, which can be only mildly symptomatic, is the presenting symptom in 10% of patients. The diagnosis is confirmed by serologic testing. Severe cases should be treated with 4–6 weeks of antibiotics.

Opportunistic infections in immunocompromised children can also be a cause of chronic cervical lymphadenopathy. For instance, *Nocardia* species are ubiquitous pathogens found in the environment that only cause infections in immunosuppressed hosts. The infections are acquired through the skin or by way of the respiratory tract. Direct skin contact may result in a localized pustule, which can be cultured to establish a diagnosis. *Nocardia* infections can also cause significant adenopathy, in which case biopsy and culture of the node itself establishes the diagnosis. Sulfonamides are the treatment of choice. *Actinomyces* species are oral commensal organisms in humans. However, in hosts with compromised defense barriers, local invasion results in craniofacial actinomycosis and cervical nodal involvement. The diagnosis is difficult to make, but sulfur granules may be seen on histologic examination of an involved lymph node. Human immunodeficiency virus in children is usually acquired by vertical transmission from mother to child. Adenopathy is often a prominent manifestation and is sometimes the presenting sign. The diagnosis is made by serology, and the treatment is medical.

Malignancy

Cervical lymphadenopathy can also be the result of neoplasia in children, although statistically this is much less common than an inflammatory cause. By far the most common etiology of neoplastic lymphadenopathy in the neck is lymphoma. The cervical lymph node chains may be the prominent lymph node basin harboring the systemic disease, or they may be associated with a mediastinal mass. Lymphomas generally fall into two histologic subtypes: Hodgkin's disease and non-Hodgkin's lymphoma.

Hodgkin's disease (HD) accounts for approximately 40% of childhood lymphomas. In the pediatric age group, HD generally occurs in adolescents, and is rare in children less than 10 years of age. It is characterized histologically by the pathognomonic Reed–Sternberg cells. The four classic subtypes include nodular sclerosing, mixed cellularity, lymphocyte predominant, and lymphocyte depleted. HD arises in the lymph node itself. Patients will often have constitutional ("B") symptoms such as fever, night sweats, or unintentional 10% or greater weight loss in the preceding 6 months. The nodes are generally nontender, firm, and rubbery. Solitary nodes are usually mobile, whereas aggregates of nodes may be bulky and fixed to the underlying tissue.

Non-Hodgkin's lymphoma (NHL) accounts for approximately 60% of childhood lymphomas. It most commonly occurs in children 7–11 years of age, and there is a 3:1 male to female predominance. NHL are divided into small-cell noncleaved (Burkitt's and non-Burkitt's), lymphoblastic, and large cell lymphomas (anaplastic and diffuse large B cell). Ten percent of patients with NHL have head and neck involvement. The neoplasm itself may or may not arise in nodal tissue. Often there is an aggressively enlarging mass causing local symptoms due to invasion of bone, nerves or soft tissue, and constitutional symptoms may be present.

Cervical lymphadenopathy in children may also be caused by metastatic disease. Metastasis from a thyroid carcinoma sometimes present as unilateral lymph node enlargement. When this occurs, it is important not to disregard the mass as ectopic thyroid tissue, and a search for a thyroid mass should be undertaken. Patients with stage 4 neuroblastoma sometimes present with cervical lymphadenopathy, often bilateral. In these cases, the diagnosis is made on biopsy of the enlarged lymph node.

Miscellaneous Causes of Cervical Lymphadenopathy

There are numerous other causes of cervical lymphadenopathy in children that a pediatric surgeon should be familiar with. When the more common inflammatory and neoplastic causes have been ruled out, one must consider some of these esoteric conditions. In general, a biopsy of an involved node is required to make the diagnosis of one of these diseases.

Uncommon infections can lead to lymph node enlargement. An infection due to *Francisella tularensis* causes tularemia ("rabbit fever"), a serious infectious disease that occurs in humans after contact with infected rodents. *Yersinia pestis* is the causative organism of the plague. The vector of infection is a flea, and bites in the head and neck region can cause regional adenopathy. *Pasteurella multocida*, an organism transmitted from animal bites, is another unusual cause of cervical adenopathy.

Sarcoidosis is a chronic granulomatous disease that can affect children. Pulmonary involvement is common, but peripheral lymphadenopathy also readily occurs. The involved lymph nodes are usually bilateral, firm, and rubbery. Children can have cervical lymphadenopathy from sarcoidosis, and the diagnosis is made by biopsy of one of the affected nodes. The treatment is medical.

Kawasaki disease, or mucocutaneous lymph node syndrome, is an acute vasculitis in which there is inflammation of small and medium-sized blood vessels throughout the body. The peak age is between 1 and 2 years and 80% of cases occur before the age of 4. The etiology of the condition is unknown. Inflammation may occur in cervical lymph nodes early in the course of the disease. The involved nodes are usually confined to the anterior triangle of the neck on one side. The nodes are sometimes large (>1.5 cm) and are tender and non-fluctuant. The disease and the adenopathy are self-limited.

Kikuchi–Fujimoto disease, also known as histiocytic necrotizing lymphadenitis, is a rare condition of unknown etiology. Patients present with bilateral, painful, enlarged lymph nodes in the posterior triangle of the neck. Constitutional symptoms are present, and children can develop splenomegaly as well as a skin rash. The diagnosis is confirmed by excisional biopsy of an affected lymph node. The treatment is supportive as the disease rarely causes significant morbidity and is self-limited.

Rosai–Dorfman disease, also known as sinus histiocytosis and massive lymphadenopathy, is a rare disease of unknown etiology that occurs in young children. Cervical lymphadenopathy commonly occurs as proliferating histiocytes accumulate in lymph nodes. The lymph nodes are initially mobile and discrete. However, as the condition progresses, there is massive enlargement of the cervical lymph nodes as well as other nodal regions. The disease may resolve spontaneously, however progression of the disease requires chemotherapy to control associated histiocytosis and plasmacytosis.

Castleman's disease, or giant lymph node hyperplasia, may cause a unicentric or multicentric adenopathy. The disease is caused by the hypersecretion of the cytokine IL-6. Excision of the involved node can be curative.

Periodic fever, aphthous stomatitis, pharyngitis and cervical adenitis (PFAPA) syndrome is a disease of unknown etiology that occurs in young children. Patients have cyclic recurrences of the above symptoms every 3–5 weeks, and are healthy in between episodes. Corticosteroids have been used to alleviate symptoms during flare-ups but the episodes generally abate with time.

Preoperative Preparation

The most important aspect of the work-up for cervical lymphadenopathy is a properly obtained history and a thorough physical examination. The history should elicit whether the adenopathy has occurred acutely or has become a chronic condition. It should be determined whether there has been a recent upper respiratory infection or if there has been contact with an individual with typical URI symptoms. Any recent travel and any contact with animals, especially cats, should be noted. The presence of other symptoms in the patient is also important. For example, the acute onset of pain and swelling should raise the suspicion of acute lymphadenitis. Related constitutional symptoms such as fever, night sweats, and weight loss might indicate a disseminated process such as a lymphoma. Physical examination, especially serial exams by the same practitioner, is of particular importance. Pertinent findings to note on exam include the laterality, size, number, and mobility of the lymph nodes. In addition, the presence of tenderness, overlying skin changes, erythema, induration, or fluctuance should be determined.

Laboratory studies are also an important aspect of the work-up for cervical lymphadenopathy. Basic studies like a complete blood count with differential and a peripheral smear should be obtained. Serologic studies can be obtained to confirm infections due to CMV, EBV, or HIV. Serologies can also confirm toxoplasmosis and cat scratch disease. If fluid can be obtained from an infected lymph node it should be sent for gram stain and culture (aerobic, anaerobic, fungal, acid-fast bacilli). Finally a PPD skin test should be applied.

Imaging studies should include at least a chest radiograph to evaluate for mediastinal lymphadenopathy, as this has important implications if a biopsy under anesthesia is being considered. If further imaging of the neck or lymph node itself is necessary, an ultrasound should be obtained. The ultrasound can give information about the lymph nodes such as size, number, and whether there is normal or abnormal architecture. Additionally, the relationship of the node to adjacent structures can be determined. It is sometimes difficult to determine whether the palpable mass is in fact a lymph node as opposed to either the parotid or submandibular salivary glands. In these cases, ultrasound is useful. Occasionally, a CT or MRI can give further information regarding the relationship of a palpable node to adjacent structures, but most of the time these costly studies do not add much information.

Fine needle aspiration is a procedure to consider in helping to make a diagnosis. It is most useful for obtaining fluid from an abscessed lymph node, and can be useful for making the diagnosis of a malignancy. An FNA should also be considered when a family is very reluctant for their child to have an anesthetic and undergo an operation. However, there is the distinct possibility that the FNA will be non-diagnostic. An open biopsy will then be required to obtain an adequate amount of tissue to make a diagnosis, for confirmation of a diagnosis that was suggested on FNA or for other studies that may be necessary such as flow cytometry. It is our preference, therefore, to forego an FNA and to proceed with a single operative intervention, whether it is a drainage procedure or a biopsy, when the decision to obtain tissue has been made.

Another very important aspect of the evaluation and management of cervical lymphadenopathy is a proper discussion with the parents of the child, particularly if the child's adenopathy has become chronic. The parents are usually aware of the possibility of an infection or a malignancy, and so their anxiety level is already high. A thorough discussion of significant history and physical findings and the possible diagnoses is essential. Also, a logical explanation of the rationale for either a period of observation or proceeding with immediate operative intervention is necessary. In general, it is our practice to observe small (subcentimeter), mobile, bilateral cervical lymph nodes that have been present for less than 2–3 weeks, particularly in the presence of recent URI symptoms or a documented exposure to cats. This allows time for a proper workup, including laboratory/serology studies, a chest radiograph, and PPD. When unilateral, large (>1 cm), firm, fixed or matted nodes are present, particularly in the posterior triangle of the neck or in the supraclavicular area, we favor biopsy. It is especially important to expedite a biopsy if constitutional symptoms such as fever, night sweats, and weight loss have been present. The workup, particularly the laboratory studies and chest radiograph, also should be done expeditiously.

Once it has been decided to proceed with operative intervention, the procedure planned must be explained to the parents. Options include an FNA only, a simple incision and drainage procedure, an incisional biopsy for large, fixed lesions, or an excisional biopsy. Risks of the operation must be discussed. These include bleeding, infection, injury to adjacent structures (such as the facial nerve for lymph nodes near the angle of the jaw), and the possible need for further treatment, including another procedure for recurrent infection, to obtain more tissue, or excision of a persistent fistulous tract in the case of an atypical mycobacterial infection. Further medical management, such as antibiotics for an infection or chemotherapy for a malignancy, may be necessary and should be thoroughly discussed.

Surgical Technique

There are several operative options available, and the appropriate technique depends on the clinical scenario. For a suspected abscessed lymph node, a simple incision and drainage procedure, either with a local or general anesthetic, is all that is required. Fluid is sent for gram stain and culture. Gentle curettage followed by irrigation and packing of the cavity to prevent premature skin closure is useful. When the abscess has been caused by typical bacteria, the cavity fills and the wound generally heals without the need for any further surgical therapy. However, in cases where the abscess has been caused by an atypical mycobacterial infection, the wound may persist and subsequently mature into a chronic draining fistula. In this case, antibiotics are generally ineffective and it is therefore necessary to reoperate for excision of the entire fistulous tract and any residual nodal tissue.

When biopsy is required, one must consider what is easiest and safest for making a diagnosis. For large or fixed lesions, an incisional biopsy may be the best choice. A nerve stimulator is useful especially when the node is located near important nerves such as the facial nerve. For smaller, easily accessible lesions that are not fixed to adjacent structures, an excisional biopsy is safe. In cases where a lymphoma is diagnosed, further excision is unnecessary, and systemic chemotherapy is instituted. This is also the case when cat-scratch disease is diagnosed, as the disease is usually self-limited.

A very important situation to consider is when a cervical lymph node biopsy is required in a patient with a large anterior mediastinal mass. This scenario is most often encountered in cases of lymphoblastic lymphoma and is one reason that a chest radiograph is an important part of the preoperative workup. In such cases, there is a significant possibility of life-threatening airway collapse upon induction of anesthesia. Once this occurs, there is little that can be done to re-establish the airway as the collapse is distal to the tip of a typical endotracheal tube. Therefore, in this situation, a CT scan is recommended preoperatively to evaluate the degree of either tracheal or bronchial compression. Some also suggest obtaining pulmonary function testing to evaluate peak expiratory flow rate (PEFR). It has been suggested that a decrease in either the tracheal cross-sectional area by one half or the PEFR by 50% of predicted for age places a patient at high risk for respiratory compromise during general anesthesia.

It is the responsibility of the surgeon and anesthesiologist to recognize this danger when a cervical lymph node biopsy is requested and to plan to perform the biopsy as an awake procedure under local anesthesia. Alternatively, if a pleural effusion is present, one can forego the lymph node biopsy and perform thoracentesis, whereupon analysis of the fluid will make the diagnosis.

Postoperative Care

The post-operative management is relatively straight forward. For incision and drainage procedures, the packing should be removed in 24–48 h. Local wound care with a topical antibiotic and gauze dressing along with frequent washing is all that is necessary. Otherwise, wounds that have been primarily closed generally heal without incident. Culture and biopsy results are shared with the parents and further therapy, if necessary, can be planned.

Cervical lymphadenopathy is common in children, and pediatric surgeons must be familiar with the evaluation and management of this condition. Lymphadenitis is the most common cause of lymph node enlargement in children. However, neoplasia and other uncommon disorders should also be considered. The patient's history, physical findings, laboratory tests and imaging studies are all important in helping to make the diagnosis and to formulate a plan of care. If acute viral cervical lymphadenitis is suspected, the enlarged lymph nodes should be closely observed for 2–3 weeks. If a severe bacterial infection, neoplasm or other unusual condition is suspected, or if the adenopathy has become chronic, then surgical intervention must be considered. The operative technique chosen is based on the characteristics of the lymph node enlargement, and one should avoid a general anesthetic when a large anterior mediastinal mass is associated with the adenopathy. Finally, it is essential to have a thorough discussion with the parents of the child regarding the rationale for the treatment plan that has been instituted.

Summary Points

- In general, neck masses in children can be congenital, inflammatory or neoplastic.
- Specifically, cervical lymphadenopathy is most commonly due to inflammation or infection and can be acute, sub-acute or chronic.
- Cervical lymphadenopathy due to neoplasia is most likely a lymphoma.
- Unusual causes of cervical lymphadenopathy should be considered once the more common inflammatory and neoplastic causes have been ruled out.

Editor's Comment

Few clinical issues create more anxiety for parents than an enlarged cervical lymph node. They need to know that it is not cancer and they need to know today. The experienced pediatric surgeon usually has a good feel for whether an enlarged lymph node is something to be concerned about or can be safely observed and the parents reassured. Unfortunately the only option for sampling a lymph node in a child is a surgical procedure under general anesthesia, which is generally safe and usually straightforward, but entails a certain amount of risk and an obligatory scar. This means that the surgeon should have a high index of suspicion before recommending a biopsy. Fortunately, a period of observation is almost always safe, even in the case of a malignant process, so, when in doubt, a brief delay can help one to make the best recommendation.

In children, FNA is simply not a good option for the evaluation of cervical masses: pediatric pathologists have little experience with the technique, most children will not let you come near them with a needle, and, most importantly, the most common neoplastic processes seen in children (lymphoma and leukemia) cannot be reliably differentiated from an inflammatory process by FNA. Likewise, a neoplastic process cannot be excluded on the basis of blood tests, serologies, or medical imaging. What we are left with then is the history, the physical examination, and the growth pattern of the node. A lymph node that is larger than 1.5 cm and continues to grow over time, especially if it is located in an unusual location (supraclavicular), should be excised. Likewise, the patient with constitutional symptoms (the presence or absence of which should be specifically documented at the initial visit) should undergo biopsy.

A typical busy pediatric surgeon will see at least one or two children with an enlarged lymph node every week. Most can be simply observed with no further studies, but nearly all should be encouraged to return for at least one follow-up visit in 2–3 weeks. At the other extreme is the rare patient with systemic symptoms and a worrisome node that clearly needs to be excised for biopsy. These patients should be scheduled for surgery and at minimum have a CBC with differential and a chest X-ray to rule out a mediastinal mass. The remainder will have clearly pathologic lymphadenopathy but no clear indication that a neoplastic process is necessarily involved. These patients should be scheduled for follow up in no more than 2–3 weeks and should undergo a work up: CBC w/diff.; serologies for cat scratch, toxoplasmosis, and mononucleosis, depending on what is endemic in the area; and a chest X-ray. If there are risk factors, a PPD might be prudent. In some cases in which a bacterial lymphadenitis is suspected, an empiric 7-day trial of antibiotics is reasonable, albeit controversial. A node involved with tumor almost never get smaller without treatment, so a node that shrinks can probably be observed. However, lymphoma can regress rapidly when the patient is given corticosteroids (for example for a coincidental asthma flare), in which case a biopsy becomes imperative.

Cervical lymph node biopsy is a delicate procedure not to be taken lightly. There is always the risk of nerve injury and attention should be paid to scar placement for cosmesis and comfort. A small transverse incision placed in a skin crease is preferred. Once the platysma has been breached, the remainder of the dissection should be by careful blunt dissection only. A curved hemostat should be used to gently push adjacent tissues away from the capsule of the lymph node and nothing should be cut or cauterized. With proper technique, the node will gently rise up to meet the incision and the vessels at the hilum can be ligated or cauterized with precision right at the capsule. The goal should be complete excision of the node, but this can be done in piece-meal fashion. Lymph nodes that surprise the surgeon by being excessively vascular can be assumed to represent metastatic thyroid carcinoma (or another even less common neoplasm). The incision should be closed only at the level of the platysma and the skin as deeper sutures are not necessary and increase the risk of nerve injury. Finally, the child with an enlarged lymph node that is highly suspicious for malignancy should be evaluated by a pediatric oncologist before surgery so that a proper work up can be initiated, including a bone marrow biopsy to be performed while the patient is under general anesthesia.

Differential Diagnosis

Acute cervical lymphadenitis

- Viral
- Bacterial

Subacute and chronic cervical lymphadenitis

- Atypical mycobacterial
- Typical or tuberculous mycobacterial
  - Cat scratch disease
  - Fungal
  - Parasitic
  - Opportunistic

Neoplasia as a cause of cervical lymphadenopathy

- Hodgkin's disease
- Non-Hodgkin's lymphoma
- Metastatic disease

Uncommon causes of cervical lymphadenopathy

- Unusual infections
- Sarcoidosis
  - Kawasaki's disease
  - Kikuchi–Fujimoto disease
  - Castleman's disease
  - Rosai–Dorfman disease
  - PFAPA syndrome

Diagnostic Studies

- Complete blood count with differential
- Peripheral blood smear
- Serology testing
- PPD
- Chest radiograph
- Ultrasound
- CT, MRI (rarely necessary)
- Consider FNA

Parental Preparation

- Frank discussion regarding possible etiologies.
- Discussion of treatment options:
  - Period of observation
  - Operative intervention
- Discussion of possible complications of surgical intervention:
  - Bleeding
  - Wound infection
  - Nerve injury
  - Recurrence
- Discussion of the possible need for further therapy:
  - Antibiotics for infection
  - Re-excision for recurrence or fistula
  - Chemotherapy for lymphoma

Preoperative Preparation

- ☐ Review results of laboratory and imaging studies
- ☐ Informed consent

Technical Points

- Consider using a nerve stimulator.
- Perform incision and drainage for an abscess.
- A large mass should be sampled by incisional biopsy.
- Perform excisional biopsy for smaller lymph nodes.
- Perform complete excision of nodes for suspected atypical mycobacterial infection.
- If a lymph node biopsy is being performed in a patient with a large mediastinal mass, strongly consider performing the biopsy awake under local anesthesia to avoid life-threatening airway compromise.

Suggested Reading

Dickson PV, Davidoff AM. Malignant neoplasms of the head and neck. Semin Pediatr Surg. 2006;15:92–8.

Gosche JR, Vick L. Acute, subacute, and chronic cervical lymphadenitis in children. Semin Pediatr Surg. 2006;15:99–106.

Moss RL, Skarsgard ED, Kosloske AM, Smith BM. Case studies in pediatric surgery. Philadelphia, PA: McGraw Hill; 2000: pp. 258–65.

Shamberger RC, Holzman RS, Griscom NT, Tarbell NJ, Weinstein HJ, Wohl ME. Prospective evaluation by computed tomography and pulmonary function tests of children with mediastinal masses. Surgery. 1995;118:468–71.

Tracy TF, Muratore CS. Management of common head and neck masses. Semin Pediatr Surg. 2007;16:3–13.

Part V
Esophagus

Chapter 29
Esophageal Atresia and Tracheo-Esophageal Fistula

Jean-Martin Laberge

Esophageal atresia may be suspected on prenatal sonography by the absence of a gastric bubble, polyhydramnios, and distension of the upper esophagus during swallowing attempts by the fetus. After birth, a child with EA presents with excessive salivation, mucus coming out of the mouth or nose, and noisy breathing with episodes of choking or cyanosis. These symptoms worsen if oral feedings are attempted. The diagnosis is confirmed when a 10F Replogle tube passed through the mouth or nose cannot be passed beyond about 10 cm. Smaller or more flexible catheters should be avoided because they can coil in the upper esophagus and give a false impression of esophageal patency. The tube is placed on suction to clear the excess secretions. An AP and lateral radiograph that includes the neck, chest and abdomen ("babygram") is then obtained while gentle pressure is maintained on the Replogle and 10 mL of air is injected through it. This delineates very well the location of the upper pouch in relation to the vertebral bodies. Routine contrast studies are not indicated and might lead to aspiration.

The X-ray is crucial in several ways: (1) The presence of abdominal gas will confirm a distal fistula (~85% of cases), while its absence usually indicates a pure atresia, to be confirmed at bronchoscopy. (2) The Replogle tip should project over the C7 to T2 vertebral body. An abnormally high or low blockage could indicate pharyngeal or esophageal perforation rather than atresia, especially in a premature baby or when there is blood-tinged aspirate from the Replogle. In such circumstances, a contrast study is indicated, using 1 mL or less of a non-ionic, iso-osmotic water-soluble agent. (3) Anomalies of vertebrae or ribs can be detected. (4) Cardiac malformations or a right aortic arch might be detected. (5) The pattern of abdominal gas excludes a duodenal atresia. (6) The lungs are assessed for pneumonia, which usually occurs in the upper lobes and is related to a delay in diagnosis, and, when the child is premature, for RDS.

The initial diagnosis may will sometimes have been made at another hospital before the infant is transferred to a tertiary care pediatric center. During transfer, it is important to keep the baby warm, to keep the head elevated with the Replogle on continuous suction, and to maintain good oxygenation. On physical examination, one will assess the pulmonary status and look for signs of associated malformations such as cardiac, anal, limb, and chromosomal anomalies. A scaphoid abdomen will suggest the diagnosis of a pure atresia. Thirty-five to fifty percent of infants with EA have other anomalies (Table 29.1). In about 10%, these occur in associations such as VACTERL (vertebral, anal, cardiac, tracheo-esophageal, renal, limb) or, less frequently, CHARGE (coloboma, heart defects, choanal atresia, growth retardation, genitourinary anomalies, ear abnormalities/deafness) syndrome.

Preoperative Preparation

We routinely obtain a CBC, electrolytes, glucose, BUN, creatinine, and a cross-match for blood. Preoperative echocardiogram and renal sonography are useful but can be performed post-operatively if the baby clinically demonstrates normal cardiac and renal function, although more and more the anesthesiologist will insist on obtaining the cardiac echo before surgery. Echocardiography is useful to determine the location of the aortic arch, which influences the surgical approach. Ampicillin and gentamicin are given preoperatively.

When life-threatening anomalies are suspected (Trisomy 13 or 18, anuria, complex cardiac malformation) it is wise to postpone surgery until appropriate investigations and consultations are obtained. In other cases, the operation should not be delayed since, despite a well-functioning Replogle tube, aspiration can occur from reflux of gastric secretions through the distal fistula. Even in premature babies with RDS, it is generally preferable to operate as soon as possible instead of waiting for the lungs to improve. These neonates usually get worse before they start to improve, with the risk that non-compliant lungs will result in most of the ventilation

J.-M. Laberge (✉)
Department of Pediatric General Surgery, McGill University, Montreal Children's Hospital of the McGill Health Care Centre,
Montreal, QC H3H 1P3, Canada
e-mail: jean-martin.laberge@muhc.mcgill.ca

P. Mattei (ed.), *Fundamentals of Pediatric Surgery*,
DOI 10.1007/978-1-4419-6643-8_29, © Springer Science+Business Media, LLC 2011

Table 29.1 Associated anomalies

System	Percentage (%)
Cardiovascular	20–30
VSD, ASD, tetralogy of Fallot, PDA, coarctation	
Gastrointestinal	15–25
Imperforate anus, duodenal atresia, malrotation, Meckel's diverticulum, distal esophageal stenosis	
Genito-urinary	10–20
Hydronephrosis, renal agenesis, hypospadias, undescended testis	
Musculoskeletal	10–15
Extremity malformations, vertebral anomalies, hip dysplasia	
Craniofacial/CNS	5–10
Cleft lip/palate, dysmorphism, eye anomalies, spina bifida, hydrocephalus	
Chromosomal	3–5
Trisomy 21, 18, Turner's syndrome	
Respiratory tract (excluding tracheomalacia)	3–5
Lung hypoplasia/agenesis, choanal atresia, laryngeal web, laryngotracheoesophageal cleft (LTEC)	
Miscellaneous	1
Omphalocele, CHARGE	

Note: Only the most frequently associated anomalies are listed; many others have been described

escaping through the distal TEF into the stomach. Not only might it become impossible to obtain adequate ventilation, but gastric perforation can occur. In such cases, a catheter may have to be placed at the bedside to decompress the pneumoperitoneum. Ideally, the distal TEF is controlled before one reaches that point.

Operative Technique

Appropriate intravenous access and monitoring devices are placed while hypothermia is prevented with heating lamps and a warming pad. We strongly advocate performing a rigid bronchoscopy before proceeding with the operation. We use a rigid ventilating bronchoscope with a Hopkins rod-lens telescope attached to a videocamera, monitor, and video recorder. Once the child is intubated and the anesthesiologist is ready, the surgeon places the bronchoscope to visualize the cords. The endotracheal tube is slowly removed, then the scope is advanced through the cords down to the level of the carina. The site of the distal fistula is clearly seen and a proximal fistula can be excluded. The side of the aortic arch can usually be appreciated from the pulsations transmitted through the tracheal wall. The scope is withdrawn slowly and then removed when the anesthesiologist is ready to reintubate. The whole procedure takes less than 5 min. Everyone in the room can see and the procedure is recorded for later

review, if questions arise. Some anesthesiologists prefer to put the baby to sleep gradually, allowing spontaneous ventilation, and proceed with bronchoscopy first, intubating later. Either way works well.

We consider bronchoscopy essential in all patients suspected of a pure atresia, since these are treated with an initial feeding gastrostomy, followed by a delayed primary esophageal anastomosis 2–3 months later. There are reports that 10–15% of babies with pure EA by the absence of gastrointestinal gas have a proximal TEF, which can result in recurrent aspiration and pneumonia during the 2- to 3-month waiting period. Furthermore, there have been reports of babies in whom a small distal TEF was obstructed by mucous, causing a gasless abdomen. Obviously, these patients are best treated with an immediate primary repair.

After bronchoscopy, patients with pure EA undergo a gastrostomy through a midline epigastric incision. Since the stomach has not been distended by swallowed amniotic fluid, it is smaller and thinner than normal, making this operation more of a challenge than usual. A Malecot or Pezzar catheter is more useful for the gastrostomy than a Foley catheter since the tip of the latter can perforate the back wall of the tiny stomach, especially in premature babies. Surgeons also must consider which of the lesser or greater curvature they favor should esophageal replacement become necessary, though in our experience a delayed primary esophageal anastomosis can be achieved in most cases. All babies are kept on H_2-blockers to prevent acid reflux.

In patients with EA-distal TEF, the bronchoscopy remains useful to: (1) eliminate a proximal TEF, which could be missed during repair; (2) eliminate other malformations such as a laryngeal web, subglottic stenosis or laryngotracheoesophageal cleft (LTEC); and (3) evaluate the site of the distal TEF. In the latter instance, if one sees a "trifurcation" (a TEF at the carina) and the Replogle blocks at C7, the surgeon knows that it will be a long-gap atresia and will prepare for it accordingly. In such cases, we would position and prep the baby with a free arm drape and include the neck in the sterile field. This allows mobilization of the upper pouch through a cervical incision and easier performance of circular or spiral esophageal myotomies if necessary.

The only situation where the risk of bronchoscopy may outweigh its benefits is in a premature baby with severe RDS; but even in this situation, the bronchoscope can be used to deliver surfactant directly in the mainstem bronchi, rather than having most of it go down the TEF. Such babies require a quick transpleural thoracotomy with control of the fistula. Alternatively, if the baby does not even tolerate the lateral decubitus position, we have successfully occluded the fistula by passing a 6 or 8 Fr Foley catheter through a gastrostomy. Even in this situation, some surgeons advocate placement of a Fogarty balloon catheter in the fistula under bronchoscopic control as a method of blocking the fistula.

A word of caution: anesthesia textbooks recommend intubating beyond the fistula to avoid ventilating through it. The problem is that this is impossible with a very low or trifurcation fistula, and even with the usual distal tracheal fistula, there is a risk that the tube could slip into it when positioning the patient for thoracotomy. Having done the bronchoscopy at the beginning, everyone can see the site of the fistula. During the case, the rigid bronchoscope should stay in the room in case ventilation becomes problematic. The quality of image even with small flexible bronchoscopes has also improved and makes this a useful tool to have during surgery. If a patient desaturates, does not have a pneumothorax or massive gastric distension, and the anesthesiologist is convinced the tube is going through the cords, the likelihood is that its tip is in the fistula. *Take it out* and use the rigid bronchoscope to ventilate the patient – using this maneuver, you could save the baby's life! In our hospital, we had a near-miss, in which the surgeon pulled the endotracheal tube out against the anesthesiologist's will, but in another case, the child died and autopsy demonstrated that the tube was in the distal TEF, which was larger than the distal trachea.

After bronchoscopy, the patient with the usual EA-distal TEF is placed in left lateral decubitus (right side up) with the right arm extended and a roll placed under the left chest. We use a limited posterolateral thoracotomy incision along the skin lines with the aim of entering the chest in the fourth intercostal space. The latissimus dorsi is divided, but the serratus anterior is simply reflected off the chest wall. The intercostal muscles are carefully divided to keep the pleura intact. We prefer an extrapleural dissection when possible; if a small postoperative anastomotic leak occurs (up to 10% incidence), it can seal spontaneously without the risk of empyema. The dissection is begun posteriorly with a wet peanut dissector, then extended with a wet finger or by gradually introducing a wet gauze into the extrapleural space. The areas where the pleura will most often tear during dissection are anteriorly, especially if the ribs are spread too rapidly before the dissection is completed, and posteriorly once the mediastinum is reached, in the area between the azygos vein and the distal esophagus. A small pleural tear is usually ignored, as it will seal rapidly after surgery. It should be noted that, throughout the operation, desaturations sometimes occur, requiring the anesthesiologist to re-expand the right lung from time to time.

The arch of the azygos vein is then divided between ties. The distal esophagus can usually be found just deep to this structure, and it enters the trachea just above it in most instances. Identification of the vagus nerve and observation of air distending the esophagus confirms its position. Palpation is important to confirm the position of the trachea, main stem bronchi and aorta. A silastic vessel loop is passed around the distal esophagus near its junction with the trachea after meticulous blunt dissection. Care is taken to avoid damage to the

vascular and nervous supply to the lower esophagus. With a small amount of cephalad dissection and more fingertip palpation, the junction between the fistula and trachea becomes clear. The fistula is divided stepwise and closed with interrupted 5-0 synthetic resorbable sutures. This should be done close enough to the trachea to avoid leaving a diverticulum, while not causing tracheal stenosis. The area is then checked for air leaks before proceeding with identification of the proximal pouch.

The upper pouch is easy to identify after the anesthesiologist is asked to gently push on the Replogle tube. A stay suture is then placed on the apex of the proximal pouch. With sharp and blunt dissection and gentle use of the cautery, the upper pouch is mobilized. It often seems to share a common wall with the posterior part of the trachea in its lower portion. After the first 1 or 2 cm, the dissection usually becomes easier, unless there is a proximal fistula. The upper pouch being thicker and better vascularized than the lower esophagus, it can be dissected as far as the pharynx, if necessary.

The anastomosis is usually performed under mild or moderate tension and yet heals adequately in most cases. If the two ends cannot be approximated after full mobilization of the upper pouch and constant traction maintained intraoperatively for 20–30 min, the next steps available are: careful mobilization of the distal esophagus while maintaining its blood supply and upper pouch circular or spiral myotomy (allows a gain of up to 1.5 cm).

If the two ends still do not meet after this, it is probably safer not to attempt an anastomosis, although some surgeons elect to mobilize the stomach through the hiatus or elongate the lower esophagus by creating a lesser curve gastric tube with the use of staplers (Collis-type). The classically used options are to close the lower esophagus and then tack it to the prevertebral fascia under some tension, or tack it to the upper pouch with the use of a heavy through-and-through silk suture. In the first case the child is fed by gastrostomy, allowing the lower esophagus to hypertrophy and elongate by the action of gastroesophageal reflux (GER), and perform a delayed anastomosis 8–12 weeks later. The latter option, called the "suture-fistula" technique, will often result in a spontaneous fistula that can be dilated without the need for reoperation. Other times a resection of the area and end-to-end anastomosis is required, but at least there will be no tension. This technique should probably not be employed in small premature babies since poor tissue healing may lead to fistulization to the mediastinum or pleural space with septic complications.

Another option that has gained popularity in the last decade is the Foker technique, whereby traction sutures are placed on both upper and lower pouches and brought out through the chest wall. Traction on the sutures is readjusted once or twice a day until radiographs confirm that the two ends, which have been marked with metal clips, are close to each other. Reoperation after 7–10 days then allows successful esophageal anastomosis. This technique has resulted in spectacular results in some hands, but has led to serious complications in others. It should not be used as a primary modality in premature babies. Whether it should be used at birth to replace the 3-month wait before attempting a delayed primary anastomosis in term babies with pure EA remains controversial. One advantage of the waiting period is that gastrostomy bolus feedings increase the gastric capacity. A disadvantage is the difficulty in initiating oral feedings once esophageal continuity is restored.

Let us return to the "usual" anastomosis under mild or moderate tension. If the two ends can be brought in contact with the use of DeBakey forceps, then the distal esophagus is inspected and gently dilated with a fine mosquito or Jake forceps to ensure an adequate lumen. There can be cartilage remnants in the wall of the lower esophagus close to the trachea and occasionally one has to resect a few millimeters of esophageal end. A transverse opening is then made in the upper pouch, and the distal esophagus can be spatulated if necessary. Two corner sutures of 4-0 or 5-0 synthetic resorbable sutures are placed in the full thickness of either end, so that the knots will be on the outside, but these are not tied yet. The posterior row of three or four sutures are placed with the knots inside the lumen to facilitate placement and tying. One must be careful during placement of the sutures, first because the mucosa tends to retract, and second to avoid trauma to the esophageal wall. Once the posterior row in place, gradual tension is applied on all sutures, while the proximal and distal esophagus are brought in apposition with DeBakey forceps. The posterior and corner sutures are tied, the Replogle is gently advanced through the anastomosis and into the stomach to check distal esophageal patency (and thus eliminate a congenital esophageal stenosis). The tube is then withdrawn to 1 cm above the anastomosis and marked by the anesthesiologist. In recent years we have passed at this point a 5F or 6F silastic nasogastric tube which is used for postoperative feeding. The anastomosis is completed with four or five interrupted sutures with the knots on the outside. Air is injected through the Replogle tube after the anastomosis is placed under saline in order to detect leaks. Mediastinal tissue, pleura or azygos vein are used to cover the tracheal side of the fistula. A small extrapleural chest tube is usually placed close to the anastomosis and may be tacked in the desired position with a catgut suture. This is connected to a sealed drainage system to avoid an extrapleural pneumothorax. Some surgeons prefer to avoid the chest tube in term babies with an "easy" anastomosis. The thoracotomy is closed in layers, avoiding excessively tight pericostal sutures that can lead to overlapping or fused ribs.

The patient is transferred intubated to the neonatal unit. Premature extubation with subsequent reintubation can lead to anastomotic disruption from neck hyperextension or inadvertent esophageal intubation.

Thoracoscopic repair has been done successfully since 1999. The main arguments of its proponents are the morbidity and scarring associated with thoracotomy, with the added benefit, according to some, that the anastomosis appears under less tension than with open repair. As we can expect, the complications of thoracotomy are often exaggerated. Significant scoliosis is unusual, except in cases complicated by a major leak, empyema, or requiring multiple reoperations. Early results of thoracoscopic repair suggest an equal or higher leak and stricture rate. While this approach appears safe in the hands of the pioneers who have described it, it remains a technically challenging operation. I have heard of 6- to 8-h ordeals, finally converted to open procedures, leading to significant morbidity. If you plan on doing one by thoracoscopy, you should be assisted or mentored by someone who has already done several with success.

Postoperative Care

The patient is managed by a team approach that includes surgeon, neonatologist, nurses, and respiratory therapists. In a near-term baby with an uncomplicated anastomosis, the anesthetic effects are allowed to wear off and extubation is achieved within 24 h. Fentanyl is used for postoperative pain, either by bolus or continuous drip. Some prefer to keep the child heavily sedated or even paralyzed for a few days, especially when the anastomosis has been done under a lot of tension, in which case extubation may be delayed for up to 6 or 7 days. Neck flexion has also been advocated to decrease tension on the anastomosis. We keep the tip of the Replogle tube above the anastomosis as marked intraoperatively and under continuous suction. Some remove the Replogle after a few days if there is minimal drainage, indicating passage of saliva through the anastomosis. Parenteral nutrition is started as soon as possible and enteral feedings are initiated through the silastic feeding tube.

The extrapleural chest tube is kept on underwater seal drainage and gentle (10 cm H_2O) suction added for the first 24 h. Usually only a minimal amount of serous drainage is noted. In a stable extubated baby, we obtain a contrast esophagram and UGI series under fluoroscopy 5–7 days postoperatively. After removing the Replogle, we usually start this study with a non-ionic isoosmolar water-soluble agent, then switch to dilute barium if there is no aspiration or anastomotic leak. We observe the swallowing reflex, esophageal motility, anastomotic site and distal esophagus. Then, if the baby is tolerating the procedure well, we fill the stomach enough to look for GER and assess gastric emptying and the position of the ligament of Treitz. It is normal for the esophageal anastomosis to appear narrowed and for the upper esophagus to appear dilated, but there should be no stasis.

As long as there is no leak and good swallowing, feedings are initiated after this study and will help to gradually dilate the anastomosis and lower esophagus. The chest tube is removed the next day and antibiotics are stopped if this is not already done. Oral feedings often progress slowly because of poor sucking or swallowing reflexes. The silastic nasogastric tube is used to complete each feeding, after the child has been offered the bottle.

The infant may be discharged when feeding well and gaining weight, occasionally with the feeding tube still in place to ensure adequate intake. Parents are warned about the signs of complications such as reflux, tracheomalacia, anastomotic stricture, and recurrent fistula. We discharge all babies on H_2-blockers until a pH probe is done at 6 months of age. Patients are followed up frequently in the first year of life, and then once or twice a year at least until school age and preferably until adulthood. It is very important to explain to the parents that there will be some permanent scarring at the anastomosis, which prevents normal distensibility of the esophagus at this site. We therefore recommend pureed food up to 12–18 months, and then only minced food until 5 years of age when the child has learned to chew well before swallowing, and has adequate teeth to do so. All those caring for such children have seen patients admitted with an impacted foreign body at the anastomotic site despite a normal appearance of the anastomosis on contrast studies. This might be food, often a piece of meat or popcorn, or a foreign body.

Complications

Although most term babies do very well after esophageal atresia repair, some even going home by 1 week of age, the potential complications are numerous. These can be related to associated problems such as prematurity and cardiac defects, to the malformation itself, or to its treatment. Our discussion will focus on the latter. These may be divided roughly into early (<30 days), intermediate (1–3 months) and late complications (Table 29.2).

Anastomotic leaks occur in 5–10% and can be suspected by the presence of frothy saliva in the chest tube drainage. Small extrapleural leaks that are well drained by the tube are treated with continued upper pouch suctioning and antibiotics and usually seal spontaneously. Some surgeons even start feedings despite a leak, but we prefer to wait until radiological resolution. Beware of anastomotic stenoses, which often develop within a few weeks after a leak. A complete hemithorax "white-out" or a massive pneumothorax is usually caused by a major leak or a total anastomotic disruption. Breakdown of the tracheal suture line should also be considered. The child can rapidly deteriorate and necessitate more chest tubes and emergency thoracotomy. If the baby is not

Table 29.2 Complications of esophageal atresia repair

Type	Timing	Rough incidence of significant/ symptomatic complication
Anastomotic leak (+/– pneumothorax, empyema)	Early	5%
Anastomotic dehiscence	Early	1%
Recurrent fistula	Early	3–5%
Anastomotic stenosis	Early/intermediate	20–30%
Swallowing incoordination, aspiration, poor suck	Early/intermediate	5% + higher in prematures
Tracheomalacia	Early – intermediate	5–10%
Gastroesophageal reflux (GER)	Intermediate/late	10–30% require surgery≥50% medical treatment
Recurrent pneumonia/ bronchitis/asthma	Intermediate/late	10–30%
Failure to thrive	Intermediate/late	10–20%
Scoliosis and chest wall deformities	Late	<5%

acutely sick, we would perform a contrast study; extravasation of most of the contrast agent indicates the need for thoracotomy, while a smaller leak can be treated non-operatively. When thoracotomy is required, it is sometimes possible to simply repair the dehiscence if the tissues appear healthy and the repair can be performed under minimal tension. Otherwise, it is wiser to ligate the distal end, create a cervical esophagostomy and a gastrostomy, with repair delayed for some months. However, as the trend has been to avoid cervical esophagostomy in recent years, some would elect to close the upper pouch and leave it decompressed with a Replogle tube, returning later for a delayed reanastomosis.

Patients who develop recurrent coughing, choking, apneic episodes, pneumonia and vomiting or regurgitation, present a diagnostic challenge. These are symptoms common to several of the complications. Choking during feedings may indicate a recurrent or missed fistula, tracheomalacia, esophageal stenosis, or swallowing incoordination with aspiration. Choking after feedings, with or without vomiting, is usually a manifestation of GER. The contrast esophagram with videofluoroscopy is the first and most important investigation. It is crucial for the surgeon and radiologist to cooperate on this study in order to evaluate swallowing coordination and esophageal motility. The patient is bottle-fed initially to study the full progression of the contrast medium.

Tracheal narrowing may occur at the tracheal suture line or with tracheomalacia, most often at the level of the upper pouch. This can often be diagnosed on the lateral views during video fluoroscopy. The tracheal diameter is evaluated during inspiration and expiration and with a bolus of swallowed contrast material. With severe tracheomalacia, the tracheal lumen may appear completely obliterated between the aortic arch and the distended esophagus, especially during expiration or crying.

A *distal congenital stenosis* might be difficult to differentiate from an acquired one due to reflux. If seen early and not responding to balloon dilations, it is more likely to be congenital and is very likely to require resection. However, this associated anomaly is more often diagnosed after a few months, when the child starts taking solids.

In order to evaluate the presence of GER, the rate of gastric emptying and the position of the ligament of Treitz, more contrast may be required. If the baby is unable to swallow enough contrast material, the existing nasogastric feeding tube is used, or one can be inserted gently under fluoroscopic control.

A *recurrent TEF* can be difficult to demonstrate. This study is best done with the patient in the prone position, injecting the contrast through a feeding tube under pressure as it is gradually withdrawn from the lower esophagus.

Depending on the results of radiological investigations, the precise symptoms and their severity, further tests may be required. Bronchoscopy is the best procedure to evaluate fistula recurrence and the presence of a tracheal diverticulum at the fistula site. The bronchoscopy can be done simply as a diagnostic procedure or as part of the definitive operation if the problem has been identified by the contrast study.

When *tracheomalacia* is severe and is associated with "dying spells" (apnea and cyanosis during feeding or following a crying spell), aortopexy is indicated. Bronchoscopy is useful before, during and after this procedure to assess the tracheal lumen. To confirm tracheomalacia, the tracheoscopy is done with the patient breathing spontaneously under light general anesthesia, since the collapsed lumen is most obvious during expiration. Rare patients with diffuse tracheobronchomalacia may require more than a simple aortopexy. The incidence of severe tracheomalacia requiring aortopexy varies from 2.5 to more than 10% in some series. This wide variation is explained in part by the fact that some patients in the past died without a diagnosis, or were treated by prolonged intubation or tracheostomy awaiting spontaneous improvement. Surgeons are now more aggressive in doing an aortopexy, which has proven to be safe and effective. It is interesting to note that tracheomalacia is unusual in cases of pure esophageal atresia, but there is no clear explanation to this observation. Another important point is that tracheomalacia may manifest itself early by the inability to extubate and CO_2 retention as the child starts to breathe spontaneously, or it may become symptomatic much later, even a few weeks after discharge with the typical dying spell described above.

Fistula recurrence is a serious complication that can lead to death, therefore aggressive investigation with fluoroscopy and bronchoscopy are essential. The identification and the surgical repair of a recurrent fistula can be facilitated by the insertion of a ureteral catheter at bronchoscopy. The classic approach is a repeat right thoracotomy, transpleural division of the fistula, and interposition of healthy tissue such as an intercostal pedicle or a pericardial flap. Some surgeons have approached this problem through a left thoracotomy or by means of a transtracheal repair. Less invasive ways to obliterate the fistula by bronchoscopy with laser, electrocoagulation or synthetic glue and sclerosing agents were initially associated with a higher recurrence rate. However, the use of fibrin glue has gained in popularity and may be an acceptable first line of treatment in a stable patient, but one must be careful not to use excessive pressure when applying the glue since an excess amount could spill over into the trachea with disastrous consequences.

GER might present with vomiting, recurrent pneumonia and asthma, failure-to-thrive, or stenosis of the lower esophagus or at the site of anastomosis. Since nearly all EA patients have some degree of GER, we make a liberal use of drugs to inhibit acid production. In patients presenting with symptoms while on H_2-blockers, we optimize the dose, use proton pump inhibitors, and use motility agents in some patients. Evaluation should include an extended pH probe study, preferably done with the tip in the mid-esophagus to pick up only the more significant refluxes.

Fundoplication is required in 10–25% of patients after esophageal atresia repair. The indications are life-threatening symptoms, recurrent esophageal stenosis refractory to dilations, and failure of medical treatment. Fundoplication is more complicated in these patients. The esophagus is often short, the gastroesophageal junction having been pulled up into the chest at the time of esophageal repair. Because of abnormal esophageal peristalsis, the wrap has more risk of causing a mechanical obstruction. Despite these complicating factors, and the fact that the long-term failure rate has been high in some series, the increased use of fundoplication combined with better techniques for esophageal anastomosis (single layer, end-to-end) has led to a marked reduction in the need for secondary esophageal surgery.

Symptomatic *anastomotic stenosis* often results from a leak. It can also be related to reflux or to an anastomosis constructed under tension. Most stenoses can be treated with balloon dilations, which is now the method preferred by most pediatric surgeons, gastroenterologists, and radiologists. It is thought to be safer than bougienage. It can performed under fluoroscopy in the radiology suite, without general anesthesia, or in the operating room, under endoscopic and fluoroscopic control. After one or two dilatations, the addition of triamcinolone injected into the stricture or mitomycin C applied topically might reduce subsequent stricture formation, increasing the success rate and decreasing the number of dilatations required. Failure to respond to repeated dilations over a period of several weeks or months despite appropriate treatment of an associated reflux indicates the need for excision of the area. With proven GER, we would usually perform a fundoplication first, then resect the anastomotic stricture if it keeps recurring after a few more dilatations.

Often several complications coexist and the treatment sequence is based upon a judgment of which is most life-threatening to the baby. Most infants after esophageal atresia repair have abnormal esophageal peristalsis, some degree of GER and tracheomalacia. When life-threatening symptoms are present, a careful history and appropriate investigation will help decide what should be addressed first. Faced with a child with severe hypoxic spells associated with feeding or crying and radiographic evidence of both GER and tracheomalacia, we would perform a bronchoscopy to exclude a recurrent or missed fistula and be prepared to perform an aortopexy during the same anesthesia if severe tracheomalacia was confirmed (apposition of the posterior and anterior tracheal walls during expiration).

Patients who are discharged from the hospital after successful restoration of esophageal continuity should not be considered cured. There is a general impression that feeding and respiratory problems completely disappear after a few years. Although it is true that most patients tend not to complain and are reluctant to return for yearly follow-ups, one must be aware of the potential problems. Late mortality can occur from associated anomalies and from complications of the disease or its treatment. In infants with a smooth initial course, unexpected death has resulted from tracheomalacia or food impaction in the esophagus. A surprisingly high incidence (>1%) of sudden infant death syndrome is noted in several large series, which gives some support to the theory of an immaturity of vagal reflexes in these patients. Tracheomalacia and GER may also contribute to these deaths.

Late morbidity can be related to the esophageal anastomosis, to abnormal esophageal motility, to GER and to respiratory problems. GER is probably the most troublesome since it can result in anastomotic or lower esophageal strictures and may be accompanied by Barrett's esophagus. Esophageal carcinoma has now been reported in six patients, 20–46 years after esophageal atresia repair. Because most children grow up with symptoms from an abnormally-functioning esophagus, they tend not to realize that they have a problem. It was formerly thought that reflux improved with time, but several studies have now shown that GER and esophagitis persist in a significant number of older children and adults, even when they are asymptomatic. Closer follow-up and more aggressive treatment of GER are therefore required. Since reflux and esophagitis do not necessarily correlate with symptoms, surveillance esophagoscopy every 3–5 years has been recommended. The development of Barrett's esophagus calls for an antireflux procedure. Reflux has also been linked to respiratory problems such as recurrent pneumonia, bronchitis and asthma.

The anastomotic scar and abnormal esophageal motility contribute to long-term dysphagia in about half the patients, although most do not complain about it. This often leads to swallowing difficulties and to food impaction requiring esophagoscopy for its removal. Patients are counseled to eat slowly, take small bites and drink a lot while eating.

Respiratory problems in the first year might be related to recurrent fistula, GER, tracheomalacia or associated anomalies such as LTEC. Any of these may lead to serious morbidity and even mortality if not promptly recognized and treated. Later in life, the respiratory symptoms tend to improve. In contrast to classical teachings, however, one study found that 40% of adults still had the typical barking cough of tracheomalacia and 24% had intermittent respiratory problems such as asthma, pneumonia and bronchitis. This finding was more common in patients who had these problems in early childhood. A daily cough was associated with symptoms of reflux and dysphagia.

Long-term growth and development have been considered within the normal range in most reviews, but in a large series of patients operated at Great Ormond Street between 1980 and 1984, one-third of patients were below the third percentile for their age when assessed at 6 months to 5 years of age, including 21% of patients in the good risk category.

Scoliosis may be secondary to vertebral or rib anomalies, anastomotic leak with pleural scarring, or an unnecessary long thoracotomy with rib excision. One must follow all the patients and actively look for any deformity.

Overall, most adults who survive esophageal atresia repair seem to enjoy a normal life and do not perceive their symptoms as significant. Several large series confirm the gradual improvement in survival in the last half century, despite the fact that smaller newborns with a higher frequency of associated anomalies are being treated. All authors agree that associated anomalies are the most significant factor affecting the prognosis, but a small number of infants who "should" survive continue to die of complications even in experienced centers. Waterston's classification has lost all its usefulness in the past two decades. The classification we have proposed (Table 29.3) highlights the fact that children with life-threatening anomalies and those with major anomalies combined with preoperative ventilator dependence, for example extreme prematures with severe hyaline membrane disease, are in a high-risk category, with an expected mortality of 40% or more, depending on the anomalies. The remainder have a good prognosis, with an expected survival of well over 90%. Other recent classifications put the emphasis on cardiac anomalies as making patients high-risk.

Table 29.3 Prognostic classification for esophageal atresia

Class I (low risk)	All patients who do not satisfy Class II criteria
Class II (high risk)	Life-threatening associated anomalies (e.g., Bilateral renal agenesis, Trisomy 13, hypoplastic left ventricle)
	Major associated anomalies with preoperative ventilator dependence

Source: Modified from Poenaru D, Laberge J-M, Neilson IR, et al. A new prognostic classification for esophageal atresia. Surgery. 1993;113:426–32, with permission from Elsevier

Tracheoesophageal Fistula (Isolated, H-Type)

Choking and coughing in association with feedings and repeated pneumonia (especially right upper lobe) suggest the possibility of an isolated congenital TEF. In some cases, asthma or impressive chronic abdominal distention are the predominant signs of the disorder. Excessive mucous or hypersalivation might also be noted. In most cases, the symptoms start from birth, but the diagnosis is often delayed because of failure to investigate the problem, or falsely negative initial studies. The presence of other anomalies, such as laryngeal or tracheal atresia or stenosis may obscure the diagnosis. In distinction to the findings in babies with esophageal atresia, a history of polyhydramnios is rare, and low birth weight is less common. Associated malformations may occur, but they are generally not as frequent and as severe as those associated with EA.

The next step in establishing diagnosis should be a contrast esophagram with video fluoroscopy. Ideally this is done in the prone or lateral decubitus position, injecting thin barium or non-ionic water soluble contrast material under pressure through a feeding tube, starting in the lower esophagus. The catheter is gradually withdrawn and boluses of contrast are injected at various levels. This eliminates confusion with aspirated contrast from swallowing incoordination or a LTEC. This technique, by distending the esophagus, also facilitates opacification of the fistula since the tracheal opening is usually proximal to the esophageal opening.

In patients with persistent symptoms and a negative esophagram done in ideal conditions, rigid bronchoscopy should be done. Special attention is paid to the posterior larynx to avoid missing a LTEC. This is followed by a thorough examination of the entire posterior tracheal wall to identify one or multiple TEF. Sometimes a small catheter is necessary to "probe" the posterior wall of the trachea, although in most instances a small dimple indicating the fistula site will easily be seen. Even with a positive contrast study, bronchoscopy is an essential part of the operation. With the telescope just above the fistula and the operating room lights dimmed, one can visualize the bronchoscope light through the skin in the lower neck, confirming that the TEF can be approached through a cervical incision (80–90% of cases). The fistula is then cannulated with a small Fogarty catheter, a ureteral catheter or a soft guidewire passed through the instrument channel. This step is essential to facilitate intra-operative identification of the fistula and minimize dissection, thereby decreasing the risk of recurrent laryngeal nerve damage. I prefer to pass a 4 Fr Fogarty, then inflate the balloon and pull it back. Esophagoscopy may be used to confirm that the balloon is up against the fistula. The ventilating bronchoscope is removed and the patient intubated by the anesthesiologist. Since the Fogarty is passed through the instrument channel of the scope, the latter has to remain on the operating table next to the patient's head. When using a ureteral catheter or guidewire, it is best to then retrieve the distal end through an esophagoscope and bring it out through the mouth. During the surgery, the surgeon can ask the anesthesiologist to pull on the looped catheter or guidewire to facilitate identification of the fistula, as simple palpation may not readily identify the catheter or guidewire.

With the head kept in hyperextension, it is now turned to the left and the right neck is prepped and draped. Even with a fistula at the thoracic inlet, it is easier to pull it cephalad with the help of the Fogarty than to work at the apex of the pleural cavity from a thoracic approach. Through a lower transverse incision along a skin fold, the sternomastoid and the carotid sheath are retracted laterally. Below the right lobe of the thyroid, the tracheoesophageal groove is exposed by blunt dissection. Palpation of the Fogarty catheter and balloon is facilitated when gentle traction is applied by the anesthesiologist. The right recurrent laryngeal nerve is identified and preserved, avoiding traction to it. The fistula is carefully dissected and encircled with a silastic vessel loop; it is always much thicker than is suggested by the contrast study. I prefer to put 5-0 absorbable stay sutures on the tracheal side on the cephalad and caudal ends of the TEF, then divide it close to the trachea as would be done in EA-TEF. Interrupted sutures are used to complete the tracheal closure, followed by esophageal closure. Ideally the tracheal suture line is then covered with healthy tissue such as the omohyoid muscle to prevent recurrence. I usually leave a 5 mm silastic drain connected to a low-pressure closed suction bulb, then close the wound in layers.

When a thoracic approach is required, a right transpleural exposure through the fourth interspace usually gives the best exposure, although thoracoscopic repair is gaining popularity. Again, the presence of the Fogarty in invaluable. Attempts at closing a congenital TEF non-operatively is less successful than with a recurrent TEF after EA-TEF repair since the former is lined with mucosa.

Immediate extubation is usually possible. The patient is maintained on parenteral nutrition until a contrast esophagram is obtained 3–5 days postoperatively. Others may choose to feed sooner and not perform a contrast study. Contrary to babies with EA, feeding difficulties are uncommon.

Intraoperative and early postoperative complications are quite common. They include accidental extubation, tracheal perforation, bradycardia and cardiac arrest, laryngeal edema, unilateral and even bilateral recurrent laryngeal nerve damage with vocal cord palsy, missed or recurrent fistula, mediastinitis, pneumothorax, and even phrenic palsy. Many of these complications can be avoided or minimized by identification and catheterization of the fistula preoperatively. Most of the reported complications were due to operations on patients who had only a clinical diagnosis, or those in whom the fistula was not catheterized. I would not perform a cervical exploration for presumed TEF if I cannot visualize the fistula by bronchoscopy. Minimal dissection with preservation of the recurrent nerves, precise suturing of the trachea and esophagus, and verification of vocal cord movement at the end of the operation are important. Postoperative intubation may be required for vocal cord palsy or airway edema; in the latter situation, racemic epinephrine and steroids may be useful.

Late complications are uncommon, but a recurrent fistula may become apparent after several months. GER and abnormal esophageal peristalsis are uncommon.

The diagnosis and treatment of isolated tracheoesophageal fistula has improved over the years, and the prognosis is excellent. The excellent results obtained with TEF approached through a cervical incision do not warrant attempts at endoscopic occlusion.

Finally, I would like to make a plea for all pediatric surgeons and those in training to stop referring to patients with esophageal atresia as "TEF" patient. It is the EA that gives the magnitude of the challenge, not the TEF. A pure TEF is a piece of cake! So let's say esophageal atresia when there is one present, not TEF.

Summary Points

- Diagnosis usually straightforward, may be suspected prenatally
- Associated anomalies and prematurity common and may affect prognosis
- Rigid bronchoscopy useful to eliminate a proximal fistula and verify location of distal fistula
- For the usual EATEF, repair usually done under some tension; if unable to approximate despite usual maneuvers, Foker technique may be considered but classic method is to close distal esophagus and tack it to prevertebral fascia, feed by gastrostomy and return later (definitely safest method in premature babies or those with major associated anomalies)
- Postoperative complications common
- Most leaks can be treated conservatively and seal spontaneously
- Strictures common, treated with balloon dilatation
- All patients should be treated medically for GER initially
- Be aware of symptoms of severe tracheomalacia ("dying spells")
- Despite these complications and the fact that all patients have esophageal dysmotility to varying degrees, long-term outcome is excellent in most.
- Final word: an esophageal atresia is not a "TEF"

Editor's Comments

Esophageal atresia with tracheoesophageal fistula is often considered the quintessential pediatric general surgical operation. It is usually straightforward, elegant, and gratifying, but only if the two ends come together easily. When they do not, it can be one of the most challenging and disheartening experiences for young and seasoned pediatric surgeons alike. The key in these situations is to always have a back-up plan and to avoid irrevocable errors: (1) excessive mobilization of the distal esophagus, which can compromise the blood supply; (2) multiple attempts to approximate the ends under tension, which results in loss of length when the sutures tear through, and (3) creation of a cervical esophagostomy, which often commits the patient to esophageal replacement and is associated with multiple complications.

I consider repair of the typical patient with EA to be a semi-elective operation, unless a patient with a distal fistula is intubated and mechanically ventilated, in which case I consider it an emergency. This is because regardless of the position of the tip of the endotracheal tube, positive pressure inevitably results in massive abdominal distension and ventilatory compromise. The thoracoscopic approach holds some promise of a better way and it is important that there are pioneers who are advancing the field, but, given the initial results, it is hard not to conclude that the leak and stricture rates are high, perhaps suggesting that the technique needs to be significantly more refined before it can become the standard approach.

For most patients, a small, posterolateral, muscle-sparing thoracotomy and extrapleural approach to the esophagus are preferable. Occasionally, one encounters a variation of the major vascular anatomy, such as double aortic arch or aberrant subclavian artery. Generally, it is possible to work around these structures but it is important to be vigilant regarding the vagus nerves and thoracic duct, whose course in the chest might be altered, exposing them to injury. When a right aortic arch is encountered, it is occasionally best to close the chest and reposition the patient for a thoracotomy on the opposite side. When approximating the two ends of the esophagus while the back-row sutures are being tied, ring forceps work well and are less traumatic than DeBakey forceps. The choice of suture material for the repair is individual, but using absorbable suture is probably better than using nonabsorbable suture, which has been known to cause foreign body reaction, granulation tissue, and, in rare cases, fistulas. The trachea can be oversewn with absorbable or nonabsorbable suture but it should probably always be a monofilament suture.

All patients with EA have reflux, but only those with failure to thrive, recurrent stricture, or complications will need a fundoplication. I still think a partial wrap, preferably done laparoscopically, better prevents dysphagia, but some surgeons insist that a loose Nissen works just as well. In patients who are difficult to extubate or who have other signs of severe tracheomalacia, one should have a low threshold for performing an aortopexy. It is a safe operation with excellent results and can be performed thoracoscopically. Finally, balloon dilatation under fluoroscopic guidance is clearly the best way to manage anastomotic strictures at any age. It is safer, more effective, and lasts longer than traditional bougienage.

Differential Diagnosis

Prenatally

- Absent/small stomach seen with neuromuscular disorders with inadequate swallowing

After birth

- Esophageal atresia with/without fistula, possibility of proximal fistula
- Esophageal perforation (especially prematures)

H-type

- LTEC, GE reflux

Diagnostic Studies

- Attempt to pass a 10 Fr Replogle (8 Fr Replogle may be adequate in premature babies)
- AP plain "babygram" with 10 mL of air injected in the Replogle
- Contrast only if Replogle blocks at unusual level or blood-tinged aspirate, especially if premature
- Bronchoscopy before positioning for thoracotomy/ thoracoscopy
- H-type: contrast injected by feeding tube in esophagus under fluoroscopy in prone or lateral decubitus; rigid bronchoscopy

Preoperative Preparation

- ☐ Replogle to suction
- ☐ Cross-match
- ☐ Prophylactic antibiotics
- ☐ Rigid bronchoscopy preop +/− flexible intraop

Parental Preparation

- Major surgery, multiple possible complications, but likelihood of a good long-term outcome in term babies without major associated anomalies.
- Pamphlet explaining frequent complications and giving addresses of useful web sites

Technical Points

- Limited posterolateral thoracotomy
  - Use flexible bronchoscopy intraop PRN if unexplained desaturations
  - Use continuous traction on esophageal ends intraop PRN if tension excessive
  - Pure EA: scope to R/O proximal fistula, gastrostomy and wait
- H-type fistula:
  - Bronchoscopy to identify location of fistula and catheterize it.
  - Cervical approach in most cases.

Suggested Reading

Bagolan P, Iacobelli B, De Angelis P. Long gap esophageal atresia and esophageal replacement: moving toward a separation? J Pediatr Surg. 2004;39:1084–90.

Benjamin B, Phan T. Diagnosis of H-type tracheoesophageal fistula. J Pediatr Surg. 1991;26:667–71.

Foker JE, Kendall Krosch TC, Catton K, et al. Long-gap esophageal atresia treated by growth induction: the biological potential and early follow-up results. Semin Pediatr Surg. 2009;18:23–9.

Healy PJ, Sawin RS, Hall DG, et al. Delayed primary repair of esophageal atresia with tracheoesophageal fistula: is it worth the wait? Arch Surg. 1998;133:552–6.

Laberge J-M, Guttman FM. Esophageal atresia and tracheoesophageal fistulas. In: Donnellan WL, editor. Abdominal surgery of infancy and childhood, vol. I. Luxembourg: Harwood Academic Publishers; 1996. p. 11/1–11/34.

Myers NA, Beasley SW, Auldist AW, et al. Oesophageal atresia without fistula – anastomosis or replacement? Pediatr Surg Int. 1987;2:216–22.

Myers NA, Beasley SW, Auldist AW. Oesophageal atresia and associated anomalies: a plea for uniform documentation. Pediatr Surg Int. 1992;7:97–100.

Ogita S, Tokiwa K, Takahaski T. Transabdominal closure of tracheoesophageal fistula: a new procedure for the management of poor-risk esophageal fistula. J Pediatr Surg. 1986;21:812–4.

Rintala RJ, Sistonen S, Pakarinen MP. Outcome of esophageal atresia beyond childhood. Semin Pediatr Surg. 2009;18:50–6.

Schullinger JN, Vinocur C, Santulli TV. The suture fistula technique in the repair of selected cases of esophageal atresia. J Pediatr Surg. 1982;17:234–6.

Spitz L, Kiely E, Brereton RJ. Esophageal atresia: five year experience with 148 cases. J Pediatr Surg. 1987;22:103–8.

Chapter 30
Long-Gap Esophageal Atresia

Pietro Bagolan and Francesco Morini

To anastomose the ends of an infant's esophagus, the surgeon must be as delicate and precise as a skilled watchmaker. No other operation offers a greater opportunity for pure technical artistry

Willis Potts, 1950

Esophageal atresia is a rare congenital anomaly that occurs in 1 in 4,500 live births. The expected outcome is close to 100% survival, though this varies depending on birth weight, degree of prematurity, and associated anomalies (especially cardiac). Ideal surgical management consists of a primary end-to-end anastomosis between the upper and the lower esophageal remnants and division of a tracheo-esophageal fistula, if one is present. The vast majority can be corrected without difficulty soon after birth. However, this goal is not always easily achievable with all anatomical variants and the management of long-gap esophageal atresia remains a major challenge to the pediatric surgeon. In addition, there is controversy regarding the definition of a "long gap" and a general lack of consensus regarding which is the best technique. This is perhaps due to the fact that attempts to bridge the gap to allow a delayed anastomosis have led to the introduction of several interesting techniques, none of which are perfect.

Definition

Patients with long-gap esophageal atresia are mainly represented by those with pure esophageal atresia (type A) or proximal tracheo-esophageal fistula (type B). Even patients with esophageal atresia and a distal tracheo-esophageal fistula (type C or D) can have a wide gap between esophageal ends. In fact, more than 40% of babies operated on for long-gap esophageal atresia, defined by the inability to perform a primary anastomosis between the two esophageal ends, have esophageal atresia with a distal fistula. In addition, a number of patients managed with primary anastomosis develop a "secondary" long gap as a result of complications of the primary procedure, often followed by cervical esophagostomy, closure of the distal stump, and gastrostomy, or development of refractory gastro-esophageal reflux and persistent long stricture.

The definition is somewhat subjective, and what is amenable to primary anastomosis for one surgeon might be considered impossible for another. Thus "long-gap" could be (and often is!) defined as any gap one cannot bridge. This is why these neonates should be referred to experienced, tertiary-care neonatal/pediatric surgical units. There are more objective ways to define the gap, measured both in centimeters and in vertebral bodies. The most commonly used cut-off value is 3 cm or three vertebral spaces, based on the fact that there is a higher complication rate associated with anything over this distance. Since the measurement is done in patients with a wide range of body weight (from below 1.5 kg to more than 3 kg) and because an absolute measure does not take into account the patient's size, the distance between the stumps is best expressed in terms of vertebral bodies.

Diagnosis

Esophageal atresia is sometimes diagnosed antenatally by experienced ultrasonographers. Prenatal ultrasound might detect the upper blind esophageal pouch or in type A and B esophageal atresia the inability to visualize the stomach, which is not being filled with amniotic fluid. This finding suggests a long-gap esophageal atresia, but false positives still occur in 15–50% of cases. Postnatally, the combination of failure to advance a gastric tube beyond 10 cm from the nose or mouth and a gasless abdomen on plain radiograph confirms esophageal atresia without distal fistula. Though many surgeons believe that the absence of a distal fistula automatically means there is a long gap, thus precluding primary repair, it is important to remember that this is not always the case. The true gap should be formally assessed before any decisions are made or irreversible procedures performed.

P. Bagolan (✉)
Department of Medical and Surgical Neonatalology, Bambino GESU Children's Hospital, Piazza S. Onofrio, 4, Roma 00165, Italia
e-mail: bagolan@opbg.net

P. Mattei (ed.), *Fundamentals of Pediatric Surgery*,
DOI 10.1007/978-1-4419-6643-8_30, © Springer Science+Business Media, LLC 2011

Once the diagnosis is made, the upper pouch should be continuously aspirated with a Replogle or similar large-bore tube. A chest X-ray is taken with a feeding tube deeply inserted into the esophagus to confirm the diagnosis of esophageal atresia and to define as exactly as possible the level of the upper pouch. An echocardiogram is performed to look for associated cardiac anomalies and, more importantly from a surgical point of view, to define the side of the aortic arch, which determines the side of thoracotomy. Broad-spectrum antibiotics and parenteral nutrition should also be initiated.

Operative Approach

Tracheoscopy

In all patients with esophageal atresia, including those with a likely long gap, the first operative step is a tracheoscopy. This procedure allows one to define the presence of an upper pouch fistula (3–4% of patients) and the level of the distal tracheo-esophageal fistula, when present. A distal tracheo-esophageal fistula at the level of the carina can be a sign of a wide gap. Moreover, tracheoscopy enables one to gather information about vocal cord motility and to exclude associated and more complex laryngo-tracheo-esophageal anomalies, such as laryngotracheal or tracheo-bronchial cleft, which would modify the approach. In our personal experience with 145 consecutive patients with esophageal atresia, regardless of the length of the gap, three patients with a gasless abdomen had a proximal fistula that would have been missed without tracheoscopy, and one had a laryngo-tracheo-esophageal cleft. Finally, tracheoscopy performed together with fluoroscopy enables one to better define the gap length even in cases with a distal fistula (type C and D), by measuring the number of vertebral bodies between the radiopaque tube in the upper pouch and the tip of the broncoscope placed at the level of the opening of the distal fistula (Fig. 30.1).

The tracheoscopy is performed with a 3.5 flexible endoscope. In the case of a proximal fistula, a guide wire passed through the fistula into the esophagus and pulled out through the mouth makes it easier to identify, minimizes necessary dissection, and allows proximal traction at the neck during

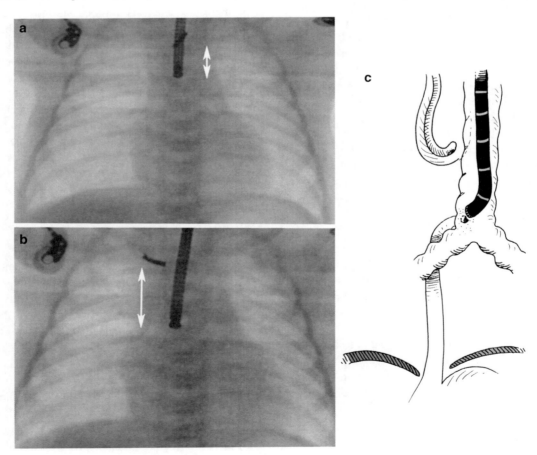

Fig. 30.1 Radioscopic measurement of the gap (*double arrows*) in type C esophageal atresia. (**a**) 1.5 vertebral bodies. (**b**) >3 vertebral bodies. (**c**) Diagram showing the tube in the upper esophagus and the endoscope at the level of the tracheo-esophageal fistula ((**c**) courtesy of Dr. Fabio Ferro, MD)

the operation. This also allows one to define the level of the fistula by fluoroscopy, indicating the best route to close it, cervical (usually) or thoracic (20%) (Fig. 30.2). Moreover, when a wide carinal fistula is found, it can be cannulated and occluded by a 3.5 Fr Fogarty catheter (the balloon is inflated with 0.2 mL of saline solution), through the rigid ventilating bronchoscope (Fig. 30.3). This is done to make mechanical ventilation easier and to avoid intra-operative gastric overd-istension and gastroesophageal reflux.

Gastrostomy with or without Cervical Esophagostomy

The classic surgical approach to infants with long-gap esophageal atresia was to perform a cervical esophagostomy and gastrostomy. We suggest to always avoid early esophago-stomy since with this procedure strongly commits the patient to esophageal replacement, effectively burning a bridge.

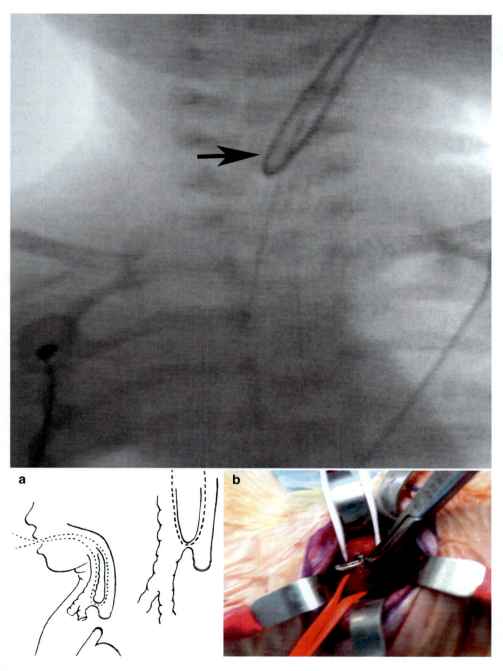

Fig. 30.2 Chest X-rays of an infant with a proximal tracheo-esophageal fistula and a radiopaque guide wire passed through it (*arrow*). *Inset A*: Diagram showing the guide wire passing through the fistula and in and out from the mouth. *Inset B*: The fistula is microdissected and the guide wire is visible

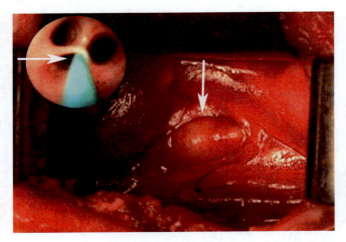

Fig. 30.3 Intra-operative picture of a Fogarty balloon catheter placed through the distal fistula in the lower esophagus. *Arrow*: The balloon inflated in the lower esophagus. *Inset*: Endoscopic view of the catheter (*arrow*) in the distal tracheo-esophageal fistula

Esophagostomy should be limited to cases with postoperative complications and after all attempts at preserving native esophagus have failed. It should be electively used only as a temporary measure while awaiting esophageal replacement. In addition, we recommend that patients referred with cervical esophagostomy and gastrostomy, as a primary approach or even after a failed attempt of primary anastomosis, should be carefully considered for an attempt at reconstruction of their native esophagus. The mandatory step in such patients will be to move the esophagostomy, usually in the left neck, to the right side (if a right thoracotomy is foreseen). In patients with type A or B esophageal atresia, a Stamm gastrostomy is performed through a periumbilical laparotomy and in those with a proximal tracheo-esophageal fistula, this is closed first, usually through a cervical approach. In patients with type C esophageal atresia gastrostomy is never considered, primary repair being the first choice. Immediate primary repair is always attempted because in these cases the lower esophagus, unlike esophageal atresia without lower fistula, usually has a thick muscular wall due to the trophic effects of the normal passage of amniotic fluid through the fistula.

Gap Measurement

As mentioned, the diagnostic criteria for long gap differ among different surgeons. Some define 2 cm as a cut-off point, others classify the gap into short (1 cm), intermediate (2.5–3.0 cm) and long (>3 cm), others define a gap more than 3–3.5 cm as long, while still others recommend an esophageal replacement if the gap exceeds the length of six vertebral bodies. There is also a lack of uniformity in the methods used to measure the gap. In addition, most reports do not indicate whether the gap was measured before or after dissection of the esophageal stumps, or whether or not it was measured under tension.

The method of gap measurement chiefly depends on the anatomical type of esophageal atresia, and is usually done under general anesthesia. In patients with type A or B esophageal atresia (as well as in those with a previous failed attempt), the gap between the esophageal ends may be measured either by injecting sufficient radio-opaque contrast into the stomach to allow it to enter the distal esophagus, or by passing a radio-opaque instrument, such as a bougie, Hegar dilator, urethral sound or flexible endoscope, through the gastrostomy site into the distal stump. At the same time, a radio-opaque tube is advanced in the upper pouch. The use of rigid tools allows measurement of the gap both under passive tension (not pushing on the rigid instruments) and with active stretch (pushing on the instruments) and gives a more precise estimate of the true gap and the degree of tension that can be anticipated after anastomosis (Fig. 30.4). Though rare in type A and B esophageal atresia at birth, a gap under tension of two vertebrae or less usually easily allows immediate primary anastomosis. For a gap of three or more vertebrae, delayed primary anastomosis should be planned, usually in 4–6 weeks. During this time, the progressive increase of bolus feeding by gastrostomy can induce distal pouch growth through shear stress caused by reflux of gastric contents into the distal pouch. Other methods of inducing esophageal pouch growth have been proposed: proximal pouch bougienage once or twice daily, electromagnetic bougienage with metallic bullets placed in the two esophageal ends, the placement of silver olives in the blind pouches that are then gradually approximated through an attached thread, and hydrostatic stretch-induced growth through an indwelling balloon catheter. Like any post-atretic intestinal loop and perhaps partially due to the lack of exposure to amniotic fluid, the lower esophagus and stomach are hypoplastic at birth. After gastrostomy, the regular feeding induces progressive gastric growth and esophageal lengthening thanks to gastro-esophageal reflux.

The gap is measured serially (every 2–3 weeks) to determine the optimal time for an attempt at delayed primary anastomosis. Esophageal reconstruction may be delayed for 8–12 weeks because it has been noted that maximal esophageal growth occurs during this period.

In patients with type-C esophageal atresia, it might not be possible to measure the gap with the method described above, due to the absence of gastrostomy. In such cases, a *preoperative* estimate of gap length can be made by measuring, under fluoroscopy, the length between the radiopaque tube deeply inserted in the blind upper pouch and the broncoscope's tip just placed at the opening of lower fistula. Otherwise an *intra-operative* (and less useful) measurement, both with and without tension on the esophageal ends, is performed after tracheo-esophageal fistula division.

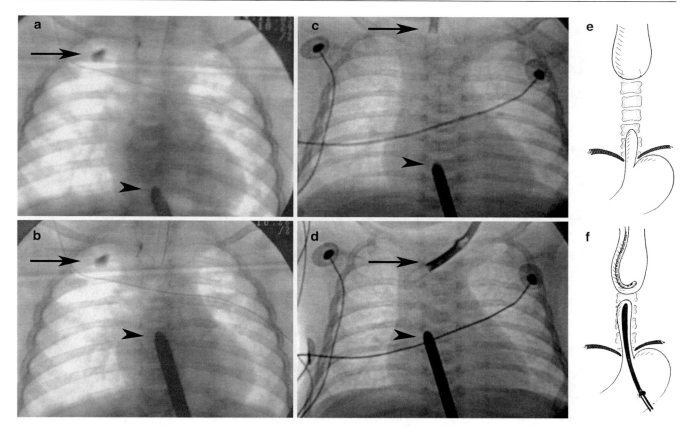

Fig. 30.4 Gap measurement (gapogram) in type A esophageal atresia. (**a**) Without tension in a patient with cervical esophagostomy. *Arrow*: Contrast media at the level of the cervical esophagostomy. *Arrowhead*: Hegar dilator passed through the gastrostomy. (**b**) Gapogram of the same patient as under tension. *Arrow*: Contrast at the level of the cervical esophagostomy. *Arrowhead*: Hegar dilator passed through the gastrostomy. Note the reduction of the gap under active tension on the lower esophagus. (**c**) Gapogram without tension. *Arrow*: Tip of the radiopaque tube inserted in the upper esophageal pouch. *Arrowhead*: Hegar dilator passed through the gastrostomy. (**d**) Gapogram of the same patient as (**c**) under tension on both esophageal pouches. *Arrow*: Tip of the radiopaque tube inserted in the upper esophageal pouch. *Arrowhead*: Hegar dilator passed through the gastrostomy. Note the reduction of the gap under active tension. (**e, f**) Diagram showing a type A esophageal atresia without tension on the pouches (**e**) and after a Hegar dilator is passed through the gastrostomy and active tension is applied on both esophageal pouches (**f**) ((**e, f**) courtesy of Dr. Fabio Ferro, MD)

Surgical Repair

Most surgeons advocate the use of patient's own esophagus to bridge the gap between the two pouches whenever possible. A delayed primary anastomosis for esophageal reconstruction seems to have better long-term results than esophageal replacement. Others believe that this is not necessary and have proposed various methods of esophageal substitution. In our experience, esophageal reconstruction is achievable in the vast majority of cases. In fact, in our series of 145 patients since 1995, esophageal substitution was never required.

Esophageal Reconstruction

A central venous line inserted in an anatomical site compatible with subsequent surgical procedures (left jugular, femoral

veins) is useful for intra-operative and postoperative care. A Hegar dilator is passed through the gastrostomy into the lower pouch and secured at the skin level in order to facilitate intraoperative identification and upward thrust of the lower esophagus (Fig. 30.5). Total body antiseptic preparation is then undertaken to allow a cervical approach to the upper pouch, if needed, and thoracotomy, centered on the appropriate intercostal space based on the results of the gapogram. The muscles are split, not divided, and the posterior mediastinum is accessed through a subperiosteal (to prevent chest/muscular deformities and costal synostosis) extrapleural approach. Both esophageal pouches are identified and extensively mobilized with gentle meticulous dissection and minimal manipulation using 4× magnification and 6-0 silk stay sutures to avoid tissue damage from forceps (Fig. 30.5). And actually, extensive dissection of both upper and lower esophagus can be performed safely, without vascular compromise. Extensive but gentle dissection is better than performing an anastomosis under extreme tension.

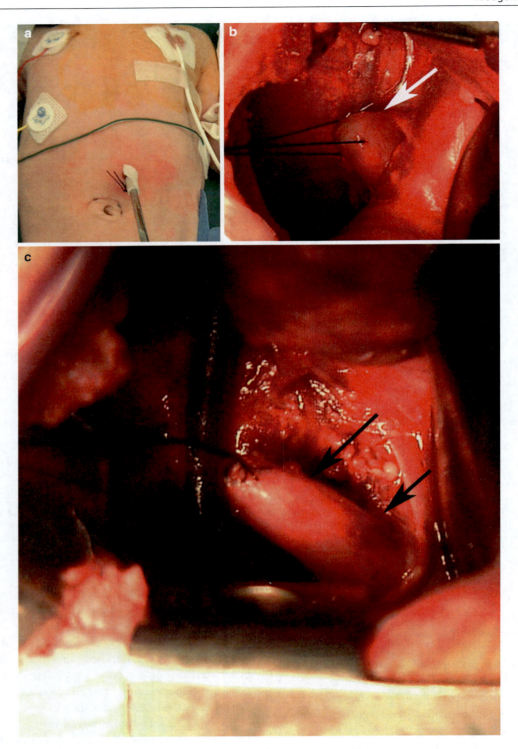

Fig. 30.5 Type A esophageal atresia repair. (**a**) After total body preparation, the Hegar dilator is passed through the gastrostomy and secured at the skin level. (**b**) Intra-operative view. Pushing on the Hegar dilator, the lower pouch (*arrow*) comes into the operative field and stay sutures are placed on the pouch. (**c**) After extensive dissection of the lower pouch, and pushing on the Hegar dilator, extra length of lower pouch (*arrows*) is obtained

Only when an anastomosis is felt to be feasible, the upper and lower pouches are opened, the posterior row of 5-0 or 6-0 polypropylene sutures is placed without tying, and then they are tied simultaneously to decrease disruptive traction forces of each single suture (Fig. 30.6). The anastomosis is performed over an 8 Fr nasogastric tube left in situ as a transanastomotic stent. If a tension-free anastomosis is not possible at this moment, a few technical refinements night help:

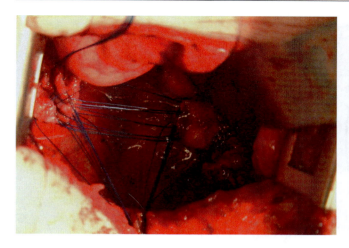

Fig. 30.6 Intra-operative view: the posterior row of sutures in placed and left untied

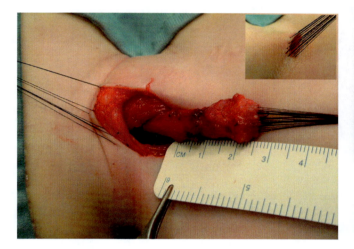

Fig. 30.7 Intra-operative view of the upper esophageal pouch after extensive esophageal dissection through a cervical approach. This was a patient with a cervical esophagostomy (*inset*). The technique is the same in patients without esophagostomy

1. A more extensive upper esophageal dissection through a cervical approach can give an extra 1–1.5 cm length (Fig. 30.7)
2. Progressive intra-operative traction for 10–15 min can be applied through the stay sutures placed on the upper and lower esophageal segments
3. The cushion underneath the patient's chest can be removed, allowing a gain of up to 1 cm (Fig. 30.8)
4. The upper posterior esophageal wall can be mobilized by making a transverse myotomy of the posterior aspect of the blind pouch (Fig. 30.9)
5. A minimal anterior flap can be used to lengthen the upper pouch though a horizontal myotomy on the anterior aspect of the proximal stump (Fig. 30.10)

If these methods do not provide sufficient length, external traction can be used. Stay sutures of 4-0 polypropylene

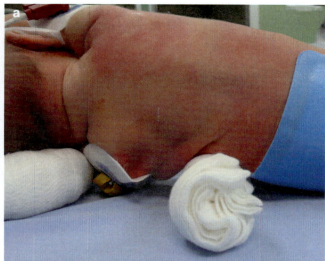

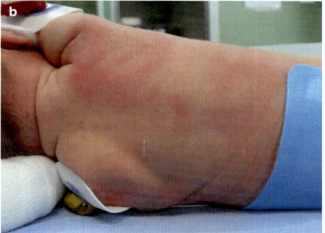

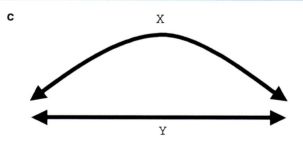

Fig. 30.8 The back of a patient with (**a**) and without (**b**) the cushion underneath his left chest. The removal of the cushion straightens the spine. (**c**) Diagram illustrating the effect on the gap of the straighten up of the spine: the gap with (*X*) and without (*Y*) the cushion. The entity of gap reduction can be calculated as the difference between the length of the arc (*X*) and the straight line (*Y*)

placed in the upper and lower segments are brought out through the skin above and below the incision and the thoracotomy is closed. Over the subsequent 4–7 days, the sutures are pulled 1–2 mm daily and when the two ends are in proximity esophageal anastomosis can be performed. This technique requires an additional 7 days of sedation,

Fig. 30.9 Diagram illustrating the principle of the esophageal slide. (**a**) An incision is made on the anterior aspect of the esophageal wall of the upper pouch. (**b**) Caudal stretching on the incised blind upper pouch leads to caudal skew of the circular muscle fibers and extra length is gained. (**c**) Esophageal anastomosis is completed and the incision is sutured (Courtesy of Dr. Fabio Ferro, MD)

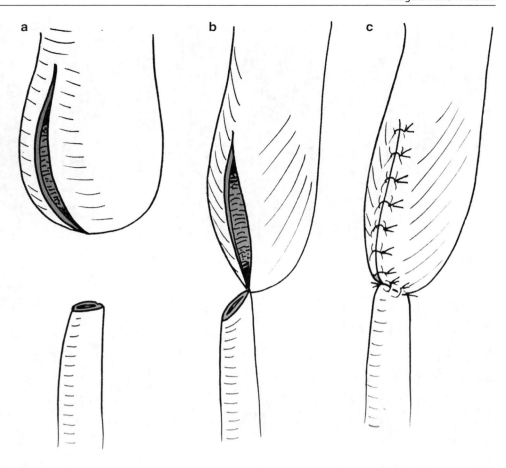

paralyzation and mechanical ventilation as well as a second thoracotomy. Even in patients referred after failed primary anastomosis, traction sutures can be used to produce significant esophageal elongation within days.

A different method of "traction and elongation" has been described, which relies on a multistaged extrathoracic esophageal prolongation technique. The proximal esophagus is translocated to the subcutaneous tissues of the anterior chest wall, essentially creating a thoracic esophagostomy. After a few months, the esophagostomy is mobilized and dissected and exteriorized a few centimeters below the previous esophagostomy. Extrathoracic elongation is repeated until esophageal length is considered sufficient to allow restoration of esophageal continuity.

At the end of the operation, just before the closure of the thorax, a chest drain is left for early detection of signs of anastomotic leak. Costal synostosis should be avoided while closing the thorax to reduce the risk of later thoracic asymmetry.

Postoperative Care

Postoperatively, the infant is kept paralyzed, sedated and mechanically ventilated for 6 days to minimize disruptive forces on the anastomosis (crying, hiccups, retching). Before

starting feeds, a contrast esophagram is performed on the sixth or seventh postoperative day to rule out a leak. When excluded, the chest drain and the trans-anastomotic tube are removed and feeding is started, orally if possible or through the gastrostomy tube if the swallowing reflex is not yet present. If an minor anastomotic leak is detected, feeding is postponed, the chest drain is left in place, and parenteral nutrition is continued. One week later, a second esophagram is performed to confirm resolution of the leak and feedings are started. In the presence of either an anastomotic disruption or persistent leak, a second-look operation should be performed. At this point, depending on the condition of the esophageal ends, options might include revision of the anastomosis, cervical esophagostomy and lower pouch closure with delayed attempt at anastomosis, or esophageal substitution.

One month after surgery, another esophagram and esophagoscopy are performed looking for strictures (esophageal diameter <5 mm) and to assess the impact of gastro-esophageal reflux. When necessary, dilatations are carried out under general anesthesia with Savary bougies over a guide wire. In the presence of signs or symptoms of gastro-esophageal reflux, specific diagnostic studies are performed. When gastro-esophageal reflux disease is confirmed, aggressive treatment, including early anti-reflux surgery (Nissen fundoplication is our preference), should be considered, due to the high rate of

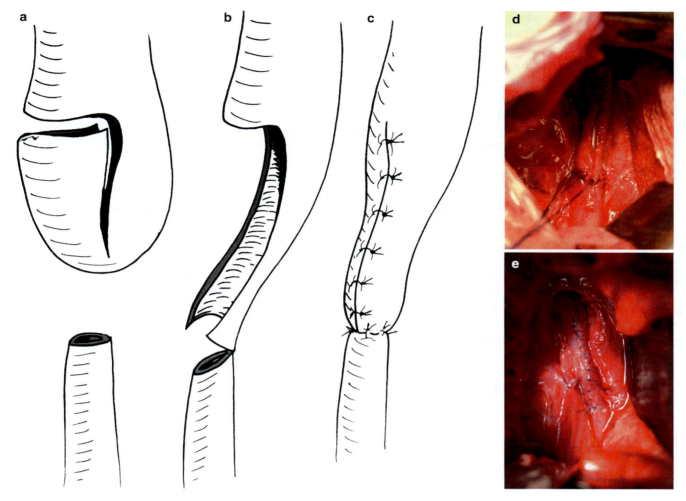

Fig. 30.10 Upper esophageal flap. (**a–c**) Diagram showing the principle of the esophageal flap. Anterior horizontal incision of the upper pouch is extended caudally on both sides (**a**), the flap is reversed, brought down (**b**), and anastomosed to the lower pouch (**c**). (**d**) Intraoperative view. The flap has been reversed, the anastomosis completed and the suture of the longitudinal incision begun. A Y-plasty of the resulting defect on upper (transverse) part of the incision is often needed. (**e**) Intra-operative view. Final appearance of the esophagus after complete closure of the longitudinal incision (Courtesy of Dr. Fabio Ferro, MD)

gastro-esophageal reflux disease in babies operated on for long gap esophageal atresia and the strong correlation between gastro-esophageal reflux and recurrent esophageal stenosis.

At 1 year of follow-up, pH monitoring and esophagoscopy are always repeated because of the high rate of gastro-esophageal reflux, esophagitis and stenosis in these patients.

Complications

The prevalence of early complications, such as minor leaks, recurrent tracheo-esophageal fistula, infections, esophageal stenosis, and gastroesophageal reflux, is related to the adequacy of blood supply to the esophageal ends, gentle handling of tissues, the degree of tension on the anastomosis, and careful postoperative care and paralysis. The incidence of complications is higher, but not all significantly, than in patients with short–long gap esophageal atresia. Other late complications include oral aversion, which depends on the length of intubation and withholding of oral feeds, and vocal cord paralysis, due to recurrent laryngeal nerve injury following extensive upper esophageal pouch dissection or cervical esophagostomy. Despite these complications, the long-term quality of life of patients operated on for long-gap esophageal atresia seems no different from that of their short-gap counterparts. Mortality, which is strongly associated with complications, tends to be higher in patients operated on for long gap esophageal atresia than in patients with a short gap.

It is our opinion, shared by many pediatric surgeons, that the long-term results of primary esophageal anastomosis are better than those with esophageal replacement. Irrespective of the type of replacement chosen, there appears to be less morbidity and fewer on-going problems. However, there are no randomized, controlled studies comparing outcomes of primary anastomosis with that of esophageal replacement. The short- and medium-term outcomes of 19 consecutive cases of long-gap atresia treated only with primary or delayed esophago-esophageal anastomosis were recently compared with that of short-gap esophageal atresia. The authors concluded that all babies with long-gap atresia can be treated successfully with primary anastomosis, that strictures and GERD represent the most frequent postoperative problems, and that the additional procedures often required (dilatations, fundoplication) are an acceptable trade-off to maintain the patient's own esophagus and avoid replacement, which should be reserved only for cases in which a previous attempt of esophageal reconstruction failed.

In our experience and that of others, primary and delayed anastomosis for long-gap esophageal atresia is always possible if one follows a systematic and well standardized approach. Esophageal anastomosis in this challenging anomaly may cause short-term problems. Esophageal dysfunction is evident early after repair of long-gap atresia but swallowing usually improves quickly, esophageal stricture and gastro esophageal reflux can usually be managed with only minor difficulties, and the function of the native esophagus continues to improve over time, making it our procedure of choice.

Esophageal Replacement

The most common indications for esophageal replacement in children are long-gap esophageal atresia and chemical injury of the esophagus. The prevalence of both indications is declining, the former as pediatric surgical and neonatology skills evolve, the latter thanks to the implementation of widespread prevention.

Some surgeons propose to avoid attempts at delayed primary anastomosis and plan esophageal replacement when the gap is felt to be unbridgeable with native esophagus, but we prefer to reserve substitution for patients with failed anastomoses. The most common approaches are to use stomach (reversed tube or whole transposition) or colon. Esophageal substitution should be delayed until the infant weighs at least 5 kg. While waiting, it is important to stimulate the swallowing reflex with sham oral feeding. The esophageal substitute may be positioned through the retrosternal, transpleural or posterior mediastinal spaces. The *retrosternal* space is easy to develop but should be the choice only when the trans-pleural or posterior mediastinal routes are unavailable due to inflammation or scarring. Disadvantages of this route are the longer length to reach the neck from the abdomen, the risk of angulation of the graft, and later problems with access if cardiac surgery is needed. The *transpleural* route is relatively easy but requires a thoracotomy and leads to lung displacement.

In addition, if the ansastomosis is in the chest, there is a high risk of empyema in the event of anastomotic leak or disruption. The *posterior mediastinal* route is probably the optimal one because it is the most anatomical and direct route, the graft is contained in the mediastinum, there is no lung compression, and thoracotomy can be avoided. However, this route is often unavailable due to previous surgery, fibrosis or inflammation.

Colon interposition has been the most common. Either the right colon placed retrosternally based on the middle colic vessels (or the ileocolic when a segment of terminal ileum is chosen) or the left colon in the posterior mediastinum, based on the left colic vessels may be used. Early complications include leaks at the proximal esophageal anastomosis (20–60%), strictures due to inadequate vascular supply or gastrocolic reflux; and excessive mucus production by the colonic mucosa. Graft failure resulting from an inadequate arterial blood supply or venous obstruction is the most catastrophic complication. In recent series, the prevalence of graft necrosis has been reported to range from 7 to 33%. To prevent this grave complication, the vessels should be clamped before division and the colon observed for at least 10 min to ensure that the blood supply is adequate. Redundancy is a frequent long-term problem, so the graft should be just long enough to bridge the gap.

The *gastric tube* may be either anti-peristaltic, based on the left gastroepiploic vessels, or iso-peristaltic, based on the right gastroepiploic vessels. Gastric tube esophagoplasty has become easier and faster due to the use of stapling devices. The tube should be sized by using a 20 or 24 Fr chest tube and can be placed either retrosternal or posterior mediastinal, although the positioning in the latter may be more difficult. After tube construction, a new gastrostomy must be sited in the anterior or posterior wall of the gastric remnant. Care must be taken to maintain the correct orientation of the vascular pedicle to avoid twisting. After the cervical esophagus is mobilized, a cervical esophago-gastric anastomosis is performed. The advantages of gastric tube esophagoplasty are the adequate length and size of the conduit, the good blood supply that can be obtained, and the rapid transit of food. On the other hand, gastric tubes have a long suture line that increases the risk of leakage, potentially reduced by wrapping the suture line with the omentum. Anastomotic leak has been reported in 16–66% of patients treated with this technique. In addition, almost all gastric tubes suffer from reflux, which could lead to the development of Barrett's esophagus.

Gastric transpositio (gastric pull-up), was developed in an effort to diminish complications associated with a long suture line and anastomotic leaks found with reversed gastric tubes and the potential leaks and motility problems associated with colon interposition. Stomach may be transposed either by a thoraco-abdominal approach or transhiatally. The stomach is mobilized after division of the gastrocolic and short gastric vessels and the duodenum is kocherized. The distal esophagus is resected, a pyloroplasty is performed, and the cervical esophagus mobilized. The retrosternal or posterior mediastinal space is developed, the stomach is transposed, and a cervical gastro-esophageal anastomosis performed. This technique usually provides an adequate conduit length, has an excellent blood supply and requires a single anastomosis in the neck. The drawbacks are that the bulk of the stomach can cause space problems in the thorax, GERD potentially leading to Barrett's esophagus, poor gastric emptying due to vagotomy, the loss of the digestive function of the stomach, dumping syndrome, and oral aversion. In addition, the extensive dissection in the soft tissues in the posterior mediastinum can lead to edema and respiratory compromise in the early postoperative period. Cervical anastomotic leaks are reported in 12% of cases but necrosis of the graft has not been reported.

Jejunum has been used for esophageal substitution in the adult, however it has not become popular in infants and children. Two methods of jejunal replacement are used: the pedicled and the free jejunal grafts. In the pedicled graft, the jejunum is prepared just distal to the duodenal-jejunal flexure. The blood supply will depend usually on the third major mesenteric branch. Before division, the vessels should be clamped to ensure a good vascular supply of the loop chosen for the graft. Usually it is necessary to sacrifice a further 30 cm of jejunum to obtain adequate length of the vascular pedicle. Bowel continuity is restored by an end-to-end jejunal anastomosis. The proximal end of the graft is then brought up through the posterior mediastinum into the neck taking care not to twist it, to be anastomosed with the upper esophageal pouch. The distal end is anastomosed to the stomach, or better, to the lower esophageal stump, which helps preventing gastro-jejunal reflux. Alternatively, one can use a free graft interposition, which requires microvascular anastomoses. The vessels that can be used include the internal mammary artery and vein, external carotid artery, internal jugular vein, hemiazygos vein, aorta, subclavian artery and brachiocephalic vein. Advantages include the more natural caliber of the substitute and the fact that peristaltic activity is preserved. The disadvantages are the precarious blood supply, the length of the operation, and the need for multiple anastomoses. In a recent series, no intra-operative mortality is reported. Graft necrosis occurs in as many as 12% of patients, anastomotic leaks in 25%, and stenosis in 5–50%.

The ideal esophageal substitute in infants with EA should have several characteristics: relative ease of surgical technique for construction in small children, no interference with cardiac or respiratory function, minimal gastric acid reflux, an efficient conduit from mouth to stomach, and the potential to grow with the child. A perfect substitute is not to be found and so reasonable compromises have to be accepted. In our personal experience, we have never needed to replace the esophagus in infants with a long-gap esophageal atresia. If we ever need to, we would prefer to use a jejunal graft.

Summary Points

- What constitutes a "long gap" has always been an arbitrary concept: almost all (*but not all*) type A and B and some type C and D esophageal atresia have a long gap between the two esophageal stumps.
- Preserving the native esophagus is almost always possible when the surgeon is committed to this goal and a well defined protocol is followed.
- In patients with esophageal atresia with and without fistula, it is important to measure the gap accurately before an operation is undertaken.
- Radiographs taken with a radiopaque feeding tube inserted deeply in the upper pouch and a sound or bougie passed into the distal esophagus through the gastrostomy should allow accurate assessment of the distance between the two ends.
- Tracheoscopy should always be performed to rule out proximal fistula. It can also be used in combination with fluoroscopy to help define the gap.
- With a long-gap esophageal atresia (≥3 vertebral bodies), experienced senior staff should be alerted or the patient referred to a tertiary care center institution.
- In types A and B, always delay the primary anastomosis 4–6 weeks (even more if necessary) to allow growth of the hypoplastic distal pouch.
- A gastrostomy is useful to immediately start feeding the patient, induce the growth of the lower esophagus and stomach, and allow serial measurement of the gap.
- In patients referred after a failed attempt at primary anastomosis, always rigorously measure the gap to define the possibility of a further attempt at esophageal anastomosis.
- Esophageal substitution is indicated only if primary anastomosis has proven impossible.
- Regardless of the technique used to bridge the gap, patients with long-gap esophageal atresia experience a higher incidence and severity of early and late complications, but this is considered an acceptable trade-off if the native esophagus can be preserved.
- Strict long term follow-up of these patients is mandatory.

Editor's Comment

The take-home message here should clearly be that retaining the native esophagus, be it imperfect or patently flawed, is almost always preferable to any of the various esophageal substitutes that have been described over the years. With experience, meticulous patience and good judgment, we should be able to achieve this goal in the vast majority of patients with esophageal atresia no matter the length of the gap. In most cases, the critical element is time: the esophageal ends will grow, but in some cases this can take many months. There should be no rush to get into the chest to try and bridge a long-gap unless the plan has been thought out very carefully and the advice of experienced pediatric surgeons has been sought.

I look forward to the day when another treasured staple of pediatric surgical history, the cervical esophagostomy, has become a banished relic of a bygone era. This gruesome spectacle of an operation generally precludes salvage of the native esophagus and should only be performed under extraordinary circumstances, never as a primary therapeutic maneuver. The alternative is to control secretions by maintaining a suction cannula in the proximal esophageal pouch for weeks or sometimes months, which usually makes it impossible for the infant to be discharged to home but in the long run is a small price to pay for saving the esophagus.

There are many tricks that have been described to help bridge a long gap. I have found that maximally flexing the neck (chin to chest) helps a great deal. It is also usually safe to mobilize the distal esophagus (and stomach) but this needs to be done carefully so as to preserve the blood supply. Likewise, up to three circumferential myotomies may be performed on the upper pouch, providing a significant amount of length. A common mistake is to begin tying the anastomotic sutures one by one, rather than parachuting them down simultaneously to distribute the tension more evenly. This commonly results in stitches being torn out and the loss of a centimeter or more of esophageal length. I use ringed bowel forceps to grasp each esophageal stump just above and below the respective suture lines and push the ends together so that the entire posterior row of sutures can be tied down under no tension. Silk and other nonabsorbable suture material should not be used on the esophagus because of the risk of foreign body reactions and fistulas, especially since some of the knots usually need to be placed within the lumen. I usually place a small nasogastric tube through the anastomosis to allow gastric decompression and then enteral feeds in the postoperative period, though a tube that is too large can create radial tension and ischemia at the anastomosis, leading to breakdown or stricture. Finally, the technique of gradual lengthening by use of external traction sutures popularized by Foker is clearly a major advance in the field, but I have also seen it fail miserably in inexperienced hands – it is not as easy as it seems and should be guided by someone with direct experience in the technique.

Differential Diagnosis

- Laringotracheal or laryngo-bronchial cleft

Diagnostic Studies

- Chest and abdominal radiographs
- Cardiac ultrasound
- Bronchoscopy under fluoroscopy, as the last diagnostic step before starting operation
- Serial gap measurement (measured in vertebral bodies) with rigid instruments, with and without pressure (repeat every 2 weeks)

Parental Preparation

- This procedure carries a much higher risk when compared to EA without a long gap.
- Multiple-step or delayed procedures might be necessary, depending on the type of EA and whether repair has been attempted previously.
- Several refinements have become available, which seem to have improved the success rate of the technique.
- After repair, expect a long period (at least 6 days) of sedation, paralyzation, and mechanical ventilation.
- Final repair might be delayed even longer (up to 14 days) when an extrathoracic esophageal elongation technique is utilized.
- There is the possibility that subsequent esophageal substitution will become necessary if primary repair is not achievable.
- Most patients have a good quality of life despite an early stormy course.

Preoperative Preparation

- ☐ Chest and abdominal radiographs visualizing the ends of esophageal stumps (even to exactly define the best intercostal space for operative approach)
- ☐ Cardiac ultrasound confirming left aortic arch
- ☐ Continuous suction of the upper pouch
- ☐ Before delayed primary repair: rigorous definition/ visualization the true gap length
- ☐ Type and crossmatch
- ☐ Informed consent

Technical Points

- Tracheoscopy first: to rule out proximal fistula, to define the gap even in type C and D, and to exclude wide laringo-tracheo-esophageal cleft.
- Measure the gap precisely, both with and without tension before deciding the timing of surgical procedure.
- Always avoid primary cervical esophagostomy (waste of time and esophageal length).
- Choose the best intercostal space for thoracotomy (looking at "gapogram" and the vertebral body where the gap falls), use a muscle-splitting technique, use a retropleural approach when possible, preferable through e subperiosteal approach.
- Use magnification.
- Don't try to perform the anastomosis immediately; perform a gastrostomy and close proximal fistula (type B). Define initial gap and re-measure it every 15 days.
- Gap <3 vertebral bodies:
- Ready to do the anastomosis, alert senior staff always.
- At anastomosis, use a Hegar dilator (4–5 mm) trough the gastrostomy into the lower esophageal stump to help intra-operative identification of the lower pouch.
- Always attempt primary anastomosis.
- Gap ≥3 vertebral bodies:
- Alert senior staff
- Close and divide the fistula
- Re-measure the gap rigorously
- If a left esophagostomy has already been done, move it to the right neck (when right thoracotomy and esophageal re-anastomosis is considered possible and planned).
- Handle tissues very gently: Use stay sutures on both esophageal ends; don't clamp esophagus with forceps.
- Mobilize both upper and lower esophageal segments extensively.
- Verify the gap is bridged before opening either lower or upper esophageal pouch.
- If the gap can be bridged, do the anastomosis.
- If the gap is still "unbridgeable," consider:
- Intra-operative traction on each end for 10 min
- Upper pouch sliding
- Further dissection of upper pouch through a cervical approach
- Upper esophageal flap (as small as possible)
- Esophageal lengthening with external traction and redo thoracotomy 6 days later
- Doing the anastomosis:
- Posterior row with 3–4 sutures (5-0 or 6-0 polypropylene) placed without tying, and then tied simultaneously
- Remove chest bump
- Drain the chest (even if extrapleural approach); avoid costal synostosis.
- Maintain the patient sedated and paralyzed for at least 6 days.
- Don't move, rotate, or hyperextend the neck during patient's transportation and for at least 6 days.
- Check the chest drain daily to exclude drainage of saliva: white with foam instead of serous or seroanguinous.
- Contrast study on post operative day 6–7, to rule out leak, before starting feeding.

Suggested Reading

Ahmed A, Spitz L. The outcome of colonic replacement of the esophagus in children. Prog Pediatr Surg. 1986;19:37–54.

Anderson KD, Randolph JG. The gastric tube for esophageal replacement in infants and children. J Thorac Cardiovasc Surg. 1973;66:333–42.

Atzori P, Iacobelli BD, Bottero S, et al. Preoperative tracheobronchoscopy in newborns with esophageal atresia: does it matter? J Pediatr Surg. 2006;41:1054–7.

Bagolan P, Iacobelli BD, De Angelis P, et al. Long gap esophageal atresia and esophageal replacement: moving toward separation? J Pediatr Surg. 2004;39:1084–90.

Bax NMA, van der Zee DC. Jejunal pedicle grafts for reconstruction of the esophagus in children. J Pediatr Surg. 2007;42:363–9.

Foker JE, Linden BC, Boyle EM, et al. Development of a true primary repair for the full spectrum of esophageal atresia. Ann Surg. 1997;226:533–43.

Puri P, Blake K, O'Donnell B, et al. Delayed primary esophageal anastomosis following spontaneous growth of esophageal segments in esophageal atresia. J Pediatr Surg. 1981;16:180–3.

Puri P, Khurana S. Delayed primary esophageal anastomosis for pure esophageal atresia. Semin Pediatr Surg. 1998;7:126–9.

Ring WS, Varco RL, L'Heureux PR, et al. Esophageal replacement with jejunum in children: an 18 to 33 year follow-up. J Thorac Cardiovasc Surg. 1982;83:918–27.

Spitz L, Kiely E, Sparon T. Gastric transposition for esophageal replacement in children. Ann Surg. 1987;206:69–73.

Chapter 31
Esophageal Replacement

Lewis Spitz

The need to replace the esophagus in pediatric surgical practice has become increasingly uncommon. The main reason for this is the improvements that have occurred in the management of esophageal atresia leading to only a minority of cases where esophageal continuity cannot be restored. Caustic esophageal injury is now rare in the developed countries; however, in the developing countries it remains a major cause of irretrievable esophageal damage. Other rare indications for esophageal replacement include tumors, extensive intractable reflux strictures and prolonged foreign body impaction.

There are four main methods for esophageal replacement: colon, stomach, gastric tube and jejunum. Each procedure has its own advantages and disadvantages (Table 31.1). Essentially, the substitution needs to function as an efficient conduit from mouth to intestine to satisfy the nutritional needs of the child and should continue to grow with the child and function well into adult life. The ideal position for the esophageal substitute is the posterior mediastinum, the bed of the native esophagus, which is the shortest distance between the neck and the abdomen. The retrosternal route is commonly used for colonic replacement, while the transpleural route is used when there is extensive scarring in the posterior mediastinum as a result of previous attempts to retain the native esophagus or due to transmural esophageal damage such as from caustic injury or perforation.

Colon Interposition

Colon interposition is the most widely used procedure for esophageal replacement (Fig. 31.1). It was first used in a child by Lumblad in 1921 and subsequently popularized by Waterston in London and Clatworthy in the United States. The largest reported series is that reported by Hamza (Egypt) in 2003.

The colon graft can consist of either the right colon based on the middle colic or ileocolic vessels, or the left colon based on the left colic vessels. Following adequate bowel preparation, the blood supply to the entire colon is inspected at laparotomy. The anatomy of the vascular supply will determine the most appropriate section of the colon for the interposition. The most commonly used segment is the left transverse and upper left colon based on the ascending branches of the left colonic vessels. The graft is brought up into the neck through the posterior mediastinum, the transpleural route or a retrosternal tunnel. The proximal end of the colon is anastomosed to the end of the cervical esophagus and the distal end to the body of the stomach or to the distal esophageal stump.

Leaks and strictures at the proximal colo-esophageal anastomosis are relatively common and directly related to the precarious blood supply of the proximal end of the colonic interposition. Most leaks will heal spontaneously. With the advent of fiberoptic instrumentation, dilatation of an anastomotic stricture is now easier and safer. Reflux of gastric contents into the colonic interposition occasionally results in peptic ulceration, which can cause hemorrhage or rarely perforation. As peristalsis is generally absent, transit of food through the colonic graft is by gravity. In the long term, one of the major problems is redundancy of the colon with resultant stasis.

Gastric Transposition

Originally described by Sweet in 1945, gastric transposition is currently the procedure of choice for adults with esophageal carcinoma (Fig. 31.2). It has only recently found favor in pediatric surgical practice (Spitz in England and Coran in Ann Arbor).

Transhiatal gastric transposition without thoracotomy is the technique of choice. The mediastinal route might not be available where there has been extensive scarring due to previous attempts at retaining the esophagus or secondary to inflammation from caustic ingestion. In these cases, a transthoracic route is usual.

The stomach is mobilized along the greater and lesser curvatures, ligating the left gastric vessels while retaining the right

L. Spitz (✉)
Department of Paediatric Surgery, Institute of Child Health, University
College, London, Great Ormond Street Hospital, London, UK
e-mail: lspitz@ich.ucl.ac.uk

P. Mattei (ed.), *Fundamentals of Pediatric Surgery*,
DOI 10.1007/978-1-4419-6643-8_31, © Springer Science+Business Media, LLC 2011

Table 31.1 Advantages and disadvantages of the various esophageal substitutions

Method	Advantages	Disadvantages
Colon	Adequate length	Blood supply may be precarious
	Relative ease of the procedure	High incidence of leaks/strictures
		Multiple anastomoses
		Slow transit
		Redundancy in the long term.
Gastric transposition	Adequate length	Reflux and dumping
	Excellent blood supply	Strictures feeding problems
	Single anastomosis	
	Ease of procedure	
Gastric tube	Adequate length	Very long suture line
	Good blood supply	High incidence of leaks and strictures
	Appropriate size	Reflux leading to Barrett's esophagitis
	Rapid transit	
Jejunum	Appropriate size	Multiple anastomoses
	Retention of peristaltic activity	Precarious blood supply
		Leaks and strictures
		Length may be a problem
		Technically difficult

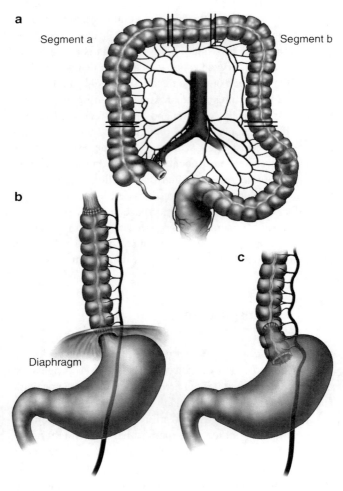

Fig. 31.1 Colon interposition. (**a**) *Segment a* Based on right/middle colic vessels or ileocolic vessels. *Segment b* Based on ascending branch of left colic vessels. (**b**) Colon graft passed retrosternally or transhiatally to posterior mediastinum or left thoracic cavity. (**c**) Distal anastomosis to distal esophageal stump or to stomach

gastric and gastroepiploic vessels and the vascular arcades. The distal esophagus is excised and the whole stomach is "pulled-up" into the lower cervical region through the esophageal hiatus and posterior mediastinum. The distal end of the cervical esophagus is anastomosed end-to-side to the highest point on the fundus of the stomach. A pyloroplasty or pyloromyotomy may be added. A jejunal feeding tube is inserted for infants with esophageal atresia who have never previously swallowed liquids. This is a temporary procedure to provide enteral nutrition while the infant is adapting to the gastric transposition.

Leaks and strictures at the esophago-gastric anastomosis are uncommon; however, feeding problems such as dumping and food refusal are troublesome, particularly for the first few months. In the long term, growth and development are relatively normal with height proceeding at around the 50th percentile and weight between 25th and 50th percentile for age. The patients tend to eat small meals more frequently but no deterioration in function has been observed over time.

We published our series of gastric transposition in 2004. A total of 192 children underwent the procedure between 1980 and 2004 with a mortality rate of 4.6%. Anastomostic leaks occurred in 12% of patients. Stricture occurred in 20%, all but three having responded to dilatation alone. The high mortality and morbidity is a reflection of the complex nature of the patients sent to our tertiary referral center.

Gastric Tube Esophagoplasty

First devised by Jianu in 1912, the gastric tube method of esophageal replacement was popularized by Gavrilou in Europe and Heinlich in the United States (Fig. 31.3). Proponents for this procedure include Ein (Toronto) and Randolph and Anderson (Washington).

Fig. 31.2 Gastric transposition. (**a**) Left gastric and gastroepiploic vessels divided. Right gastric and gastroepiploic vessels preserved vascular arcades on greater curvature preserved. Stump of esophagus excised. *xy* highest point on the stomach. (**b**) Cervical esophagus anastomosed to top of fundus of stomach; pylorus below the diaphragm

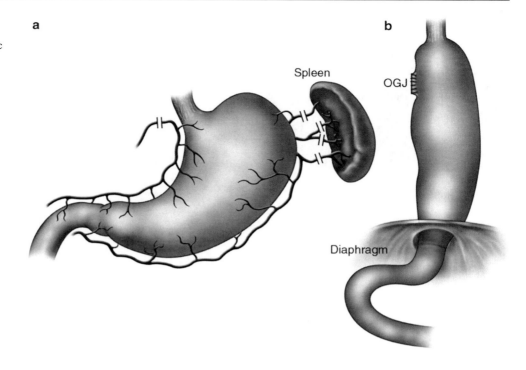

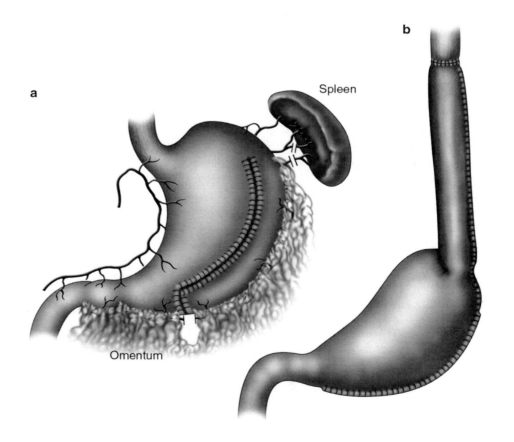

Fig. 31.3 Gastric tube esophagoplasty. (**a**) Reversed antiperistialtic tube fashioned from the greater curvature of the stomach. (**b**) Gastric tube swung up to meet end of esophagus in neck or upper thorax. Note long suture lines

Fig. 31.4 Jejunal interposition.
(**a**) Isolating a section of jejunum
with its vascular arcade.
(**b**) Jejunal segment with blood
supply passed through diaphragmatic hiatus. Anastomosed
end-to-end to proximal and distal
esophagus

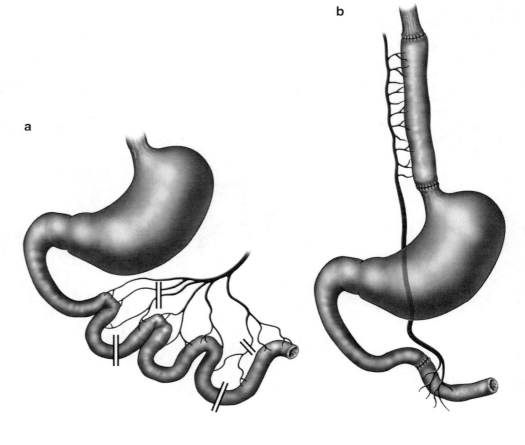

An antiperistaltic tube of appropriate size is fashioned
from the greater curvature of the stomach, ensuring an adequate blood supply from the gastroepiploic arcade of vessels.
The gastric tube is placed either retrosternally or transpleurally and anastomosed end-to-end to the cervical esophagus.
This procedure involves two very long suture lines, one on
the neo-esophagus and the other on the greater curvature of
the stomach, with a resultant high rate of anastomotic leaks
and stricture.

Peristalsis is absent in the tube but emptying occurs rapidly by gravity. In long-term follow-up, a high incidence of
Barrett's esophagitis has been reported.

Jejunal Interposition

Roux (1906) reported the first success with jejunum placed
intrathoracically in a 12-year-old child following caustic
ingestion (Fig. 31.4). The patient died of an unrelated cause

at age 53 years. Bax in 2007 reported on a large number of
children undergoing the procedure.

The most suitable segment of jejunum of sufficient length
is selected for the interposition. This is entirely based on the
vascular supply to the segment being of adequate mobility to
reach the cervico-thoracic region without compromise. The
isolated segment of jejunum is passed through the esophageal hiatus and the proximal end is anastomosed to the end of
the cervical esophagus in the superior mediastinum. The distal end of the jejunal graft is anastomosed either to the distal
esophagus or to the stomach.

Transit through the jejunal interposition is rapid as it
appears to maintain its peristaltic activity, but the procedure
is very demanding and attended by considerable morbidity,
especially in the early postoperative period.

While it is important, in order to achieve the best results,
to master one technique, the surgeon should be conversant
with the various alternative methods of esophageal substitution in the event of the favored technique not being feasible
in a particular circumstance.

Summary Points

- There are four operations described for replacement of the esophagus in children: colonic interposition, gastric transposition, gastric tube esophagoplasty and jejunal interposition.
- For most esophageal replacement operations, the best location for placement of the graft is the posterior mediastinum (the bed of the native esophagus), providing the shortest distance between the neck and abdomen.
- When the posterior mediastinum is not available, usually due to severe scarring of the native esophagus, other options include the retrosternal space and the transpleural route.
- The pediatric surgeon should have experience with at least one technique but should be familiar with all available techniques.
- Colonic interposition is technically the most straightforward but the graft has a tendency to elongate as the child grows, creating symptoms that are sometimes debilitating.
- The gastric transposition operation is increasingly being used as a useful alternative to the colonic transposition procedure.

Editor's Comment

In general, when several different operations, each with its own vocal proponents and detractors, are described for a single clinical problem, one can be fairly certain that not one of them is the ideal solution for every patient. Nevertheless, it is clearly important for the pediatric surgeon to have confidence and experience with at least one of the operations and its various permutations and have some familiarity with the other options that are available so that patient care can be individualized and optimized.

Historically in the United States, the colonic interposition has been the most popular. It is perhaps the easiest to perform and patients generally do quite well for several years. The problem is that over time, the colon continues to grow in length and diameter, so that eventually it becomes huge, tortuous and poorly functioning. This has led to fairly widespread dissatisfaction with the technique and a recent intensification in the search for a better alternative. The gastric transposition ("gastric pull up") is now increasingly being used for this reason. It is safe, technically straightforward and though the initial postoperative phase can be trying, the long-term results appear to be quite acceptable. Most surgeons prefer to perform a pyloroplasty, although a pyloromyotomy is also reasonable. It is also preferable, though not mandatory, to place the graft in the posterior mediastinum and if possible to avoid a thoracotomy. Regardless of the approach, it is essential to preserve the blood supply of the stomach and to create a tension-free anastomosis. Leaks are relatively common but usually easily managed, especially when the anastomosis is in the neck.

The jejunal conduit is the most appealing option in that the diameter of the graft approximates that of the esophagus, transit should be better since peristalsis is preserved, and the long-term issues seen with the other types of graft should be eliminated. However, the operation is technically challenging and the blood supply to the cephalad portion of the graft is often tenuous.

Differential Diagnosis

- Caustic injury of the esophagus
- Long-gap esophageal atresia
- Esophageal neoplasm
- Impacted foreign body
- Iatrogenic/traumatic injury of the esophagus
- Reflux-associated stricture
- Barrett's esophagitis with dysplasia

Diagnostic Studies

- Upper GI contrast study
- Contrast enema
- Intra-operative hand-held Doppler probe to assess vascular anatomy of graft
- Postoperative contrast study to rule out anastomotic leak and assess transit through the conduit

Parental Preparation

- There is no "perfect" replacement for the esophagus.
- This is a big operation with a high risk of complications, especially anastomotic leak and stricture.
- Leaks usually heal spontaneously.
- Strictures usually respond to dilatation.
- Revision is sometimes necessary.
- There is a risk of reflux, feeding intolerance, or dumping syndrome, but the children usually eventually do well and grow normally.

Preoperative Preparation

☐ Informed consent
☐ Type and cross
☐ Mechanical bowel preparation
☐ Meticulous surgical planning, with contingency plan in anticipation of a surprise
☐ Prophylactic antibiotics
☐ Anticipate need for alternative means of providing nutrition (jejunostomy tube or central venous catheter)

Technical Points

• The portion of colon used for interposition is determined by the blood supply of the colon but is usually the transverse/left colon or the right colon.
• To maintain viability of the stomach during a gastric transposition, it is important to preserve the right gastric and right gastroepiploic vessels as well as the vascular arcades.
• A gastric tube can be created by serial application of a gastrointestinal stapling device but the long suture line that results is prone to leaks and stricture.
• A jejunal interposition graft is perhaps the most appealing because of it appropriate diameter and the fact that it maintains peristaltic activity, but the procedure is technically challenging and the overall morbidity is high.

Suggested Reading

Anderson KD, Randoph JGL. The gastric tube for esophageal replacement in infants and children. J Thorac Cardiovasc Surg. 1973;66:333.

Bax WM, Van der Zee DC. Jejunal pedicle grafts for reconstruction of the esophagus in children. J Pediatr Surg. 2007;42:363.

Ein SH, Shandling B, Stephens CA. Twenty-one year experience with the pediatric gastric tube. J Pediatr Surg. 1987;22:77.

German JC, Waterston DJ. Colon interposition for replacement of the esophagus in children. J Pediatr Surg. 1976;11:227.

Hamza AF, Abdelhay S, Sherif H, Hasan T, Soliman H, Kabesh A, et al. Caustic esophageal strictures in children: 30 years' experience. J Pediatr Surg. 2003;38:828.

Hirschl RB, Yardeni D, Oldham K, Sherman N, Siplovich L, Gross E, et al. Gastric transposition for esophageal replacement in children: experience with 41 consecutive cases with special emphasis on esophageal atresia. Ann Surg. 2002;236:531.

Ring WS et al. Esophageal replacement with jejunum in children: an 18 to 33 year follow-up. J Thorac Cardiovasc Surg. 1982;83:918.

Spitz L. Gastric transposition via the mediastinal route for infants with long-gap esophageal atresia. J Pediatr Surg. 1984;19:149.

Spitz L, Kiely E, Pierro A. Gastric transposition in children – a 21-year experience. J Pediatr Surg. 2004;39:276.

Chapter 32
Esophageal Injuries

Kristin N. Fiorino and Petar Mamula

Injuries to the esophagus in children are often due to accidental ingestions or traumatic injuries as young children have a tendency to explore the world with their hands and mouth. Childhood curiosity, lack of complete dentition, limited oromotor control, and immature judgment or carelessness each contribute to foreign body or caustic ingestion. Although ingestion of foreign bodies, batteries, coins, and drugs are accidental in most instances, child abuse, psychiatric illness, suicide, or Munchausen by proxy should be considered. Once having passed through the esophagus, most ingested foreign bodies, including sharp or pointed objects, will pass spontaneously through the alimentary tract.

Most children who ingest foreign bodies are between the ages of 6 months and 6 years. Coins are the most common, while meat or food impactions are more common in adolescents and adults. Nearly 90% of ingested foreign bodies pass uneventfully through the digestive system, but some become lodged in the esophagus. Up to 20% require endoscopic removal, and less than 1% require surgical intervention. Although deaths due to ingestion of foreign bodies have been reported, mortality rates are extremely low, with a recent large series reporting no deaths among 852 adults and 1 death among 2,206 children.

Diagnosis

Older children and adults are usually able to identify the swallowed object and area of discomfort or pain. Localization of the level of impaction, however, is often unreliable. In many instances, the ingestion is not witnessed and is only reported with the onset of symptoms. Retrosternal chest pain, dysphagia, hypersalivation, stridor, and retching are typical symptoms of esophageal injuries, but in young children symptoms are not always obvious. Children present with a variety of symptoms including drooling, hoarseness, choking, refusal to eat, or respiratory distress secondary to tracheal compression or esophageal erosion. Less frequent complaints include odynophagia and chest pain. The presence of cervical swelling, erythema or crepitus raises concern for an oropharyngeal or proximal esophageal perforation. Occasionally, children present with life-threatening gastrointestinal hemorrhage secondary to aortoesophageal fistula.

Esophageal foreign body impactions should be investigated and removed as soon as possible to prevent aspiration and perforation. If the patient is asymptomatic, the foreign body should be removed within 12–24 h of ingestion, in which case radiographic confirmation should be repeated immediately prior to endoscopy as the object might have migrated. Coins that reach the stomach, depending on their size and patient's age, are likely to pass without complication and can usually be simply followed radiographically. Button batteries, sharp objects, and objects causing bleeding, acute or severe airway compromise, or significant pain or dysphagia require emergent removal. In general, foreign body or food impaction should not remain in the esophagus beyond 24 h.

In considering the outcome of ingested foreign bodies, the composition, shape, size, and number of ingested bodies should be taken into account. The anatomic barriers of the gastrointestinal tract also need to be recognized. Impaction, perforation, or obstruction most often occurs at areas of acute angulation or physiologic narrowing. The main anatomic locations for esophageal foreign body retention are the levels of the cricopharyngeus muscle, the aortic arch, left main stem bronchus, and the lower esophageal sphincter. Transit is also delay at the pylorus, duodenal curve, ligament of Treitz, Meckel's diverticulum, ileocecal valve, and rectosigmoid junction. Children with a history of prior gastrointestinal operations, congenital intestinal malformations, (esophageal atresia), achalasia, or strictures secondary to prior caustic ingestions, are at an increased risk for obstruction and perforation.

Antero-posterior and lateral radiographs of the neck, chest and abdomen are often useful in identifying both the location and shape of the foreign body, as well as sequelae: an esophageal

K.N. Fiorino (✉)
Department of Pediatric Gastroenterology, Children's Hospital of Philadelphia, Philadelphia, PA, USA
e-mail: fiorino@email.chop.edu

P. Mattei (ed.), *Fundamentals of Pediatric Surgery*,
DOI 10.1007/978-1-4419-6643-8_32, © Springer Science+Business Media, LLC 2011

Fig. 32.1 AP and lateral radiographs demonstrating a coin lodged in the esophagus. Coins usually become lodges at the level of the cricopharyngeus, the aortic arch, the left mainstem bronchus, or the distal esophagus. This is a somewhat unusual location and raises the possibility of an underlying stricture

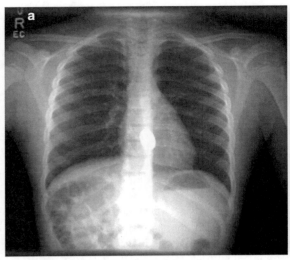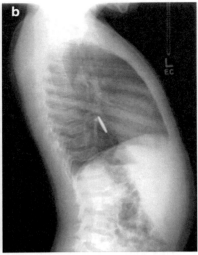

fluid level, pneumomediastinum, or pneumoperitoneum. Flat objects, such as coins or batteries lodged in hypopharynx are oriented on edge in a lateral view, whereas if lodged in the upper airway, appear on edge in the frontal view (Fig. 32.1). In the AP projection, batteries present as a double-density shadow, and on lateral have a step-off at the junction of the anode and cathode. The lateral film sometimes reveals the presence of multiple ingested objects. Non-visualization of an object on X-ray, however, does not rule out the presence of a foreign body such as a fish bone or objects made of plastic, glass, wood, or thin metal. Radiologic signs suggestive of perforation include extraluminal foreign bodies, retropharyngeal air, or widening of the retropharyngeal soft tissue.

A barium esophagogram usually demonstrates the presence of a non-radiopaque foreign body and might identify an underlying stricture or stenosis. Water-soluble contrast is indicated if a fistula or perforation is suspected; however, because of the risk of aspiration and the issue of barium coating the foreign body and mucosa and compromising endoscopy, a contrast examination should not be routinely performed. CT is sometimes useful but less so when the object is radiolucent. Hand-held metal detector scanning has been shown to be an accurate, radiation-free method of detecting metallic objects in children. Persistent symptoms should be pursued with endoscopy even if the radiologic evaluation is negative.

Anatomy/Technical Approach

The diameter of the esophagus is normally reduced at four points: the cricopharyngeus, the crossing of the aorta, the crossing of the left mainstem bronchus, and at the diaphragm. A fifth narrowing of the esophageal lumen occurs at the thoracic inlet, probably due to crowding by the many parallel and adjacent structures in this area.

Both rigid and flexible esophagoscopy are effective methods for removing foreign bodies. Flexible esophagoscopy with mirror examination is often used in identifying an object in the oral cavity or hypopharynx. Direct laryngoscopy can be used to identify an embedded object. Esophageal foreign bodies can be removed with a rigid endoscope with forceps, especially if located in the upper third of the esophagus. Magill forceps are commonly used to extract coins in the upper esophagus under direct visualization. Most foreign body forceps used with rigid endoscopy can be classified into four types. Alligator forceps have straight jaws and serrations to add friction when grasping the foreign body. They are useful in removal of vegetable matter, irregular hard objects, coins, or objects with a sharp point, such as pins and needles. Globular grasping forceps with curved blades are useful for spherical objects when serrated forceps can slip. Rotational forceps are useful in extracting pins, needles, tacks, and nails. A hollow cylinder in the esophagus or bronchus is a difficult extraction for which hollow object forceps are used. Serrations are on the outside of the forceps to aid in grasping the object with minimal mucosal damage.

The flexile esophagogastroduodenoscopy (EGD) performed by a gastroenterologist allows for visualization of the gastrointestinal tract including the distal esophagus and beyond. The commonly used pediatric gastroscope has an 8.6 mm outer diameter insertion tube with an inner channel diameter of 2.8 mm. Four-way angulation (210° up, 90° down, and 100° right/left) and a 140° field of view allow for a complete and comprehensive view of the gastrointestinal tract. The neonatal endoscope has a 5.9-mm outer diameter insertion tube, an inner channel diameter of 2 mm, four-way angulation (180° up, 90° down, and 100° right/left), and a 120° field of view. The adult endoscope has an 8.8 mm outer diameter insertion tube and an inner channel diameter of 2.8 mm. The 2.8 mm inner channel diameter in the adult and pediatric endoscopes allow for the use of the accessories needed for foreign body retrieval.

Equipment that should be readily available for foreign body removal include rat tooth, alligator, and grasping forceps, Pelican grasping forceps, three-prong polypectomy snare, polyp grasper (3, 4, or 5 prong), Roth retrieval net, retrieval basket, overtubes of esophageal and gastric lengths, and a foreign body protector hood. To grasp a foreign body during flexible endoscopy, the forceps are inserted beyond the tip of the endoscope before they are opened and may be used to push surrounding mucosa away from the foreign body. Sharp and pointed foreign bodies, as well as elongated objects, can be difficult to manage and are associated with a higher complication rate. Sharp objects should be sheathed, or rotated so that the point trails. An overtube offers airway protection during retrieval, allows for multiple passes of the endoscope during removal of the foreign body, and protects the esophageal mucosa from sharp objects. The overtube is not as frequently used as it is in adults because of the risks of esophageal injury during overtube insertion. The foreign body protector hood is preferred when removing sharp objects from the esophagus.

Treatment

The management of esophageal foreign bodies is influenced by the child's age and weight as well as the composition and number of ingested objects, the anatomic location in which they are lodged, and the skill of the endoscopist. Generally, children undergoing endoscopy for foreign body removal should be intubated and under general anesthesia, allowing control of the airway, optimal conditions for therapeutic endoscopy, and less time pressure.

Urgent endoscopic intervention is required when a sharp object or disc battery is lodged in the esophagus or if an object is located in the upper third of the esophagus. Urgent intervention is also required to prevent aspiration when there is a high-grade obstruction or if the child is unable to manage his or her secretions. Those without a high-grade obstruction or able to handle oral secretions can be managed less urgently because the likelihood of spontaneous passage is higher. If the object lies in the middle to lower esophagus, a repeat film should be obtained and endoscopy performed within 12–24 h if the child is asymptomatic. Foreign body or food impaction should not remain in the esophagus beyond 24 h. Foreign bodies in the stomach are likely to be eliminated within 30 days. If the object is below the diaphragm and has not passed in the feces, an abdominal radiograph should be obtained; if it has not passed in 4–6 weeks, endoscopy is recommended for removal.

Specific Foreign Bodies

Most objects less than 2 cm in diameter pass through the esophagus spontaneously. Small coins (15–20 mm) are less likely to get retained in esophagus, whereas larger coins (20–35 mm) usually lodge at the cricopharyngeus (60–65%), aortic arch (10–15%), and at or above lower esophageal sphincter (20–25%). There is a higher incidence of complications with objects larger than 5 cm in length and 2 cm in diameter, sharp-ended objects and batteries.

Blunt Objects

Coins are the most commonly ingested foreign body in children. If lodged in the hypopharynx or upper esophagus, coins should be removed under direct visualization with Magill forceps or rigid or flexible esophagoscopy. If lower in the esophagus, blunt objects can usually be removed with a flexible endoscope using rat-tooth or grasping forceps, a snare, retrieval net, or basket. The forceps are a very efficient way to ensure coin retrieval and will allow the foreign body to swivel in the plane of least resistance. All coins produced in the United States have a rim, facilitating the endoscopist's ability to grasp them. Smooth, round objects are best secured with a retrieval net or basket. It is advised not to push objects into the stomach since distal stricture or other pathology can increase the risk of esophageal injury.

If objects are left in the stomach and are less than 2 cm in diameter and 5 cm in length, they should pass within 6 days, although some may take as long as 4 weeks. On occasion, a coin can overlie the pylorus, causing intermittent obstruction, in which case endoscopic removal is warranted. Children should resume a regular diet and the stool should be strained for passage of the foreign body. In the absence of symptoms, weekly radiographs are sufficient to follow the progression of blunt objects that are not observed to pass spontaneously. If an object is beyond the stomach but remains in the same location for more than 1 week, surgical removal should be considered. Fever, vomiting, abdominal pain or peritoneal signs are indications for immediate surgical removal.

Large Objects

Objects that are long or large pose a considerable risk of complications when ingested. Knives, chopsticks, screwdrivers, toothbrushes, or spoons have difficulty passing the esophagus, pylorus (which does not easily allow passage of objects greater than 15 mm in diameter), and the duodenal sweep (which will not allow the passage of objects greater than 10 cm in length). In patients with normal rotation, the ileocecal valve is usually the final location of such ingested objects. In addition, a combination of length and caliber precludes the passage of objects greater than 5 cm in length and 2 cm in thickness in an adolescent.

Urgent endoscopy is warranted if the patient is symptomatic. If the patient is asymptomatic, endoscopy may be performed after an appropriate period of fasting, but within 24 h. A polypectomy snare, retrieval net, or basket is helpful in retrieving long and large foreign bodies. Long objects are to be removed parallel to the plane of the esophagus. All toothbrushes require removal as they will not pass the duodenal sweep (Fig. 32.2). Gastric overtubes (>45 cm) can also be used with removal of the entire apparatus in one motion, avoiding losing the grasp of the object in the overtube itself. Complications of retained large or long foreign bodies include perforation and obstruction (Fig. 32.3).

Sharp Objects

Morbidity and mortality are higher after ingestion of sharp or pointed foreign bodies. The most commonly ingested problematic objects are chicken and fish bones, straightened paperclips, razor blades, toothpicks, needles, bread bag clips, and dental bridgework. Many sharp pointed objects are not visible radiographically; therefore endoscopy should follow a negative radiographic exam.

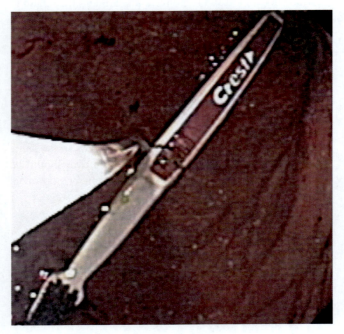

Fig. 32.2 Toothbrush in the stomach. Although perhaps narrow enough to pass through the GI tract, the length of this foreign body makes passage through the duodenal C-loop unlikely

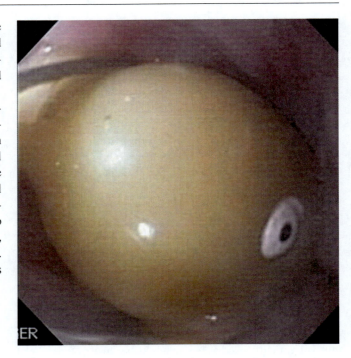

Fig. 32.3 Plastic toy duck lodged in the esophagus. Large and smooth-walled objects can be difficult to grasp and extract

If an object is lodged in the hypopharynx or at the cricopharyngeus muscle, rigid endoscopy with forceps or direct laryngoscopy is recommended. If the object is below this area, flexible endoscopy may be used with retrieval forceps or a polypectomy snare; baskets, or retrieval nets should be avoided in most cases, as they offer less control of the sharp object and increase the risk of mucosal injury.

Straight-pin ingestion represents a special circumstance in the management of sharps. Pins tend to follow Chevalier Jackson's axiom that "advancing objects puncture, trailing objects do not." Straight-pins usually pass uneventfully as the blunt head usually passes first. However, if longer than 5 cm, straight pins sometimes fail to pass through the duodenum and carry the risk of perforation, hepatic hemorrhage or infection.

Sharps other than straight-pins (Fig. 32.4) require endoscopic, or, at times, surgical, removal. If not removed, perforation is likely, the majority of which are near the ileocecal valve. Management of sharp objects includes the use of a foreign body protector hood or an overtube to help prevent esophageal injury. If followed with daily radiographs, objects that fail to migrate for three consecutive days and are beyond reach of an endoscope should be considered for surgical removal. Fever, vomiting, abdominal pain or peritoneal signs are indications for immediate surgical removal.

If an open safety pin is in the esophagus with the open end proximal, it is best managed with a flexible endoscope and a foreign body hood. Some advocate pushing the pin into the stomach, turning it, and then grasping the hinged end,

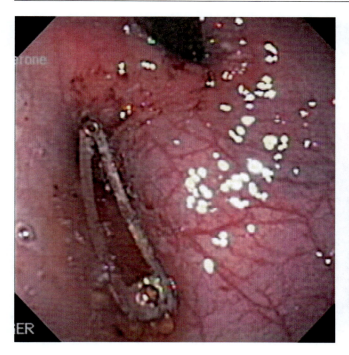

Fig. 32.4 Safety pin in the fundus of the stomach. It is closed and would have likely passed uneventfully through the GI tract

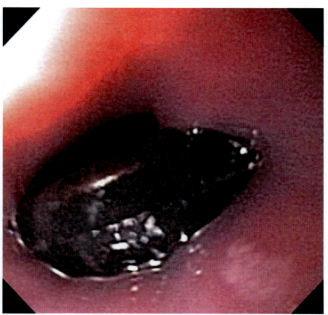

Fig. 32.5 Button battery in the upper esophagus. These can cause severe and penetrating injuries to the esophagus in a matter of hours and therefore need to be extracted emergently in all cases

pulling it out first; however, care should be taken if pushing an object into the stomach as there might be a distal stricture or underlying esophageal pathology. An alternative is to close the safety pin with a polypectomy snare. A closed safety pin in the stomach should pass the gastrointestinal tract without complications.

Razor blades can be managed with a rigid endoscope by pulling the blade into the instrument. The endoscopist can alternatively use a rubber hood on the end of the endoscope to protect the esophagus.

Batteries

Button batteries (Fig. 32.5) can cause significant injury when lodged in the esophagus. Each contains caustic alkalis similar to crystalline lye with a potential for leakage, significant burns, and pressure necrosis. Liquefaction necrosis and perforation can occur rapidly and therefore removal is always an emergency. Esophageal mucosal burns have been noted within 1 h of ingestion, with involvement of all layers within 4 h after ingestion, and perforation as soon as 6 h. Emetics should not be used for risk of aspiration, retrograde advancement of battery from the stomach to esophagus, or perforation if mucosal injury has occurred. Administration of neutralizing agents or charcoal has not been of benefit. A delay in diagnosis can result in aorto-esophageal fistula.

A retrieval basket, retrieval net, or polyp snare is usually successful. One can also use the "through-the-scope" balloon under direct vision. It is not recommended to push the battery into the stomach as there might be a distal stricture or underlying esophageal pathology. Once in the stomach, however, batteries usually pass without consequence. Batteries that have passed beyond the esophagus do not need to be retrieved unless the patient experiences symptoms, if a large-diameter battery (greater than 20 mm in diameter) remains in the stomach for more than 48 h, or if the battery contains lithium. Once beyond the duodenal sweep, 85% pass within 72 h. Batteries greater than 15 mm in size that do not pass the pylorus within 48 h are less likely to pass spontaneously and thus generally require removal. In children less than 6 years of age, batteries larger than 15 mm are not likely to pass spontaneously. Failure to be recovered in the stool within 7 days requires serial radiographic evaluation and retrieval by endoscopy. If the patient develops peritoneal signs, surgical removal is required. If there is evidence of tissue damage, follow-up barium study within 10–14 days is recommended to rule out stricture or fistula formation.

The battery should be identified by size and imprint code, or by evaluation of a duplicate, measurement of the battery compartment, or examination of the product, packaging, and instructions. If the chemical system cannot be identified from packaging or product instructions, it can be determined from the imprint code by calling the National Button Battery Ingestion Hotline at 202-625-3333. The Poison Control Center can also be called at 800-222-1222 for both ingestion of batteries and caustic materials. Lithium batteries produce more severe injury than alkaline batteries, with damage occurring within minutes. If mercuric oxide cells are ingested and the cell is observed to split in the gastrointestinal tract or radiopaque droplets are evident in the gastrointestinal tract, blood and urine mercury levels must be followed.

Food Impaction

Esophageal food impaction occurs in children with an esophageal stricture, esophageal dysmotility disorder, or eosinophilic esophagitis. Impaction of meat or food is the most common cause of accidental ingestion in adolescents and adults. Children who are in severe distress or unable to handle their own secretions require urgent attention. If the patient is not symptomatic, endoscopy may be postponed up to 12 h as food impactions often pass. Endoscopic intervention should not be delayed more than 24 h as the risk of complications increases. Rigid endoscopy with alligator forceps is often more successful in removal of food impactions or vegetable matter than flexible endoscopy. With the flexible endoscope, removal can be en bloc or piecemeal with rat tooth forceps, tripod or pentapod forceps, or retrieval net. The use of cautery current applied to a bipolar snare to cut into, grasp or retrieve the food bolus has been reported. An overtube can be used to protect the esophagus and decrease the risk of aspiration. However, there is a risk of esophageal injury with overtube insertion. Once the food impaction is reduced in size, if needed, it can be pushed into the stomach only under endoscopic visualization and direction. The endoscope should be steered around the food bolus, into the stomach and then pulled back to gently push the contents in to the stomach. Care should be taken not to push the food into the stomach without visualizing the distal esophagus.

The use of proteolytic enzymes, such as papain, is not recommended. There is a high association with hypernatremia, erosion, and esophageal perforation. Glucagon, a smooth muscle relaxant, is generally not recommended because it can cause retching, vomiting, and chest pain.

Magnets and Lead

The ingestion of magnets poses a danger to children. The number of magnets is thought to be critical. If a single magnet is ingested, there is the least likelihood of complications. If two or more magnets are ingested, the magnetic poles are attracted to each other and create the risk of obstruction, fistula development, and perforation. After biplane radiographs are obtained, endoscopic removal is urgent when multiple magnets are ingested and are within endoscopic reach. If the

magnets are beyond the reach of the endoscope, careful monitoring or surgical consultation for removal are options that should be made on an individual basis. Abdominal pain or peritoneal signs require urgent surgical intervention.

Lead-based foreign bodies can cause lead intoxication. Early endoscopic removal is indicated if an object is suspected to contain lead and lead level should be measured. Gastric acid might promote dissolution of the lead with subsequent duodenal absorption.

Narcotic Packets

Body bagging or body packing is a way to smuggle drugs. Narcotic wrapped in plastic or contained in latex condoms can usually be seen CT. Drug bags should be removed surgically if they fail to progress or rupture, or if there are signs of intestinal obstruction. Endoscopic retrieval is not recommended because of the risk of rupture, which can be fatal.

Postoperative Care

Following uncomplicated removal of an asymptomatic foreign body, most patients can be fed after having recovered from anesthesia. In the case of an atypical foreign body, difficult extraction, or significant underlying disease, patients should be observed for some time. A chest radiograph should be obtained to evaluate the possibility of free mediastinal air or pleural effusion, infiltrate or pneumothorax. Either one or both hemithoraces can be affected. If perforation is suspected, contrast esophagography should be performed with water-soluble contrast.

Alternative Methods

The use of an endoscope is considered the gold standard for evaluating and removal of foreign bodies. However, other methods have been advocated and may be useful in selected circumstances. Pharmacologic agents such as nifedipine have been used with varying degrees of success to facilitate the passage of an impacted foreign body by manipulating esophageal muscular tone, but have not been generally successful in children. Glucagon does not appear to be effective in the dislodgement of esophageal coins in children. Enzymatic digestion of a meat bolus with papain has largely been abandoned because of an unacceptable complication rate including hypernatremia, erosion and esophageal perforation. Emetic agents are ineffective and unsafe. Blind bougienage with Maloney dilators and nasogastric tubes to push the object into the stomach are occasionally used, but current opinion favors abandoning these methods as lacking safety and efficacy. Non-endoscopic removal of foreign bodies does not allow evaluation of esophageal injury or visualization of multiple or radiolucent foreign bodies. An endoscopist can use a Foley balloon catheter to remove esophageal coins and blunt objects. The catheter is placed orally under fluoroscopy to keep the foreign body out of the nasopharynx. This technique should not be used if the foreign body has been present for more than 24 h or if there is edema. It is recommended only if endoscopy is not available.

Some newer techniques include a double snare technique for long objects, a friction adapter for meat impactions, and combined forceps-snare technique for safety pins. A suture technique has been described in which a surgical suture is placed through the biopsy channel and a loop of suture is placed around the foreign body. The suture is tightened and the suture, foreign body and endoscope are removed together. It also allows for parallel removal of an object with respect to the esophagus. The use of a banding device, which is routinely used for esophageal variceal ligation, has been described in the literature for removal of food impactions. In such cases, the food impaction is drawn into the cylinder with suction and removed from the esophagus.

Pitfalls

Foreign bodies should be removed from the gastrointestinal tract only under general anesthesia with the patient intubated. To avoid perforation, the endoscope and instruments should only be advanced when the esophageal lumen is visible, and the distal end of the instrument is visible within the esophageal lumen.

A suction channel can be used to aspirate secretions that interfere with visualization. Foreign bodies are sometimes surrounded and obscured by granulation tissue, and some that escape detection during prograde endoscopy can sometimes be found while slowly withdrawing the endoscope. After foreign body removal, it is reasonable to repeat endoscopy to evaluate the possibility of mucosal erosions or additional foreign bodies, as well as underlying strictures or other lesions, especially if the object was atypical.

Complications

Sharp objects have a perforation rate of 15–35%, but even blunt objects can cause stridor, esophageal erosions, aorto- or tracheoesophageal fistulas, mediastinitis, or paraesophageal abscess.

Other complications of esophageal foreign bodies include esophageal edema, laceration or erosion, hematoma, granulation tissue, retropharyngeal abscess, migration of foreign body into the fascial spaces of the neck, arterial-esophageal fistula with massive hemorrhage, respiratory problems, strictures, and proximal esophageal dilation. Nickel dermatitis and associated gastritis as well as copper and zinc toxicity have been reported after coin ingestion.

Food-related esophageal trauma is rare. In adults, esophageal hematoma or laceration has followed ingestion of tortilla chips, taco shells, bagels, and bay leaves. Esophageal burns have been associated with hot pepper sauce. Inflammation is associated with significant increase of esophageal peristalsis.

Esophageal perforation can occur as a consequence of ulceration or erosion of the esophageal wall from the foreign body. Perforations most commonly occur at the weakest points of the esophageal wall, such as the area just below the cricopharyngeus, the distal one-fifth, or the site of any local lesion that weakens the wall. Symptoms include retrosternal pain, back pain, and fever. Subcutaneous emphysema might be evident on physical examination. Because the retrovisceral space and the superior mediastinum have few tissue barriers, infection following rupture spreads rapidly and extensively and can result in septic mediastinitis.

Perforation caused by endoscopy can often be managed by prohibiting oral intake, and administering antibiotics and intravenous fluids. A feeding jejunostomy is occasionally indicated. If the tear is large or there is evidence of infection in the pleural space or mediastinum, surgical repair and drainage should be performed urgently. A pleural effusion necessitates drainage. The associated mortality rate is high and is greater in patients under 10 years of age or if recognition is delayed 24 h or longer.

Other potential complications of endoscopy include crico-arytenoid joint dislocation and bleeding. Insufflation used during endoscopy can cause abdominal distention, contributing to respiratory compromise. Judicious choice of instrument diameter and length, maintaining visualization of the esophageal lumen, and gentle technique help to prevent complications.

Most patients who have undergone atraumatic removal of asymptomatic esophageal coins do not require additional follow-up; however, children with atypical impactions often have a predisposing condition such as esophageal strictures or neuromuscular disturbance. Patients are instructed to return for follow-up if they have risk factors for esophageal stricture or have dysphagia or signs or symptoms of esophageal perforation, in which case a barium swallow or additional swallowing evaluations may be useful. If there is evidence of tissue damage, follow-up barium study within 10–14 days is recommended to rule out stricture or fistula formation.

Caustic Ingestion

Caustic ingestions remain a significant health concern. The frequency of admission for caustic ingestion ranges from 1,000 to 20,000 per year in industrialized countries, the majority of which are children. Caustic ingestions are the leading toxic exposure in children and are surpassed only by analgesic drugs in adults. Children account for the majority of poison exposures, 75% of which are ingestions. The most frequent exposures in children are mild alkalis, such as household bleach. The age distribution is bimodal, occurring as accidental ingestions in children younger than 5 years and as suicide attempts in those older than 20 years.

The ingestion of corrosive agents can cause devastating injury to the esophagus and stomach (Fig. 32.6). The extent of injury depends on the type, concentration, and quantity of corrosive and the duration of exposure. Caustic ingestions are most often strong alkali or acidic agents. Liquid forms cause more significant injuries than solid products. Household bleach, liquid laundry detergents, and ammonia usually result in mild esophageal burns since they are weak bases at low concentrations. Ammonia, also results in chemical pneumonitis and pulmonary edema. Ingestions of strong alkalis such as liquid lye, dishwasher cleaner, oven or toilet bowel cleaner, Clinitest tablets, or button batteries are associated with the most deaths since they represent the highest concentration of a strong base (Table 32.1). Clinitest tablets also cause a thermal injury leading to deep burns. Lye is odorless

Table 32.1 Caustic agents	
Chemical agent	Source
Alkaline	
Ammonia	Toilet bowel cleaners
	Hair dyes
	Floor strippers
	Glass cleaners
Sodium hydroxide	Clinitest tablets
	Detergents
	Laundry powders
	Paint removers
	Drain cleaners
	Oven cleaners
	Button batteries
Sodium borates, carbonates, phosphates	Detergents
	Electric dishwashers
	Water softeners
Sodium hypochlorite	Bleaches
	Cleaners
Acid	
Hydrochloric acid	Swimming pool cleaners
	Metal cleaners
	Toilet bowel cleaners
Hydrofluoric acid	Antirust products
	Liquid refrigerant
Sulfuric acid	Automobile batteries
	Drain cleaners

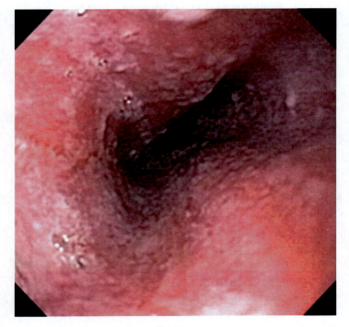

Fig. 32.6 Esophagoscopy after liquid lye (drain cleaner) ingestion. Note the presence of an exudate but apparently intact and viable mucosa, suggesting a superficial injury, at least in this location

and tasteless and its high viscosity results in a slow transit time with prolonged exposure and deeper tissue penetration.

The physical form and pH of the corrosive agent play a significant role in the resultant injuries. Alkalis produce a liquefactive necrosis with rapid tissue penetration. The most significant injuries occur at pH exceeding 11, and pH >12.5 causes esophageal ulceration. An alkaline ingestion causes violent regurgitation against a closed cricopharyngeus, typically re-exposing the esophageal mucosa to further injury after the initial insult. Lye tends to adhere to the oropharynx, where it causes most of its damage, whereas high density drain cleaners cause more injuries to the lower esophagus and stomach. In contrast, the odor and bitter taste of strong acids induce a rapid expectoration that is somewhat protective. The lack of viscosity of acids is associated with a rapid transit time and relative esophageal sparing. Thus, acids usually spare the oropharynx and esophagus, causing skip lesions and a higher incidence of distal perforations. Any acid with a pH <2 should be considered capable of causing severe damage.

Acids cause a coagulation necrosis and a superficial eschar. This coagulum limits the extension of further mucosal penetration beyond the surface burn. Strong acids are found in battery fluids, antirust compounds, and swimming pool cleaners. A caveat is that the ingestion of highly concentrated sulfuric or hydrochloric acid causes esophageal injury in about half of cases. Hydrofluoric acid is another notable exception because it produces liquefactive necrosis and immediate life-threatening disturbances of calcium metabolism.

Following the ingestion of either acid or alkali, hemorrhage, thrombosis, or a marked inflammatory response with significant edema are present within the first 24 h after ingestion (early acute phase). Inflammation can extend through the muscle layer, and perforation can occur. After several days, the necrotic tissue is sloughed, edema decreases, and neovascularization occurs. This subacute phase usually last through the second week after injury, and with minor burns, esophageal function returns. The cicatrisation phase begins when fibroblast proliferation replaces the submucosa and muscularis mucosa. It is at this stage that stricture formation occurs. Reepithelization begins around the third week and is not complete until the sixth week after injury.

Presentation

The clinical presentation of corrosive ingestion varies from a normal physical examination without symptoms to respiratory distress and shock. The most common features of ingestions are oropharyngeal burning, odynophagia, dysphagia, and chest pain. Clinical symptoms are poor predictors of the degree of injury. Stridor is indicative of laryngeal and epiglottal edema. Drooling in the setting of stridor is highly suggestive of esophageal injury. Dysphagia and hematemesis are further suggestive of esophageal injury. Retrosternal pain radiating to the back and acute epigastric pain herald a full-thickness injury to the esophagus and stomach, respectively. Sloughing of the esophageal mucosa elicits hematemesis. Hemodynamic instability with systemic signs such as a change in mental status, fever, and tachycardia typically follow massive ingestion. Severe injuries with peritoneal signs, cervical crepitance, and retrosternal pain radiating to the back are ominous findings, consistent with esophageal perforation and impeding mediastinitis.

In corrosive injuries, intense pylorospasm and gastric atony limit passage into the duodenum, which results in pooling of the material in the antrum and fundic sparing. Large volume ingestions can overcome the reflex pylorospasm and extend into contiguous structures beyond the duodenum. All areas of esophageal anatomic narrowing or sites of pooling are potential areas of prolonged contact resulting in circumferential injuries and severe strictures. Such areas of narrowing or pooling include the hypopharynx, cricopharyngeus, aortic arch, tracheal bifurcation, and distal esophagus.

Serious esophageal burn, including perforation, can occur in the absence of oropharyngeal burns or abdominal pain. On the other hand, burns to the mouth do not provide evidence of an esophageal burn.

Immediate Intervention

The primary goals of management are to identify the severity of injury and minimize the extension of injury. The type and amount of corrosive ingested should be identified in the history if possible. The initial priority is airway assessment and stabilization with fluid resuscitation. Direct visualization of the oropharynx is the initial step in evaluating the extent of injury. Stridor strongly suggests laryngeal insult and mandates orotracheal intubation. If there are signs of laryngeal edema or changes in mental status, an airway should be established by orotracheal intubation or, less commonly, tracheostomy. Blind passage of the nasogastric tube or blind nasopharyngeal intubation is contraindicated.

Measures to dilute or neutralize the corrosive agent are contraindicated. Ingestion of water or milk can stimulate vomiting which results in re-exposure. Alkalis cause such rapid tissue penetration that immediate attempts at dilution are unsuccessful. With concentrated acid injuries, large volumes of water may dilute and successfully neutralize the acid only if given immediately after the ingestion; however, attempts to neutralize acids or alkalis cause an exothermic reaction, enhancing the destruction of surrounding tissue. Therefore, all oral intake should be prohibited.

Activated charcoal interferes with endoscopy and further compromises management. Emetic agents are also contraindicated. Biplane radiographs of the chest and abdomen readily identify specific operative indications such as pneumoperitoneum, pneumomediastinum, and pleural effusions, all associated with full thickness injury and necessitating immediate operative intervention.

The ingestion of concentrated hydrofluoric acid can cause significant gastritis and life-threatening calcium disturbances. The risk of perforation by passage of a nasogastric tube is markedly lower than the risk of systemic absorption of hydrofluoric acid. Uniquely in this exposure, blind nasogastric decompression to evacuate the stomach is acceptable because these exposures are otherwise universally fatal.

Early endoscopy is the gold standard for the evaluation of caustic injuries and should occur within the first 12–24 h. The reason for early endoscopy is that most perforations occur in a delayed fashion around the second to third day after injury. It is unlikely that a significant burn will be missed if endoscopy is performed only 12 h after ingestion. Endoscopy is indicated in all instances of stridor, all intended suicidal ingestions, and any symptomatic child. Endoscopy is not essential in patients already meeting operative criteria with evidence of esophageal or gastric perforations or mediastinitis.

Based on endoscopic criteria, caustic esophageal injuries should be classified by grade (Table 32.2). No evidence of esophageal damage is grade 0. First degree injuries include

Table 32.2 Classification of caustic injuries

Grade	Degree of injury	Endoscopic characteristics
0	None	Normal esophagus
I	Superficial mucosal burn	Mucosal edema and hyperemia
IIA	Transmucosal injury	Noncircumferential, patchy, superficial ulcerations, exudates, mucosal sloughing over <1/3 esophagus length
IIB	Transmucosal injury	Circumferential injury, deeper ulcerations, exudates, mucosal sloughing over >1/3 esophageal length
IIIA	Transmural injury, periesophageal or perigastric extension	Deep ulcerations, black of gray discoloration, full-thickness necrosis over < 1/3 of esophagus
IIIB	Transmural injury, periesophageal or perigastric extension	Deep ulcerations, black of gray discoloration, full-thickness necrosis over > 1/3 of esophagus
IV	Transmural injury, periesophageal or perigastric extension	Deep ulcerations, black of gray discoloration, full-thickness necrosis associated with shock, coagulopathy, or metabolic acidosis

superficial erythema and edema, and mucosal sloughing without scar or stricture. Grade II-A are non-circumferential superficial mucosal ulcerations with necrotic tissue and white plaques extending over less than one-third of the esophageal length. Grade II-B are the same as grade II-A, but with deep or circumferential ulcerations extending over more than one-third of the esophagus. Grade III injuries involve full-thickness esophageal injury with perforation into or through the muscle layers. Grade III-A injuries include mucosal ulcerations and areas of necrosis in a circumferential pattern extending over less than one-third of the esophageal length. Grade III-B injuries include extensive necrosis over more than one-third of the esophageal length. Some authors include a Grade IV, indicative of signs of transmural necrosis, shock, coagulopathy, and metabolic necrosis. Grade I and IIA injuries do not evoke strictures. Other authors do not take into account the circumferential appearance of the lesion. Distinguishing grade II from grade III lesions can therefore be difficult. Most grade III injuries and more than 70% of grade IIB injuries have some degree of progression to strictures.

The limitations of endoscopy include (a) the presence of circumferential burns that preclude full visualization, (b) the unrecognized progression of caustic injuries resulting in delayed perforation at 7–14 days, and (c) the difficulty in reliably distinguishing grade IIB from grade III injuries. Differentiation between second and third-degree injuries is often difficult, but third-degree injuries are usually associated with gray, friable tissue, thrombosed submucosal vessels, and extensive black eschar.

Endoscopy up to the site of maximal esophageal injury provides the ideal evaluation to direct therapy and minimizes the risks of iatrogenic perforation. Contrast radiography is a method of identifying grade III injuries and is performed first with water soluble contrast followed by thin barium contrast. Dye extravasation is diagnostic for perforation. Because endoscopy is limited to superficial mucosal evaluation only, laparoscopy can assist in documenting full-thickness injury.

Treatment

The severity of the endoscopic grade of injury correlates with the expected incidence of subsequent strictures. Endoscopic grades of injury exceeding grade IIA are associated with esophageal perforation, infection, and stricture. Limiting the severity of injury is important because esophageal replacement can be problematic and is less satisfactory than retention of a damaged but functional esophagus.

Most investigators recommend the judicious use of broad spectrum antibiotics to cover oropharyngeal flora, because tissue disruption provides a source of bacteremia. Tissue turnover and remodeling for caustic burns is significant, and delayed perforation of the esophagus can occur between seven and 14 days post-ingestion. Fever and impending perforation can be partially masked by prophylactic antibiotics. However, the use of antibiotics is advocated for all patients also receiving corticosteroids to decrease the higher incidence of associated infection.

The role of corticosteroids was purported to arrest inflammation and prevent strictures. In the 1960s, the introduction of steroids to reduce the inflammatory response combined with antibiotics to reduce infection resulted in reduced mortality; however, most recent control studies have shown no benefit. In grade I and IIA injuries strictures are rare and steroids provide no benefit. Grade III injuries evolve into strictures regardless of therapy; thus steroids do not provide a definitive long-term benefit. In grade IIB injuries, they are of unproven efficacy and might have a detrimental effect by masking an evolving perforation or delaying the diagnosis of infection. Future randomized studies that focus on grade II injuries might help clarify the value of steroids.

Acid suppression is recommended to decrease acid reflux, and possibly decrease stricture rates. Intravenous alimentation is essential in those with perforations and delayed enteric feedings. A nasogastric tube is often left in place for 6 weeks for circumferential second and all third degree burns. Gastrostomy, jejunostomy, or a nasogastric tube provides a nutritional conduit. Gastrostomies are placed in children with severe injuries to provide enteral feedings and a route for retrograde dilatations. If a grade I or IIA injury is found, the patient may be started on liquids in 48 h. Grade IIB and III injuries should be observed for at least 48 h and started on hyperalimentation. Vigilant observation is essential to detect delayed perforations and acute aorto-esophageal fistulas.

Early identification of patients with full-thickness injuries to the upper digestive tract is critical for immediate resection of devitalized organs and limiting further extension of the corrosive injury. The decision to perform emergent surgery is dictated by radiographic signs of perforation, the presence of peritoneal signs, or endoscopic stigmata of a full-thickness injury. Delaying surgical repair has been associated with increased morbidity and mortality. Identifying the subtle evolution of corrosive injuries in patients who have not manifested evidence of significant tissue damage initially is challenging. The overall mortality rate is high, but has been reduced from 20 to 3% over the past 20 years due to improved and timely surgery and the early introduction of parental nutrition and antibiotics. Full-thickness esophageal necrosis is associated with high morbidity and a 20% mortality rate. A depressed or agitated mental status, shock, persistent acidemia, or coagulation disorders are usually associated with severe findings intraoperatively. Some surgeons advocate routine laparotomy or laparoscopy for patient with grade IIB and III burns of the esophagus for evaluation of serosal surfaces to determine full-thickness injury.

The operative field should span from the mandible to the pelvis to accommodate cervical, thoracic, and abdominal approaches. Emergent operative intervention is best approached through the abdomen with complete visualization of the stomach and contiguous structures. Black eschar and thrombosis of the submucosal vessels indicate full-thickness gastric injury and warrant consideration of a total gastrectomy. Severe gastric injury is often associated with an equally severe esophageal injury. An emergent esophageal resection can be performed though a transhiatal approach, thus avoiding a thoracotomy. A transhiatal dissection for a total esophagogastrectomy is facilitated by the extensive acute periesophageal edema. A cervical esophagostomy is created, and a feeding jejunostomy is placed for enteral feeds. Delaying resection in the setting of third-degree burns and perforation is associated with 100% mortality. Tracheoesophageal fistulas can occur within the first week of injury and usually necessitate tracheostomy, cervical esophagostomy, and gastrostomy. After immediate and urgent resection, reconstruction is delayed for several months.

Esophageal reconstruction is challenging and requires the use of a substernal isoperistaltic colon interposition with the right or transverse colon or a reversed gastric tube. Gastric tubes may be of inadequate length, usually due to the original injury, associated stricture, or gastrostomy. Other disadvantages are dumping symptoms following the usual pyloroplasty and reflux esophagitis occurring above the esophagogastric anastomosis. A colon interposition is still probably the most widely used anatomic reconstruction. It provides a similar anatomic reservoir and dependable blood supply. Redundancy and stasis are common late complications. Microvascularized free tissue jejunal grafts are excellent reconstructive bridges for minimal defects, particularly those in the hypopharynx, and can be used in conjunction with other surgical techniques.

Late Sequelae

Long-term complications from a caustic ingestion include esophageal stricture and the potential for malignant transformation. Stricture formation can be up to 15%, mainly from grade III lesions and 70% from grade IIB. Acute inflammatory strictures appear by 3 weeks and complete stricture at by 4–6 weeks. Progressive dysphagia usually indicates a stricture, which can be documented radiographically or endoscopically. Bougienage is useful in the setting of a documented stricture more than 4 weeks after ingestion. Earlier dilations carry a higher risk for iatrogenic perforations.

Persistent strictures or iatrogenic perforation may necessitate esophagectomy with esophagogastric anastomosis or colonic interposition. An esophageal bypass leaves the native esophagus in situ with the reconstruction of a new esophageal conduit and risks the formation of a mucocele in the isolated remnant.

Lye ingestion is associated with esophageal motor dysfunction, which is delayed for days to years after ingestion. Motor dysfunction is manifested as weak to absent peristaltic contractions, non-propulsive contractions, gastroesophageal reflux, and dysphagia. Pyloric stenosis can occur after gastric injury, especially those due to acidic agents. Other sequelae include achalasia and bradyesophagus.

In general, caustic esophageal burns are regarded as premalignant. The risk for carcinomatous degeneration in the strictured residual esophagus is said to be up to 1,000-fold higher than the expected frequency in the general population. Carcinoma is most commonly seen after lye ingestion. The interval between injury and development of cancer is unknown but averages more than 40 years. Tumors are usually squamous cell cancers and typically develop in the mid-esophagus. Long-term annual follow-up of patients with grade IIB and III injuries is warranted. Persistent or recurrent dysphagia after a caustic ingestion should be evaluated annually, with both endoscopy and barium swallow. Periodic endoscopic biopsies are essential in evaluating the retained segment or documented stricture.

Summary Points

- Although ingestion of foreign bodies are usually accidental, child abuse, psychiatric illness, suicide, or Munchausen by proxy should be considered.
- Retrosternal chest pain, dysphagia, hypersalivation, stridor, and retching are typical symptoms of esophageal injuries in older children, but in young children, symptoms are not always obvious.
- If the patient is asymptomatic, an esophageal foreign body in the lower esophagus should be removed within 12–24 h of ingestion, in which case radiographic confirmation should be repeated immediately prior to endoscopy.
- The main anatomic locations for esophageal foreign body retention are the cricopharyngeus, the aortic arch, left main stem bronchus, and the lower esophageal sphincter.
- Following the ingestion of either acid or alkali, hemorrhage, thrombosis, and a marked inflammatory response with significant edema are present within the first 24 h after ingestion (early acute phase).
- Serious esophageal burn, including perforation, can occur in the absence of oropharyngeal burns or abdominal pain, and burns to the mouth do not provide evidence of an esophageal burn.
- After caustic ingestion, most recommend the judicious use of broad-spectrum antibiotics, but corticosteroids probably have little benefit in most cases.
- Caustic esophageal burns are regarded as pre-malignant (squamous cell carcinoma).

Editor's Comment

Esophageal foreign bodies can remain in place for a surprisingly long time before coming to the attention of a clinician. By then, the object can become deeply embedded in the wall of the esophagus, often surrounded by a considerable mass of granulation tissue and phlegmonous reaction. Some will have partially eroded through the wall and into adjacent tissues, usually walled off by several layers of inflammation. A pediatric thoracic surgeon will be asked in these situations to remove the foreign body at thoracotomy, although in some cases thoracoscopy might also be a reasonable option. A pre-operative CT scan helps with planning the approach and anticipating complications. The key elements of such an operation, as always, include: wide exposure, protection of adjacent structures (especially nerves and vessels), primary repair of the esophagus and, most importantly, adequate drainage. The wall of the esophagus itself is rarely able to be identified; rather, suture repair simply involves approximating layers of inflammatory tissue, arguably with little actual benefit. Most esophageal injuries will heal spontaneously if adequate drainage is achieved, essentially creating a controlled fistula. This means a large sump-type nasogastric tube to continuous suction in addition to a well-placed chest tube. Placement of a second suction catheter in the upper esophagus more proximal to the injury is unlikely to function as desired and adds significantly to the discomfort of the patient. Antibiotics that cover oral flora should be continued until the fistula has closed completely. After five to 7 days of *nil per os*, a contrast esophagram should be obtained and, if no leak is identified, the patient may resume oral intake. A leak will usually heal after another week or so of fasting. A cervical esophagostomy should almost never be required, except perhaps in the extremely rare case of uncontrolled mediastinal soiling and life-threatening sepsis.

Children with esophageal atresia and tracheo-esophageal fistula are at life-long risk of esophageal foreign body and food impaction due to either an actual stricture or an area of relative narrowing created by an inelastic ring of scar. Many pediatric surgeons will therefore continue to follow these patients into adulthood and prefer to perform foreign body removal and esophageal dilatation themselves.

Caustic injuries of the esophagus have thankfully become rare in most developed countries but remain a huge public health dilemma in the third world. The worst offenders are sodium hydroxide-based drain cleaners, as they are viscous and strangely palatable to young children. All patients, regardless of symptoms or severity of clinical presentation should undergo a careful esophagoscopy by an experienced endoscopist, who should conclude the examination as soon as a severe injury is identified. Nearly every patient should receive a gastrostomy tube, which should be placed in a location on the stomach that does not preclude the use of the stomach as a replacement, should this option eventually become necessary.

The very rare full-thickness esophageal injury with mediastinal extension is associated with a high risk of death and therefore mandates urgent esophagectomy. Nearly all other injuries can be observed and allowed to heal, which can take up to 4–6 weeks. Superficial injuries will usually heal without sequelae, while deeper burns inevitably result in strictures. Corticosteroids should be administered with caution, if at all, while antibiotics are probably of some benefit. All esophageal replacement operations are huge undertakings with a very high incidence of early complications and long-term problems; thus the adage that retaining a damaged native esophagus is almost always preferable to reconstructing the esophagus. For isolated strictures of the esophagus, balloon dilation under radiographic guidance is the safest and most effective technique. For long or multiple strictures, bougienage using tapered dilators passed over a wire or heavy suture that loops into the nose and out through a gastrostomy is still probably the best approach.

Esophageal replacement operations are chosen mostly on the basis of the surgeon's experience. Colonic interposition is the easiest, safest, and most popular operation; however the problem of long-term redundancy and stasis remains an unresolved issue – nearly every patient will develop recurrent symptoms and require multiple surgical revisions as an adult. Gastric pull-up and gastric tube operations are popular in some centers, but are also fraught with complications and the need for further surgery in the long term. The most anatomic replacement in terms of size and function appears to be the jejunum, but issues related to the blood supply of the graft and the relatively high risk of ischemia make it another less-than-perfect choice. Self-expanding wire stents have been tried but are associated with life-threatening complications (septic mediastinitis, esophago-aortic fistula) and are extremely difficult to remove once they become incorporated into the soft tissue of the esophageal wall. Their use outside of a carefully designed study and truly extreme circumstances should be condemned.

Differential Diagnosis

- Foreign body impaction
- Esophageal perforation
- Caustic ingestion

Diagnostic Studies

- Plain radiographs (chest X-ray)
- Contrast esophagram
- Flexible esophagoscopy
- Rigid esophagoscopy

Preoperative Preparation

- ☐ Prophylactic antibiotics
- ☐ Repeat radiograph prior to endoscopic retrieval of foreign body
- ☐ For surgical intervention, wide sterile preparation (neck, chest, abdomen)

Parental Preparation

- With endoscopy, there is a very small risk of esophageal perforation.
- There is no ideal surgical replacement for the esophagus so we will make every attempt to preserve the native esophagus, even if it is damaged.
- With foreign bodies that have become embedded in the wall of the esophagus, it is sometimes necessary to retrieve them by thoracotomy.

Technical Points

- Both rigid and flexible esophagoscopy are effective methods for removing foreign bodies.
- Urgent endoscopic intervention is required when a sharp object or disc battery is lodged in the esophagus, if an object is located in the upper third of the esophagus, if there is a high-grade obstruction, or if the child is unable to manage secretions.
- Esophageal mucosal burns have been noted within 1 h of caustic ingestion, with involvement of all layers within 4 h after ingestion, and perforation as soon as 6 h.
- Early endoscopy is the gold standard for the evaluation of caustic injuries and should occur within the first 12–24 h.
- Early identification of patients with full-thickness injury is critical for immediate resection of devitalized tissue and limiting further extension of the corrosive injury.

Suggested Reading

Ayantunde AA, Oke T. A review of gastrointestinal foreign bodies. Int J Clin Pract. 2006;60:735–9.

Cordero B, Savage RR, Cheng T. Corrosive ingestion. Pediatr Rev. 2006;27:154–5.

Eisen GM, Baron TH, Dominitz JA, et al. Guidelines for the management of ingested foreign bodies. Gastrointest Endosc. 2002;7:802–5.

Ginsberg G. Management of ingested foreign objects and food bolus impactions. Gastrointest Endosc. 1995;41(1):32–7.

Kay M, Wyllie R. Pediatric foreign bodies and their management. Pediatr Gastroenterol. 2005;7:212–8.

Mehta DI, Attia MW, Quintana EC, Cronan KM. Glucagon use for esophageal coin dislodgement in children: A prospective, double-blind, placebo-controlled trial. Acad Emerg Med. 2001;8:200–3.

Seikel K, Primm PA, Elizondo BJ, Remley KL. Handheld metal detector localization of ingested metallic foreign bodies. Accurate in any hands? Arch Pediatr Adolesc Med. 1999;153:853–7.

Smith CS, Miranda A, Rudolph CD, Sood MR. Removal of impacted food in children with eosinophilic esophagitis using Saeed banding device. J Pediatr Gastroenterol Nutr. 2007;44:521–3.

Chapter 33
Foregut Duplications

Pablo Laje

Foregut duplications are cystic or tubular malformations that arise from the cephalic segment of the primitive gastrointestinal tube. The foregut is an embryonic structure from which several respiratory and digestive structures originate: trachea, lungs, pharynx, esophagus, stomach, proximal duodenum, the parenchyma of the liver and pancreas. Most of these structures arise from the original tube as simple buds that then branch repeatedly. Foregut duplications are thought to be the result of abnormal additional buds that do not undergo a branching process and remain as simple blind cysts. They can occur at any level of the foregut, from the pharynx to the duodenum, but the vast majority develops from the tracheobronchial tree and the esophagus.

Foregut duplications are classified according to their location and organ of origin. Less than 3% are located in the neck, 60% are intra-thoracic, 30% are located in the upper abdomen and about 7% are thoraco-abdominal. The organ of origin determines the nature of the mucosal lining of the cyst: pharyngeal, esophageal, gastric, duodenal, or bronchogenic. Interestingly, the origin does not always correlate with the location: duodenal duplications can be found in the thorax, colonic duplications have been described in the neck, bronchogenic cysts have been found in the abdomen, and so on. Rarely, two or more foregut duplications have been described in a single patient. While the majority of foregut duplications do not communicate with the lumen of organ of origin, such a feature needs to be ruled out in the preoperative imaging work up. Despite sharing a common embryologic pathophysiology, duplications of the hepato-bilio-pancreatic tract are generally discussed separately because the clinical and therapeutic implications are substantially different.

P. Laje (✉)
Department of General Pediatric and Thoracic Surgery,
Children's Hospital of Philadelphia, Aapt K-1103,
Philadelphia, PA 19144, USA
e-mail: laje@email.chop.edu

Diagnosis

Symptomatic foregut duplications are generally identified during childhood, although some can remain silent for many years and present during adulthood. Thoracic foregut duplications can cause a variety of symptoms, most of which are related to a space-occupying effect. The esophagus can be compressed, causing dysphagia and regurgitation. The lungs can be compressed and resulting in either air trapping or atelectasis, which can be severe enough to produce respiratory symptoms such as dyspnea, cough, or wheezing. In some cases, a major airway can be compromised, causing severe respiratory distress that requires positive pressure ventilation and immediate surgical intervention. Foregut duplications typically contain a sterile mucoid fluid, but infections can occur, especially if there is a communication with the esophageal or respiratory lumen.

In rare cases, the mucosa of a duplication can bleed and produce hemoptysis or hematemesis, but again, only if there is a patent communication. Pain is hardly ever a symptom of a thoracic foregut duplication in children. In very rare cases, the major mediastinal veins can be compressed, but signs of venous congestion are exceptional. Despite the wide range of potential clinical manifestations, foregut duplications are for the most part asymptomatic and are usually incidentally found on imaging studies obtained for other reasons. In addition, the widespread use of prenatal screening ultrasound has significantly increased the detection of foregut duplications in utero, which allows the development of a prompt plan of care after birth.

On plain chest radiographs, foregut duplications appear as well-defined tissue-density structures, due to the high density of the mucoid content. However, since most of them are located in the mediastinum, the overlapping of multiple structures often makes them barely discernible. Occasionally, bronchogenic cysts are distant from the major airway and appear within the lung fields, away from the mediastinum. On lateral films, foregut duplications are generally seen in the middle or posterior mediastinum. Air–fluid levels indicate an open

P. Mattei (ed.), *Fundamentals of Pediatric Surgery*,
DOI 10.1007/978-1-4419-6643-8_33, © Springer Science+Business Media, LLC 2011

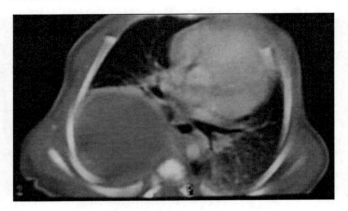

Fig. 33.1 Large foregut duplication in the right posterior thorax, displacing and compressing the airway, heart and great vessels

communication with the digestive or respiratory tract. A barium swallow is usually obtained to determine the proximity of the lesion to the esophagus and the degree of compression, and to rule out an open communication. The typical image is that of a concave indentation on the esophageal silhouette.

The next study in the work up process is usually computed tomography. Foregut duplications are discrete, well-circumscribed masses of homogeneous content that do not enhance with intravenous contrast (Fig. 33.1). The density of the content can vary according to the amount of protein in the fluid. In terms of location and relationship with surrounding structures, CT provides the best characterization of a foregut duplication, which is crucial when it comes to deciding the optimal surgical approach. The extent of compression exerted on surrounding structures can also be accurately determined by CT. Moreover, high resolution CT scans can help in ruling out communication between the lesion and the digestive or respiratory tracts. Finally, although not always necessary, three-dimensional CT reconstructions can provide very accurate information regarding the relationship between the mass and the great vessels. Other imaging studies are usually obtained only when there is concern for a certain differential diagnosis. MRI is particularly useful in assessing the spinal cord and canal, which is sometimes needed when an intrathoracic cyst is suspected to be of neural origin. An echocardiogram can help in cases of suspected pericardial cyst, and also provides dynamic cardiac information, which is useful when signs of venous congestion are present (superior vena cava syndrome).

duplications, bronchogenic cyst), but also a number of entities of diverse nature. While the final diagnosis can only be determined by the anatomic pathology, a highly precise presumed diagnosis can generally be made by a thorough examination of the preoperative imaging studies. When the cyst is in close proximity with the heart and does not have a clear dissecting plane with it, a *pericardial cyst* must be considered. Even though most of them have an irregular shape that conform to the contour of the heart, they can be fairly round and resemble a true foregut duplication. An echocardiogram can be of help to determine whether the cyst is intra- or extrapericardial. *Lymphatic malformations* can resemble foregut duplications on imaging studies, however most of them are irregular and have an infiltrative pattern of growth. Defects in the closure of the anterior aspect of the neural tube can result in a condition known as *anterior meningocele* (herniation of the meninges through a vertebral defect), which is most frequently found in the sacral region, but can be intra-thoracic. The key anatomical feature in these cases is a severe defect in one or more vertebral bodies. When this is found on a CT scan, an MRI is recommended to further characterize the relationship between the cyst and the spinal subarachnoid space, which are generally communicating. If such a communication is left untreated, a cerebrospinal fluid leak is guaranteed.

Vertebral defects can also be associated with true foregut duplications that are in direct contact with the spinal cord components. These have a complex embryologic pathogenesis, and are referred to as *neuroenteric cysts*. *Congenital cystic adenomatoid malformations* are usually solid-cystic masses, but occasionally they can consist of a large single cyst that mimics a foregut duplication. They develop within the parenchyma of the lung, so they tend to be located off the midline. *Cystic germ cell tumors* and *cystic thymic tumors* are very rare and generally located in the anterior or middle mediastinum, but can resemble a foregut duplication if they are clearly demarcated and homogeneous. If abnormal endocrine features are clinically present in conjunction with a cystic mediastinal mass, a germ cell origin must be suspected. Among other rare diagnoses in the differential, *pulmonary hydatid cysts* can mimic a thoracic foregut duplication, especially if they are located close to the midline. A positive epidemiologic background and the coexistence of similar cysts in other organs should raise the suspicion of these rare lesions.

Differential Diagnosis

There are several diagnoses to be considered when a thoracic cystic mass is discovered, not only all the variants of a true foregut duplication (esophageal, gastric and duodenal

Treatment

All foregut duplications must be resected. If they are symptomatic, they must be resected to relieve the symptoms, and if they are asymptomatic, they must be resected for several reasons: (1) space-occupying masses are likely to eventually compress adjacent structures, compromising their function; (2) if there is an open communication with the lumen of the respiratory or digestive tract, infections can occur, which are difficult to clear and make the eventual surgical resection technically much more difficult; (3) in young children, all thoracic space-occupying masses must be resected to allow adequate compensatory lung growth; and (4) malignant degeneration of the mucosa of foregut duplications has been reported and the timing is unpredictable. Partial resection, aspiration of the cyst contents, marsupialization or simple unroofing of the cyst are never recommended because the recurrence rate is extremely high and because they do not eliminate the potential for malignant transformation.

Foregut duplications can be resected using an open or minimally invasive approach. The MIS approach is feasible in the majority of cases, with the exception of the few that produce massively distended lung lobes due to air trapping, in which case an adequate thoracoscopic view is impossible to obtain. The size of the foregut duplication, on the other hand, is never a limiting factor, because partial decompression can always be accomplished with a needle inserted percutaneously under direct vision. In order to optimize the operative space, single-lung ventilation should always be used. In addition, a CO_2 pneumothorax through valved trocars is always of great help and can be rapidly released should the patient develop hypercarbia or diminished venous return.

Since the location of the cyst is variable, the patient's position must be determined on a case-by-case basis. As a general rule, for cysts that are located in the para-vertebral posterior mediastinum, the patient should be placed in a lateral decubitus position (with the side of the lesion up), leaning slightly forward with the upper arm extended over the head, and with the surgeon and assistant standing at the patient's front facing a monitor located at the patient's back. The size of the instruments to be used depends on the size of the patient: neonates should be operated on with 3-mm instruments, older children with 5-mm instruments. As for any minimally invasive procedure performed in the thoracic cavity, thirty-degree scopes are preferred over zero-degree scopes. In general, three trocars are required to safely and effectively resect a foregut duplication, but in some cases a fourth trocar may be necessary. The position of the trocars must be determined by the location of the cyst. It is recommended to place the initial trocar in a neutral site, insert the scope, and decide the position of the remaining trocars according to what is determined by direct visualization. The trocars can be placed in a linear orientation, which is ergonomically better, but with lower versatility to interchange the scope and instruments, or a triangular orientation.

After all trocars have been inserted and secured, the thoracic cavity must be thoroughly inspected. Once the foregut duplication is identified, it must be gently dissected off the surrounding structures. Preferably, it should not be decompressed until the end of the procedure because the tension helps with the dissection and the spillage can compromise proper visualization. In general, foregut duplications are loosely attached to most of the surrounding structures, and firmly attached to the organ from which they arise, so, in the thorax, the dissection between the cyst and the esophagus or the tracheobronchial tree must be precise. The original pathophysiologic theories claimed that foregut duplications must, by definition, have a common muscular wall with the organ of origin. While this statement has been recently disputed because this feature is not present in all cases, it is indeed observed frequently. Once the cyst has been entirely dissected and the content aspirated, it is extracted through a slightly enlarged port site.

If there is a known open communication between the duplication and the originating organ, it must be identified and repaired. An opening in the esophagus must be treated with interrupted stitches, post-operative nasogastric decompression (to avoid the high intra-luminal pressure associated with vomiting), chest-tube drainage, and a contrast study after the fifth post-operative day. An opening in a major airway must be treated with interrupted stitches and a chest tube drain, which should remain in place for a minimum of 24 h in the absence of an air leak or pneumothorax. If an air leak is present, the chest tube should prevent the development of a pneumothorax, and will allow monitoring of its evolution. Thoraco-abdominal foregut duplications can also be treated by a MIS approach. After the thoracic component has been thoroughly dissected all the way down to the trans-diaphragmatic stalk, the patient can be turned to a supine position for a laparoscopy and completion of the resection.

The classical open approach for the treatment of foregut duplications is through a postero-lateral thoracotomy at the level of the 4th or 5th intercostal space. A muscle-sparing thoracotomy should always be attempted. The abdominal component of thoraco-abdominal foregut duplications can be treated through a phrenotomy from the thorax, or through a formal laparotomy.

Postoperative Care

The recovery for an elective resection of a foregut duplication is generally fast. Pain management is usually straightforward in patients after a thoracoscopic resection, usually including less than 24 h of intravenous analgesia followed by oral non-narcotic agents. For patients who undergo open surgery, thoracic epidural analgesia, if available, is the best option for immediate post-operative management. Enteral alimentation should be resumed promptly, except in those patients with an esophageal suture line, who should wait until the barium swallow confirms that there is no esophageal leak. Antibiotic treatment is only required perioperatively, unless an infection of the cyst is encountered, in which case cultures should be sent and treatment extended accordingly.

The postoperative course for cases not involving repair of the esophagus or airway is usually uneventful. Small air leaks from a tiny lung injury are somewhat common and resolve spontaneously within 24–72 h. Significant air leaks from tears in the major airway generally require surgical re-exploration and repair. Esophageal leaks are dangerous due to the risk of mediastinitis, and should be closely monitored. Adequate chest drainage, broad antibiotic coverage and appropriate nutrition are critical for a successful outcome. If there are no signs of mediastinitis and there is adequate drainage, a temporizing non-operative approach is the best option. On the other hand, if mediastinitis is suspected, operative intervention may be required.

The long term post-operative course is uneventful in the vast majority of patients. Only those with severe immediate complications are at risk for long-term complications (esophageal strictures or airway strictures) and require a closer follow-up.

Summary Points

- Foregut duplications are aberrant cystic or tubular malformations that arise from the cephalic segment of the primitive gastrointestinal tube. The majority are located in the thorax.
- The primitive gastrointestinal tube, or foregut, is an embryonic structure from which several respiratory and digestive structures originate: trachea, lungs, pharynx, esophagus, stomach, proximal duodenum, and the parenchyma of the liver and pancreas.
- The term "foregut duplication" comprises a wide group of entities that share a common embryologic pathophysiology. The most common ones are esophageal duplications, duodenal duplications, gastric duplications and bronchogenic cysts.
- The organ of origin (usually determined by the type of mucosa lining the inner surface of the duplication) does not always correlate with the location of the malformation.
- The majority is asymptomatic, and found on imaging studies obtained for other reasons. Symptoms are generally associated with a space-occupying effect and the compression of adjacent organs.
- All foregut duplications must be resected. If they produce symptoms, the resection is intended to relieve them. If they are asymptomatic, they must be resected due to the high likelihood of becoming symptomatic, due to the potential for infections, to allow for compensatory lung growth, and due to the potential for malignant degeneration.

Editor's Comment

In clinical practice, foregut duplications include bronchogenic cysts and esophageal duplications. Nearly all can and should be excised thoracoscopically. Exceptions include some that communicate with or involve a long segment of the esophagus or airway, and those that were infected at one time and therefore likely to be extremely difficult to excise easily. As with all operations performed in the mediastinum, careful attention to avoid injury to adjacent structures (especially the phrenic and vagus nerves and the thoracic duct) is paramount, though fortunately these lesions typically separate from all important structures by gentle blunt dissection, until, of course, you reach the organ of origin, when patience and meticulous technique are critical. Spillage of the sterile contents of the cyst does not appear to increase the risk of recurrence or infection and is often performed deliberately to aid in the dissection of a large cyst or to remove it from the chest. When dealing with an especially adherent or fibrotic cyst wall, it is acceptable to enter the lumen and to strip the mucosa completely, leaving the fibrotic wall behind, but it is especially important to identify and repair communication with the lumen in these cases. Except when a lumen has been breached or frank infection is present, routine placement of a drains or chest tube is generally unnecessary.

Long, tubular thoraco-abdominal esophageal duplications can also be approached thoracoscopically, by mobilizing the thoracic portion first and then completing the dissection in the abdomen by laparoscopy or laparotomy. Extensive preoperative imaging with three-dimensional reconstruction is very useful in planning these challenging operations.

Differential Diagnosis

- Pericardial cyst
- Lymphatic malformations
- Anterior myelomeningocele
- Neuroenteric cyst
- Cystic congenital adenomatoid malformation
- Cystic teratoma
- Hydatid cyst

Diagnostic Studies

- Plain chest radiograph
- Esophagogram
- Computed tomography scan
- Echocardiogram
- Magnetic resonance imaging

Parental Preparation

- Possible opening of the esophagus
- Possible opening of the major airway
- In general, satisfactory outcome

Preoperative Preparation

- ☐ NPO/IV hydration
- ☐ Type and screen
- ☐ Blood on hold
- ☐ Informed consent

Technical Points

- Open or minimally invasive approach are feasible
- Thorough examination of the thoracic cavity
- Gentle blunt dissection of the duplication
- Careful dissection of the plane between the duplication and then organ of origin
- Careful search for a patent communication with the esophagus or airway

Suggested Readings

Azzie G, Beasley S. Diagnosis and treatment of foregut duplications. Semin Pediatr Surg. 2003;12(1):46–54.

Holcomb III GW, Gheissari A, O'Neill Jr JA, et al. Surgical management of alimentary tract duplications. Ann Surg. 1989;209(2):167–74.

Martinez-Ferro M, Laje P, Piaggio L. Combined thoraco-laparoscopy for trans-diaphragmatic thoraco-abdominal enteric duplications. J Pediatr Surg. 2005;40(9):e37–40.

Nobuhara KK, Gorski YC, La Quaglia MP, et al. Bronchogenic cysts and esophageal duplications: common origins and treatment. J Pediatr Surg. 1997;32(10):1408–13.

Chapter 34
Achalasia

J. Duncan Phillips

Achalasia is an uncommon disorder of esophageal dysmotility, with an annual incidence of only 1 in 100,000 individuals. Although usually thought of as being simply a failure of normal relaxation of the lower esophageal sphincter (LES) during swallowing, it is actually part of a more diffuse disease of esophageal function. Because treatment for diminished or absent esophageal peristalsis is so poorly developed at this time, clinicians tend to focus on the LES, which is the only part of esophageal anatomy that lends itself to intervention.

Normal swallowing is a complex process that involves antegrade propulsion of ingested liquids and solids by coordinated peristaltic contractions of the esophageal body and a transient relaxation of the LES from its normal resting pressure. In patients with achalasia, this normal relaxation fails to occur.

Although the precise etiology of achalasia is uncertain, the primary cause is likely an abnormality of the esophageal myenteric plexus. Patients with achalasia often have a reduced number of ganglion cells and the ganglion cells are surrounded by an inflammatory infiltrate. Unlike Hirschsprung disease, which is thought to be due to failure of normal migration of ganglion cells during fetal life, the etiology of achalasia might involve an autoimmune mechanism, with progressive partial destruction of the ganglion cells and the inhibitory neurons that normally mediate LES relaxation.

Achalasia in children has been associated with trisomy 21, triple-A syndrome (achalasia, alacrima and ACTH insensitivity) and familial dysautonomia, but most appear to be sporadic. Although the disease has rarely been described in toddlers, the typical pediatric patient is a teenager between the ages of 13 and 17.

Diagnosis

Patients typically present with a history of progressively worsening dysphagia that begins with solid foods and then progresses to soft foods and eventually even liquids. Most describe food getting stuck in the cervical region and point to the base of the neck. They usually discover that they can propel that food into the stomach by swallowing liquids frequently throughout their meals. Most also experience intermittent regurgitation of undigested food that occurs immediately or up to a few hours after meals. They and their parents frequently describe this as "vomiting" but careful questioning usually reveals that the vomitus is nonbilious and composed of only chewed-up food.

Substernal chest pain is another very common symptom. This pain is typically described as "heartburn" and often incorrectly attributed to gastroesophageal reflux disease, leading to empiric treatment with acid blocking medications or promotility drugs. These agents are typically of no benefit in patients with achalasia. Most children with achalasia will experience weight loss that ranges from mild to severe (10–20% of body weight). The weight loss is gradual and often subtle.

The initial diagnostic test in the child with dysphagia is usually a contrast esophagram. It is important that the study be performed in both the supine and upright positions, to properly assess esophageal emptying. It is also helpful to take video recordings with emphasis on the pattern of esophageal contractions. Classic findings include a dilated, dysmotile esophagus and a "bird's beak" deformity at the gastroesophageal junction (Fig. 34.1). Early in the course of the disease the radiographic findings can be subtle, while in cases of long-standing disease the progressively redundant esophagus can adopt a sigmoid shape. Careful observation by the radiologist will usually reveal the absence of relaxation of the GEJ.

Probably because GERD is so much more common, most children with achalasia are initially thought to have lower esophageal spasm or stricture due to GERD. Following the esophagram, most physicians will usually then recommend a flexible esophagogastroduodenoscopy. Endoscopy may

J. Duncan Phillips (✉)
Department of Surgery, University of North Carolina, Chapel Hill, North Carolina Children's Hospital, Chapel Hill, NC, USA
e-mail: duncan_phillips@med.unc.edu

P. Mattei (ed.), *Fundamentals of Pediatric Surgery*,
DOI 10.1007/978-1-4419-6643-8_34, © Springer Science+Business Media, LLC 2011

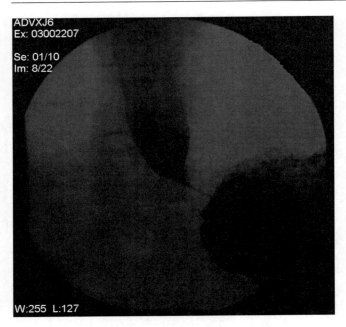

Fig. 34.1 Esophagram demonstrating the "bird's beak" deformity at the gastroesophageal junction, indicating long-standing esophageal achalasia. This 16-year-old girl had dysphagia for over 1 year. Resting lower esophageal sphincter pressure was 42 mmHg

demonstrate pooling of retained fluid within the esophagus and esophageal inflammation related to stasis. The endoscopist might encounter mild resistance but can usually pass the endoscope into the stomach, essentially ruling out a fibrotic stricture.

The gold-standard test for esophageal achalasia remains esophageal manometry. Pressure recordings show absent or diminished peristalsis in the upper esophagus, elevated LES pressures, and minimal or absent LES relaxation. It is important to note that these pressure differences are typically not as impressive as they might be in adults, affected children having resting LES pressures only about two-thirds that of adults.

Preoperative Preparation

Current treatment strategies for achalasia are directed specifically at the LES. Balloon dilatation of the LES under general anesthesia is the most common non-operative technique utilized in children. Symptomatic relief is unfortunately almost always transient and thus repeated dilatations are required. Dilatation also carries with it the risks of general anesthesia and approximately a 3% risk of esophageal perforation. It is useful mostly as a diagnostic tool to help children and their parents understand the potential benefits of Heller myotomy.

An alternative non-surgical treatment for esophageal achalasia is endoscopic intra-sphincteric injection of botulinum toxin, which lowers LES pressure by inhibiting acetylcholine

release from nerve endings. This effect is also transient, requiring repeated injections for long-term success. Several investigators have found that a repeated botulinum toxin injection induces scarring within the wall of the distal esophagus. As a result, the risk of esophageal perforation during subsequent Heller myotomy is increased. For this reason, many pediatric gastroenterologists do not advocate botulinum toxin injections for their patients and most experienced pediatric laparoscopic surgeons are recommending against it.

The occasional patient with achalasia will present with severe weight loss and malnutrition. These children benefit from preoperative supplemental feeds delivered by nasogastric tube. Positive nitrogen balance is associated with decreased peri-operative morbidity but can take several weeks to achieve.

Treatment

Esophageal myotomy, originally including longitudinal incisions on both anterior and posterior sides of the LES, was described by Ernest Heller in 1913. Since essentially all authors now utilize a single anterior myotomy, a more accurate term for the operation as it is performed today is the modified Heller myotomy. Nevertheless, most authors consider "the Heller" the procedure of choice for the surgical treatment of children with achalasia. Excellent results have been reported with long-term follow up of children treated with this procedure.

Controversy regarding specific technical aspects of the Heller myotomy include: (1) whether it is better to approach the LES through the chest or the abdomen, (2) to what degree balloon dilatation or botulism toxin injection increases the complication rate of the operation, (3) whether one should also perform an antireflux operation, and (4) whether minimally invasive techniques are as good as the traditional open approach.

Heller originally performed the myotomy through a left thoracotomy. It was felt that this allowed better visualization of the esophagus and that the myotomy could more easily be extended superiorly to the level of the inferior pulmonary veins. In fact, until the late 1980s this was the standard approach at most centers. More recently however, most have found that the abdominal approach allows for an adequate myotomy, is associated with less perioperative pain and morbidity, and makes fundoplication easier to perform.

Nonoperative treatments such as balloon dilatation and injection of botulinum toxin offer at best a transient improvement in symptoms and are associated with a small risk of significant complications. In addition, extensive scarring within the wall of the esophagus can make subsequent myotomy difficult or even dangerous. Therefore, most pediatric surgeons experienced with the laparoscopic technique recommend against both dilatations and injections.

After disruption of the LES by myotomy, many patients develop GERD, which may or may not be clinically apparent. Most surgeons therefore advocate a concomitant antireflux operation when performing the Heller procedure. This is mainly due to the concern that long-standing GERD places the patient at risk for Barrett's esophagus and esophageal carcinoma. No single technique is clearly favored and various authors have advocated the Nissen, Dor, Toupet and Thal procedures.

Both laparoscopic and thoracoscopic Heller myotomy have been described. The thoracoscopic approach was initially more popular, but it soon became clear that up to 60% of patients have significant gastroesophageal reflux. Since most surgeons felt that concomitant fundoplication was exceedingly difficult to do thoracoscopically, there was interest in developing a practical laparoscopic approach that would accommodate both operations.

Surgical Technique

The patient is positioned in the supine position with the surgeon standing to the patient's right side and the assistant on the left. Older children may have the legs extended on stirrups with the knees flexed 20–30° so that the surgeon can stand between the legs. We prefer to place a Foley catheter to evacuate the bladder and a nasogastric tube to decompress the stomach. A single dose of intravenous antibiotic is given prior to incision.

Five trocars are standard, with initial access at the umbilicus. We use a 5-mm trocar and a 5-mm/30° telescope but initial access with a larger trocar is preferred by some. We then place four more trocars under laparoscopic view. We have found it best to insert these trocars fairly high, along the costal margins, for optimal advantage.

A trocar along the right anterior axillary line allows for introduction of a liver retractor. We use a "snake" retractor to elevate the left lateral segment, exposing the anterior gastric wall and gastroesophageal junction. A telescope holder can be attached to the operating room table to hold this liver retractor, thus freeing up the surgeon and assistant to each use both hands during the remainder of the procedure.

The three additional trocars are usually inserted in the right mid-clavicular line for insertion of a grasper, in the left anterior axillary line for the assistant's grasper, and in the left mid-clavicular line. The assistant can move the laparoscope to the left mid-clavicular trocar and control the camera with the left hand. This allows the surgeon, standing at the patient's right side, to operate with the left-hand instrument inserted via the right mid-clavicular trocar and the right hand to control instruments via the umbilical trocar.

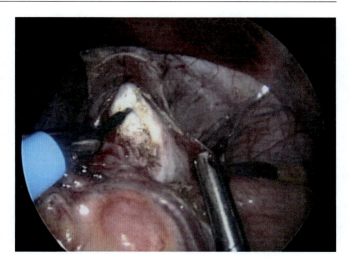

Fig. 34.2 Laparoscopic Heller myotomy. Peritoneum overlying the intra-abdominal esophagus has been divided. The hook cautery is used to begin the myotomy on the anterior surface of the esophagus

The dissection is typically started by incising the gastrohepatic ligament to expose the right crus of the diaphragm. We then incise the peritoneum overlying the intra-abdominal esophagus, just superior to the phreno-esophageal fat pad. One can use the hook cautery or Harmonic Scalpel for most of this dissection. As during a Nissen fundoplication, we typically also incise the peritoneum along the anterior surface of the right crus. The anterior and poster vagus nerves are usually visible on the surface of the esophagus and should be carefully protected. If one has chosen to perform an anterior fundoplication, the posterior esophageal attachments may be left intact.

The myotomy is typically performed with the monopolar hook cautery at the 10 or 11 o'clock position, just to the right of the anterior vagus nerve (Fig. 34.2). We usually start this just cephalad to the phreno-esophageal fat pad, which is sometimes quite thick, and extend this cephalad for about 5 or 6 cm. The surgeon typically uses the left-hand instrument to grasp the right edge of the myotomy and the assistant typically uses a gentle grasper to control the left edge of the myotomy so that the muscle edges can be gently separated. We find that 5 mm Hunter bowel graspers work quite well for this step. To avoid thermal injury to the underlying esophageal submucosa, it is important to not set the current too high and avoid arcing of the current. The myotomy incision must be carried through the outer longitudinal muscle and also through the inner circular muscle, exposing the submucosal vascular plexus. Gentle downward traction on the cut muscle edges allows the surgeon to extend the myotomy well up into the lower mediastinum. The myotomy is then extended 1–1.5 cm onto the anterior gastric wall (Fig. 34.3). In anticipation of the fundoplication, we typically divide the short gastric vessels at this point, using either cautery or the Harmonic Scalpel.

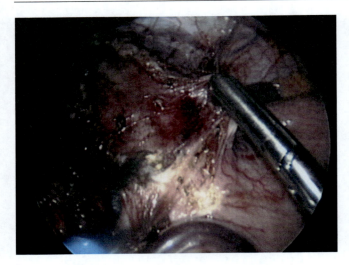

Fig. 34.3 Laparoscopic Heller myotomy. The myotomy of the distal esophagus has been completed and is being extended onto the stomach for 1–2 cm

Due to the risk of causing significant dysphagia, most surgeons prefer to avoid creation of a 360° Nissen fundoplication in patients with disorders of esophageal motility. To create an anterior 180° fundoplication (Dor), two rows of permanent sutures are used. We prefer to use 2-0 braided nylon or a similar multifilament coated suture. To help the needles pass through the 5 mm trocars, they need to be straightened slightly into a canoe or ski shape.

The first row of sutures secures the gastric fundus to the left edge of the myotomy. Three or four interrupted sutures are typically needed (Fig. 34.4). The stomach is then "folded over" the myotomy site (from patient's left to right) and a second row of interrupted sutures secures the fundus to the right edge of the myotomy. The uppermost stitch on each side usually includes the crus. We typically place one or two additional sutures between the fundus and the diaphragm anteriorly.

Many authors have described the intra-operative use of a flexible esophagoscopy to aid in myotomy assessment and suture placement. As an alternative, we pass a 6 Fr Fogarty catheter by mouth, inflate the balloon with air or water, and pull it retrograde from stomach to esophagus under laparoscopic visualization. This allows assessment of myotomy completeness. Some authors inject dilute methylene blue dye to exclude occult inadvertent esophageal perforation.

If one has chosen to perform a posterior 180° (Toupet) fundoplication, one must make sure that the posterior esophageal attachments at the esophageal hiatus have been completely divided during the initial esophageal dissection. Following completion of the myotomy, the surgeon reaches posterior to the esophagus with a left-hand instrument to grasp the mobilized fundus and pulls it from the patient's left to right toward the caudate lobe of the liver. If the short gastric vessels have been properly divided, there should be no significant tension on the fundus and it does not snap back toward the patient's left.

Three rows of interrupted sutures are typically placed to complete the Toupet: an interrupted row securing the fundus to the right edge of the myotomy, a second row securing the fundus to the right crus of the diaphragm, and a final row securing the stomach to the left edge of the myotomy. In the Montupet modification of the Toupet, a crural stitch is placed posterior to the esophagus, to approximate the crura in the midline.

To perform the Heller myotomy using an open approach, most surgeons prefer an upper midline incision, beginning at or just to the side of the xiphoid process and extending to just above the umbilicus. A Thompson or Buckwalter retractor is extremely helpful for improved exposure of the GEJ. The left lateral segment of the liver can be detached from the undersurface of the left hemidiaphragm using electrocautery and retracted to the patient's right with a smooth blade of the retractor. The remainder of the intra-abdominal portion of the procedure is similar to that described above.

A thoracoscopic approach may useful in certain circumstances. For left-sided thoracoscopic procedures, single lung ventilation can often be achieved via right mainstem intubation or by the use of a bronchial blocker. In older children, a double-lumen endotracheal tube can be used. An alternative is the use of valved trocars and gentle CO_2 insufflation with pressures of 5–8 mmHg.

Typically, a four-trocar technique is utilized: in the sixth intercostal space in the midaxillary line, in the fourth intercostal space approximately 2 cm posterior to the posterior axillary line, in the fifth intercostal space in the anterior axillary line, in the eighth intercostal space in the posterior axillary line. With the lung retracted anteriorly and superiorly, the inferior pulmonary ligament may be divided as high as the inferior pulmonary vein. The mediastinal pleura is incised to expose the distal thoracic esophagus. This can be facilitated by the placement of a flexible esophagoscope.

The myotomy is then performed in a fashion similar to that described for the laparoscopic procedure, using 5-mm hook cautery. The myotomy is typically extended just beyond the GEJ. A chest tube is usually placed through one of the port sites.

Postoperative Care

Most surgeons at our institution obtain an esophagram on the first postoperative day prior to beginning oral feedings to verify proper esophageal emptying and to rule out the presence of a leak. It should be noted that the esophagram will not reveal any significant change in esophageal dilatation and often shows a somewhat long area of apparent esophageal narrowing at the myotomy site. This is often quite

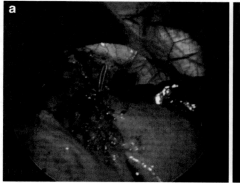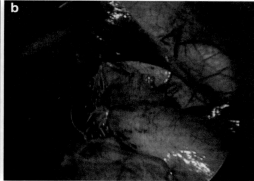

Fig. 34.4 Laparoscopic Heller myotomy with Dor fundoplication. (**a**) The first row of sutures (*arrows*) secures the fundus to the left edge of the myotomy. (**b**) The second row of sutures (*arrows*) helps to "fold" the fundus over the anterior wall of the esophagus at the level of the myotomy to secure the fundus to the right edge of the myotomy

confusing or even alarming to those unfamiliar with the typical early postoperative radiographic appearance.

Following minimally invasive surgery, diet can usually be resumed immediately following the esophagram. Intake of soft foods is preferable to hard foods, such as crusted breads. Some authors recommend a "no-chunk" diet for 2–4 weeks after surgery. Most surgeons continue empiric acid blocking medications for a period of approximately 6 weeks, though there is little evidence that this is necessary. Most patients can be discharged home within 1–2 days of the minimally invasive operation.

Since achalasia is just one part of a more diffuse esophageal disorder, affected patients should be followed indefinitely by an experienced gastroenterologist. The association between long-standing achalasia and esophageal carcinoma is well-established. Surgical treatment of achalasia during childhood would be expected to reduce this risk but long-term follow-up data are lacking.

Summary Points

- Achalasia is a motility disorder that affects the entire esophagus, but its most prominent and directly treatable component is spasm of the lower esophageal sphincter complex.
- The clinical presentation of achalasia includes dysphagia that progresses slowly over the course of many months or years, chest pain, and regurgitation of undigested food.
- Patients are frequently erroneously treated for GERD.
- Esophagram classically reveals a dilated and sometimes tortuous esophagus that tapers down to a sharp "bird's beak" appearance at the level of the diaphragm.
- Most patients should undergo esophagoscopy to rule out the presence of a mass or stricture.
- The gold-standard diagnostic test is esophageal manometry, which reveals minimal peristalsis of the esophageal body, high resting LES pressure, and failure of relaxation of the LES after swallowing.
- Balloon dilatation and injection of botulinum toxin offer at best temporary relief and both cause significant scarring that can make operative myotomy more difficult and dangerous.
- Heller myotomy offers the best chance for long-standing relief of symptoms and should be considered first-line therapy.
- Heller myotomy can be performed open or minimally invasively, through the chest or the abdomen.
- Many pediatric surgeons favor the laparoscopic approach, in which a fundoplication is usually performed concomitantly.

Editor's Comment

Achalasia rarely affects children and the clinical presentation, though often insidious, is distinctive: dysphagia, chest pain, and regurgitation of undigested food. Nevertheless, patients frequently present for surgical consultation only after many months of misery, failed interventions, ineffective medical therapy. This is unfortunate, not only because the patient suffers needlessly, but because there is a safe and effective operation available that becomes more arduous and more perilous when the patient presents late after having been dilated or injected. Primary physicians and gastroenterologists should be encouraged to refer these patients to an experienced surgeon early in the course of the disease rather than as a "last resort."

Laparoscopic Heller myotomy is an advanced minimally invasive technique but is generally safe in the hands of an experienced laparoscopist. I feel the operation can be done safely with the patient in the supine position and the surgeon standing to the right, which avoids the inherent delay and added risk of placing the patient in stirrups. Some have touted the use of intra-operative adjuncts like manometry or endoscopy to assess the adequacy of the myotomy, but these are unproven and generally unnecessary. To protect the exposed submucosa and to avoid unnecessary dissection posterior to the esophagus, I always perform an anterior fundoplication, but this is certainly open to debate. A postoperative esophagram is admittedly overkill but avoiding even a single rare case of unrecognized perforation seems like adequate justification for this generally harmless exercise.

The key to the success of the Heller myotomy, like most complex operations, is proper management of expectations. Patients naturally, but inappropriately, expect instantaneous relief of their symptoms and the ability to eat anything and everything immediately after the operation. In most cases, this is unrealistic and patients should be counseled to expect that some degree of dysphagia will persist for some time after the operation. This is because the disease affects the motility of the entire esophagus, the chronically dilated esophagus is ineffective at peristalsis, and there is a partial functional obstruction at the LES after myotomy. The esophagus drains principally by gravity and pressure from the advancing bolus of swallowed food or liquid. These symptoms resolve gradually over the course of several weeks or months; but in the meantime patients should be encouraged to avoid food with large chunks (meat, bread crust), to chew their food well, and to drink fluid frequently during meals. Some patients can develop intermittent painful episodes of esophageal spasm that usually eventually cease. This has been treated with variable results using calcium channel blockers and medications that counter smooth muscle spasm.

Intra-operative perforations should be primarily repaired and then "patched" with the fundoplication, in which most patients should be able to tolerate oral intake after a brief (48–72 h) period of observation and a negative esophagram. The rare patient with an esophageal perforation noted on postoperative esophagram is treated initially with bowel rest, antibiotics, and careful observation. The leak usually seals spontaneously in 5–7 days but occasionally will require percutaneous drainage or reoperation for local or systemic sepsis. Perforation should be an extraordinarily rare event.

Differential Diagnosis

- Gastroesophageal reflux disease
- Esophageal stricture (reflux-induced, caustic ingestion)
- Diffuse esophageal spasm
- Chagas disease
- Esophageal tumor (carcinoma or leiomyoma)

Diagnostic Studies

- Contrast esophagram
- Esophagogastroduodenoscopy
- Esophageal manometry

Parental Preparation

- Achalasia is a diffuse esophageal motility disorder.
- The child might benefit from preoperative nasogastric nutritional supplementation.
- Risks of surgery include esophageal perforation, gastroesophageal reflux, and recurrent dysphagia.
- Relief will likely not be sudden and dramatic; rather it will come over the course of several weeks or months after the operation.

Preoperative Preparation

- ☐ Type and screen
- ☐ Intravenous antibiotics
- ☐ Nasogastric tube, consider Foley catheter
- ☐ Informed consent

Technical Points

- Laparoscopic Heller myotomy is approached in much the same way as a fundoplication, with the patient either in the supine position and the surgeon to the right or modified lithotomy with the surgeon at the foot of the operating table.
- Many surgeons prefer to perform a concomitant antireflux procedure, which can be complete or partial, anterior or posterior.
- The myotomy should extend 5–6 cm onto the thoracic esophagus and 1–2 cm onto the anterior stomach.
- Be sure to visualize and protect the anterior vagus nerve.
- Perforations should be repaired primarily and covered by the fundoplication.
- Consider a postoperative esophagram within 24–48 h before allowing oral intake.

Suggested Reading

Ballantine TVN, Fitzgerald JF, Grosfeld JL. Transabdominal esophagomyotomy for achalasia in children. J Pediatr Surg. 1980;15:457–61.

Hurwitz M, Bahar RJ, Ament ME, et al. Evaluation of the use of botulinum toxin in children with achalasia. J Pediatr Gastroenterol Nutr. 2000;30:509–14.

Mehra M, Bahar RJ, Ament ME, et al. Laparoscopic and thoracoscopic esophagomyotomy for children with achalasia. J Pediatr Gastroenterol Nutr. 2001;33:466–71.

Paidas C, Cowgill SM, Boyle R, et al. Laparoscopic Heller myotomy with anterior fundoplication ameliorates symptoms of achalasia in pediatric patients. J Am Coll Surg. 2007;204:977–86.

Patti MG, Feo CV, Arcerito M, et al. Effects of previous treatments on results of laparoscopic Heller myotomy for achalasia. Dig Dis Sci. 1999;44:2270–6.

Patti MG, Albanese CT, Holcomb III GW, et al. Laparoscopic Heller myotomy and Dor fundoplication for esophageal achalasia in children. J Pediatr Surg. 2001;36:1248–51.

Phillips JD, Weiner T. Laparoscopic Heller myotomy and Dor fundoplication for pediatric esophageal achalasia: recent technical modifications of an established procedure. Pediatr Endosurg Innov Tech. 2004;8:229–35.

Rothenberg SS, Partrick DA, Bealer JF, et al. Evaluation of minimally invasive approaches to achalasia in children. J Pediatr Surg. 2001;36:808–10.

Spiess AE, Kahrilas PJ. Treating achalasia: from whalebone to laparoscope. JAMA. 1998;280:638–42.

Waldhausen JHT, Horgan S, Pellegrini C. Laparoscopic Heller myotomy and Dor fundoplication for achalasia in children. Pediatr Endosurg Innov Tech. 1999;3:23–7.

Part VI
Thorax and Mediastinum

Chapter 35
Patent Ductus Arteriosus

Stephanie Fuller and Peter J. Gruber

The ductus arteriosus is a normal fetal structure arising from the left sixth aortic arch. It is a vascular connection between the main pulmonary artery and the upper descending thoracic aorta that penetrates the pericardium and just distal and opposite to the origin and insertion of the left subclavian artery. The anatomy of the thorax is essential to identifying and safely closing a PDA as several important structures surround the ductus. The left vagus trunk enters the chest from the root of the neck in a groove between the left subclavian artery and the left common carotid artery, crosses the aortic arch as well as the ductus and continues downward. The recurrent laryngeal branch curves around the ductus arteriosus posteriorly and extends back upward into the neck over the surface of the esophagus. The left phrenic nerve enters the thorax medial to the vagus nerve and continues downward on the pericardium. The pericardium encompasses the pulmonary artery end of the ductus arteriosus.

Patent ductus arteriosus accounts for 5–10% of all congenital heart defects. It is twice as common among females, occurs in approximately 1 in 1,600 term live births, and is much more common in preterm infants. The overall incidence of PDA in preterm infants is approximately 20–30%. The incidence rises sharply with earlier gestational age and lower birth weight. In infants at gestational age 34–36 weeks, the approximate incidence of PDA is 20%, at 31–33 weeks 50%, and at 28–30 weeks 75%. This is due in part to decreased sensitivity of immature ductal tissue to O_2-mediated constriction and increased sensitive to prostaglandin in preterm infants.

The origin and insertion of the ductus is somewhat variable, especially in the setting of a congenital heart anomaly. In cases of a right-sided aortic arch due to persistence of right sided embryological structures, the ductus usually arises from the right-sided proximal descending aorta. When there is persistence of both right and left embryonic attachments, bilateral ductuses can occur but are rare. The ductus also varies in its position and angle of take off from the aorta. In isolated cases, the angle between the superior margin of the ductus and aorta is most often acute, and the ductus is in smooth continuity with the descending aorta. In patients with ductal-dependent circulation and additional cardiac anomalies, the proximal angle is usually less acute and may even be obtuse. The ductus is present in many other congenital cardiac anomalies, with the prominent exception of Tetralogy of Fallot with absent pulmonary valve.

During fetal development, approximately 60% of the right ventricular blood flow is diverted from the high-resistance pulmonary vascular bed through the ductus arteriosus into the aorta. Local and circulating prostaglandins actively maintain ductal patency during the fetal period through endothelial-smooth muscle signaling pathways. At birth, an elevated arterial partial pressure of O_2, generated after the infant's first few breaths, inhibits prostaglandin synthetase, resulting in decreased prostaglandin levels, which in turn stimulates ductal constriction. In addition, increased pulmonary blood flow enhances metabolism of prostaglandin subsequently leading to decreased prostaglandin levels and ductal constriction. Ductal closure occurs in three well-described phases: (1) initial smooth muscle constriction narrowing the ductal lumen, (2) loss of ductal responsiveness to prostaglandin vasodilation, and (3) irreversible anatomic remodeling resulting in permanent occlusion. Initial constriction of the ductus produces a zone of hypoxia in the media leading to local smooth muscle cell death and production of vascular endothelial growth factor. Once fibrosed, the ductus is referred to as the ligamentum arteriosum. In term infants, functional closure of the ductus usually occurs within a few hours of birth and is permanently closed within 6 weeks.

Patent ductus arteriosus causes morbidity in one of two ways. The first is a low flow state induced by the steal of systemic blood flow that results from a significant left-to-right shunt across the ductus. This manifest by necrotizing enterocolitis, abnormal cerebral blood flow, and endocarditis. The second harmful effect of a PDA is heart failure and pulmonary overcirculation, which causes respiratory distress and, if unchecked, chronic lung disease. Retrograde blood flow in the descending aorta in diastole leads to decreased systemic flow

S. Fuller (✉)
Department of Cardiothoracic Surgery, Children's Hospital of Philadelphia, 34th Street & Civic Center Boulevard, Ste. A2NWAD, Philadelphia, PA 19103, USA
e-mail: fullers@email.chop.edu

P. Mattei (ed.), *Fundamentals of Pediatric Surgery*,
DOI 10.1007/978-1-4419-6643-8_35, © Springer Science+Business Media, LLC 2011

and predisposition to end-organ ischemia. In the setting of low pulmonary vascular resistance, a large, nonrestrictive ductus without concomitant defects results in a substantial left-to-right shunt with increased pulmonary return to the left atrium. This results in left atrial dilation, left ventricular volume overload, and progressive congestive heart failure. Left untreated, a large PDA may lead to pulmonary arteriolar hypertension with the eventual development of a right-to-left shunt and Eisenmenger's physiology as early as 6 months of age.

The first ligation of a PDA was performed by Robert E. Gross in 1938 at Boston Children's Hospital and is considered the first successful congenital heart operation. It is also the first congenital cardiac lesion approached using a transcatheter technique when, in 1967, Porstmann used a polyvinyl alcohol foam plug to close a PDA.

Indications for PDA closure are still somewhat controversial and generally based on the likelihood of complications developing as a result of leaving it open. First-line therapy in most centers is indomethacin, which is a prostaglandin inhibitor that usually induces closure of the ductus. Most agree that a moderate to large PDA that has failed to close in response to medical treatment with indomethacin places the infant at significant risk of congestive heart failure and pulmonary hypertension and should therefore be surgically ligated.

Diagnosis

Symptoms and physical findings are dependent on the size of the PDA, associated intracardiac defects, and the degree of pulmonary vascular resistance. Typically, a small ductus with minimal shunting is restrictive and the child is asymptomatic. The diagnosis is frequently made in a toddler when a continuous machinery murmur is heard near the left second intercostal space. With a moderately large PDA, the shunt increases significantly over the first few months of life as the pulmonary vascular resistance falls. These children often develop failure to thrive, recurrent upper respiratory tract infections, and fatigue with exertion. On physical examination there is typically a continuous murmur and an overactive cardiac impulse. Infants with a large PDA develop heart failure within the first few weeks of life. They typically demonstrate tachypnea, tachycardia, and failure to thrive. Physical findings include a widened pulse pressure, prominent precordial pulse, and hepatomegaly. Preterm infants exhibit respiratory distress resulting from heart failure and pulmonary overcirculation. They often require intubation and have ventilator-dependent respiratory failure that can eventually cause bronchopulmonary dysplasia. With these physical findings, the differential diagnosis includes shunting lesions above the semilunar valves including aortopulmonary window, sinus of Valsalva fistula, and aorto-left ventricular tunnel.

Signs associated with persistent PDA are relative to the degree of left-to-right shunting. A large PDA results in enlargement of the left atrium and left ventricle, increased pulmonary vascular markings, and interstitial pulmonary edema on chest radiograph. Electrocardiographic changes indicative of left ventricular hypertrophy and left atrial enlargement are present. If chronic pulmonary hypertension has developed, there may also be evidence of right ventricular enlargement.

Transthoracic echocardiography is the diagnostic method of choice and can accurately identify ductal anatomy and characterize shunt flow. The vast majority of children with "classic" physical findings and an echocardiogram indicating isolated PDA do not require further diagnostic testing. Additionally, a complete study is essential to ensure the absence of concomitant lesions that require ductal patency for either systemic or pulmonary blood flow. The most common echocardiographic scenario is a PDA with flow directed all left-to-right, no significant intracardiac abnormalities (with the exception of a patent foramen ovale), occasional left atrial or left ventricular dilation, and a left-sided aortic arch with a normal branching pattern. The exceptions are those patients in whom echocardiographic data suggest severe pulmonary hypertension or cyanosis resulting in a right-to-left shunt at ductal level. If elevated pulmonary artery pressures are present, oxygen and pulmonary vasodilators are administered during cardiac catheterization to determine the reactivity of the pulmonary bed. Patients with fixed pulmonary hypertension >75% of systemic resistance can exhibit differential cyanosis with systemic desaturation. These patients are not considered candidates for ductal closure because of the high risk of right ventricular failure. Although rarely indicated, MRI or CT angiography can also help to evaluate the PDA, aortic arch anatomy, and the degree of shunting.

Treatment

There are a number of available treatment strategies available for PDA. In pre-term neonates, the mainstay of therapy is pharmacologic. Indomethacin is an inhibitor of prostaglandin synthetase and has been applied clinically since 1976 to constrict the ductus and facilitate closure in premature infants. A schedule of three doses of 0.1–0.2 mg/kg administered intravenously every 12–24 h is widely used prior to consideration for surgical therapy. Echocardiography is used to document the size of the patent ductus before and after the administration of indomethacin. The efficacy of indomethacin is well documented. Its use is associated with an approximately 80% incidence of duct closure in premature infants. Contraindications to indomethacin therapy include hyperbilirubinemia, sepsis, thrombocytopenia or coagulopathy, intracerebral hemorrhage, and renal insufficiency. Risks of therapy include renal insufficiency and gastrointestinal perforation. In the pre-term population, if indomethacin is contraindicated or if treatment is unsuccessful following three courses of therapy, conversion to a surgical strategy is recommended. Although successful cases have been reported, indomethacin is rarely effective in full-term infants.

Premature infants who fail indomethacin therapy or who have uncontrolled congestive failure with significant deterioration in pulmonary function are candidates for ductal ligation within a few days of diagnosis. However, it is never a surgical emergency. Early surgical closure of PDA in preterm infants carries a low operative morbidity and mortality. Compared with medical management for treatment of congestive heart failure with digoxin and diuretic therapy, surgical ligation reduces the need for mechanical ventilation and oxygen therapy, shortens hospital stay, and decreases the incidence of necrotizing enterocolitis. Our choice is to perform pre-term neonatal PDA ligation at the bedside in the neonatal intensive care unit with the services of cardiac anesthesia. Prior to intervention, it is crucial to obtain an echocardiogram to confirm a patent ductus with all left-to-right flow, a left aortic arch with normal branching, and adequate ventricular function. Importantly, one must also confirm that there are no additional cardiac lesions besides a patent foramen ovale. All patients are typed and cross matched for the appropriate blood type and blood is available at the bedside for all procedures. For all cases, it is necessary to confirm endotracheal tube placement with a chest radiograph. Adequate intravenous access for potential volume resuscitation in case of massive hemorrhage is also required.

For open surgical ligation of a patent ductus arteriosus in the preterm infant, attention of the operating team must also be directed at maintaining adequate ventilation and preventing hypothermia. The infant is identified, anesthetized, and placed in the right lateral decubitus position with the left arm raised over the head to elevate the left scapula. The ductus arteriosus is exposed through a left posterolateral thoracotomy through the fourth intercostal space. The lung is gently retracted anteriorly using a moist gauze sponge and malleable retractor. The parietal pleura is divided longitudinally posterior to the vagus nerve. Great care is used in dissecting the ductus and the aortic arch. It is easy to mistake a large ductus for the aortic arch or to mistake the aortic isthmus as the left subclavian artery. Extensive dissection of the ductus in pre-term infants is not advised as the tissue is friable and may lead to life-threatening hemorrhage. Caution is used to identify the recurrent laryngeal nerve and sweep it inferiorly away from the operative site. Once the ductus is identified, it is dissected with a blunt, right-angled clamp both superiorly and inferiorly, creating a plane for ligation.

We prefer to place an appropriately sized surgical clip. Most ductuses will take a medium clip. Great care must be used

when applying the clip. Scissoring can injure the ductus and result in hemorrhage. We usually avoid dissecting the deeper aspect of the ductus as it is often adherent to the surrounding tissues and can be easily torn in the process of mobilization. In cases when a surgical clip is not appropriate, the posterior aspect of the ductus must be exposed in order to encircle the ductus with a single strand of 2-0 silk suture for ligation. This is accomplished by retracting the aorta medially with gentle traction on the aorta both above and below the ductus. We prefer 2-0 silk suture for ductus ligation as finer suture material can cut through the friable ductus and result in hemorrhage.

Alternative methods of interrupting ductal flow include ligation and division. In these cases, it is possible to either to place several 2-0 silk ties around the ductus and sharply divide in between these ties or to place vascular clamps on either side of the ductus and oversew it with polypropylene suture. However, these procedures are rarely necessary, especially in the preterm infant. In older patients, we favor division of the ductus, as recanalization has been reported to occur, albeit rarely. The lowest risk of residual ductus or recanalization follows division and oversewing of the PDA.

During the ligation procedure, lower extremity saturations or blood pressure is assessed to assure that the PDA was not associated with critical coarctation. The parietal pleura is usually left open as it thin and friable. The chest is closed with absorbable pericostal sutures, as are the muscle layers and skin. Prior to closure, the pleural space is irrigated with saline solution. Under direct visualization using the Seldinger technique, a pleural catheter is placed in the left pleural space and left in place for approximately 24 h. Hemodynamic changes seen immediately after ligation of the ductus include a significant increase in systolic and diastolic blood pressure. A post operative chest radiograph confirms endotracheal tube placement in neonates, no evidence of hemo- or pneumothorax, and both clip and chest tube position. In 1994, Mavroudis et al. from Children's Memorial Hospital in Chicago described the traditional surgical management for 1,108 patients who underwent surgery between 1947 and 1993. A total of 98% of the patients had interruption of the ductus by ligation and division. There were no deaths. The recurrence rate was zero and the authors reported a transfusion rate of less than 5%.

The first video-assisted thoracoscopic surgical closure of a PDA was reported in 1991. The technique was first published by Laborde in 1993 and has been widely used in neonates as well as infants and children. VATS is performed utilizing three to four small thoracostomy incisions for introduction of instruments. As with open ductal ligation, dissection of the ductus is performed above and below the aortic end of the ductus. The duct is closed with a single vascular clip. Again, great care is used not to trap the recurrent laryngeal nerve in the medial end of the clip. In 2004, the Laborde group updated their experience and published the largest series available on

703 patients who underwent PDA ligation via VATS from September 1991 to March 2003. Indications for operation were persistent clinically significant patency or failure to close in older children. Exclusion criteria included PDA diameter >8 mm, previous thoracotomy, infection and aneurysm. Mean age was 3.0 ± 3.8 years (5 days to 33 years) and the smallest patient weighed 1.2 kg. Only 3.1% of the procedures were performed on low birth weight (<2.5 kg) neonates. Operative and 30-day mortality was 0 though recurrent laryngeal nerve injury was noted in 3%. However, only 0.4% had persistent dysfunction. Incidence of conversion to thoracotomy was 1%. Low birth weight infants were identified as at increased risk for transfusion requirement and bleeding and residual ductal patency was detected in 1.4% of cases.

In children, interventional catheter closure is sometimes used for ductus closure. A number of different catheter delivered devices have been used and currently Dacron-coated steel coils are popular. Performed by interventional cardiologists, interventional catheterization closure offers the advantage of no incision in infants greater than 5 kg. Disadvantages of the technique include potential embolization of the device, residual ductal flow as high as 41% intermediate ductal patency, projection of the device into either the aorta or the pulmonary artery resulting in potential obstruction, and expense. No extensive cost/effectiveness comparisons of open surgery versus VATS versus transcatheter techniques are available in the literature.

Complications

As with all cardiac procedures, a thorough preoperative discussion with parents detailing risks, benefits, and possible complications of the procedure takes place. Risks and complications include but are not limited to infection, bleeding, pneumothorax, prolonged chylothorax, injury to the heart or lungs, injury to the phrenic or recurrent laryngeal nerves, recurrent PDA, potential coarctation of the aorta, and death. Chylothorax may occur when lymphatics crossing the parietal pleura overlying the duct and in the periaortic adventitia are divided. Risk is increased in patients with recent upper respiratory infections when lymphatics are engorged and more difficult to seal with electrocautery. When detected, leaking lymphatics can sometimes be controlled with cautery or vascular clips.

Bleeding from a torn ductus arteriosus can be torrential. Because of the friability of the ductal tissue, it is often difficult to control. In the event of hemorrhage, it is often necessary to obtain distal and proximal control of the aorta for volume resuscitation and arterial repair as well as entry into the pericardial space to control bleeding from the pulmonary artery.

Accidental ligation of the aorta or left pulmonary artery has been described in patients with a large ductus overlying the aortic arch. Great care should be used in removing surgical clips accidentally placed on adjacent vessels. For this reason, proper monitoring during the procedure is essential with either a blood pressure cuff or pulse oximetry documenting flow in the lower extremities. A postoperative chest radiograph can demonstrate interrupted pulmonary blood flow.

It is important to inform parents that although ductal ligation might be expected to improve cardiac function and thus ameliorate heart failure and pulmonary overcirculation, improvement in pulmonary status does not necessarily follow. This is due to the fact that these infants typically have several other risk factors for pulmonary disease including intrinsic lung disease, surfactant insufficiency, and primary pulmonary hypertension.

Summary Points

- PDA must be considered in the newborn with failure to thrive, evidence of pulmonary overcircualtion, and a continuous murmur.
- Plain radiographs can give clues (pulmonary congestion) but are not diagnostic.
- Transthoracic echocardiography is diagnostic of a PDA.
- One must be sure that there are no additional cardiac defects that require the patency of the ductus arteriosus and that ductal flow is left-to-right, *not* right-to-left.

Editor's Comment

Although surgical closure of the patent ductus arteriosus in premature newborns is technically straightforward and generally safe, there are several well-recognized potential complications including: bleeding, recurrent laryngeal nerve injury, and erroneous ligation of a major vessel such as the left pulmonary artery. The operation is best performed with the patient in the NICU with proper anesthesiology support and monitoring, preferably including an arterial cannula, secure intravenous access, and at least one blood volume (80–100 mL/kg) of packed red blood cells warmed and ready to infuse at a moment's notice.

Indications for surgery are well-established and there is usually consensus among the clinicians involved in the patient's care regarding the need for intervention. It is preferable for the patient to have had an echocardiogram performed less than 48 h before the proposed operation to be certain that the ductus is still large enough to warrant ligation. Indomethacin might make the ductus more friable and could make bleeding more difficult to control due to its effect on platelet function, but its recent use is not a contraindication to an operation.

The thoracoscopic approach to ductus ligation in premature newborns appears to be safe and effective and will likely eventually become standard. Nevertheless, the open approach is still acceptable and does not require a large incision. A small left posterolateral muscle-sparing incision, rarely more than 3 cm in length, is made near the tip of the scapula and the chest is entered through the fourth intercostal space. In general, the more posterior the incision, the smaller it needs to be. An extrapleural dissection provides optimal exposure, allows easier containment of bleeding should it occur, and obviates the need for a chest tube. The lung is gently retracted anteriorly using a small malleable Deaver retractor bent at 90° and fixed to the Finochietto retractor by means of an Allis clamp. Although proximal and distal control of all major vascular structures is risky and unnecessary, all structures should be clearly identified with certainty, including the aortic arch, the descending aorta, the subclavian artery, the pulmonary artery, the ductus arteriosus, and, perhaps most importantly, the vagus and recurrent laryngeal nerves. Identification of the nerves helps to ensure that the structure to be divided is in fact the ductus and helps to avoid vocal cord paralysis, a morbid complication to be avoided if at all possible. The ductus can usually be safely dissected circumferentially to allow passage of two 2-0 silk ligatures; however many have proposed that the risk of bleeding is lessened by only partially dissecting the ductus and only to the degree necessary to allow placement of a hemoclip.

Erroneous ligation of a vascular structure other than the ductus is surprisingly easy to do, but should be quite rare for the experienced surgeon. The risk is minimized by identifying the vagus and recurrent laryngeal nerves and all pertinent vascular structures clearly. It is also important to test-clamp the structure to be ligated to confirm that post-ductal blood pressure improves (an arterial cannula with continuous pressure tracing is helpful), oxygen saturation remains high, and lower extremity perfusion is intact. If errant ligation does occur, it must be recognized early and the ligature or clip removed as soon as possible if there is any hope of survival.

Bleeding from an injured ductus can be astonishingly brisk. It is important to maintain poise and to use a careful approach to control the bleeding. It is important to have excellent suction, a second pair of hands, and good exposure. Blind placement of a hemoclip on the proximal ductus can be effective in slowing down the bleeding but must be done with care as injury of the ductus at the aortic take-off can make things much worse. Frantic attempts to control the bleeding almost invariably result in recurrent laryngeal nerve injury. Parents need to be aware of the potential for bleeding and that it can sometimes result in death of the infant.

Parents should be warned that the infant's clinical condition will likely not improve immediately after ligation of the ductus. Instead, they usually become relatively fluid overloaded and require ongoing support until they can diurese. Most will begin to improve by the third or fourth postoperative day.

Differential Diagnosis

- Shunt above semilunar valves
- Aorto-pulmonary window
- Sinus of Valsalva fistula
- Aorto-left ventricular tunnel

Diagnostic Studies

- Plain chest radiograph
- Transthoracic echocardiography
- MRI or CT angiogram, rarely necessary

Parental Preparation

- Likelihood of change in clinical course
- Risks include bleeding and recurrent laryngeal nerve damage
- It is possible a coarctation of the aorta could be identified intra-operatively
- It is likely that congestive heart failure can be avoided or improved with ligation but pulmonary disease may persist or progress

Preoperative Preparation

- ☐ Intravenous hydration
- ☐ Type and crossmatch for blood
- ☐ Informed consent

Technical Points

- Left posterolateral thoracotomy usually provides the best exposure for safe repair.
- During the procedure, always monitor lower extremity saturations or blood pressure.
- Always be certain to identify the recurrent laryngeal nerve and sweep it away from the operative site to avoid injury and subsequent vocal cord paralysis.
- Ductal division is not required in neonates and infants.
- The ductus should be dissected carefully and only enough to apply a clip or 2-0 silk ligature.
- A left pleural catheter may be placed selectively.

Suggested Reading

Gould DS, Montenegro LM, Gaynor JW, et al. A comparison of on-site and off-site patent ductus arteriosus ligation in premature infants. Pediatrics. 2003;112:1298–300.

Gross RE, Hubbard JP. Surgical ligation of a patent ductus arteriosus. Report of first successful case. JAMA. 1939;112:729.

Heymann MA, Rudolph AM, Silverman NJ. Closure of the ductus arteriosus in premature infants by inhibition of prostaglandin synthesis. N Engl J Med. 1976;295:530–3.

Mavroudis C, Backer CL, Gevitz M. Forty-six years of PDA division at Children's Memorial Hospital of Chicago. Standards for comparison. Ann Surg. 1994;220:402.

Villa E, Eynden FV, Le Bret E, et al. Paediatric video-assisted thoracoscopic clipping of patent ductus arteriosus: experience in more than 700 cases. Euro J Cardiothor Surg. 2004;25:387–93.

Wagner HR, Ellison RC, Zierler S, et al. Surgical closure of patent ductus arteriosus in 268 preterm infants. J Thorac Cardiovas Surg. 1984;87:870.

Chapter 36
Vascular Compression Syndromes

Mark L. Wulkan

Vascular compression syndromes consist of vascular rings, pulmonary artery slings, and innominate artery compression syndrome. Vascular rings cause the majority of vascular compression syndromes. A double aortic arch and a right aortic arch with an aberrant left subclavian artery constitute approximately 85–95% of all thoracic vascular compression syndromes. There are no demographic predispositions to vascular compression syndromes. These anomalies occur equally in both males and females. Complete vascular rings encircle the trachea and esophagus causing compressive symptoms. Younger children tend to present with respiratory symptoms such as noisy breathing, stridor, cyanosis, apnea, respiratory distress, or a brassy cough. Patients might also have a history of reactive airway disease or recurrent pneumonias. It is not uncommon for children with a complete vascular ring to have some feeding difficulty, however formula and breast milk usually pass easily through the compressed esophagus. It is more common for older children to have symptoms of dysphagia and difficulty feeding. Patients with complete rings tend to present earlier and have more severe symptoms.

Pulmonary artery sling occurs when there is an abnormal take off of the left pulmonary artery from the posterior aspect of a normally positioned right pulmonary artery. A pulmonary artery sling can cause compression of the distal trachea and right mainstem bronchus. The left pulmonary artery then courses between the esophagus and trachea. Repair is usually accomplished with reanastomosis of the left pulmonary artery on cardio-pulmonary bypass. Pulmonary artery sling is often associated with tracheobronchial abnormalities such as complete tracheal rings.

Innominate artery compression is thought to occur when there is compression of the trachea by an abnormal leftward take off of the innominate artery. True innominate artery compression syndromes are rare.

Diagnosis

Delays in diagnosis of vascular compression syndromes are not uncommon. Often they are discovered during a work up for respiratory symptoms or dysphagia. There can be suggestive findings on a plain radiograph of the chest, including an abnormal aortic knob or deviation of the trachea or esophagus. Definitive diagnosis can often be made by contrast esophagram (Fig. 36.1). On esophagram there are distinct impressions on the esophagus caused by adjacent vascular structures. An astute radiologist can often distinguish the various types of vascular ring based solely on the pattern of these impressions.

Diagnosis is also sometimes made by bronchoscopy in a patient being evaluated for airway symptoms. Bronchoscopic findings include vascular compression and tracheomalacia, often with obvious narrowing of the airway.

Patients with evidence of a vascular compression syndrome by contrast esophagram or bronchoscopy are usually referred for echocardiography to better define the anatomy and rule out associated cardiac defects, though three-dimensional imaging with computed tomography or magnetic resonance provides much better anatomic detail for proper surgical planning.

Treatment

Once the diagnosis is made, the symptomatic patient should be considered for an operation. Non-operative observation is sometimes warranted in patients who are asymptomatic. There is some evidence that patients who only have minor symptoms can eventually outgrow them. However, it is recommended that symptomatic vascular rings be divided.

Once the decision is made to surgically divide a vascular ring, many surgeons obtain either a CT- or MR-angiogram. If the lesion is to be approached through a thoracotomy, an esophagram confirming the diagnosis is sufficient as complete dissection of the structures is warranted during the procedure. On the other hand, if a thoracoscopic approach is to

M.L. Wulkan (✉)
Department of Surgery, Children's Healthcare of Atlanta at Egleston,
Emory Children's Center, 2015 Uppergate Drive, NE,
Atlanta, GA 30322, USA
e-mail: mark.wulkan@choa.org

P. Mattei (ed.), *Fundamentals of Pediatric Surgery*,
DOI 10.1007/978-1-4419-6643-8_36, © Springer Science+Business Media, LLC 2011

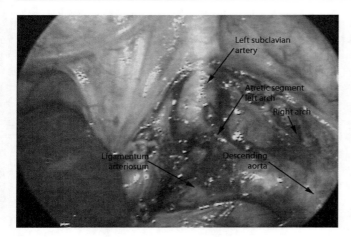

Fig. 36.1 Thoracoscopic view of a double aortic arch, with an atretic segment of the left arch between the left subclavian artery and the descending aorta

be considered, it is best to define the anatomy further to determine if the patient is a good candidate for such an approach.

Monitoring of blood flow to the extremities is essential when dividing a vascular ring. This is typically accomplished with a *left* radial arterial line as well as pulse oximeter on the left upper and lower extremities. The principles of the operation are the same whether one is using a thoracoscopic or open approach. Thoracoscopic division is considered for patients with a right aortic arch, aberrant left subclavian artery, and left-sided ligamentum arteriosum, and for patients with a double aortic arch with an atretic or very small segment to be divided. We currently do not recommend dividing true double aortic arches thoracoscopically due to the potential for catastrophic bleeding.

Double Aortic Arch

The patient is approached through either a left thoracotomy or thoracoscopically. The pleura overlying the aorta is opened from the descending aorta to the level of the take-off of the left subclavian artery. The pleura is reflected medially as the left arch and ductus arteriosis are identified. The left arch is dissected free from surrounding structures with particular attention paid to the area over the esophagus. The right arch is also identified. If there is an atretic segment of the arch as identified on preoperative studies, this area can be used for division. Otherwise, the arch is typically divided between the take-off of the left subclavian arch and descending aorta. If there is a large discrepancy between the arches, with a much smaller right arch, the right arch may need to be divided.

Again, this is usually done at the junction with the descending aorta. Care must be taken when dividing a right posterior arch, as the right arch can retract and bleed quite briskly into the right mediastinum upon division. We typically oversew the aorta to prevent any accidents. Plastic interlocking clips are used for small atretic or stenotic segments if the double arch is approached thoracoscopically. The ligamentum is also typically divided. Once the arch is divided, the tissues overlying the esophagus are dissected free to make sure there are no constricting bands.

Right Sided Arch with Aberrant Left Subclavian Artery

A right-sided arch with an aberrant left subclavian artery and a left ligamentum arteriosum is approached in a similar fashion (Fig. 36.2). The goal is to divide the ligamentum arteriosum. Complete dissection should still be done to verify that there is not an atretic double aortic arch, which, if left untreated, can leave the patient symptomatic. During the course of the dissection, the recurrent laryngeal nerve must be carefully identified and preserved (Fig. 36.3). Although the ligamentum theoretically has no blood flow, it should still be suture ligated. Again, care is taken to dissect the tissues overlying the esophagus in order to completely release the ring.

Placement of a chest tube is optional. The typical postoperative stay is 2–3 days for thoracotomy and 1–2 days for thoracoscopy. Patients are started on a diet immediately postoperatively. We do not routinely place patients in the ICU.

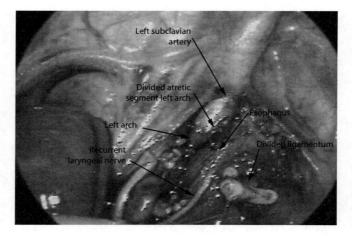

Fig. 36.2 Thoracoscopic view of the double aortic arch and ligamentum arteriosum divided. Note the space between the divided segments

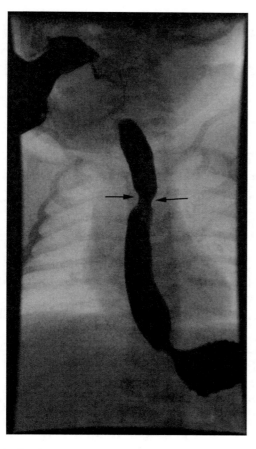

Fig. 36.3 Esophagram showing lateral and posterior indentations from a double aortic arch (*arrows*)

While patients will commonly have immediate relief of their constricting symptoms, there is often residual tracheomalacia that can take some time to resolve. This is especially true of younger children with a double aortic arch. Symptoms of dysphagia may take some time to resolve as well. Of note, there still may be what appears to be vascular compression on an esophagram due to the presence of the blood vessels in an abnormal position.

Complications

During the course of the procedure and especially when ligating the vessels, the surgeon should always be prepared for potential bleeding. Catastrophic bleeding should first be prevented. Survival is only likely if the surgeon has a plan already formulated for control. Initially this includes proximal and distal control of the vessels prior to division. In the case of thoracoscopic division, a thoracotomy tray should be readily available for rapid entry into the chest.

Chylothorax is a rare complication of division of a vascular ring. In addition to preparation for catastrophic bleeding, the surgeon should be aware of and identify the course of the vagus nerve and the recurrent laryngeal nerve.

Summary Points

- Vascular compression syndromes should be considered for children with noisy breathing, recurrent pneumonias and older children with dysphagia.
- Work-up consists of a plain chest radiograph followed by an echocardiogram.
- An esophagram can be confirmatory, if echocardiography is not available.
- A magnetic resonance arteriogram or computed tomographic arteriogram is very helpful to define the anatomy for surgical planning.
- Bronchoscopy is usually not necessary; however, the diagnosis is sometimes made during bronchoscopy for an airway work-up.
- Consider thoracoscopic division to divide the ligamentum arteriosum or to divide a narrow or atretic segment of a double aortic arch.

Editor's Comment

In many tertiary care pediatric centers, pediatric cardiac surgeons are responsible for the care of patients with a vascular compression syndrome. Nevertheless, pediatric surgeons need to be aware of the signs and symptoms of these uncommon anomalies and should be familiar with the basic anatomy and principles of management. It is not uncommon to encounter a vascular anomaly during a thoracotomy or thoracoscopy being performed for esophageal atresia or other mediastinal lesion, in which case it is important to know what to do and, perhaps more importantly, what not to do. Such a finding usually prompts an immediate review of available imaging to see if something was missed on the initial reading. The next step is to carefully dissect and define all structures, including those on the opposite side of the mediastinum, being very careful not to injure important adjacent structures. No vessel should be divided unless it is clear that a true ring exists and that there is brisk flow in the descending aorta after test occlusion of the vessel in question.

For certain vascular anomalies, the thoracoscopic approach is safe in experienced hands. Vessels can be ligated with a variety of techniques and most surgeons prefer to use at least two for added safety. In small children, most vessels can be clipped and then divided with bipolar electrocautery or the harmonic scalpel. Other options include simple suture ligation and oversewing the end with a running permanent monofilament suture. Stapling devices would probably work well but there is rarely enough space to manipulate the device and fire it properly without fear of inadvertently incorporating an important adjacent structure or nerve.

Bleeding is the most feared complication as these are large, high-pressure, high-flow vessels that have a tendency to retract and become extremely difficult to control. Even when the bleeding is stopped, much to the relief of all present, the risk of injury to other structures (recurrent laryngeal nerve) is significant. A contingency plan must be prepared in advance, especially if the procedure is being performed thoracoscopically, with the ability to perform a rapid thoracotomy at a moment's notice. Proximal and distal control of all vessels can be difficult and time-consuming but it is time well invested.

Finally, chylothorax is a particularly distressing complication and one that is often frustrating to manage. It is best prevented by using meticulous technique and staying close to all vessels being dissected. At the conclusion of the operation, one should take a moment to observe the operative field closely for signs of a chyle leak and place sutures to repair a leak if one is found. Some have suggested that application of a commercially available fibrin sealant works well to help small chyle leaks to seal. If a chylothorax occurs, management includes establishing drainage with a chest tube, initial bowel rest, and a great deal of patience. If the leak persists after 3 or 4 weeks, operative management should be considered, which can be difficult given that this entails a redo operation in the chest.

Differential Diagnosis

- Tracheomalacia
- Laryngomalacia
- Complete tracheal ring
- GERD

Diagnostic Studies

- Plain chest radiograph, consider confirmatory esophagram
- Echocardiography
- CT-angiogram
- MR-angiogram

Parental Preparation

- Possible conversion to thoracotomy for thoracoscopic procedures
- Possible catastrophic breathing
- Symptoms might take time to resolve, mostly due to persistent tracheomalacia

Preoperative Preparation

- ☐ Two large-bore IVs
- ☐ Type and crossmatch
- ☐ Arterial line monitoring
- ☐ Pulse-oximeter on the left upper extremity and one lower extremity
- ☐ Thoracotomy tray open for thoracoscopic procedures
- ☐ Informed consent

Technical Points

- Most vascular compression anomalies are approached from the left side.
- All vascular structures should be carefully dissected and visualized before any structure is ligated and divided.
- The vagus, recurrent laryngeal, and phrenic nerves should be carefully identified and protected throughout the procedure.
- One must be prepared for the possibility of catastrophic bleeding and have a plan for dealing with it should it occur.
- The best treatment for hemorrhage is prevention: proximal and distal control of vessels, ability to convert rapidly to open thoracotomy, all instrumentation available at a moment's notice.
- Thoracoscopic plastic interlocking clips can be used to control vascular structures that are to be divided.
- Chest tubes are optional.

Suggested Reading

Alsenaidi K et al. Management and outcomes of double aortic arch in 81 patients. Pediatrics. 2006;118(5):e1336–41.

Backer CL et al. Trends in vascular ring surgery. J Thorac Cardiovasc Surg. 2005;129(6):1339–47.

Hernanz-Schulman M. Vascular rings: a practical approach to imaging diagnosis. Pediatr Radiol. 2005;35(10):961–79.

Humphrey C, Duncan K, Fletcher S. Decade of experience with vascular rings at a single institution. Pediatrics. 2006;117(5):e903–8.

Koontz CS et al. Video-assisted thoracoscopic division of vascular rings in pediatric patients. Am Surg. 2005;71(4):289–91.

Chapter 37
Congenital Lung Lesions

Bill Chiu and Alan W. Flake

Congenital lung anomalies include congenital cystic adenomatoid malformation (CCAM), congenital lobar emphysema (CLE), bronchopulmonary sequestration (BPS), and bronchogenic cyst. Lesions may contain a mixture of these elements or communicate with the gastrointestinal tract. Diagnosis is now commonly made by routine prenatal ultrasound and patients are frequently referred to a fetal diagnosis and treatment center before birth. The discovery of these anomalies should be followed by full ultrasonographic evaluation, and, in some cases, fetal MRI to search for coexisting anomalies.

The key prognostic indicator is the size of the lesion, not necessarily the etiology. A large mass compresses the normal lung or the esophagus, and can cause mediastinal shift. The heart and great vessels can also be compressed, resulting in hemodynamic instability and hydrops fetalis. Hydrops portends a grave situation but may be successfully treated in selected cases with steroids, early delivery, or in utero intervention.

Congenital Cystic Adenomatoid Malformation

Congenital cystic adenomatoid malformation is characterized by a lack of normal alveoli and an excessive proliferation and cystic dilation of terminal respiratory bronchioles. There have been various histologic classifications of CCAM. However, from a clinical perspective, the impact of the size of the mass on normal pulmonary development and physiology is a more important consideration. Most CCAMs receive only pulmonary arterial blood supply. A lesion containing CCAM histology that is found to have a systemic feeding vessel, which is characteristic of bronchopulmonary sequestration, is referred to as a hybrid lesion. Hybrid lesions are relatively common and represent 23% of asymptomatic

congenital lung lesions in our most recent series. In up to 3% of cases, CCAM is present in more than one lobe of the lung.

CCAM is now frequently diagnosed on routine prenatal ultrasonography. Other lesions that have a similar appearance include congenital diaphragmatic hernia, foregut duplication cyst, bronchogenic cyst, congenital lobar emphysema, lobar or segmental bronchial atresia, unilateral lung agenesis, and mediastinal cystic teratoma. Fetal MRI can help to distinguish between these entities. In addition, we always perform a karyotype analysis and fetal echocardiogram to identify the rare associated anomaly or genetic syndrome.

CCAMs have a predictable prenatal growth pattern with maximal growth occurring between 20 and 28 weeks. Thereafter, the majority of CCAMs plateau in size or regress during the third trimester. Postnatally, patients are often asymptomatic or can present with respiratory distress from large lesions that compress the mediastinum or adjacent lung tissue. Significant pulmonary hypoplasia related to CCAM is rather uncommon. Older patients with undiagnosed CCAM may present with recurrent infections from abnormal drainage of tracheobronchial secretions, or, rarely, with malignant degeneration. We perform computed tomography on all patients within the first 6 weeks of life to confirm the diagnosis and guide surgical treatment.

Due to the risks of infection, spontaneous pneumothorax, and malignant degeneration (pleuropulmonary blastoma, rhabdomyosarcoma), we advocate resection of all CCAMs. For microcystic CCAMs prior to 28 weeks gestation with associated hydrops, we offer a trial of corticosteroids, followed by fetal lobectomy if the hydrops does not resolve (Fig. 37.1). Macrocystic CCAMs causing hydrops are best treated by thoraco-amniotic shunts. In our series, survival after open fetal surgery and thoraco-amniotic shunting is 60 and 75% respectively. CCAMs that remain massive with associated mediastinal shift but not causing hydrops are best delivered by ex utero intrapartum treatment (EXIT procedure), in which uteroplacental circulation is maintained while the lobectomy is performed. Lesions that are symptomatic at birth are best resected within the first few days of life and the asymptomatic CCAM can be electively resected

B. Chiu (✉)
Department of Surgery, Children's Hospital of Philadelphia,
Philadelphia, PA, USA
e-mail: chiub@email.chop.edu

P. Mattei (ed.), *Fundamentals of Pediatric Surgery*,
DOI 10.1007/978-1-4419-6643-8_37, © Springer Science+Business Media, LLC 2011

Fig. 37.1 Algorithm for the management of prenatally diagnosed congenital lung lesions

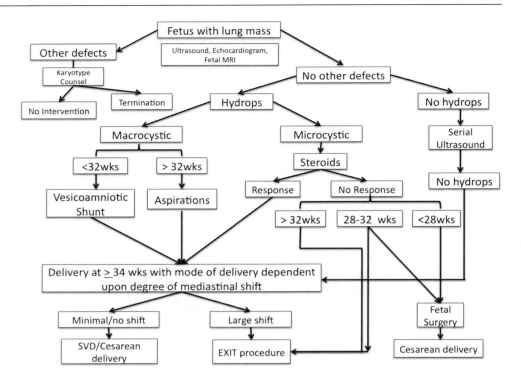

by open or thoracoscopic techniques within the first 3 months of life. Using this algorithm, the vast majority of infants with CCAM have an excellent outcome and can ultimately expect to have a normal quality of life.

Congenital Lobar Emphysema

Congenital lobar emphysema (CLE) is defined as the abnormal inflation of a histologically normal lobe of the lung. The most common cause is an intrinsic defect in bronchial cartilage, leading to airway collapse on expiration and progressive air trapping. Other types of extrinsic or intrinsic compression of a lobar bronchus, such as a bronchogenic cyst, may present as CLE, as can acquired forms of lobar air trapping caused by extrinsic compression of bronchi from mediastinal masses or by loss of elasticity of lung parenchyma related to prolonged ventilatory support.

CLE occurs most frequently in the left upper lobe, followed by the right middle lobe and the right upper lobe. Typically, infants are asymptomatic after birth, but respiratory distress and tachypnea develop within the first few days of life due to progressive air trapping.

CLE appears on chest radiographs as lobar hyperinflation, with flattening of the ipsilateral diaphragm and mediastinal shift. In some newborns, it is identified radiographically as delayed clearance of lung liquid from a single lobe. Other entities

with similar radiographic appearance include pneumothorax, macrocystic CCAM, and bronchogenic cyst. In premature infants with bronchopulmonary dysplasia, regional cystic degeneration can sometimes be confused with congenital CLE. Computed tomography or nuclear medicine ventilation/perfusion scan can be helpful in establishing the diagnosis. CT can also evaluate whether a mediastinal structure is compressing the otherwise normal lung. Echocardiography is necessary to rule out associated cardiac anomalies.

All lung lobes affected by CLE should be surgically resected. Overexpansion of the lung needs to be avoided, especially after endotracheal intubation for surgery. The progressive air trapping sometimes requires emergent decompressive thoracotomy. The outcome after resection is generally excellent.

Bronchopulmonary Sequestration

Bronchopulmonary sequestration (BPS) is an abnormal, nonfunctioning portion of lung tissue that does not communicate with the tracheobronchial tree. It is extralobar if the mass has its own pleural investment, intralobar if it is contained within the normal pleura. Extralobar BPS are frequently associated with congenital diaphragmatic hernia and can be found postero-medially in the left lower chest or occasionally below the diaphragm. Newborns with extralobar BPS often have respiratory distress or feeding intolerance, whereas intralobar BPS can be clinically silent until recurrent infections occur later in life. Most intralobar BPS are located in the lower lobes and are rarely associated with other anomalies. Both types of BPS can communicate with the gastrointestinal tract, most commonly the lower esophagus.

Extralobar BPS diagnosed antenatally sometimes have a non-cystic echogenic appearance similar to microcystic CCAM, but color Doppler imaging will usually demonstrate a systemic feeding vessel. On postnatal chest radiograph, extralobar BPS appears as a retrocardiac density, while infected intralobar sequestration appears as a consolidated area of lung tissue, often with an air-fluid level due to abscess formation.

Antenatally, extralobar BPS can create a mass effect on normal lung development or tension hydrothorax from lymphatic fluid exudation. In our series of 41 prenatally diagnosed lesions, three fetuses developed tension hydrothorax and required thoraco-amniotic shunting or thoracentesis. Twenty-eight lesions regressed during gestation and did not require postnatal resection. Seven patients had postnatal resection and one with hydrops died after delivery despite postnatal ECMO.

The arterial supply of BPS is commonly from the aorta, and in 20% of cases comes from below the diaphragm. This anomalous systemic blood supply can lead to arteriovenous fistula physiology, resulting in high-output cardiac failure or hemorrhage. The venous drainage of extralobar sequestration is via the azygous system, while intralobar lesions drain via the pulmonary veins. The blood supply usually enters through the inferior pulmonary ligament, and as many as 15% have more than one feeding vessel.

Surgical resection is indicated for all intralobar BPS and those extralobar lesions presenting a mass effect or with high systemic blood flow. Both types of sequestration can be resected via thoracotomy or thoracoscopy. Intralobar lesions should be resected using a formal lobectomy, since segmental resection has a high risk of recurrence and subsequent infection.

Bronchogenic Cyst

Bronchogenic cysts are fluid-filled cysts derived from abnormal budding of the foregut. They can arise anywhere along the tracheobronchial tree and can cause compression of lung, trachea, or esophagus. During development, obstruction of a lobar bronchus will be manifest as lobar hyperplasia beyond the obstruction, which appears as an echogenic lung mass. Most patients are initially asymptomatic but because of the potential for producing respiratory distress, pneumonia, or dysphagia, they should always be excised.

Detecting bronchogenic cyst prenatally can be difficult and is always considered in the context of a cystic chest lesion associated with lobar echogenicity, often with a similar appearance to CCAM or CLE. On chest radiograph, bronchogenic cysts appear as a smooth mass and may contain an air-fluid level if there is a communication with the airway or the gastrointestinal tract. Computed tomography is useful in confirming the diagnosis.

Excision of a bronchogenic cyst can be accomplished via thoracotomy or thoracoscopy. Depending on the extent of pulmonary involvement, a segmentectomy or lobectomy may rarely need to be performed. Bronchogenic cysts within the mediastinum should be excised, not simply drained, and a course of preoperative antibiotics are required if the patient presents with an infected cyst.

Surgical Technique

In the absence of significant intrinsic lung disease or prematurity, major pulmonary resection is generally well tolerated by young children, who can usually achieve impressive compensatory lung growth following surgery. Access to the chest may be through a standard posterolateral thoracotomy, but a muscle-sparing or axillary thoracotomy is preferred. We have increasingly used thoracoscopy for lobectomies and other complex procedures. Fusion of the normal anatomic fissures is frequently encountered, especially with large CCAMs, and is a significant risk factor for hemorrhage and conversion to thoracotomy. Distortion of the usual anatomy should also be expected. When resecting a sequestration, it is important to identify and control the systemic feeding vessel early and carefully, especially if it arises from below the diaphragm. These vessels are large but delicate and they can retract, essentially disappearing into the mediastinum or below the diaphragm, and cause a very rapid exsanguination. Pulmonary arteries and veins should also be dissected carefully to avoid hemorrhage, especially during thoracoscopy. We prefer to ligate each vessel twice and use a hemoclip or precise application of bipolar electrocautery. Control of the pulmonary vein is especially challenging as it is usually very wide, very short, and, of course, very thin-walled. We close the bronchus with a proximal ligature and distal suture ligation using fine monofilament suture, but because of the small size of the bronchus in small infants, we do not use a stapling device. We also leave a thoracostomy tube, which can be removed as early as postoperative day 1 if there is no evidence of an air leak or significant effusion.

Meticulous intra-operative technique and epidural analgesia can expedite the postoperative recovery course. We try to have all stable infants extubated before leaving the operating room or, if possible, within 24 h of the operation. Most can advance diet as tolerated. In most cases, prophylactic antibiotics should be discontinued within 24–48 h.

The most common major complication is prolonged air leak, which will usually seal on their own, but occasionally require reoperation for repair of a bronchial stump leak. Other complications include infection, thoracotomy-related scoliosis, and recurrent disease, presumably due to inadequate resection.

Congenital lung anomalies consist of a diverse group of lesions that share a common embryologic origin and have similar clinical presentations. Many are now diagnosed prenatally. Fetal or perinatal intervention can affect outcome in selected cases, especially when the fetus develops hydrops. Postnatally, babies can present with compression of the normal lung, infection from failure to clear secretions or, in rare cases, malignant degeneration. Complete excision of the lesion is well tolerated and represents definitive therapy.

Summary Points

- Most congenital lung anomalies can be diagnosed in utero by ultrasonography.
- The primary prenatal prognostic factor is size of the mass rather than the specific type of lung anomaly.
- Fetal CCAMs have a predictable prenatal growth pattern with maximal growth between 20 and 28 weeks and frequent regression but not disappearance of the mass in the third trimester.
- All CCAMs should be resected because of their propensity for infection and malignant degeneration.
- CLE typically becomes symptomatic in the first few days of life and requires resection due to progressive lobar expansion from air trapping.
- BPS may be intralobar or extralobar and these two types have different clinical manifestations.
- Extralobar BPS can cause a mass effect during fetal development or a tension hydrothorax from lymphatic exudation. After birth, large extralobar BPS or those representing a large AV shunt should be resected.
- Intralobar BPS are typically asymptomatic until infection or a large AV shunt becomes apparent. Intralobar BPS should nearly always be resected by lobectomy.
- Bronchogenic cysts can cause compression of the lung, major airways, or esophagus and should always be resected.

Editor's Comment

Most congenital lung lesions need to be excised, but the timing varies depending on the clinical circumstances: in utero, at birth using an EXIT strategy, urgently or semi-urgently in the newborn period, or after a several-month period of maturation and close observation. A CCAM might regress in the third trimester and for a time after birth, but it will rarely disappear completely. Most cases of true congenital lobar emphysema will present acutely in the newborn period and need to be excised urgently or emergently. In the rare case of a CLE under tension, a decompressive thoracotomy performed at the bedside can be a life-saving maneuver. Fetuses that develop hydrops clearly require some form of intervention: induction and delivery for near-term infants with severe hydrops, thoraco-amniotic shunting for macrocystic lesions, thoracotomy with EXIT, or, rarely, fetal surgery. Asymptomatic patients with a CCAM, sequestration, or hybrid lesion can be safely observed for a period of weeks or even months after birth, which makes general anesthesia somewhat safer and the operation technically more straightforward.

The thoracoscopic approach is an advanced minimally invasive procedure that is being offered only at selected centers, but in the absence of an indication for urgent intervention or a contraindication to the approach, parents should be offered the option of having their baby's care transferred to a center where there is experience with this technique. In preparation for any operation that might involve lung lobectomy, it is always sensible to review the relevant anatomy beforehand. The operation itself should be done with single-lung ventilation, usually best accomplished in an infant by main-stem intubation under fluoroscopic guidance. The most significant hurdle to successful thoracoscopic resection is an incomplete major fissure, the dissection of which frequently results in bleeding and troublesome air leaks. Because the tissues are so delicate and the vessels so prone to tearing, the most important technical aspects of the operation are patience and absolutely meticulous dissection. Most importantly, the surgeon needs to resist the temptation to use aggressive blunt dissection, which, although it is the trademark of the accomplished laparoscopist, can quickly lead to exsanguinating hemorrhage.

Differential Diagnosis

- CCAM, BPS, CLE, bronchogenic cyst
- Bronchial atresia or stenosis
- Lung agenesis (with contralateral compensatory hypertrophy)
- Congenital diaphragmatic hernia
- Pneumothorax
- Bronchial foreign body
- Cystic lung disease
- Bronchiectasis/lung abscess

Diagnostic Studies

- Level II ultrasound
- Fetal MRI
- Fetal echocardiogram
- Chest radiograph
- CT scan
- MRI/MRA

Parental Preparation

- Prenatal counseling in the context of size of lesion/gestational age
- Occasional prenatal intervention or delivery by EXIT procedure
- Major operative procedure – thoracotomy or thoracoscopy
- In most cases, the outcome is excellent

Preoperative Preparation

- ☐ IV hydration
- ☐ Prophylactic antibiotics
- ☐ Type & screen
- ☐ Informed consent

Technical Points

- Muscle sparing, axillary, or thoracoscopic approach
- Meticulous dissection of hilar structures
- Awareness of anatomic variation
- Techniques for dividing parenchyma and bronchial structures are age-dependent

Suggested Reading

Adzick NS, Flake AW, Crombleholme TM. Management of congenital lung lesions. Semin Pediatr Surg. 2003;12:10–6.

Crombleholme TM, Coleman B, Hedrick H, et al. Cystic adenomatoid malformation volume ratio predicts outcome in prenatally diagnosed cystic adenomatoid malformation of the lung. J Pediatr Surg. 2002;37:331–8.

Mann S, Wilson RD, Bebbington MW, Adzick NS, Johnson MP. Antenatal diagnosis and management of congenital cystic adenomatoid malformation. Semin Fetal Neonat Med. 2007;12:477–81.

Tsai AY, Liechty KW, Hedrick HL, et al. Outcomes after postnatal resection of prenatally diagnosed asymptomatic cystic lung lesions. J Pediatr Surg. 2008;43:513–7.

Chapter 38
Thoracoscopic Biopsy and Lobectomy of the Lung

Sanjeev Dutta and Craig T. Albanese

Thoracoscopic surgery is now the preferred method of both lung biopsy and lobectomy in children. This is supported by a number of studies from multiple institutions that demonstrate reduced pain and hospital stay, superior cosmesis, and avoidance of the potentially morbid sequelae of posterolateral thoracotomy such as scoliosis, winged scapula, shoulder muscle girdle weakness, and chest wall deformity. While still technically demanding, cooperation from the anesthesiologist, appropriately sized minimal access instrumentation, and novel energy devices have facilitate this procedure for surgeons with advanced laparoscopic experience.

Indications for lung biopsy are the same regardless of the surgical approach. A biopsy for a diffuse interstitial lung disease may be requested, or a more directed biopsy for discrete lesions of infectious or malignant origin may be needed. Thoracoscopy might be contraindicated in unusual circumstances in which the child cannot tolerate partial collapse of the affected lung, there is extensive obliteration of the pleural space and a workspace cannot be achieved, or the target lesion is centrally located, placing the mainstem bronchus at risk for injury.

The majority of thoracoscopic lobectomies are performed for congenital cystic lesions, including cystic adenomatoid malformations (CCAM), bronchopulmonary sequestration (BPS), or hybrid lesions. Sequestrations can be intralobar, typically requiring complete resection of the involved lobe, or, less commonly, extralobar. Less common indications include bronchiectasis, congenital lobar emphysema (CLE), and malignancies such as metastatic sarcoma. Standard indications for resection of congenital cystic lesions include potential for infection and the long-term risk of malignant transformation. Mass lesions occupying greater than 50% of the hemithorax are amenable to thoracoscopic biopsy but often provide insufficient workspace for safe thoracoscopic resection.

Diagnosis

Lesions for biopsy are typically discovered as part of a workup for respiratory symptomatology, or as part of imaging for malignancy at other sites. Discrete lesions with a diameter less than 10 mm and subpleural depth greater than 5 mm are sometimes difficult to identify by thoracoscopic inspection, or by instrument probing, necessitating conversion to thoracotomy and manual palpation. A number of preoperative CT-guided localization strategies have been developed to address this challenge including hook wire placement (similar to breast tumor localization) or tattooing with methylene blue or the patient's own blood. These have variable success, and are dependent on the institutional interventional radiology expertise. An emerging method, still experimental, is the use of endoscopic ultrasound with the lung collapsed and the instillation of intrathoracic saline to improve acoustic coupling. The role and success rate of this technique is not well established, but as experience increases it seems more and more promising.

Increasingly, congenital cystic lung lesions are identified antenatally by ultrasound or MRI. While some progress to mediastinal compression, hydrops and fetal demise, most continue to term, typically asymptomatic at birth. In these cases, a repeat CT scan is obtained a few months postnatally prior to a planned surgical resection. Some surgeons recommend observation of asymptomatic cystic lung lesions because some will spontaneously regress and one might be able to avoid the morbidity of a thoracotomy. However, the ongoing risk of infection and malignancy, and the fact that thoracoscopy minimizes the morbidity, increasingly weaken the argument for a nonoperative approach. Furthermore, infection is most likely to occur in the first 2 years of life

S. Dutta (✉)
Department of Surgery, Stanford University, Lucile Packard Children's Hospital, 780 Welch Road, Suite 206, Stanford, CA 94305, USA
e-mail: sdutta@stanford.edu

P. Mattei (ed.), *Fundamentals of Pediatric Surgery*,
DOI 10.1007/978-1-4419-6643-8_38, © Springer Science+Business Media, LLC 2011

and can complicate subsequent surgical resection due to inflammation and scarring and can increase the risk of a bronchopleural fistula.

Surgical Technique

Lung Biopsy

Preoperative preparation includes correction of coagulopathy and thorough assessment of anesthetic risk. Critically low respiratory reserve is a contraindication to thoracoscopy. For patients with severe interstitial lung disease, an intensive care hospital bed should be arranged in advance. Appropriate instrumentation for thoracotomy should be available during the operation should there be the need for urgent conversion. Single-lung ventilation is desirable but not absolutely necessary. For larger children, this is easily achieved with a selective mainstem bronchial intubation, a bronchial blocker, or a double lumen endotracheal tube. Lung collapse is aided by low-flow, low-pressure insufflation of carbon dioxide, and for babies it is all that is necessary to maintain adequate collapse of the ipsilateral lung. Thus for infants, we prefer standard tracheal intubation.

The patient is positioned in a standard thoracotomy position with bolsters or on a bean bag, with the surgeon and assistant at the patient's back and the monitor placed across the table (Fig. 38.1). Secured to the table, the patient can be tilted back and forth to optimize ergonomics and exposure.

We prefer to use a Veress needle in a trocar sheath with insufflation tubing attached, which is slowly advanced into the chest cavity through a 5-mm incision in the midaxillary line at the fifth or sixth intercostal space. While the Veress needle is being advanced, a CO_2 insufflation pressure of 4–8 mmHg with a flow rate of 1 L/min is maintained. This allows the lung to collapse away as the needle is introduced. After a minute of insufflation, the Veress is removed from the

sheath and a 5 mm trocar introduced. One or two additional ports are placed under direct visualization. Ports can be placed along the mid-axillary line, but placement a little off midline can improve triangulation around the operative site (Fig. 38.2). For children who weigh more than 10 kg, one of the port sites, most commonly closest to the axilla, is enlarged to a 12-mm size to accomodate an endostapler containing a vascular cartridge (2.5-mm staple height).

For biopsy, the diseased tissue is held with an atraumatic grasper and excised with multiple stapler firings. The specimen is retrieved directly through the 12 mm port with an endo retrieval bag or one fashioned from the finger of a surgical glove. Staple line hemostasis is achieved with the hook cautery as necessary.

In children too small to accomodate a stapling device, the tissue is grasped and two endoloops are applied around the affected parenchyma, which is then sharply excised. A chest tube is left in place through one of the port sites and attached to 10–15 cm-H_2O suction. Skin incisions are reapproximated with absorbable suture, and intercostal nerve blocks with 0.25% bupivacaine are placed.

Lobectomy

Preoperative preparation, patient positioning, and port placement are the same as for biopsy. Occasionally, a fourth port is necessary. In larger children, one 12-mm port is placed to accomodate an endostapler that is used for completing the fissure and transecting vessels and bronchus. In smaller children with insufficient workspace to introduce and maneuver a stapler, a 5-mm Ligasure (Valleylab, CO) device with a curved "Maryland"-type grasper (non-bladed) is used to

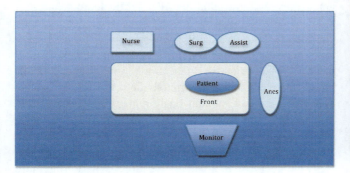

Fig. 38.1 Optimal layout of the positioning in the OR for thoracoscopic lung biopsy. Note that the surgeon and the assistant are at the patient's back and on the same side of the operating table. The patient is in a standard thoracotomy position

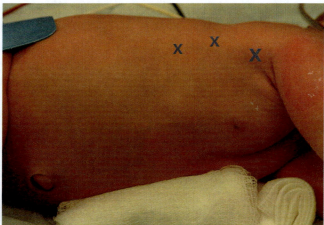

Fig. 38.2 Infant positioned in the right-side-up thoracotomy position for lung biopsy. Note the roll of gauze used as an axillary roll and another roll of gauze used to keep the patient from rolling forward. The incisions are placed so as to triangulate, with the largest incision, if necessary, placed nearest to the axilla for cosmetic reasons

complete the fissure and divide pulmonary vessels, obviating the need for a 12-mm port. The Ligasure utilizes radiofrequency energy to create a tissue seal, and can be used to safely seal and divide pulmonary vessels less than 7 mm in diameter. We will sometimes apply the device at adjacent points on the vessel to achieve a longer sealed length prior to dividing sharply. Multiple applications of the Ligasure at one point can be used to achieve sealing and division. Space-occupying cysts such as CCAM or CLE can be addressed prior to resection by puncture or reduction with Ligasure application, allowing for a larger workspace.

The lower lobes are most frequently resected due to the high frequency of cystic lesions at this location. Dissection begins with careful division of the inferior pulmonary ligament. For BPS, a systemic arterial vessel is usually present, and is isolated by exposing it within the lung parenchyma. A combination of silk sutures tied intracorporeally and 5 mm clips and are used to control and divide this often friable, calcified, high-pressure vessel. If less than 5 mm diameter, the vessel can be divided with the Ligasure. The pulmonary vein is then isolated. If feasible, this vessel is left undivided to prevent lobar congestion, however it can be divided at this time if it facilitates exposure of the other structures. The Ligasure device is used from an anterior to posterior direction to complete the fissure and dissect out the pulmonary arterial branches. The main branch supplying the lower lobe is divided at the hilum, or segmental branches are divided, depending on the individual anatomy. With arterial supply divided, the pulmonary vein is divided, and the bronchus is divided with a stapler in larger children, or suture-ligated using an absorbable monofilament suture and divided sharply. The specimen is removed intact through a slightly enlarged axillary port site, or piecemeal from a retrieval bag. Postoperative care is usually straightforward.

Upper lobes are more challenging due to tight anatomic proximity of the hilar structures to the lobar vascular and bronchial branches. The superior pulmonary vein is first divided, exposing the main pulmonary artery. Progressing in a cephalocaudal direction, the lobe is stripped off the main trunk, dividing segmental branches as encountered. The major fissure is completed, and then the bronchus divided.

The right middle lobe is approached by completing the minor and major fissures, after which the lobar vessels and bronchus are divided.

Chest tubes are not placed for cases of extralobar sequestration, or select cases where there is a well-defined fissure and easy bronchial closure. Otherwise, an appropriate size chest tube is placed through one of the port sites, intercostal nerve blocks with 0.25% bupivacaine are placed, and the skin is closed with absorbable suture.

Postoperative Care

Chest tubes are removed within 24–48 h, after air leak is ruled out on underwater seal and a normal chest radiograph obtained. Analgesic requirements are usually minimal: narcotics (patient-controlled when possible) for 1 or 2 days, followed by acetaminophen. Radiographs after chest tube removal are not routinely obtained. Patients are instructed not to immerse wounds in water for 5 days.

Complications include prolonged air leak, which is commonly due to parenchymal air leak from a completed fissure, and typically resolves with chest tube suction alone. This can be avoided intra-operatively by application of fibrin glue to the retained fissure surface. Bronchopleural fistula is rare but can result especially after resection of a previously infected lobe and may require reoperation to correct.

Thoracoscopic lung biopsy and lobectomy are feasible, safe and effective in the hands of experienced minimal access pediatric surgeons. They are enabled by the use of novel technologies such as endostaplers and radiofrequency energy devices. The benefits include reduced pain and scarring, reduced hospital stay, and avoidance of the musculoskeletal deformity sometimes seen after thoracotomy. The future challenge is to educate trainees in the safe application of these techniques.

Summary Points

- The inability to manually palpate lung lesions during thoracoscopic biopsy sometimes necessitates the use of adjunct localization procedures such as CT-guided hook wire placement, CT-guided tattooing, or endoscopic ultrasound.
- Pulmonary lobar lesions traditionally removed by thoracotomy can now be resected thoracoscopically, using valved ports, low pressure CO_2 insufflation, laparoscopic instrumentation, endostaplers, and radiofrequency energy devices such as the Ligasure.
- Thoracoscopic resection avoids the potential long term musculoskeletal deformity associated with thoracotomy in the young.
- Contraindications to thoracoscopic resection include: inability to tolerate one lung ventilation, extensive thoracic adhesions, or centrally located lesions with hilar involvement.

Editor's Comment

In the small child with diffuse or military disease, a true "mini" anterolateral thoracotomy incision (2 cm, in the fifth or sixth intercostal space) can be used to gain access to the lingula or lower lobe. Done well, this is less invasive than a thoracosopic procedure. In the absence of an absolute contraindication, most lung biopsies should be performed using a minimally invasive technique.

Thoracoscopy works best for patchy disease or when the nodules are large and peripheral. but with one-lung ventilation, 5–8 mmH$_2$O CO$_2$ insufflation, and extreme patience to let the lung become completely atelectatic (20–30 min), lung lesions as small as 2–3 mm in diameter and up to 2 cm deep to the pleura may be "palpated" at thoracoscopy. The trick is to use the smooth shaft of a 5-mm grasper or suction cannula to "squeegee" the lung surface while applying gentle downward pressure until the instrument "catches" on the lesion. The parenchyma near the lesion is grasped and lifted so that the stapling device can pass deep to the lesion. The vascular cartridge should always be used on the lung and, even if the device is being used extracorporeally, the endoscopic stapling device is superior to the standard hand-held stapling device because it places three rows of staples instead of just two.

I always place three incisions, one in the anterior axillary line in the fifth or sixth intercostal space (I enter the chest with a hemostat as for a chest tube), a second 5-mm trocar posteriorly in the eighth or ninth intercostal space, and 10/12-mm port in the midaxillary line in the lowest transverse axillary skin crease. Placing the last port within the axilla might be better cosmetically but the arm will prevent you from getting enough leverage to direct the stapler towards the diaphragm. It is important to minimize unnecessary grasping of the parenchyma as this creates small parenchymal hematomas that can mask the lesion or result in air leaks. Though the risk of pneumothorax is very low, I always leave a chest tube whenever I take a lung biopsy to prevent even one case in a hundred of tension pneumothorax. I use a 16 or 20 French tube, place it throught the camera port site, and take it out on the first postoperative day while still on suction if there has never been an air leak. The tube does not always need to be sutured in place and the incision, if properly "Z"-tracked (obliquely through the tissues), can be closed with cyanoacrylate glue or a small occlusive dressing when the tube is pulled. The other incisions are closed at the level of the deeper fascia and the skin and covered with cyanoacrylate skin adhesive.

The thoracoscopic approach should be used to sample suspicious nodules in children with cancer, but I do not recommend the technique when a careful and through search for small nodules needs to be made in a potentially therapeutic scenario, such as in the rare patient with a small number of metastatic lung nodules due to osteogenic sarcoma who is still considered curable with surgery. In these situations, bilateral staged thoracotomy or sternotomy with bimanual palpation of each lung is still considered standard.

Differential Diagnosis

Biopsy

- Interstitial lung disease
- Infection
- Metastasis

Lobectomy

- Cystic adenomatoid malformation
- Bronchopulmonary sequestration
- Bronchiectasis
- Congenital lobar emphysema
- Malignancy

Diagnostic Studies

- Antenatal U/S
- Antenatal MRI
- Chest X-ray at birth
- CT
- MRI

Parental Preparation

- There is always the potential for conversion to thoracotomy.
- We will very likely need to place a chest tube, usually for no more than 1–3 days postoperatively.
- Risks include: bleeding (uncommon), infection (rare), prolonged air leak (rare), or death (extremely rare).

Preoperative Preparation

- ☐ Appropriate imaging
- ☐ Preoperative localization, if necessary
- ☐ Coagulopathy work up
- ☐ Intensive care bed for severe interstitial lung disease or infection

Technical Points

- For large patients, lung collapse is achieved with mainstem intubation, a bronchial blocker, or double lumen tube, in addition to CO_2 insufflation at pressure 4–8 mmHg, flow 1 L/min.
- For infants, adequate lung collapse is achieved with CO_2 insufflation alone.
- Hemithorax must be 5 cm in minimal diameter to accomodate an endostapler, used for completing fissures and dividing vessels and bronchus.
- In children under 10 kg, the biopsy can be taken by placing an endoloop proximal to the lesion and dividing the lung parenchyma distal to the ligature.
- In smaller children, the Ligasure can be used to complete fissures, and divide vessels; bronchi are suture ligated.
- In suspected pulmonary sequestration, look for systemic feeding artery.
- Upper lobes are more difficult to resect than lower lobes.

Suggested Reading

Albanese CT, Rothenberg SS. Experience with 144 consecutive pediatric thoracoscopic lobectomies. J Laparoendosc Adv Surg Tech. 2007;17:339–41.

Albanese CT, Sydorak RM, Tsao K, Lee H. Thoracoscopic lobectomy for prenatally diagnosed lung lesions. J Pediatr Surg. 2003;38: 553–5.

Ponsky TA, Rothenberg SS. Thoracoscopic lung biopsy in infants and children with endoloops allows smaller trocar sites and discreet biopsies. J Laparoendosc Adv Surg Tech. 2008;18:120–2.

Rothenberg SS. First decade's experience with thoracoscopic lobectomy in infants and children. J Pediatr Surg. 2008;43:40–5.

Vu LT, Farmer DL, Nobuhara KK, Miniati D, Lee H. Thoracoscopic versus open resection for congenital cystic adenomatoid malformations of the lung. J Pediatr Surg. 2008;43:35–9.

Chapter 39
Diseases of the Pleural Space

Keith A. Kuenzler

Air, blood, chyle, or infected fluid may inappropriately accumulate in the pleural space, resulting in acute or chronic clinical manifestations of varying severity.

Chylothorax

Lymphatic fluid in the pleural space originates from an injury or anomaly of the thoracic duct or its tributaries. While the medical management of chylothorax has improved with advances in pharmacology and nutrition, its surgical management has evolved as well, with more frequent use of minimal access surgical techniques. Regardless of the cause of chylothorax, the general treatment algorithm is the same: (1) drain the effusion, which relieves respiratory embarrassment and collects the fluid for analysis; (2) support the patient by replacing fluid and nutritional losses; (3) slow and then stop the leak by dietary, medical, or surgical means; and (4) consider a pleuroperitoneal shunt if the leak remains persistent. The vast majority of patients are successfully treated without surgery.

The anatomy of the thoracic duct is quite variable (Fig. 39.1). Abdominal lymphatics coalesce as the cysterna chyli at about the level of L2. The thoracic duct enters the chest through the aortic hiatus, and then travels cephalad through the posterior mediastinum along the right side of the spine and behind the esophagus. At the T4–T5 level, it travels left and through the superior mediastinum on its way into the neck, where it empties into the venous system at the junction of the left internal jugular and subclavian veins. The presence of the duct behind the aortic arch places it at high risk for injury during cardiac surgery, which often results in left chylothorax. Chyle contains greater than 80% of ingested fat in the form of chylomicrons and is also quite rich in protein. High-output chylothorax can therefore result in gradual protein loss which must be replaced by parenteral nutrition. Additionally, chyle carries a large number of white blood cells, primarily lymphocytes, which explains not only why a persistent loss of chyle can result in an immunocompromised state, but possibly why these effusions seem to be particularly resistant to bacterial infection.

Chylothorax can be traumatic or spontaneous (Table 39.1). It is the most common fetal pleural effusion. In fact, antenatal sonographic evidence of chylous effusions helped to dispel the notion that neonatal chylothorax always resulted from birth trauma. Like any space-occupying mass causing shift of the fetal mediastinum, a large chylothorax can cause pulmonary hypoplasia and *hydrops fetalis*. In cases of rapidly expanding effusions causing hydrops, thoraco-amniotic shunting has been used with success. Chyle leak in newborns is probably related to congenital anomalies of the thoracic duct or trauma during childbirth.

Most cases result from direct injuries to the thoracic duct or a major feeding channel. The most common setting for traumatic chylothorax is following cardiac surgery, but it has also been described after esophageal operations, mediastinal tumor resections, and in reoperative chest surgery. In addition to iatrogenic injury, the thoracic duct can also rupture with severe hyperextension of the spine, vigorous coughing, and nonaccidental trauma (child abuse). Spontaneous chyle leaks, presumably related to increased pressure within the duct, arise in the setting of superior vena cava thrombosis or large mediastinal neoplasms. Anomalies of the duct such as those associated with lymphangioma may also predispose to spontaneous leaks.

Diagnosis

Clinically, as with any pleural effusion, patients with chylothorax often present with acute respiratory distress, dyspnea, or cyanosis. On physical examination, one can expect to find decreased breath sounds and dullness to percussion. A chest radiograph will demonstrate the presence of pleural fluid which layers out on decubitus films. Though one usually has a high index of suspicion due to the clinical scenario, analysis of a fluid sample will make the definitive diagnosis.

K.A. Kuenzler (✉)
New York University Medical Center, 530 First Avenue,
New York, NY 10016, USA
e-mail: Keith.Kuenzler@nyumc.org

P. Mattei (ed.), *Fundamentals of Pediatric Surgery*,
DOI 10.1007/978-1-4419-6643-8_39, © Springer Science+Business Media, LLC 2011

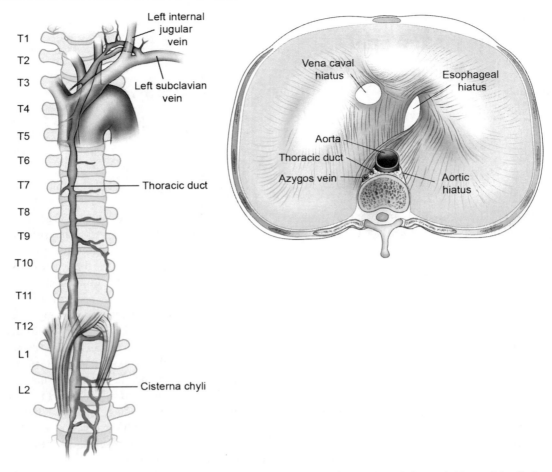

Fig. 39.1 (**a**) The typical course of the thoracic duct. (**b**) Orientation of structures coursing through the aortic hiatus of the diaphragm

Table 39.1 Causes of chylothorax

Traumatic	Spontaneous
Cardiothoracic surgery	Superior vena cava thrombosis
Hyperextension of the spine	Lymphangioma
Vigorous coughing	Mediastinal neoplasms
Child abuse	Congenital lymphatic malformations

Table 39.2 Fluid composition confirming chylothorax

Total fat > 400 mg/dL
Triglycerides > 110 mg/dL
Total protein > 5 g/dL
Lymphocytes > 80% of total white blood cell count

If a chest tube is in place (after cardiac surgery) the fluid can easily be observed and collected. Otherwise, we prefer to insert a small pigtail catheter using the Seldinger technique. These small-caliber (8.5 French) tubes will adequately drain the fluid, serving both to treat the symptoms and provide fluid for analysis. In a fasting patient, chyle grossly appears clear or straw-colored, whereas after a meal, chyle has the characteristic milky-white appearance. Demonstrating elevated levels of total fat, triglyceride, protein, and lymphocyte content confirms the diagnosis (Table 39.2).

Treatment

Placement of a thoracostomy tube allows for the alleviation of respiratory symptoms, confirmation of the diagnosis, and the means to quantify the daily fluid output. Lung re-expansion alone may facilitate thoracic duct healing by allowing the visceral pleura to appose the mediastinal leak. Fluid, lipid, and protein losses must be replaced. Attempts to stop the leak begin with the initiation of either a no-fat or high medium-chain triglyceride diet, which should decrease chyle flow through mesenteric lymphatics. In many patients, however, any oral intake (even clear liquids) sustains chyle flow and can prevent cessation of the leak. In such cases, bowel rest and parenteral nutrition should be prescribed. In addition to dietary alterations, subcutaneous injections of the somatostatin analog octreotide (10–20 µg/kg/day divided in three doses) is sometimes a useful adjunct due to its ability to inhibit gastrointestinal secretions.

There are no absolute indications for surgery. We define a failure of nonoperative therapy as a significant leak (greater than 10 mL/kg/day) that persists for more than 3 weeks. Certainly, one might elect for earlier operation in patients unable to tolerate the nutritional or immunologic effects of continued chyle loss.

The value of preoperative localization techniques by lymphoscintigraphy or radioactive isotope scanning is debatable, since the precise site of the leak is often difficult to visualize directly in surgery with or without these studies. Feeding the patient 30–60 mL of cream approximately 30 min before surgery can increase visible chyle flow and aid with intraoperative localization. Currently, thoracoscopy provides excellent visualization transpleurally on the side of the effusion; thoracotomy is almost never indicated. Exposure is optimized by single lung isolation and turning the patient into a modified prone position, which allows access to the mediastinum while allowing gravity to assist in moving the lung anteriorly.

Although often easier to describe than to accomplish, the surgical objective is the direct suture ligation of the leak, provided that this specific region of the thoracic duct or one of its tributaries is apparent. However, the leak is not always able to be definitively localized. When faced with this scenario in the right chest, the surgeon should ligate the origin of the thoracic duct at the aortic hiatus, usually found on the right lateral portion of the spine. The pleura adjacent to the azygous vein just above the diaphragm is opened to identify the duct medially and posterior to the esophagus. A careful attempt to dissect the delicate duct circumferentially is made, but if the duct is entered or injured, clips or suture ligatures must be placed above and below this area. In the left chest, the thoracic duct is often not visible, and one must make a concentrated effort to identify the leaking tributary. Following suture ligation, it is probably efficacious to apply fibrin sealant over the area. The addition of talc or mechanical pleurodesis, especially when the precise leak has not been identified with certainty, might also increase the success rate.

Patients with large, mediastinal lymphatic malformations and those with conditions causing elevated central venous pressures (such as superior vena cava syndrome) have the most challenging form of chylothorax. When refractory to aggressive medical and surgical therapy, these rare patients are candidates for a pleuroperitoneal shunt.

Pneumothorax

Spontaneous pneumothorax is managed in two phases: the initial treatment and prevention of recurrence. All general and pediatric surgeons are familiar with the acute management of pneumothorax. However, there is not universal agreement regarding the algorithm for long-term prevention of recurrent pneumothorax.

Patients are typically tall, thin adolescents who present with the sudden onset of chest pain and varying severities of dyspnea. Obviously, if there is clear evidence of tension pneumothorax by initial physical exam (absent breath sounds, jugular venous distension, tracheal shift, severe dyspnea, hypoxia, hypotension) the first responder must provide immediate relief with needle decompression or tube thoracostomy. In our institution, we prefer small-caliber pigtail catheters that readily available in the emergency department for rapid insertion (Fig. 39.2). These small caliber tubes are especially useful for the evacuation of air as they can be placed anteriorly and apically within the thorax.

More commonly, spontaneous pneumothorax presents without severe symptoms or tension physiology. Initial evaluation includes a history including the precise onset of symptoms, severity of discomfort over time, previous history of pneumothorax, the presence of underlying chronic lung diseases (cystic fibrosis), and the distance the patient lives from the nearest emergency department. Physical examination typically reveals decreased breath sounds on the affected side. Chest radiograph confirms the diagnosis.

The next step is predicated on the duration and severity of the symptoms and the size of the pneumothorax. Patients who describe the onset of discomfort greater than 24 h prior to presentation, who have minimal or resolving symptoms, and whose chest X-ray reveals only a small pneumothorax, may be successfully treated with supplemental oxygen and observation. Once the pneumothorax has resolved clinically and radiographically, these patients can be discharged without ever requiring tube thoracostomy. In contrast, patients with larger pneumothoraces who present within a short time of the onset of more severe symptoms are best served with prompt catheter placement. In the majority of these cases, there is rapid resolution. An air leak, if present, usually stops once the pleural space is evacuated, bringing the visceral and parietal pleura in apposition. We then place the chest tube to water seal drainage and obtain a follow-up radiograph in 4–6 h. If the lung remains fully expanded, the tube is removed and the patient is discharged to home.

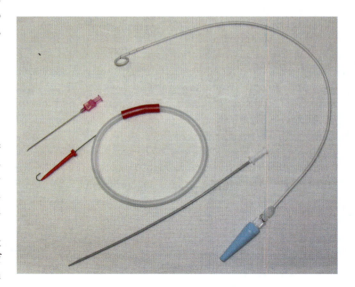

Fig. 39.2 A pigtail catheter kit allows an 8.5 Fr catheter to be easily placed by the Seldinger technique with local anesthesia and sedation

Surgical Therapy

Patients with persistent air leak (greater than 5 days duration) or with recurrent pneumothorax are candidates for surgery. One objective of the operation is the excision of apical lung tissue in an attempt to remove the bullae responsible for the inciting air leak. The other goal is a thorough mechanical pleurodesis to obliterate the pleural space and minimize the chances for future lung collapse. The operation is effectively performed with video-assisted thoracic surgery (VATS). One 12-mm and two 5-mm ports are used to accommodate a 30-degree thoracoscope, an atraumatic grasper, and an endoscopic stapling device. Because bullae are not always visible thoracoscopically (even when evident by CT scan), a few centimeters of lung apex are excised empirically. In some cases, this resection may remove the blebs, while in other patients it might simply encourage the formation of apical adhesions. The 12-mm port is then removed so that instruments may be directly inserted into the thorax for mechanical pleurodesis. We wrap small pieces of the cautery scratch pad around a Kelly clamp for abrasion of the parietal pleura. One chest tube positioned apically is usually adequate. Recurrence rates for spontaneous pneumothorax after VATS are less than 5%.

There is some debate regarding the utility of CT scan to guide therapy and whether surgery should be recommended after one or two episodes of pneumothorax. Some surgeons believe that the presence of ipsilateral bullae visible by CT after a single episode of spontaneous pneumothorax should prompt recommendation for VATS. However, most agree that CT evidence of bullae on the asymptomatic, contralateral side is not an indication for operation. Because of the unclear benefit of surgery after a single episode of spontaneous pneumothorax, we prefer to spare these adolescents the radiation of CT and recommend clinical observation and close follow-up. We offer VATS after a second episode of ipsilateral pneumothorax. In fact, for stable surgical candidates who present with recurrent pneumothorax, it is acceptable to spare them the additional thoracostomy procedure in the emergency department, and proceed with prompt VATS. Surgery is also strongly indicated in rare cases of bilateral pneumothorax, or if the patient resides a significant distance from the nearest medical facility.

Patients with cystic fibrosis who may be candidates for lung transplantation require special consideration. If these patients present with recurrent pneumothorax, the dense adhesions created by mechanical pleurodesis or talc poudrage place the patient at high risk for blood loss during the subsequently difficult pneumonectomy. Therefore, in this population, we limit our treatment to thoracostomy and apical resection whenever possible, especially if patients are end-stage and likely to need lung transplantation.

Empyema

In children, empyema most commonly results from infection of a parapneumonic effusion, although infection of thoracic structures other than lung can also spread to fluid in the pleural space. Common organisms implicated in empyema include *Staphylococcus aureus*, *Haemophilus influenzae*, and *Streptococcus pneumoniae*. However, the responsible organism rarely grows in culture, perhaps because the early initiation of antibiotic therapy sterilizes the fluid prior to collection. As most surgeons are aware, empyema progresses through a continuum of three phases. During the initial exudative phase, the fluid is thin and acellular. In the fibrinopurulent phase, the deposition of fibrin and large numbers of neutrophils render the effusion increasingly gelatinous and prone to loculation. In the final, or organizing, phase there is marked fibrosis and the theoretical risk of lung entrapment. The mainstay of treatment remains the medical management of the underlying infection. The surgeon's focus in empyema is the extrapulmonary pleural space. Evacuating the empyema during the first two phases provides immediate symptomatic relief by removing a volume of infected material, and also indirectly helps to treat the underlying pneumonia by allowing lung re-expansion. The aims of surgery are a reduction in the overall length of illness and a shorter in-hospital stay (Fig. 39.3).

Diagnosis

The accumulation of significant fluid in the pleural cavity may complicate up to a third of children diagnosed with pneumonia. Children with pneumonia should be suspected of having an infected parapneumonic effusion when they fail to have an appropriate resolution of their symptoms after a course of antibiotics. Dyspnea, an oxygen requirement, or persistent fever should prompt a chest X-ray with decubitus views.

At this point, many pediatricians and surgeons opt for CT scan. Indeed, CT is an excellent means by which to differentiate between consolidated, infected lung parenchyma and extrapulmonary pleural disease (Fig. 39.4). However, for patients referred relatively early in their course, we prefer to use ultrasound, which is rapidly obtained and avoids unecessary radiation exposure. If ultrasonography reveals only a trace amount of fluid, then the antibiotics, chest physiotherapy, and supportive care should be continued with no surgical intervention. On the other hand, if a significant amount of fluid is seen in the pleural space, operative intervention should be considered, and the next step is predicated on the suspected stage of the empyema. Early in

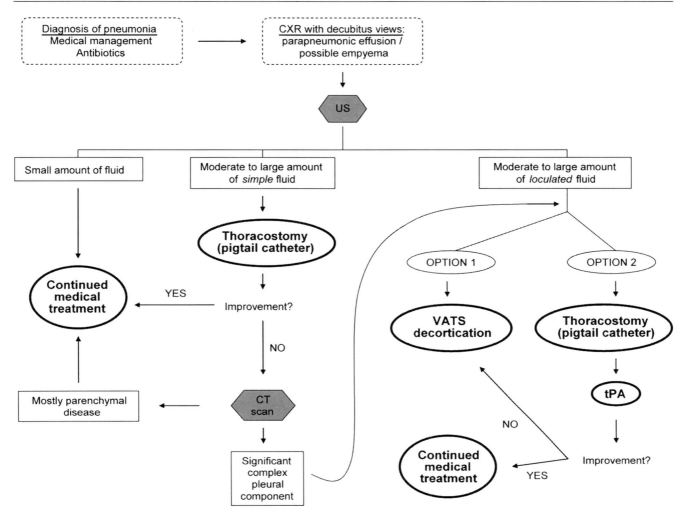

Fig. 39.3 Proposed algorithm for the treatment of empyema. *CXR* chest X-ray; *US* ultrasound; *tPA* tissue plasminogen activator

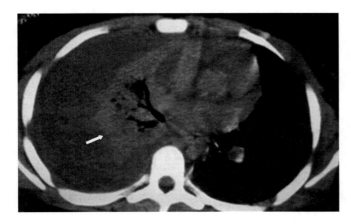

Fig. 39.4 Chest CT scan demonstrating significant right empyema and collapsed, consolidated lung with air bronchograms

the clinical course, simple effusions that "layer out" on decubitus chest radiographs may be assumed to be in the first phase, and thus amenable to thoracostomy drainage.

This approach is further supported by ultrasound evidence of an effusion that lacks septations or loculations. Placement of a pigtail catheter with local anesthesia and sedation can be accomplished in a designated procedure room or in the pediatric intensive care unit. This obviates the need for an operating room, general anesthesia, and intubation of a patient with respiratory compromise. If patients improve clinically (decreased work of breathing, diminishing oxygen requirement), medical treatment of pneumonia should continue. Chest tubes are then removed when the drainage is less than 30 mL daily. If the initial return of fluid is much less than expected, or if there is a rapid decrease in chest tube output without clinical improvement, the empyema may be in a more advanced stage than originally expected. Here, CT can be very helpful in quantifying pleural vs. parenchymal disease.

A moderate to large amount of loculated fluid with septations suggested by ultrasound or CT implies that simple tube drainage will be unsuccessful. The fibrinopurulent phase represents the most common presentation of empyema in pediatric patients, probably because most children present to their primary physicians several days into the course of their illness and are then treated with antibiotics for a period of time before the effusion is discovered. The treatment options for these patients are either VATS or catheter-directed fibrinolytic therapy. There is growing evidence that each of these methods is effective in reducing the duration of illness and in-hospital stay. Currently, surgeons choose one therapy or the other based upon their experience, institutional resources (the availability of conscious sedation and treatment rooms), and possibly the bias of referring primary care physicians.

Thoracoscopic decortication uses a minimal access approach to evacuate the pleural disease. Advantages include the ability to visualize and operate in all regions of the pleural space and to remove the fibrinous peel from the entire surface of the pleura, which often allows immediate re-expansion. In institutions where conscious sedation (for chest tube placement) on the pediatric ward or intensive care unit is difficult or impossible, surgeons argue that VATS enables prompt, definitive treatment with a single anesthetic. In other words, if a trip to the operating room is necessary for chest tube placement, one could argue that proceeding directly to VATS is more sensible.

In most patients, VATS employs three incisions (two 5 mm and one 12 mm) for the thoracoscope and working ports. In smaller toddlers (1–2 years old), we have had success with a single 2-cm incision, through which we can simultaneously pass the scope, grasping instruments for decortication and larger suction catheters. Resection of 1 cm of rib can dramatically facilitate the mobility of these instruments; performing a subperiosteal dissection allows the rib to regenerate.

A number of recent studies have shown that fibrinolytics provide the same clinical benefits. Similar to reports from centers in both North America and Europe, our group has seen promising early results with this modality, specifically with tissue plasminogen activator (tPA). Using 4 mg in 30 mL of normal saline (2 mg in 15 mL for children less than 1 year old), a total of six doses are instilled through the chest tube every 12 h. So far, overall success rates, duration of illness, and hospital course have been similar to the experience with VATS. We have been impressed to see large, complex empyemas successfully drain through catheters as small as 8.5 French after tPA therapy.

Advocates of tPA point out the benefits of avoiding VATS: obviating general anesthesia and endotracheal intubation, using one small-caliber tube instead of three incisions, and the lower overall hospital cost. Additionally, the pigtail catheter for tPA can be placed very quickly on a supine patient, while VATS patients are committed to a longer procedure in lateral decubitus position (with the "good lung" dependent). Proponents of VATS as first-line therapy counter that surgery allows more immediate evacuation of the pleural space. We currently view VATS and tPA as equivalent (Fig. 39.3), though we continue to also offer VATS when patients do not improve after attempts at fibrinolysis. The goal is for children to have more rapid resolution of dyspnea, hypoxia, and fever within a few days, but those with severe pneumonia sometimes remain symptomatic for a time despite adequate treatment of the empyema. Commonly, radiographic abnormalities persist for a number of weeks. Preoperatively, these expectations must clearly be communicated to parents and primary-care physicians, who should be prepared for the possibility of escalating respiratory support immediately following the operation and the likelihood that fevers and radiographic abnormalities will persist for some time.

The optimal management of empyema continues to be debated by pediatric surgeons, probably because long-term outcomes are excellent no matter which treatment modality is chosen. In addition, we lack a set of absolute clinical criteria to define success. In the past, evacuation of empyema and decortication were accomplished via thoracotomy. The advent of minimal access approaches moved pediatric surgeons to more readily offer VATS drainage and decortication. Now, as randomized, prospective studies imply that thrombolytics may be equivalent in efficacy to surgery, we may be in the midst of yet another paradigm shift in the surgical treatment of empyema.

Summary Points

- Chylothorax is readily diagnosed by clinical situation and fluid composition.
- Chylothorax is usually treated effectively by dietary changes and medicine, not surgery.
- Prevention of recurrent pneumothorax by VATS and apical resection should be offered to adolescents following their second spontaneous pneumothorax.
- If possible, pleurodesis should be avoided in potential lung transplant candidates (cystic fibrosis).
- The treatment of empyema is the subject of ongoing debate, but evacuation of the pleural space either by VATS decortication or catheter-directed fibrinolytics can shorten the course of illness and hospital stay.

Editor's Comment

Chylothorax will usually resolve spontaneously, but this can take weeks. Whether dietary changes, special formula, or octreotide make any difference is doubtful but there appears to be little potential downside to trying them. If the effusion persists for more than 3 weeks, it is usually time to consider surgical intervention, though parents need to be warned that it is a very tricky business and the success rate is not 100%. The thoracoscopic approach is excellent and thoracotomy should rarely, if ever, be necessary. A small amount of dairy cream can be given by gastric tube intra-operatively to improve the likelihood of visualization but even when clearly identified, repair of the leak can be extremely difficult. Direct suture repair should be attempted using fine monofilament suture and precise technique to avoid simply obscuring the leak from view with adjacent tissue. The application of fibrin sealant is probably useful and is simple to apply through a port site. If the leak cannot be controlled adequately with direct suture repair, ligation of the thoracic duct is the most effective maneuver. This can be difficult, especially from the left side of the chest. Though it might seem dramatic or even dangerous, it has proven to be safe and highly effective.

Most children who present with a spontaneous pneumothorax can and should be simply observed without having a chest tube placed, unless they are very symptomatic or the pneumothorax is enlarging on follow-up chest radiograph. Most will resolve spontaneously and at follow up a decision needs to be made whether to recommend pleurodesis or continued observation. It seems reasonable to offer pleurodesis after the second episode or if obvious bullae are seen on chest CT, which should not be done at the initial visit while a pneumothorax is still present as the bullae might be collapsed and therefore not visible. Pleurodesis might also be offered to children whose lifestyle would be compromised by an unexpected pneumothorax (travel, varsity athletics, high-level academics). Apical bleb resection (blebs are usually identified at operation even when the CT did not) and mechanical pleurodesis is a straightforward thoracoscopic procedure that should not need to be done by thoracotomy. It is helpful to resect the apex using at least three firings of the stapling device so as to recreate the tapered shape of the apex. A flat top creates a large air space when the lung is re-expanded, potentially compromising the effectiveness of the pleurodesis. Postoperatively, maintaining the chest tube to suction for 72 consecutive hours without fail before pulling it usually prevents that frustrating tiny pneumothorax that occurs frequently when the suction is broken in the early postoperative period and which is then practically impossible to get rid of, again, potentially compromising the effectiveness of the pleurodesis. The recurrence rate for this procedure should be very low.

Ultrasound is usually sufficient to make the diagnosis of empyema in a child. Progression can be rapid and imaging often needs to be repeated within 24 h. The decision to recommend intervention is usually based on symptomatology (tachypnea, fever, oxygen requirement) or the presence of a very large effusion. Children with empyema respond so well and so quickly to a timely thoracoscopic debridement that it is puzzling why some pediatricians and many pediatric surgeons still prefer to continue antibiotics for weeks or attempt painful and labor-intensive thrombolytic therapy. Thoracoscopy is safe and, if done properly, straightforward and quick. It should rarely take more than 20 min, it does not require lung isolation, and it can be done with two incisions: one 5-mm incision for the camera port (and chest tube) and one 10-mm incision in the axilla for alternate passage of a curve sponge clamp and large plastic Yankhauer suction cannula. An attempt should be made to remove all of the fibrinous exudate from the parietal pleura and to break up all loculations (especially the subpulmonic effusion) but it is usually best to manipulate the lung as little as possible to avoid tears, bleeding, and the possibility of a subsequent fistula. Despite an irrational fear expressed by some surgeons, bronchopleural fistula is exceedingly rare and the presence of necrosis, pneumatocele, or even a pneumothorax on preoperative imaging should not be considered a contraindication to a thoracoscopic debridement.

Parental Preparation

- Resolution of chylothorax may take several weeks or longer.
- Surgery for recurrent pneumothorax is aimed at preventing future dangerous episodes of lung collapse, but is not 100% effective.
- The surgeon's target in empyema is the extrapulmonary pleural disease; respiratory symptoms, fevers, and radiographic abnormalities will likely persist while the parenchymal disease resolves.

Suggested Reading

Gates RL, Hogan M, Weinstein S, et al. Drainage, fibrinolytics, or surgery: a comparison of treatment options in pediatric empyema. J Pediatr Surg. 2004;39(11):1638–42.

Sonnappa S, Cohen G, Owens CM, et al. Comparison of urokinase and video-assisted thoracoscopic surgery for treatment of childhood empyema. Am J Respir Crit care Med. 2006;174:221–7.

St. Peter SD, Tsao K, Spilde TL, et al. Thoracoscopic decortication versus tube thoracostomy with fibrinolysis for empyema in children: a prospective, randomized trial. J Pediatr Surg. 2009;44(1):106–11.

Thomson AH, Hull J, Kumar MR, et al. Randomised trial of intrapleural urokinase in the treatment of childhood empyema. Thorax. 2002;57:343–7.

Chapter 40
Pectus Deformities

M. Ann Kuhn and Donald Nuss

Chest wall malformations can be present at birth or become evident in infancy, childhood or early adolescence. Congenital chest wall deformities fall into two groups: those with overgrowth of the rib cartilages causing a depression or protrusion of the sternum, and those with varying degrees of aplasia or dysplasia. The most common chest wall malformations are the depression or protrusion abnormalities called pectus excavatum and pectus carinatum. The excavatum defect constitutes about 88% of the deformities while the carinatum deformity makes up another 5%.

Pectus excavatum defects were recognized as early as the sixteenth century and a genetic predisposition was first noted in the 1800s. The first attempt at surgical correction was by Meyer in 1911. In the 1920s, Sauerbruch first performed a repair that used the bilateral costal cartilage resection and sternal osteotomy technique with external traction. Ravitch advocated even more radical mobilization of the sternum and wide resection of the costal cartilage with transection of all sternal attachments including the intercostal bundles, rectus muscles, diaphragmatic attachments and excision of the xiphisternum hoping to avoid external traction. However, this technique resulted in an increased recurrence rate. Wallgren and Sulamaa introduced internal support in 1956 with a bar passed through the sternum and subsequently Adkins and Blades proposed passing a straight stainless steel bar behind the sternum. Controversy existed about the resection of rib cartilages in young patients and Haller documented the risk of acquired asphyxiating chondrodystrophy as a result of the repair in early childhood. In 1998, Nuss et al. published their 10-year experience with a minimally invasive technique that required neither resection nor sternal osteotomy.

Pectus Excavatum

Pectus excavatum is the most common anterior chest wall deformity with an incidence of between 1 and 3 per 1,000. It is usually noted in early childhood and progresses, especially during puberty, when the defect can worsen significantly in as little as 6 months. It is more frequent in boys than girls by a 4:1 ratio. It is rare in African Americans.

The cause of pectus excavatum has not been established. A theory has been proposed that the deformity results from unbalanced overgrowth in the costochondral regions. Cartilage segments from pectus deformities show disorderly arrangement of cartilage cells, perichondritis and areas of aseptic necrosis. There is association with other musculoskeletal abnormalities, particularly scoliosis and Marfan syndrome. There is also a high genetic predisposition with a family history of pectus excavatum in more than a third of patients. Congenital heart disease occurs in 1.5%.

Pectus excavatum is characterized by posterior displacement of the body of the sternum that varies significantly between affected individuals. The defect typically involves the lower half of the sternum, with the deepest point being just above the xiphisternum, and the lower costal cartilages. The depression is characterized by posterior angulation of the body of the sternum beginning just below the insertion of the second costal cartilage and posterior angulation of the costal cartilages to meet the sternum. The depression is sometimes worse on the right or the left side, or the sternum may be rotated. The Haller index is calculated by dividing the transverse diameter of the chest (today usually based on measurements on a CT scan) by the antero-posterior diameter at the deepest point of the depression (Fig. 40.1).

Anatomic classifications have been developed to describe the variable appearances of pectus excavatum. These include a small localized deep deformity that is "cup shaped"; a diffuse, wide shallow deformity that is "saucer-shaped"; and a long asymmetric defect involving the left or right chest which is longitudinal or transverse and sometimes referred to as the "grand canyon" type. The "horseshoe deformity" is a mixed

M.A. Kuhn (✉)
Children's Hospital of the King's Daughters, 601 Children's Lane, Suite 5B, Norfolk, VA 23507, USA
e-mail: Ann.Kuhn@chkd.org

P. Mattei (ed.), *Fundamentals of Pediatric Surgery*,
DOI 10.1007/978-1-4419-6643-8_40, © Springer Science+Business Media, LLC 2011

excavatum and carinatum defect with anterior protrusion of the manubrium and posterior displacement of the body of the sternum (Fig. 40.2). The majority of young children are asymptomatic, but as they become older the deformity becomes more severe and the chest wall more rigid, which results in decreased exercise capacity. They have difficulty keeping up with their peers when engaged in aerobic activities, causing most affected children to stop participating in sports. In addition, they are usually embarrassed by the deformity and will avoid situations in which they have to take their shirts off. Withdrawal from social activities leads to feelings of worthlessness, causing some to become extremely depressed and, in rare cases, even suicidal.

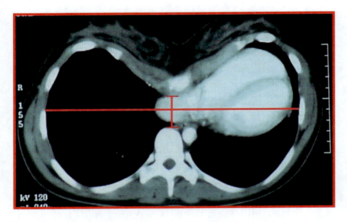

Fig. 40.1 Chest CT showing, severe, symmetric pectus excavatum with significant cardiac compression and displacement, secondary left lung compression and Haller index of 8.0 (Transverse diameter of 80 mm divided by A.P. diameter of 10 mm)

The pectus posture frequently seen in these patients is a result of associated thoracic kyphosis, forward sloping shoulders and a relaxed, protuberant abdomen, which aggravates the condition. For this reason we recommend aggressive posture exercises and a breathing program. The exercise program may halt the progression of the deformity but it is unlikely that it will correct a severe deformity. In addition, rapid growth during puberty almost always accelerates the progression.

The earliest complaints are shortness of breath and lack of endurance with exercise. As the defect progresses, chest pain and palpitations can occur especially with exercise. Other symptoms that can occur are frequent and prolonged respiratory tract infections and asthma. The children often have poor body image and diminished self worth. It is therefore important to correct the deformity before it affects the ability to function normally.

The depth of the deformity determines the degree of cardiac and pulmonary compression. A systolic ejection murmur is often noted. There is a large amount of data reporting the cardiac and pulmonary effects of pectus excavatum. Some studies have shown a significant compromise of cardiac and pulmonary function. Other studies have been unable to demonstrate significant variation from predicted values. There are several factors that need to be taken into account when testing cardiopulmonary function, including the severity of the deformity, the inherent physical fitness of the individual, age-associated conditions, and whether the tests are done supine or erect, at rest or during exercise.

Cardiac effects fall into three categories: decreased cardiac output, mitral valve prolapse, and arrhythmias. Compression of the heart results in incomplete filling and

Fig. 40.2 Classification of pectus excavatum morphology. (**a**) Localized deep depression – "cup shaped" deformity. (**b**) Diffuse shallow depression – "saucer shaped" deformity. (**c**) Asymmetric long funnel shaped deformity – "grand canyon" deformity. (**d**, **e**) Mixed carinatum/excavatum deformity – Currarino–Silverman deformity, also called "pouter pigeon," "horns of steer," and horseshoe deformity ((**b** and **c**) reprinted with permission from Ashcraft KW, Holcomb GW, Murphy JP, eds. Congenital chest wall deformities. In: Pediatric surgery, 4th ed. Philadelphia, PA: Elsevier, 2005. Copyright Elsevier 2005)

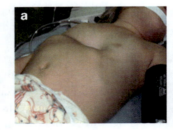
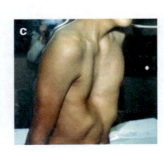
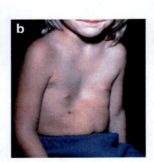
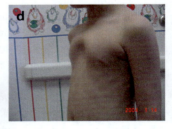
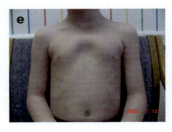

decreased stroke volume and can alter right ventricular morphology and function. Compression also interferes with normal valve function. Prolapse is present in 17% of patients compared to 1% in the normal population. A functional systolic cardiac murmur is often present along the upper left sternal border from turbulence due to compression of underlying structures. Dysrhythmias including first degree heart block, right bundle branch block, and Wolff Parkinson White syndrome have been documented in 16% of our patients. The physical work capacity at a given heart rate is significantly lower in the sitting compared to the supine position. Stroke volume is limited so an increase in cardiac output can only be achieved by increasing heart rate (upright vs. supine).

The pulmonary effects of pectus excavatum fall within three categories: restrictive lung disease, atelectasis, and increased airway resistance due to lung compression; paradoxical respiration; and a predilection for prolonged respiratory infections and asthma. Children with severe deformities from birth tend to compensate by increasing the diaphragmatic component of respiration. They can thus compensate somewhat and are able to achieve low-normal pulmonary function studies. It is documented that they often lack endurance during exercise, apparently due to a very low reserve lung volume. Stress testing reveals an increase in oxygen consumption and increased work of breathing. In some instances, a severe excavatum defect can cause significant tracheal compression.

Preoperative Evaluation

The most important aspect of the evaluation is to perform a complete history and physical exam. Photographs of the deformity should be obtained for documentation. A mild or moderate pectus excavatum is generally asymptomatic and is treated with an exercise and posture program. This exercise program is an intervention that attempts to halt the progression of the pectus excavatum and includes deep breathing with breath holding, posture exercises, and aerobic exercise. These patients are also seen at least annually to reinforce the value of the exercise program and to check for progression of the defect. Particular attention is paid to worsening of symptoms. Severe pectus excavatum occurs in approximately one third of cases. These children are started on the exercise and posture protocol but also undergo cardiac evaluation, pulmonary function testing, and computed tomography to determine whether they are candidates for surgical correction.

The CT scan allows a three-dimensional evaluation of the anterior chest wall and usually demonstrates the degree of cardiac and pulmonary compression or displacement. The CT also allows assessment of the severity of sternal torsion, costal flaring, asymmetry, abnormal ossification, and scoliosis. It is important to estimate the length of the pectus excavatum, which determines how many support bars might be needed. A Haller index greater than 3.25 generally constitutes a severe depression and one that should be considered for surgical correction.

Pulmonary function testing is done in patients old enough to understand and cooperate, generally over age 7. Published studies of the effects of pectus excavatum on pulmonary function vary considerably. Some have shown a decrease in vital capacity, total lung capacity, and maximal breathing capacity. Exercise pulmonary function studies might demonstrate a limitation of oxygen uptake (VO_2 max) and decreased ability to do cardiopulmonary work. Data from our population of over 900 patients show that of those evaluated for primary surgery, the forced vital capacity (FVC) was below average (80–100% of predicted) in 51%, below 80% of predicted in 26%, and normal or above normal in only 23%. The FEV1 was below 80% of predicted in 32% of the patients and the FEF25–75% was below 80% of predicted in 45% of the patients. The bell shaped distribution curve for FVC should peak at 100% of predicted but in our series it peaked at 80% of predicted, suggesting the presence of a significant restrictive component in the majority of these patients.

Electrocardiogram and echocardiogram sometimes reveals conduction pathway abnormalities, mitral valve prolapse, right ventricular wall abnormalities, or other effects of cardiac compression. These are used to determine whether the patient is a reasonable candidate for operation. Specific abnormalities commonly found on ECG are right axis deviation and depressed ST segments caused by rotation of the heart. Echocardiogram shows mitral valve prolapse in 17% and is especially common in patients with Marfan syndrome.

Characteristics of a severe pectus excavatum and the need for repair include two or more of the following: (1) a Haller index greater than 3.25; (2) pulmonary function studies indicating restrictive or obstructive airway disease or both; (3) cardiac evaluation that shows signs of compression (murmur, mitral valve prolapse, cardiac displacement, or conduction abnormalities); (4) progression of the deformity with associated symptoms; (5) a failed Ravitch procedure; (6) a failed minimally invasive procedure.

The optimal time for performing pectus excavatum repair depends on the type of procedure used. The more invasive procedures interfere with growth plates so should not be done at a young age. The minimally invasive repair can be done at any age since it does not interfere with growth plates and has been applied in patients between the ages of 17 months and 50 years. Our experience has shown that the optimal age is between 11 and 14 years because in this age range the chest is still very pliable, allowing for a quick recovery with rapid return to normal activities, and excellent results due to the fact that the musculoskeletal system matures while the support bar is in place, which reduces the risk of recurrence. Young patients who undergo minimally invasive repair with removal of the bar before puberty have an increased risk of recurrence with subsequent growth, while older patients often require two or, rarely, three bars. All patients treated with an operation are also treated with the aerobic exercise, deep breathing, and posture program starting at their first consultation and are encouraged to continue with the exercise program until 1 year after bar removal.

Surgical Technique

Prior to surgical repair it is necessary to review all studies and to check for allergies. If the patient is allergic to metal (usually nickel or copper), a titanium bar should be used. To determine correct bar length, the chest is measured from the right to left mid-axillary line and 1 in. is subtracted from this length to account for the fact that the bar takes a shorter course than the tape measure.

General endotracheal anesthesia and epidural catheter insertion are undertaken by the anesthesiologist. After induction of anesthesia, the patient is positioned supine with both arms abducted at the shoulder. We obtain a photograph of the chest prior to beginning the procedure to document the excavatum defect. The bar is bent into a smooth semi-circle leaving a 2-cm flat section in the middle to support the sternum. The arch shape of the bar allows sustained load bearing of the bar. If the central flat section of the bar is too long, the pectus excavatum will be under corrected. The bar should fit loosely on each side without pressing on the chest wall muscles.

The deepest point of the pectus excavatum is marked with a surgical marking pen. If the deepest point of the pectus is inferior to the sternum, the distal sternum is marked instead. At least one support bar should be under the bony sternum otherwise the excavatum defect will not be corrected. The deepest point determines the horizontal plane for bar insertion. The intercostal spaces that are in the same horizontal plane as the deepest point of the pectus excavatum are marked with an "x." These points on each side of the sternum should be medial to the top of the pectus (costochondral) ridge. Lines are drawn for the bilateral chest wall incisions in the same horizontal plane. It might be necessary to add a second bar superiorly or inferiorly, especially if the deepest point of the depression is at the xiphisternum or at the more inferior costal cartilages.

A thoracoscope is inserted into the right lower chest one or two interspaces inferior to the proposed right lateral thoracic skin incisions. Carbon dioxide is insufflated to a pressure of 6 mmHg, which causes the right lung to collapse and improves visualization. The right hemithorax and mediastinum are inspected to ensure there is no contraindication to repair. The scope is used to correlate the internal anatomy with the external markings. Pressure is applied over the pro-

posed entry and exit sites to ensure that these line up well with the deepest point of the pectus excavatum. Once it has been confirmed that the internal and external anatomy match, the bilateral thoracic skin incisions are made in the region of the mid-axillary line. A skin tunnel is raised anteriorly toward the intercostal space marked with an "x," medial to the top of the pectus ridge. A subcutaneous pocket is also created for the stabilizer. The chest must not be entered lateral to the pectus ridge because then the bar has only the intercostal muscles to oppose the strong posterior force on the bar, and they will tear under the load. The load must instead be borne by the ribs as they curve in toward the sternum. Under thoracoscopic guidance, the appropriate size Lorenz introducer (Biomet Microfixation, Jacksonville, FL) is inserted through the right intercostal space at the top of the pectus ridge at the previously marked "x" (Fig. 40.3). The ECG volume is turned up so the heartbeat is clearly audible. The pericardium is gently dissected off the under-surface of the sternum. The introducer is slowly advanced across the mediastinum under thoracoscopic guidance with the point always facing anteriorly and in contact with the sternum. When the substernal tunnel has been completed, the tip of the introducer is pushed through the contralateral intercostal space at the previously marked "x," and advanced out through the skin incision.

Occasionally it is impossible to see the dissection with a thoracoscope. There are several interventions that can aid in visualizing this important step: a 30° scope can be used, a short subxiphoid incision can permit passage of a finger between the sternum and pericardium to guide the dissector, a clamp can be used to pull the xiphisternum anteriorly, or a suction device can be applied to the anterior chest wall to elevate the sternum.

After being advanced out through the left lateral incision with only the handle protruding on the right side, the introducer is then used to elevate the sternum by lifting it in an anterior direction. The surgeon lifts the introducer on the right side and the assistant lifts the introducer on the left side. The lifting is repeated until the sternum has been elevated out of its depressed position and the pectus excavatum has been corrected. Loosening up the chest wall in this manner prevents excessive torque on the pectus bar when turning it over. An umbilical tape is attached to the introducer and the introducer is withdrawn from the chest cavity, pulling the umbilical tape through the substernal tunnel. The previously prepared pectus bar is tied to the umbilical tape and guided through the substernal tunnel under thoracoscopic guidance using the umbilical tape for traction. The bar is inserted with the convexity facing posteriorly. With the bar in position, it is rotated 180° using the bar flipper.

Pressure effects often cause the bar to straighten out when it is turned over and it may require further bending to fit well against the chest wall. If necessary, the bar is turned over and

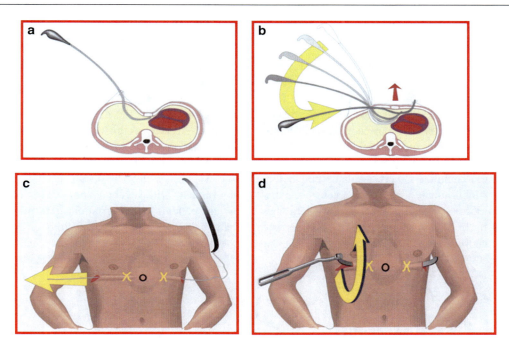

Fig. 40.3 Substernal tunnel correction and pectus bar insertion. (**a**) Insertion site of introducer and dissection phase. (**b**) Exit site on contralateral side after completion of substernal tunnel. (**c**) Bar insertion using tape for guidance. (**d**) 180° bar rotation after insertion. ((**a**) printed with permission from Nuss D. Chest wall deformities. In: Stringer MD, Oldham KT, Mouriquand PDE, eds. Pediatric surgery and urology long-term outcomes. 2nd ed. New York: Cambridge University Press; 2006. (**b–d**) reprinted with permission from Ashcraft KW, Holcomb GW, Murphy JP, eds. Congenital chest wall deformities. In: Pediatric surgery, 4th ed. Philadelphia, PA: Elsevier, 2005. Copyright Elsevier; 2005)

molded where required with the small Lorenz bar bender. If one bar is not enough, then a second bar is inserted one interspace above or below the first one. Two bars give better and more stable correction, especially in older patients. Slight overcorrection is necessary to prevent recurrence after the bar is removed.

A stabilizer is attached to the left end of the bar and wired to the bar with No. 3 surgical steel wire. If the bar does not seem stable, a second bar, rather than a second stabilizer, is probably required. Heavy absorbable peri-costal sutures of heavy (0 or 1) monofilament absorbable suture are placed around the bar and underlying rib using an "endo-close" laparoscopic needle under thoracoscopic visualization on the right side. In addition, several 0 Vicryl sutures are placed to secure the fascia of the lateral chest wall to the holes in the bar and stabilizer. The incisions are closed in layers over the steel bar and stabilizer and the skin is closed with subcuticular sutures. Once the incisions are closed, the thoracoscope is reinserted into the chest and a thorough inspection is done to ensure that there is no bleeding from the mediastinum, bar entry and exit sites, or pericostal suture sites. The scope is withdrawn, the CO_2 tubing is cut and the proximal end is placed in a basin of saline to create a water seal. The patient is placed on PEEP of 5–6 cm of water pressure while the operating table is placed in Trendelenburg position and the anesthesiologist re-inflates the lungs until there are no more air bubbles escaping. The lungs are held in full inflation when the trocar is

withdrawn and the incision is closed. A chest X-ray is obtained in the operating room to check for a residual pneumothorax.

All patients are started on antibiotics at the beginning of surgery and these are continued until they are afebrile and have no signs of a respiratory tract infection. Betadine is used for skin preparation prior to surgery. In over 1,000 cases, our infection rate has been 1.1%. To avoid bar displacement due to agitation during emergence from general anesthesia, we administering morphine and midazolam. Adequate pain control after surgery usually requires the use of several drug classes. We have found that the use of an epidural with fentanyl and bupivacaine for 3–4 days and intravenous ketorolac for 4–5 days is a very effective regimen. We administer NSAIDs, diazepam, and Robaxin after discontinuation of the epidural and codeine is prescribed on as needed. Patients are required to undergo vigorous pulmonary toilet. Constipation is a predictable outcome of pain management and this is treated with daily laxatives. Hemorrhagic gastritis is a risk and we routinely administer an H_2 blocker. Patients must sleep on their back for 6 weeks. The patient is weaned off analgesics during the first 2 postoperative weeks. We encourage walking and deep breathing and patients usually return to school by 3 weeks. No sports are permitted for 6 weeks. Normal activities are slowly resumed and breathing and posture exercises are done twice daily. Aerobic sports such as soccer, basketball, and swimming are encouraged. Follow-up care is done at 6, 12 and 24 months and we plan bar removal at 36 months.

Complications

Early complications of minimally invasive repair include pneumothorax requiring chest tube drainage, occurring in less than 4%. Hemothorax requiring drainage is rare (0.4%). We have had only three patients with postoperative pleural effusion requiring drainage. Pericarditis has occurred in 0.5%, pneumonia in 0.6%. Late complications include bar displacement in 58 (5%) patients, of which 43 (4.3%) required revision. Most of these occurred before stabilizers were available and before pericostal sutures were routinely used. More recently, the displacement rate has decreased to less than 1%. Bar allergy has been documented in 29 (2.8%) of 1,015 patients. Other late complications include overcorrection and recurrence. At our institution, the overall wound infection rate is 1.1%.

Open Technique

The open technique of pectus excavatum repair is used in some centers for patients with severe deformities (Fig. 40.4). There is a risk of interference with the growth plates in young children and the development of acquired thoracic chondrodystrophy, so this repair is usually undertaken after patients have undergone their pubertal growth spurt. Most surgeons now prefer to delay surgery until the chest has achieved full growth. The open procedure is better suited to older patients with severe asymmetric or eccentric deformities and patients with carinatum deformities. The surgical repair involves various modifications of the original procedure described by Brown and modified by Ravitch and Welch. Internal sternal support minimizes the occurrence of

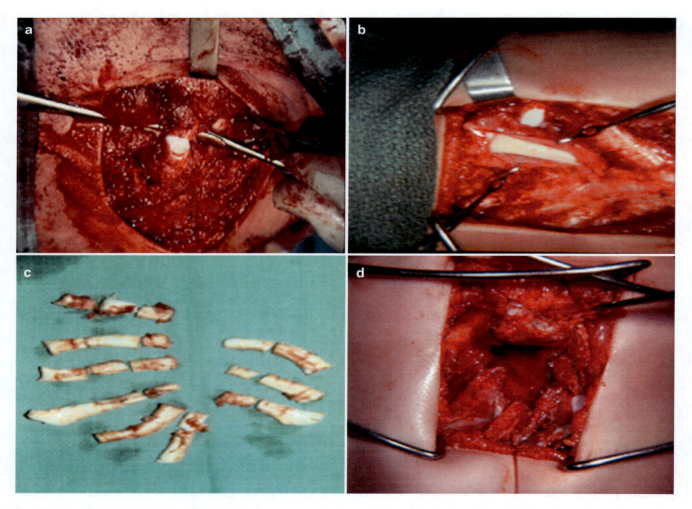

Fig. 40.4 The open ("Ravitch") procedure. (**a**) The large anterior thoracic incision needed for mobilization of the pectoralis major and minor muscles and the malformed ribs. (**b**) The extent of the subperitoneal mobilization of the rib cartilage. (**c**) The rib cartilages that required removal. (**d**) The anterior chest wall after removal of the costal cartilages and complete mobilization of the sternum and the retro-sternal space

postoperative respiratory distress caused by paradoxical chest wall motion, decreases the recurrence rate, and maximizes the extent to which the defect is corrected.

The open technique involves making an anterior thoracic transverse incision in the inframammary crease to provide adequate exposure of the entire sternum. Cutaneous and pectoralis muscle flaps are elevated with electrocautery to expose the depressed portion of the sternum and the costal cartilages. All costal cartilages from T3 to T6 should be exposed. The perichondrium is incised longitudinally and the deformed cartilages are either partially or completely removed with preservation of the perichondrial sheaths. If the xiphoid cartilage is angled anteriorly and would protrude when the position of the sternum is corrected, it is divided from its attachment to the sternum. An anterior table, wedge-shaped sternal osteotomy is performed at the cephalad transition from the normal to the depressed sternum, usually at the level of the insertion of the second or third costal cartilages. The sternum is elevated and the posterior table of the sternum is fractured by the upward traction. Once the lower sternum is elevated to the desired position, the osteotomy is closed with nonabsorbable sutures. A straight pectus bar is inserted under the sternum to bridge the gap between the ribs and the sternum and to prevent the sternum from sinking back into the chest. The bar is attached on each side to the ribs just lateral to the costochondral junction to give the sternum maximal support. Care is taken to maintain a good blood supply to the lower sternum and to avoid complete transection at the site of the osteotomy to prevent necrosis of the distal segment. The perichondrium is resutured and a drain is placed below the muscle flaps. The muscle flaps are sutured back into position and the incisions are closed.

Frequent deep inspirations with incentive spirometry are done during the postoperative period to minimize the occurrence of atelectasis. Patients are usually hospitalized for 2 or 3 days. Patients are required to refrain from contact sports for at least 3 months. Complications of surgery include pneumothorax, which occurs in less than 10% of patients, hemopneumothorax, infection, bar migration, and recurrence. The recurrence rate is between 5 and 15%. Patients can also develop hypertrophic scarring at the incision site.

Pectus Bar Removal

Bar removal is done as an outpatient procedure. The patient undergoes general endotracheal anesthesia with 5–6 cm of PEEP. The position is supine with both arms abducted at the shoulder and the chest X-rays are reviewed to confirm the position of the stabilizers. The old scar is identified and pal-

pated to see if the bar and stabilizer are close to the old scar. If the hardware is not palpable, fluoroscopy can be used to determine the exact site of the bar and stabilizer. The old scars are used for the incision when removing the bar and stabilizer. The bar ends and stabilizers are mobilized and the wire is cut in two places and removed.

When the bar and stabilizer have been released from the surrounding scar tissue, the inferior wing of the stabilizer is delivered out of the incision followed by the end of the bar and finally the superior wing of the stabilizer. The stabilizer is removed from the bar. The bar is unbent with the bar flippers or the small bar bender. An orthopedic bone hook is passed through the hole in the end of the bar and gentle traction is used to extract the bar. The patient is kept on PEEP until the incision is closed.

Pectus Carinatum

Pectus carinatum occurs approximately ten times less frequently than excavatum. Overall it constitutes 5% of patients with chest wall deformities. The most common protrusion deformity that occurs is protrusion of the lower sternal body (gladiolus) and is called chondrogladiolar. An associated lateral depression of the ribs (runnels or Harrison's grooves) is often present. A prominence in the upper manubrium of the sternum is called chondromanubrial. The protrusion may be unilateral, bilateral, or mixed. The ratio of boys to girls is approximately 4:1.

The etiology of this defect is unknown but it has been shown that excessive growth of the ribs or costal cartilages can produce either pectus carinatum or excavatum defects. A genetic component has been proposed and roughly one-fourth of patients have a family history of chest wall defects. Carinatum has been reported to occur after treatment for pectus excavatum.

Pectus carinatum is initially recognized in childhood usually in conjunction with a growth spurt. Symptoms are minimal but some patients complain of shortness of breath with exercise and lack of endurance probably due to the fact that they do not exhale adequately since the chest is "barrel shaped" as in COPD. Tenderness at the protruding site may be present. There are associated findings of congenital heart disease, marfanoid habitus, scoliosis (15%), kyphosis, and musculoskeletal defects. Mitral valve disease has been reported to be associated but in patients without congenital heart disease, cardiopulmonary limitation due to pectus carinatum has not been reported.

In the last 10 years, orthotic (pressure) bracing has become a very popular alternative to surgical correction. These reports describe correction by means of a brace exerting pressure in the anteroposterior direction. We have used bracing for the past several years and have shown success with the bracing technique.

Surgical treatment involves either a minimally invasive technique (Abramson procedure) or the same open resection used for the excavatum repair with resection of the more severely involved costal cartages while preserving the perichondrium. The transverse osteotomy across the anterior table of the upper sternum is filled with a wedge of costal cartilage to secure it in a more downward position with transsternal sutures that cover the deformity.

Postoperative problems are not common but include infection, pneumothorax, and pneumonia or wound separation. Recurrence is reported rarely in centers with a large experience.

Summary Points

- Pectus excavatum is the most common (90%) congenital chest wall deformity, occurring in between 1 and 3 in 1,000 individuals.
- In addition to poor body image, many patients with pectus excavatum describe symptoms of poor exercise tolerance and shortness of breath, presumably due to compression or displacement of the heart and lungs.
- Pectus excavatum mainly involves the lower portion of the sternum below the insertion of the second costal cartilage and can be symmetric or asymmetric.
- The Haller index (transverse diameter of chest divided by the antero-posterior diameter at the deepest portion of defect) is a measure of severity of pectus excavatum, >3.25 being a typical indication for surgical correction.
- Patients with pectus excavatum should be screened for Marfan's disease, scoliosis, and congenital heart disease.
- The minimally invasive approach to the correction of pectus excavatum has been proven to be safe, effective, and durable.
- Pectus carinatum (5% of pectus deformities) is corrected using an external brace that gradually reshapes the sternum posteriorly.

Editor's Comment

The "Nuss" procedure has revolutionized the treatment of pectus excavatum. It is very effective, has a low complication rate, and is associated with minimal external scarring when compared to the traditional "Ravitch" operation. The principal drawback is extreme pain, which is usually effectively managed in the immediate postoperative period with a thoracic epidural catheter, and for the first 2–3 weeks with narcotic analgesics. Narcotic addiction is a significant concern but should be rare with ethical and appropriate pain management techniques and conversion of non-narcotic analgesics as soon as possible after the operation.

Whether pectus excavatum produces measurable deficits in cardiac or respiratory function is controversial. Although many believe it is purely a cosmetic defect, patients frequently describe significant symptoms before surgery and many report considerable (albeit subjective) improvement in their stamina and comfort after the operation. Especially in active teenagers, flipping of the bar remains a constant worry but is thankfully rare, especially with the current widespread use of bar stabilizers.

The Ravitch repair done well is elegant and effective in its own right, but should only be offered when there are contraindications to the minimally invasive approach. Rather than remove all the costal cartilages, Dr. Haller described a technique whereby some of the cartilages are bisected at an angle (anteromedial to posterolateral) and the medial half is brought anterior to the lateral half, thus helping to push the sternum anteriorly. They should be stitched in this position to avoid postoperative slippage. A bar is not always necessary, but recommended for severe defects especially in older teenagers and adults.

In many cases, pectus carinatum is even more of a cosmetic concern than pectus excavatum. The operations described for correction of this defect are more invasive and perhaps less effective than those available for pectus excavatum. The external bracing technique, in which external pressure is applied to the sternum, appears to be very effective; however, compliance remains a significant hurdle.

Differential Diagnosis

- Pectus excavatum
- Pectus carinatum
- Mixed pectus deformity

Diagnostic Studies

- Thoracic CT scan with calculation of Haller index
- Pulmonary function testing
- EEG/echocardiogram, where appropriate

Parenteral Preparation

- The minimally invasive approach to correction of pectus excavatum is painful but we have a plan to make your child comfortable, including a thoracic epidural catheter for the immediate postoperative period.
- The stabilizer bar(s) passes between the sternum and the heart, but we will use thoracoscopy to help avoid serious injuries.
- The bar(s) will need to be removed in a second procedure 2–3 years after the initial operation.

Preoperative Preparation

- ☐ Medical imaging
- ☐ Preoperative photographs
- ☐ Complete blood count
- ☐ Type and crossmatch

Technical Points

- Patient is positioned supine with the arms abducted at the shoulder (at no more than 90° to avoid a brachial plexus nerve injury).
- The bar should be placed at the deepest point of the defect, no lower than the distal sternum.
- The incisions are made laterally on a line that goes through the deepest point of the defect.
- The bar length should be 1 in. less than the distance between the axillary lines measured with tape.
- The bar should be bent into the shape of a semicircle with a 2-cm flat section at the apex, creating a slight over-correction.
- For older children with severe defects, two (or even three) bars might be necessary.

- The chest is entered under thoracoscopic guidance at the *top* of the pectus ridge, never lateral to the ridge, so that the load is borne by the ribs, not the intercostal muscles.
- Stabilizer bars are useful to prevent flipping of the bar.
- Bars are left in place for 3 years.
- The open ("Ravitch") technique involves removal of the costal cartilages while preserving the perichondrium, a transverse anterior osteotomy of the sternum, and, sometimes, a straight support bar.

Suggested Reading

Croitoru DP, Nuss D, Kelly RE, Goretsky MJ, Swoveland B. Experience and modification update for the minimally invasive Nuss technique for pectus excavatum repair in over 303 patients. J Pediatr Surg. 2002;37:437–45.

Haller JA, Colombani PM, Humphries CT, et al. Chest wall constriction after too extensive and too early operations for pectus excavatum. Ann Thorac Surg. 1996;61:1618–25.

Kelly Jr RE, Shamberger RC, Mellins RB, et al. Prospective multicenter study of surgical correction of pectus excavatum. J Am Coll Surg. 2007;205:205–16.

Lawson ML, Cash TF, Akers R, et al. A pilot study of the impact of surgical repair on disease specific. Quality of life among patients with pectus excavatum. J Pediatr Surg. 2003;38:916–8.

Lawson ML, Mellins RB, Tabangin M, Kelly Jr RE, Croitoru DP, Goretsky MJ, et al. Impact of pectus excavatum on pulmonary function before and after repair with Nuss procedure. J Pediatr Surg. 2005;40:174–80.

Martinez D, Stein JJ, Pena A. The effect of costal cartilage resection on chest wall development. Pediatr Surg Int. 1990;5:70–3.

Martinez-Ferro M, Fraire C, Bernard S. Dynamic compression system (DCS) for the correction of pectus carinatum. Semin Pediatr Surg. 2008;17:201–8.

Nuss D. Minimally invasive surgical repair of pectus excavatum. Semin Pediatr Surg. 2008;17:209–17.

Nuss D, Kelly Jr RE, Croitoru DP, Katz ME. A 10 year review of a minimally invasive technique for the correction of pectus excavatum. J Pediatr Surg. 1998;33:545–52.

Ravitch MM. The operative treatment of pectus excavatum. Ann Surg. 1949;129:429–44.

Rushing GD, Goretsky MJ, Gustin T, Morales M, Kelly Jr RE, Nuss D. When it's not an infection: metal allergy after the Nuss procedure for repair of pectus excavatum. J Pediatr Surg. 2007;42:93–7.

Chapter 41
Mediastinal Masses

Richard D. Glick

Mediastinal masses are varied and present at all ages, from newborn to adolescence. There is a wide spectrum of pathology that may include congenital, inflammatory, infectious, and neoplastic processes. Because of the limited space and confined geometry of the region, masses can interfere with both the respiratory and cardiovascular systems, sometimes with grave results. Urgent consultations from oncologists and pediatric intensivists are common, and most of these patients will require some form of surgical intervention, such as biopsy, resection, or venous access. Applicable techniques range from minimally invasive procedures to large thoracotomy or sternotomy. Expertise with these procedures as well as a detailed knowledge of the anatomy and wide range of pathology of the region are essential. An in-depth understanding of the decision-making regarding pre-anesthetic work-up and management can help prevent potentially disastrous complications.

The mediastinum is defined most simply as the space that lies between the two pleural cavities. It is bounded by the sternum and by the vertebral bodies, and extends from the thoracic inlet to the diaphragm. Most importantly for pediatric surgeons, the region is divided into anterior, visceral (or middle), and posterior (or paravertebral) (Fig. 41.1). The anterior compartment is bounded anteriorly by the sternum and posteriorly by the pericardium and anterior aspect of the great vessels. Normally it contains the thymus, lymph nodes, and fat but can also house thyroid or parathyroid tissue. The middle mediastinum contains the heart, great vessels, esophagus, large airways, and major nerves (vagus and phrenic), and is populated with lymph nodes as well. The thoracic duct is often difficult to clearly identify and thus susceptible to injury during mediastinal surgery. It ascends through the mediastinum just anterior to the vertebral column and posterior to the esophagus and pericardium. Inferiorly, it is found more towards the right. It then curves toward the left side at the level of the fifth thoracic vertebra and ascends through the upper aspect of the mediastinum behind the aortic arch and left subclavian artery intimately associated with the left posterior esophagus. The posterior mediastinum is essentially the paravertebral space, defined by the costovertebral sulcus, and contains the sympathetic chain. Various lesions arise from these tissues and thus differential diagnoses can be narrowed significantly by anatomic location. It is important to recognize, however, that when a lesion gets large enough, it can extend from one region into another. This is especially true of lymphomas. It can sometimes be difficult to tell if such a mass originates in the anterior or middle compartment.

Anterior mediastinal masses are most often neoplastic. The most common lesion found in the anterior mediastinum in the pediatric population is lymphoma. However, germ cell tumors, thymomas, and thyroid tumors can occur as well. The middle mediastinum is more likely to be involved with a more congenital anomaly, such as a foregut duplication or bronchogenic cyst. The posterior mediastinum is a characteristic location for neurogenic tumors. Lymphatic and vascular malformations can be present in any of these spaces and are sometimes contiguous with a cervical component.

Diagnosis

Symptoms of a mediastinal mass are usually a direct result of compression of surrounding structures, mainly the airway and large blood vessels. This can manifest as noisy breathing, dyspnea, shortness of breath on exertion, or orthopnea. Orthopnea is considered the most worrisome symptom, especially when caused by an anterior mediastinal mass. Children can present with true respiratory distress, in which case the diagnosis and treatment become emergent. In younger patients, these symptoms can sometimes be more subtle. Constitutional symptoms can also occur, especially with the lymphomas. One should always inquire specifically about fever, chills, weight loss and night sweats. Incidentally found mediastinal masses are most commonly found in the posterior

R.D. Glick (✉)
Department of Pediatric Surgery, Albert Einstein College of Medicine, Schneider Children's Hospital, 269-01 76th Avenue, Suite 158, New Hyde Park, NY 11040, USA
e-mail: rglick@nshs.edu

P. Mattei (ed.), *Fundamentals of Pediatric Surgery*,
DOI 10.1007/978-1-4419-6643-8_41, © Springer Science+Business Media, LLC 2011

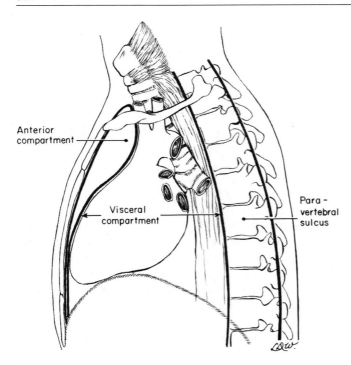

Anterior
compartment

Visceral
compartment

Para-
vertebral
sulcus

Fig. 41.1 The mediastinum can be divided into three compartments: anterior, visceral (or middle), and posterior (paravertebral) (From Sheilds T. Mediastinal surgery. Philadelphia: Lea & Febiger; 1991. Reprinted with permission from Lippincott Williams & Wilkins)

compartment because of their distance from the airways. As well, it is important to note that both non-Hodgkin's lymphoma (NHL) and Hodgkin's disease (HD) can present with cervical adenopathy only and a related mediastinal mass found only on work-up.

Physical examination should be thorough. Examination of the head and neck should focus on cervical masses as well the presence of venous distension. A careful respiratory and chest exam is important. One should palpate the abdomen for organomegaly and masses.

Because of the diversity of the lesions seen in the mediastinum, one needs to take into account the patient's age, history, symptoms, and signs. The work-up not only involves making the diagnosis but also assessing the child for an anticipated general anesthetic. The chest X-ray (two views) is usually the first imaging study to investigate a mediastinal mass and often provides a great deal of important information in this regard. The anatomic location of the mass can usually be identified, which helps narrow the differential. The association of the mass with adjacent structures is important to note, especially if there is displacement or luminal compromise of the trachea or mainstem bronchi. Related phenomena such as pleural effusion, lung consolidation, or air trapping should be noted and carefully documented.

Most patients will then proceed to computed tomography with intravenous contrast. This study typically provides

accurate images to help assess the nature of the mass, its anatomy, whether or not it is calcified, and its relationship to the critical structures of the mediastinum. Airway and vascular impingement can be quite clearly seen. Magnetic resonance imaging is most often used for posterior mediastinal masses. This is because most of these are of neural origin and this study nicely defines extension into the spinal canal. Also, posterior lesions rarely cause respiratory issues and these patients can tolerate MRI scans quite easily. An echocardiogram is obtained if there is any suspicion of heart or great vessel impingement and is often obtained at the insistence of the anesthetist prior to a planned surgical procedure. Other imaging studies are rarely necessary initially.

Laboratory studies should be tailored to the possible diagnoses. All patients should have a complete blood count with peripheral smear and a chemistry panel. Tumor-specific markers should be sent depending on clinical suspicion. For example, anterior mediastinal tumors suspected of being of germ cell origin warrant sending human chorionic gonadotropin (HCG) and alpha fetoprotein (AFP). In a young child with a posterior mediastinal mass where there is suspicion of neuroblastoma, urine studies for homovallinic acid (HVA) and metanephrines should be sent. Most other lesions require no specific laboratory testing.

The key to the diagnosis and subsequent treatment usually lies in obtaining a tissue diagnosis. This involves biopsy in some cases and surgical resection in others. A close relationship with both a pediatric oncologist and experienced pathologist is important. Educated decision making will allow for the safest and most efficacious plan of action. If time permits, new cases should be discussed at a multi-disciplinary tumor board.

When caring for a patient with a mediastinal mass, any procedure requiring general anesthesia can be extremely hazardous. The potential for airway compromise must always be in the mind of the surgeon. A discussion of airway assessment in patients with large lesions must always occur. The safest approach is usually the least invasive procedure available. Blasts seen on peripheral smears can sometimes help in the diagnosis of acute leukemia with mediastinal involvement. Pleural effusions or bone marrow sampling can yield diagnostic cells. Quite often with HD and less so with NHL, cervical or other easily accessible lymph node masses might be amenable to biopsy and thus avoid the need for a more invasive and potentially very dangerous procedure. Patients with an anterior mediastinal mass are at the greatest risk for respiratory or cardiac arrest during general anesthesia or even deep sedation and consideration should therefore be given to the possibility of performing a diagnostic procedure under local anesthesia with minimal, if any, sedation. For example, percutaneous core biopsies performed by an interventional radiologist commonly yields excellent diagnostic results and can often be done with only a local anesthetic. Nonetheless, if less invasive steps are not possible or fail to yield a diagnosis, biopsy of the mediastinal mass itself is indicated.

Preoperative Preparation

This is a commonly discussed topic among pediatric surgeons and anesthesiologists. It is well-recognized that life-threatening airway obstruction can develop in these patients when undergoing anesthesia. Impingement on the heart and great vessels can also produce deleterious effects that are acutely exacerbated by general anesthesia. Tumor bulk and size as well as tracheal and vascular compression have all been implicated as factors associated with adverse anesthetic outcomes. In addition, NHL imparts a greater risk than other tumors. The reason for respiratory collapse on induction of general anesthesia in these patients is multi-factorial. Anesthesia reduces functional residual capacity and decreases lung compliance. Relaxation of the chest wall musculature and diaphragm and the institution of positive pressure ventilation results in a loss of the normal negative intrathoracic pressure transmitted to the airways. Narrowed regions can progress and become critical. Positive pressure disrupts the normal resistance-lowering effect of laminar airflow and worsens the ability to move air. Unfortunately, the critical compression commonly occurs at or near the carina, distal to the end of the endotracheal tube where even a surgical airway may not be of any help. There have been numerous reports in the literature of death under these circumstances.

Assessment of anesthetic risk commences at the bedside with an appropriate history and physical examination, but predictions based solely on clinical findings have been known to be inaccurate. Two widely available tests have been shown to fairly useful in determining risk: assessment of cross-sectional area of the trachea by CT scan and pulmonary function tests. The trachea is measured at its narrowest point and in the appropriate radiographic window. This value is then compared to expected values for age and patients with areas less than 50% of expected are considered to be at risk for significant airway compromise. Intrathoracic tracheal compression affects flow-volume loops mainly at the maximum expiratory flow rate. The peak expiratory flow rate (PEFR) can be assessed with a handheld device at the bedside and correlates with central airway size. PEFR less than 50% of predicted is concerning. These two criteria have been used together to define anesthetic risk. If both studies are less than 50% of predicted, general anesthesia should be considered too risky. If either is less than 50% of predicted, general anesthesia is risky and local anesthesia or other means of obtaining diagnosis should be considered if at all possible. If the values are both greater than 50%, general anesthesia is considered a safe option.

Biopsy Techniques

The least invasive technique to achieve a diagnostic biopsy or resection should always be entertained. In general, a suspected lymphoma should be biopsied while likely germ cell tumors, neural tumors, thymic masses, and congenital anomalies should be treated by resection. There are various ways to gain access to the mediastinum, almost all of which require general anesthesia.

Mediastinoscopy is uncommonly used in children but has been shown to be useful and safe as technique to sample pre- and paratracheal lymph nodes in the retrovascular plane. The mediastinoscope is inserted through a transverse incision in the suprasternal notch and tunneled just anterior to the trachea. Thoracoscopy allows excellent access to all three compartments of the mediastinum with superb visualization of difficult areas. Fig. 41.2 shows the CT scan of a 9-year-old boy with persistent constitutional symptoms and a small mass just superior to the right pulmonary hilum. It was biopsied successfully thoracoscopically and found to be HD.

The Chamberlain procedure is a small anterior mediastinotomy used to biopsy lesions in the anterior mediastinum. A transverse incision is made over the second intercostal space, the underlying pectoralis major muscle is split, and the second costal cartilage is resected, providing access to the anterior mediastinum. This can be done under local anesthesia if necessary. For patients with airway issues, the head of the bed should be elevated.

For larger tumors, such as germ cell tumors and neuroblastoma, thoracotomy or sternotomy is indicated. Advances in single lung ventilation in smaller patients have helped achieve success in thoracic procedures. Double-lumen endotracheal tubes for older children, selective bronchial intubation, and

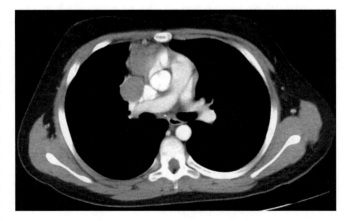

Fig. 41.2 Nine-year-old boy with persistent constitutional symptoms. A small mass can be seen on the right side of the mediastinum adjacent to the superior vena cava and superior right hilar structures. This was biopsied thoracoscopically. Pathology revealed nodular sclerosing Hodgkin disease

bronchial blockers are techniques commonly used by pediatric anesthesiologists. Also, during thoracoscopy, the application of pneumothorax with carbon dioxide can help keep the lung deflated. A detailed discussion with the anesthesia team pre-operatively about each particular patient is very important.

Treatment

Anterior compartment lesions make up almost half of medi-astinal masses and are malignant 80% of the time. These most commonly include lymphomas, germ cell tumors, and thymic masses. Both non-Hodgkin's lymphoma (NHL) and Hodgkin's disease (HD) will be quite frequently seen in this location by the pediatric surgeon. More than half of all chil-dren with lymphoblastic lymphoma present with an anterior mediastinal mass, while over a third of all NHLs have their primary sites in the mediastinum. NHL tends to occur in a younger age group (mean age 9 years) and can often be dra-matic with a rapid onset of symptoms and a large mass (Fig. 41.3). Doubling rates can be as short as 12 h. There is often a pleural effusion. Symptoms due to local compressive effects are more than twice as common as in HD patients (Fig. 41.4). The two most common types of NHL affecting the pediatric mediastinum are lymphoblastic and large cell lymphoma. Sampling a pleural effusion is a quick and mini-mally morbid procedure that can often achieve diagnosis. HD is slower growing and occurs more frequently in adolescents.

For the lymphomas, the issue of permanent central venous access will need to be discussed with the oncology

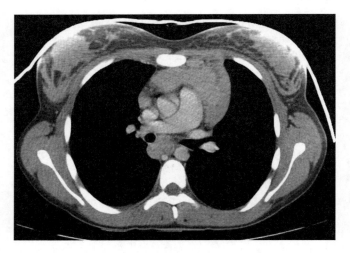

Fig. 41.4 CT scan of a typical HD patient with a moderate-sized medi-astinal mass and no compressive symptoms. On physical examination, she had enlarged cervical lymph nodes and the diagnosis of nodular sclerosing HD was obtained quite easily by cervical lymph node biopsy

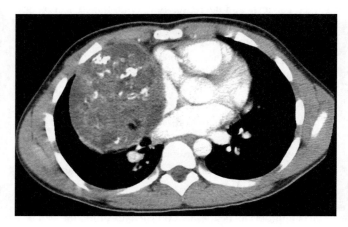

Fig. 41.5 CT scan shows a large heterogeneous anterior mediastinal mass (12 cm) in a 9-year-old boy containing both fat and calcifications. This was completely resected by median sternotomy and found to be a malignant germ cell tumor containing endodermal sinus tumor as well as immature teratoma

team. When a mass is large and there is airway or vascular compression, peripherally inserted central venous catheters are an excellent way to be able to administer therapy with less risk. After the lesion has decreased in size, a mediport or other permanent access can be placed in a much safer fashion.

The anterior mediastinum is a common location for germ cell tumors. Teratomas and endodermal sinus (yolk sac) tumors predominate. These lesions can be very impressive in size and have a characteristic appearance on CT scan. They are heterogeneous, containing fat, calcifications, cysts, and soft tissue (Fig. 41.5). Pre-operative work-up must include the tumor markers AFP and β-HCG. Surgical removal is indicated. Although surgeons have approached small germ

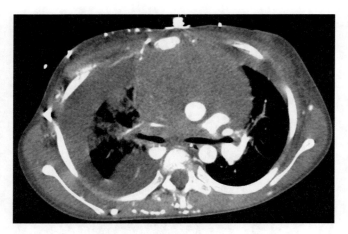

Fig. 41.3 Nine-year-old girl with dramatic symptoms that came on rap-idly. She was unable to lie flat and had her CT done in the prone position. It revealed complete obstruction of the superior vena cava, compression of the heart, large airways, and right pulmonary artery, as well as a large right pleural effusion. The diagnosis of T-cell lymphoblastic lymphoma was made by sampling the pleural effusion

cell tumors thoracoscopically with success, most will require a thoracotomy or, for a very large tumor, a median sternotomy. Avoidance of tumor rupture is important. In general, teratomas can be treated with surgical resection alone while malignant germ cell tumors require platinum-based adjuvant chemotherapy.

Thymic masses in the pediatric population are quite uncommon and diagnostic confusion may occur, though most are benign. Cysts should be resected because of the risk of bleeding and infection. Although rare, thymomas do occur in the pediatric population and about half are malignant. These are treated primarily by resection. Both thoracoscopy and median sternotomy have been used safely and effectively to remove tumors of the thymus.

Posterior mediastinal masses are most commonly of neural origin with ganglioneuroma and neuroblastoma predominating. They arise from the sympathetic chain in the paravertebral sulcus. Ten to twenty-five percent of neuroblastomas are found in this location. They are often found incidentally but can produce respiratory symptoms. Neurologic symptoms can occur because of extension through the neural foraminae into the spinal canal. Neuroblastomas are usually found in children under the age of 2 years. For these tumors, near-complete surgical resection is the primary goal and is often possible. Those patients with extension into the spinal canal may require neurosurgical decompression or chemotherapy prior to an attempt at resection. Pre-operative chemotherapy is also indicated if a primary resection is thought to be too morbid. The prognosis for these children is significantly more favorable than for abdominal neuroblastomas, with overall survival around 75%. Ganglioneuromas predominate in older children and are most often found incidentally on a chest X-ray (Fig. 41.6). Because there is no absolutely reliable way to distinguish ganglioneuromas from neuroblastomas, resection is usually indicated.

Benign foregut cysts are congenital anomalies most commonly found in the middle compartment of the mediastinum. They are thought to arise from abnormal budding of the forming esophagus or tracheobronchial tree. They are most often divided into two groups: bronchogenic cysts and enteric duplications.

Patients with bronchogenic cysts are frequently asymptomatic and the abnormalities are often found incidentally. If a cyst is very close to the airway and causing compression, respiratory symptoms may be present. They can produce respiratory distress in newborns and recurrent pulmonary infections in older children. Imaging reveals a non-enhancing, homogeneous, smooth-walled, cystic lesion. Bronchogenic cysts are most often found near the carina but can also be found in the pulmonary hilum or parenchyma. Only rarely do they communicate with the tracheobronchial tree. The cysts are lined by a respiratory epithelium and contain thick mucous. The treatment is complete excision. Frequently, they can be removed safely thoracoscopically. If the cyst is adherent to the airway, one can leave a small part of the cyst wall in place but the mucosa should be stripped.

Enteric duplications include esophageal duplications and neuroenteric cysts. Esophageal duplications (Fig. 41.7) are found intimately associated with the esophageal wall, arising within a muscular layer. They may produce esophageal obstructive symptoms as they slowly grow and can impinge on the lumen. They typically have muscular walls lined with gastric or intestinal mucosa, although respiratory epithelium may be found. Most can be resected thoracoscopically with careful dissection to excise the cyst from the esophagus without entering the lumen. Neuroenteric cysts are rare anomalies that communicate posteriorly with the meninges. Their removal is more complex and requires the assistance of a neurosurgery team.

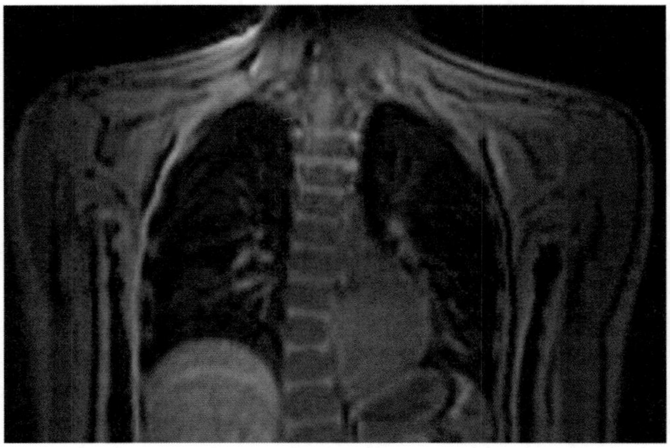

Fig. 41.6 Chest MRI of a large posterior mediastinal/paravertebral mass found incidentally by CXR. It was resected by thoracotomy and found to be ganglioneuroma

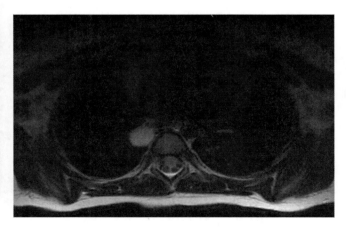

Fig. 41.7 Chest MRI was performed as part of a neurologic work-up. Esophageal duplication was found incidentally

Postoperative Care

The most feared complication of surgery for mediastinal masses is respiratory collapse, as discussed above. The obvious potential risks with resection or biopsy of mediastinal masses involve inadvertent injury of neighboring structures. A detailed pre-operative discussion with the family is important and parents should be informed of the likelihood of a chest tube and how long it may need to be in place. These lesions can be intimately associated with the great vessels and bleeding can be very difficult to control. This is particularly true for mediastinoscopy. Injury to the lung or bronchus can result in air leak. Injury is often not readily apparent at the time of surgery and presents post-operatively as a chylothorax. With chest tube drainage and enteral nutritional support, most of these will seal. The phrenic and recurrent laryngeal nerves are also susceptible to injury with resulting diaphragmatic and laryngeal dysfunction.

Summary Points

- Pediatric surgeons must be well-versed in the anatomy and range of pathology in the mediastinum.
- The lesion must be assessed by plain radiographs, CT, and sometimes MRI to help with differential diagnosis.
- Consultation with an experienced pediatric radiologist can be very helpful with creation of a differential diagnosis, assessing airway patency, and surgical planning.
- Close interaction with pediatric oncology team is important to formulate a cohesive plan for biopsy or resection.
- For biopsy, always search for least morbid procedure to achieve desired result.
- The pre-anesthesia work-up is key to avoid serious airway complication prior to any operative intervention involving anesthesia.
- Operative strategies include minimally invasive (thoracoscopy, mediastinoscopy) or open (thoracotomy, median sternotomy).

Editor's Comment

Mediastinal masses are quite variable in their origin, diagnostic work up, and therapeutic approach. There are a handful of lesions that we commonly see in children but there are also many that are unusual and require a thoughtful and often multidisciplinary approach to management. Regardless of the diagnosis, it is extremely important for the pediatric surgeon to have absolute command of the intricate anatomy of the mediastinum, including all known variations thereof, especially before embarking on an attempt at resection. Biopsy or removal of apical paraspinous lesions places the stellate ganglion at risk, which can result in Horner syndrome (ipsilateral enophthalmos, small pupil, ptosis, dry eye). This is sometimes unavoidable and expected (neuroblastoma resection) and parents need to be warned in advance that it is likely to be permanent. The phrenic nerve is always at risk and should be clearly identified and protected throughout the course of any operation in the chest. The recurrent laryngeal nerve can also be injured and its anatomic course should be anticipated. Finally, thoracic duct injury can occur unexpectedly and results in significant postoperative morbidity. After resection of a mass or dissection anywhere in the mediastinum, the tissue bed should be examined carefully for leakage of lymphatic fluid, which will be clear in the patient who has fasted. If the source is not visible, infusing a small amount of cream into the GI tract by nasogastric gastric tube can be helpful.

Rapidly expanding lymphoma that presents as an anterior mediastinal mass can be challenging due to the risk of sudden airway collapse after induction of anesthesia or even sedation. An alternate means of obtaining diagnostic material should be sought: cervical lymph node biopsy, drainage of pleural fluid for cytology, bone marrow biopsy, US- or CT-guided percutaneous core needle biopsy under minimal sedation and local anesthetic. If general anesthesia is truly the only option, which is rarely the case, contingencies should be made for possible cardio-pulmonary bypass or ECMO should airway collapse become a reality. Clearly, this is a situation that is best avoided if at all possible.

Foregut duplications, thymic masses, and paraspinous ganglioneuromas are nearly always safely resectable by thoracoscopy and this should be the standard approach for each of these lesions. Likewise, biopsy of almost any mediasatinal lesion, including paratracheal and subcarinal lymph nodes, can be performed safely using a minimal-access approach. Because the resultant scar is frequently cosmetically unappealing, the Chamberlain operation should only be used if there is truly no other approach available. For large lesions or malignant lesions, the posterolateral thoracotomy is standard, but a muscle-sparing approach should always be used. The pediatric general surgeon should also be comfortable with performing a sternotomy when necessary for large midline lesions (mediastinal teratoma). It is safe, offers excellent exposure, provides for a very stable closure, and is extremely well-tolerated (in most cases, better than a large thoracotomy!). The only real disadvantage is the scar. Finally, the axillary approach can be useful in certain cases, especially when dealing with lesions near the apex. A transverse incision is placed in the lowest axillary skin crease between the pectoralis major and latissimus dorsi muscles and the chest is entered through the third intercostal space. An extra-pleural approach can be used in some cases. The principle limitations of this approach are limited exposure and the inability to extend the incision.

Differential Diagnosis

Anterior (often neoplastic)

- Lymphoma
- Germ cell tumor
- Thymic cyst/thymoma

Middle (often cystic)

- Congenital foregut malformation

Posterior: usually neural

- Ganglioneuroma
- Neuroblastoma

Diagnostic Studies

- Chest X-ray
- CT scan
- ± MRI (depending on location)
- Pulmonary function tests for anterior mediastinal mass
- Appropriate tumor markers as indicated by clinical suspicion
  - AFP
  - HCG
  - Urine for catecholamines and metanephrines

Preoperative Preparation

- ☐ Airway assessment
- ☐ Type and screen
- ☐ Informed consent regarding potential injury to great vessels, airway, thoracic duct, nerves, likelihood and duration of chest tube

Suggested Reading

Glick RD, LaQuaglia MP. Lymphomas of the anterior mediastinum. Semin Pediatr Surg. 1999;8:69–77.

Grosfeld JL, Skinner MA, Rescorla FJ, et al. Mediastinal tumors in children: experience with 196 cases. Ann Surg Oncol. 1994;1:121–7.

King RM, Telander RL, Smithson WA, et al. Primary mediastinal tumors in children. J Pediatr Surg. 1982;17:512–20.

Ricketts RR. Clinical management of anterior mediastinal tumors in children. Semin Pediatr Surg. 2001;10:161–8.

Shamberger RC. Preanesthetic evaluation of children with anterior mediastinal masses. Semin Pediatr Surg. 1999;8:61–8.

Shields TW. The mediastinum and its compartments (Chapter 1). In: Shield TW, editor. Mediastinal surgery. Philadelphia, PA: Lea & Febiger; 1991. p. 3–5.

Part VII
Stomach and Small Intestine

Chapter 42
Gastroesophageal Reflux Disease

Thane Blinman

Few topics in pediatric surgery spark more disagreement and foster more misunderstandings about pathophysiology and management than gastroesophageal reflux disease. The picture is confounded by the differences between small children and adults, the vastly higher energy (and volume) requirements of babies, the preponderance of non-acid reflux, the poorly defined accuracy of the diagnostic tests for reflux, the questionable effectiveness of "anti-reflux" medications, and the variations of technique and experience of surgeons. Further, there are sometimes troubling complications that can occur after anti-reflux surgery, often made worse by feckless attempts to manage the postoperative patients without regard for the mechanical constraints fundoplasty imposes on the performance and regulation of the gastrointestinal tract. It is important to consider GERD as a mechanical disease and surgical treatment of reflux as a way to provide a specific mechanical solution, and to take into account the biomechanics of reflux and its amelioration.

GERD is a foregut disease: the physiology originates in the stomach and esophagus, but the more serious pathology lies within the airway and lungs. It results from the passive flow of stomach contents retrograde through the GE junction because of failure of the lower esophageal sphincter. This definition excludes emesis, which is the forceful ejection of stomach contents initiated by the vagal nuclei of the medulla and driven by retrograde peristalsis. All humans reflux; not all reflux is disease. GER becomes GERD when it causes comorbidities. In children, "acid reflux" (heartburn, esophagitis) can certainly be pathologic, but in young patients and babies, non-acid reflux can be just as troublesome and harder to diagnose.

Symptoms and signs of GERD in children stem not only from the retrograde flow of acid, but from chronic micro-aspiration of milk and enzymes (in particular, pepsin and related gastric peptidases). Barrett's esophagus is rare in children, but pain (manifested as arching, post-feeding irritability, food fear) is common. Some children complain of a sour or bitter taste in the mouth ("throw up throat"), and babies will be relentless "spitters." But, as long as growth is good and the lungs are healthy, the "spitty baby" more likely simply has GER. Others however, even non-spitters, may manifest GERD as failure to thrive, stemming from some combination of decreased oral intake and increased work of breathing.

The upper respiratory problems are the most dangerous and it is with these that we find the most compelling reasons to intervene surgically. Asthma has been posited as stemming from GERD in as many as half of children labeled with the disease. Chronic ear infections, hoarse voice, bad breath, and even tooth decay can all be signs of reflux with ongoing damage to the larynx, pharynx, and airways. In hospitalized patients with severe disease such as pulmonary hypertension (as seen with CHD and omphalocele) or congenital cardiac disease or even chronic lung disease of prematurity, GERD may manifest as failure to wean from the ventilator or from supplemental oxygen. Failure to thrive despite more than adequate calories results directly from the increased work of breathing. Of course, chronic lung disease is not the only respiratory manifestation of GERD: while is has been difficult to demonstrate a causal link between GERD episodes and apneic spells, it is plain that reflux and aspiration can be implicated in some cases of pneumonia, especially in neurologically impaired children, and even acute life-threatening events (ALTE).

Reflux is a function of fluid, pressure, viscosity, and the mechanisms of the so-called lower esophageal sphincter. The lower two third of the esophagus is not under voluntary control. It automatically propagates a peristaltic wave initiated by a swallow, and the last few centimeters of the esophagus normally hold intrinsic tone that relaxes in response to a peristaltic wave from above. But the lower esophageal tone is also lost in events known as transient lower esophageal sphincter relaxations (TLESR), during which most reflux episodes happen. Other mechanical effects are also in play. In particular, there must be a pressure gradient from abdomen to chest (or more particularly between stomach and lower esophagus). The viscosity of the gastric contents also play a part. Early treatment of GERD in babies consisted largely of thickening the feeds, a practice that increased the viscosity,

T. Blinman (✉)
General, Thoracic and Fetal Surgery, Children's Hospital of Philadelphia, 34th and Civic Center Boulevard, 5 Wood, Philadelphia, PA 19104, USA
e-mail: blinman@email.chop.edu

P. Mattei (ed.), *Fundamentals of Pediatric Surgery*,
DOI 10.1007/978-1-4419-6643-8_42, © Springer Science+Business Media, LLC 2011

although studies have not been able to demonstrate a strong effect. Some negative studies may have failed to show results because the viscosity of the feeds was only raised about 20%, which would, in theory, decrease GER by only 20%, at most, too fine a difference to discern. The expected effect of viscosity and pressure as well as the radius of the esophagus are seen in the equation: $Flux \propto \Delta P R^4 / cL\eta$, where ΔP = the pressure gradient between stomach and lower esophagus, R = the radius of the esophagus, c = a constant, L = the length of the LES (essentially, the distance from crura to GE junction), and η = the fluid viscosity. This equation figures strongly in the treatments for GERD, both in what measures might be expected to work and in the technical aspects of the repair.

But first, let's examine the mechanisms that the normal, non-refluxing human uses to prevent reflux. Understand that there is no true "lower esophageal sphincter" in the human. Instead, a complex arrangement of at least five mechanical mechanisms protects from reflux: (1) muscular tone (elastance) of the lower esophagus ($\downarrow R$, $\square \Delta P$), (2) the muscular "pinch cock" effect of the diaphragmatic crus muscles ($\square R$, $\square \Delta P$), (3) the length of the esophagus below the diaphragm ($\uparrow L$), (4) an acute angle of His (cardiac angle, $\square \Delta P$), and (5) normal gastric emptying (decreased dwell time, or average intragastric pressure = $\square \Delta P$).

Any problem causing reflux and any proposed solution for treating reflux, must work through one of the variables in the equation, as do all five mechanisms of a working fundoplasty. Notice that pH is not among the factors affecting reflux! All five mechanisms are disrupted in hiatal hernia: the esophageal elastance is diminished, the crura are ineffective and dilated, there is no length of esophagus below the diaphragm, and even gastric emptying may be effected. Other conditions also lead to reflux through one or more of these mechanisms: CDH leads to ineffective crura, TEF produces diminished esophageal length and function, omphalocele increases ΔP via decreased gastric emptying and often leads to hiatal hernia (just as it often leads to giant inguinal hernias), premies have decreased gastric emptying or increased dwell time ($T_{1/2}$ around 75 min instead of 45 min for term babies), and all babies need to consume large feeding volumes relative to body mass to achieve growth (dwell time). Even malrotation can mimic reflux symptoms by slowing gastric emptying from Ladd's bands. Critically, any therapy for effective control of reflux (surgical, endoluminal, medical) must work to restore at least some of these mechanical protections to be effective.

Diagnosis

Like most tests in medicine, studies for diagnosis of reflux in children are more specific than sensitive. That is, if a given test demonstrates reflux, it is probably present; if does not, you may know nothing. Nevertheless, the broad differential

diagnosis for GERD-type symptoms plus the penalty for intervening for the wrong diagnosis make it important to have objective evidence of GER. While the pH probe is claimed by many to be a gold standard, it is relatively insensitive in children and especially babies who tend to have non-acid reflux. Impedance probes work rather like a pH probe but use the drop in resistance (impedance) during a reflux event instead of the pH change, and might be more sensitive, but are also trickier to use. The same goes for manometry, perhaps most clearly indicated to diagnose achalasia but also helpful to demonstrate uncoordinated esophageal peristalsis. It too is tricky to use properly in the small patient. Nuclear medicine scans are claimed to be both sensitive and specific, but experience calls this into question: they tend to over-call reflux and under-call aspiration, and even their ability to accurately quantify gastric emptying is questionable.

Ultimately, the diagnosis is best made on clinical grounds. The only test that must be done before proceeding with surgical intervention is the upper GI contrast study. Though poorly sensitive for reflux, it is the best test to reveal hiatal hernia, microgastria, achalasia, and malrotation. Of these, malrotation is the most important to exclude before proceeding with repair. Other tests are added on a case-by-case basis to resolve whatever specific uncertainty remains, particularly to exclude mimics of GER: a highly atopic patient with dysphagia or odynophagia would be well served by esophagoscopy and biopsy to investigate eosinophilic esophagitis (or even Candidal esophagitis). The most likely outcome for any treatment (such as operative fundoplasty) applied without clear indication is a complication.

Nonoperative Therapy

Non-surgical treatment of reflux includes prokinetics, acid blockade, and feeding modifications. In general, prokinetics include metoclopramide, bethanechol, and erythromycin. Metoclopramide, a dopamine receptor (D_2) antagonist, is expected to increase emptying and improve lower esophageal tone, but no evidence for improving any objective measure of reflux in children can be demonstrated (but it is a known cause of dystonic reactions). Bethanechol, a parasympathomimetic, may have some use for thinning viscous secretions and improving gastric emptying, but randomized trials have shown no effect and experience demonstrates that it is at best weakly effective. Erythromycin given at low doses (typically around 20% of antimicrobial doses) is an analog of motilin. It has demonstrable effects in improving gastric emptying, but the effect begins to fade within 2 weeks (and seems to have no effect after 4 weeks).

Prokinetics offer at least the possibility of promoting a mechanical solution for GER, while acid blockade does not. It is unsurprising then that H_2 blockers such as ranitidine have so little demonstrable effect and even PPIs do not demonstrate any decrease in the volume of refluxate. Still, strong acid blockade from proton pump inhibitors may improve reflux in at least three ways. First, decreased acid certainly diminishes the noxious sensation from GER by reducing acid injury to the esophagus and allowing esophagitis to heal. Second, it is posited but not proved that chronic low-pH microaspiration increases the reactivity of bronchioles, and removing this acid decreases the tendency toward bronchospasm. Finally, chronic acid blockade produces a reactive hypergastrinemia, and since gastrin has known prokinetic effects in the stomach, it could improve motility even as the antisecretory effect diminishes the volume that must be emptied. This effect of hypergastrinemia has not been shown, but rebound gastritis after sudden discontinuation of PPIs has been observed and the effect appears to persist for up to 6 weeks.

What and how the baby is fed can also have an effect. Choice of formula certainly affects gastric emptying and therefore GER in babies. Breast milk has the best emptying profile, followed closely by Good Start (Nestlé). Regular, nonspecialized formulas empty around one third slower than breast milk. Unfortunately, children with persistent severe reflux are often started on expensive, unpalatable "elemental" formulas based on the mistaken notion that reflux is somehow an allergy or other "intolerance." But these formulas have the highest osmolarity of any available feed, and high osmolarity is plainly shown to drastically retard gastric emptying, making these formulas in fact counterproductive. Meanwhile, thickening agents, although working to diminish reflux by increasing viscosity (doubling viscosity should, all other things being equal, halve reflux), also tend to decrease gastric emptying; the sum effect is probably a wash. Another way to decrease ΔP is to use gravity: Parents are instructed to keep the babies upright after feeds in a car seat or have them sleep on a wedge.

Often, transpyloric or jejunal feeds are used, via naso-duodenal tubes, naso-jejunal tubes, or gastro-jejunal tubes. These can offer some protection from GER by leaving the stomach mostly empty and decreasing the ΔP. But it is not true that the pylorus offers much GER protection; the pylorus is not a true valve, since, rather than holding tonic pressure, it only generates pressure in response to a gastric peristaltic wave. Transpyloric tubes probably decrease pyloric tone and certainly provide a conduit for biliary reflux. Meanwhile, these strategies have a few other problems. First, aside from the bothersome requirement for near-around-the-clock pump feedings, reflux protection cannot be demonstrated in studies and tube complications (dislodgement, perforation, pnuematosis, sinusitis) are well-known. Second, GJ tubes do not close the hiatus, restore esophageal length, restore the angle of His, improve esophageal tone, or improve gastric motility. Transpyloric feeds may diminish the amount of milk seen in the mouth, but do not decrease acid or protease micro-aspiration, and in sick patients, tube feeds plus strong acid blockade raise the risk of aspiration pneumonia (probably by allowing bacterial and fungal overgrowth of the stomach). In the critically ill patient, transpyloric feeds may have some justification; GJ tubes should not be considered a first line GERD treatment. Instead, they serve far better in cases that mimic reflux, but for which a fundoplasty would be disadvantageous (severe gasroparesis, microgastria, dysmotility, perhaps cerebral palsy). No child with a demonstrated hiatal hernia should be considered for a GJ tube.

Surgical Principles

Surgical treatment of GERD in children in indicated whenever three conditions have been met: (1) objective demonstration of reflux, (2) at least one comorbidity, and (3) failure of maximum medical treatment. The surgeon sees those babies for whom the medical measures alone have been inadequate, and this is as it should be. With the exception of a reflux-related ALTE or rare indications such as preservation of lung transplants, surgery should be the last option.

Any operation intended to control reflux should restore LES function: repair the hiatus, restore length of esophagus beneath the diaphragm, create a zone of low compliance (or high elastance) between the diaphragm and GE junction, restore an acute angle of His, and improve gastric emptying. All successful anti-reflux operations share these mechanisms. Moreover, the anti-reflux operation should accomplish these goals without causing dysphagia. And the repair should last.

First, a word about terminology: here, we do not describe a Nissen (Nissen's original wrap was long, tight, and did not mobilize the short gastric vessels and dysphagia was a major complication); the Nissen–Rosetti (a shorter, looser wrap); or the so-called Collis–Nissen (both cut and un-cut versions appear to yield poor results); but the "Floppy Nissen" fundoplication (FNF). This fundoplasty is a 360° wrap that is loose, short, and takes advantage of a fully mobilized fundus. In general, while most surgeons still perform the operation using an open technique, fundoplication seems to be going the way of appendectomy and cholecystectomy: laparoscopy is the method of choice, even in children as small as 2.5 kg. Toupet's operation, a 270° posterior wrap, works according to the same principles as the FNF.

To restore intra-abdominal esophageal length, it is important to move the GE junction below the level of the diaphragm. In infants with severe reflux, the GE junction is often at, or just above, the hiatal opening. In hiatal hernia, it is well above the hiatus. In either case, the distal 2 or 3 cm of esophagus need to be mobilized into the abdominal cavity. Some disagreement exists among experts about the degree of mobilization that is needed. Some advocate an extensive mobilization into the chest while others just as adamantly condemn this practice. Some emphasize that the key to reducing recurrent hiatal hernias is to minimize dissection at the anterior, or posterior, part of the hiatus. All agree that the vagus nerves should be preserved. In general, a "just enough" dissection allows free movement of the esophagus into the abdominal cavity while still preserving some anterior and most posterior phrenoesophageal attachments. During this dissection, it is also critical to preserve the peritoneal coverings of the crura, without which the ability to create a lasting repair of the diaphragmatic hiatus will be diminished.

Without an intact hiatus, the LES cannot function. The surgical objective is to "take out the slack" by gently tightening the hiatus, typically by reapproximating the posterior hiatus. In the case of a large hiatal hernia, prevention of recurrence appears to depend upon removing any hernia sac that has formed. In these cases, there is often a massive hiatal aperture, and only closing posteriorly will create a kink or bump in the esophagus, risking dysphagia (and a more fragile repair). In this circumstance, the extra "slack" can be taken up by placing a series of collar stitches, re-establishing new phreno-esophageal attachments well proximal of the GE junction. Some have also tried pledgets or biocompatible mesh, but this practice has yielded uneven results. Experts also disagree about whether an esophageal bougie is needed to guide the sizing. Most warn against placement of anterior cruciate sutures, which seem to increase the risk of stricture at the hiatus. The unifying principle seems to be to make a snug, but not tight, closure using permanent sutures.

The angle of His, or "cardiac angle," should be acute in order to prevent reflux. As the stomach fills, the fundus expands and, if the angle is sharp, the fundus will tend to close the LES. On the other hand, an obtuse angle encourages overflow from the distended fundus up into the esophagus. In both Nissen and Toupet (as well as Dor and Thal, for that matter), careful attention should be paid toward creating a new cardiac angle. In the case of the Nissen, this is achieved automatically by simply ensuring that the entire wrap lies above the GE junction. In the Toupet, the angle is made by positioning the last suture on the left portion of the wrap precisely at the GE junction.

Many mistakenly believe that the wrap creates some sort of choke-resistor at the LES to prevent GERD. If it were true (and it is true in badly constructed wraps), then dysphagia would always accompany fundoplasty. As it is, dysphagia is a complication that the surgeon guards against by making a loose wrap. The idea of the wrap is not to create a choke point, but rather to bolster the lower esophageal tone, to create a segment of decreased compliance that counters transient LES relaxations. Both the Nissen and Toupet appear to do this well, with no measurable difference in outcome between them in adult patients. Observe that the other, possibly more important, purpose of the wrap is to maintain the gap (length) between the hiatus and the GE junction.

However, some caveats are in order. First, in the floppy Nissen, the fundus should be fully mobilized from the splenic short-gastric vessels, at least along the upper third of the greater curvature, and including the attachments and vessels that lie between the tail of the pancreas and the left crus. Some surgeons omit this step, but failure to do this risks a twisted or high tension wrap. Second, a Nissen should be relatively short, around 2–2.5 cm from crus to GE junction. Longer wraps increase the risk of dysphagia and shorter wraps tend to be less effective. Meanwhile, Toupet fundoplasties need to be longer than the Nissen, around 3 cm, to create good reflux protection. Of course, the pediatric surgeon should scale these lengths down a little for the smallest patients, but the converse is not true: larger patients apparently do not need longer wraps.

Fundoplasty is thought to improve gastric emptying by at least two mechanisms: by pulling the fundus around the esophagus, the reserve capacity of the stomach is diminished and gastric relaxation in response to food in the lumen is also diminished. Both effects produce a stiffer stomach that contracts more forcefully while the gastric pacemaker and vagal nerve-mediated peristaltic waves are undiminished, or even enhanced. The experience of experienced surgeons supports the notion that fundoplasty improves gastric emptying even without pyloroplasty, which inordinately risks development of early dumping syndrome and therefore should rarely if ever be done. Moreover, the changes in the gastric lumen capacity and function bear directly on the proper management of feeds and complications. Meanwhile, it is wise to always check for incomplete rotation where a high riding cecum drapes tight Ladd's bands across the duodenum, producing resistance to emptying.

Postoperative Management

In general, fundoplasty is extremely successful at alleviating symptoms of GERD, with a relatively low rate of complications. However, significant problems can be seen after fundoplasty, and these can be exacerbated by a clinician unaware of the risks or of the altered state of the stomach after fundoplasty. Fundoplasty may be successful in improving the nutrition and lungs of the child with bad GERD, but the surgeon who cedes all postoperative management to others does his patients a disservice. Like imperforate anus, many patients require ongoing gentle attention from a clinician who understands the mechanical constraints imposed by the operation.

Feeding

The normal human stomach holds around 20 mL/kg of body weight. After fundoplasty, tube fed babies usually can handle bolus feeds of only about 15 mL/kg. This is certainly adequate for growth, but ignoring this limit is one of the prime causes of retching in the early postoperative period. In general, feeds can be started within 12 h of fundoplasty (the delay allows anesthetic-associated nausea to resolve). In children who do not have a gastrostomy, it is reasonable to recommend at least 2 weeks (and up to 6 months) of a "soft, slimy, slick and slippery" diet, avoiding foods that exacerbate dysphagia such as meat, doughy bread and hard-edged chips. Babies that are formula-fed can be rapidly advanced to ad libitum feeds, and because of the vagally-mediated accommodation reflex originating in the pharynx, tend to be less volume limited than gastrostomy fed babies.

Medications

Once the fundoplasty is completed, antireflux medications can be stopped. Ranitidine has no rebound associated with it and continuing metoclopramide after fundoplasty is pointless since the mechanical repair of fundoplasty dwarfs any small effect this drug could provide while still risking side effects (diarrhea, dystonic reactions). Proton pump inhibitors should generally be weaned off. If the patient has been on a PPI for months, there will be elevated serum gastrin levels. This hypergastrinemia can persist for up to 6 weeks, raising the risk of hypersecretion of acid in the stomach with subsequent erosive gastritis. In general, this problem is not seen if PPIs are weaned off over 2–4 weeks. In rare cases, PPIs should be continued, say in a patient taking steroids or with severe gastritis or esophagitis preoperatively.

Gas Bloat

Gas bloat syndrome is a somewhat-poorly defined "syndrome" in which air introduced into the GI tract either from the tube or aerophagia is trapped in the stomach. Instead of burping, the child can only handle the air two ways: by venting via the gastrostomy, or by passing the air distally. The resulting distension, cramping, and pain are the manifestations labeled as "colic" and the irritated child may cry inconsolably or retch. The best way to treat gas bloat is good venting. Some favor the use of a Farrell valve, but this long thin tube tends to have uneven performance in small babies and is not the path of least resistance for ingested air. Often, better results are obtained by use of "chimney" venting. Other adjuncts include the use of simethicone, "tummy time," and avoidance of fiber or other feedings that promote gas formation in the colon.

Dumping

When clinicians talk about "dumping" they often refer to two distinct phenomena after gastric surgery. Here, we will refer to so-called "early dumping" syndrome, in which relatively high osmotic foods enter the small bowel and induce a period of intestinal hypermotility. The exact pathogenesis is not known, but links to GLP-1, renin-angiotensin, VIP, cholesystokinin, and other mediators have been demonstrated or proposed. The manifestations include pain, cramps, flushing, tachycardia, and watery diarrhea in response to a bolus feed. Of the two syndromes labeled as dumping, this is the more rarely seen in practice. Treatment consists of changing to lower osmotic feeds, slowing the rate of delivery and administration of octreotide. Meanwhile, because of the risk of this syndrome, rarely (if ever) should a pyloroplasty be done at the same time as a fundoplasty.

Post-Prandial Hypoglycemia

Also still referred to as "late dumping," post-prandial hypoglycemia (PPHG) can occur after any gastric procedure, but as a practical matter it is seen in children virtually exclusively after fundoplasty. Because the reactive hypoglycemia can be critical, this complication is arguably the most dangerous complication of fundoplasty. Because it can be asymptomatic, the method and criteria of diagnosis is in doubt, and awareness is poor, estimates of its prevalence range from 2 to 30%. In practice, we screen every patient for this syndrome by checking a series (30, 60, 90, and 120 min) of post-prandial glucose levels (d-sticks) once the children are at full feeds, or anytime they exhibit unexplained lethargy, somnolence, irritability or retching. A very high (>180 mg/dL) followed by a very low (<50 mg/dL) sugar is diagnostic. Some premies will exhibit low sugars after feeds without a spike; this is not true PPHG, and more likely represents relatively poor hepatic sugar mobilization. Evidence suggests that PPHG is a feedback-control failure, and over-secretion of incretins GLP-1 and GIP is posited as responsible for a inappropriate insulin response to a high blood glucose, leading to a precipitous and dangerous fall in blood glucose.

Treatment of PPHG is aimed at decreasing the rate and magnitude of the rise in glucose after a feed. Obviously, continuous feeds will avoid cyclic blood glucose levels, but also tie the child to a pump and can exacerbate bloating and retching. Other options include use of any combination of acarbose (which blocks intestinal alpha glucosidase to slow absorption of intraluminal polysaccharides), uncooked cornstarch, microlipid, or even a simple change from formulas containing "corn-syrup solids" (pure glucose) to those containing maltodextrin (a triose) or other more complex sugars. Whatever strategy is employed, ongoing home monitoring of post-feed sugars is essential to safe management (and eventual weaning of the interventions used).

Retching

Of all of the complications after fundoplasty, retching is one of the most distressing to parents. Clinicians often mistake retching for evidence of new reflux after fundoplasty, and restart anti-reflux medications to treat this mistaken diagnosis. But wrap failure is actually a very unlikely cause of retching. Retching is not reflux; it is frustrated emesis. Any noxious stimulus that provokes emesis in a baby can cause retching when an intact wrap prevents this active retrograde flow. While mechanical problems such as a herniated wrap or esophageal obstruction certainly can cause retching, more commonly retching is, in fact, evidence that the wrap is intact!

The approach to treating retching is to remove the noxious stimuli, the most common of which is over-large feeds. Dropping feeding boluses below 15 mL/kg/bolus usually removes this stimulus. Meanwhile, high osmolarity either of feeds (such as elemental formulas) or drugs (especially KCl) decrease emptying while also directly stimulating vagal afferents in the stomach and duodenum. It is also important to look beyond the stomach. For example, some children retch because they cannot handle their post-nasal drip, or because they have an acute exacerbation of pulmonary hypertension, or because they have an occult infection, or because they have unstable blood sugar. In general, a "whole-patient" approach to retching may be required to solve post-fundoplasty feeding intolerance. To solve retching, the doctor must find and eliminate the triggers of nausea, intestinal irritability, and vomiting that are the real sources of retching.

Dysphagia

Dysphagia (and odynophagia) occur more often after Nissen than Toupet, but is reported after any type of wrap in around 1 in 20 patients. But these reports probably fail to capture the mild dysphagia often seen in the immediate postop period. While a surgeon can make a proper loose wrap over a large guide, one cannot control inflammation, edema and related esophageal dysmotility as a result of surgical manipulation. As a result, patients may have a transient period (usually no more than 2 weeks, but some as long as 6 months) of dysphagia. For this reason, most surgeons recommend a soft diet free of hard-to-swallow meats or breads initially. In some cases of persistent dysphagia, a short burst of solumedrol or other corticosteroid can relieve the swelling, while others may require gentle dilatation. Dysphagia that persists requires further workup (endoscopy, manometry) to determine if the wrap needs to be revised, or if actually there was another diagnosis (achalasia, eosinophilic esophagitis, etc) that was mimicking GERD.

Recurrent GERD

In general, it is thought that surgical fundoplasty provides excellent control of GERD in >95% of pediatric patients. The wrap should also be intact and functioning in 90% of patients at 5 years. However, those numbers still leave many children who will have a wrap failure, which usually manifests as herniation of the wrap, slipping of the wrap onto the stomach ("napkin ring"), or unwrapping of the wrap. Herniation of the wrap usually requires re-operation since these children often have both dysphagia and insufficient reflux protection in addition to what is, essentially, a paraesophageal hernia. Other wrap failures may not need revision if the child has "outgrown" his reflux or if medical treatment is sufficient. Diagnosis of a failed wrap is best made via upper gastrointestinal series that includes an esophagram in order to show the entire wrap. Revision of a Nissen or other fundoplasty via a laparoscopic approach (regardless of initial approach) is feasible, but requires a patient, meticulous method and complete undoing and rebuilding of the wrap. Surgeons who have a large redo referral practice report that long-term results are similar to initial results.

Summary Points

- GERD is a mechanical disease that responds best to mechanical solutions.
- The mechanical disease of GERD involves the lower esophageal sphincter, but the principal medical consequence of GERD in children is damage to the airway and lungs.
- Surgical treatment of reflux is considered when (1) there is objective evidence of GER, (2) medical treatment is inadequate, and (3) there is at least one comorbidity.
- Retching is not reflux. Management of postoperative complications requires a mechanical understanding of the changes to the GI tract after surgery as well as a "whole-patient" approach.

Editor's Comment

Gastroesophageal reflux disease is still one of the most frequent indications for referral to a pediatric surgeon. Gastroesophageal reflux is quite common in all humans but there are certain children for whom reflux is severe and intractable, or associated with complications such as pain, failure to thrive, aspiration pneumonia, or reactive airways disease. It is extremely important to distinguish reflux, which is effortless, and emesis, which is forceful, as fundoplication in the setting of forceful vomiting will always fail eventually. The decision to operate should be based on clinical grounds. Ideally, there should be a consensus among the primary physician, gastroenterologist, pediatric surgeon, and, perhaps most importantly, the parents. Objective testing is useful in some borderline cases, but available tests are insensitive and nonspecific, and therefore cannot be used as the sole factor in making the decision. The only preoperative test considered mandatory by most pediatric surgeons is an upper GI contrast study, which is useful not to confirm or exclude GER but to rule out achalasia, esophageal stricture, gastric anomalies, and malrotation.

Children being considered for fundoplication generally fall into one of two broad categories: neurologically intact and neurologically impaired. Children who are neurologically impaired often need feeding access (gastrostomy), frequently have moderate-to-severe reflux that could be made worse with gastric feeds, and, most importantly, are sometimes unable to protect their airway. This combination strongly supports the use of fundoplication when gastrostomy is felt to be indicated, but some families may choose to proceed only with gastrostomy, especially if the child has been tolerating nasogastric feeds. This might be reasonable, especially considering that these children also have the highest incidence of postoperative complications, retching, feeding intolerance, hiatal hernia, wrap failure, and recurrent reflux.

There are several time-tested surgical principles that should be adhered to when performing a fundoplication in a child: (1) Perform a complete (360°) wrap whenever feasible. Partial wraps are not as effective or as durable, though they are useful in certain situations, such as esophageal atresia, when esophageal motility is known to be poor. (2) Close the hiatus by approximating the crura posterior to the esophagus. Anterior repair of the hiatus is ineffective and these stitches are doomed to pull through and fail. The use of pledgets or mesh is associated with a significant incidence of erosion and esophageal perforation and so should only be used if there is truly no alternative. (3) The wrap should be loose ("floppy") and care must be maintained to avoid simply twisting the stomach around the lower esophagus, which can cause severe dysphagia. A bougie is very useful to prevent over-tightening of the hiatus and the wrap. There are published guidelines as to how large a bougie should be used based on the weight of the child, but, in general, one should use the largest bougie that the esophagus will comfortably accommodate. (4) Mobilize at least 3 cm of esophagus into the abdomen and make the wrap 2.0–2.5 cm in length. Use at least three stitches (permanent braided are best) and include a bite of esophagus with each stitch. Try to identify and protect both vagus nerves throughout the procedure to prevent gastric emptying problems. (5) It is generally unnecessary to place collar stitches between the esophagus and hiatus, "rip-stop" stitches (fundus to fundus below the lowest wrap stitch), or stitches between the fundus and diaphragm, but these can be potentially useful in certain situations. (6) Always divide at least some of the upper short gastric vessels. This allows more of the fundus to be wrapped and allows the creation of a tension-free wrap, which is very important. (7) Despite the lack of long-term outcome data, the laparoscopic approach is preferable to the open because of the many advantages of minimal-access surgery, but the steps of the operation must be performed exactly how they would be for the open operation. The open approach is preferred by many surgeons for very small infants and patients undergoing re-do fundoplication.

Intra-operative complications are rare but can be serious. One should be wary of an accessory or replaced left hepatic artery. If a particularly large vessel is "in the way" it makes sense to test-clamp it to be sure the liver does not demarcate. Passing the bougie should be considered the most dangerous part of the operation as esophageal perforation has been described. The surgeon and anesthesiologist must agree that the bougie should be advanced slowly and only when both parties are aware of it. Most perforations are low and small and best repaired primarily and covered with the wrap. If it occurs higher in the chest, adequate drainage, a period of bowel rest, and a contrast study 5–7 days post-op are in order. Re-do Nissen fundoplication can be an extremely tedious procedure, mostly due to the dense adhesions typically formed in this region of the body. This is considered by some surgeons to be an added advantage to the laparoscopic approach: revising the wrap is somewhat easier and can often be done again laparoscopically. The vagus nerves are at high risk for injury during revision fundoplasty but performing an empiric pyloroplasty is no longer recommended due to the high risk of producing the dumping syndrome. Finally, when revising a fundoplication, it is important to take it down completely first, rather than simply reinforcing the part that has loosened. This allows proper closure of the hiatus, identification of the reason for failure, and creation of a tension-free and hopefully more durable wrap.

Postoperative dysphagia occurs in approximately 10% of patients after fundoplication, but only about 10% of these persist for more than 6 weeks. Those that persist should be considered for dilatation of the fundoplication, best done using a balloon dilator under fluoroscopic guidance. Refractory dysphagia could require revision, conversion to a partial wrap, or reversal of the wrap, but surgical intervention of any kind is rarely indicated.

Differential Diagnosis

- Vomiting
- Malrotation
- Achalasia
- Gastric anatomic abnormality

Preoperative Studies

- Thorough history
- Upper GI contrast study
- Nuclear medicine reflux scan
- pH probe acid reflux study
- Impedance probe reflux study

Parental Preparation

- Fundoplication is a big operation but a generally safe and well-tolerated study.
- Laparoscopy offers the advantages of less postoperative pain, faster recovery, and less scarring, but the long-term results are not known.
- Besides the generis risks of any operation (infection, bleeding, injury to adjacent structures, recurrence) there is a risk of gas-bloat, dumping syndrome, dysphagia, esophageal perforation, and a gradual return of GERD, sometimes requiring a second operation to revise the fundoplication.
- After fundoplication, the child may not be able to burp or vomit, but this is almost never a dangerous or painful problem.

Preoperative Preparation

- ☐ Upper GI contrast study
- ☐ Informed consent

Technical Points

- Division of at least some of the short gastric vessels allows creation of a complete wrap with less tension.
- Approximate the crura posteriorly.
- Create a wrap that is 2–2.5 cm in length.
- Complete wraps (360°) are more effective at preventing reflux but must be loose to avoid dysphagia.
- Partial wraps (posterior or anterior) might not be as effective at preventing reflux but allow patients to belch and vomit and appear to result in less postoperative dysphagia.
- The laparoscopic approach is purported to result in less postoperative pain, quicker recovery, and less scarring.

Suggested Reading

International Pediatric Endosurgery Group Standards and Safety Committee. IPEG guidelines for the surgical treatment of pediatric gastroesophageal reflux disease (GERD). J Laparoendosc Adv Surg Tech A. 2008;18(6):x–xv.

Lindeboom MYA et al. Function of the proximal stomach after partial versus complete laparoscopic fundoplication. Am J Gastroenterol. 2003;98(2):284–90.

Lobe TE. The current role of laparoscopic surgery for gastroesophageal reflux disease in infants and children. Surg Endosc. 2007;21:167–74.

Pandolfino JE et al. Esophagogastric junction distensibility: a factor contributing to sphincter incompetence. Am J Physiol Gastrointest Liver Physiol. 2002;282:G1052–8.

Spitz L, McLeod E. Gastroesophageal reflux. Semin Pediatr Surg. 2003;12(4):237–40.

Stylopoulos N, Rattner DW. The history of hiatal hernia surgery, from Bowditch to laparoscopy. Ann Surg. 2005;241(1):185–93.

Chapter 43
Hypertrophic Pyloric Stenosis

Marjorie J. Arca and Jill S. Whitehouse

Hypertrophic pyloric stenosis (HPS) is an acquired disorder that presents in infants between 3 and 8 weeks of age. The radial smooth muscle of the pylorus undergoes concentric hypertrophy, which causes narrowing of the pyloric channel and produces a gastric outlet obstruction. The obstruction results in progressive, projectile, nonbilious emesis, which can lead to dehydration, metabolic alkalosis, weight loss, and hypoglycemia.

The incidence is approximately 1 in 800 births. Male infants are affected four times as frequently as females and there appears to be a multifactorial familial inheritance. The risk of developing HPS if either parent was affected is about 5–7%. Although the belief that first-born males are at a higher risk has never been proven, there is a documented decline in risk with increasing birth order up to the fourth child. It is two- to threefold more common in Caucasians compared to Asians or Blacks.

Diagnosis

When an infant presents with recurrent vomiting, the primary care physician often changes the formula as a treatment for gastroesophageal reflux or formula intolerance. If the emesis persists or progresses, then further diagnostic testing is warranted. On physical examination, one should look for evidence of dehydration (sunken fontanelle, dry mucous membranes, lethargy). Severe dehydration is almost never seen in children with reflux or lactose intolerance.

The classic diagnostic tool is physical examination by a skilled clinician. The hypertrophied pylorus has been described as an "olive" palpable in the epigastrium. An optimal examination is elicited by decompressing the stomach with a nasogastric tube, then allowing the infant to suck on a small bottle of Pedialyte or a pacifier soaked in sugar water. The examiner gently palpates deep in the epigastrium through the child's relaxed abdominal wall using just the fingertips, starting just below the xiphoid and sliding downward, feeling the "olive" rolling beneath.

If the hypertophic pylorus is palpated by an experienced examiner, no further test is needed. If the examination is equivocal, an abdominal ultrasound or upper GI contrast study should be performed. An ultrasound performed by a skilled technician has a sensitivity and specificity approaching 100% and is the diagnostic procedure of choice. Ultrasound criteria confirming HPS include: a pyloric muscle thickness of 4 mm and a channel length of 16 mm or greater (Fig. 43.1) An UGI study is used primarily when both the physical exam and ultrasound results are equivocal. This study will characteristically show a narrowed pyloric channel with corresponding "string" sign of contrast within the lumen and bulging "shoulders" of the pyloric muscle protruding into the antrum (Figs. 43.1– 43.3) Although an UGI can reveal other sources of infantile vomiting such as foregut atresias, webs, malrotation, or gastroesophageal reflux, it does have the disadvantage of filling an obstructed stomach with contrast, which should be decompressed prior to induction of general anesthesia.

Preoperative Preparation

Although surgical correction of HPS offers a complete cure, the operation is not an emergency. Correction of dehydration and electrolyte abnormalities is obligatory before bringing the infant to the operating room. A metabolic panel is drawn and intravenous access is obtained. All enteral feedings are held prior to surgery but nasogastric decompression is no longer de rigueur.

The classic electrolyte abnormality associated with pyloric stenosis is hypokalemic, hypochloremic metabolic alkalosis, presumably due to ongoing gastric acid loss from vomiting. Paradoxical aciduria is sometimes noted because the kidney excretes protons in exchange for sodium in an attempt to

M.J. Arca (✉)
Department of Surgery, Medical College of Wisconsin, Children's Hospital of Wisconsin, Milwaukee, WI, USA
e-mail: marca@chw.org

P. Mattei (ed.), *Fundamentals of Pediatric Surgery*,
DOI 10.1007/978-1-4419-6643-8_43, © Springer Science+Business Media, LLC 2011

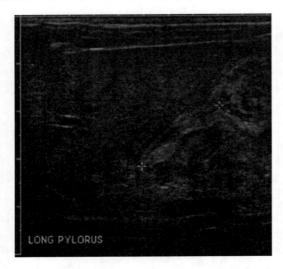

Fig. 43.1 Ultrasound image of a hypertrophied pyloric channel in a longitudinal plane. The channel measures 21 mm (between the two white crosses), far exceeding the diagnostic threshold of 16 mm

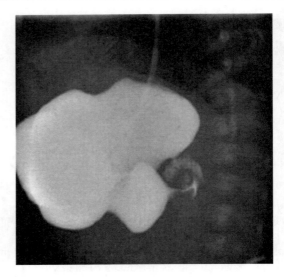

Fig. 43.3 An UGI contrast study in a patient with HPS. The stomach is dilated and filled with contrast material, with a classic "string sign" just to the right of the stomach, representing the narrowed lumen of the pyloric channel

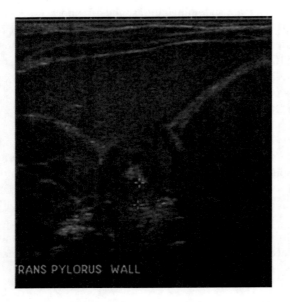

Fig. 43.2 An ultrasound image in cross-sectional view of the same hypertrophied pylorus. The thickness of the pyloric wall is 4.5 mm

in a baby whose renal function might be compromised by decreased intravascular volume. The baby's glucose should also be monitored during the initial resuscitation and maintenance fluids should contain dextrose. Close attention is paid to urinary output, overall perfusion and repeat laboratory values. If the initial laboratory values are within normal limits, fluids are then switched to a maintenance regimen until the operation. Once the infant is hemodynamically stable and has acceptable electrolyte levels, a pyloromyotomy is performed at the earliest convenience.

Surgical Technique

Ramstedt described the practice of longitudinal pyloromyotomy in 1911. The first pyloromyotomy described suture closure of the cut edges of the pyloric muscle, which caused significant bleeding. The current practice omits this unnecessary step.

conserve fluid. Prior to general anesthesia, the serum chloride level should be greater than 90 mEq/L and the serum bicarbonate should be below 29 mEq/L. A child with uncorrected metabolic alkalosis will hypoventilate to normalize serum pH (compensatory respiratory acidosis). Clinically, this translates to an inability to wean from mechanical ventilation post-operatively.

I bolus every infant with pyloric stenosis with 20 mL/kg of 0.9 normal saline while waiting for the electrolyte results. If there is evidence of hypoperfusion or an ongoing metabolic derangement, aggressive isotonic resuscitation is continued. Replacing potassium initially should not be attempted

Pyloromyotomy can be performed using an open or laparoscopic approach. The traditional open pyloromyotomy is performed through a right upper quadrant incision with a transverse fascial opening, but this has largely been replaced by the supra-umbilical approach, which utilizes a curvilinear skin incision and a vertical fascial opening. A V-Y-plasty closure can be used instead. A laparoscopic pyloromyotomy typically involves an umbilical incision for visualization and two tiny stab incisions in the right and left upper quadrants.

Regardless of the approach, the principles of the pyloromyotomy remain the same. Once the infant is anesthetized,

I place an orogastric catheter to be used later for injecting air into the stomach at the conclusion of the pyloromyotomy. A knife is used to score the serosa. The muscle is split with a blunt tip dissector from the serosa to the submucosa. The muscle is separated until the intact mucosa and submucosa are visualized bulging outward. To ensure adequate relief of the obstruction, the myotomy should be continued for a short distance onto the stomach, until the circular muscle fibers are visualized. Each exposed edge of the pyloromyotomy is grasped with instruments and then moved in opposite longitudinal directions. If they do not move independently from one another, the pyloromyotomy should be extended. Finally, the duodenum is occluded using an atraumatic grasper and approximately 50 mL of air is injected through the orogastric tube into the stomach. The pyloromyotomy site is examined for signs of a leak (air bubbles) and if air passes into the duodenum it is assumed that the pyloromyotomy is adequate.

In the open procedure, the pylorus is stabilized between the surgeon's thumb and forefinger. After the initial cut in the serosa, the muscle fibers are split using the back end of a scalpel handle, a hemostat to gently break the muscle fibers, or a pyloric (Benson) spreader is used to pry open the split halves of the muscle. In the laparoscopic technique, abdominal access is gained by an umbilical incision and the abdomen is insufflated through a trocar (5 mm or less). An angled scope is inserted and two stab incisions are made to the right of the umbilicus and in the left upper quadrant. An atraumatic grasper is inserted directly through a stab incision without the use of a trocar and used to steady the pylorus by grasping either the duodenum or the stomach. A retractable arthrotomy knife, inserted through the other stab incision, makes the incision through the serosa. The knife is withdrawn into its sheath and this blunt instrument is used to shimmy between the cut edges of the muscle. The knife is then removed and a laparoscopic pyloric spreader is introduced to complete the myotomy along the length of the muscle.

Postoperative Care

Complications from a pyloromyotomy include mucosal perforation, postoperative wound infection, emesis, incisional hernia, dehiscence, and recurrent pyloric stenosis, usually due to an incomplete pyloromyotomy. Mortality is extremely rare, with reported rates worldwide of less than 0.5%. When the operation is performed at institutions experienced in the technique, duodenal perforation, recurrence, and wound infection each occur at a rate of 1–3%. Duodenal perforation is best identified at the time of the operation, at which time it should be repaired immediately.

Most surgeons convert to an open procedure at this point but the repair can be done laparoscopically. The traditional recommendation was to repair the entire pyloromyotomy in layers, rotate the pylorus 90°, and redo the pyloromyotomy; however, most surgeons simply repair the perforation with absorbable mattress stitches (for a small perforation a single U-stitch is usually sufficient) and make the baby NPO for 12–24 h before restarting feeds. Children with a delayed diagnosis of perforation can become quite ill with peritonitis, dehydration and frank sepsis usually developing within 24 h. Aggressive resuscitation and prompt re-exploration are clearly indicated. Recurrence (persistence) of pyloric stenosis should be treated with operative revision as soon as possible, but confirming the diagnosis can be surprisingly difficult. A contrast study or nuclear medicine gastric emptying scan is usually necessary as ultrasound is not useful in this setting (even when clinical symptoms resolve muscle thickness and channel diameter remain abnormal for 8–12 months). A complication unique to the laparoscopic approach is vascular injury during trocar insertion. In infants less than 3 weeks of age, injection of carbon dioxide into a patent umbilical vessel can cause a gas embolus, which is why I only offer laparoscopy to patients older than 3 weeks of age.

A typical postoperative course after any approach to pyloromyotomy involves rapid resolution of emesis, a short duration of analgesic requirement, and significant improvement in feeding tolerance. Postoperative feeding advancement is still somewhat controversial. No single method has proven to be superior. One regimen advances to goal feeds in a step-wise fashion, starting at 15 or 30 mL per feed several hours after the conclusion of the operation. This is the method utilized in our institution. Over the course of 18–24 h, the infant is back to feeding *ad libitum* and discharged to home. A different regimen used successfully at other institutions reinstates *ad libitum* feeds immediately after surgery. Retrospective studies suggest no significant differences in postoperative emesis or length of hospital stay between these methods, and therefore both are widely practiced and accepted. If a baby has persistent emesis while in the hospital, giving H2-blockers or proton pump inhibitors often helps. Upon discharge, we advise the parents that the baby may have occasional emesis or "wet burps" but that persistent feeding intolerance warrants return to hospital. A single routine postoperative office visit is performed 3–4 weeks after surgery.

Studies comparing the various pyloromyotomy methods tend to focus on cost-effectiveness, cosmesis, pain control, infections, length of hospital stay, and duration of surgery. The supraumbilical approach is associated with a slightly higher risk of wound infection (1.8–7%), but excellent cosmetic results. Cosmesis is improved further by using the laparoscopic approach. The largest prospective randomized controlled series comparing open vs. laparoscopic pyloromyotomies showed less postoperative pain and emesis and fewer complications in the laparoscopic group, but no difference in length of hospital stay or operating time. Several studies have shown a definite learning curve in performing laparoscopic pyloromyotomy. Once the learning curve plateaus, operative times and complications both decrease. Outcomes have been shown to be better when pediatric operations such as pyloromyotomy are done in specialty centers by surgeons with a great deal of experience.

Summary Points

- Hypertrophic pyloric stenosis is an acquired gastric outlet obstruction.
- The etiology is unknown but there appears to be a genetic basis.
- It typically affects predominantly male infants between 3 and 8 weeks of age.
- A palpable "olive" in epigastric region is diagnostic.
- If physical exam is equivocal, ultrasound is usually the best diagnostic procedure.
- US criteria: muscle thickness ≥4 mm, muscle length ≥17 mm.
- Normalize volume status and electrolyte abnormalities before surgery.
- Treatment is surgical by open or laparoscopic pyloromyotomy.
- An early post-operative feeding regimen, either gradual or *ad libitum*, shortens length of hospital stay.
- Complications are rare and include: duodenal perforation (1–3%), wound infection (1–3%), post-operative emesis (3%), incomplete/recurrent pyloromyotomy (<1%), incisional hernias/dehiscence (<1%), and death (very rare).

Editor's Comment

To the chagrin of the surgical purist, physical examination is no longer the favored test for confirming the diagnosis of pyloric stenosis. This might be another example of the lost art of medicine, but in reality it has become impractical for several reasons: to be successful it requires the use of a nasogastric tube, which is painful, distressing and no longer routine in infants with HPS; it is time-consuming for the clinician and uncomfortable for the infant; it is not especially accurate; the alternative (US) is quick, painless, accurate, and relatively inexpensive; and, perhaps most importantly, the pediatric surgeon is almost never called upon anymore to make the diagnosis, but rather is almost invariably called after the US has been done and the diagnosis is known. Nevertheless, surgeons should examine every infant after induction of anesthesia to confirm the diagnosis and gain experience with the technique. An upper GI should only be performed if the diagnosis is in serious question (possibly bilious emesis, atypical presentation) or if the US is equivocal. Idiopathic hyperbilirubinemia was considered commonplace in infants with HPS but is now rarely seen, perhaps because patients present much earlier now. Prior to induction of general anesthesia, gastric contents should be aspirated thoroughly to prevent massive aspiration, still a significant cause of morbidity (hypoxic brain injury) and even mortality in this population of vulnerable infants.

The right upper quadrant incision was commonly employed in the past, perhaps because infants presented very late and their hugely dilated stomachs displaced the pylorus into the RUQ. But because the pylorus is actutally a midline structure and the RUQ scar becomes very large and unsightly in adulthood, in this day and age one should *never* use a RUQ incision for pyloromyotomy in an infant. The laparoscopic and the periumbilical approaches are essentially equal in every respect, which means either is acceptable; however, I believe that when two approaches are considered equal, the minimally invasive approach should de facto be the preferred approach. Regarding the laparoscopic technique, insufflation with a Veress needle should not be needed as every infant has a patent umbilical ring that can be gently dilated with a hemostat to allow passage of a small trocar under direct vision. And many feel that grasping the stomach with the right hand and incising the pylorus with the left hand is safer than grasping the more delicate duodenum with one's non-dominant hand. Finally, the most common serious error is overly aggressive splitting of the pyloric muscle fibers adjacent to the duodenum, where the bowel wall is thin and the bulging of the muscle into the lumen creates an angle that is prone to perforation (Fig. 43.4). Remember: recurrence occurs on the gastric side (incomplete myotomy), perforation occurs on the duodenal side (aggressive myotomy).

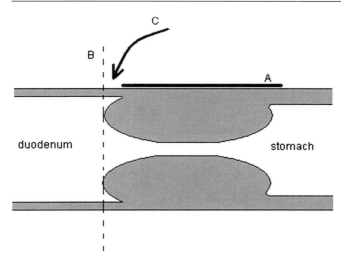

Fig. 43.4 Schematic diagram of the hypertrophic pylorus in longitudinal cross-section. *A* represents the correct length of the pyloromyotomy. *B* is the apparent end of the pylorus based on where the bulge of the muscle is perceived when viewed externally. *C* is the point where the mucosa can be injured if the pyloromyotomy is extended too far onto the duodenum. There is less of a risk of perforation on the gastric side because the gastric wall is thicker and the angle between the mucosa and the intraluminal portion of the pylorus is less acute

Differential Diagnosis

- GERD
- Duodenal web/stricture
- Malrotation ± volvulus
- Lactose/ formula intolerance

Diagnostic Studies

- Physical exam
- Abdominal ultrasound
- Contrast UGI

Parental Preparation

- Preoperative IV fluid resuscitation is crucial – surgery is not emergent!
- Pyloromyotomy, though not completey risk-free, has a very high success rate and a very low complication rate.
- Duodenal mucosal injury is possible and requires repair
- Post-operative emesis might occur at first but usually resolves within 24–48 h.

Preoperative Preparation

- ☐ IVF hydration
- ☐ Corrected electrolyte abnormalities (bicarb < 28 mEq/L, chloride >90 mEq/L)
- ☐ Gastric decompression, aspiration of residual gastric contrast if UGI obtained
- ☐ Informed consent

Technical Points

- Laparoscopic incisions: Umbilical ≤5-mm port for insufflation and camera, one stab incision in right abdomen and left upper quadrant for working instruments.
- Pyloromyotomy extending distally from the duodenopyloric junction proximally onto the gastric antrum.
- At conclusion of pyloromyotomy, opposite sides of pylorus should be grasped and moved in opposite longitudinal directions independently of one another, confirming complete disruption of hypertrophied fibers.
- Inject air into stomach to test for perforation.

Suggested Reading

Everett KV, Chioza BA, Georgoula C, Reece A, Capon F, Parker KA, et al. Genome-wide high-density SNP-based linkage analysis of infantile hypertrophic pyloric stenosis identifies loci on chromosomes 11q14-q22 and Xq23. Am J Hum Gen. 2008;82(3):756–62.

Hulka F, Harrison MW, Campbell TJ, Campbell JR. Complications of pyloromyotomy for infantile hypertrophic pyloric stenosis. Am J Surg. 1997;173(5):450–2.

Kim SS, Lau ST, Lee SL, Schaller R, Healey PJ, Ledbetter DJ, et al. Pyloromyotomy: A comparison of laparoscopic, circumbilical, and right upper quadrant operative techniques. J Am Coll Surg. 2005;201(1):66–9.

Ly DP, Liao JG, Burd RS. Effect of surgeon and hospital characteristics on outcome after pyloromyotomy. Arch Surg. 2005; 140:1191–7.

MacMahon B. The continuing enigma of pyloric stenosis of infancy. Epidemiology. 2006;17(2):195–201.

Muramori K, Nagasake A, Kawanami T. Ultrasonographic serial measurements of the morphologic resolution of the pylorus after Ramstedt pyloromyotomy for infantile hypertrophic pyloric stenosis. J Ultrasound Med. 2007;26(12):1681–7.

St Peter SD, Holcomb III GW, Calkins CM, Murphy JP, Andrews WS, Sharp RJ, et al. Open versus laparoscopic pyloromyotomy for pyloric stenosis: A prospective, randomized trial. Ann Surg. 2006; 244:363–70.

Vegunta RK, Woodland JH, Rawlings AL, Wallace LJ, Pearl RH. Practice makes perfect: Progressive improvement of laparoscopic pyloromyotomy results, with experience. J Laparoendoc Adv Surg Tech. 2008;18(1):152–6.

Chapter 44
Surgical Enteral Access

Tim Weiner and Melissa K. Dedmond

The creation of surgical access to the gastrointestinal tract for the direct administration of food and medications or for decompression is a common procedure and familiar to most surgeons. While the technical aspects are straightforward, some degree of critical thinking in the selection of patients as well as close attention to surgical details will reward the patient, the family, and the surgeon with fewer post-operative "nuisance" problems.

The indications for placement of a gastrostomy tube are varied and increasing: (1) inability to take sufficient oral nutrition or failure to thrive; (2) presence of pharyngeal or esophageal pathology; (3) the need to carefully titrate enteral feeds; (4) excessive metabolic demands or risks of oral feeding; (5) the need to administer unpalatable diets or medications over a long period; (6) the need to decompress a portion of the GI tract.

Often, the decision to place a gastrostomy in a child has been more or less finalized by a non-surgical colleague. In these situations we have found it appropriate to carefully review the indications, frankly discuss contraindications, and extensively prepare the patient and family for the operation and post-operative care. To this end, we ask the family to review a short video that discusses the G-tube from their perspective and provides them with a resource to review when they encounter questions or problems at home. In addition, our nurses provide extensive one-on-one teaching. We find that this intensive pre-operative preparation has made families much more independent in the care of their child's G-tube and significantly decreased the number of phone calls and visits to the surgical clinic.

Diagnosis

The decision to place a GT immediately raises questions of anatomy and pathology and a limited but focused investigation is recommended. Typically, an upper GI contrast study is performed to characterize the foregut anatomy. Esophageal lesions, microgastria, gastric outlet obstruction or malrotation might necessitate modification of the operative plan. Most surgeons also prefer to assess whether the child has clinically significant gastroesophageal reflux disease. Although a thorough clinical history and UGI is usually sufficient to resolve these issues, in some cases a pH-probe or impedence study is felt to be necessary.

Assuming the work-up is unremarkable, the patient is prepared in a routine manner for either open, laparoscopic, or percutaneous endoscopic gastrostomy. If there are concerns about GER, an anti-reflux procedure or a more distal feeding access, such as a surgical jejunal tube, should be discussed. While some surgeons feel that placement of a gastrostomy can alter the gastric anatomy in ways that create or worsen GER, there are no data to support the need for an antireflux operation with every gastrostomy. Should the GER become more significant after G-tube placement, a subsequent fundoplication can still be performed, though the gastrostomy may have to be re-sited to allow for a full fundoplication.

Surgical Technique

In our practice, we prefer an open or laparoscopic technique and usually attempt to place a low-profile (MIC-KEY) button as the initial access. Unless the tube is being replaced through an established tract, we do not routinely use the PEG technique in order to avoid the rare but significant misadventures that can occur, such as passage through the liver, gastrocolic fistula, tube misplacement, or dislodgement into the peritoneal cavity.

In children for whom more distal enteral access is needed, we generally use a Roux-Y feeding jejunostomy for ease of care and durability. A Witzel-type jejunostomy is a functional option but presents more challenges for long-term use: balloon obstruction, malposition, kinking within the bowel lumen, and loss of the access tract.

T. Weiner (✉)
Department of Surgery, University of North Carolina, UNC Hospitals, Chapel Hill, NC, USA
e-mail: tweiner@med.unc.edu

P. Mattei (ed.), *Fundamentals of Pediatric Surgery*,
DOI 10.1007/978-1-4419-6643-8_44, © Springer Science+Business Media, LLC 2011

Open (Stamm) Gastrostomy

First described in the late 1800s, the Stamm gastrostomy remains a technically simple and safe operation for uncomplicated enteral access in children. A 2-cm upper midline or left subcostal incision is made and the anterior aspect of the stomach is identified. Our preference is to site the gastrostomy to the left of the incisura and near the greater curve of the stomach body. This position limits tension on the gastric outlet and gastroesophageal junction, reduces the likelihood of inadvertent placement of the tube across the pylorus and into the duodenum, allows for a better trajectory if a post-pyloric feeding tube is required, and does not fix the stomach at a difficult angle should a fundoplication be needed later. We find that a single 3-0 purse-string suture at the gastrotomy site is sufficient in most cases and does not compromise a small gastric lumen. A 5–8-mm stab incision is made in the left upper abdomen without "window shading" the abdominal tissue planes at the tube exit site. The exit site is chosen to avoid apposition of the tube on the coastal cartilages; in infants, one finger breadth from the lowest rib and one finger breadth from the midline incision works well. A 10-14 French low-profile device with a stem length estimated to account for abdominal and stomach wall thickness (usually 1.2 or 1.5 cm in infants) is carefully brought through the incision. A Malecot or Pezzar tube is used if a low-profile device cannot be placed at the initial surgery. A small gastrostomy is made with electrocautery within the pursestring suture, entry into the gastric lumen is confirmed, and the tube is maneuvered into the stomach, taking care to avoid a submucosal dissection. The balloon is filled (or the tube flange is "snugged" against the inner stomach wall) and the purse string is secured. Two to four 3-0 seromuscular stitches are placed close to the gastrostomy, being careful to avoid puncturing the balloon and then to the tube exit site within the abdomen in order to bring the anterior stomach and peritoneal surfaces into secure apposition. One or two nylon sutures are used to secure the tube to the skin and removed between the fourth and seventh postoperative day.

We typically test the tube for proper function in the operating room under direct observation before closing the incision. Use of the tube begins the following morning. Malecot or Pezzar tubes are replaced with a low-profile device after the tract has matured for 3–4 weeks.

Laparoscopic Gastrostomy

Laparoscopy can be used to guide the placement of a gastrostomy tube as a stand-alone procedure or as an adjunct to an endoscopic approach. It is also performed as part of a laparoscopic fundoplication.

The anticipated exit site is determined and marked prior to insufflation, which distorts the surface anatomy. A 3- or 5-mm port and 30° laparoscope are introduced through a small umbilical incision. A second incision is made at the pre-determined tube exit site and a 3 or 5-mm atraumatic grasper is passed directly through the abdominal wall. As in the open technique, the gastrotomy site is selected near the greater curvature on the stomach body and the mobility of this area to the abdominal wall is tested.

While pre-loaded, single-use T-stabilizers may be used, we prefer the placement of two heavy polypropylene U-stitches through the abdominal wall to capture the anterior stomach. This maneuver requires some degree of finesse in order to properly position the sutures lateral to the anticipated gastrotomy while traversing the seromuscularis of the anterior stomach wall with enough purchase to hold it under tension. A pronounced supination-pronation as the needle is driven in a cephalad to caudad direction helps considerably. Using the stomach grasper to position the stomach as a target helps place the sutures (Fig. 44.1). These sutures are then tagged with a clamp and a needle-Seldinger technique is used to cannulate the stomach lumen between the U-stitches. The tract is then enlarged sequentially with dilators up to a 16 or 20 French caliber. An appropriately-sized button is then loaded over the smallest dilator or within the peel-away device and passed into the stomach lumen. Successful placement is often registered with a distinct "pop" or "give" when the balloon enters the stomach. The balloon is inflated, the sutures are tied over the external flanges of the button and the tube is tested with air under laparoscopic visualization to confirm intraluminal position.

The tube can be used within 24 h and the sutures can be removed between 4 and 7 days after placement, before

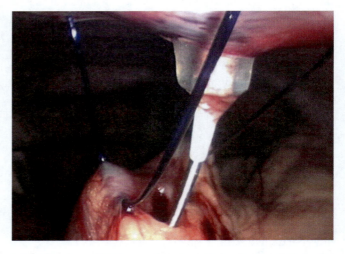

Fig. 44.1 Laparoscopic placement of a MIC-Key button device. Notice the transabdominal monofilament tacking sutures and the Seldinger technique using the small dilator to guide the button into the gastrotomy

foreign body irritation occurs. If a peel-away system was used, some surgeons suggest confirmation of stomach cannulation by passage of the scope through the peel-away sheath. Endoscopy can also be used to confirm proper GT positioning.

Jejunostomy Tubes

In situations where post-pyloric enteral access is indicated, a surgically placed tube can be created either as a side-entry (Witzel) tube, a Roux-Y, or by a laparoscopic technique. As noted, the Roux-Y is felt by our group to be the best option in terms of ease of care, replacement, and durability.

The Witzel technique is familiar to most surgeons and simply involves placing a small caliber tube, such as a 10 or 12 French Malecot catheter through a proximal jejunal enterotomy on the anti-mesenteric side of the bowel. A 3-0 purse string is used to hold the tube in place and advancing the tube into the lumen for an additional 4–10 cm helps to secure it and prevent dislodgment. Some surgeons recommend creating a short serosal tunnel with imbricating sutures over the tube and along the long axis of the bowel. The tube then exits the abdominal wall at a selected site and the bowel serosa adjacent to the tube is tacked to the peritoneum of the exit site.

The Roux-Y is typically done through a midline epigastric incision. The orientation of the small bowel is determined and a jejunal loop 10–20 cm from the duodenal-jejunal junction is located. The small bowel is divided at this point and an end-to-side anastomosis is created distally. We find that a 5–10-cm Roux limb is usually sufficient. A 3-0 purse string suture is then placed adjacent to the staple line at the blind end of the Roux limb. A Malecot tube or button device is then brought through the abdominal wall, an enterotomy is made within the purse string, and the tube is passed into the bowel lumen as the purse string is secured. Tacking sutures are placed and the tube is secured externally with a nylon suture.

The Roux-Y has the advantages of creating a straight trajectory for tube replacement and poses little risk of bowel occlusion with a balloon device. Overfilling a balloon, however, can precipitate pressure necrosis of the bowel wall and caregivers should be carefully advised to avoid this hazard. There is also a risk of volvulus around the Roux limb, which can present as a bowel obstruction, or in the neurologically impaired child with bowel necrosis and profound sepsis.

Laparoscopic Witzel and Roux-Y using a combination of the Seldinger technique and extracorporeal anastomoses have been described. These are technically feasible and follow the same principles of an open technique but may entail the usual laparoscopic learning curve.

Percutaneous Endoscopic Gastrostomy (PEG)

In our practice, we rarely use the endoscopic-assisted approach. The endoscopist views the anterior aspect of the stomach and places the camera light against the anticipated entry site. This is confirmed externally with the operating room lights dimmed. Insufflation of the stomach also facilitates the exclusion of colon and liver from the intended cannulation trajectory. A needle is passed through the intended gastrostomy site and visualized by the endoscopist. Premade kits include a wire which is passed through the needle and a snare used by the endoscopist to capture the wire. The wire is then drawn out through the patient's mouth by the scope and a mushroom-flanged PEG tube is passed over the wire in a "push" technique through the patient's mouth, captured at the tube exit site and pulled through the abdominal wall. The tube is secured by placing an outer flange against the skin while the endoscopist confirms the tube's position. The tube can be replaced with a low-profile button device when the tract is mature, usually at 4–6 later.

Postoperative Care

Optimal management of surgical gastrostomies is achieved through a coordinated approach involving the surgical team, nursing staff, and patient caregivers. Routine maintenance includes ensuring the child has a properly fitted, functioning gastrostomy device and careful peristomal skin care. Approximately 85% of children will eventually have a low profile or skin-level balloon device placed after surgery. Gastrostomy tubes come in a variety of diameters and stem lengths, depending on the manufacturer. The tube should be able to rotate freely within its tract, with at least a few millimeters between the patient's abdomen and the outer flange. Tube size and stem length are adjusted according to the thickness of the abdominal wall and depends on weight gain and activity level, typically requiring frequent adjustments in the first year.

Low profile balloon devices typically last 4–6 months with replacement being necessary due to the patient outgrowing the tube, a slowly-leaking balloon, or rupture of the balloon, all of which can cause leakage, a loose tube, or dislodgement. Patients with balloon devices benefit from periodic assessment of the amount of water in the balloon: 5 mL of water is typically recommended for toddler age and above; a small infant might need less depending on their size. Balloon devices can be replaced easily in the office setting; caregivers can also learn how to perform replacements at home. Alternatively, the non-balloon devices with soft silicone domes (Bard buttons) are advantageous because they can last a year or more, are much more difficult to dislodge accidentally, and their flatter external appearance is more appealing to some adolescent patients. However, they are more difficult and painful to replace, malfunction more often, and the one-way valve tends to leak more.

Minor gastrostomy complications are common but usually respond to interventions that can be safely performed at home: gastrostomy leakage, accidental dislodgement, granulation tissue, and skin erosion. Educating caregivers on preventive strategies, can result in fewer clinic visits and improved quality of life for patients with long-term enteral access.

Leakage from the gastrostomy site can occur for a variety of reasons including improper tube fit, inadequate volume of water in the balloon, enlargement of stomal site due to poor wound healing, or excessive tension on the site. If the cause of the leakage is due to an enlarged stoma, the tube should be replaced with a *smaller* Foley catheter (two French sizes smaller) into the site for 24–48 h, which allows the hole to contract creating a more secure fit of the gastrostomy tube. Another option is removal of the tube for as long as several hours to allow downsizing of the tract. Some caregivers are comfortable doing this at home, although this is most safely performed in the office or inpatient setting. Infants and children with poor gastric motility or small stomach size can experience gastric distension with high volume enteral feeds or bolus feeds; formula may take the path of least resistance and seep out around the gastrostomy site. This problem can be alleviated with low-volume continuous feeds, which is better tolerated by many patients. Additionally, leakage coming from the opening of the gastrostomy device, indicates malfunction of the one-way valve and warrants replacement of the device. Regardless of the cause of the leakage, the surrounding skin should be protected with a good barrier cream along with a gauze dressing that is changed frequently to keep the skin dry.

Accidental tube dislodgement can occur if there is little or no water in the balloon, or if the tube is forcefully jerked or accidentally caught on another object. Proper education on what to do if the tube comes out can be extremely helpful in preventing frantic caregivers facing this situation. Sending patients home with an emergency kit can lessen caregiver anxiety, and moreover, prevent partial or complete closure of the gastrostomy tract, which can occur within several hours. The emergency kit should include Foley catheters that are smaller in diameter than the gastrostomy device. If the tube becomes dislodged in the initial post-operative period, the tube should be gently reinserted as soon as possible and, because a mature tract may not have been established yet, surgical consultation should be obtained prior to resuming enteral feeds. After the tube is replaced, a radiologic tube study should be performed to verify correct positioning within the stomach. Replacement of a tube in a mature tracts does not require radiologic confirmation, as long as the tube is replaced into the gastrostomy site without

resistance, enteral feeds flow into the stomach by gravity, and gastric contents can be aspirated to confirm correct positioning. Tubes that have been dislodged for a long time often require serial dilation of the tract with smaller diameter tubes, until the previous gastrostomy tube can be reinserted easily.

Granulation tissue is at the insertion site is a common problem. Although the exact etiology is not entirely clear and likely multifactorial, it is likely to be a foreign body reaction to the tube itself. Granulation tissue is commonly seen with new gastrostomies, in patients with poor wound healing, and in patients who have excessive tension or moisture at their gastrostomy site. Chemical cautery with silver nitrate applicator sticks is the traditional treatment for granulation tissue; this can be performed once daily or every other day with the use of topical anesthetic prior to treatment if necessary. Triamcinolone steroid cream is a less traumatic alternative, although more tedious as the cream is applied 3 times a day until the granulation tissue resolves. Severe overgrowth of granulation tissue unresponsive to the above measures might need to be debrided in the operating room using electrocautery for more definitive therapy. Decreasing tension at the gastrostomy site by securing extension tubing with tape over the rib area, prevents trauma to peristomal region when the tubing is accidentally tugged or pulled. Moreover, keeping the site clean and dry, and ensuring proper tube fit, are important techniques to aid in prevention of granulation tissue.

Skin erosion is often due to excessive tension or leakage from the gastrostomy, as gastric secretions can excoriate the surrounding skin. Skin barrier creams with zinc oxide provide a good barrier to protect against constant moisture and acidic drainage. Over-the-counter zinc oxide cream works well; we prefer Critic-Aid barrier cream. Calmoseptine cream, a zinc oxide and menthol mixture that promotes skin healing, can be particularly helpful on chapped, excoriated skin. Antifungal creams and powders (Nystatin) are useful when patients develop an erythematous, yeast-like rash with multiple satellite lesions extending outward from the G-tube site. Many caregivers are inclined to apply antibiotic ointments to the gastrostomy site, however, gastrostomies rarely become infected. Tender erythema surrounding the gastrostomy site suggests the possibility of G-tube cellulitis, which is most commonly seen in the initial post-operative period, particularly when the nylon sutures are still in place. This can be effectively treated with short-term oral or IV antibiotics and suture removal as early as possible. An additional problem, although rare, is gastric mucosal prolapse at the gastrostomy site. Gastric mucosa is sometimes difficult to distinguish from granulation tissue, and often requires operative management. A reddened g-tube site is often a reminder that a child has an ill-fitting device or that proper site care needs to be reinforced with the caregiver.

Tube Removal

When an enteral feeding tube is no longer needed, it can usually be removed safely in the office and the site allowed to close spontaneously. Tubes that have been in place for more than about a year sometimes fail to close on their own, in which case they might need to be closed surgically. Techniques vary, but the gastrocutaneous fistula is usually excised and the wound closed in layers, essentially the same approach used for any enterostomy.

Tracts that are allowed to close prematurely need to be replaced. Though this might need to be done surgically, the tract can usually be cannulated or a wire can be passed under fluoroscopic guidance and the tract dilated sequentially until a tube can fit through the tract. If the hole is big enough, a very small Foley catheter can be placed in the office or the Emergency Department and then the tract can be dilated with a series of gradually larger catheters until a gastrostomy tube can be placed safely. Naturally, if there is *any* question as to the proper placement of the tip of the catheter, a tube contrast study must be performed prior to starting feeds.

The key to achieving exceptional gastrostomy care and function is comprehensive caregiver education, which begins in the preoperative phase. We use a 30-min teaching video to help caregivers gain a better understanding of what to expect during their child's hospital admission and postoperative management and to demonstrate core skills related to site care and the best way to trouble-shoot complications. This video has played an integral role in reducing the number of clinic and emergency room visits, as it empowers caregivers and gives them the knowledge to handle many of the low-acuity complications at home.

Summary Points

- Careful and thorough pre-operative and post-operative hands-on teaching will enable the caregiver to troubleshoot and solve many minor gastrostomy-related problems.
- A GER evaluation is typically done before a GT is placed.
- If a surgical jejunostomy tube is need for an extended period, a Roux-Y technique is recommended for ease of care and durability.
- Tube misplacement into the peritoneal cavity or balloon occlusion of the pylorus, duodenum or more distal bowel are rare but significant complications of enteral access tubes. A radiologic study with contrast should be done promptly if these are of concern.

Editor's Comment

The decision to allow a gastrostomy or jejunostomy tube to be placed is often very difficult for parents, especially given the huge emotional and psychological implications involved. For the surgeon it might be technically no more than a minor procedure, but caregivers should be approached with an appropriate level of empathy and patience as they grapple with what for them might be a life-changing event.

The laparoscopic approach has been refined and is probably the safest and most comfortable approach. I use absorbable U-stitches that are buried under the skin, which tracks the stomach securely to the fascia and obviates the need for external stitches around the flange of the button. In this day and age, there is no reason to use an old-fashioned Malecot or Pezzar catheter. They are made of latex, they need to be secured to the skin with complex contraptions involving adhesives and a large wafer, and they are not user friendly. There is no reason to avoid placement of a primary button and if, usually for some technical reason a button can't be placed, a silastic gastrostomy tube with a balloon and proper valves and connectors should be used instead. A cleanly placed gastrostomy requires, at most, a simple 2×2 split-gauze dressing; tape and bulky dressings are not necessary.

Contrary to conventional teaching, G-tube cellulitis does occur on occasion, but the signs and symptoms are easily dismissed as being due to skin irritation or local trauma and the diagnosis is nearly impossible to confirm objectively. A G-tube site that is erythematous, indurated, and tender should be assumed to be infected and treated empirically with oral or intravenous antibiotics. Some surgeons are uncomfortable with this admission of a possible complication without hard evidence but appropriate patient care obviously supersedes all other concerns. Leakage is also a common and frustrating problem that is rarely due to the tube itself. It can be due to poor positioning of the gastrostomy (too close to the pylorus) but is more often due to poor gastric emptying or distal obstruction. Placing a smaller tube will sometimes allow the hole to contract down but a larger tube almost always makes the hole bigger and the leakage worse. When the site becomes enlarged and leaks heavily, closure and resiting the tube is necessary.

Closure of a gastrocutaneous fistula should be a simple outpatient procedure without having to resort to a laparotomy or even laparoscopy. The fistula can be excised using a transverse elliptical incision, dissected down to just below the fascia, and ligated at its base (on the stomach). The fascia is then closed over it and the wound closed in layers.

It is important not to place the gastrostomy too close to the costal margin and to recall that the costal margin advances inferiorly as we grow. Tubes that are right up against the lowest rib cause pain and often need to be re-sited. Usually at or inferior to a point midway between the umbilicus and the costal margin and just lateral to the rectus sheath works well.

Surgical jejunostomies are fraught with complications and should be avoided unless all other options have been exhausted. The Roux-Y is more practical than the Wetzel, but there is a significant risk of volvulus around the Roux limb, which has been lethal for patients who are impaired and unable to alert others about abdominal pain.

Preoperative Preparation

□ Prophylactic antibiotics
□ Informed consent
□ Upper GI contrast study

Parental Preparation

– Like any mechanical device, gastrostomy tubes can be associated with technical problems, most of which are easily dealt with.
– There are several techniques available for placement of an enteral feeding device and we will explain the advantages and disadvantages of each one and tell you why we prefer one over the others.
– We recognize that dealing with a feeding tube can be intimidating at first, but we will help you to be more comfortable over the next several weeks or months if necessary.

Diagnostic Studies

– Upper GI contrast study
– If GER is clinically moderate or severe, consider pH probe study or nuclear medicine scan
– In case of tube dislodgement or dysfunction, consider a tube contrast study to confirm intragastric position.

Technical Points

• Place the gastrostomy tube too close to the pylorus can cause obstruction.
• Placement too close to the fundus can limit a subsequent fundoplication.
• The ideal location is usually near the level of the incisura and near the greater curvature of the stomach.
• For an open operation, a small midline incision or left upper quadrant transverse incision can be used with good effect.

Suggested Reading

Borkowski S. G tube care: managing hypergranulation tissue. Nursing. 2005;35(8):24.

Browne NJ, Flanigan LM, McComiskey CA, Peiper P. Care and management of patients with tubes and drains. In: Farber LD, editor. Nursing care of the pediatric surgical patient (2nd ed). Sudbury, MA: Jones and Bartlett Publishers; 2007. p. 90–3.

Crosby J, Duerksen DR. A prospective study of tube- and feeding-related complications in patients receiving long-term home enteral nutrition. J Parent Ent Nutr. 2007;31(4):274–7.

Jones VS, La Hei ER, La Shun A. Laparoscopic gastrostomy: The preferred method of gastrostomy in children. Pediatr Surg Int. 2007; 23:1085.

Raval MV, Phillips JD. Optimal enteral feeding in children with gastric dysfunction: Surgical jejunostomy vs image-guided gastrojejunal tube placement. J Pediatr Surg. 2006;41(10):1679–82.

Chapter 45
Duodenal Atresia

Keith A. Kuenzler and Steven S. Rothenberg

Duodenal atresia is a congenital bowel obstruction, usually located between the first and second portions of the duodenum. The overall incidence is approximately 1 in 6,000 births. Approximately one-third of patients with neonatal duodenal obstruction also have trisomy 21. Other frequently associated anomalies include congenital heart disease, annular pancreas, and malrotation. The widely accepted theory regarding the embryogenesis of duodenal atresia is a failure of recanalization of the solid portion of the gastrointestinal lumen rather than a mesenteric vascular accident or interruption, which is the prevailing theory as to the pathogenesis of other intestinal atresias. The number of infants born with duodenal obstruction appears to be declining, but survival is increasing. These trends might be due to the increasing frequency of early prenatal diagnosis and elective termination of pregnancies when major cardiac or chromosomal anomalies are identified.

Diagnosis

Most cases of duodenal atresia are discovered antenatally. The classic double-bubble appearance can be recognized on fetal ultrasound (Fig. 45.1). A proximal intestinal obstruction may also be suggested by polyhydramnios. When the diagnosis is made antenatally, a meeting should be scheduled with the expectant parents to discuss the initial management and operative course. This discussion allows parents the opportunity to deliver their baby in an institution with experienced neonatal and pediatric surgical staff. Shortly after birth, a confirmatory abdominal radiograph should be obtained (Fig. 45.2), followed by prompt nasogastric decompression.

When an antenatal diagnosis has not been made, feeding intolerance and bilious emesis in the immediate newborn period should raise the suspicion for duodenal atresia, stenosis,

or web. The proximal location of the obstruction makes it uncommon for infants to have significant abdominal distention; in fact, the classic finding is that of a scaphoid abdomen. A plain radiograph will usually demonstrate a double-bubble sign with no distal bowel gas, confirming a complete duodenal obstruction. Air provides excellent contrast, and so additional studies using barium or water-soluble contrast are usually unnecessary. When there is distal bowel gas, the diagnosis is less certain and might need to be confirmed with a contrast study. On the other hand, the presence of distal bowel gas does not rule out the diagnosis as there are two plausible explanations for the passage of distal bowel gas in the setting of a true duodenal atresia: high-grade but incomplete obstruction due to a duodenal web with a tiny central aperture, or passage of air through the ampulla of Vater, which often bifurcates to open on both sides of a duodenal web. Of course, the surgeon must always ensure that the bilious vomiting is not a sign of malrotation with midgut volvulus. One should be confident of the diagnosis of duodenal atresia in newborns who are not in distress and who present with vomiting shortly after birth. In babies with delayed presentation of bilious vomiting, especially in the setting of acidosis or systemic illness, an emergent upper GI contrast study must be done to definitively rule out malrotation, or one must perform an immediate laparotomy to rule out midgut volvulus.

Preoperative Preparation

Once the diagnosis of congenital duodenal obstruction has been confirmed, semi-elective operation is planned in the first few days of life. Placement of a nasogastric tube decompresses the stomach and rules out concomitant esophageal atresia, seen in a small subset of patients. Stable intravenous access must be secured for ongoing fluid replacement. Close monitoring of urine output ensures that the infant is well hydrated, and serum electrolytes should be corrected. We also favor the early placement of a peripherally inserted central catheter (PICC), which can be used preoperatively for maintenance of normoglycemia and will

K.A. Kuenzler (✉)
Minimally Invasive Pediatric Surgery, NYU Langone Medical Center, New York, NY 10016, USA
e-mail: Keith.Kuenzler@nyumc.org

P. Mattei (ed.), *Fundamentals of Pediatric Surgery*,
DOI 10.1007/978-1-4419-6643-8_45, © Springer Science+Business Media, LLC 2011

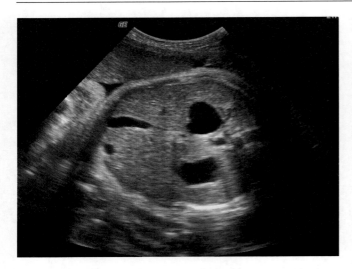

Fig. 45.1 Prenatal ultrasound in a mother with polyhydramnios demonstrating a double bubble: fluid-filled stomach and dilated first portion of duodenum

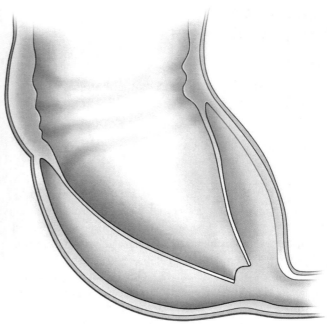

Fig. 45.3 Diagram of duodenal web illustrating that the proximal duodenum may be dilated beyond the origin of a windsock-type web

Operative Management

The traditional repair of duodenal atresia begins with a right upper quadrant transverse laparotomy. The abdomen is entered approximately halfway between the liver edge and the level of the umbilicus. One expects to find decompressed jejunum, ileum, and colon. The first investigation should be whether the bowel is normally rotated. If normal rotation is observed, the hepatic flexure is mobilized medially and a generous Kocher maneuver performed. If malrotation is encountered, Ladd's bands should be divided, the mesentery widened, the colon repositioned to the left side of the peritoneum, and the appendix removed or inverted. Finally, the duodenum is examined for an atresia or other form of obstruction unrelated to Ladd's bands.

Regarding the duodenal examination, if there is continuity of the serosa between the dilated and decompressed segments, a duodenal web (also known as Type 1 atresia) should be suspected. We recommend passing a nasogastric tube into the proximal duodenum so that the proximal extent of the web may be demonstrated. Because the duodenum is sometimes dilated right to the end of the web, yet the web may originate considerably more proximally (Fig. 45.3), one must take care not to mistakenly perform the duodenoduodenostomy entirely distal to the actual cause of the obstruction. This error is also avoided by observing the nasogastric tube in the dilated duodenum proximal to the obstruction.

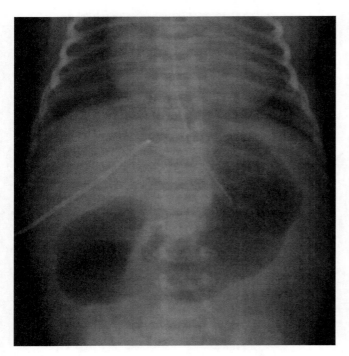

Fig. 45.2 Abdominal radiograph shortly after birth demonstrating a double bubble

almost certainly be needed for parenteral nutrition during the postoperative period. In addition, consultation with a pediatric cardiologist should be requested and an echocardiogram reviewed promptly. Congenital heart disease must be identified and corrected when appropriate. The repair of duodenal atresia should be performed in a hemodynamically stable, euvolemic newborn.

Once the anatomy is understood, the web can either be excised or bypassed. Excision is best accomplished via a longitudinal duodenotomy. Careful observation of bile flow allows the surgeon to avoid injury to the ampulla of Vater during web excision. The duodenotomy is then closed transversely to prevent subsequent stenosis. Our preference is to perform a duodenoduodenostomy so as to avoid injury to the ampulla.

In the case of a type 2 atresia (solid cord between segments), a type 3 atresia (total discontinuity between segments), or annular pancreas, bypass of the obstruction is required. In the majority of patients, this is accomplished by duodenoduodenostomy with the double-diamond method, originally described by Kimura (Fig. 45.4). When the duodenal segments are too far apart for a reasonable anastomosis, a retrocolic, side-to-side duodenojejunostomy can be done. If annular pancreas is encountered, no attempt should be made to divide pancreatic parenchyma or visualize the underlying duodenum, as this may result in a ductal injury.

In the standard repair, after opening the distal duodenum, our preference is to pass a small rubber catheter intraluminally. By gently injecting saline, the distal bowel can be distended to rule out the rare additional atresia. A soft feeding catheter (or Broviac catheter) is tied to the nasogastric sump tube for passage to the level of the anastomosis by the anesthesiologist. After the posterior wall of the anastomosis is completed, the soft tube is advanced beyond the anastomosis into the jejunum. This allows for early postoperative enteric feeds to be delivered beyond the anastomosis in the case of delayed emptying. The tip of the sump tube is left in the stomach for postoperative decompression. We place a surgical gastrostomy only in infants who are expected to be poor oral feeders, such as those with trisomy 21 or congenital heart disease.

Laparoscopic Repair

Standard neonatal 3-mm laparoscopic instruments are used. The patient is placed supine at the end of the operating table, with the surgeon standing at the feet. The abdomen is insufflated through an umbilical ring incision and a 4-mm port is inserted. Two other ports, one 3-mm and one 5-mm, are placed in the right lower quadrant and left mid-abdomen respectively (Fig. 45.5). The 5-mm port will accommodate the introduction of needles and suture. Alternatively, a 3-mm port may be used for instruments, and sutures can be passed into the peritoneum through the abdominal wall. Because of the decompressed distal bowel, there is usually abundant intra-abdominal space and excellent visualization (Fig. 45.6). If necessary for liver retraction, a fourth port can be added in the right upper quadrant.

The duodenum is then Kocherized and the site of the obstruction visualized. When a web is suspected, a longitudinal duodenotomy is made across the area of apparent transition. The web is resected and a transverse closure performed with

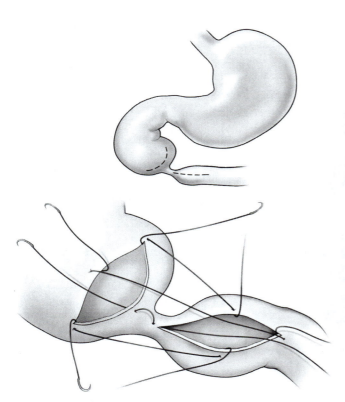

Fig. 45.4 Opening the proximal duodenum transversely and the distal duodenum longitudinally allows one to create a double-diamond anastomosis

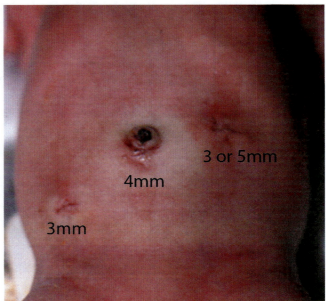

Fig. 45.5 Infant after laparoscopic repair; port size and location is demonstrated

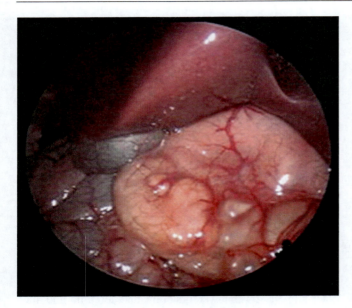

Fig. 45.6 Clear, magnified view during laparoscopic repair

running suture. In clear cases of atresia, proximal (transverse) and distal (longitudinal) duodenotomies are created, and the standard double-diamond anastomosis is performed using 4-0 sutures. Traction sutures are placed at each corner to orient the anastomosis. The apical traction stitch can be exteriorized and placed on slight tension to stabilize the bowel. The posterior and anterior walls are sewn individually in running fashion. The distal bowel can then be examined using atraumatic laparoscopic bowel graspers for distal atresias. A trans-anastomotic feeding tube is generally not employed during the laparoscopic repair. However, results from our early experience appear to indicate that feeding by mouth is usually possible within 4–7 days.

Postoperative Care

Initially, all infants are maintained on bowel rest and parenteral nutrition. Nasogastric aspirates are monitored and fluid losses replaced. If a trans-anastomotic feeding tube is in place, continuous jejunal feeds are initiated on the first or second postoperative day. Once nasogastric drainage is no longer bilious and bowel function returns, the tubes are removed and oral feeds are gradually increased. This typically occurs over the course of 1–3 weeks.

Short-term complications are uncommon in infants with duodenal atresia and include anastomotic leak, wound infection, and delayed gastric emptying. Long-term complications include adhesive bowel obstruction and anastomotic stenosis causing proximal duodenal dilatation. The latter may result in chronic feeding difficulties and stasis. In these older children, tapering duodenoplasty for luminal narrowing or balloon dilatation of an anastomotic stricture may aid in alleviating symptoms.

Duodenal atresia is a cause of newborn bowel obstruction usually identified antenatally and easily confirmed by plain abdominal radiograph. Trisomy 21 and congenital heart disease should be ruled out. Following gastric decompression and fluid resuscitation, corrective surgery should be done in a hemodynamically stable baby. Successful outcomes can be achieved by creating a bypass of the obstruction by duodenoduodenostomy, accomplished via traditional laparotomy or with minimally invasive techniques. A minority of patients suffer from progressive duodenal dilatation and emptying difficulties, which may respond to medical therapy or nutritional changes, but can persist in the long term. Nevertheless, the overwhelming majority of children recover promptly and enjoy normal lives.

Summary Points

- In the newborn with proximal bowel obstruction, one must consider: malrotation with midgut volvulus, duodenal atresia, duodenal stenosis, duodenal web.
- Patients with duodenal atresia may have congenital heart disease and/or trisomy 21.
- When the diagnosis has been suggested antenatally or clinical suspicion is high, plain radiographs will usually confirm duodenal atresia by demonstrating a double-bubble sign.
- Cardiac anomalies should be ruled out, and repair of duodenal atresia should be performed in stable infants after preoperative preparation with IV fluids.
- Long-term outcomes are excellent.

Editor's Comment

The repair of the straightforward duodenal atresia is relatively simple and in many centers is routinely being performed laparoscopically. However, not every case is clear-cut, and there are many potential pitfalls: what to do with a duodenal web (resection or duodenoduodenostomy); recognizing and managing the windsock deformity; ruling out a distal atresia; performing a proper Ladd procedure when malrotation is found; whether to taper a dilated duodenum;

and when and how to do a proper duodenojejunostomy. Annular pancreas is not included here, because the treatment is the same as for a simple duodenal atresia. The pediatric surgeon needs to be prepared for every variation and even unique anatomic variants that have yet to be clearly defined.

There is some disagreement over the proper management of the duodenal web, namely the question as to whether one should resect the web or simply bypass it. This is because of the risk of injury to the ampulla, which always enters the medial portion (mesenteric side) of the web. Though either approach is acceptable, I prefer to excise the web, being careful to preserve the medial aspect, but only after identifying the ampulla. The ampulla is identified by compressing the gallbladder and looking for the flow of bile.

The windsock deformity is a web that is stretched out distally for a variable distance. The circumferential origin of the web is still way back at the level of the ampulla while the central portion can be several centimeters downstream, where the obstruction appears to be. These can be extremely difficult to recognize and are easily missed. It is important to remember that duodenal obstruction almost always arises at the level of the ampulla (at the junction of the first and second portion of the duodenum) so that an obstruction that appears to be involving the third portion of the duodenum should be investigated further to rule out a windsock. Treatment involves excision or bypass once the anatomy has been properly sorted out.

It is important to rule out the presence of a second more distal obstruction, typically by passing a red rubber catheter distally and injecting saline to ensure flow through the lumen. This currently poses a problem for laparoscopists, but I suspect that this will be resolved creatively in the near future.

A significant number of infants with duodenal atresia also have malrotation and this needs to be addressed at the time of the duodenoduodenostomy by performing a proper Ladd procedure. The anatomy can be confusing and the unused small bowel is often very delicate and of small caliber, demanding patience and gentle technique.

Even when the bowel is normally rotated, the duodenum can be quite dilated, which creates the potential for dysmotility and stasis. It is usually best to taper the duodenum, as there is very little risk involved and it appears to be effective. The technique is well-described elsewhere, but it is a good idea to use a 20 Fr red rubber catheter within the lumen as a guide, a series of Babcock clamps on the antimesenteric border, and a gastrointestinal stapling device fired sequentially around the circumference of the dilated duodenum.

If a duodenoduodenostomy cannot be performed with minimal tension and in such a way that the proper flow of intestinal contents can be ensured (long-gap between duodenal ends, bulky annular pancreas), there should be a low thresh-

old to perform a duodenojejunostomy, which is generally straightforward and well-tolerated. Given the small caliber of the jejunum, it is important to make the anastomoses long and with precise technique to ensure patency.

Finally, the postoperative care of these infants can be long and difficult, mostly due to duodenal stasis and prolonged ileus. All infants should be given parenteral nutrition through a PICC line and most with trisomy 21 or significant associated anomalies benefit from having a gastrostomy tube placed at the initial operation. The usual indication of normal bowel function, namely a transition to nonbilious gastric aspirates, might never occur in these infants even when their ileus has resolved, presumably due to the fact that their pylorus is incompetent and they tend to reflux bile into their stomachs for a very long time. If the patient is extubated and stable on the sixth or seventh day, I will empirically clamp the nasogastric tube and start a slowly advancing trial of water or glucose-electrolyte solution. Most infants are ready to feed at this point but some will need another 3 or 4 days before starting another trial. Infants who cannot feed beyond 2–3 weeks should have a contrast study to rule out a stricture or other form of obstruction.

Parental Preparation

- It is probably best to deliver the baby at a center with experienced neonatologists, cardiologists, anesthesiologists and surgeons available.
- Surgery is required in the first few days of life.
- There is the possibility of a delay in oral feeding for 1–3 weeks.
- We might recommend placement of a gastrostomy if congenital heart disase or trisomy 21.
- There is a low probability of long-term problems with duodenal dilatation and emptying.

Differential Diagnosis

- Malrotation with midgut volvulus
- Pyloric stenosis or atresia
- Meconium aspiration syndrome

Preoperative Preparation

- ☐ Echocardiogram
- ☐ PICC line
- ☐ IV Hydration
- ☐ Type and screen
- ☐ Informed consent

Technical Points

- Right upper quadrant incision or laparoscopic approach
- Double-diamond duodenoduodenostomy or retro-colic duodenojejunostomy
- Rule out distal intestinal atresia
- Consider transanastomotic tube for early postoperative jejunal feedings

Suggested Reading

Kimura K. Diamond-shaped anastomosis forduodenal atresia: an experience with 44 patients over 15 years. J Pediatr Surg. 1990;25:977–8.

Ladd WE. Congenital obstruction of the duodenum in children. N Engl J Med. 1931;206:277–83.

Rothenberg SS. Laparoscopic duodenoduodenostomy for duodenal obstruction in infants and children. J Pediatr Surg. 2002;37(7): 1088–9.

Valusek PA, Spilde TL, Tsao K, et al. Laparoscopic duodenal atresia repair using surgical u-clips: a novel technique. Surg Endosc. 2007;21:1023–4.

Chapter 46
Intestinal Atresias

Peter F. Nichol and Ari Reichstein

Intestinal atresia is a congenital obstruction of the intestine, sometimes associated with a loss of tissue, resulting in a disruption of intestinal continuity. An atresia can occur anywhere throughout the gut, including the esophagus, pylorus, pancreatic duct, bile duct and rectum. The incidence of intestinal atresia is approximately 1 in 4000 live births. The two principal hypotheses regarding the etiology of intestinal atresia are: failure of recanalization of the initial solid-core phase of intestinal development, and *in utero* vascular accident. Neither of these theories has been proven and this is an area of active interest and ongoing scientific scrutiny.

Atresias present with varying degrees of severity, ranging from a mucosal web with a small hole in it to a complete loss of intestinal continuity and mesentery. Less frequently there can be multiple atresias throughout the bowel. Intestinal atresias can occur anywhere along the intestinal tract including the duodenum, jejunoileal region and colon. Duodenal atresias are frequently seen in association with Down syndrome and can also be seen in combination with imperforate anus and heterotaxy. Jejunoileal atresias can occur anywhere from the ligament of Treitz to the ileocecal valve, and are seen in association with a number of conditions, including cystic fibrosis and malrotation. Colonic atresias are somewhat unusual in that they occur with great consistency in the same anatomical region of the colon (transverse colon) and with the same degree of severity (loss of intestinal lumen and mesentery) in most instances.

Diagnosis

The presentation of an intestinal atresia is largely determined by the anatomic location of the defect. Newborns with atresia of the duodenum present with vomiting and inability to tolerate feeds within the first 24 hours of life. A plain abdominal film will often demonstrate the classic double-bubble sign. If a plain radiograph is indeterminate, the diagnosis can often be clarified with an upper GI contrast study. The presentation is sometimes more nuanced, particularly when the patient has a mucosal web with a small opening that permits the passage of intestinal contents. These patients present days or even years later with failure to tolerate feeds or gain weight. In these cases, an upper GI series may be required for diagnosis. The UGI will demonstrate two large collections of contrast in the stomach and duodenum with or without a small string-like defect distally. It is essential to note that although 100% of patients with duodenal web will demonstrate these findings, neonates with volvulus can present with identical findings on UGI. For this reason, the surgeon should always evaluate radiographic studies with a provisional diagnosis of duodenal atresia with this in mind.

Infants with atresias of the jejunum, ileum or colon present with signs of obstruction, including abdominal distension, bilious emesis, and often a failure to pass meconium. Other congenital anomalies that must be considered as part of the differential diagnosis include imperforate anus, congenital small left colon syndrome, meconium plug syndrome, meconium ileus, and Hirschsprung disease. After completing a through physical examination, the surgeon should review plain radiographs of the abdomen: the presence of extremely dilated loops of bowel with a paucity of distal bowel gas are considered by some to be pathognomonic of intestinal atresia. Nevertheless, in most cases, a contrast enema is usually the best study to obtain next. The presence of a small, unused colon (microcolon) and failure of the contrast to reflux into dilated proximal bowel indicate an anatomic obstruction and the need for an operation. It is worth noting that, in the case of a distal atresia, nasogastric suction often fails to adequately decompress the distended bowel. Since the proximal intestine will continue to distend and dilate, it is important to proceed with haste to the operation. Delaying surgical correction can lead to ischemia of the distal most portion of the proximal limb, perforation, and spillage of meconium, making the intraoperative and postoperative management more challenging.

P.F. Nichol (✉)
Department of Surgery, University of Wisconsin School of Medicine and Public Health, 608 Highland Avenue, CSC H4/785c, Madison, WI 53792, USA
e-mail: nichol@surgery.wisc.edu

P. Mattei (ed.), *Fundamentals of Pediatric Surgery*,
DOI 10.1007/978-1-4419-6643-8_46, © Springer Science+Business Media, LLC 2011

Treatment

All patients with atresia should be adequately hydrated and have a nasogastric tube placed pre-operatively. Prophylactic antibiotics should be administered. Typically, neonates less than 24 hours old have not had time to colonize their intestinal tract, and therefore a second generation cephalosporin is usually sufficient. If the patient is presenting after a period of oral feeding, then anaerobic coverage should be added. Given the well-recognized association of duodenal atresia with Down syndrome and congenital cardiac anomalies, pre-operative cardiology consultation and echocardiogram are strongly recommended.

The surgical strategy for all intestinal atresias is to re-establish intestinal continuity. If this is not technically possible, one should temporize with an ostomy and mucus fistula so that the patient can receive enteral nutrition. Refeeding the distal limb through the mucus fistula has the added advantage of facilitating its growth, reducing the proximal-distal size mismatch at the time of definitive repair.

Duodenal Atresia

Duodenal atresias are optimally treated by re-establishing intestinal continuity by primary repair. Despite numerous reports of laparoscopic repairs of duodenal atresia, we do not favor the minimally invasive approach for several reasons. First, a significant number of these patients will have malrotation or additional more distal atresias and the failure to recognize and correct intestinal malrotation or a second atresia is a potential pitfall with the laparoscopic approach. Furthermore, the laparoscopic repair of duodenal atresia is technically challenging because the distal limb can be completely retroperitoneal making dissection and subsequent anastomosis very difficult. Given these limitations, many minimally invasive surgeons favor using surgical clips instead of sutures for the anastomosis. Naturally, we would recommend that one should use whichever approach one is most comfortable with.

Several approaches have been described for the repair of duodenal atresia, including tapering the proximal limb and the long-favored practice of fashioning a diamond anastomosis. Tapering the proximal limb is unnecessary unless the patient has demonstrated a long term problem with overgrowth and motility. In this case, imbrication of the antimesenteric side can be performed without resection of the intestine.

The abdomen is entered through a supra-umbilical transverse incision made on the right side. The umbilical vein is taken between ties. The proximal and distal limbs may need to be Kocherized depending on the location of the atresia. A transverse incision is made on the proximal limb and a longitudinal incision on the distal limb. The initial sutures are placed so that the cornering sutures in one incision come through the mid-point of the opposite incision. The back wall is completed in interrupted fashion with the knots on the inside. Often, the wall of the proximal limb is thick, whereas the wall of the distal limb is thin and hypomorphic. The placement of suture on the distal limb therefore must be done with great precision so that the needle fully follows its curve and the end of the needle is not pulled through the tissue obliquely. Failure to do so will create larger needle holes than is necessary in the delicate tissue, which can potentially lead to a leak or stricture. A naso-jejunal feeding tube is passed by anesthesia and positioned distal to the anastomosis and beyond the duodeno-jejunal junction and gently injected with saline to rule out more distal mucosal defects. A small, soft flexible tube that will not exert pressure on the anastomosis is preferred. The front wall of the anastomosis is then competed in interrupted fashion with the knots on the outside. The integrity of the anastomosis is tested by occluding proximally and distally to the repair and injecting the proximal limb with normal saline using a 27 gauge needle.

A contrast study is obtained on the fifth postoperative day to confirm patency of the anastomosis. Most patients will establish gastro-duodenal motility adequate for oral feeds within several days of the operation. However, patients with Down syndrome or heterotaxy in some cases take weeks for the ileus to resolve. Frequently this subgroup of patients will have normal distal intestinal motility and poor gastric emptying. In this setting we will advance them to full naso-jejunal feeds and then gradually transition to gastric or nasogastric feeds. Before assuming dysmotility as the primary cause of impaired gastric emptying, however, it is advisable to rule out an anastomotic stricture in these patients. We recommend obtaining an UGI if the patient has persistently prolonged gastric emptying more than two weeks after the repair.

Jejunoileal Atresias

In contrast to duodenal atresias, jejunoileal atresias can frequently be repaired in a laparoscopic-assisted manner in a way that benefits the patient (smaller incisions, less pain, quicker recovery) without compromising the repair. However, many surgeons still favor a transverse supraumbilical incision. In the laparoscopically assisted approach, the peritoneal cavity is entered through the center of the umbilicus using blunt dissection with fine forceps. A Veress needle is passed into the peritoneum and the position is confirmed by water drop test. A pneumoperitoneum is established to 8-10 mmHg pressure. A 3-mm port is deployed through this site and secured with 3-0 vicryl suture at the skin. Two-mm incisions are made on the right and left on a line one finger breadth above the umbilicus and lateral to the rectus on either side. These tracts are bluntly stretched with a Jacobsen forceps. Small graspers are passed through these incisions. The patient is placed in a gentle reverse Trendelenberg position to facilitate identification of the ligament of Treitz. The bowel is run proximally to distally until the atresia is encountered. The proximal and distal ends are grasped and the pneumoperitoneum is released. The umbilical incision is extended superiorly in the vertical midline so that it is 1-1.2 cm in length. The limbs of bowel are delivered to the incision by the graspers and brought through the wound into the field. Thereafter, the principles of the operation are the same as for the open approach. The proximal limb is decompressed and evacuated of all meconium to facilitate handling. Approximately 5 to 8 cm of proximal limb is resected and the remainder is tapered over a red rubber catheter that more closely matches the luminal diameter of the distal limb of bowel. We perform the tapering with a gastrointestinal stapling device using a vascular cartidge. We prefer this stapler because of its hemostatic properties, which are achieved without crushing the tissue, and because the cutting mechanism can easily come through a staple line if necessary. A single-layer, end-to-end anastomosis is performed with 5-0 absorbable monofilament sutures in interrupted fashion. After testing the anastomosis, the mesenteric defect is closed. The intestine is then returned to the peritoneal cavity and the incision is closed.

Notably, there are several scenarios where the open approach though a supraumbilical transverse incision is preferred. If the patient has intestinal perforation, the degree of bowel dilation and peritoneal inflammation make the laparoscopic approach prohibitively difficult. Type 3b atresias (apple-peel lesions) are best addressed with an open approach because the distal limb is coiled and needs to be carefully uncoiled prior to repair. It becomes very difficult to maintain proper orientation of the vasculature when trying to uncoil the distal limb with the laparoscopic-assisted approach. Furthermore, the mesenteric defect in these patients is quite large and cannot be satisfactorily repaired by a laparoscopic approach or through a keyhole incision. Type 4 atresias may be amenable to a laparoscopic-assisted approach provided all of the atresias can be identified and brought out through the incision for repair. Finally, the open approach is excellent in patients with very proximal jejunal defects, since the proximal limb can be very difficult to deliver through the incision.

In most scenarios, a limited resection of the proximal limb with more proximal tapering is preferred. Histological studies indicate that the enteric nervous system of the dilated bowel is abnormal. Although neuronal dysplasia is most severe at the site of the defect, the optimal amount of proximal bowel that should be resected is unknown.

Patients with meconium peritonitis present a technical dilemma. While an ostomy with mucus fistula is preferred, the mesentery in these patients may be foreshortened, limiting the ability to mobilize and mature the ostomy. The alternative is to perform a primary anastomosis in an extremely inflamed peritoneum. If the defect is fairly distal in a critically ill child, it is safest to bring up an ostomy. For proximal defects, a mucus fistula permits refeeding of the distal limb effluent. This serves to minimize fluid and electrolyte derangements as well as promote intestinal growth, allowing for a reasonable size match at the time of definitive repair.

Colonic Atresia

Colonic atresias often present as type IIIb lesions with a long mesenteric gap. There usually is a significant size mismatch of the proximal and distal ends as well. The patients have a full complement of small bowel which is usually not dilated. The right colon functions to absorb water and sodium but in most patients is not essential for survival. Therefore the easiest way to deal with this defect is to resect the proximal colon and perform an ileo-colic anastomosis. This usually does not require tapering as the small bowel is not dilated and is a good size match for the distal colon. Because of the diminutive nature of the unused distal colon, these patients can have significant problems re-establishing intestinal motility.

Postoperative Care

Patients should be monitored closely in a neonatal intensive care unit in the immediate postoperative period. A nasogastric tube should be left in place for gastric decompression. The cessation of large-volume, bilious, nasogastric output indicates the return of intestinal motility and function at which point the NG tube is discontinued and oral feeds are initiated. Parenteral nutrition via central or peripheral route should be considered for infants and children expected to have a delayed return of bowel function.

Summary Points

- Intestinal atresias can occur anywhere along the intestinal tract including the duodenum, jejunum, ileum, and/or colon.
- Duodenal atresia is commonly associated with other congenital anomalies, including Down syndrome, heterotaxy, annular pancreas, and malrotation.
- The presentation and management of intestinal atresia is dictated by the anatomic location of the lesion.
- Intestinal malrotation is commonly found in patients with intestinal atresia and should be sought out in patients with atresia.
- The goal of surgery for intestinal atresia is the restoration of intestinal continuity.
- Postoperative anastomotic stricture can be ruled out with a contrast study of the intestine.

Editor's Comment

The stable newborn with bilious emesis, abdominal distension, and dilated loops of bowel on plain abdominal x-ray nearly always has one of four diagnoses: meconium plug syndrome, meconium ileus, Hirschsprung disease, or intestinal atresia. This is one of the few exceptions to the "every child with bilious emesis needs either an urgent upper GI or an emergent laparotomy" rule. Proximal obstruction due to duodenal or pyloric atresia does not present with abdominal distension or dilated loops and although malrotation with volvulus can present with a comparable clinical picture, it quite rarely does so and an experienced examiner can recognize the differences. Rather than an upper GI, a contrast enema is the diagnostic study of choice in these situations: it is therapeutic for meconium plug syndrome and some cases of meconium ileus, it allows identification of a transition zone in many patients with Hirschsprung disease, and it confirms the diagnosis of intestinal atresia. With the confidence that comes with experience, one might eventually be able to recommend surgery for intestinal atresia based simply on the plain radiographic findings but there is no shame in requesting a contrast enema to be more certain of the correct diagnosis.

The treatment should be primary anastomosis in most cases, even in the rare case of colonic atresia in which the size discrepancy between the proximal and distal ends can be quite dramatic. Whether to resect or taper the bowel is a decision best determined after assessing the length of viable intestine and how much bowel would be lost if the dilated portion were resected. In most cases, a limited resection of the most severely dilated bowel followed by tapering of the bowel just behind this segment is the best approach. Imbrication is more difficult to perform and tends to undo itself over time, thus defeating the purpose of the tapering. Even after tapering, some infants will develop a pseudo-obstruction and require resection of a dysmotile segment.

The apple-peel lesion (type 3b jejunal atresia) can be tricky to manage. One finds a proximal atresia, a large mesenteric defect with loss of the primary trunk of the SMA, and the entire ileum and distal jejunum remaining viable on the basis of the marginal artery and a tiny remnant of the distal SMA. Some of these patients do quite well after simple primary repair, but many have long-term motility or absorption problems and need parenteral nutrition for a long time after repair. It is important to untwist the bowel carefully, close the mesenteric defect without compromising the remaining blood supply, and inject saline through the distal bowel to rule out a second stricture or web.

Diagnostic Studies

- Plain radiograph
- Upper GI
- Water-soluble contrast enema

Differential Diagnosis

- Intestinal malrotation with midgut volvulus
- Intestinal duplication cyst
- Internal hernia
- Congenital small left colon syndrome
- Meconium plug syndrome
- Meconium ileus
- Hirschsprung disease
- Imperforate anus

Parental Preparation

- Possible bowel resection
- Potential ostomy and mucus fistula placement
- Possible long term gastrointestinal dysmotility
- Possible associated congenital anomalies requiring initial echocardiogram and possible multidisciplinary follow-up

Preoperative Preparation

☐ IV resuscitation
☐ Type and Screen
☐ Echocardiogram and Cardiology consultation
☐ IV antibiotics
☐ Informed Consent

Technical Points

- Rule out intestinal malrotation
- Delicately handle tissue
- If the patient with duodenal atresia is a candidate for primary repair, create a diamond anastomosis with monofilament suture
- If primary repair is contraindicated, create an end-ostomy, with mucus fistula to facilitate refeeding of the distal limb
- Test anastomosis with contrast injection intra-operatively
- Leave orogastric and trans-asnastomotic naso-jenunal feeding tubes
- Inject saline through proximal and distal feeding tubes to check for additional atretic segments

Suggested Reading

Schoenberg RA, Kluth D. Experimental small bowel obstruction in chick embryos: Effects on the developing enteric nervous system. *J Pediatr Surg* (2002) 37: 735-740.

Sweeney B, Surana R, Puri P. Jejunoileal atresia and associated malformations: Correlation with the timing of in utero insult. *J Pediatr Surg* (2001) 36:774-776.

Dalla Vecchia LK, et al. Intestinal atresia and stenosis: A 25 year experience with 277 cases. *Arch Surg* (1998) 133: 490-497.

Escobar M, et al. Duodenal atresia and stenosis: Long-term follow-up over 30 years. *J Pediatr Surg* (2004) 39: 867-871.

Chapter 47
Abdominal Cysts and Duplications

Patricia A. Lange

Many intra-abdominal cystic masses are being detected by prenatal imaging. They are often asymptomatic but those that cause symptoms usually do so in the first year or two of life. Symptoms are usually the result of compression or obstruction due to enlargement of the cyst as it gradually fills with fluid, or bleeding and ulceration due to gastric or pancreatic lining of the cyst. Cysts can arise from solid or hollow organs and various imaging modalities can help to distinguish the specific site of origin. Enteric duplication cysts are sometimes associated with intestinal atresias whereas tubular colonic or rectal duplications are commonly associated with genitourinary malformations. Optimal treatment usually involves complete resection of the cyst; but in some situations asymptomatic cysts detected prenatally can be observed clinically and radiographically.

Enteric duplications are rare and represent only about one in 4,500 autopsies. About two thirds of alimentary tract duplications are in the abdominal cavity, and more than half are in the jejuno-ileal segments. Three quarters of duplications are cystic with no communication to the adjacent alimentary tract while the remaining are tubular, sometimes communicating with the intestinal lumen. By definition, duplications share a blood supply with the intestine and lie in close proximity to the alimentary tract. Typical histopathologic features include distinct muscle wall layers and an epithelial lining, which is often gastric or pancreatic epithelium. Several theories exist that attempt to explain the formation of enteric duplications and intra-abdominal cysts but the exact etiology is poorly understood. Embryologic signaling errors might lead to abnormal diverticularization of the intestinal endoderm. Other theories suggest failure of regression of the diverticular process resulting in cyst formation. No single theory works to explain all of the variety of cysts and duplications found in the thorax or abdomen.

The differential diagnosis for intra-abdominal cystic masses is broad and includes duplication cysts, ovarian cysts, lymphangiomas, liver cysts, pancreatic cysts, omental cysts, extralobar pulmonary sequestration, genitourinary abnormalities, tumors, traumatic cysts, and pseudocysts.

Adnexal Cysts

Neonatal ovarian cysts are being detected with increasing frequency given the widespread use of perinatal ultrasonography. In general, simple ovarian cysts less than 4 cm in diameter can be observed and followed with serial US, as most of these will resolve spontaneously. Those that have complex features on US or are larger than 4 cm should be electively excised to prevent torsion and to rule out neoplasm.

Older children with a simple ovarian cyst can also be observed unless the cyst is larger than 5 cm, enlarging on serial US, or causing symptoms. Complex cysts that contain calcifications usually represent mature teratomas but any complex cyst should be considered to potentially harbor a malignancy. Ovarian cysts can also bleed or rupture. Fallopian (para-ovarian) cysts are usually asymptomatic but they can cause torsion.

Lymphangioma

Abdominal lymphangiomas are rare as most cystic lymphatic malformations occur in the head and axilla. They usually arise within the retroperitoneum and are sometimes extensive. Those in the abdomen occur presumably due to lack of lymphatic connection of the intestine or retroperitoneum to the normal lymphatic channels. US is a good initial study, but CT or MRI is usually necessary to confirm the diagnosis and assess the extent of the cyst, which can be extensive. It usually appears as a thin-walled, multicystic mass with homogenous fluid. Treatment is complete resection, which sometimes involves resection of the adjacent intestine (Fig. 47.1). These lesions are benign but frequently recur and can be locally infiltrative.

P.A. Lange (✉)
Department of Surgery, University of North Carolina, Chapel Hill, UNC Hospitals, Chapel Hill, NC 27599-7223, USA
e-mail: patricia_lange@med.unc.edu

P. Mattei (ed.), *Fundamentals of Pediatric Surgery*,
DOI 10.1007/978-1-4419-6643-8_47, © Springer Science+Business Media, LLC 2011

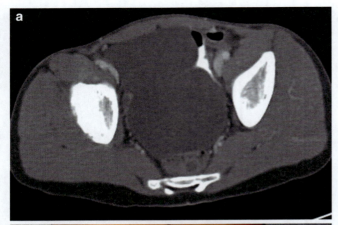

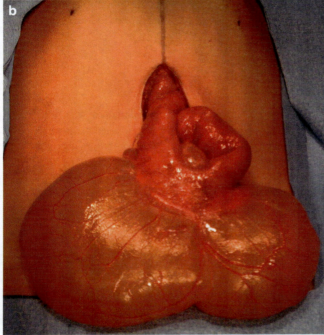

Fig. 47.1 (**a**) CT scan of a 7-year-old girl who presented with a several-month history of intermittent abdominal pain. (**b**) Intra-operative photograph of small bowel lymphangioma. A segmental resection of the ileum to include the entire cyst was performed

Mesenteric and Omental Cysts

Mesenteric and omental cysts probably represent a form of lymphangioma. Mesenteric cysts are more common but both are rare, occurring in only 1 in about 20,000 children. Mesenteric cysts can occur anywhere in the small bowel or colonic mesentery but are most common in the ileal or distal sigmoid region. Both omental and mesenteric cysts can be simple or complex and contain a variety of fluid including serum, blood, chyle or infected fluid. Often these cysts are found incidentally but can cause symptoms due to obstruction, segmental volvulus or intussusception. Computed

tomography and ultrasonography are the preferred imaging modalities to investigate the masses or symptoms. Ideal treatment is complete surgical excision but for large cysts or those at the base of the mesentery, drainage and marsupualization can be performed.

Liver Cysts

Liver cysts are rare and are usually asymptomatic. They include simple cysts, abscesses, hydatid cysts, neoplastic cysts or associated with the biliary system, such as choledochal cysts or Caroli's disease. The work up generally includes imaging such at CT or MRI to better define the cyst characteristics. Symptoms and laboratory values sometimes aid in the diagnosis. Patients with fever, elevated white blood cell count, and pain are more likely to have an abscess rather than a simple cyst.

Management depends on the etiology of the cyst. Simple cysts that are asymptomatic need no further treatment. Abscesses often respond well to percutaneous drainage and intravenous antibiotics. Cystic neoplastic lesions need to be excised with clear margins. Echinococcal (hydatid) cysts should be surgically excised or percutaneously drained and treated with anti-hydatid agents (such as albendazole and mebendazole).

Pancreatic Cysts

Congenital foregut duplication cysts of the pancreas are extremely rare but are also sometimes detected by prenatal imaging. True cysts have an epithelial lining. Other pancreatic cysts found in children include papillary cystic neoplasm, primitive neuroectodermal tumors, pancreatic blastomas, serous cystadenomas, and pancreatic pseudocysts. These can be treated with cyst aspiration, partial pancreatectomy or enucleation.

Splenic Cysts

Splenic cysts can be due to trauma, in which case they are probably pseudocysts and usually resolve spontaneously. True cysts are presumably congenital in origin and usually grow slowly over time. If smaller than 5 cm and asymptomatic, they can be observed but serial US (every 6 months to a year) should be performed. Cysts that are larger than about 5 cm or are causing symptoms (they can also rupture, but this is exceedingly rare) should be excised.

Genitourinary Abnormalities

Obstruction of the lower genitourinary structures can lead to cystic changes in more proximal structures and present as a cystic abdominal mass. Often these are discovered on prenatal ultrasound during routine screening or for workup of oligohydramnios or fetal growth retardation. Abnormalities include polycystic kidneys, isolated renal cysts, hydronephrosis, ovarian cysts, ureterocele, urachal cysts, abdominoscrotal hydroceles and duplications of the vagina/uterus. Most of these abnormalities can be treated postnatally and specific treatment is aimed at relieving obstructions or removing cysts.

Tumors

Complex cystic abdominal masses should be considered neoplasms until proven otherwise (Fig. 47.2). Ultrasound, CT and MRI are used to evaluate for cystic neoplasms and possible metastases or synchronous lesions. Tumor types include intra-abdominal sacrococcygeal teratoma, ovarian germ cell tumors, pancreatic neoplasms, mucinous cystic neoplasms, and renal or genitourinary tumors.

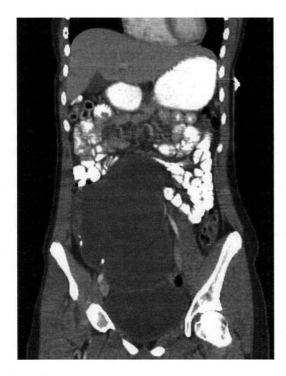

Fig. 47.2 CT scan to evaluate a palpable abdominal mass in a 14-year-old girl. Note the calcifications in the RLQ. The mass was resected and revealed a mature teratoma of the left ovary

Trauma/Pseudocysts

Blunt force injury to the abdomen most commonly involves solid organs. Trauma to the abdomen can also cause rupture of preexisting cysts (hydatid, renal, choledochal, splenic) or the formation of pseudocysts. Hematomas around the liver and spleen, the two most common organs injured in blunt abdominal trauma, can also mimic intra-abdominal cysts. Acute and chronic inflammation of the pancreas sometimes leads to leakage of pancreatic enzymes that ultimately develops into a pseudocyst. Ventriculoperitoneal shunts sometimes result in the formation of a cerebrospinal fluid pseudocyst, which can become infected, cause a small bowel obstruction, or result in shunt malfunction. Cyst and pseudocyst formation due to abdominal trauma can be completely asymptomatic or they can cause pain, distension, and obstruction. In some cases, the workup for blunt trauma leads to the discovery of a preexisting intra-abdominal cyst.

Diagnosis

Though enteric duplications are sometimes found unexpectedly at laparotomy, many are identified preoperatively by medical imaging techniques. Ultrasonography can often detect alimentary tract duplications by their signature appearance – a hyperechoic mucosa and hypoechoic outer smooth muscle layer (Fig. 47.3). Peristalsis within the abnormal structure further supports the diagnosis. Cystic structures in the abdomen detected by prenatal US should be followed up by a postnatal study. If asymptomatic, these structures can usually be followed with serial US until the child is older and elective surgery is deemed safer.

Additional imaging is sometimes necessary to determine the origin of the cystic structure as this can alter management. Computed tomography provides more detail and information about the relationship to nearby structures. Spiral CT is especially useful for identifying feeding vessels, especially when an extralobar pulmonary sequestration is thought to be present. CT scans are also better able to detect synchronous lesions in the chest or abdomen.

Magnetic resonance imaging is being performed more frequently in the prenatal period and can often detect asymptomatic intra-abdominal cystic structures. This modality is also useful in delineating bilio-pancreatic abnormalities and can help to distinguish intestinal duplication cysts, choledochal cysts, and pancreatic cysts. MRI has the additional advantage of avoiding radiation in children but often requires the use of general anesthesia in young children.

Contrast studies (upper GI with small bowel follow-through, contrast enema) are sometimes used to investigate

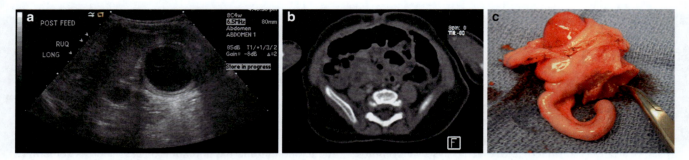

Fig. 47.3 (**a**) Abdominal US showing cystic structure in upper abdomen. (**b**) CT scan showing cystic structure in right lower quadrant. This is in a different location than the cyst seen on abdominal US indicating mobility either outside or within the intestine. (**c**) Resection of terminal ileum and cecum for cecal duplication cyst that had caused intermittent intussusception

Fig. 47.4 (**a**) Air-contrast enema to evaluate for intussusception. A persistent mass is seen in the ileocecal valve area with no air refluxing into the terminal ileum. (**b**) Abdominal US showing intussusception of ileal duplication cyst

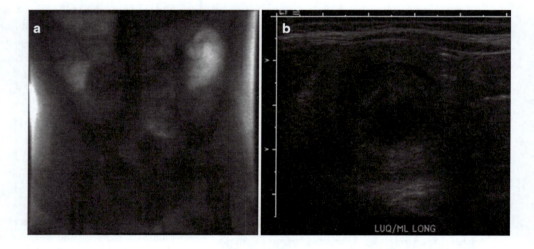

particular symptoms. A child with bilious emesis undergoing an UGI to rule out malrotation might instead be found to have a duodenal duplication. Barium or air enemas to diagnose and treat intussusception might reveal a persistent cystic structure in the cecum or terminal ileum that on exploration is confirmed to be an enteric duplication cyst (Fig. 47.4).

Endoscopic retrograde cholangiopancreatography and MRCP are useful diagnostic adjuncts when cysts are located in close proximity to the biliary or pancreatic systems. They should also be used when patients present with jaundice or have symptoms of pancreatitis.

Although advancements in radiographic technology are rapidly improving, the final diagnosis is often not determined until surgical resection and histopathologic examination.

Treatment

When treating a patient with a symptomatic enteric duplication or intra-abdominal cyst, the primary goal should be complete resection. For the simple cysts, excision can be relatively straightforward. Tubular duplications are often intimately associated with the normal bowel, making simple excision impossible. Segmental intestinal resection can be performed for cysts confined to a short segment. Because most upper abdominal cysts have gastric or pancreatic ectopic mucosa, bleeding and ulceration can occur if the cyst is not removed or if the mucosa is left intact. For this reason, long small bowel duplications require mucosal stripping and marsupialization of the cyst wall.

For certain locations, different techniques are employed. Gastric duplications are commonly found on the greater curve of the stomach and usually do not communicate with the gastric lumen. Children with gastric duplications might be completely asymptomatic or they can present with non-bilious vomiting, failure to thrive, or hematemesis. Removal of these cysts is recommended to prevent bleeding, ulceration and, although extremely rare, malignant degeneration. The cyst can usually be removed without having to remove any of the stomach. Simply excising the cyst and the common wall and closing the serosal defect should be adequate. If there is communication with the gastric lumen and the cyst is small, a segmental resection can be performed. For larger cysts, resection of the common wall followed by repair of the gastrotomy is necessary.

Duodenal duplications are less common than gastric or small bowel duplications. These are typically found on the mesenteric side of the first or second portion of the duodenum. Presenting symptoms include vomiting, abdominal mass, failure to thrive, pancreatitis, jaundice or bleeding. Diagnosis can be made with abdominal US, UGI or CT. ERCP can also be used to confirm the diagnosis and is sometimes be therapeutic, if a window can be created between the cyst and duodenal lumen. Most duodenal cysts contain duodenal mucosa but up to 20% have gastric mucosa and therefore can cause ulceration and bleeding. Removal of the cyst or stripping the mucosa will prevent these complications. Care must be taken not to injure the common bile duct or pancreatic duct during cyst resection.

Small bowel duplication cysts are the most common variety and can be either cystic or tubular. Tubular duplications share all or part of their wall with the intestine and can have a shared or separate blood supply. They are usually on the mesenteric side and present with bleeding, obstruction, intussusception, perforation, or a palpable mass. The diagnosis is rarely made pre-operatively. Treatment involves removal of small cysts by enucleation, larger cysts by segmental resection, and long tubular duplications by mucosal stripping.

Colonic duplications present in a similar fashion to small bowel duplications: vomiting, obstruction, volvulus or perforation. Making the diagnosis preoperatively is challenging and often these cysts are not discovered until laparotomy or laparoscopy. Like their small bowel counterparts, these can be cystic or tubular. They can be found on the mesenteric or the antimesenteric side of the normal colon and can end blindly or as a separate anus or as a fistula to the genitourinary tract. The proximal end of the duplication usually connects to the normal colon and can thus become filled with stool. If the distal end has no fistula or colonic connection, the duplicated tube can fill with stool and compress the normal rectum.

Colonic duplications have a high association with other intestinal and genitourinary anomalies. Children with double penis, bifid scrotum, double vagina or didelphic uterus should be evaluated for possible colonic duplication. Since the mucosa of the duplication is usually colonic and not at risk for bleeding, complete resection is not usually required. The distal portion of the duplication can be connected to the normal colon to relieve buildup of stool within the duplicated segment.

Rectal duplications are very rare and are more common in females. They are typically located posterior to the normal rectum. Many have a fistulous connection to the rectum or skin and are confused with perirectal abscess or fistula-in-ano. Rectal duplications present with pain, constipation, bleeding, fistula or prolapse. Workup typically includes contrast enema, CT or MRI. These studies will also help to rule out spinal cord anomalies such as myelomeningocele. Complete resection of a rectal duplication can be achieved by a transanal or posterior sagittal approach. Occasionally, an unresectable duplication will need to be addressed by mucosectomy.

Many intra-abdominal cysts and duplications are amenable to minimal access surgery. The same principles are applied: complete resection or partial resection with mucosectomy. Any cystic structure suspected of being a malignancy should be left intact with avoidance of spillage of cyst contents. As with an open approach, laparoscopic exploration should be thorough enough to evaluate for synchronous intra-abdominal cysts and associated anomalies.

Children with intussusception who require surgical exploration should be examined intra-operatively for intraluminal masses. A duplication or mesenteric cyst can cause intussusception and will need to be excised, usually with a segmental resection of the involved intestine (Fig. 47.3).

Postoperative Care

The postoperative care of children undergoing resection of duplication cysts is no different that used after other intestinal procedures. The timing of initiation of enteral feeds is determined by the surgical procedure. If a simple cyst is entirely removed and the intestinal lumen remains intact, feeds can start in the immediate postoperative period. Those children undergoing intestinal resection with primary anastomosis or marsupialization of a cyst might need to wait until adequate return of bowel function. Following resection of upper abdominal cysts such as those found in the stomach and duodenum, patients usually require nasogastric tube decompression for 1 or 2 days. Antibiotics are generally not needed in the postoperative period and need only be given prior to the surgical incision.

Children should be monitored for recurrent bleeding following excision or mucosectomy of duplication cysts, especially if any mucosa was left behind. Resection of cysts lying in close proximity to the pancreas can induce postoperative pancreatitis that will usually resolve with bowel rest. Patients who undergo resection of rectal duplication cysts and develop fecal incontinence should undergo anal manometery and should be considered for biofeedback therapy. Duplication cysts that are found in adulthood need to be removed due to the risk of malignant degeneration. Nevertheless, routine follow-up imaging is usually not necessary in the asymptomatic patient.

The overall prognosis for children with duplication cysts is generally excellent. As many of these are now being discovered prenatally, earlier detection and treatment can often be carried out before symptoms or complications occur.

Summary Points

- Intestinal duplications are extremely rare, only about 1 in every 4,500 autopsy cases.
- The majority of duplications are found in the jejuno-ileal region (44%); other areas more rare-stomach 7%, duodenum 5%, colon 15%, rectal 5%, thoracic 4%, cervical very rare.
- Synchronous abdominal and thoracic cysts/duplications may occur (approximately 15%).
- Many cysts and duplications are asymptomatic and are discovered by prenatal imaging.
- Diagnosis can be made by radiographic imaging but often duplications are discovered intra-operatively.
- Treatment goal is complete removal of cyst/duplication for gastric and small bowel duplications due to risk of bleeding. May need to consider mucosal stripping and/or marsupialization for longer duplications.
- Prognosis – overall prognosis is excellent, especially for isolated, small duplication cysts. Malignant degeneration of duplication cysts is a rare but serious complication.

Editor's Comment

Ovarian cysts identified antenatally or at birth are almost always the result of antenatal torsion. They are usually asymptomatic and can be safely observed but many will fail to resolve by serial US and should be removed. The contralateral ovary should be inspected, however oophoropexy is unnecessary and probably ineffective. Simple ovarian cysts in older girls should be excised if they are large, growing or symptomatic. The inner lining can usually be stripped cleanly, preserving the parenchyma and the ovarian capsule, where the ova reside. Simple unroofing or marsupialization results in a high recurrence rate and should only be done if stripping is impossible due to hemorrhage or inflammation.

Nearly every true cyst can be treated by stripping its epithelial lining, though complete excision is often easier and less morbid. By definition, enteric duplication cysts have a mucosal lining but removal of just the lining is a challenge. It is usually safer to simply excise it. Since they almost always arise from the mesenteric side of the bowel wall, this usually entails bowel resection. This approach is not used for long tubular duplications or duodenal duplications, which should be stripped, if possible, or the common wall between the cyst and the adjacent bowel lumen can be obliterated to create a single lumen. This is not ideal in that it essentially creates a diverticulum but it might be the only alternative to an extensive and dangerous bowel resection (Whipple procedure, esophagectomy).

A simple liver cyst should be observed and will usually remain stable, unless it represents an echinococcal cyst or abscess. Simple pancreatic cysts are rare and can be excised if located in the tail but should probably be treated like a pseudocyst if located in the head or neck of the pancreas. Splenic cysts must always be completely excised by partial or total splenectomy, as the lining is never able to be stripped or obliterated. Some have tried using sclerotherapy, the argon beam coagulator to destroy the epithelium, or marsupialization, but each of these techniques is associated with an unacceptable recurrence rate.

Omental cysts can torse, bleed or rupture, in some cases mimicking appendicitis. They can be simply excised by laparoscopic partial omentectomy. Mesenteric cysts are more difficult to deal with as they can insinuate extensively within the mesentery and retroperitoneum. Ideally they should be excised, but this might not be feasible, in which case the only option is partial excision and marsupialization.

Most abdominal cysts and duplications can and should be approached laparoscopically, at least at first. Preoperative planning must include high-resolution three-dimensional imaging such as a CT or MRI. The goal should be to effectively eradicate the cyst, either by excision, epithelial stripping, or marsupialization, in that order of preference, but to minimize postoperative discomfort and scarring.

Differential Diagnosis

- Mixed solid/cystic tumors
- Choledochal cysts
- Splenic cysts
- Genitourinary dilatation
- Pancreatic cysts/pseudocysts
- Dilatation of normal structures (hydroureter)
- Traumatic hematoma
- Ovarian cysts/tumors

Diagnostic Studies

- Plain radiographs
- Abdominal US
- Upper GI contrast study
- Contrast enema
- CT
- MRI
- ERCP/MRCP

Parental Preparation

- Possible bowel resection
- Possible stoma
- Risk of recurrence (lymphangioma)
- Possible oophorectomy or salpingectomy

Preoperative Preparation

- ☐ IV hydration
- ☐ Informed consent
- ☐ Foley catheter if pelvic cyst

Technical Points

- Laparoscopy vs. open
- Leave cyst intact if suspect malignancy
- Bowel resection if cyst/duplication involves mesentery
- Mucosal stripping if unable to remove entire cyst/duplication
- Connect colonic duplications distally to normal colon
- Exploration for synchronous duplications

Suggested Reading

Azzie G, Beasley S. Diagnosis and treatment of foregut duplications. Semin Pediatr Surg. 2003;12(1):46–54.

Cauchi JA, Buick RG. Duodenal duplication cyst: beware of the lesser sac collection. Pediatr Surg Int. 2006;22(5):456–8.

Charlesworth P, Ade-Ajayi N, Davenport M. Natural history and long-term follow-up of antenatally detected liver cysts. J Ped Surg. 2007;42(3):494–9.

Foley P, Sithasanan N, McEwing R, et al. Enteric duplications presenting as antenatally detected abdominal cysts: is delayed resection appropriate? J Pediatr Surg. 2003;38(12):1810–3.

Foley P, Ford W, McEwing R, et al. Is conservative management of prenatal and neonatal ovarian cysts justifiable? Fetal Diagn Ther. 2005;20(5):454–8.

Katara A, Shah R, Bhandarkar D, et al. Laparoscopic management of antenatally-diagnosed abdominal cysts in newborns. Surg Laparosc Endosc Percutan Tech. 2004;14(1):42–4.

Laje P, Martinez-Ferro M, Grisoni E, et al. Intraabdominal pulmonary sequestration. A case series and review of the literature. J Pediatr Surg. 2006;41(7):1309–12.

McCollum M, Macneily A, Blair G. Surgical implications of urachal remnants: presentation and management. J Pediatr Surg. 2003;38(5): 798–803.

Menon P, Rao K, Vaiphei K. Isolated enteric duplication cysts. J Pediatr Surg. 2004;39(8):e5–7.

Mobley III L, Doran S, Hellbusch L. Abdominal pseudocyst: predisposing factors and treatment algorithm. Pediatr Neurosurg. 2005;41(2): 77–83.

Schenkman L, Weiner T, Phillips J. Evolution of the surgical management of neonatal ovarian cysts: Laparoscopic-assisted transumbilical extracorporeal ovarian cystectomy (LATEC). J Laparoendosc Adv Surg Tech. 2008;18(4):635–40. doi: 10.1089/lap. 2007.0193.

Spellman K, Stock JA, Norton KI. Abdominoscrotal hydrocele: a rare cause of a cystic abdominal mass in children. Urology. 2008;71(5): 832–3.

Tawil K, Crankson S, Emam S, et al. Cecal duplication cyst: a cause of intestinal obstruction in a newborn infant. Am J Perinatol. 2005; 22(1):49–52.

Chapter 48
Anomalies of Intestinal Rotation

François I. Luks

Rotational anomalies of the intestinal tract refer to the failure of the primitive midgut to establish its normal anatomical relationships and attachments as it develops into duodenum, small bowel, and proximal colon. The incidence of isolated malrotation in the general population is estimated at 1 in 500 live births, but it is much more common in a number of genetic, chromosomal, and congenital disorders. The term malrotation is most commonly used to describe *nonrotation*, whereby the duodenum fails to form its characteristic C-loop and instead runs in a straight cephalocaudal line into the proximal jejunum. Other rotational anomalies include *incomplete rotation*, where the normal rotational process of the midgut has been interrupted, *reverse rotation*, and *errors of intestinal fixation*, typically of the cecum and the ascending and descending colon.

Embryology

The final anatomic arrangement of the midgut follows a complex series of events that starts around the fourth week of gestation, when the straight intestinal tube rapidly elongates and the embryo develops left–right differentiation. Midgut rotation has been artificially divided into three stages, representing the various positions of the distal duodenum and the cecum as they follow a 270° counter-clockwise path. The exact understanding of this intricate four-dimensional process is less important than the final anatomic relationships between the various components of the midgut, the mesentery and the vascular pedicle of the superior mesenteric artery. The key features of normal intestinal rotation include: (1) the duodenum describes a C-loop with concavity to the

patient's left and the third portion of the duodenum (at the ligament of Treitz) to the left of the midline; (2) the superior mesenteric artery runs in front of the third portion of the duodenum, which is in a retroperitoneal position; (3) the mesentery is attached posteriorly along a broad line that runs from the ligament of Treitz in the left upper quadrant to the cecum in the right lower quadrant, thereby preventing torsion of the mesentery on its axis (Fig. 48.1), and (4) the colon describes a frame with the cecum and ascending colon fixed along the right side of the abdomen and the descending colon fixed along the left side.

The initial mechanisms of normal intestinal rotation are still poorly understood, but likely involve the same genes that are responsible for other aspects of asymmetrical development, the most important of which is the infolding of the primitive heart to form a four-chamber structure with clear separation between systemic and pulmonary circulations. Several disorders of left–right differentiation, such as the heterotaxia syndromes, are therefore often associated with some form of anomalous intestinal rotation, abnormal budding of the endodermal appendages (polysplenia or asplenia, biliary anomalies, preduodenal portal vein), and varying degrees of cardiac anomalies. In immotile cilia disorders such as Kartagener syndrome, 50% of patients have situs inversus/ambiguus or anomalous intestinal rotation. All these disorders may be related to abnormal expression or differential signaling of the Hedgehog genes, transforming growth factor (TGF) β, and tyrosine kinase receptor pathways, all of which play a crucial role in establishing left–right asymmetry in the early embryo.

As the intestinal tract rapidly elongates around the fourth week of gestation, it temporarily leaves the abdominal cavity through a wide umbilical ring, while it also undergoes its rotational changes: both the duodenum and the colon rotate 270° counter-clockwise to lie in their final configuration. The last stage of intestinal rotation is completed as the midgut returns to the abdominal cavity. Any event that interferes with this process can result in incomplete rotation or nonrotation of the midgut. Thus, congenital diaphragmatic hernia and abdominal wall defects are associated with malrotation. It should be noted that while the visual image of moving and rotating intestinal loops can be illustrative, the process is

F.I. Luks (✉)
Warren Halpert Medical School of Brown University, Providence, RI, USA
and
Division of Pediatric Surgery, Hasbro Children's Hospital, 2, Dudley Street, Suite 180, Providence, RI 02905, USA
e-mail: francois_luks@brown.eduv

P. Mattei (ed.), *Fundamentals of Pediatric Surgery*,
DOI 10.1007/978-1-4419-6643-8_48, © Springer Science+Business Media, LLC 2011

Fig. 48.1 Cut-out view of the mesentery in normal rotation (*left*) and non-rotation (*right*). Normally, the posterior attachment of the mesentery stretches from the ligament of Treitz to the ileocecal valve (ICV), preventing torsion of the mesenteric vessels. In non-rotation, the posterior mesenteric attachment (between duodenum and ICV) is narrow, placing it at risk of volvulus around the superior mesenteric artery

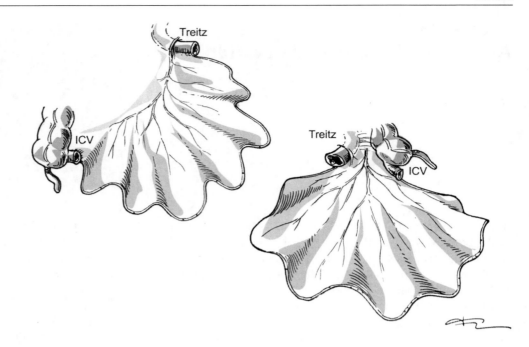

more likely one of differential growth and proliferation of specific portions of the primitive intestinal tube, as elegantly demonstrated by Kluth and Lambrecht in their scanning electron microscopy studies of the fetal rat.

In the absence of normal intestinal rotation, the duodenum fails to cross the midline and its third portion lies to the right of the spine. The SMA never crosses the duodenum and lies within a narrow mesenteric base that connects the duodenojejunal junction with the cecum (Fig. 48.1). The cecum is in a left paramedian location and congenital bands between duodenum and cecum keep the mesenteric root attached in a single narrow pedicle rather than the broad base seen in normal rotation. This configuration places the mesentery at risk for complete volvulus, which results in vascular cut-off at the root of the SMA and ischemic necrosis of the entire midgut from duodenum to proximal transverse colon.

Two other features of nonrotation or incomplete rotation can become clinically significant. The cecum is normally fixed to the right lateral abdominal wall by peritoneal folds. These bands (Ladd's bands) are frequently present in malrotation and cause varying degrees of duodenal or proximal jejunal obstruction as they cross from the cecum to the right peritoneal wall. In addition, the anomalous location of the appendix can create diagnostic uncertainty in patients presenting with acute appendicitis and left-sided abdominal pain.

There are other, less common forms of rotational anomalies. These include reverse rotation, whereby the duodenum comes to lie in front of the colon, and fixation anomalies of the colon. When either the ascending or the descending colon

fail to adhere to the posterior abdominal wall, small bowel loops can herniate through these mesocolic gaps and cause an intestinal obstruction. These conditions are not only rare, but very difficult to accurately diagnose preoperatively.

Diagnosis

The majority of children with malrotation present in infancy, but since abnormal intestinal rotation is often asymptomatic, its true incidence is unknown. The most dramatic presentation of malrotation is midgut volvulus. This must be suspected in any infant who presents with bilious vomiting, and prompt diagnosis is important to avoid ischemic loss of intestine. Midgut volvulus and other intestinal catastrophes are easily differentiated from hypertrophic pyloric stenosis, where vomiting is non-bilious and occurs in an otherwise well and hungry child. Bilious vomiting is seen in half of the infants and one third of those older than 1 month who present with malrotation or midgut volvulus. Bilious vomiting is not pathognomonic for malrotation and is seen with other forms of intestinal obstruction, such as duodenal atresia, annular pancreas, small bowel atresia, meconium ileus, and Hirschsprung disease. While these conditions are all surgical, they do not require immediate surgical exploration. Initial treatment consists of bowel rest, intravenous hydration, and nasogastric decompression. Midgut volvulus, on the other hand, demands rapid operative correction, as it is associated with extensive intestinal ischemia. Initially, the infant with midgut volvulus has a scaphoid abdomen, since the point of obstruction is so proximal. However, gastric distention can obscure this clinical finding. As venous and lymphatic congestion progress toward ischemia, the intestinal loops become thickened and fluid-filled, and abdominal distention develops. By then, the child appears sick, with significant hypovolemia from third-space fluid losses and vomiting. Sloughing of intestinal mucosa can occur, leading to bloody stools. Clinical features include tachycardia, oligo- or anuria, poor capillary refill, metabolic acidosis and, ultimately, vascular collapse.

Imaging plays a central role in the diagnosis of malrotation. A plain abdominal radiograph is non-specific, but may sometimes suggest the diagnosis. In the presence of tight Ladd's bands, duodenal obstruction may be seen as a "double bubble," similar to that seen in patients with duodenal atresia. Unlike the usual situation with duodenal atresia., there is usually some distal intestinal gas, unless a complete midgut volvulus is present. In that case, the abdomen is gasless, save for the gastric and duodenal bubbles. In advanced volvulus, intestinal ischemia may result in breaches in the mucosal barrier, and the clinical and radiographic signs may be indistinguishable from those of necrotizing enterocolitis. These include intestinal pneumatosis and portal vein gas. It is important to realize that more than one cause of proximal intestinal obstruction may be present in the same infant: duodenal atresia and duodenal web can be associated with malrotation, as can jejunal atresia.

If the child's condition permits, malrotation is most reliably diagnosed with an upper gastrointestinal contrast study. As contrast leaves the stomach, the duodenum and proximal jejunal loops opacify to the right of the midline (Fig. 48.2). Normal rotation of the midgut includes a duodenal C-loop that crosses the midline and the ligament of Treitz (duodenojejunal junction) that is located to the left of the spine and at least as high as the pylorus. These are important landmarks, because even a nonrotated duodenum may be tortuous (particularly if Ladd's bands partially occlude the duodenal outlet). This may give the impression of a C-loop, but an incomplete one, whereby the duodenojejunal junction does not quite reach the level of the gastric outlet. Other features of malrotation on UGI include right-sided position of the majority of small bowel loops and absence of a typical colonic frame. Instead, ascending and transverse colon are all located to the left of the spine (Fig. 48.3). A contrast enema may show the colonic anatomy better, but this is a less reliable test – even a partially or completely rotated colon does not rule out malrotation or, more importantly, a narrow-based mesenteric attachment and its associated risk of volvulus.

In recent years, ultrasound has been increasingly accurate in detecting abnormal rotation. If the duodenum is clearly seen, it can be followed as it is supposed to cross the spine. The relationship of the superior mesenteric vessels is the most typical ultrasonographic feature of malrotation. Normally, the SMA is posterior and to the left of the vein. In malrotation, the SMA lies to the right of the vein. In midgut volvulus, the further torsion of the vessels can be clearly seen as a swirl, or whirlpool pattern, on Doppler ultrasound (Fig. 48.4). The duodenal obstruction may be clearly visible

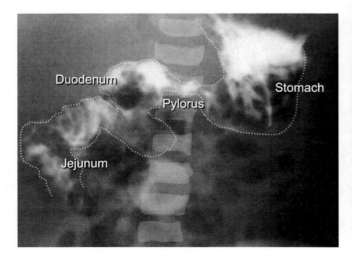

Fig. 48.2 Upper gastrointestinal contrast study (UGI) in an infant with malrotation: the duodenum does not cross the midline (enhanced vertebral bodies) and the duodenojejunal junction lies to the right of the spine

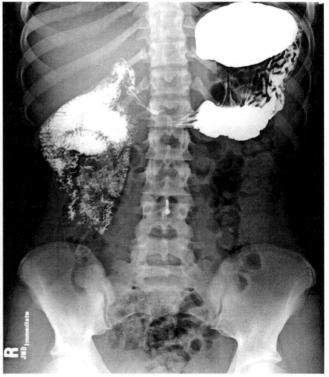

Fig. 48.3 UGI in an older child with malrotation. Note duodenum and small bowel on the *right* and colon on the *left*

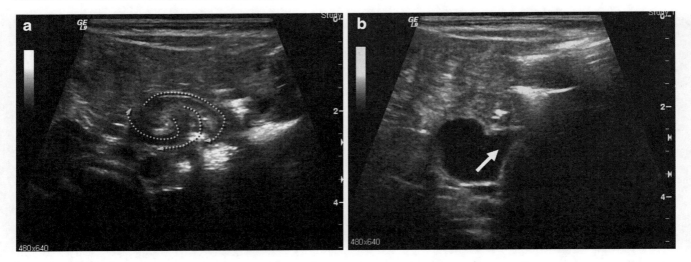

Fig. 48.4 Ultrasonographic signs of midgut volvulus. *Top*: "swirling" pattern of the superior mesenteric vessels due to volvulus of the mesentery. *Bottom*: beak-like obstruction of the duodenum (*arrow*)

and the torsion may give it a bird's beak appearance (Fig. 48.4). Other ultrasonographic signs of advanced midgut volvulus include free peritoneal fluid, intestinal wall edema, pneumatosis, and portal vein gas. While often accurate, ultrasonography is not as reliable as UGI in the diagnosis of malrotation. The right-sided course of the duodenum and the mesenteric vessel inversion may be missed, and false-positive results may be seen with any process that pushes the root of the mesentery to the right, such as acute gastric distention, splenomegaly or a splenic hematoma. The whirlpool sign and duodenal obstruction can also be seen on abdominal CT, however CT is not the diagnostic procedure of choice for either malrotation or midgut volvulus.

While it is the diagnostic cornerstone of malrotation, one should forgo the UGI study if midgut volvulus is suspected, particularly in the very young infant. Any delay in surgical intervention can result in irreversible ischemic damage to the entire midgut, which in turn may lead to short bowel syndrome or death. The combination of bilious emesis, a scaphoid abdomen (after gastric decompression), and shock require prompt exploration. If the presentation is less dramatic, it may be reasonable to obtain an UGI, as long as surgical delay is kept to a minimum. The typical appearance of midgut volvulus on UGI is a corkscrew or apple-peel appearance of the first jejunal loops, best seen in a lateral view (Fig. 48.5).

The management of asymptomatic malrotation is the subject of some debate. In the past, many have argued that malrotation is never asymptomatic, since its discovery follows an imaging study that was obtained for a reason. However, the symptoms ascribed to malrotation are often vague and nonspecific, including gastroesophageal reflux, chronic emesis, colicky abdominal pain, malabsorption, chronic diarrhea, or failure to thrive. Moreover, the presence of certain pathologies (heterotaxia syndromes) will often lead to a search for

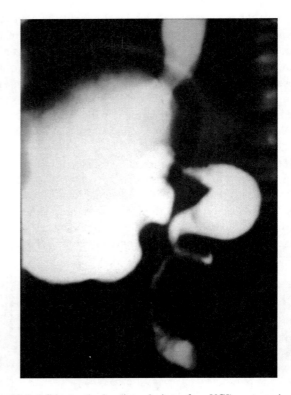

Fig. 48.5 Midgut volvulus (lateral view of an UGI): note corkscrew appearance of the duodenum and proximal jejunum

associated malrotation – and the increased use of medical imaging has led to the incidental finding of malrotation in patients who truly have minimal to no symptoms. The diagnostic criteria for malrotation in older or asymptomatic patients are the same as in infants. Malabsorption and failure to thrive may be a result of chronic or intermittent volvulus and lymphatic congestion; vomiting and reflux symptoms may be secondary to partial duodenal obstruction by Ladd's bands.

Treatment

Midgut volvulus is a surgical emergency. Aggressive intravenous hydration is important to counteract the hypovolemia due to vomiting and third spacing, but this should not delay intervention. Antibiotics are administered prophylactically. A laparotomy is performed through a right transverse incision above the level of the umbilicus. Viscera are gently exteriorized and examined. Because of the volvulus, the colon (which now lies posteriorly) is obscured by the small bowel loops. While maintaining the intestinal loops moist and warm, the volvulus is untwisted by turning the intestinal mass in a *counter-clockwise* fashion. The torsion may be more than 360°, and the intestinal mass must be gently and methodically untwisted until the colon comes into view. This should release vascular constriction and allow the ischemia to improve. In reality, a midgut volvulus is often confusing at first and care must be taken not to cause additional bowel damage during detorsion. In some patients, further confusion may be caused by the presence of situs ambiguus or situs inversus, whereby the stomach may be on the right and the liver midline or on the left. In these cases, the duodenum may be on the left and the colon on the right.

Once the intestinal torsion is corrected, viability of the loops is assessed. A period of observation, during which tension on the mesenteric root is alleviated and the viscera are kept warm, may allow some return of perfusion. If necessary, a hand-held Doppler probe or fluorescein may be used to assess vascular status. Only if bowel loops are frankly necrotic should they be resected – in some cases, it may be better to preserve borderline viable intestine and perform a second-look operation in 12–24 h. Overly aggressive resection can result in short bowel syndrome.

After the volvulus has been corrected, the malrotation itself needs to be addressed. It is also important to confirm the patency of the intestinal tract, particularly in very young infants: a newborn who presents acutely with midgut volvulus may also have a duodenal web. This is best ruled out by passing the nasogastric tube through the duodenum. As the duodenum is straight, this is easier than with normal rotation.

Surgical correction of malrotation *without* midgut volvulus is not an emergency, and may even be unnecessary in some cases. The main purpose of intervention is to prevent future midgut volvulus. This implies that the anatomic condition of the patient predisposes to torsion. While most patients with malrotation have a very narrow mesenteric pedicle caused by the close proximity of the duodenum and the ascending colon, the mesenteric attachment in some patients may be wide enough so as to be essentially normal. In congenital diaphragmatic hernia, for example, the intrathoracic migration of small and large intestinal loops allows the posterior mesenteric attachment to stretch sufficiently to prevent future volvulus. The same probably holds true for abdominal wall defects as well, although cases of midgut volvulus have been described in these patients. It has been speculated that the presence of intra-abdominal adhesions (particularly in gastroschisis) may limit the risk of volvulus, but objective evidence is lacking. Some surgeons will contemplate a Ladd procedure during laparotomy for the repair of congenital diaphragmatic hernia if the patient's condition warrants additional operative time. In all other patients with malrotation, surgical exploration should be considered.

The classic surgical treatment of malrotation is the Ladd procedure. Its goals are to relieve any duodenal or jejunal obstruction and decrease the risk of future midgut volvulus by widening the mesenteric base. The viscera are carefully examined, and any bands crossing anteriorly to the duodenojejunal junction are divided (Fig. 48.6). These Ladd's bands are avascular, but care must be taken not to damage the underlying mesentery. The root of the mesentery is then exposed, and the avascular connections between the duodenum and the ascending colon are carefully dissected with Metzenbaum scissors. Cautery should be kept to a minimum as mesenteric injury is a real risk (particularly at the level of the SMA take-off). The duodenum is then gently teased toward the patient's right side of the abdomen, while the cecum and ascending colon are pushed to the left. This fully exposes the superior

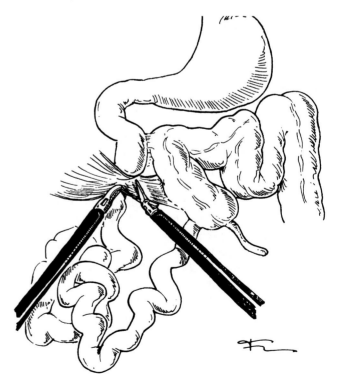

Fig. 48.6 Laparoscopic take-down of Ladd's bands between cecum and right lateral abdominal wall (from Lessin MS and Luks FI. Laparoscopic appendectomy and duodenocolonic dissociation (LADD) procedure for malrotation. Pediatr Surg Int 1998, Springer. Used by permission)

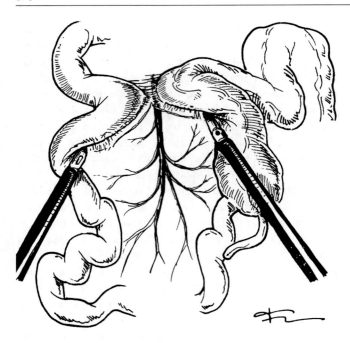

Fig. 48.7 Laparoscopic division of duodenocolonic bands to expose the root of the superior mesenteric artery and widen the posterior attachment of the mesentery (from Lessin MS and Luks FI. Laparoscopic appendectomy and duodenocolonic dissociation (LADD) procedure for malrotation. Pediatr Surg Int 1998, Springer. Used by permission)

mesenteric vessels and their proximal branches (Fig. 48.7). The separation of duodeno-colic bands is all that is needed to widen the mesenteric base: duodenal fixation and cecopexy in their respective location is unnecessary. Again, in some patients the base of the mesentery is already wide enough. If the root of the SMA is clearly splayed between the duodenum and the cecum, no further dissection is required. Appendectomy completes the Ladd procedure as the appendix lies in an abnormal location, making diagnosis of acute appendicitis difficult. Some surgeons prefer to perform an inversion appendectomy, citing a lower risk of infection, since the intestinal tract is not opened: the mesoappendix is divided, and the appendix is inverted into the colon. An absorbable tie is used to ligate the appendix at its base. Now devascularized, the appendix will auto-amputate within days and be eliminated in the stool. Of course, classic appendectomy is simpler, fast, and actually very safe.

All the steps of the Ladd procedure, except detorsion of a midgut volvulus, can be safely performed laparoscopically as well (Figs. 48.6 and 48.7). An increasing number of surgeons are now choosing this approach, particularly in the older,

asymptomatic patient. Placement of the trocars is straightforward: a 5-mm telescope is introduced through the umbilicus. Instrument cannulas may be placed in the inguinal regions, which is cosmetically superior. Because the area of interest lies in the mid-abdomen, it is not easy to establish a classic diamond-shaped configuration between telescope, instruments and target. This lack of adequate triangulation and the short distance between telescope and target introduce a degree of difficulty to the laparoscopic procedure. Performing the operation with only two instruments may be challenging as well, since sharp division of the congenital bands requires adequate tension between duodenum and colon. If necessary, a third instrument port should be placed. The appendix lies in a periumbilical location and can be easily exteriorized through the trocar incision for "open" removal at the end of the laparoscopic procedure.

Postoperative Care

The postoperative course primarily depends on the intraoperative findings. In cases with volvulus and significant intestinal ischemia, a prolonged ileus is typically seen. If bowel resection was performed, parenteral nutrition might be required and the chronic treatment of short bowel syndrome may be difficult. If the operation was performed electively for malrotation alone, prompt recovery can be anticipated.

The long-term results of Ladd's procedure are believed to be excellent. However, postoperative small bowel obstruction occurs in up to 14% of patients, similar to the cumulative risk of small bowel obstruction after laparotomy for other indications. Moreover, recurrent midgut volvulus has been described. Its true incidence is not known but probably occurs in less than 2% of patients. The laparoscopic approach is too new to provide reliable recurrence rates, but the minimally invasive approach appears to be at least as efficient as the classic operation. While operative treatment of midgut volvulus is very effective, it is important to note that chronic symptoms believed to be associated with malrotation (malabsorption, failure to thrive, vague abdominal complaints) are less often corrected. Thus, patients and parents must be warned preoperatively that the operation is mainly aimed at preventing future midgut volvulus, and that some or all symptoms may still be present postoperatively.

Summary Points

- Bilious vomiting in the newborn is a surgical emergency and suggests intestinal obstruction or midgut volvulus until proven otherwise.
- If the infant's condition allows it, a diagnostic upper gastrointestinal series (UGI) may be obtained, but one should be ready to perform a rapid surgical exploration without imaging.
- Initially, infants with midgut volvulus have a scaphoid abdomen (if the stomach is decompressed).
- Delay in recognition and treatment of midgut volvulus may lead to necrosis of the entire small bowel and part of the colon.
- Malrotation carries the risk of midgut volvulus at any age – therefore, surgical exploration and a Ladd procedure is recommended even in the older and asymptomatic patient.
- The main goals of the Ladd procedure are to widen the basis of the mesentery to avoid torsion of the mesenteric vessels, relief of duodenal obstruction by congenital bands and appendectomy, to avoid future confusion if appendicitis were to develop.

Editor's Comment

Many people confuse the terms *malrotation* and *volvulus*; they are not interchangeable. *Malrotation* describes a specific anatomy that is in and of itself harmless and usually asymptomatic; however, patients with malrotation are at risk for midgut *volvulus,* which is potentially catastrophic. In addition to signifying that the duodenum does not pass behind the SMA, *malrotation* also implies that the cecum and jejunum are adjacent to each other and that the entire midgut is based on a narrow mesenteric pedicle. *Nonrotation* also indicates that the duodenum does not pass behind the SMA, but it suggests that the mesentery is sufficiently broad that the risk of volvulus is minimal – it is the anatomic configuration that remains after a properly performed Ladd procedure and occurs naturally in most patients with congenital diaphragmatic hernia and other anomalies that associated with rotational abnormalities.

Infants and children with bilious emesis (and no prior abdominal surgical history) should be presumed to have malrotation with volvulus until proven otherwise. If they are septic or have peritonitis, they should be prepared for immediate laparotomy. Time is of the essence. If the patient is stable, an upper GI contrast study should be performed urgently – it cannot wait until morning! If the findings are consistent with volvulus, the patient goes to the OR immediately. If there is malrotation without volvulus, most pediatric surgeons make plans to operate within 24 h but this can wait until the light of day. It is important to note that the picture of a well-appearing child and a totally benign abdomen (even if laboratory values and radiographs are within normal limits) does not rule out the possibility of volvulus with ischemic bowel.

The Ladd procedure can be performed laparoscopically or open. Most useful when the procedure is being performed non-emergently, the laparoscopic approach is often quite difficult and there is a significant rate of conversion to open even for experienced laparoscopists. Regardless of the approach, the steps are the same: (1) detorse the bowel in a counter-clockwise direction ("turn back the hands of time"): if bowel is frankly necrotic it should be excised, which places the child at risk for short gut syndrome and intestinal failure, but if the bowel is of questionable viability, a second-look operation should be planned for 48–72 h; (2) divide Ladd's bands; (3) straighten the duodenum (lyse all adhesions and undo its typical accordion configuration); (4) broaden the mesentery – separate the colon and duodenum, open the anterior mesenteric peritoneum, and fan out the vessels of the mesentery; (5) remove the appendix; (6) establish a nonrotation configuration: place the small bowel on the right side of the abdomen with the duodenum along the right lateral side wall, and place the colon on the left side with the cecum in the left lower quadrant. Cecopexy and duodenal fixation sutures are unnecessary and create sites around which a volvulus could occur. When it comes the Ladd procedure, novices always place undue importance on the lysis of the Ladd bands; but the most important steps are the broadening of the mesentery, which is what prevents volvulus, and the straightening of the duodenum, which relieves many of the GI symptoms patients with malrotation have (emesis, reflux, failure to thrive). Turbid fluid at operation is almost always chylous ascites due to lymphatic congestion from partial volvulus and not evidence of bowel perforation. Postoperatively, many patients have a prolonged ileus. Some will have protracted symptoms of duodenal dysmotility or pseudo-obstruction.

There are many variants of malrotation, including partial rotation, and right and left paraduodenal hernia. All are treated by trying to establish the nonrotation configuration – the steps of the Ladd procedure are modified as necessary but the final anatomy should be the same. The exception is reverse rotation, which often requires that a portion of the bowel be divided to relieve entrapment. The rotational anomalies displayed by patients with heterotaxy are also often quite challenging to deal with. The goal in these cases is to do whatever you have to do to leave the patient with a mesentery that is as broad as possible and therefore unlikely to volvulize.

The upper GI is the gold standard for the diagnosis of malrotation but in clinical practice is frustratingly imprecise. To avoid missing a single case of malrotation, pediatric radiologists adhere to very strict criteria to define normal. Any variation, no matter how clinically insignificant, will be read out as the dreaded "cannot rule out malrotation." Exploratory surgery has historically been the only way to decide if the intestine was truly malrotated; however, newer imaging modalities (US, MR) are becoming increasingly useful ways to confirm the retroperitoneal sweep of the duodenum and the absence of a narrow root of the mesentery. The ligament of Treitz can also be displaced by gastric or colonic distension and simply repeating the upper GI after a few weeks might yield a different result. Because 15% of patients with duodenal malrotation have normal colonic anatomy, contrast enema is not an accurate test for malrotation. Finally, there are some children who have an abnormally low ligament of Treitz. If the duodenum passes behind the SMA and the mesentery is sufficiently broad, these children are at minimal risk of volvulus and can be safely observed.

Preoperative Preparation

☐ Avoid delays
☐ Intravenous hydration
☐ Prophylactic antibiotics
☐ Type & screen
☐ Informed consent

Technical Points

- Right upper quadrant transverse incision
- Careful exteriorization and examination of the bowel
- Detorsion of the midgut volvulus in a counter-clockwise fashion
- Assess and reassess viability of the bowel
- If bowel resection is unavoidable, limit its extent – if necessary, re-explore after 12–24 h
- Divide Ladd's bands (crossing duodenum), if present
- Widen mesenteric base by dividing avascular duodenocolonic bands
- Fully expose root of superior mesenteric artery and its first branches
- Adequate peri- and postoperative hydration to reverse third-spacing and fluid losses

Differential Diagnosis

- Pyloric stenosis
- Duodenal atresia
- Annular pancreas
- Small bowel atresia
- Meconium ileus
- Hirschsprung disease

Diagnostic Studies

- Plain radiograph
- Upper gastrointestinal (UGI) contrast series (diagnostic test of choice)
- Contrast enema
- Ultrasonography

Parental Preparation

- Possible extensive bowel necrosis, bowel resection
- Possible short bowel syndrome
- Possible stoma

Suggested Reading

Ladd WE. Congenital obstruction of the duodenum in children. N Engl J Med. 1932;206:277–83.

Kluth D, Kaestner M, Tibboel D, Lambrecht W. Rotation of the gut: fact or fantasy? J Pediatr Surg. 1995;30:448–53.

van den Brink GR. Hedgehog signaling in development and homeostasis of the gastrointestinal tract. Physiol Rev Surg Int. 2007;87: 1343–75.

Seashore JH, Touloukian RJ. Midgut volvulus: an ever-present threat. Arch Pediatr Adolesc Med. 1994;148:43–6.

Patino MO, Munden MM. Utility of the sonographic whirlpool sign in diagnosing midgut volvulus in patients with atypical clinical presentations. J Ultrasound Med. 2004;23:397–401.

Spigland N, Brandt ML, Yazbeck S. Malrotation presenting beyond the neonatal period. J Pediatr Surg. 1990;25:1139–42.

Lessin MS, Luks FI. Laparoscopic appendectomy and duodenocolonic dissociation (LADD) procedure for malrotation. Pediatr Surg Int. 1998;13:184–5.

Chapter 49
Necrotizing Enterocolitis

Cynthia A. Gingalewski

Necrotizing enterocolitis (NEC) is the most common diagnosis that requires emergent operation in the neonate. Since first described by Touloukian in 1966, the pathophysiology of this disease remains an enigma. The disease involves the culmination of three factors: a premature infant, an immature immune system, and a gastrointestinal tract colonized with pathologic bacteria (Fig. 49.1). When these three factors are present in the setting of feeding an immature intestinal tract, an unknown trigger or series of events occur that together create the "perfect storm" that is NEC.

The premature infant lacks a mature barrier defense: mucosal cells are poorly developed, the goblet cells produce scant mucus, and gastric, pancreatic and intestinal secretions are reduced. In addition, secretory IgA levels are low or absent. This allows bacteria to gain access to the macrophages and dendritic cells of the innate immune system, which recognizes pathogenic bacteria via pattern recognition receptors, the toll-like receptors (TLR). The two main TLRs are TLR2, which recognizes lipoproteins of gram positive bacteria and mannans of yeast, and TLR4, which recognizes the lipopolysaccharide component of all gram negative bacteria. Based on the results of experiments in cell culture and in mice, it appears that NEC is a TLR4-driven process.

Diagnosis

Necrotizing enterocolitis is predominantly a disease of premature infants. The incidence in infants weighing less than 1,500 g is 10%. The risk of mortality is inversely proportional to birth weight, with infants less than 750 g having a mortality of more than 50%. Necrotizing enterocolitis causes 15% of infant deaths after 1 week of life and one third of all infectious disease-associated late deaths.

The disease is rare in full-term infants and those who have never been fed. Typically, several days after feeds are started, NEC is suspected when the abdomen becomes distended and a large or bilious gastric residual is produced. Physical findings include a distended abdomen, palpable bowel loops, and lethargy. An erythematous abdominal wall is ominous and usually suggests underlying gangrene of the bowel or frank perforation. The erythema occurs because the thin abdominal wall and lack of subcutaneous fat of the premature infant allow the inflammatory reaction to produce cellulitis of the overlying abdominal wall. Laboratory values that are corroborative but not pathonomonic include anemia, thrombocytopenia, neutropenia, and acidosis.

The hallmark of NEC is pneumatosis intestinalis seen on an abdominal X-ray (Fig. 49.2). Portal venous air is sometimes present and usually signifies extensive intestinal injury, although by itself it is not necessarily an indication for operation (Fig. 49.3).

Preoperative Preparation

Initial treatment for NEC includes bowel rest, antibiotics, and supportive care. All feeds should be held, a sump-type oro- or nasogastric tube should be placed to intermittent suction. Broad-spectrum antibiotics should be given to cover both gram negatives and gram positives. Coverage for anaerobes with metronidazole or clindamycin is usually unnecessary but this decision is usually made based on institutional preferences. Supportive care should include intravenous fluid resuscitation, transfusions of red blood cells and platelets, and, if necessary, endotracheal intubation and blood pressure support with dopamine.

The timing of operative treatment is based on experience and good judgment and as such is often somewhat subjective. Intra-abdominal free air, a discolored abdomen due to meconium peritonitis, and abdominal wall erythema are the only universally agreed-upon indications for operative intervention. The combination of persistent or worsening thrombocytopenia or acidosis despite adequate resuscitation,

C.A. Gingalewski (✉)
Department of General Surgery, George Washington University, Children's National Medical Center, Washington, DC, USA
e-mail: CGingale@cnmc.org

P. Mattei (ed.), *Fundamentals of Pediatric Surgery*,
DOI 10.1007/978-1-4419-6643-8_49, © Springer Science+Business Media, LLC 2011

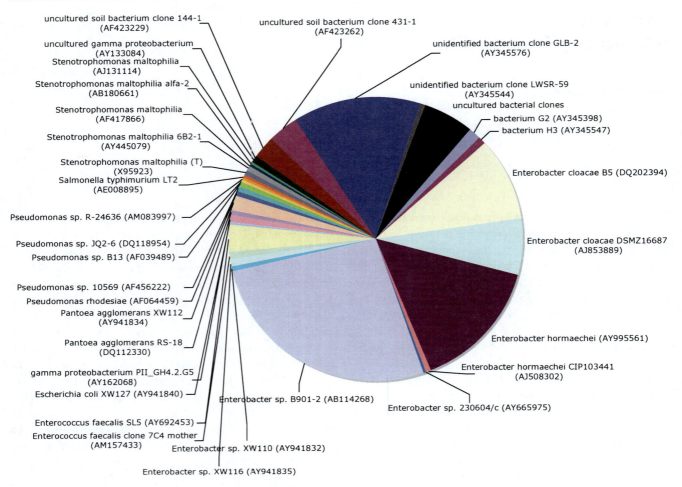

Fig. 49.1 Bacterial microbiome in rectum of NICU infants. Rectal swabs taken from neonates in NICU for routine culture assessment for MRSA were then analysed by identifying bacterial genomic sequences.

This reveals numerous bacteria that cannot be identified by conventional culture mechanisms. Results shown for a single infant and include numerous pathogenic bacteria

especially in the presence of a fixed loop (which is likely severely ischemic) on X-ray, would prompt most pediatric surgeons to operate (Table 49.1). It is important to stress that surgical intervention does not halt the disease process, but rather treats the end result of the process of NEC.

Surgical Technique

Peritoneal Drainage

If the infant cannot be stabilized, bedside exploration should be considered. These infants are also good candidates for peritoneal drainage, which is not usually definitive but can facilitate ongoing resuscitation efforts. In general, unstable infants weighing less than 1,000 g are the best candidates for peritoneal drainage. These drains can be placed at the bedside with local anesthesia or with intravenous sedation. The skin

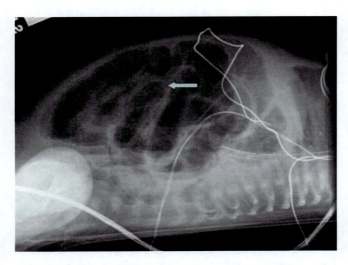

Fig. 49.2 Pneumatosis intestinalis in necrotizing enterocolitis. Abdominal cross table radiograph of infant with NEC. Note severe pneumatosis intestinalis identified by *arrow*

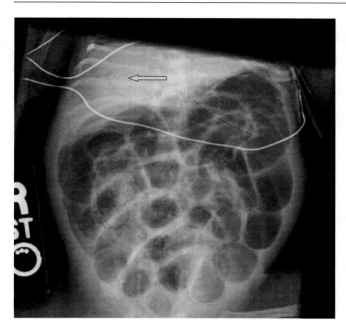

Fig. 49.3 Portal venous air in severe necrotizing enterocolitis. AP abdominal X-ray of infant with NEC demonstrating portal venous gas (*arrow*)

Table 49.1 Indications for operation in necrotizing enterocolitis

Absolute indications
Free intraperitoneal air
Abdominal wall erythema
Discolored abdomen
Meconium in processus vaginalis
Relative indications
Persistent or worsening acidosis or thrombocytopenia
Fixed loop on abdominal radiograph

of the abdomen is prepared and a small skin incision is made in the right lower quadrant. The abdominal cavity is entered bluntly using a curved hemostat and the meconium and air are evacuated. Warm saline irrigation can be used as an aide to remove intraperitoneal meconium. Using a red rubber catheter, 10–15 mL/kg can be used to wash out the peritoneal cavity. A ¼-in. penrose drain is then placed into the peritoneal cavity aiming for the left upper quadrant. The drain is sutured in place including the muscle of the abdominal wall using a nylon suture. The infant is then monitored and resuscitation is continued. If the infant shows no further improvement over the next 8–24 h, laparotomy should be performed.

In a prospective randomized trial, Moss et al. showed that in infants less than 34 weeks gestation and weighing less than 1,500 g with NEC complicated by perforated viscus, the type of operation performed, drain or laparotomy, did not influence overall survival, length of hospital stay, or need for parenteral nutrition at 90 days after surgery. Despite the fact that the study groups were relatively small and therefore true differences between treatment groups may not have been borne out, this study has attempted to answer an important and still

somewhat controversial question in neonatal surgery. For most pediatric surgeons, peritoneal drainage remains an option that is potentially useful in selected cases.

Laparotomy

In the stable infant, laparotomy is ideally performed in the operating room. A transverse supra-umbilical incision provides access to the entire abdominal compartment in these small infants. One must be cautious with the premature liver. Because the liver capsule is poorly developed, incidental injury can easily lead to life-threatening exsanguination. If there are no umbilical lines in place, the falciform ligament should be transected and ligated to avoid inadvertent liver injury.

The bowel is usually distended and care should be taken while entering the peritoneal cavity. Bloody ascites is frequently encountered and usually indicates the presence of gangrene. The bowel should be delivered from the abdomen and thoroughly examined. The goal of operative treatment of NEC should be to preserve intestinal length. Only bowel that is clearly gangrenous should be removed.

There are several approaches in these infants to preserve length and avoid more than one stoma. If only a single segment of bowel is involved, the best option is to resect the clearly dead bowel and create an ostomy of the proximal end. These stomas are typically brought out through one end of the primary incision and do not need to be formally matured. The stoma should be sutured to the fascia of the abdominal wall and the edges of the stoma will roll back on their own over time. If the resected bowel is in the proximal jejunum, one might elect to close it with a large hemaclip and return several days later to perform a primary anastomosis if no further diseased bowel is encountered and the baby is hemodynamically stable. Any infant instability or additional bowel compromise should warrant an ostomy, regardless of how proximal it might be.

In an infant with multiple sites of involvement, the "clip and drop back" technique championed by Jay Grosfeld is an excellent option: the gangrenous bowel segments are resected and the ends of each segment are closed with a large hemaclip. The abdomen is closed *en masse* and the baby is brought back to the NICU for further resuscitation. The abdomen is re-explored between 24 and 72 h later, depending on the physiologic status of the infant. Those who remain persistently acidotic, thrombocytopenic, or hypotensive likely have additional gangrenous intestine and should return promptly to the OR. Those who improve should return in 48 or 72 h. At the time of the second-look procedure, if the bowel is viable, a proximal ostomy is created and all distal segments are reanastomosed. This leaves the infant with only one ostomy to close at a later date. The more proximal the ostomy, the sooner the bowel should be put back in continuity (usually 4–6 weeks) to avoid parenteral nutrition-associated cholestasis and ongoing liver damage.

The most common sites of involvement are the terminal ileum and colon and 44% of infants have involvement of both. Twenty percent of infants have NEC totalis, which is involvement of more than 75% of the intestine. Most pediatric surgeons would deem this condition nonsurvivable, but there are those who believe that intestinal transplantation is an increasingly viable option.

Postoperative Care

The postoperative care of these infants requires the collaboration of neonatologists and surgeons. It consists of supportive care with IV fluids and parenteral nutrition and treatment of sepsis with antibiotics and, if necessary, vasopressors. Intestinal decompression is continued with a nasogastric tube until return of bowel function. Antibiotics are generally continued for 7 days postoperatively, but there are no good data to support how long to continue antibiotics after resection.

Ongoing hemodynamic instability, thrombocytopenia, and acidosis warrant re-exploration in these infants, especially if there are concerns regarding bowel of questionable viability left at the first exploration.

A frequent early complication is necrosis of the ostomy. This can be due to ongoing intestinal ischemia at the level of the ostomy, a fascial defect that is too small, postoperative edema or use of epinephrine for blood pressure support. If the ostomy becomes necrotic below the level of the skin, early revision is warranted if the infant is stable. The goal should be to achieve the ability to enterally feed the infant.

Recurrent NEC is a rare event, occurring in approximately 5% of cases. It generally occurs 5–6 weeks postoperatively and one must rule out the presence of an intestinal stricture as a contributing factor. Intestinal strictures occur in one third of infants with NEC. Symptoms include feeding intolerance, abdominal distention, and intestinal obstruction. Strictures can also occur in the defunctionalized colon, most commonly in the sigmoid. Routine radiographic examination of the colon is necessary prior to reversal of any ostomy.

Terminal ileal strictures can be harder to define and are also best diagnosed by a barium enema with a specific attempt to reflux barium into the terminal ileum. This should be discussed ahead of time with your pediatric radiologist. These should be resected and a primary anastomosis can usually be safely performed.

Other complications can occur, the most severe of which is short bowel syndrome. This is generally defined by the length of bowel remaining after resection, and the bowel length should be routinely measured in these babies to determine the likelihood of insufficient bowel length. Traditionally, the likelihood of eventually achieving full enteral feeds is good if there are 15 cm bowel remaining with the ileocecal valve, or 30 cm bowel without the ileocecal valve. Though preservation of questionable intestine is commonly done, one must keep in mind that there is normally an increase in intestinal length with age and the younger the infant, the more overall growth there is yet to occur.

If there is colon remaining, all infants should undergo a contrast enema prior to stoma reversal to rule out a distal stricture. An upper intestinal contrast series is not necessary if the infant is tolerating feeds. However, if full feeds are not achieved the better part of valor is to perform a contrast follow through to make sure there are no other anatomic problems in the proximal intestinal tract.

Other ostomy complications include prolapse, bleeding, and peristomal hernias. It is critical to have a nurse trained in ostomy care for these infants given their fragile thin skin. Most late complication of ostomy creation can be addressed at the time of ostomy reversal.

Liver failure due to prolonged exposure to parenteral nutrition is a significant problem for these infants, especially in the setting of short bowel syndrome. Studies have demonstrated that up to one half of infants requiring surgical intervention for NEC remain on TPN more than 90 days after surgical intervention. This requires indwelling catheters, which also places the infants at risk for catheter related sepsis events.

Late outcomes are also common, including an unexpectedly high incidence of neurodevelopmental impairment. Infants recovering from NEC have a 25% chance of developing microcephaly and serious developmental delays, especially in psychomotor development (hypotonia, spasticity). This is thought to be in part secondary to the effect of lipopolysaccharide on developing white matter of these infants via TLR4 activation.

We have seen steady improvements in survival of premature infants, most notable in those who weigh less than 1,000 g and those born at a gestational age of less than 28 weeks. This can be attributed to progress in the critical care of very low birth weight infants. Unfortunately, the overall survival for infants with NEC remains largely unchanged from 30 years ago: for those treated medically it is between 65 and 90%, while for those requiring surgery it is between 50 and 75%.

Summary Points

- NEC is most common intra-abdominal emergency in infants.
- The is a lower incidence in babies who are breast fed.
- Medical management is first line therapy: bowel rest and decompression, IV fluids, antibiotics.
- Infants who require surgery have a worse prognosis.
- The goal of surgery is to preserve intestinal length.
- There are numerous surgical options: bowel resection, ileostomy, clip and drop back, placement of drains.
- In a single randomized prospective study, infants treated by peritoneal drain or laparotomy had the same outcomes.
- Malabsorption, liver failure, line infections, stricture, ostomy complications, TPN dependence, short bowel syndrome and neurodevelopmental delays are common.
- There is a need to identify preventive strategies for NEC (probiotics, toll-like receptor blockade).

Editor's Comment

Primary therapy for the infant with NEC is medical. Surgery is indicated only for complications: perforation, bowel necrosis, overwhelming sepsis. Nevertheless, the decision to operate or continue observing can be difficult. In general, it is better to err on the side of performing an operation, rather than waiting until it is too late to make a difference. Though some have attempted to use ultrasound or paracentesis to improve the accuracy of the decision-making process, ultimately the decision is based on the good judgment that comes with experience.

Drainage has fallen into disfavor of late, but it is still occasionally useful, specifically for the extremely critically ill micropremie with an obvious perforation who cannot be transported safely, needs more time for resuscitation, or has other anomalies that need to be sorted out. In these cases, peritoneal drainage can buy some time. But drainage is rarely definitive and one can justify performing a laparotomy within 48–72 h whether the patient has improved (able to safely undergo a more formal surgical procedure) or deteriorated (requires an escalation in therapy). It is useful to make small bilateral lower quadrant incisions, irrigate with warm normal saline solution, and place three ¼-in. Penrose drains: one that passes between the two incisions, one that reaches into the pelvis from the right-sided incision, and one that passes into the left upper quadrant from the left side. In this way, the abdomen is widely drained, injury to the liver is avoided, and the drains can be sutured to themselves rather than the patient.

We have all seen infants months after a laparotomy for NEC with a huge and misshapen scar that crosses the entire upper abdomen and is usually cross-hatched with suture scars. Some surgeons question why such an incision is ever necessary. A small right lower quadrant incision that rarely needs to cross the midline, unless there is bowel to be dealt with

near the ligament of Treitz, is all that is necessary. The entire abdomen in a small premature is available through this incision and the ultimate appearance is far superior. The stoma and mucous fistula can be brought out in the corners of the wound and the incision can be closed at the level of Scarpa's fascia and steri-strips or cyanoacrylate glue. There is also a tendency to wait an excessively long time to close the stoma in these infants, which puts them at risk for parenteral nutrition-associated liver failure. Closing the stoma usually allows them to tolerate enteral nutrition sooner. If the patient is stable, one should consider closing the stoma within 2 weeks of resection. There is even a trend towards performing a primary anastomosis at the original operation and avoiding a stoma altogether. At any rate, continuity should be re-established no more than 4–6 weeks after resection.

The most difficult situations arise when the there is loss of nearly the entire small intestine. Despite recent advances in the field of intestinal transplantation, it is still very unlikely that an infant with essentially no intestine can be made to survive long enough to undergo a successful transplant. Nevertheless, it will likely soon be a viable option and every case should be assessed individually and with intimate involvement of the parents. It is also important to remember that the length of the remaining intestine does not tell the whole story: some of it was likely ischemic and though now viable, it might be dysmotile or otherwise dysfunctional.

Differential Diagnosis

- Isolated ileal perforation

Diagnostic Studies

- Abdominal X-rays, including an AP and either x-table lateral or decubitus view.
- Contrast studies to rule out stricture formation if fails feeding advancement.
- Contrast enema to rule out a stricture of colon prior to ostomy takedown.

Parental Preparation

- Gut rest and antibiotics may fail to halt the progression, but surgery might be required.
- This is a major operation requiring bowel removal and stoma formation, with the possibility of short bowel syndrome and death.
- May require second-look operation.
- Short bowel syndrome and its nutritional consequences.
- Prolonged use of parenteral nutrition.
- Intubation and mechanical ventilation will be required in the postoperative period, possibly for a prolonged period.

Preoperative Preparation

- □ Type and crossed for blood and platelets
- □ Informed consent

Technical Points

- A decision regarding peritoneal drainage vs. laparotomy needs to be made.
- Supraumbilical transverse incision for laparotomy.
- Caution with liver, divide falciform ligament.
- Intestine is friable and distended, and requires careful handling to avoid injury to the viable portion.
- To preserve bowel length, resect only obviously gangrenous or otherwise nonviable bowel.
- Create a single stoma, if possible.

Suggested Reading

Ein SH, Marshall DG, Girvan D. Peritoneal drainage under local anesthesia for perforation from necrotizing enterocolitis. J Pediatr Surg. 1977;12:963–7.

Gribar SC, Richardson WM, Sodhi CP, et al. No longer an innocent bystander: epithelial toll-like receptors signaling in the development of mucosal inflammation. Mol Med. 2008;14(9–10):645–59.

Ishihara S, Rumi MA, Ortega-Cava CF, et al. Therapeutic targeting of toll-like receptors in gastrointestinal inflammation. Curr Pharm Des. 2006;12(32):4215–28.

Lin HC, Hsu CH, Chen HL, et al. Oral probiotics prevent necrotizing enterocolitis in very low birth weight preterm infants: a multicenter, randomized, controlled trial. Pediatrics. 2008;122(4):693–700.

Moss RL, Dimmit RA, Barnhart DC, et al. Laparotomy versus peritoneal drain for necrotizing enterocolitis and perforation. N Engl J Med. 2006;354(21):2225–34.

Salhab WA, Perlman JM, Silver L, et al. Necrotizing enterocolitis and neurodevelopmental outcome in extremely low birth weight infants <1000 g. J Perinatol. 2004;24:534–40.

Touloukian RJ. Ischemic gastroenterocolitis in infants:clinical aspects and thoughts on its etiology. Conn Med. 1973;37(5):229–34.

Touloukian RJ, Smith GJ. Normal intestinal length in preterm infants. J Pediatr Surg. 1983;18(6):720–3.

Chapter 50
Short Bowel Syndrome

Thomas Jaksic, Brian A. Jones, Melissa A. Hull, and Shimae C. Fitzgibbons

To appreciate the complexities of short bowel syndrome, the disease should be thought of as a functional disorder rather than a simple anatomical abnormality. For this reason, many experts in the field now prefer the term intestinal failure (IF) as a more appropriate description of this syndrome. The true definition of IF is a reduction of the functional gut mass below the level needed to allow adequate digestion and absorption of enteral fluids, electrolytes, and nutrition to sustain hydration, electrolyte balance, and growth.

Attempts have been made to identify a length of bowel that can be used to define the disorder. Though 35 cm of small bowel in the neonate is often cited as the minimum amount of intestine needed to attain enteral autonomy, rare case reports describe children with less than 20 cm of small bowel who have been fully weaned from parenteral nutrition. Therefore, while still a valuable tool in the overall management of these children, measured bowel length is not always the most reliable predictor of rehabilitative potential. The duration of parenteral nutritional therapy is a common way of stratifying severity, with children who need it for more than 90 days typically considered to have severe disease.

The most common causes of short bowel syndrome in children are a reduction in the overall length of functional bowel due to necrotizing enterocolitis (NEC), intestinal atresia, gastroschisis (with or without volvulus), or malrotation with midgut volvulus. Less common surgical causes include cloacal extrophy, and segmental volvulus. There are other causes of intestinal failure, in which the overall length of intestine is normal, but its absorptive capacity or motility is altered. These include Hirschsprung disease involving the small intestine, chronic intestinal pseudo-obstruction, congenital intestinal epithelial dysplasia (tufting enteropathy), and microvillus inclusion disease. Regardless of the initial insult, the functional result is the same, namely an inability to sustain nutrition and hydration in an enterally autonomous fashion.

Pediatric surgeons are often among the first physicians to encounter these patients. It is important to maintain a sense of vigilance in the operating room when treating infants with illnesses that can lead to short bowel syndrome. Every effort should be made to preserve the maximum amount of viable small intestine. With long-term multidisciplinary therapy and aggressive bowel rehabilitation, many infants with very short lengths of remnant bowel can eventually be transitioned from parenteral nutrition.

Diagnosis

The first diagnostic test that should be performed whenever possible in a patient with short bowel syndrome is an accurate intra-operative measurement of the viable small bowel. This should be done at the time of any major bowel resection. This measurement should incorporate any and all small bowel, from the ligament of Trietz to the ileocecal valve in normally rotated patients, or from the duodenum to the ileocecal valve in malrotated patients. By convention, this is measured along the antimesenteric border. It is important to document the presence or absence of the ileocecal valve and the type of bowel resected, as ileal resections carry the risk of unique micronutrient and vitamin deficiencies more so than jejunal resections. Finally, a detailed diagram of anastomoses and stomas is a valuable resource for others who will assist in the care of these patients.

Once patients are out of the initial postoperative resuscitation period, are hemodynamically stable, and have demonstrated some return of bowel function, slow enteral advancement should be started. As feeding tolerance will vary, this trial will serve both diagnostic and therapeutic functions. Excessive stool output is common and should prompt stool studies to assess for carbohydrate and fat malabsorption. Typically, this involves checking the stool for reducing substances, pH, and fecal fat. Reducing substances greater than 1% and pH below 5.5 are indicative of carbohydrate malabsorption. Because infectious sources of diarrhea are also common in patients with short bowel syndrome, stool viral and bacterial cultures and testing for *Clostridium*

T. Jaksic (✉)
Department of Pediatric Surgery, Children's Hospital Boston, Boston, MA, USA
e-mail: tom.jaksic@childrens.harvard.edu

P. Mattei (ed.), *Fundamentals of Pediatric Surgery*,
DOI 10.1007/978-1-4419-6643-8_50, © Springer Science+Business Media, LLC 2011

difficile toxin should be routine whenever stool output is greater than 8–10 stools per day or 2 mL/kg/h.

Feeding intolerance that manifests itself as emesis or high gastric output should prompt an investigation for an anatomic source of obstruction. As a majority of children with short bowel syndrome have undergone prior laparotomy, they carry a risk of adhesive bowel obstructions. This is especially true in children with a history of NEC, as this condition is known to be associated with tenacious adhesions. In addition, children with multiple resections and anastomoses are at risk for anastomotic stricture formation. Gastroschisis especially is associated with poor motility. Upper GI with small bowel follow-through is a standard study used to delineate the remnant anatomy of children with short bowel syndrome. It can be helpful for gross estimation of bowel length and assessment of stricture formation, bowel dilation, or possible adhesive obstruction. A contrast enema is helpful in visualizing the colon if no stricture is seen by upper GI. Very rarely, a child could have another process, such as Hirschsprung disease, responsible for a more distal obstruction. Suction rectal biopsy can be used to confirm the presence of ganglion cells in the rectum. A contrast enema should also be done in every patient with a stoma prior to restoration of bowel continuity.

The initial laboratory work up of a patient with short bowel syndrome should be comprehensive and include: a complete blood count, serum chemistries, liver function tests, and coagulation profile. These studies should be monitored weekly in a child who is hospitalized on parenteral nutrition. As a patient transitions to outpatient care, it is important to monitor labs on a schedule that allows problems to be detected and treated early, while minimizing blood draws.

Recent studies have found serum citrulline concentrations to be a reliable biomarker of intestinal failure in children with short bowel syndrome. Citrulline levels have been shown to correlate with bowel length, enterocyte mass and the ability to achieve independence from parenteral nutrition. All studies to date have shown that a child with a persistent citrulline concentration of less than 12 μmol/L is very unlikely to wean from parenteral nutrition. Serum citrulline is not a static measurement and can increase significantly during bowel adaptation, therefore repeat measurements should be obtained every 3–6 months.

Treatment

The medical management of children with short bowel syndrome can be quite complex, with an array of nutritional strategies and medications now available. Having a team of clinicians dedicated to the care of these children is an integral factor in their success. Recently published data have shown significantly improved survival (90 vs. 70%) in a group of patients treated by a multidisciplinary intestinal rehabilitation program when compared with a control group. This study highlighted the importance of having a team of nutritionists, pharmacists, social workers, nurses, gastroenterologists, and surgeons to care for these medically complex children.

Nutrition

Neonates and children with short bowel syndrome should be placed on parenteral nutrition early, typically within 1–2 days after surgery, when post-operative fluid requirements and electrolytes have stabilized. Though parenteral nutrition is a life-saving intervention in children with short bowel syndrome, most children will experience some degree of liver dysfunction if it is used for a long time. Steps to reduce the risk of parenteral nutrition-induced cholestasis include avoiding overfeeding, cycling parenteral nutrition when possible to allow cyclic release of enteric hormones, meticulous central venous catheter care to minimize infections, and rapid transition to enteral feedings. Another strategy that appears effective is reducing the amount of lipid given parenterally to 1 g/kg/day.

Once liver dysfunction has developed, the most successful strategy for reversing it is a transition to full enteral feeding, with most patients normalizing direct bilirubin within 3–4 months. When this is not possible, children with cholestasis (direct bilirubin >2 mg/dL) should receive a reduced amount of lipid (typically 1 g/kg/day) or be switched to an omega-3-based lipid formulation dosed at 1 g/kg/day. Both of these reduced lipid strategies have been shown to be effective in reversing parenteral nutrition-associated liver dysfunction. Omega-3 lipids might also result in a decrease in peroxidative hepatic damage. It is important to continue to monitor liver function in children after reaching parenteral nutrition independence as the ALT has been shown to remain elevated despite full enteral tolerance and normalization of direct bilirubin. This sometimes indicates ongoing or fixed liver injury that is not reflected by direct bilirubin alone.

Enteral nutrition should be started postoperatively only after the patient is hemodynamically stable and has evidence of bowel function. If possible, we try to begin with breast milk. Continuous feeds tend to be better tolerated in children with intestinal failure. We start enteral feeding rates at 10 mL/kg/day of continuous feeds with a goal of advancing by 10 mL/kg one to two times a day. The rate of feed advancement, however, is highly individual and often limited by signs of high stool output, gastric residuals, or signs of malabsorption. If a child's stool output exceeds 2 mL/kg/h when averaged over a 6-h period, feeds should be held until output decreases, then resumed at the rate most recently tolerated. Children with a very proximal stoma can have very high output as feeds are advanced. If a mucous fistula or loop ostomy is present, it is often possible to place a small feeding tube into the distal loop of bowel and refeed the proximal output through this tube. This can allow the child to reach full enteral nutrition while conditions for ostomy closure are not ideal.

Feeds should be advanced to the rate required to maintain hydration. When this rate has been reached, the caloric density of the enteral formula can be increased sequentially by 2 kCal/kg/day until consistent weight gain is attained. Caloric requirements for children with short bowel syndrome are higher than those for weight-matched healthy controls due to obligate malabsorption. Once a child reaches enteral feeds of 20 mL/kg/day, parenteral nutrition volume can be reduced by a rate proportional to feeding increases. It may be necessary to give more concentrated parenteral nutrition during this time to meet caloric requirements. Intravenous lipids are the most calorie-dense portion of parenteral nutrition, and are usually the final parenteral solution to be stopped.

Due to the high incidence of disordered intestinal motility in children with short bowel syndrome, even those patients who tolerate a significant portion of enteral calories can have high G-tube losses or outputs that make fluid supplements necessary. Replacement fluids may be in the form of a fixed intravenous amount per day if the output is consistent, or can be a portion of the output replaced every few hours (0.5 mL replacement for every 1 mL of gastric output). The replacement fluid should be similar in electrolyte composition to the fluid lost. Thus, it is sometimes beneficial to measure gastric fluid or stomal electrolytes.

Once a child has reached full enteral nutrition on continuous feeds, transition to bolus feeds can be attempted. Children who are able to eat by mouth are allowed to take as much of the feed as possible orally, after which the remainder is given as a bolus through a feeding tube. Because many of these children have an oral aversion, it is important to involve feeding specialists in the multidisciplinary team as early as possible. They can evaluate for coordinated swallowing and make recommendations regarding the consistency of food that can be tolerated without aspiration. As children develop the ability to tolerate oral feeds, we often allow ad libitum feeding throughout the day, and then supplement the remaining needed calories by continuous overnight feeds through a feeding tube. If a child has been tolerating full enteral nutrition without difficulty and does not have lactose intolerance, it might be possible to convert to cow's milk once the child is at least 12 months corrected gestational age.

Medications

During the course of enteral advancement, and even after reaching full enteral nutrition, a variety of medications may be needed to facilitate enteral tolerance.

Histamine-2 blockers and *proton pump inhibitors* are routinely used in this population to suppress gastric fluid secretion. As small bowel resection often results in gastric hypersecretion and hypergastrinemia, all patients should be started on an H_2 blocker while NPO after surgery. The H_2 blocker can be replaced with a proton pump inhibitor if there is evidence of persistent reflux or heme-positive gastric output. These medications are typically stopped after the patient is on enteral nutrition and has no evidence of reflux.

Cholestasis and liver dysfunction are frequent and potentially deadly complications of prolonged parenteral nutrition. Though the best method of reversing cholestasis is a transition to full enteral nutrition, there is a medication that can help to reduce liver damage in these children. In small studies, *ursodeoxycholic acid* has been shown to reduce transaminase levels and hyperbilirubinemia in children with early liver dysfunction. We start children on ursodeoxycholic acid at the first biochemical signs of liver dysfunction, and continue this medication until normalization of serum bilirubin and transaminase levels.

As intestinal adaptation progresses, many children with short bowel syndrome develop dilated bowel loops. This can worsen motility and increase gastric output. If a child with short bowel syndrome is unable to advance on feeds due to vomiting or high gastric output and an anatomic cause such as stricture has been excluded, a prokinetic agent such as metoclopramide or erythromycin should be started. If this fails, it might be necessary to switch to post-pyloric feeds, leaving a gastrostomy tube or nasogastric tube in place to decompress the stomach. Once a child reaches full feeds in this manner, an attempt should be made to convert back to gastric feeding. It is crucial to closely monitor hydration status, including electrolytes and renal function, as children with a large amount of gastric output frequently require additional fluid replacement.

Cisapride is a pro-kinetic agent initially approved in 1993 for refractory GERD, but also found to be effective in short bowel syndrome. Serious potential side effects including prolongation of the QT interval and death due to cardiac arrhythmias led to its removal from the market in 2000. It is currently only available for compassionate use.

Antimotility agents, such as loperamide (Immodium), can be quite useful to slow transit time in children with short bowel syndrome. These are typically begun once a patient has shown a pattern of intolerance to enteral advancement, with stool output rising above 2 mL/kg/h. Antimotility agents should be started at a low dose and increased until stool output falls to acceptable levels. It is important to rule out infection (rotavirus, *C. difficile*) prior to starting therapy with antimotility drugs.

The addition of *fiber* to the diet in patients with the colon in continuity has several benefits. Fiber serves as an energy source for colonocytes and enhances sodium and water absorption, thereby reducing fluid losses.

Surgical Technique

Central Venous Access

At the time of the initial procedure, careful thought should be given to inserting a central venous catheter if the patient will tolerate placement and is not septic. Children with short bowel syndrome require long-term central access for parenteral nutrition and so a tunneled line (Broviac catheter) is preferred. Infants, especially prematures, often require a cutdown to access the vein (saphenous, external or internal jugular). Preferably, this procedure should be done without ligating the vein, as these children tend to have central venous access problems throughout their lives. The importance of good hygiene and line care cannot be overemphasized, as these children are already at high risk for central line infections due to bacterial translocation.

Enteral Feeding Access

Most children with short bowel syndrome will require a feeding tube and placement should be considered if the child is undergoing another surgical procedure. In children with a very short length of bowel who are unlikely to wean quickly from parenteral nutrition, a gastrostomy tube facilitates continuous enteral feeding and is less prone to dislodgement than a nasogastric tube. If necessary, a gastrostomy tube can later be converted to a gastrojejunal tube.

Restoration of Bowel Continuity

Depending on their location, stomas can contribute to electrolyte imbalance and dehydration. In order to facilitate bowel rehabilitation, restoration of continuity is a necessity. The ideal timing for restoration of bowel continuity will vary for each patient. Often surgeons wait at least six weeks after the most recent laparotomy to minimize the vascularity of adhesions. Respiratory and hemodynamic stability, as well as optimal nutritional status, are all pre-requisites for re-operation. At the time of surgery, the distal intestinal specimens should be examined by a pathologist for the presence of ganglion cells.

Bowel Lengthening Procedures

Two bowel lengthening procedures, the Bianchi or Longitudinal Intestinal Lengthening and Tapering (LILT) and Serial Transverse Enteroplasty (STEP), are used in patients with short bowel syndrome who have failed enteral advancement despite maximal medical management. Both procedures require a segment of dilated bowel to be technically feasible. These procedures can significantly increase intestinal length and have been shown to facilitate parenteral nutrition independence and decrease bacterial overgrowth in a dilated segment, though the intestine tends to re-dilate after either procedure. Ongoing research is being performed to best identify those patients who will garner maximum benefit from intestinal lengthening procedures. Neither procedure should be done in the setting of severe liver disease as these patients should be directed toward combined liver/intestine transplantation.

The Bianchi procedure is a bowel lengthening procedure first described in 1980. The mesentery of the dilated segment of bowel must be carefully separated into two leaves. The dilated bowel is then bisected longitudinally along the axis of the mesenteric border. This creates two concentric bowel segments, which are then anastomosed in an end-to-end handsewn fashion. It requires symmetrical bowel dilatation.

The STEP procedure is a bowel lengthening procedure first described in 2003. A small window is created in the mesentery through which a gastrointestinal anastomosis stapler is placed, perpendicular to the longitudinal axis of the mesentery and fired partly across the bowel. This is repeated at measured intervals, with each staple line approaching from the direction opposite to the preceding one, creating a zigzag channel which is of constant diameter throughout. It has three primary indications: as a bowel lengthening procedure in patients with short bowel syndrome who have failed to progress to enteral autonomy despite maximal medical therapy, to reduce refractory bacterial overgrowth in a dilated intestinal segment, and at the time of the initial procedure in neonates with intestinal atresia and a dilated proximal bowel loop who are at significant risk for developing short bowel syndrome as an alternative to traditional tapering or resection. The STEP procedure is advantageous because it requires no bowel anastomoses (thus has a reduced risk of leak or stricture), it can be used on a bowel segment with varying degrees of dilatation, and it can be used after a prior Bianchi, or even after a prior STEP. Both Bianchi and STEP procedures have equivalent outcomes, with over 50% of patients reaching enteral autonomy, although in a single-center study comparing the two procedures, STEP was associated with fewer post-operative complications.

Small Bowel and Multivisceral Transplantation

Transplantation is an established salvage strategy for children with short bowel syndrome who fail bowel rehabilitation. Although transplantation can be a life-saving procedure for these patients, it still has many complications, including a high rate of rejection and infectious complications from the high level of immunosuppression required. Currently, graft and patient survival following transplantation of the intestine with or without liver transplantation is approximately 70% at 3 years.

Postoperative Care

The long-term management of short bowel syndrome involves close monitoring of growth and nutritional status, while employing strategies to minimize complications. The adaptive phase of bowel rehabilitation can be a lengthy process, particularly in children, extending from months to years following their most recent surgery. Bowel adaptation, including increased bowel surface area, enterocyte and villous hyperplasia, and increased crypt depth, can lead to gradually increasing enteral tolerance in children who were once dependent on parenteral nutrition.

During this long course of bowel adaptation, however, the clinician must remain alert to signs and symptoms of vitamin and mineral deficiencies. The loss of the distal ileum can lead to deficiencies in the fat-soluble vitamins A, D, E and K. Deficiencies in vitamin A cause corneal ulcerations, night blindness, and growth delay, while vitamin D deficiency leads to poor growth and bowing of the extremities. Extreme vitamin E deficiency causes retinopathy and nerve symptoms, including paresthesias, ataxia and depressed deep tendon reflexes. Vitamin K deficiency results in coagulopathy, causing petechiae, ecchymosis or frank bleeding. Finally, zinc is an important constituent of many enzymes involved in most major metabolic pathways, including nucleic acid synthesis. Signs of deficiency include growth failure, skin changes, hair loss, and delayed wound healing.

Essential fatty acid deficiency can result from long-term dependence on parenteral nutrition. Linoleic and linolenic acid deficiency can manifest as dermatitis and alopecia, ultimately resulting in overall growth retardation. Finally, micronutrient levels should be checked frequently in this population, as poor enteral absorption may require supplementation in the parenteral nutrition.

Persistent anemia is another potential problem in patients with short bowel syndrome. The GI tract is a common site of blood loss and this should always be ruled out as a source with gastric aspirate and stool studies for occult blood. Endoscopy is often helpful in identifying bacterial overgrowth, ulceration, or allergic enteritis. Without an obvious GI source of blood loss, further work up, including reticulocyte count, iron studies, and copper and B12 levels should be checked to identify a possible micronutrient deficiency as a source of the anemia.

Low levels of calcium and vitamin D can cause metabolic bone disease, resulting in osteopenia and bone fractures. Close monitoring of vitamin levels in addition to bone density testing is recommended. If a patient is found to be osteopenic by dual X-ray absorptiometry, treatment with supplemental calcium and vitamin D should be initiated. In certain cases, consultation with an endocrinologist is clearly warranted.

Central venous catheter infections remain a frequent and deadly complication of short bowel syndrome. Great care must be taken to ensure sterile technique with each catheter placement and subsequent access. While signs and symptoms such as change in mental status, spiking fevers, erythema, and purulent drainage from the catheter insertion site are clear indicators of catheter related infection, the clinical presentation is often more subtle. Increased fussiness might be the only indication and therefore a high index of suspicion must be maintained.

We recommend checking blood cultures both peripherally and through the catheter, in addition to a CBC. An elevated C-reactive protein level is sometimes an early sign of line infection. If any question remains as to the patient's stability, we proceed with admission to the hospital and administration of broad spectrum intravenous antibiotics while the lab processes the blood cultures. Failure to respond to broad spectrum antibiotics should prompt additional cultures, altering the antibiotics, and possibly the addition of anti-fungal agents. Recurrent fevers or progressing signs of sepsis despite adequate antibiotic therapy should prompt removal of the catheter. Fungal infections usually warrant prompt line removal. The catheter tip can be sent for culture to confirm the diagnosis and obtain specific speciation and antibiotic sensitivities.

Maintaining this low threshold for catheter infections will allow early treatment initiation and possibly prevent the need for line replacement. Often, treatment with intravenous antibiotics for 14 days results in a sterilized line. This approach will help minimize the need for multiple catheters and subsequent exhaustion of access sites over a lifetime.

The use of tunneled catheters and the avoidance of catheter placement in the groin have been associated with a decreased rate of infection. The standardization of sterile technique has also been beneficial. The use of ethanol locks on a daily or every-other-day regimen has shown promise in further limiting central line infections.

Intestinal infections, including *C. difficile* and Rotavirus, occur relatively frequently in children with short bowel syndrome. Stool studies should be sent routinely when patients present with increased stool output or worsening abdominal symptoms. It is important to note that the infection can occur within the patient's remaining small intestine in addition to the more common site within the colon. Many children with short bowel syndrome are chronically colonized with

C. difficile, but if it is present without symptoms, treatment is not indicated. As with non-short bowel syndrome patients, the mainstay of treatment for symptomatic *C. difficile* disease is metronidazole or oral vancomycin.

Bowel adaptation usually results in bowel dilation presumably to increase absorptive surface area. This, combined with disrupted intestinal motility, leads to the development of bacterial overgrowth. In turn, bacterial overgrowth may worsen a patient's already compromised intestinal absorption. Presenting signs and symptoms include abdominal distension, vomiting, diarrhea, abdominal pain, central venous catheter infection, fatigue, and growth failure. Esophagogastroduodenoscopy with sampling of duodenal fluid for culture and sensitivity can be helpful in targeting antimicrobial therapy. Treatment typically involves the initiation of a rotating schedule of oral antibiotics. Common regimens include metronidazole and ciprofloxacin, with time off between treatment. Caution is advised with the use of probiotics, as bacterial translocation of *Lactobacillus acidophilus* has been reported.

Short bowel syndrome, or intestinal failure, is a complicated medical and surgical condition that is best treated with a comprehensive multidisciplinary approach. Although it is still has substantial associated morbidity and mortality, many recent improvements in therapy promise to improve the outcomes and quality of life for these children.

Summary Points

- "Intestinal failure" is gradually replacing "short bowel syndrome" as the preferred term, as it includes those with poor intestinal function and poor motility.
- Intestinal failure results from a variety of congenital and acquired conditions, especially necrotizing enterocolitis, intestinal atresia, and malrotation with volvulus.
- Morbidity and mortality result from nutritional deficiencies, infectious complications, and end-stage liver disease.
- A multidisciplinary approach to care is critical for successful intestinal rehabilitation.
- A lifetime of close follow-up is warranted in any child with short bowel syndrome.

Editor's Comment

Surgeons who care for patients with short bowel syndrome need experience, creativity, and patience, as the first several months of life for these infants are often marked by frustrating trial and error, frequent complications, unexpected downturns, and extremely slow progress, with the added pressure of trying to "beat the clock" vis-à-vis parenteral-nutrition induced liver failure. Although a multi-disciplinary approach appears to be best, it is important that the team have a unifying philosophy regarding the care of these children. Frequent changes in course or abandoning a particular therapy before giving it a chance to work only worsens the frustration and can further harm the child.

As a general rule of thumb, newborns with more than 60 cm of intestine are likely to wean from parenteral nutrition, those with less than 40 cm are unlikely to become independent enteral feeders without intervention, and those between 40 and 60 cm have an intermediate prognosis. Children with intestinal failure due to NEC are the most difficult to predict as the bowel that remains after resection is often injured due to ischemia and therefore dysfunctional. Most also seem to be able to tolerate more feeds when bowel continuity has been established, making it desirable to close an enterostomy as soon as possible. While full-length bowel dilatation is a welcome sign of bowel adaptation and allows the child with short gut to have a bowel-lengthening procedure, segmental bowel dilatation can be the result of a specific problem (stricture, adhesion, segmental dysmotility) and the cause of a problem (bacterial overgrowth, pseudo-obstruction, pain), and upper GI contrast and motility studies are not especially accurate in distinguishing a true obstruction from a pseudo-obstruction. Given the pressure to advance enteric feeds, one should have a low threshold to explore the abdomen and perform a lysis of adhesions in these children when the possibility of a stricture or adhesion remains and antibiotics are not effective in relieving symptoms.

Most pediatric surgeons trained in a certain era are partial to the Bianchi bowel-lengthening procedure, and, in the right patient, it clearly works – children are often able to wean from parenteral nutrition and they generally do well. But it is becoming increasingly clear that the STEP operation is easier to perform, is probably better tolerated, and also has excellent results. The STEP has clearly become the bowel-lengthening procedure of choice for children with short bowel syndrome who have developed adequate adaptation-associated bowel dilatation.

Preoperative Preparation

☐ Labs, including liver function tests, PT/INR, PTT, type and screen.

☐ Consider concomitant medical issues as many of these patients are premature and have chronic lung disease.

☐ Broad spectrum preoperative antibiotics.

☐ UGI/barium enema to rule out stricture prior to re-anastomosis.

☐ Consider liver biopsy during any abdominal procedure in a patient on parenteral nutrition >90 days or with evidence of liver dysfunction.

Technical Points

• Accurately document residual bowel length – the measurement should incorporate any and all small bowel from the ligament of Trietz to the ileocecal valve, measured along the anti-mesenteric border.

• Document presence or absence of the ileocecal valve, and type of bowel resected (ileum or jejunum).

• Create a loop ostomy or mucous fistula if possible (rather than Hartmann's pouch) to allow for distal refeeding.

• To conserve access sites when placing a cutdown CVC, do not ligate the vein.

Diagnostic Studies

– Contrast enemas and upper GI studies with small bowel follow-through are often part of the initial work up.

– Upper and lower endoscopy with quantitative cultures and biopsies are also useful, particularly after the development of specific complications.

– Manometry may be helpful in certain cases of suspected dysmotility.

Parental Preparation

– Parents should expect a long hospitalization and the potential for multiple complications.

– Though seemingly "unnatural," continuous tube feeds are often the only way to facilitate bowel rehabilitation and adaptation.

– Small bowel transplantation might someday be the treatment of choice for children with intestinal failure but the complication rates and long-term survival are not yet at the levels that would make it an acceptable first-line therapy.

– Parenteral nutrition is often the only way to keep patients alive while enteral feeding is advanced to gola, but it is associated with many complications and because of liver disease cannot be relied upon for the long term.

– Bowel-lengthening procedures are available but cannot be attempted until the bowel is sufficiently dilated, which usually takes several months.

Suggested Reading

Andorsky DJ, Lund DP, Lillehei CW, Jaksic T, Dicanzio J, Richardson DS, et al. Nutritional and other postoperative management of neonates with short bowel syndrome correlates with clinical outcomes. J Pediatr. 2001;139(1):27–33.

Buchman AL. Etiology and initial management of short bowel syndrome. Gastroenterology. 2006;130:S5–15.

Ching YA, Gura K, Modi B, Jaksic T. Pediatric intestinal failure: nutrition, pharmacologic, and surgical approaches. Nutr Clin Pract. 2007;22(6):653–63.

Goulet O, Ruemmele F. Causes and management of intestinal failure in children. Gastroenterology. 2006;130:S16–28.

International STEP Data Registry. http://www.childrenshospital.org/cfapps/step/index.cfm. Accessed 25 Jan 2010.

Modi BP, Langer M, Ching YA, Valim C, Waterford SD, Iglesias J, et al. Improved survival in a multidisciplinary short bowel syndrome program. J Pediatr Surg. 2008;43(1):20–4.

Spagnuolo MI, Iorio R, et al. Ursodeoxycholic acid for treatment of cholestasis in children on long-term parenteral nutrition: a pilot study. Gastroenterology. 1996;111:716–9.

Chapter 51
Meconium Ileus

Peter Mattei

Meconium ileus is a small bowel obstruction in newborns caused by inspissated meconium. It is associated with cystic fibrosis in nearly all cases, and up to 20% of newborns with cystic fibrosis present with meconium ileus. Pancreatic enzyme insufficiency leads to extremely viscous meconium that cannot pass through the ileum, although why some infants with cystic fibrosis develop meconium ileus and others do not remains unclear. While often treatable by nonoperative means, many of these infants require laparotomy and can have life-long difficulty with bowel function related to their cystic fibrosis.

As with other causes of bowel obstruction, meconium ileus also can give rise to volvulus, ischemia and perforation. This form of "complicated" meconium ileus can occur in utero and may result in intestinal atresia, short bowel syndrome, or meconium peritonitis, which itself can cause ascites, intraperitoneal calcifications, or meconium pseudocysts. Antenatal ultrasonography may detect dilated loops of bowel or ascites, but except for the occasional case of polyhydramnios related to a more proximal volvulus or atresia, most are not detected before birth.

Diagnosis

Meconium ileus must be considered in the differential diagnosis of any newborn infant with a bowel obstruction or failure to pass meconium in the first few days of life. Most are otherwise well-appearing newborns who present with feeding intolerance or bilious emesis and progressive abdominal distension. The remainder of the physical examination is often unremarkable, and the family history is positive for cystic fibrosis in less than one third of cases. The differential diagnosis of newborn bowel obstruction includes intestinal atresia, volvulus, meconium plug syndrome and Hirschsprung disease.

The next step in the diagnostic workup is plain radiography of the abdomen. This usually demonstrates dilated air-filled loops of bowel consistent with a distal obstruction. A large amount of retained meconium with a ground-glass or soap bubble appearance (Neuhauser's sign) is highly suggestive of meconium ileus (Fig. 51.1). On the other hand, the presence of air-fluid levels makes the diagnosis less likely, given that the highly viscous meconium does not layer out very easily. The presence of peritoneal calcifications suggests the diagnosis of complicated meconium ileus with in utero perforation and subsequent meconium peritonitis.

Patients who are clinically well with no evidence of perforation or ischemic bowel should have a contrast enema. Prophylactic antibiotics (ampicillin and gentamicin) are given before the study is undertaken. A contrast study will confirm and treat meconium plug syndrome and might suggest the diagnosis of Hirschsprung disease or small left colon syndrome. If the findings include a microcolon, then a diagnosis of intestinal atresia or meconium ileus is most likely. It is in this situation that the pediatric radiologist should attempt to reflux the contrast material into the ileum. If there are filling defects in the terminal ileum consistent with pellets of meconium, then the diagnosis of meconium ileus is confirmed. Further retrograde progress of the contrast column will reveal a dilated segment of ileum filled with meconium (Fig. 51.2). The contrast itself may help to evacuate the meconium and thus alleviate the obstruction.

The choice of contrast material probably matters very little, although the traditional recommendation is diatrizoate meglumine (Gastrografin, Schering Diagnostics, Berlin, Germany). Gastrografin formulations in the past included a wetting agent, polysorbate 80 (Tween-80, Unigema, New Castle, Delaware), which perhaps made it a superior solvent for evacuation of inspissated meconium. Current formulations do not contain Tween-80 and although its high osmolarity (1,900 mOsm/L) might give it a theoretic advantage, many experienced pediatric radiologists feel that other agents are just as effective. Others have added Tween-80 or acetylcysteine to the contrast material and feel that this improves their results. Nevertheless, most of us are bound by the

P. Mattei (✉)
Department of General Surgery, Children's Hospital of Philadelphia, Philadelphia, PA 19140, USA
e-mail: mattei@email.chop.edu

P. Mattei (ed.), *Fundamentals of Pediatric Surgery*,
DOI 10.1007/978-1-4419-6643-8_51, © Springer Science+Business Media, LLC 2011

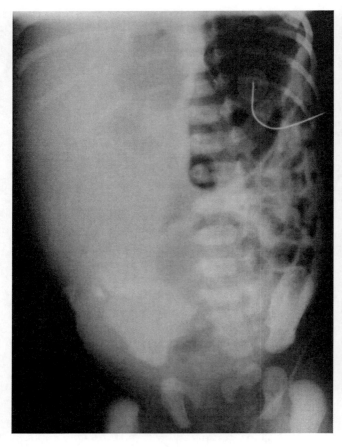

Fig. 51.1 Plain radiograph of a newborn infant with meconium ileus. Note the dilated loops suggestive of obstruction, the paucity of gas in the right lower quadrant and ground-glass appearance of meconium (Neuhauser's sign)

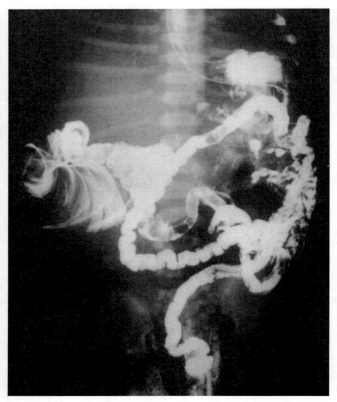

Fig. 51. 2 Contrast enema in an infant with meconium ileus. Note the small caliber of the unused microcolon, the filling defects in the ileum (meconium pellets) and the hugely dilated bowel proximal to the obstruction

preferences and experience of the radiologists at our respective institutions, which I suspect is the most important factor. Some radiologists are comfortable with the technique and are therefore more aggressive, whereas others are less likely to keep trying due to a concern about the potential for a bowel perforation. Up to half or more of the babies with meconium ileus may have a successful clean-out with the contrast enema, although in most centers the actual success rate is probably lower.

Total colonic aganglionosis (long-segment Hirschsprung disease) may present with a clinical and radiographic picture indistinguishable from meconium ileus. If the obstruction is alleviated by contrast enema, aganglionosis should be ruled out by suction rectal biopsy. If a laparotomy is performed, the appendix can be evaluated for the presence of ganglion cells, which will rule out colonic aganglionosis with rare exception. Not all babies with meconium ileus have cystic fibrosis, although the proportion who do not is unknown and likely varies considerably between populations. It is especially in these infants that aganglionosis coli needs to be ruled out with certainty.

The diagnosis of cystic fibrosis is best made by measurement of sweat chloride after the collection of sweat using pilocarpine iontophoresis, but the test is not always useful in the first few weeks of life. Genetic testing can be performed on a buccal smear or blood sample, but current genetic testing only detects approximately 97% of all mutations. Some state newborn screens include measurement of immunoreactive trypsinogen using standard blood collection blots, however the results often take weeks to process and need to be confirmed with more definitive tests because of a high false positive rate. Nonetheless, all infants with meconium ileus should be treated as though they have cystic fibrosis until the diagnosis can be ruled out with sweat chloride testing. General support and genetic counseling should be available for the families while the diagnosis is being confirmed.

Treatment

Nonoperative therapy is possible if the contrast enema is successful in clearing a significant amount of meconium, though sometimes the enema needs to be repeated. These patients are maintained on bowel rest initially. Adequate intravenous hydration is provided and is especially important if high-osmolarity enema solutions have been used. A typical management regimen is 10% acetylcysteine (Mucomyst) administered by orogastric tube at a dose of 10 mL every 6 h for 7–10 days. Acetylcysteine is a mucolytic that is very effective in loosening the viscous meconium in infants with meconium ileus. The contrast enema should be repeated if signs of obstruction recur. These infants also need to be assessed frequently for evidence of bowel perforation related to the obstruction or the enemas. When all signs of obstruction have resolved, enteral feedings can be started and advanced carefully. Pancreatic enzyme supplements are provided after feedings have started.

Some babies with meconium ileus complicated by in utero perforation can be treated nonoperatively, although most require laparotomy. An operation can be avoided in infants with peritoneal (or scrotal) calcifications on radiography who are presumed to have had meconium peritonitis but who show no signs of obstruction and are passing meconium without difficulty. A cautious feeding trial may be started while the cystic fibrosis work up continues. More often the calcifications are identified in an infant being evaluated for obstruction, in which case laparotomy is indicated without further studies.

Patients who fail nonoperative therapy should undergo laparotomy. The parents are informed that the goal is to remove the inspissated meconium but that a bowel resection, stoma, or tube ileostomy may be necessary depending on the operative findings. I prefer to make a transverse right lower abdominal incision, through which the ileum can be easily delivered and an ileostomy and mucous fistula can be brought out if necessary (Fig. 51.3). The cecum may need to be gently

mobilized, and the peritoneum should be protected from contamination with moistened gauze packs. Simple meconium ileus, with no evidence of perforation, volvulus, or atresia, is best treated by irrigation. An enterotomy is made on the antimesenteric border of the dilated ileum for instillation of irrigation solution and evacuation of the meconium. Although saline solution is used by some surgeons with good results, I prefer to use acetylcysteine. Acetylcysteine comes in 10 and 20% solutions and can be diluted with saline or water to a final concentration of 4%. A 10 or 12 French catheter is used to instill the irrigation solution, which usually allows the tar-like meconium to be removed easily from the bowel lumen through the enterotomy (Fig. 51.4). The acetylcysteine also should be instilled distally to allow further evacuation of meconium from the colon. After removal of the inspissated meconium, the enterotomy is closed transversely and an appendectomy is performed. The pathologist should be made aware that the appendix needs to be evaluated specifically for the presence of ganglion cells. Histologic examination of the appendix might also reveal mucous plugging of the crypts and exuberant intraluminal mucinous material, which are suggestive of cystic fibrosis. At the conclusion of the procedure, especially if a large amount of meconium was seen to pass into the colon, a gentle anal dilatation and rectal irrigation should be performed.

Although enterotomy and bowel irrigation is a useful approach in most cases of simple meconium ileus, a modified technique is occasionally necessitated by the operative findings. In the past, it was common practice to treat all infants with meconium ileus with an ileostomy. This was felt to be necessary to facilitate postoperative irrigation and evacuation of meconium. Although no longer used routinely, the various stoma operations described should be part of the armamentarium of the pediatric surgeon (Fig. 51.5). The Bishop-Koop ileostomy is a Roux-en-Y construct in which the distal limb is brought out as an end stoma and the

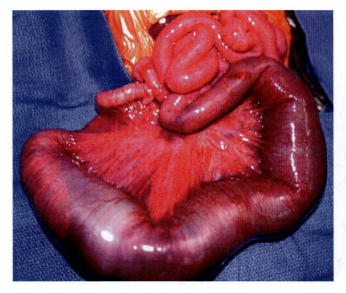

Fig. 51.3 Operative findings in a patient with meconium ileus. There is gradual tapering of the ileum, which is filled with inspissated meconium

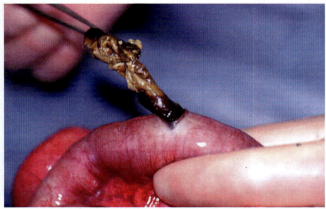

Fig. 51.4 The meconium has the consistency of tar and can be pulled out through the enterostomy in large pieces

Fig. 51.5 The operations described in the past for meconium ileus are mostly of historical importance but are occasionally useful in selected patients today. (**a**) The Mikulicz operation after resection of the dilated ileum. (**b**) The Bishop-Koop operation. (**c**) The Santulli-Blanc operation. (**d**) Tube ileostomy for postoperative irrigation (Reprinted with permission from Rescorla FJ, Grosfeld JL. Contemporary management of meconium ileus. World J Surg. 1993;117(3):318)

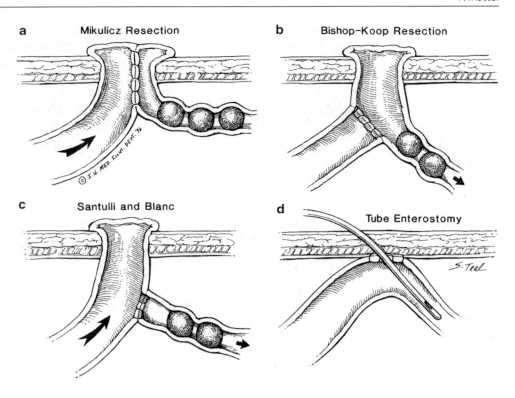

proximal bowel is anastomosed end-to-side. This procedure was commonly used in the past and produced excellent results. The Santulli-Blanc operation creates a proximal stoma and the distal bowel is sewn to it end-to-side. The Mikulicz operation was widely used at one time for various indications and consists of a double-barrel stoma in which the two ends are sutured together side to side for some length proximal to the end of the stoma. It was designed for bedside stoma closure in which the common wall was crushed and obliterated with a specially designed clamp and the bowel ends were closed over the top. This operation is rarely used today. A useful option is a tube ileostomy. A small-caliber rubber tube is placed through a small enterotomy and secured with a purse-string suture. The bowel is tacked to the fascia in standard fashion with the tube exiting through a small stab incision. This allows instillation of irrigant solution directly into the ileum without the creation of an ileostomy. Of course, a conventional end or loop ileostomy may be necessary if peritonitis or obstruction precludes a safe anastomosis after bowel resection or volvulus.

The approach to complicated meconium ileus is the same as for any complicated intestinal process and includes: an extensive lysis of adhesions, careful inspection of the bowel, possible bowel resection, if necessary, and evacuation of inspissated meconium. Perforations may be amenable to primary repair if a distal obstruction can be safely excluded. If a bowel resection is felt to be necessary, a judgment is made whether primary anastomosis is feasible or a stoma is necessary, based on the condition of the bowel, the likelihood of a distal obstruction and the overall condition of the patient. The fibrous wall of the pseudocyst is debrided without sacrificing viable intestine. Meconium peritonitis can cause obstruction due to adhesions, requiring extensive adhesiolysis. The adhesions are typically dense and very vascular. It is not necessary to perform a radical debridement of all meconium or calcified plaque that is encountered, as long as the obstruction is relieved. Appendectomy should be performed to rule out long-segment Hirschsprung disease and to avoid diagnostic confusion in the future. A gastrostomy should be considered in infants with complicated meconium ileus, especially if extensive bowel resection is necessary. Most infants will also need central venous access for parenteral nutrition during the postoperative period.

Postoperative Care

Patients are initially on bowel rest and are given acetylcysteine by gastric tube as described above for nonoperative management. Rectal irrigations may be necessary as well. Most eventually establish a normal stooling pattern and can be advanced on feedings within 1–2 weeks. Patients should be maintained on parenteral nutrition in the meantime.

Recurrence is uncommon and treatment can be attempted using contrast enema, if necessary. Reoperation may suggest the need for ileostomy and a more definitive workup for Hirschsprung disease.

Infants with meconium ileus require an extensive workup involving multiple pediatric subspecialists including: gastroenterologists, geneticists, pulmonologists, and pediatric surgeons. Family support should include access to counseling services and social work assistance. Patients are initially followed in the surgery office as after any major abdominal procedure, and the surgeon may need to become involved again later for issues related to feeding access, central venous access and stoma care. Stomas can be taken down after the customary 4–6 weeks, according to the usual criteria of adequate weight gain and resolution of symptoms. A distal contrast study should be performed to rule out obstruction prior to reanastomosis.

Short-term complications are uncommon in infants with simple meconium ileus. Long-term complications are generally those common to patients with cystic fibrosis. Patients also may present years later with bowel obstruction. Those with a history of meconium peritonitis or laparotomy may have obstruction due to adhesions or segmental volvulus, but other diagnoses need to be considered. For example, patients with cystic fibrosis are more susceptible to intussusception. The intussusception can be of the conventional ileocolic variety seen in patients under the age of 3 years, but also may be ileo-ileal and can occur in older children. Appendicitis appears to be more common in patients with cystic fibrosis, and when associated with perforation and phlegmon can be a cause of bowel obstruction or severe ileus. Inguinal hernias are also more common in this population and, as in other patients, can be a cause of obstruction due to incarceration. High-dose pancreatic enzyme supplementation has been associated with the development of colonic strictures. These are diagnosed by contrast enema and are usually treated with resection and anastomosis. Finally, older patients may develop meconium ileus equivalent, an obstruction caused by inspissated stool in the ileum and colon. Many of these patients can be treated initially with decompression and enemas, although some will require laparotomy. The cause is unknown but is presumably related to the high viscosity of intestinal mucus.

In summary, meconium ileus is a cause of bowel obstruction in the newborn and mainly affects infants with cystic fibrosis. The diagnosis is confirmed with contrast enema, which can sometimes also be therapeutic. Patients with complications related to the obstruction, including volvulus, perforation, or atresia, and those who fail nonoperative management require operative intervention. At laparotomy, the conventional approach for simple meconium ileus is to irrigate the bowel lumen with acetylcysteine through a small enterotomy, which facilitates evacuation of the highly viscous meconium. Patients with complicated disease may require bowel resection, tube enterostomy, or creation of a stoma, many varieties of which have been described over the years for management of the disease. Most patients respond well to therapy in the short-term but need to be followed closely for complications related to their underlying disease. This includes bowel obstruction, which has many potential causes in these patients.

Summary Points

- In the newborn with bowel obstruction, one must consider: meconium ileus, meconium plug syndrome, Hirschsprung disease, ileal atresia, and malrotation with midgut volvulus.
- Plain radiographs can give clues (e.g. large amount of stool in the right lower abdomen) but are often not diagnostic.
- Water-soluble contrast enema is diagnostic and may be therapeutic.
- If contrast enema fails to relieve the obstruction, laparotomy should be the next step.
- Technical points: right lower (or upper) quadrant incision, enterotomy with irrigation (4% acetylcysteine or saline), enterotomy closed transversely.
- Consider tube ileostomy for postoperative irrigations or ileostomy with mucous fistula.
- Nearly always associated with cystic fibrosis: sweat chloride analysis in *all* cases.
- Patients are best served by a team approach: neonatology, gastroenterology, genetics, pulmonology, and pediatric surgery.

Editor's Comment

Meconium ileus is nearly always due to cystic fibrosis and associated with the abnormal secretion or function of pancreatic digestive enzymes. The diagnosis needs to be considered in the differential diagnosis in any infant who presents with a clinical picture of intestinal obstruction in the immediate newborn period. After a thorough physical examination and baseline radiograph, the first step should include a water-soluble contrast enema performed by an experienced pediatric radiologist. This study is diagnostic and often therapeutic in infants with meconium ileus. It can also rule out other important conditions that are in the differential diagnosis. If the obstruction is not relieved by the enema then an operation is indicated. At laparotomy the meconium is evacuated through a small enterotomy, usually with the help of a solvent such as acetylcysteine, which is said to break the disulfide bonds that make the meconium especially glutinous. In the modern era, an ileostomy is rarely necessary and is avoided whenever possible. Children with cystic fibrosis who present with meconium ileus generally have a phenotype that includes mild respiratory illness but significant gastrointestinal difficulties throughout their lives.

Differential Diagnosis

- Meconium plug syndrome
- Hirschsprung disease
- Ileal atresia
- Malrotation with midgut volvulus

Diagnostic Studies

- Plain radiograph
- Water-soluble contrast enema
- Sweat chloride test for cystic fibrosis

Parental Preparation

- It is possible we will need to perform a bowel resection.
- A temporary ileostomy is sometimes necessary.
- There is a very high likelihood that the baby has cystic fibrosis, but we will need to confirm it with a sweat chloride test.
- Even if all goes well with this operation, there is the possibility of ongoing problems with constipation or recurrent obstruction later in life.

Preoperative Preparation

- ☐ IV hydration
- ☐ Type & screen
- ☐ N-acetylcysteine solution
- ☐ Informed consent

Technical Points

- A right lower quadrant transverse incision provides excellent exposure and can be used for an ileostomy should one become necessary.
- If an operation is indicated (contrast enema fails to relieve the obstruction), a procedure that includes enterotomy and irrigation with saline or dilute acetylcysteine should be considered first.
- The enterostomy should be placed in the dilated segment of bowel and closed transversely.
- If ongoing access to the bowel lumen is felt to be necessary for postoperative irrigations, consider placing an ileostomy T-tube.
- If there is no other available option, an ileostomy can be created, preferably a standard loop ileostomy or a Bishop-Koop type.

Suggested Reading

Del Pin CA, Czyrko C, Ziegler MM, et al. Management and survival of meconium ileus, a 30-year review. Ann Surg. 1992;215: 179–85.

Ein SH, Shandling B, Reilly BJ, et al. Bowel perforation with nonoperative treatment of meconium ileus. Pediatr Surg. 1987;22: 146–7.

Kao SCS, Franken Jr EA. Nonoperative treatment of simple meconium ileus: a survey of the Society for Pediatric Radiology. Pediatr Radiol. 1995;25:97–100.

Mak GZ, Harberg FJ, Hiatt P, et al. T-rube ileostomy for meconium ileus: four decades of experience. Pediatr Surg. 2000;35: 349–52.

Noblett H. Treatment of uncomplicated meconium ileus by Gastrografin enema: a preliminary report. Pediatr Surg. 1969;4:190–7.

Rescorla FJ, Grosfeld JL. Contemporary management of meconium ileus. World Surg. 1993;17:318–25.

Ziegler MM. Meconium ileus. Curr Prob Surg. 1994;31:731–77.

Chapter 52
Intussusception

John H.T. Waldhausen

Intussusception is a telescoping of the intestine into itself. It is one of the most common causes of abdominal pain in children under 5 years of age. The disease occurs most commonly in children between 6 and 18 months of age, but has been described in all age groups including babies in utero and in adults. Approximately half of all cases occur in the second 6 months of life, and 90% of all cases occur before 3 years of age.

Ileocecal intussusception is the most common form of the disease, though entero-enteric intussusception can also occur (Fig. 52.1). In all age groups, the etiology of ileocecal intussusception is most commonly unknown. Pathologic lead points such as a Meckel's diverticulum, intestinal polyp, lymphoma or other malignancy are more common in older children with intussusception. Likewise, entero-enteric intussusceptions are usually the result of another disease process such as cystic fibrosis (CF), Henoch-Schönlein purpura (HSP) or a pathologic lead point.

Diagnosis

Intussusception is often suspected by history and physical examination alone. Children with intussusception classically present with intermittent episodes of colicky abdominal pain. One minute the child is playing normally, and the next he or she is crying and in pain. This can often mystify the physician who is called to see a reported acutely ill child, only to find that the child appears quite well. Babies and younger children, who are less able to communicate verbally, might draw their knees up to the chest as the primary physical sign that they are experiencing abdominal pain. As the condition intensifies, the pain becomes more constant. Eventually the clinical picture progresses to that of a small bowel obstruction and, if not treated promptly, the child might develop the classic sign of "currant jelly" stools caused by mucosal sloughing. Vomiting often occurs and can result in dehydration. Another classic though less common (5–10%) presentation is the child with lethargy or somnolence, which can be a sign of dehydration but can also occur early in the course of the disease for reasons that are unclear.

On careful physical examination, an abdominal mass is palpable up to 85% of the time, though the abdomen is usually soft and otherwise benign. Rarely, the intussusceptum can protrude through the anus and resemble a prolapsed rectum (Fig. 52.2). The two entities are distinguished by digital examination. With intussusception, probing alongside the prolapsed mucosa will reveal mucosa of the rectum on the outside of the digit and mucosa of the intussusceptum medially. Rectal prolapse only allows the central lumen of the prolapsed mucosa to be probed. Peritonitis is a late finding and indicates intestinal necrosis or perforation.

Plain abdominal radiographs are often read as normal and therefore not very useful in either making or excluding the diagnosis. The classic finding of an adipose rose, which represents concentric rings of fat interspersed with air, is unusual; more frequently however a soft-tissue density is detected (Fig. 52.3). In some cases, the initial presentation includes evidence of a small bowel obstruction. These children present with vomiting and abdominal distension and have dilated loops of small bowel on X-ray. This presentation might alter the management of the patient as some radiologists are reluctant to attempt enema reduction in a child under 6 months of age who presents with obstruction because they are more prone to intestinal perforation. Likewise, plain radiographs cannot be relied upon to exclude the diagnosis of intussusception. They can occasionally suggest that the diagnosis of ileocecal intussusception is unlikely, but only when the cecum is completely filled with air or stool. However, even in this situation more definitive exclusion of the diagnosis might be necessary based on the clinical suspicion. If the history or physical examination findings support the diagnosis, the appropriate course of action should be another diagnostic test.

Ultrasound has become increasingly popular for making the diagnosis of intussusception and to determine whether

J.H.T. Waldhausen (✉)
Department of Surgery, University of Washington, Children's Hospital and Regional Medical Center, Seattle, WA, USA
e-mail: john.waldhausen@seattlechildrens.org

P. Mattei (ed.), *Fundamentals of Pediatric Surgery*,
DOI 10.1007/978-1-4419-6643-8_52, © Springer Science+Business Media, LLC 2011

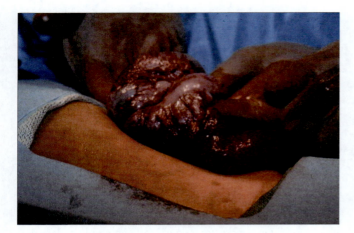

Fig. 51.1 Ileocolic intussusceptions

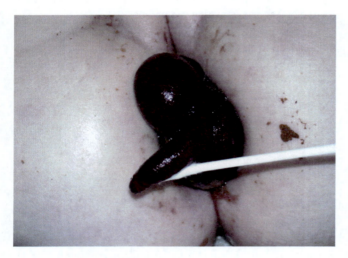

Fig. 51.2 Intussusception protruding from anus with intussuscepted appendix

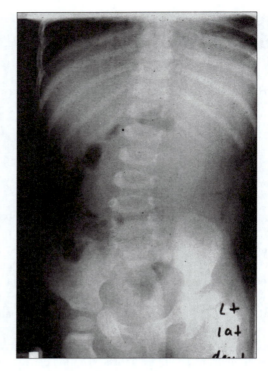

Fig. 51.3 Plain radiograph showing opaque mass associated with intussusceptions

the intussusceptum has been successfully reduced after attempts at air or hydrostatic reduction. If the diagnosis is confirmed by ultrasound, then a therapeutic contrast enema is usually the next step. The ability to reduce an intussusception is radiologist-dependent and there are several large studies showing that these children are less likely to need surgery if the radiologists are very experienced at achieving reduction. Rates of pneumatic reduction are reported as high as 94%, while success with hydrostatic reduction is usually somewhat less, typically in the 50–80% range.

Radiographic reduction is the procedure of choice in almost all children with ileocolic intussusception, unless there is a clear indication for laparotomy. Peritonitis, for example, is an absolute contraindication to enema reduction and is an unequivocal indication for laparotomy. On the other hand, reduction of an intussusception is possible even when the intussusceptum has prolapsed through the anus and in those who appear to have a bowel obstruction. There is

literature to suggest that radiographic reduction is less likely to be successful in children under 6 months of age, in those with symptoms for longer than 48 h, and in children who present with a bowel obstruction. However, we have had frequent success even in these groups of children.

There is often concern that the attempt at reduction will cause perforation, though the risk of perforation during enema reduction is actually quite small, reportedly on the order of 0.16–2.8%. If perforation does occur, it is most often due to a necrotic or already-perforated section of bowel becoming unmasked as the intussusception is reduced. This obviously mandates urgent operative intervention (Fig. 51.4).

Contrast studies are excellent at confirming the diagnosis, but it can be difficult to discern whether the intussusceptum has been completely reduced. The key finding needed to ascertain successful reduction is passage of contrast or air into the ileum. If this is not documented, reduction of the intussusceptum remains uncertain. A competent ileocecal valve adds to the confusion, particularly if the valve is edematous secondary to the intussusception. This presents as a residual, unreduced mass, which complicates the decision regarding the next step of care. In cases where the child already has a significant amount of air in the gastrointestinal tract before the application of an air enema, confirmation can be difficult. It may then be necessary to use barium contrast to track reflux back into the small bowel more effectively or to proceed with an ultrasound examination.

R/O Intussusception

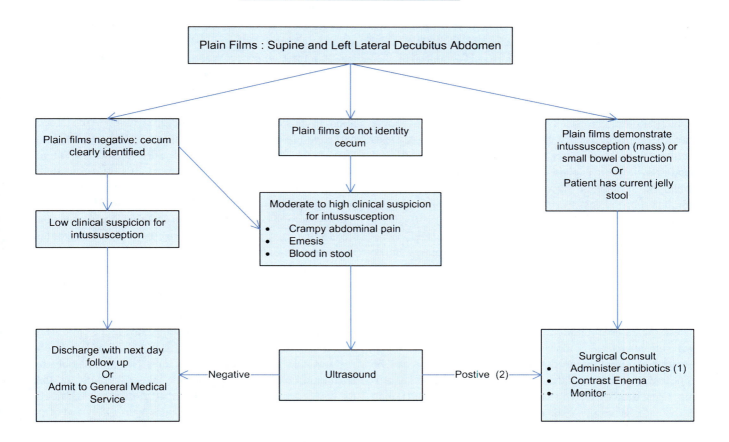

R/O Intussusception
-Start IV; give bolus NS 20cc /kg
    then run D5½ NS @1.5 maintenance

Plain Films : Supine and Left Lateral Decubitus Abdomen

Plain films negative: cecum clearly identified

Plain films do not identity cecum

Plain films demonstrate intussusception (mass) or small bowel obstruction
Or
Patient has current jelly stool

Low clinical suspicion for intussusception

Moderate to high clinical suspicion for intussusception
• Crampy abdominal pain
• Emesis
• Blood in stool

Discharge with next day follow up
Or
Admit to General Medical Service

Ultrasound

Negative

Postive (2)

Surgical Consult
• Administer antibiotics (1)
• Contrast Enema
• Monitor

(1) Antibiotic Administration
• If US **not** obtained:
      Patient < 6 months- administer cefoxitin **before** contrast enema
      Patient >6 months- administer cefoxitin **after** contrast enema
      if study is positive for intussuception
• If US positive for intussuception :
      Administer cefoxitin **before** contrast enema, regardless of age
(2) IF US positive, patient goes directly for contrast enema.

Fig. 51.4 Algorithm for treatment of intussusceptions

Children who present with a clinical picture suggestive of intussusception but whose imaging studies are negative are usually treated empirically for viral gastroenteritis. The differential diagnosis also includes various forms of infectious colitis, such as that caused by *Escherichia coli* 0157:H7, the cramping and bloody diarrhea of which can suggest the possibility of intussusception.

Treatment

Idiopathic Ileo-Colic Intussusception

All children with suspected intussusception should receive intravenous hydration. In most cases, it is appropriate to give intravenous antibiotics to cover colonic flora (second generation cephalosporin) prior to attempting radiographic reduction. However, the use of antibiotics in children with *E. coli* 0157:H7 is more likely to induce hemolytic uremic syndrome (HUS); therefore, in geographic areas such as the Pacific Northwest where there is a high incidence of *E. coli* 0157:H7-associated colitis, we recommend withholding antibiotics until the diagnosis of intussusception has been confirmed. We make an exception for children under 6 months of age, based on studies from the Hospital for Sick Children in Toronto that show intestinal necrosis and perforation are more likely to occur in this age group than in the older child. In regions where *E. coli* 0157:H7-induced bloody diarrhea is less common, administration of antibiotics prior to the contrast enema is appropriate and recommended.

The decision as to which method of intussusception reduction should be done is best left to the radiologist. Some have better experience with liquid contrast media such as barium while others prefer to use air. In some cases, clinical factors will influence the decision. Pneumatic reduction might be difficult in the child who presents with a large amount of bowel gas or evidence of a bowel obstruction. The air already filling the intestinal loops makes it difficult to visualize the air column placed by the radiologist and to adequately determine successful reduction. In these cases, liquid contrast is often more useful. Air enemas are typically performed to insufflation pressures of 80 mmHg for younger infants and 110–120 mmHg for older infants and children. As the child cries during the study, pressures fluctuate widely. These increases in intraluminal pressure may be one reason why air reduction is more often successful. If the initial attempt at reduction is not successful, the study can be repeated several hours later. Liquid contrast material is usually introduced by placing a catheter in the rectum and taping it in place. A secure seal is crucial for attaining adequate pressure without leakage from the anus. Gentle inflation of a balloon and tightly taping the buttocks around the tube usually provides a tight seal. Pressures are generated by elevating the bag of contrast up to 4 ft above the child. Several attempts should be made with the bag at this height, allowing the contrast to drain between attempts.

Successful reduction in the radiology suite is defined as the observation of contrast passing freely into the small bowel. If this is noted, the child should be admitted overnight for antibiotics and observation. We usually do not feed the child until the next morning in order to allow the swelling that accompanies the intussusception to reduce. This delay in feeding usually prevents the cramping abdominal pain that some children experience due to the swollen Peyer's patches and bowel wall edema, both of which can mimic an obstruction or recurrent intussusception. Once feeds are restarted and advanced to goal diet, the child can be discharged, usu-

ally the same day. The parents are informed that there is 5–7% risk of recurrent intussusception and encouraged to return if the abdominal pain recurs. If the child's symptoms return despite an apparently successful reduction, the child is taken back to radiology and the study is repeated to ascertain whether the intussusception has recurred. In the event it has, then hydrostatic or pneumatic reduction is again attempted.

If reflux back into the small bowel is not seen during radiographic reduction, the assumption is either that the intussusception is not completely reduced or that the child has a competent ileocecal valve. A key observation is that the ileocecal valve might be edematous and can appear to be a small, residual intussusception. Repeating the contrast study several hours after the first study might help clarify this situation, because this allows time for the swelling in the ileocecal valve to resolve. If intussusception reduction is still not discernible, the surgeon must decide whether to simply observe the child, operate, or perform a radiographic study such as ultrasound or an upper GI contrast study with small bowel follow through. Each of these avenues has its own merits and might depend in part on experience with, and confidence in the radiologist performing the study and his or her interpretation of the findings.

If an obstruction persists, then the child will need operative reduction. This is typically performed with an open technique, but is increasingly being done laparoscopically. Laparoscopy is especially useful when reduction cannot be confirmed radiographically, potentially saving the child from an unnecessary laparotomy. Historically, the standard teaching was that the intussusception must be reduced only by pushing on the leading edge of the intussusceptum and that the bowel should never be pulled apart. Nevertheless, laparoscopic surgeons routinely pull the ends apart safely and often successfully.

When performing the open operation, it is important to know how far the radiologist was able to reduce the intussusceptum. This knowledge informs the placement of the incision, which is optimally placed in the right upper or right lower quadrant, depending on the size of the child and how far the intussusceptum was reduced. During an open operation, the intussusceptum must usually be delivered outside of the abdominal cavity in order to reduce it effectively. Once the intussusceptum is delivered, the leading portion of the intussusceptum is gently squeezed in order to push it toward the ileocecal valve for eventual reduction. Careful monitoring for serosal splitting during this reduction is essential, as this is a prelude to perforation and might indicate the need for resection. Once the bowel is reduced, it is quite common for the terminal ileum to be purple and hemorrhagic, and for an enlarged Peyer's patch to be present. This "patch" feels like a thickened disc of tissue on the antimesenteric surface of the terminal ileum. To the uninitiated, this might appear to be a tumor or other pathologic lead point and will often foster the urge to biopsy or resect the mass. The enlarged Peyer's patch, however, is probably the cause of the intussusception and is likely due simply to a viral illness. Given time, the swelling will resolve and no treatment is necessary. The ischemic appearance of the bowel will usually begin to abate within 10–20 min. Keeping the bowel warm and moist helps hasten the process. If the bowel appears necrotic or there is a perforation, than a resection and primary anastomosis is needed.

When the bowel is successfully reduced, many surgeons are taught to remove the appendix, because the abdominal incision could cause confusion by suggesting that an appendectomy had been performed. It is also important to look for pathologic lead points such as a Meckel's diverticulum or intestinal polyp or duplication, especially in the older child. Any of these findings would require excision or resection depending on the lesion. The post-operative management is similar to that of any child undergoing a laparotomy.

Recurrence of intussusception occurs in 5–7% of radiographically reduced cases and in roughly 2% of surgically reduced patients. If the intussusception was originally reduced radiographically, a repeat attempt at radiographic reduction is made. If the child was surgically reduced and the recurrence occurs fairly soon after the operation, it can be somewhat disconcerting to send the child back for a contrast enema or pneumatic reduction while the appendiceal stump is still fresh. In our experience however, if the radiologist is appropriately informed about the recent operation, then rupture of the stump is unlikely.

A delayed recurrence suggests the possibility of a pathologic lead point, but this remains somewhat controversial. Most occur within 6 months of the original intussusception. Some surgeons allow three or four recurrences before considering operative intervention; some might allow even more recurrences if considerable time elapses between episodes because idiopathic intussusception is the most common root cause even in the older age group. But if the episodes are closely spaced over the course of days or weeks, the probability of a lead point increases and should prompt a more rapid decision to operate.

When a child returns to the operating room for recurrent intussusception after having been operatively reduced the first time, the surgeon will again attempt to reduce the intussusceptum without bowel resection. If successful, a search is then launched to seek a pathologic lead point. The terminal ileum can be sutured to the side of the cecum for four to five centimeters in cases of surgical recurrence after an initial surgical reduction in order to fix the bowel and prevent further ileocolic intussusception.

Entero-Enteric Intussusception

While most commonly occurring in the terminal ileum and cecum, intussusception can occur anywhere in the small intestine. A more proximal intussusception usually cannot be diagnosed or reduced with a contrast enema. In this case, ultrasound is clearly more useful. Unlike classic ileo-cecal intussusception, the entero-enteric intussusception is not usually due to a viral illness. Various other disease processes such as CF or HSP might predispose the child to small bowel intussusception. Intussusception in the CF population usually occurs between 4 and 16 years of age. The diagnosis of HSP is usually made by identifying the purpuric rash that occurs in 95% of cases. In our experience, ultrasound is sensitive and accurate in confirming the diagnosis in these patients, whereas CT is not. What appears on CT to be a clear case of small bowel intussusception is not always confirmed in the operating room, which can be disconcerting. Consequently, in cases where CT suggests intussusception, a confirmatory ultrasound is appropriate and allows for the patient's symptoms to be evaluated before going to the operating room. In some instances, a contrast small bowel follow-through study is needed to determine whether or not there is a bowel obstruction. Occasionally, cases of intussusception due to HSP or CF may be reduced by barium or air, however most require operative reduction.

There are other situations in which intussusception is rare but can nevertheless occur. Postoperative intussusception accounts for between 1 and 6% of all reported cases of intussusception, particularly following the resection of Wilms tumor or other retroperitoneal tumors and is usually located in the small bowel. Though the pathophysiology is not clear, some evidence suggests that it may be due to altered intestinal peristalsis after surgery. Postoperative intussusception typically occurs after the first week post-operatively. A pathologic lead point is seldom the cause. Intussusception can also occur in neonates, 75% of which are associated with a lead point. Enema reduction is unusual for these cases, and most require an operation to reduce the intussusceptum and resect the lead point. Intussusception can also occur in adults, and, in the developed world, the cause is due to a lead point up to 90% of the time. Approximately one half of these lead points are due to malignancy. Colo-colonic intussusception has such a high incidence of associated malignancy that some reports suggest that no attempt at intussusception reduction should be made, and that these malignant lesions should undergo resection.

Summary Points

- Ninety percent of cases occur in children under 3 years of age.
- Ileocecal intussusception is the most common form, most commonly caused by a viral illness.
- In older children, idiopathic/viral is still the most common cause, but the presence of a pathologic lead point needs to be considered.
- History and physical examination suggest the diagnosis: intermittent severe abdominal pain (every 15–20 min) with intervening periods of being asymptomatic.
- Bowel obstruction and currant jelly stool are late findings.
- Either barium or air contrast studies confirm the diagnosis and are often therapeutic. Antibiotics are given prior to or just after the radiographic study depending on the regional concern for *E. coli* 0157:H7 infection. Ultrasound is gaining increased use as a screening tool and may be better at discerning the enteroenteral intussusception.
- If the intussusception is successfully reduced by radiology, the child is admitted overnight for antibiotics and has feedings advanced the next morning.
- If the intussusception is not reduced hydrostatically or pneumatically, the child must be operatively reduced.
- Intussusception recurs in 5–7% of children radiographically reduced and 1% of those surgically reduced.

Editor's Comment

Intussusception is impossible to exclude with certainty by history, physical examination, laboratory studies or plain radiographic images either alone or in combination. In fact, if intussusception has been mentioned as a possibility and no other diagnosis can been confirmed, some feel very strongly that it absolutely must be ruled out using either ultrasound or contrast enema. If intussusception is confirmed, the next step is contrast enema, the type of which (air or liquid) should be determined by the radiologist, not the surgeon. Some radiologists insist that a surgeon be present "just in case" of a perforation, even though this is never an indication to perform surgery in the radiology suite or to take a child directly to the OR without first being resuscitated and properly prepared. Perhaps the most important role of the surgeon in these situations is to maintain a calm and commanding presence while patient and parents are being prepared for a trip first back to the ED or ward and then soon thereafter to the OR. Even after a perforation, ileostomy should almost never be necessary, as a primary anastomosis, except in the most extraordinary of circumstances, is almost always able to be done quickly and safely.

I routinely perform surgical reduction laparoscopically and feel that it is enormously preferable to laparotomy. Besides the usual benefits of smaller incisions, quicker recovery, and less conspicuous scarring, perhaps the thing I like most about the approach is that it nicely disproves yet another formerly sacrosanct surgical dictum ("never *ever* pull the bowel apart"). I still perform an appendectomy, possibly out of habit, but I believe there is little harm done and that it might prevent recurrence or appendiceal colic (due to scarring in the appendix) in the future. Performing a biopsy

(or, worse, a resection) when one encounters an edematous or hemorrhagic "mass" in the wall of the cecum or ileum is a common "rookie mistake," though it should not discourage one to look carefully for a potential lead point.

Children over the age of five with classic ileo-colic intussusception pose a challenge, as do children of any age who develop more than one recurrence. A diligent search for a lead point (US, CT, endoscopy) is reasonable, but I do not believe either is an absolute indication for laparotomy or bowel resection. Obviously, a great deal of clinical experience and good judgment is needed in such cases. On the other hand, small bowel intussusception is always pathologic and should prompt at least a diagnostic laparoscopy to rule out lymphoma, Meckel's diverticulum, polyp, tumor, or vascular malformation (blue rubber bleb syndrome is an example). A short period of observation (12–24 h, if there are no signs of sepsis or peritonitis) is reasonable when a small bowel intussusception occurs in patients who have recently undergone a retroperitoneal dissection (Wilms tumor) or those with HSP, as it can occasionally resolve spontaneously in these patients.

Differential Diagnosis

- Appendicitis
- Viral illness and gastroenteritis
- Hemolytic uremic syndrome
- Rectal prolapse

Preoperative Preparation

☐ Intravenous antibiotics (second generation cephalosporin):
- If <6 months old, give before contrast enema.
- If >6 months old in geographic areas where *E. coli* 0157:H7 is endemic, give only after intussusception has been confirmed; in other areas, give before.

☐ If radiographic reduction is unsuccessful, consider another attempt in 4–6 h, or proceed with operative reduction.

☐ Intravenous hydration.

☐ If there is vomiting or evidence of obstruction, place a nasogastric tube.

☐ Informed consent.

Technical Points

Laparotomy

- Right-sided transverse incision above or below level of umbilicus
- Deliver the mass from the abdomen
- Reduce intussusception by pushing on the intussusceptum
- Warm moist packs for 10–20 min to assess perfusion and viability
- Check for pathologic lead point. (Don't be fooled by hypertrophied Peyer's patch!)

Laparoscopy

- Standard techniques
- Gently pull the bowel apart to reduce the intussusception
- If unable to reduce, bowel resection and primary anastomosis.
- Ileostomy should rarely, if ever, be necessary.

Parental Preparation

- Possible bowel resection due to necrosis or perforation
- Probable primary anastomosis
- Possibility that the intussusception reduced simply by placing child under anesthesia
- Small chance of recurrence
- The appendix will likely be removed empirically.

Suggested Reading

Bratton SL, Haberkern CM, Waldhausen JHT, Sawin RS, Allison JW. Intussusception, hospital size and risk factors for surgery. Pediatrics. 2001;107:299–303.

Daneman A, Navarro O. Intussusception. Part 1: a review of diagnostic approaches. Pediatr Radiol. 2003;33:79–85.

Daneman A, Navarro O. Intussusception. Part 2: an update on the evolution of management. Pediatr Radiol. 2004;34:97–108.

Kaiser AD, Applegate KE, Ladd AP. Current success in the treatment of intussusception in children. Surgery. 2007;142:469–77.

Meyer JS, Dangman BC, Buonomo C, et al. Air and liquid contrast agents in the management of intussusception: a controlled, randomized trial. Radiology. 1993;188:507–11.

Navarro O, Daneman A. Intussusception. Part 3: diagnosis and management of those with an identifiable or predisposing cause and those that reduce spontaneously. Pediatr Radiol. 2004;34:305–12.

Navarro O, Daneman A, Chae A. Intussusception: the used of delayed repeated reduction attempts and the management of intussusceptions due to pathologic lead points in children. AJR Am J Roentgenol. 2004;182:1169–76.

Wong CS, Jelacic S, Habeeb RL, et al. The risk of hemolytic uremic syndrome after antibiotic treatment of Escherichia coli 0157:H7 infections. N Engl J Med. 2000;342:1930–6.

Chapter 53
Meckel's Diverticulum

Melvin S. Dassinger, III

In 1809, the German anatomist Johann Meckel the Younger described the structure that now bears his name and postulated its embryologic origin. The embryonic midgut is connected ventrally to the yolk sac via the vitelline duct, also known as the omphalomesenteric or omphaloenteric duct. Normally regressing between the fifth and seventh weeks of gestation, persistence of a portion of the vitelline duct on the antimesenteric side of the intestine results in one of several anomalous structures either alone or in combination. Meckel's diverticulum is probably the most common, but others include vitelline sinuses, cysts, fibrous cords from the intestine to umbilicus, and omphaloenteric fistulas. The right and left vitelline arteries originate from the primitive dorsal aorta and travel with the omphalomesenteric duct. The left involutes while the right becomes the superior mesenteric artery and provides a terminal branch to the diverticulum. Obliterated vitelline artery remnants can persist as fibrous bands from the mesentery to the abdominal wall, providing a potential focus of volvulus or obstruction.

Meckel's diverticulum (Fig. 53.1) represents the most common congenital anomaly of the gastrointestinal tract. It is a true diverticulum, containing all layers of normal intestine, and is frequently seen in patients with other congenital anomalies such as cardiac defects, esophageal atresia, malrotation, duodenal atresia, Hirschsprung disease, or omphalocele. For reasons that are unclear, males have a higher incidence and are more likely to become symptomatic.

The "rule of 2s" is a mnemonic often applied to Meckel's diverticulum. Two percent of the population has this anomaly and most manifest symptoms before 2 years of age. The diverticulum measures roughly two inches in length and is located within two feet of the ileocecal valve, although this distance is variable. Two types of heterotopic mucosa are commonly found within the diverticulum: gastric and pancreatic; however, colonic mucosa, endometriosis, and hepatobiliary tissue have been found as well. More than half of patients who are symptomatic have gastric mucosa within the diverticulum.

Presentation

More than 95% of patients with Meckel's diverticula remain asymptomatic. When symptoms occur, they are primarily related to hemorrhage, obstruction or inflammation and these symptoms usually correlate with age. The most common presentation is painless gastrointestinal bleeding in an infant or young child. Meckel's diverticula account for nearly 50% of cases of lower gastrointestinal bleeding in children. Although the hemorrhage often ceases without intervention, it can be massive and transfusion is frequently required. The source of the bleeding is a peptic ulcer resulting from direct exposure to the acid produced by ectopic gastric mucosa. The ulcer is frequently found at the base of the diverticulum near the junction of the heterotopic gastric mucosa and normal ileum. *Helicobacter pylori* does not play a significant ulcerogenic role in Meckel's diverticula.

Bowel obstruction is the second most common complication of Meckel's diverticula and the most common manifestation of a vitelline duct anomaly in infants. The obstruction can occur by one of several mechanisms: intussusception, volvulus, internal hernia, prolapse through a patent vitelline duct, or simple inversion of the diverticulum. As with other forms of intussusception, patients present with colicky abdominal pain, emesis, and bloody stools. Ultrasound confirms the diagnosis but is unlikely to identify the cause. Contrast enema is unable to fully reduce the intussusceptum, prompting operative intervention. Volvulus can occur around an omphalomesenteric duct or fibrous remnant as it attaches to the undersurface of the umbilicus, or an internal hernia can be created by an obliterated vitelline artery remnant. When this occurs in utero, the result can be intestinal atresia or perforation and meconium peritonitis. Intestinal prolapse through a patent vitelline duct creates an obstructive picture as well as the characteristic "ram's horn" visible externally at

M.S. Dassinger (✉)
Division of Pediatric Surgery, University of Arkansas for Medical Sciences, Arkansas Children's Hospital, Little Rock, AR, USA
e-mail: DassingerMelvinS@uams.edu

P. Mattei (ed.), *Fundamentals of Pediatric Surgery*,
DOI 10.1007/978-1-4419-6643-8_53, © Springer Science+Business Media, LLC 2011

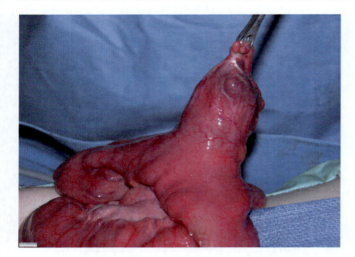

Fig. 53.1 The diverticulum always arises from the antimesenteric border of the ileum

the umbilicus. Rarely, incarceration of a Meckel's diverticulum in an inguinal or femoral hernia (Littre's hernia) can cause a bowel obstruction.

Inflammation of a Meckel's diverticulum usually presents later in childhood and is often clinically indistinguishable from acute appendicitis. If a normal appendix is found at operation, a careful search for a Meckel's diverticulum is imperative. The pathophysiology is similar to that of appendicitis with inflammation and edema leading to congestion, luminal obstruction, mucosal injury and bacterial overgrowth and invasion. The inflammation is often associated with ectopic gastric and pancreatic tissue. Because the diagnosis is usually delayed, perforation occurs often. If the diagnosis is made preoperatively, antibiotics and aggressive intravenous hydration should be initiated prior to laparotomy.

There have been reports of foreign bodies (fish bones, toothpicks, coins, seeds) becoming lodged in a Meckel's diverticulum. Rare parasite infections such as schistosomiasis and ascariasis of the diverticulum have also been described.

Primary gastrointestinal tract tumors arising from the Meckel's diverticulum occur infrequently. Carcinoids are the most common, while adenocarcinomas, sarcomas, stromal tumors, lipomas and desmoplastic tumors have all been reported. In these cases, resection of the ileal segment and its accompanying mesentery is recommended.

Diagnosis

Diagnosis of a persistent vitelline duct remnant begins with a thorough history and physical examination. Presence and character of drainage from the umbilicus should be elicited from the parents. A patent urachus produces straw-colored drainage

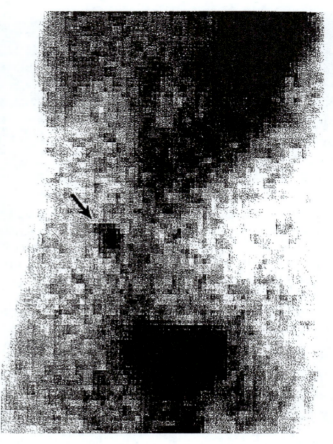

Fig. 53.2 Concentration of the [99m]Technetium pertechnetate in ectopic gastric mucosa, presumed to be within a Meckel's diverticulum (*arrow*). Also note uptake in gastric mucosa of the stomach and excreted radionucleotide in the bladder (from Grosfeld JL, et al. Pediatric surgery. 6th ed. Philadelphia: Mosby; 2006. Reprinted with permission from Elsevier)

(urine), and can be confirmed by documenting elevated creatinine levels in the fluid. Drainage of succus entericus suggests the presence of an omphalomesenteric duct remnant. The presentation is often more subtle with only intermittent drainage reported and a granuloma seen on physical exam. A sinus tract might be present, in which case the drainage is mucoid and periodic. If the lesion remains or copious drainage persists despite ligation or repeated cauterization with silver nitrate, one must assume that a visceral connection exists. The lesion should be gently catheterized and a fistulogram performed by injecting water-soluble contrast. The appearance of contrast material in the bowel or bladder confirms the diagnosis and distinguishes between urachal and omphalomesenteric duct anomalies. Ultrasound can also be a useful tool for demonstrating vitelline duct remnants or cysts.

The "Meckel's scan" ([99m]Technetium pertechnetate scinitgraphy) is the study of choice for children with gastrointestinal bleeding when a Meckel's diverticulum is considered a potential source (Fig. 53.2). The isotope is taken up and secreted by goblet cells and thus identifies ectopic gastric mucosa. Pretreatment with pentagastrin, H2 blockers or glucagon improve the sensitivity of the study. Pentagastrin 6 μg/kg given 20–30 min prior to the isotope administration stimulates gastric secretions and increases the uptake of pertechnetate. Histamine blockers, on the other hand, prevent the secretion of pertechnetate once it is taken up by the target cell, while glucagon relaxes smooth muscle, decreasing peristalsis and increasing retention of pertechnetate within the diverticulum. The overall accuracy for detecting heterotopic gastric mucosa is between 90 and 100%, with at least 85% sensitivity and 95% specificity. Because the isotope is excreted in the urine, Foley catheter placement might be necessary to decompress the bladder. Occasionally, scintigraphy needs to be repeated if bleeding persists and suspicion for a Meckel's diverticulum remains high despite a prior negative scan. If suspicion remains high despite a negative scan, laparoscopy is often a logical next step.

In cases of Meckel's diverticulum that are symptomatic due to inflammation, a CT scan might demonstrate an inflamed, blind-ending structure in the mid-abdomen that is not the appendix. Ultrasound can also be used but is technically challenging and somewhat operator-dependant. Tagged red blood cell scans have lower sensitivity and specificity than Meckel's scans and are of little utility in children with gastrointestinal bleeding. Angiography might be diagnostic in patient who are briskly bleeding, but bleeding from a Meckel's diverticulum, like most gastrointestinal bleeding, is intermittent and unpredictable. Upper and lower endoscopy are sometimes useful to rule out other sources of bleeding but usually cannot identify a Meckel's diverticulum as the source. Contrast studies have little role in the work up.

Treatment

Though the therapeutic approach varies depending on the presentation, all patients should receive adequate fluid resuscitation and intravenous antibiotics before an operation, especially in the presence of infection or perforation. Children with a bowel obstruction should have a nasogastric tube placed and electrolyte status monitored closely.

Operative resection is recommended for all patients with a symptomatic Meckel's diverticulum or vitelline duct abnormality. In neonates who present with prolapse or omphaloenteric fistula, a curvilinear peri-umbilical incision provides excellent exposure and is cosmetically acceptable. The diverticulum can usually be managed by simple diverticulectomy and transverse closure of the resultant enterotomy or resection of the involved bowel with primary anastomosis. Care must be taken in either case to control the blood supply to the diverticulum, which typically arises directly from the small bowel mesentery. Neonates who present with obstruction or meconium peritonitis will require a formal laparotomy and lysis of adhesions. In older children with intussusception due to a pathologic Meckel's lead point, complete operative reduction is often difficult, in which case resection of the bowel with primary anastomosis is required. Perforation can usually be managed by resection and primary anastomosis at initial operation. However, significant peritoneal contamination in a critically ill child might dictate creation of a temporary enterostomy. Laparoscopy is a reasonable operative approach for the patient with a bleeding Meckel's diverticulum both for diagnosis and definitive therapy. If the diverticulum is long with a narrow base, diverticulectomy by application of an endoscopic gastrointestinal stapler yields good results. A short diverticulum with a broad neck is best managed by small bowel resection and primary anastomosis. Enlarging the umbilical trocar site and performing the diverticulectomy or resection extracorporeally enables the surgeon to complete the operation without the need for formal laparotomy.

Management of the asymptomatic Meckel's diverticulum found incidentally during an abdominal procedure remains somewhat controversial. The incidence of complications from a symptomatic Meckel's diverticulum appears to decrease with age. In one large retrospective review of cases from a single institution, the cumulative lifetime risk of needing an operation for complications of a Meckel's diverticulum was 6.4%, compared to the 2% lifetime risk of a complication related to diverticulectomy. On the other hand, the results of a recent large meta-analysis suggested that there is a significantly higher incidence of complications in patients who underwent incidental diverticulectomy when compared to patients in whom the Meckel's diverticulum was left in situ. Furthermore, this same group calculated that 758 patients would need to undergo resection to prevent a single mortality from a complication due to a Meckel's diverticulum. Both of these studies included both adults and children. More moderate, selective criteria have been proposed, advising diverticulectomy in male patients under 50 years of age, when the diverticulum is greater than two centimeters in length, and when a mass or abnormality is detected within the diverticulum. Complication rates for Meckel's diverticulectomy remain low and include bowel obstruction, prolonged ileus, anastamotic dehiscence and wound infection. Mortality rates after resection of symptomatic lesions are less than 2% and approach zero for asymptomatic lesions.

Summary Points

- The spectrum of vitelline duct anomalies includes Meckel's diverticulum (most common), vitelline duct cyst, fibrous band, and omphalomesenteric duct fistula.
- Meckel's diverticula are located in the distal ileum but the exact location is highly variable.
- There is often heterotopic gastrric mucosa or pancreatic tissue within the Meckel's diverticulum.
- The most common presentations of Meckel's diverticula are bleeding, obstruction, and inflammation (diverticulitis).
- A careful history and physical examination are the best way to identify persistent umbilical drainage, which can suggest the presence of an omphalomesenteric duct fistula or urachal remnant.

Editor's Comment

Meckel's diverticulum is a relatively common congenital anomaly that only rarely causes symptoms. Except when it causes gastrointestinal bleeding, the diagnosis is usually made in the operating room when a child undergoes an exploration for bowel obstruction, intussusception, volvulus or an acute inflammatory process that looks very much like acute appendicitis. Nevertheless, the presence of this interesting and often insidious embryological leftover should be considered in any patient with an atypical presentation and should be carefully sought for at celiotomy when the findings are anything other than what was expected. The distal meter or so of ileum should be inspected carefully, as the structure is not always easily apparent and its location is highly variable.

The laparoscopic-assisted approach is generally best, as the diverticulum can be mobilized after its blood supply is divided laparoscopically and then delivered through the periumbilical incision. Whenever I suspect the presence of a Meckel's diverticulum, I always place my first laparoscopy trocar away from the midline, as it is common for the diverticulum to be adherent to the undersurface of the umbilicus where it can be easily injured by the Veress needle or trocar. Most can be excised by firing a gastrointestinal stapler across the base, making sure to orient the staple line transversely to avoid narrowing the ileal lumen. Bowel resection with primary anastomosis is necessary for the short diverticulum with a large mass of ectopic tissue or when an inflammatory process involves the base of the diverticulum. It is also generally recommended for bleeding Meckel's diverticula to ensure that the portion of the adjacent ileum containing the ulcer is removed with the specimen. Ileostomy is almost never necessary when dealing with a complication of a Meckel's diverticulum as even in the setting of a perforation the peritoneal soilage is due to succus entericus, not stool, and creating an ostomy is rarely quicker than a stapled bowel anastomosis.

Differential Diagnosis

- Bleeding: infectious colitis, anal fissure, intussusception, hemolytic uremic syndrome, duplication cyst, peptic ulcer disease, polyps.
- Obstruction: adhesive small bowel obstruction, intussusception, causes of neonatal bowel obstruction (intestinal atresia, meconium ileus, Hirschsprung disease, meconium plug syndrome).
- Inflammation: appendicitis, inflammatory bowel disease, mesenteric adenitis, gastroenteritis.

Diagnostic Studies

- [99m]Technetium pertechnetate scintigraphy (Meckel's scan) may be useful in identifying a Meckel's diverticulum as a source of gastrointestinal bleeding.
- Pentagastrin, H2 blockers, and glucagon can improve the accuracy of a Meckel's scan.

Parental Preparation

- Bowel resection with primary anastomosis might be necessary.
- There is a very small possibility that creation of a temporary ileostomy will be necessary.
- There is the potential for negative laparoscopy.

Preoperative Preparation

- ☐ Adequate intravenous hydration
- ☐ Intravenous antibiotics
- ☐ Correction of electrolytes in cases of obstruction
- ☐ Type and screen

Technical Points

- Presence of a symptomatic diverticulum mandates resection, which can be accomplished laparoscopically in most cases.
- Simple diverticulectomy is appropriate for longer diverticula with a narrow neck, while a short, broad-based diverticulum requires small bowel resection.
- Management of an incidentally found asymptomatic diverticulum remains controversial.

Suggested Reading

Cullen JJ, Kelly KA, Moir CR, et al. Surgical management of Meckel's diverticulum. An epidemiologic, population-based study. Ann Surg. 1994;220:564–9.

Ford PV, Bartold SP, Fink-Bennett DM, et al. Procedure guideline for gastrointestinal bleeding and Meckel's diverticulum scintigraphy. J Nucl Med. 1999;40:1226–32.

Menezes M, Tareen F, Saeed A, et al. Symptomatic Meckel's diverticulum in children: a 16-year review. Pediatr Surg Int. 2008;24:575–7.

Skandalakis PN, Zoras O, Skandalakis JE, et al. Littre hernia: surgical anatomy, embryology, and technique of repair. Am Surg. 2006;72:238–43.

St. Vil D, Brandt ML, Panic S, et al. Meckel's diverticulum in children: a 20-year review. J Pediatr Surg. 1991;26:1289–92.

Vane DW, West KW, Grosfeld JL. Vitelline duct anomalies: experience with 217 childhood cases. Arch Surg. 1987;122:542–7.

Yahchouchy EK, Marano AF, Etienne JCF, et al. Meckel's diverticulum. J Am Coll Surg. 2001;192:658–62.

Zani A, Eaton S, Rees CM, et al. Incidentally detected Meckel diverticulum: to resect or not to resect? Ann Surg. 2008;247:276–81.

Chapter 54
Bariatric Surgery

Joy L. Collins

Adolescent obesity is reaching near-epidemic proportions in the United States, lagging behind but following the trend of adult obesity. In some regions, nearly 40% of adolescents are obese, and many are developing severe obesity-related comorbid conditions that result in a reduced quality of life and can be progressive and life-threatening. Although nutritional counseling and behavioral modification programs have been moderately successful for overweight and obese children in the younger age groups, medical management appears to be less effective in the adolescent and young adult populations. It is estimated that up to 80% of obese teenagers will go on to become obese adults, with a pattern of continued weight gain as they enter adulthood. Bariatric surgery has been demonstrated to be a safe, effective and durable weight-loss method in adults, but its widespread application in the pediatric population remains controversial. Nevertheless, data increasingly show a similar safety and efficacy in adolescents.

Defining obesity in children and adolescents is not as straightforward as it is in adults. In younger children, obesity is defined as the 95th percentile of body mass index (BMI) for age from the reference charts constructed from extensive data collected by the National Health and Nutrition Evaluation Surveys (NHANES). In 18 year olds, the 95th percentile of BMI for age corresponds to a BMI of 30 kg/m^2. For adolescents, in the absence of a more epidemiologically accurate method to define severe obesity for age, the BMI seems to be a clinically useful correlate of adiposity.

Patient Selection

Most surgeons have adopted a BMI-based algorithm for determining candidacy of adolescents for bariatric surgery. The National Institutes of Health (NIH) defines an adult bariatric surgery candidate as having a BMI ≥ 40 or a BMI ≥ 35 with a severe obesity-related comorbidity. However, many believe that even stricter criteria should be applied before performing bariatric surgery in an adolescent. In our practice, patients with a BMI ≥ 50 or BMI ≥ 40 with an obesity-related comorbid condition are considered for evaluation. According to guidelines established by the NIH, the American College of Surgery, and the American Society for Metabolic and Bariatric Surgery, patients being considered for bariatric surgery should be evaluated at a specialized center by a multidisciplinary bariatric team who has expertise in dealing with adolescents and can provide appropriate comprehensive long-term follow up. This requires the collaborative efforts of a variety of specialists, and should include: surgeons with bariatric training, bariatric nurse specialists or other bariatric clinicians, anesthesiologists with special interest and expertise in caring for obese patients, adolescent medicine physicians, nutritionists, exercise physiologists, and adolescent psychologists and psychiatrists.

Preoperative Workup and Education

Preoperative assessment consists of a comprehensive evaluation by the surgeon and other specialists with discussion of the results among team members. The main components of the preoperative assessment and education include the nutritional, psychological and medical evaluations. The patients' families are included in each portion of this process.

The initial medical evaluation is often conducted by the surgeon, with a complete history and physical examination and initial extensive discussion and education regarding potential bariatric surgery. The medical evaluation consists of two to three visits with our surgical team in addition to assessment by adolescent medicine specialists. Medically treatable causes of obesity are initially ruled out by pediatric endocrinologists, who also screen for insulin resistance, diabetes mellitus and polycystic ovarian syndrome. Sexual and skeletal maturity are assessed by physical examination and by bone X-rays, and are confirmed by our endocrinology colleagues before each patient

J.L. Collins (✉)
Department of Pediatric General and Thoracic Surgery,
University of Pennsylvania, Children's Hospital of Philadelphia,
Philadelphia, PA, USA
e-mail: collins@email.chop.edu

P. Mattei (ed.), *Fundamentals of Pediatric Surgery*,
DOI 10.1007/978-1-4419-6643-8_54, © Springer Science+Business Media, LLC 2011

is considered for surgery. Additional comorbid medical conditions and risk factors are identified, with referrals for further testing and evaluation by specialists as necessary.

The recommended minimal preoperative laboratory studies includes a chemistry panel, hepatic function panel, lipid profile, complete blood count, hemoglobin A1C, fasting blood glucose and insulin levels, thyroid-stimulating hormone, thiamine, folate and iron levels, urinalysis, and a pregnancy test for girls. Because unrecognized sleep disorders are prevalent in the severely obese, a complete sleep history is obtained, with referral to Pulmonology for evaluation and formal polysomnography. We have uncovered severe obstructive sleep apnea in at least one patient who had no history of snoring, irregular breathing or increased daytime somnolence. An upper GI series is performed in patients with symptoms to confirm normal anatomy and rule out significant hiatal hernia or gastroesophageal reflux disease. A right upper quadrant ultrasound is performed to rule out cholelithiasis (patients without gallstones who undergo surgery are treated with ursodiol for 6 months to reduce the risk of developing gallstones during the initial period of rapid weight loss).

The nutritional evaluation focuses on detailed weight and dietary histories, the identification of environmental cues that encourage or promote inappropriate eating behavior, screening for protein and vitamin deficiency, and education regarding the appropriate postoperative nutritional and exercise programs required for success. A nutritionist educates the patient and family extensively about necessary postoperative dietary changes and evaluates the patient's ability to cooperate with postoperative requirements. It is expected that such preoperative education will be done over three to five visits, but it can require several more.

A comprehensive psychological evaluation is crucial and is conducted by an expert in adolescent development. In order to be considered for surgery, the patient is required to demonstrate an acceptable level of emotional and cognitive development, reasonable expectations of the surgery, an understanding of risks and possible outcomes, and the motivation and ability to comply with postoperative follow-up and recommendations. Certain red flags are sought, such as active emotional, behavioral or eating disorders, and alcohol or drug use. Any substance abuse or psychiatric disorders must be adequately treated and stable before consideration for surgery. Additional goals of the psychological evaluation session are to provide counseling and education regarding the lifestyle changes following bariatric surgery and to determine the existence of social and family supports which are essential for success. There is a particular focus on potential psychological stressors, both for the adolescent and his or her family, which would make compliance difficult. Family support and commitment are essential, and both the patient and family must agree to the necessary long-term lifestyle changes and follow-up. In addition, the adolescent must have no plans for pregnancy for 2 years after surgery, at which time weight loss will usually have stabilized.

Collaborative discussions involving all relevant specialists about each candidate are essential, with the goal of determining suitability for bariatric surgery and an individual plan for pre- and postoperative management. In the weeks before the operation, the patient has a final visit with the surgeon and nutritionist, as well as a final evaluation by an anesthesiologist. An extensive informed consent discussion is conducted with the adolescent and his or her family, and a final review of the perioperative regimens and instructions is completed.

Surgical Options

Bariatric procedures can be loosely divided into two main categories: purely restrictive, and restrictive plus malabsorptive. Purely restrictive operations include (1) vertical banded gastroplasty (Fig. 54.1), (2) adjustable gastric band (Fig. 54.2), and (3) vertical sleeve gastrectomy (Fig. 54.3). Combination restrictive and malabsorptive procedures include (1) the roux-en-Y gastric bypass (Fig. 54.4), and (2) the partial biliopancreatic bypass with duodenal switch, which is primarily malabsorptive (Fig. 54.5). Unfortunately, outcome data regarding adolescents remain scarce, and no procedure has been studied in a controlled fashion.

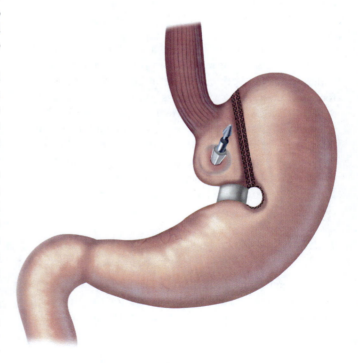

Fig. 54.1 Vertical banded gastroplasty. Adapted from Atlas of Metabolic and Weight Loss Surgery published by Cine-Med Publishing, Inc., 2010, www.cine-med.com

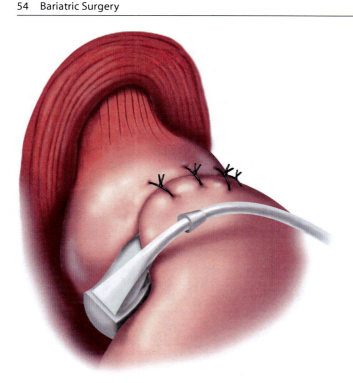

Fig. 54.2 Adjustable gastric band. Adapted from Atlas of Minimally Invasive Surgery published by Cine-Med Publishing, Inc., 2007, www.cine-med.com

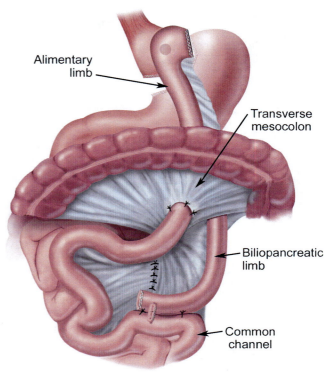

Fig. 54.4 Roux-en-Y gastric bypass. Adapted from Atlas of Minimally Invasive Surgery published by Cine-Med Publishing, Inc., 2007, www.cine-med.com

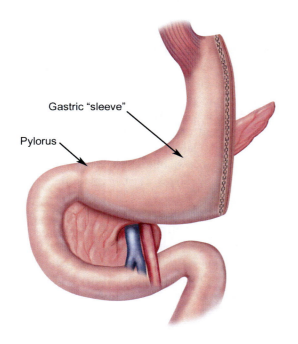

Fig. 54.3 Sleeve gastrectomy. Adapted from Atlas of Metabolic and Weight Loss Surgery published by Cine-Med Publishing, Inc., 2010, www.cine-med.com

The vertical banded gastroplasty has fallen out of favor in even the adult population due to a high rate of weight regain and reflux symptoms. Likewise, although the biliopancreatic bypass with duodenal switch results in excellent weight loss in super-morbidly obese adults, it has a higher rate of operative complications and severe postoperative nutritional deficiencies. For this reason, many surgeons feel that this is an inappropriate operation for adolescents.

The Roux-en-Y gastric bypass, which consists of a small gastric pouch (restrictive component) and a bypassed segment of stomach, duodenum and proximal jejunum (malabsorptive component), is generally considered the gold standard bariatric procedure in adults. This is also the most commonly performed procedure in adolescents; many studies with limited numbers of patients have supported its safety and efficacy in this population. In the adolescent population, the primary concerns are efficacy and long-term safety. The 0.5–1% mortality rate associated with the Roux-en-Y gastric bypass in adults is considered unacceptable by most who work with pediatric patients. For this reason, some clinicians feel that only purely restrictive procedures such as the adjustable gastric band and the sleeve gastrectomy are the most appropriate for this age group.

The gastric band is an attractive option because it is adjustable and reversible, while its purely restrictive nature make

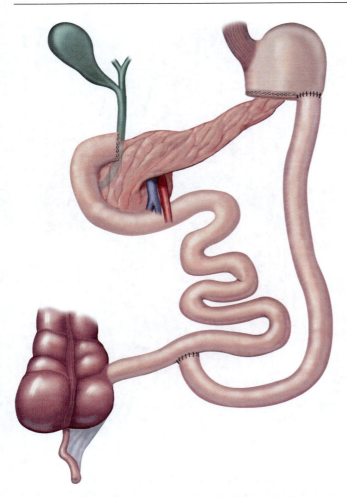

Fig. 54.5 Biliopancreatic diversion. Adapted from Atlas of Metabolic and Weight Loss Surgery published by Cine-Med Publishing, Inc., 2010, www.cine-med.com

nutritional deficiencies less likely (though these operations still significantly impair the intake of vitamins and nutrients). In addition, although the procedure has a unique set of complications, a number of which require re-operation, overall it is associated with fewer technical complications and less nutritional risk. Some surgeons feel that the vertical sleeve gastrectomy is an attractive option, because there is no gastrointestinal bypass; however there is still a risk of leak from the staple line and there is a paucity of long-term outcome data.

Perioperative Management

Patients are restricted to clear liquids for 48 h prior to the surgery date and arrive in hospital on the morning of operation. There are data to suggest that super-obese adult patients (BMI > 50) who are placed on a very low-calorie diet for 2 weeks before the operation have a decrease in liver volume

and less dense mesenteric fat, facilitating the technical aspects of the operation and potentially reducing operative complications. This might be a helpful preoperative strategy in extremely large adolescents with an android body habitus and extreme central obesity.

Prior to surgery, patients are given an injection of low-molecular-weight heparin (40 mg subcutaneously), which is continued twice daily after the operation. A dose of a second-generation cephalosporin is also administered preoperatively and continued for 24 h postoperatively. Sequential compression devices are placed preoperatively and are used for the duration of the surgical procedure and postoperative hospital stay.

Surgical Procedure

Laparoscopic Roux-en-Y Gastric Bypass

Any of the current bariatric procedures can be completed either laparoscopically or through a standard laparotomy incision, and certain technical details may vary depending on an individual surgeon's training. Initial access to the abdomen is gained by a carefully placed left upper quadrant Veress needle, followed by insufflation to a pressure of 15 mmHg and placement of a non-bladed 5-mm trocar. Two 12-mm trocars and three additional 5-mm trocars are placed. The left lobe of the liver is retracted with a flexible triangular or D-shaped retractor. The jejunum is divided 40 cm beyond the ligament of Treitz using a linear endoscopic gastrointestinal anastomosis stapling device, and one or two firings of the vascular-load stapler are used to divide the mesentery to provide length for creation of the gastrojejunal anastomosis. A Roux limb of either 75 cm (for patients with BMI < 50) or 150 cm (for patients with BMI ≥ 50 or with diabetes mellitus) is created. The length of the Roux limb is measured visually, and a stapled jejuno-jejunal anastomosis is created with the linear stapler after the two limbs of jejunum are transfixed to one another with stay sutures. The mesenteric defect is closed with a running suture.

The Roux limb can then be passed in a retrocolic or antecolic position. If passed through a retrocolic tunnel, closure of this mesenteric defect is crucial. I typically bring the limb up in an antecolic fashion after dividing the omentum, unless the Roux limb is of insufficient length to perform a tension-free gastrojejunal anastomosis. A small (10–15 mL) lesser curve gastric pouch is created with care to dissect the angle of His and exclude the gastric fundus entirely. A 35 mm endoscopic linear stapler is used to create the gastrojejunal anastomosis after a posterior layer of braided nylon suture is placed. The remaining enterotomy is then closed in two layers: an inner layer of absorbable suture and an outer layer of non-absorbable suture. An endoscope is passed into the Roux limb from above and acts as a bougie to prevent inadvertent gastrojejunal stoma narrowing during the two-layer closure. The endoscope then allows for inspection of the completed anastomosis with intraluminal air insufflation under saline to ensure that the anastomosis is air-tight. The endoscope is then used to evacuate air from the pouch and Roux limb. A closed-suction drain is placed near the anastomosis and brought out through the right upper quadrant 5-mm port site. If an anastomotic leak is identified with air insufflation, the leak is repaired and reinforced with fibrin glue, and a gastrostomy tube is placed in the bypassed gastric remnant.

There are certainly many different ways of performing these anastomoses, including entirely hand-sewn techniques or the use of an end-to-end anastomosis stapler to create the gastrojejunal anastomosis. Some surgeons prefer to use a bougie instead of an endoscope when creating this anastomosis. No controlled studies have been performed to demonstrate the superiority of any of these methods over the other, and it is reasonable for each surgeon to modify certain details based on training and experience.

Laparoscopic Adjustable Gastric Banding

Over time, the technique of adjustable gastric band placement has evolved into a method called the *pars flaccida technique*, which emphasizes minimal retro-esophageal dissection and placement of the band out of the lesser sac. This has resulted in placement of the band higher on the stomach and lower rates of postoperative gastric herniation and band slippage. Patient positioning and port placement vary based on surgeon's preference, but trocar placement similar to that used to perform a laparoscopic Nissen fundoplication is recommended. Many surgeons use port placement similar to that of the laparosopic Roux-en-Y gastric bypass. Once access is gained and the abdomen insufflated, a liver retractor is placed through a 5-mm trocar in the right subxiphoid or upper quadrant region. Additional ports are placed, including a 12 or 15-mm port in the left paramedian region. The band is primed with saline and may be placed into the abdomen early in the procedure or after dissection is completed.

A grasper is used to retract the fat between the greater curvature and the spleen downward, placing the fundus of the stomach on stretch. A cautery device is used to carefully dissect the fat pad off of its location at the angle of His and incise the peritoneum lateral to the gastroesophageal angle. Gentle blunt dissection is used to free the fundus from its attachment to the diaphragm. The nearly-transparent gastrohepatic ligament overlying the caudate lobe (pars flaccida) is then incised, with care taken to spare the hepatic branch of the vagus nerve and an accessory hepatic artery, if encountered. The right crus and vena cava should now be identified, as one can be mistaken for the other in morbidly obese patients. The peritoneum just medial to the right crus is incised just at the beginning of the lesser curve of the stomach, and the grasper is passed very gently through the scored peritoneum behind the stomach. No force should be used, and if all dissection has been correctly done, the tip of the grasper will emerge just to the left of the angle of His.

The saline-primed adjustable band is now passed through the incision of a 12 or 15 mm trocar site, if it has not already been placed within the abdomen. The end-tag of the band is placed in the jaws of the retroesophageal grasper and is pulled through to encircle the stomach. The band is locked into place, and should be loose enough to allow the placement of the tip of a 5-mm instrument between the band and the stomach. Gastric-to-gastric sutures of non-absorbable material are then placed to approximate the stomach above and below the band without tension. Sutures are carried as far posterolateral as possible, but it is important not to suture the stomach over the buckle of the band, as this promotes erosion. These sutures, along with the minimal retroesophageal dissection, have been demonstrated to minimize slippage of the band.

The liver retractor is then removed and the abdomen desufflated, after the port tubing is pulled through the left abdominal 12- or 15-mm port site. This port site is extended laterally in each direction and dissection is carried down to expose the rectus sheath. The tubing is connected to the access port, and the access port is fixed in four places to the fascia using non-absorbable suture. Once all sutures are placed, the access port is parachuted down to the fascia and the sutures tied. Any excess tubing is replaced into the abdomen, and the fascial opening is not approximated. All wounds are then closed. No fluid is placed in the balloon of the band at the time of initial placement; band adjustments ("fills") are commenced approximately 6 weeks after the operation.

Postoperative Management

Postoperatively patients are placed in a monitored setting on a surgical ward. Maintenance intravenous fluids are administered and postoperative discomfort is managed with patient controlled analgesia. Sequential compression devices are utilized, subcutaneous low-molecular weight heparin is administered, incentive spirometry is emphasized, and ambulation is commenced on the evening of surgery. Early warning signs of a complication include tachycardia, tachypnea, fever, oliguria, worsening abdominal pain, or an increasing oxygen requirement. The most dreaded postoperative complication in patients who have undergone Roux-en-Y gastric bypass is leak at the gastrojejunal anastomosis, which, if not identified and dealt with immediately, can be life-threatening. Mild tachycardia is sometimes the only sign of an anastomotic leak, and the surgeon should have a very low threshold for returning a patient to the operating room to investigate this possibility. No study is 100% sensitive for a gastrojejunal leak in the early postoperative period and an extensive work up will delay diagnosis and treatment. In the event that a leak is identified in the operating room, the area should be widely drained and a gastrostomy tube placed in the bypassed gastric remnant to allow for enteral feeds until the leak is healed.

On the first postoperative day, patients undergo a water-soluble contrast upper gastrointestinal study to rule out anastomotic leak or obstruction. Patients with a normal study are started on a clear liquid diet and can usually be discharged on the second postoperative day with a follow-up appointment in 1 week. At this first visit, the drain is removed and if all is well, the patient is advanced to a full liquid, high-protein, pureed diet. Follow-up visits are then scheduled monthly for 6 months, every 3 months for 18 months, and yearly thereafter. Laboratory evaluation is performed every 6 months, and includes iron and vitamin levels.

At each follow-up visit, the diet history is reviewed with emphasis on protein, fluid, and vitamin compliance. Weight loss is assessed and laboratory results and changes in comorbid conditions reviewed. Dietary advancement after the first month is performed with the close supervision of our bariatric nutritionist and involves gradual introduction of solid food items. The goal is a well-balanced, high protein (0.5–1 g/kg of ideal body weight per day), small-portion diet. The consumption of a minimum of 64 ounces of non-carbonated, non-caloric, non-caffeinated beverages is emphasized, as this prevents dehydration and facilitates weight loss. Non-steroidal anti-inflammatory medications are avoided to reduce the risk of marginal ulcer formation. Ursodiol is prescribed for 6 months in patients who had a normal right upper quadrant ultrasound preoperatively. The required postoperative vitamin and mineral supplementation includes: (1) a multivitamin (one adult or two children's chewable tablets); (2) calcium 500 mg TID; (3) iron 150–325 mg daily; (4) vitamin B_{12} 500 µg PO daily or 1,000 mg IM monthly; and (5) vitamin C 500–1,500 mg daily. Zinc 10–20 mg daily is optional and might prevent hair loss.

We also emphasize the importance of at least 30 min of exercise per day. Any difficulties or non-compliant behaviors result in counseling by the surgeon and referral to the appropriate specialist, such as the nutritionist or exercise physiotherapist. Our office staff make pre-visit phone calls to remind patients and their parents of the upcoming appointment, and follow-up calls when patients miss their appointments.

Complications

Complications can be intra-operative, early postoperative, or late postoperative. Some complications are unique to the type of procedure performed (Table 54.1). The most feared intra-operative complications during performance of either operation involve inadvertent perforation of the esophagus, stomach or intestine, which may or may not be recognized at the time of surgery. Additional intra-operative complications include airway mishaps and anesthetic complications, as well as bleeding from the abdominal wall, spleen, mesentery or staple line. It is important to inform patients that any of these complications could require conversion to laparotomy.

Among the postoperative complications, perhaps the most serious is a staple line leak, which can be life-threatening and requires urgent re-operation. An intestinal obstruction can occur at any time and is usually due to an internal hernia,

Table 54.1 Potential complications following Roux-en-Y gastric bypass and adjustable gastric banding

Roux-en-Y gastric bypass	Adjustable gastric band
Operative	Operative
Gastrointestinal perforation	Perforation of stomach or esophagus
Bleeding	
Twist or kink in Roux limb	Bleeding
Devascularization of biliopancreatic or Roux limb	Damage to band or tubing during placement
Anastomotic leak	
Early postoperative	Early postoperative
Emesis/dehydration	Emesis/dehydration
Food impaction	Food impaction
Anastomotic leak	Esophageal obstruction by band
Anastomotic bleed	Trocar site/band port infection
Wound infection	Deep venous thrombosis
Deep venous thrombosis	Pulmonary embolus
Pulmonary embolus	Other pulmonary complication
Other pulmonary complication	
Dumping syndrome	
Late postoperative	Late postoperative
Emesis/dehydration	Emesis/dehydration
Food impaction	Food impaction
Anastomotic stricture	Gastric herniation (band "slippage")
Marginal ulcer	Gastroesophageal reflux
Bowel obstruction	Esophageal dilation
Internal hernia	Band erosion in to esophagus
Incisional hernia	Abdominal abscess
Gallstone formation	Port infection
Nutritional deficiency	Port displacement or malfunction
– Iron deficiency anemia	
– Vitamin D deficiency	
– Beriberi	
– Neuropathy due to B-vit deficiency	
Dumping syndrome	
Nephrolithiasis	

volvulus, or adhesions. Any patient with bilious emesis must be assumed to have an obstruction distal to the jejunojejunal anastomosis until proven otherwise, which requires exploration and must be dealt with expeditiously. Pulmonary embolus is a particularly devastating and life-threatening complication in this population, and prophylactic measures must be undertaken as described. In individuals with clotting disorders or a prior history of pulmonary embolus, preoperative vena cava filter placement may be beneficial.

In adults, bariatric surgery is associated with a mortality of approximately 0.5%. Although the reported surgical mortality rate in adolescents is lower than in adults, the patient, his or her family, and all care providers must be aware of this risk and have a high suspicion for early studies or interventions when necessary.

Outcomes

Although no prospective studies have been done to evaluate bariatric surgical approaches in adolescents, the limited experience described in several small retrospective series suggests that gastric bypass and adjustable gastric banding are safe and effective in this population. Weight loss after gastric bypass has been similar to that seen in adults, with several series reporting excess weight loss of 56–80%. If the appropriate dietary and exercise regimen is followed, this dramatic weight loss seems to occur with preservation of visceral protein and a low incidence of postoperative complications.

Similarly good outcomes have been described after adjustable gastric banding, with up to 60% excess weight loss at 2 years and excellent resolution of obesity-related comorbid conditions. The most common complications in this series were mild nutritional and vitamin deficiencies, which resolved with supplementation.

Although early data suggest that adolescents can achieve significant weight loss following bariatric procedures, it remains to be seen whether or not such weight loss and comorbidity resolution is sustainable over the adolescent's lifetime. It is also unclear what potential unforeseen negative consequences may arise. However, at this time when we are faced with an increasingly growing population of obese adolescents who are facing severe and life-threatening complications of their obesity, bariatric surgery may be the best solution that we have to offer at this time. Because of this, adolescent bariatric surgical programs are being developed to meet the needs of these patients. These programs should be comprised of a multidisciplinary team of highly trained individuals with the experience to assess and meet the unique needs of the morbidly obese adolescent. Until long-term outcome data is available, surgical criteria should remain relatively conservative, the selection process rigorous, and centers should be committed to frequent, long-term patient follow-up and data collection for clinical research.

Summary Points

- Careful patient selection is crucial.
- Extensive preoperative counseling and evaluation by a multidisciplinary team of experts is essential.
- The patient and family must understand that bariatric surgery is a weight-loss tool, not a cure, and that permanent lifestyle changes must be made to ensure success.
- A variety of surgical weight-loss options exist. The most commonly applied in adolescents are the Roux-en-Y gastric bypass and adjustable gastric banding.
- Surgical weight loss can provide significant improvement or resolution of most obesity-related comorbid conditions.
- Compliance with postoperative vitamin, dietary, and exercise regimens are essential for success and prevention of complications.
- Postoperative follow-up with the bariatric team should be lifelong, in order to assure the best long-term success.

Editor's Comment

There remains a great deal of controversy regarding the use of bariatric surgery in children, largely because of the significant risks involved, the uncertain long-term effects, and the perception that obesity is largely behavioral or psychogenic in origin. However, the risks are currently acceptable, especially when weighed against the risks of ongoing obesity; the long-term effects appear to be largely correctable; and it is increasingly clear that the morbidly obese have a genetically-based metabolic disorder that happens to manifest itself in the form of a specific behavior (excessive oral intake of food) rather than simply a psychological or emotional disorder. It seems reasonable, therefore, to offer these children some relief of their illness and the hope that they can prevent the substantial sequelae that come with morbid obesity. On the other hand, the operation is clearly not an immediate or permanent cure and it also does not address the underlying cause. Success depends on an extraordinary amount of work and commitment on the part of these kids and their families and friends.

Naturally, the most effective operations also carry the highest risk and, as a result, there is still resistance to letting these operations become widely popular. The less invasive laparoscopic gastric banding operation is perhaps less effective in the long term, but it is adequate for most patients and clearly safer. Nevertheless, although it is probably the best choice for the morbidly obese teenager at this time, there is a great deal of difficulty in obtaining FDA approval for the use of the device outside of a few select centers in the US. We await the results of several well-conducted studies before it can become widely available.

Bariatric operations differ from most other surgical procedures in that a surgeon cannot expect to see a patient in the office, make a decision regarding the indications and risk, and schedule the operation if the patient agrees to proceed. The key to the success of a bariatric surgical program is the large number of clinicians that form part of the team including psychologists, nutritionists, gastroenterologists, endocrinologists, and surgeons. Protocols must be clearly designed and continually modified to achieve the best results and the least morbidity.

The operations are technically quite challenging, partly due to the body habitus of the patients. Special operating tables and instruments are needed to support the weight of the patients and allow proper access to the abdominal cavity. Careful dissection and respect of natural tissue planes are difficult to achieve due to the anatomic distortion caused by excessive adipose tissue but are critical to the success of the operation. Staple lines must be secure but visual confirmation can be difficult. Intra-operative endoscopy and testing anastomoses for leaks with air insufflation are critical adjuncts that have been shown to reduce the risk of dehiscence and death. Postoperative vigilance for even the slightest indication of a problem (unexplained tachycardia) and a low threshold for urgent reoperation are also key to mitigating the effects of an anastomotic leak.

Children who undergo bariatric surgery must be considered patients for life, as the morbidity and recurrence rates are high in the absence of an ongoing program to monitor weight loss and overall health status. Eventual transfer to an adult program might be a suitable option, making it important to foster a good relationship between the pediatric and adult programs so that patient care is seamless.

Diagnostic Studies

Preoperative

- Chemistry panel, hepatic panel, lipid profile, blood glucose and insulin levels, CBC, TSH, vitamin levels
- Screening for polycystic ovarian syndrome and pregnancy test
- Upper-GI contrast study
- Hand/wrist X-rays
- Right upper quadrant ultrasound
- Polysomnography

Postoperative

- Upper-GI contrast study
- Preoperative PreparationPreoperative bowel prep or 48 h period of clear liquid diet
- Prophylactic antibiotics
- Subcutaneous heparin and sequential compression devices

Parental Preparation

- Parents should participate in each aspect of the preoperative evaluation and counseling sessions.
- There is a risk of infection, bleeding, anastomotic leak, malnutrition, vitamin deficiency, recurrence, and death.
- Parents should receive counseling regarding the dramatic lifestyle changes that both the patient and the family will undergo and be willing to commit to support their child in making these changes.

Technical Points

- Most bariatric procedures can be completed laparoscopically.

Roux-en-Y gastric bypass.

- Roux limb of either 50 or 75 cm in length is created, depending on BMI and comorbid conditions.
- Anastomoses may be stapled or hand-sewn.
- Roux limb may be brought up in either retrocolic or antecolic fashion.
- Mesenteric defects must be closed.
- Gastrojejunal anastomosis can be performed over endoscope or Bougie stent to ensure patency and standard stoma size.
- Insufflation of gastric pouch under saline is helpful to assess for anastomotic leak.

Adjustable gastric banding

- Pars flaccida technique associated with fewer technical complications
- Gastric-to-gastric sutures essential to preventing band slippage

Suggested Reading

Collins J, Mattar S, Qureshi F, et al. Initial outcomes of laparoscopic Roux-en-Y gastric bypass in morbidly obese adolescents. Surg Obes Relat Dis. 2007;3:147–52.

Inge TH, Daniels SR, Garcia VF. In: Ashcraft KW, Holcomb GW, Murphy JP, editors. Pediatric surgery. 4th ed. Philadelphia, PA: Elsevier Saunders; 2005. p. 1116–25.

Inge TH, Krebs NF, Garcia VF, et al. Bariatric surgery for severely overweight adolescents: concerns and recommendations. Pediatrics. 2004a;114:217–23.

Inge TH, Xanthakos SA, Zeller MH. Bariatric surgery for pediatric extreme obesity: now or later? Int J Obes. 2007;31:1–14.

Inge TH, Zeller M, Garcia VF, et al. Surgical approach to adolescent obesity. Adolesc Med. 2004b;15:429–53.

Lawson ML, Kirk S, Mitchell T, et al. One-year outcomes of Roux-en-Y gastric bypass for morbidly obese adolescents: a multicenter study from the Pediatric Bariatric Study Group. J Pediatr Surg. 2006;41:137–43.

Nadler EP, Youn HA, Ginsburg HB, et al. Short-term results in 53 US obese pediatric patients treated with laparoscopic adjustable gastric banding. J Pediatr Surg. 2007;42:137–42.

Nadler EP, Youn HA, Ren CJ, et al. An update on 73 US obese pediatric patients treated with laparoscopic adjustable gastric banding: comorbidity resolution and compliance data. J Pediatr Surg. 2008;43: 141–6.

Chapter 55
Chronic Abdominal Pain

Frazier W. Frantz

Chronic abdominal pain, loosely defined as recurrent episodes of pain occurring at least weekly for 1–2 months, is a common complaint, estimated to affect approximately 20% of school-age children. It results in school absenteeism, family disruption and sometimes depression and anxiety. In the majority of children, chronic abdominal pain is thought to be "functional," which means there is no objective evidence of an underlying organic disease. Whereas surgeons are the principle caretakers for children with acute abdominal pain, pediatricians and gastroenterologists provide the bulk of care for those with chronic abdominal pain. The primary role for surgeons is to identify and treat the 10–15% of these children who have an underlying organic disorder. Even a surgical evaluation that fails to reveal an organic cause has merit because it provides reassurance to the family and allows the primary care provider to transition from a diagnostic mode to formulation of a treatment plan.

Functional Abdominal Pain

Historically, functional abdominal pain was a diagnosis of exclusion, invoked only after a battery of biochemical and radiographic testing and, in some cases, non-therapeutic surgical procedures, had been exhausted. Thanks to the efforts of the American Academy of Pediatrics Subcommittee on Chronic Abdominal Pain, the Rome criteria have evolved as a classification system based on gastrointestinal symptomatology to allow categorization and standardization of treatment and to obviate the need for extensive diagnostic testing in children who meet inclusion criteria for a functional gastrointestinal disorder (Table 55.1). While the Rome criteria have not been universally adopted by pediatricians and gastroenterologists in clinical practice, they are helpful in providing understanding and reassurance to families that their child's symptoms correspond to a real, albeit non-organic, diagnosis.

The exact etiology and pathogenesis of functional abdominal pain is not well understood, but it is believed to result from dysregulation of brain–gut communication. Specific aspects believed to contribute to this process include: (1) *abnormal bowel reactivity* to physiologic stimuli (meal, gut distension, hormonal changes), noxious stimuli (inflammatory processes), or psychologically stressful stimuli (parental separation, anxiety), (2) *visceral hyperalgesia*, a decreased threshold for pain in response to changes in intraluminal pressure associated with infection, inflammation, intestinal trauma or allergy, and (3) *abnormal central processing* of afferent signals at the level of the central nervous system.

The typical presentation of the child with a functional GI disorder (FGID) includes a history of recurrent, episodic abdominal pain that is vaguely localized in the midline. The pain is characterized as aching or cramping and is usually non-radiating. It is sometimes associated with nausea, vomiting, dizziness or diaphoresis, but there is characteristically no temporal correlation of pain with activity, meals, or bowel habits. Interference with normal daily activities, including school attendance, is common. Between episodes, the child feels well. On physical examination, there are usually no significant abnormal findings, specifically no localizing signs of abdominal tenderness. Laboratory studies are usually normal.

Treatment for patients diagnosed with FGID is predominantly carried out by primary care providers, but, in difficult cases, requires the skills of a multi-disciplinary team, including a gastroenterologist and a mental health professional. The primary goals of treatment are to reassure and educate the family, to address psychological factors, and to focus on the return to normal functioning, rather than on complete disappearance of pain. An array of psychological treatments for pain management, including cognitive-behavioral therapy, have been employed with some success. Medications are sometimes prescribed for symptom relief. Several medications with documented efficacy in appropriate situations include peppermint oil or anticholinergics such as dicyclomine (Bentyl) and hyoscyamine (Levsin) for

F.W. Frantz (✉)
Department of Pediatric Surgery, East Virginia Medical School, Children's Hospital of The King's Daughters, Norfolk, VA, USA
e-mail: kidfixer@cox.net

P. Mattei (ed.), *Fundamentals of Pediatric Surgery*,
DOI 10.1007/978-1-4419-6643-8_55, © Springer Science+Business Media, LLC 2011

Table 55.1 Rome III child and adolescent diagnostic criteria for abdominal pain-related functional gastrointestinal disorders (FGIDs)

Functional dyspepsia

Must include all of the following, experienced at least once per week for at least 2 months

1. Persistent or recurrent pain or discomfort located in the upper abdomen (above the umbilicus)
2. Not relieved by defecation or associated with the onset of a change in stool frequency or stool form (not irritable bowel syndrome)
3. No evidence of an inflammatory, anatomic, metabolic, or neoplastic process that explains the subject's symptoms

Irritable bowel syndrome (IBS)

Must include all of the following, experienced at least once per week for at least 2 months

1. Abdominal discomfort (an uncomfortable sensation not described as pain) or pain associated with two or more of the following at least 25% of the time
   a. Improves with defecation
   b. Onset associated with a change in frequency of stool
   c. Onset associated with a change in form or appearance of the stool
2. No evidence of an inflammatory, anatomic, metabolic, or neoplastic process that explains the subject's symptoms

Abdominal migraine

Must include all of the following, experienced two or more times in the preceding 12 months

1. Paroxysmal episodes of intense, acute periumbilical pain that lasts for 1 h or more
2. Intervening periods of usual health lasting weeks to months
3. The pain interferes with normal activities
4. The pain is associated with two or more of the following
   a. Anorexia
   b. Nausea
   c. Vomiting
   d. Headache
   e. Photophobia
   f. Pallor
5. No evidence of an inflammatory, anatomic, metabolic, or neoplastic process that explains the subject's symptoms

Childhood functional abdominal pain

Must include all of the following, experienced at least once per week for at least 2 months

1. Episodic or continuous abdominal pain
2. Insufficient criteria for other FGIDs
3. No evidence of an inflammatory, anatomic, metabolic, or neoplastic process that explains the subject's symptoms

Childhood functional abdominal pain syndrome

Must include childhood functional abdominal pain at least 25% of the time and one or more of the following, experienced at least once per week for at least 2 months

1. Some loss of daily functioning
2. Additional somatic symptoms such as headache, limb pain, or difficulty sleeping

Source: Reprinted from Rasquin A, et al. Childhood functional gastrointestinal disorders: child/adolescent. Gastroenterology 2006;130:1527–37, with permission

irritable bowel syndrome (IBS); H-2 blockers/proton pump inhibitors for dyspepsia; fiber supplements, laxatives and/or stool softeners for constipation; and, if necessary, tricyclic anti-depressants.

Although it is counter-intuitive for surgeons that a child with debilitating chronic abdominal pain will not benefit from an extensive work-up and eventual therapeutic operation, it should be noted that the Rome classification system have been evolving for nearly 10 years, and extensive follow up has revealed that, in children clinically diagnosed with FGID, only 2% are eventually found to have an organic abnormality. In addition, when evaluation of a child with chronic abdominal pain yields findings consistent with FGID, it is advisable to closely involve the child's primary care provider and necessary subspecialists as a multidisciplinary team, particularly if this diagnosis was not previously considered. When the surgeon is also the treating physician, the expectations of the patient and family are that a surgical procedure will eventually lead to pain resolution. Finally, it is not uncommon for patients diagnosed with FGID to present with acute abdominal pain. If nothing has changed in the history or examination, this might represent a flare of their functional abdominal pain and reassurance is indicated. If, however, there is a change in the symptomatology or focal findings on examination, a work-up for potential underlying organic causes is warranted.

Abdominal Pain of Organic Etiology

Abdominal pain can be caused by one of any number of inflammatory, anatomic, metabolic, or neoplastic processes, many of which are treatable with appropriate medical treatment and do not require surgical intervention (Table 55.2). The challenge implicit in working with these patients is identifying who might benefit from a diagnostic and/or therapeutic procedure and who can avoid an unnecessary intervention.

Diagnosis

The initial central focus in evaluating children with chronic abdominal pain is determining whether the cause is functional or organic, which directs subsequent diagnostic and therapeutic considerations. Unfortunately, there are no clear-cut diagnostic markers to differentiate the two. While children with chronic abdominal pain and their parents are more likely to be anxious or depressed, the presence of behavior problems or recent negative life events does not appear to be useful in distinguishing functional from organic abdominal pain. Likewise, while children with chronic abdominal pain are more likely to have headache, joint pain, nausea, vomiting or altered bowel habits, these associated symptoms are also not particularly helpful. On the other hand, the presence of certain symptoms or signs increase the likelihood of

Table 55.2 Differential diagnosis of organic causes of chronic abdominal pain in childhood

Gastrointestinal	Genitourinary
Acid peptic disease	Urinary tract infection (pyelonephritis, cystitis)[M]
Esophagitis[M]	Nephrolithiasis[M]
Gastritis (including *H. pylori*)[M]	Ureteropelvic junction obstruction/ hydronephrosis[M]
Peptic ulcer disease[M]	Dysmenorrhea[M]
Gastroesophageal reflux[M]	Ovarian cyst[S]
Infectious/inflammatory	Pelvic inflammatory disease/ tubo-ovarian abscess[C]
Infectious colitis/ gastroenteritis (parasitic, bacterial, viral)[M]	Fitz–Hugh–Curtis syndrome (perihepatitis)[M]
Inflammatory bowel disease[C]	Pregnancy (intrauterine or ectopic)[C]
Chronic appendicitis[S]	Endometriosis[C]
Anatomic/congenital	Genital tract obstruction[S]
Malrotation (Ladd's bands or intermittent volvulus)[S]	Sexual abuse[M]
	Mittelschmerz[M]
Intestinal duplications[S]	**Metabolic/genetic**
Meckel's diverticulum (obstruction, intussusception, diverticulitis)[S]	Hypercalcemia[C]
	Lead poisoning[M]
	Acute intermittent porphyria[M]
Chronic/recurrent intussusception[S]	
Hernias (abdominal wall, diaphragm)[S]	Familial Mediterranean fever[M]
Lymphatic malformation (including mesenteric & omental cysts)[S]	Hereditary angioedema[M]
Mechanical/dysmotility	**Hematologic/vasculitis**
Constipation[M]	Sickle cell disease[M]
Appendiceal colic[S]	
Bezoar or foreign body[C]	Henoch–Schonlein purpura[M]
	Systemic lupus erythematosus[M]
Intra-abdominal adhesions[S]	**Neoplastic**
Intestinal pseudo-obstruction[M]	Lymphoma (obstruction, perforation)[C]
Malabsorptive	Solid tumors – neuroblastoma, kidney, ovary, liver, rhabdomyosarcoma, hepatoblastoma-compression, hemorrhage, rupture, torsion[S]
Lactose intolerance[M]	**Musculoskeletal**
Celiac disease[M]	Trauma[C]
Hepatobiliary/pancreatic	Rectus hematoma[C]
Chronic hepatitis[M]	Discitis[M]
Cholelithiasis/chronic cholecystitis[S]	
Biliary dyskinesia[C]	
Choledochal cyst[S]	
Chronic pancreatitis[M]	
Pancreatic pseudocyst[S]	

M medical management; *S* surgical management; *C* combined medical and surgical management

Table 55.3 Alarm symptoms and signs for organic causes of chronic abdominal pain

History
Age of onset before 5 years old
Involuntary weight loss
Deceleration of linear growth
Unexplained fever
Gastrointestinal blood loss
Protracted or bilious emesis
Chronic, severe diarrhea
Pain that awakens the child from sleep
Pain well-localized away from the umbilicus (especially persistent right upper or right lower quadrant pain)
Referred pain to the back, shoulders, or extremities
Dysuria, hematuria, or flank pain
Family history of inflammatory bowel disease or peptic ulcer disease

Physical examination
Localized tenderness in the right upper or right lower quadrants
Localized fullness or mass effect
Hepatomegaly
Splenomegaly
Costovertebral angle tenderness
Tenderness over the spine
Perianal abnormalities – skin tags, fissures, fistulas, ulceration

organic disease and therefore justifies more extensive diagnostic testing (Table 55.3).

A detailed history, including dietary, psychological and social factors, and a complete physical examination are the most important elements in the evaluation of children with chronic abdominal pain. When possible, the history should

be obtained directly from the patient. Pertinent aspects that characterize the pain, such as location, quality, timing, and frequency, as well as precipitating factors or events, should be elicited. The goal is to identify signs or symptoms that might suggest an organic etiology and, if these are absent, to construct a patient profile for comparison with the defined FGID profiles. If the patient fits one of these profiles and does not demonstrate alarm symptoms or signs, extensive diagnostic testing is not necessary and treatment for functional abdominal pain can be initiated.

Specific questioning should be directed to antecedent viral illness, as a considerable percentage of patients can develop IBS-like symptoms after a viral gastroenteritis. Associated symptoms, such as nausea, vomiting, diaphoresis, dizziness, or pallor should be noted. Patients presenting with an infectious picture associated with persistent diarrhea should be queried regarding recent international travel. In post-menarchal females, questioning regarding menstrual irregularity, pain associated with menstruation or the presence of a vaginal discharge might suggest an underlying gynecologic problem. Prescription and over-the-counter medications being taken by the child should be recorded. In particular, NSAIDs can cause gastritis and mucosal ulcerations. It may also be helpful to inquire about medications the child may have taken to try to relieve the abdominal pain and how efficacious they were.

The physical examination should be performed in a comfortable environment for the child with the parents present. All clothing should be removed and the child dressed in a hospital gown. Physical findings of underlying organic diseases can be subtle and should be carefully sought out (Table 55.3). The child's growth parameters should be measured and plotted on standard charts to assess growth failure or weight loss. Potential clues on generalized exam include the presence of jaundice, rashes, joint tenderness/swelling or clubbing. Aphthous ulcerations or stomatitis suggest IBD, bruising or other injuries suggests abuse or trauma, and pain that is exacerbated with movement, particularly if it is well-localized and associated with superficial tenderness suggests a musculoskeletal cause. The abdominal examination should focus on the presence of a palpable mass, localized tenderness, organomegaly or hernias. The presence of localized tenderness in the right upper or right lower quadrant, especially if this correlates with the site of reported pain, has the highest correlation with underlying organic disease of surgical import. The costovertebral angles should be assessed for tenderness. The perianal area should be carefully inspected for skin tags, fissures, fistulas, ulcerations or signs of sexual abuse. Digital rectal examination, performed in a gentle and reassuring manner, allows assessment of the volume and consistency of stool in the rectal vault and provides for sampling of stool for occult blood testing. Pelvic examination is particularly important in pubertal females, especially those who are sexually active, to look for signs of infection or a mass. In prepubertal females, palpation for sacral or pelvic masses is probably best accomplished by concomitant digital rectal and abdominal wall palpation.

There is no consensus regarding initial diagnostic testing for patients with chronic abdominal pain. The laboratory and radiographic diagnostic evaluation should be driven by an index of suspicion based upon pertinent alarm symptoms and signs in the history and physical exam. A reasonable approach is to order a limited lab panel initially: CBC, urinalysis and stool occult blood test. Screening laboratory abnormalities that should raise suspicion for an underlying organic disease include: anemia, leukocytosis, abnormal urinalysis, or occult blood in the stool. Once the patient has reached the subspecialty level of consultation, especially if alarm symptoms and signs are present, a complete set of labs should be obtained to investigate several of the more common organic causes of chronic abdominal pain. This lab panel should include a CBC with differential, comprehensive metabolic panel (including liver chemistries), erythrocyte sedimentation rate, amylase, lipase, and urine culture. A pregnancy test should be obtained in adolescent girls. If diarrhea is present, stool samples should be analyzed for occult blood, leukocytes, and ova and parasites and sent for culture. A history of precedent antibiotic use warrants analysis for *C. difficile*. Additional laboratory studies to investigate specific diagnoses should be based on abnormalities in the history and physical exam.

Diagnostic imaging should be considered when the pain is localized, when symptoms of GI tract obstruction are present (vomiting, constipation, obstipation), or to confirm or characterize abnormalities discovered on physical exam. The decision of which diagnostic studies to employ should be based on a risk vs. reward/yield assessment. In general, the least invasive studies should be used first and they should be used liberally. Focal abdominal or pelvic ultrasound is probably the most frequently utilized modality. Ultrasound is particularly useful for imaging the hepatobiliary and genitourinary tracts and should always be performed when focal symptoms or examination findings suggest underlying disease of gallbladder, renal or adnexal origin. It is effective for retroperitoneal tumor screening and is also sensitive for intussusception and cystic anomalies, such as intestinal duplications. Plain films of the abdomen are appropriate for patients presenting with symptoms of GI tract obstruction. These might identify abnormalities in the bowel gas pattern, a radiopaque stone in the urinary tract or gallbladder, an appendicolith, a potential GI foreign body or fecal retention. Barium contrast upper GI series with small bowel follow-through is indicated for patients who present with symptoms of GI tract obstruction, and to rule out malrotation. It is also useful for evaluating the ileum in patients suspected of having Crohn's disease. It is not helpful in identifying peptic ulcer disease in children.

Computed tomography provides the most information regarding the intra-abdominal organs but exposes the child to ionizing radiation. Unless the study is being done specifically to detect a stone in the urinary tract, intravenous and enteral contrast should be used to optimize the diagnostic yield. Measures that minimize the radiation exposure risk, including weight-based dose adjustment and lead shielding, should be employed routinely.

For patients who present with chronic abdominal pain associated with alarm symptoms and suspected organic disease of gastrointestinal origin, early consultation with a gastroenterologist is recommended. This applies to patients with symptoms of either acid peptic disease or altered bowel patterns (IBS, IBD). Esophagogastroduodenoscopy is the gold standard for diagnosing inflammatory and infectious disorders of the upper GI tract and should be considered in patients with alarm symptoms, for those who fail to respond to gastric acid reduction therapy for presumed functional dyspepsia, and when symptoms recur after discontinuation of effective therapy. It allows accurate diagnosis of *H. pylori* gastritis by confirming the presence of both the causative organism and mucosal injury. In patients with suspected celiac disease, EGD allows sampling of small intestinal tissue to look for evidence of villi flattening with lymphocytic infiltration. Colonoscopy should be considered for patients with chronic abdominal pain and altered bowel patterns who manifest any of the alarm symptoms and signs, any extra-intestinal manifestations of potential IBD on exam, or an elevated ESR.

It certainly is not mandatory for all pediatric patients with chronic abdominal pain to undergo extensive diagnostic imaging, especially for those in whom surgical intervention is planned. Some surgeons would argue that these studies carry a low diagnostic yield, lead to patient and family anxiety and may detect abnormalities that are not causally related to the pain. The diagnostic accuracy and effectiveness of proceeding directly to diagnostic laparoscopy without imaging, especially for patients with focal RLQ pain and/or tenderness is well-documented. My own preference in these circumstances is to obtain either an ultrasound or CT to exclude tumors or other pathology of the retroperitoneum prior to diagnostic laparoscopy because the retroperitoneum is not well visualized with laparoscopy. Additionally, in patients who have warning symptoms or signs of apparent GI origin, I prefer to employ endoscopic evaluation prior to laparoscopy to exclude GI mucosal disease as the source of pain.

Surgical Approach

A thorough work-up, including physical examination, appropriate diagnostic testing, and any necessary subspecialty consultation, will typically identify one of three groups of patients with chronic abdominal pain of organic etiology for treatment:(1) those with a non-surgical organic cause;(2) those with an etiology that requires surgical intervention; and (3) those with non-localizing abdominal pain and a presumed organic cause that remains unidentified despite diagnostic testing (with or without endoscopy). Treatment for the first group is straight-forward and requires subspecialty referral if not obtained earlier. Although it is still possible that these patients will require surgical intervention if their medical treatment fails or if their disease progresses, the initial focus of treatment for these patients will be medical.

In most circumstances, surgical treatment for patients with focal pain or an identified organic cause can be carried out using laparoscopy: cholelithiasis, chronic appendicitis, or ovarian cyst. An open or laparoscopic-assisted surgical procedure might be more appropriate for tumors, malrotation with intermittent volvulus, or intestinal resection. A significant subset of this group of patients is represented by children who present with recurrent RLQ pain of unknown origin. Diagnostic laparoscopy with planned elective appendectomy has proven to be an effective intervention in this patient population. Besides gross findings of chronic appendicitis, laparoscopy has allowed detection of other significant intra-abdominal findings, such as Meckel's diverticulum, adhesions, hernias, or ovarian cysts. Histologic examination of the appendix has revealed abnormalities in up to 80% of cases. Most importantly, the majority of patients treated in this fashion, including those in whom no pathologic abnormality was detected, experienced considerable reduction in their abdominal pain.

Patients with non-localizing abdominal pain comprise the most challenging group because the expectation is that a considerable number of these patients will have no obvious pathology and therefore are likely to derive little benefit from the procedure. Performing a safe operation with minimal morbidity is paramount. Reasonable expectations should be communicated to the patient and family prior to operation. These patients are well-suited for diagnostic laparoscopy and entails a thorough and systematic examination of the abdominal wall and all contents of the intra-abdominal cavity. Initial attention should be paid to areas of more frequent pathology, such as the RLQ and pelvis. The ileum should be examined to detect changes of ileitis or the presence of a Meckel's diverticulum. The pelvic organs should be carefully inspected. Intraperitoneal fluid, if present, should be sampled and sent for analysis and culture. Visualized pathology should be documented and, if possible, addressed. Once the diagnostic portion of the procedure is completed, empiric removal of the appendix should be undertaken. Trocar sites should be injected with generous amounts of local anesthetic to minimize pain in the immediate postoperative period.

Specific Disorders

In general, the medical and surgical treatment of specific organic causes of chronic abdominal pain will be very similar to the treatment exercised for these entities in the acute setting.

Anatomic/Congenital GI Disorders

Intestinal malrotation is more difficult to diagnose in older children because, unlike the typical infant with malrotation, they rarely present with bilious emesis. Instead, they often present with recurrent abdominal pain that is usually postprandial, transient, and diffuse, and only sometimes associated with emesis. Alternatively, the pain might be associated with diarrhea or evidence of malabsorption associated with mesenteric lymphatic stasis from intermittent volvulus. Because of the risk of midgut volvulus, a high index of suspicion needs to be exercised to ensure that the diagnosis is not missed. While screening abdominal ultrasound can suggest malrotation based upon SMA/SMV vessel inversion (SMA normally to left of the SMV), the diagnostic study of choice is a contrast upper GI series. Computed tomography with enteral contrast that demonstrates all of the proximal small intestine on the right side is also suggestive of the diagnosis. Treatment entails an open or laparoscopic Ladd's procedure, which includes appendectomy. While more recent literature suggests that older patients who are asymptomatic and found to have incidental malrotation are reasonable candidates for observation, patients who present with chronic abdominal pain require surgical intervention.

Intestinal duplications are cystic or tubular structures that are intimately attached to segment of the alimentary tract and share a common muscular wall and vascular supply. The most common site of involvement is the ileum. Some are lined with ectopic gastric or pancreatic mucosa. Presentation includes abdominal pain, gastrointestinal hemorrhage, or obstruction due to mass effect or intussusception. The diagnosis can be established using ultrasound or CT. Surgical treatment involves complete surgical excision, which, because of the shared blood supply, sometimes requires a bowel resection. For duplications that cannot be safely resected due to the risk of injury to adjacent structures or for tubular duplications that would require resection of a long segment of intestine, treatment options include removing only the mucosa of the cyst or, for colonic duplications (which rarely contain ectopic mucosa), opening the common wall between the cyst and adjacent intestine to allow internal drainage.

In the chronic setting, patients with Meckel's diverticulum present with obstruction, intussusception, or diverticulitis. It is often not be possible to confirm Meckel's diverticulum as the actual pathology until operation. This entity should always be considered in patients who present with chronic RLQ pain. Treatment entails resection of the diverticulum or bowel resection and primary anastomosis.

Older children with chronic intussusception present with colicky abdominal pain and symptoms of intermittent obstruction. Unlike infants who present with idiopathic intussusception, a large percentage of these patients will have a lead point (Meckel's diverticulum, tumor, polyp, duplication cyst) that requires surgical intervention. The diagnosis will usually be made on CT or contrast studies obtained to rule out obstruction, but ultrasound is also a reasonable screening study. Treatment should include reduction of the intussusception and resection of the lead point. If a polyp is discovered as the lead point, consider screening the entire colon to exclude additional lesions. On occasion, the site of a chronic, non-obstructing intussusception will be found to have "healed" as a circumferential, fibrotic ring, which should be excised or treated with stricturoplasty to avoid a subsequent stricture.

Intra-abdominal lymphatic malformations can develop within the mesentery, omentum, or retroperitoneum. They are congenital and progressively enlarge due to underlying lymphatic obstruction. Presenting symptoms depend on the location of the malformation and its size. Generally, those originating in the omentum or retroperitoneum present with vague abdominal pain and abdominal distension when they are large enough to compress surrounding structures. Those in the mesentery present more acutely with signs of obstruction

or abdominal pain due to compression, torsion, or infection. The diagnosis is made by US, CT or MRI. Treatment consists of complete surgical resection. For those located in the mesentery, which are often multiloculated and wrapped circumferentially around the intestine, segmental intestinal resection is necessary. Those malformations originating from the retroperitoneum have the highest risk of recurrence.

Inflammatory Bowel Disease

Chronic abdominal pain is common in children with IBD. For patients with Crohn's disease, characteristic symptoms are nonspecific and include abdominal pain, anorexia, weight loss, growth failure and diarrhea. Patients with ulcerative colitis demonstrate hematochezia, diarrhea, tenesmus and abdominal cramping. Laboratory findings suggestive of IBD include anemia, elevated ESR, thrombocytosis, hypoalbuminemia and heme-positive stool. Since the pathophysiology and treatment of these diseases is very different, it is important to differentiate Crohn's disease from UC. One of the most distinguishing clues on physical exam is the presence of perianal disease, which occurs in up 50% of children with Crohn's disease. The ultimate distinction is going to depend on histologic findings from tissue obtained via endoscopy, radiographic findings of small intestinal disease (Crohn's), and pertinent serum markers for these diseases. Anti-Saccharomyces cerevisiae antibodies (ASCA) and perinuclear anti-neutrophil cytoplastmic auto-antibodies (pANCA) have been found to be strongly associated with Crohn's disease and UC, respectively. In the chronic setting, the treatment for these illnesses is predominantly medical in nature. The most common indications for surgical intervention involve patients with Crohn's disease who have a fixed stricture or severe chronic abdominal pain due to intractable disease. Stricturoplasty or segmental resection (typically ileocecectomy with primary anastomosis) is appropriate for these patients. Less common indications involve treatment of complications of Crohn's disease: symptomatic fistula or bowel obstruction that fails to response to medical therapy, abscess formation that fails antibiotic therapy or percutaneous drainage, symptomatic perianal disease.

Gallbladder Disease

Biliary tract disease of surgical import in children with chronic abdominal pain includes gallstone disease and biliary dyskinesia. The clinical patterns of cholelithiasis are similar to those seen in adults and patients achieve uniformly good results with laparoscopic cholecystectomy. Many have evidence of chronic cholecystitis on histologic examination. The diagnostic triad for patients with biliary dyskinesia includes: postprandial right upper quadrant or epigastric pain, nausea, and a gallbladder ejection fraction below 35% on CCK-HIDA scan. Multiple studies have documented that more than 75% of these patients treated with laparoscopic cholecystectomy achieve good short- and long-term pain relief. However, relief after surgery did not correlate with preoperative ejection fraction values and this same response rate has been observed in patients who did not undergo surgery, some of whom were trialed on a bland diet. The result is that some surgeons will now recommend a 4–6 week course of bland diet therapy and repeat the HIDA scan prior to proceeding with laparoscopic cholecystectomy. Others have tightened the threshold for abnormal gallbladder ejection fraction to 10%. Prior to removing the gallbladder for biliary dyskinesia, my practice is to perform multiple investigations (EGD, liver chemistries, amylase/lipase) to exclude other potential causes of epigastric or RUQ pain.

Pancreatic Disease

Chronic abdominal pain of pancreatic origin is uncommon in children and can be due to chronic pancreatitis or pancreatic pseudocysts. Chronic pancreatitis is most commonly familial. It is progressive and irreversible, causes exocrine and endocrine pancreatic insufficiency, and produces severe chronic pain. The disease can be broadly classified as obstructive (due to a focal, fibrotic narrowing or stenosis from previous acute pancreatitis) or calcifying (due to stone formation with "chain of lakes" strictures). While treatment for this disease is predominantly medical with enzyme replacement therapy and analgesics, surgical intervention should be considered when these fail to relieve pain. Central to operative planning is delineation of pancreatic duct anatomy by ERCP or MRCP, based on which appropriate intervention with ductal drainage (either endoscopic or surgical) or pancreatic resection can be planned. Two of the most commonly utilized procedures include longitudinal pancreaticojejunostomy (modified Peustow procedure) and local resection of the pancreatic head combined with longitudinal pancreaticojejunostomy (Frey procedure). These are effective in relieving pain and reducing narcotic dependence and sometimes slows progressive pancreatic insufficiency.

Most pancreatic pseudocysts in children result from trauma. When these persist, a variety of symptoms and potential complications can occur including persistent abdominal pain, nausea, vomiting and infection or rupture of the pseudocyst. Treatment options include operative and expectant management. Due to the rarity of this disease in children, there are no clear-cut treatment guidelines and therefore care is based on extrapolation of adult guidelines. Based on analysis of children with persistent pseudocysts, it appears that those pseudocysts arising from non-traumatic etiologies are more likely to require surgical interventions, while pseudocysts due to trauma are more likely to resolve with conservative management. For pseudocysts associated with familial pancreatitis, surgical intervention must not only focus on drainage of the pseudocyst but also on treating underlying pancreatic ductal abnormalities.

Bezoar/Foreign Body

Bezoars present as an abdominal mass in children with chronic abdominal pain or are detected by EGD or contrast studies obtained because of obstructive symptoms. Trichobezoars (hair) are the most common and typically require surgical removal via laparotomy with gastrotomy or enterotomy. If they are small, endoscopic fragmentation and removal might be possible. When removing these from one segment of the proximal GI tract, it is important to exclude additional distal bezoars. Phytobezoars (vegetable matter) can usually be managed with chemical dissolution and endoscopic fragmentation. Among the risks of foreign body ingestion are intestinal obstruction or perforation. Radiopaque foreign bodies are easy to identify on plain films, but those that are radiolucent are not easily appreciated until operation is performed for complications. Perforations often occur by gradual erosion over time, resulting in at least partial containment and subtle clinical signs.

Intra-Abdominal Adhesions

Although patients sometimes complain of recurrent pain after intra-abdominal surgery and it is sometimes attributed to postoperative adhesions, it is unclear whether adhesions can actually cause abdominal pain. More importantly, it is difficult to advise surgical intervention for adhesiolysis for pain control alone, especially considering the potential morbidity and the fact that adhesions will reform after each operative intervention. For children who present with these complaints, reassurance that the discomfort should abate as the adhesions soften over the next 6–12 months is sometimes helpful. Consideration for open or laparoscopic adhesiolysis is warranted in patients who complain of chronic pain associated with nausea or vomiting and evidence of partial intestinal obstruction on contrast studies.

Intra-Abdominal Tumors

Tumors are usually detected incidentally or during investigation prompted by systemic signs or symptoms. However, when these tumors achieve a certain size or compromise local organ function, they can produce abdominal pain. For lymphoma, these symptoms are usually those of bowel obstruction or intussusception. The potential for perforation due to tumor infiltration into the bowel wall or as a result of chemotherapy is also present. Symptoms caused by the more common solid tumors (neuroblastoma, Wilms tumor, ovarian tumors, liver masses, rhabdomyosarcoma, hepatoblastoma) are usually due to compression of adjacent structures, hemorrhage within the lesion, or rupture. Ovarian tumors also carry the risk of torsion. Diagnosis can be confirmed with US or CT. If additional information related to vascular anatomy or spinal cord involvement is necessary, MRI is an excellent adjunctive study. In the absence of an urgent need for operation (hemorrhage, bowel obstruction, torsion) it is important to resuscitate the patient and perform a proper staging work-up in accordance with standardized protocols.

Ureteropelvic Junction Obstruction

Unlike infants with UPJ obstruction who present with an abdominal mass or urinary tract infection, the majority of older children present with chronic abdominal pain. The symptoms are often nonspecific, which can lead to diagnostic delay and loss of renal function. Clues to the diagnosis include pain that is referred to the groin or flank, an abdominal mass, and microscopic hematuria. Unfortunately, the absence of these findings does not exclude UPJ obstruction. A high index of suspicion and liberal use of ultrasound to look for evidence of hydronephrosis is necessary to establish a timely diagnosis.

Ovarian Cysts

Girls with symptoms caused by ovarian cysts usually present with pelvic pain due to capsular stretch of the enlarging lesion or peritoneal irritation by fluid or blood within the pelvis from cyst rupture. Pelvic ultrasound will confirm the diagnosis and can usually exclude ovarian torsion as the source of pain. Most of these lesions are functional ovarian cysts of either follicular, corpus luteum (hemorrhagic), or theca lutein origin. These cysts are typically observed for spontaneous resolution, which occurs within 4–8 weeks. Indications for surgical intervention include persistent pain, size greater than 6 cm in diameter, persistence

beyond 8 weeks, cyst enlargement during observation, and ultrasound evidence of ovarian torsion. Ovarian cystectomy with preservation of the remaining ovarian tissue is the preferred operative management and can usually be performed laparoscopically. Residual fluid or blood in the pelvis should be aspirated. To prevent spillage and perform proper staging, laparotomy should be considered for cysts larger than 8 cm in diameter and when malignancy is a concern based on ultrasound findings.

Pelvic Inflammatory Disease/Tubo-Ovarian Abscess

A sexually-transmitted infection of the female pelvic organs, PID is caused by ascending polymicrobial infection with micro-organisms from the vagina and cervix to the upper genital tract, most commonly involving *Neisseria gonorrhea* and *Chlamydia trachomatis*. When chronic, the diagnosis has been missed due to mild symptomatology or the disease has recurred due to continued sexual activity or treatment non-compliance. Affected patients present with a wide variety of nonspecific complaints, including bilateral lower abdominal pain that is exacerbated with movement, purulent vaginal discharge, urethritis, vaginitis and fever. The presence of RUQ pain in this setting (Fitz–Hugh–Curtis syndrome) is due to perihepatitis from transperitoneal or vascular dissemination and signifies a considerable pathogenic inoculation. Physical findings supporting the diagnosis of PID include mucopurulent discharge, cervical motion tenderness, adnexal tenderness, and fever. Laboratory evaluation should include a pregnancy test, CBC, ESR, endocervical cultures, and an HIV screening test. Pelvic ultrasound is useful to confirm the diagnosis and to exclude TOA. Empiric treatment with broad-spectrum antibiotics should be started. Patients with mild to moderate PID can receive outpatient therapy with a single dose of an intramuscular third-generation cephalosporin and oral doxycycline (and sometimes metronidazole) for 14 days. Inpatient therapy is recommended for those who have severe PID, a tubo-ovarian abscess, high fevers, vomiting, or who have failed outpatient therapy. Recommended parenteral regimens include cefotetan or cefoxitin combined with doxycycline or clindamycin combined with gentamicin. When a TOA is present, clindamycin or metronidazole should be added for improved anaerobic coverage. Surgical intervention should be considered if the TOA fails to resolve on follow-up imaging, if the clinical picture fails to improve after 48–72 h of intravenous antibiotics, or if there is a high suspicion of an alternative diagnosis. This is typically accomplished with laparoscopy and entails confirmation of diagnosis with incision and drainage of the TOA or, in some cases, unilateral salpingo-oophorectomy.

Alternatively, the TOA can be drained percutaneously under CT or US guidance.

Endometriosis

Endometriosis is defined as the presence of functioning endometrial tissue (glands and stroma) outside of the uterine cavity. These ectopic implants are believed to result from retrograde menstruation and can be found on the ovaries, parietal peritoneum, broad and uterosacral ligaments, or in the cul-de-sac. They can invade the serosa of the intestinal wall and have also been reported at distant sites. In the pediatric population, adolescents are affected and present with dysmenorrhea and severe perimenstrual lower abdominal and pelvic pain. Those with genital tract obstruction from imperforate hymen or vaginal septum are at higher risk. Physical exam findings that support the diagnosis include retroversion of the uterus with tenderness and nodularity, tenderness or decreased mobility along the uterosacral ligaments, the presence of an adnexal mass (endometrioma), or induration or nodularity of the rectovaginal septum. There are no specific laboratory tests or imaging studies to confirm the diagnosis. Pelvic ultrasound can demonstrate findings of an ovarian endometrioma.

Definitive diagnosis requires laparoscopy or laparotomy with tissue biopsy and pathologic confirmation. The classic description is of a dark-pigmented lesion attributed to hemosiderin deposition. First-line therapy for mild disease includes NSAIDs, with oral contraceptive agents used for more severe disease. If these are ineffective at relieving pain, laparoscopy should be undertaken to confirm the diagnosis and potentially to remove or ablate any visible lesions and adhesions. In general, surgical intervention should probably be undertaken earlier in adolescents in hopes of preserving fertility. Once the diagnosis is confirmed, treatment with gonadotropin-releasing hormone analogs (Lupron) can be utilized but should be reserved for patients who have completed pubertal maturation (16 years of age) because of bone mineral density loss associated with this drug.

Sickle Cell Disease

Abdominal pain and ileus are common during acute crises in children with SCD. Surgeons are frequently called upon for the challenging task of ensuring that these symptoms are not due to a surgical cause. The absence of bone or pleuritic pain might suggest the presence of an underlying primary intra-abdominal source, but there are usually few other differentiating factors. Physical exam findings are often equivocal as well.

Children in the midst of a painful crisis often have an acute drop in their hemoglobin, hyperbilirubinemia, and leukocytosis, but these are nonspecific findings. Because of the potential morbidity associated with missing an intra-abdominal surgical source, imaging should be used liberally, consisting primarily of abdominal CT. After initial consultation, close follow-up of the patient is necessary as symptoms associated with sickle cell crises usually resolve within 4 days. Persistence beyond this time should raise suspicion for another organic cause.

Hypercalcemia

Children with hypercalcemia can present with chronic abdominal pain as part of a symptom complex including nausea, constipation, polydipsia, polyuria, fatigue, lethargy, weakness, and cognitive difficulties. There might be a history of nephrolithiasis. Potential underlying causes include primary hyperparathyroidism (HPT), vitamin D intoxication, milk/alkali syndrome, familial hypocalciuric hypercalcemia, William's syndrome, prolonged immobilization, thyrotoxicosis, and malignancy (much rarer compared to adults). Once the level of hypercalcemia is determined, attention should be focused on rehydration and medical treatment to correct calcium levels. A work up to determine the underlying cause, including measurement of intact parathyroid hormone to rule out primary HPT, should be undertaken. If primary HPT is present, consideration should be given to investigating for other findings of the multiple endocrine neoplasia-1 (parathyroid hyperplasia, pancreatic islet cell tumors, pituitary adenoma) or MEN2A (parathyroid hyperplasia, pheochromocytoma, medullary thyroid cancer).

Lead Poisoning

Lead poisoning results from chronic exposure, most commonly from lead-based paint exposure. The diagnosis should be considered in patients who present with abdominal complaints and a history of environmental exposure. Potential symptoms at presentation include severe colicky abdominal pain, anorexia, constipation, stocking-glove paresthesias, hyperactivity, and seizures. Physical exam might reveal oral ulcerations, a gingival lead line, and peripheral neuropathy. Laboratory analysis often demonstrates microcytic anemia with basophilic stippling of RBCs. Bone films might exhibit lead lines of the distal femur, tibia, and fibula. The diagnosis is confirmed with findings of elevated serum lead levels (recent exposure) or elevated 72-h urine lead levels after calcium disodium edetate administration. Treatment involves oral or parenteral chelating agents.

Acute Intermittent Poryphyria

The porphyrias are a group of inherited metabolic disorders that are caused by specific enzyme deficiencies in the heme biosynthetic pathway, resulting in the accumulation in the tissues of excess metabolic precursors. These are inherited in an autosomal dominant manner with low clinical penetrance. The incidence is between 1 and 10/100,000 population. Presentation is rare before puberty, and many carriers develop symptoms only after exposure to precipitating factors, such as certain drugs, menstruation or physical/emotional stress. The acute porphyrias, of which acute intermittent porphyria is the most common, are characterized by attacks of severe abdominal pain with nausea, vomiting and constipation; signs of sympathetic overactivity with tachycardia and hypertension; peripheral motor neuropathy that can progress to weakness and paralysis; and neuropsychiatric symptoms including seizures, anxiety and mental status changes. These symptoms can last for days to months. The diagnosis might be suspected on the basis of port wine urine and confirmed with measurement of urinary porphobilinogen and porphyrins. More specific quantitative and enzyme tests are subsequently employed. The abdominal exam in these patients typically reveals findings of underlying ileus with distension and decreased bowel sounds, but evidence suggestive of peritoneal irritation might be present.

Treatment involves carbohydrate loading with intravenous glucose infusion, intravenous hemin infusion and removal of identified precipitating factors.

Familial Mediterranean Fever

Familial Mediterranean fever (FMF) is an autosomal recessive disorder that manifests in childhood as self-limited and recurrent attacks of fever, peritonitis, synovitis and pleuritis that last for 1–2 days and occur once or twice monthly. The exact cause of the disorder is unclear, but the pathophysiology appears to be related to a pyrin gene mutation affecting regulation of inflammation in neutrophils. It is common in populations of Eastern Mediterranean origin (1 in 2,700 in Israel). The abdominal examination can be impressive, with findings of an acute abdomen. Laboratory tests reveal leukocytosis with an acute phase reaction (elevated CRP and ESR). Plain films demonstrate bowel wall edema and air-fluid levels. The diagnosis is suspected based on ethnic background and demonstration of the typical clinical profile. The diagnosis can be confirmed and at-risk family members can be screened by detection of the FMF-susceptibility/pyrin gene, *MEFV*, on 16p13. Colchicine is effective treatment for prevention of acute febrile attacks. Long-term complications from this disease include amyloidosis, degenerative arthritis, renal vein thrombosis, and narcotic addiction.

Hereditary Angioedema

Hereditary angioedema is an autosomal dominant inherited deficiency of activated C1 inhibitor (C1-INH), a protein which regulates the intravascular activation of complement. The incidence is approximately 1 in 50,000–150,000 population. The disorder mainly affects the respiratory and GI tracts and is characterized by episodes of self-limited swelling of the face, larynx, extremities and GI tract. Attacks usually begin in childhood and are often heralded by a prodrome consisting of tingling in the area of an impending attack or the appearance of a rash. Gastrointestinal symptoms due to mucosal edema include colicky abdominal pain, nausea, vomiting, and diarrhea and can occur in the absence of swelling at other sites. The swelling can be severe enough to cause intestinal obstruction. Upper GI series might demonstrate "thumbprinting" due to mucosal edema. Measurement of serum C4 levels can be used to screen for this disease, and an assay demonstrating low or poorly-functioning C1-INH confirms it. Treatment for acute attacks includes transfusion with FFP (to supply C1-INH) and epinephrine administered by nebulizer, and intramuscular injection. A concentrate of C1-INH has been used successfully in Europe but is only available in conjunction with clinical trials in the United States. Prophylaxis to prevent recurrent attacks includes therapy with attenuated androgens (Danazol), antifibrinolytic agents (aminocaproic acid), and FFP transfusion.

Vasculitis

It is not uncommon to encounter chronic or recurrent abdominal pain as part of the presenting symptom complex for vasculitic disease. These are systemic illnesses that involve multiple organ systems, including the intestines and solid organs. Two prototypical diseases in this category include Henoch–Schonlein purpura and systemic lupus erythematosus. For HSP, the abdominal pain is attributed to intramural bowel wall hemorrhage with intussusception, while in SLE there are multiple potential intra-abdominal sources of pain. The important point to appreciate from the surgical standpoint is that these are predominantly medical diseases that respond to appropriate medical therapy with immunosuppression and optimization of hemodynamic and hematologic parameters. While surgery does not have a central role in therapy, surgical intervention is necessary in the event of severe GI compromise or intestinal ischemia, intestinal obstruction (intussusception), perforation, or hemorrhage. Surgeons are also sometimes asked to perform a diagnostic laparoscopy with biopsy of the omentum or intra-abdominal lymph nodes to aid in confirming the diagnosis.

Summary Points

- Functional gastrointestinal pain syndromes are specific but poorly understood disorders of the neuron-enteric axis and can cause pain and significant debility.
- The Rome classification is a recently developed clinical tool that has helped us to better understand patients with chronic abdominal pain and to help determine which might benefit from surgical intervention.
- The most common chronic abdominal pain syndromes that come to the attention of the pediatric surgeon include biliary dyskinesia, appendiceal colic, and various other congenital anatomic anomalies (Meckel's diverticulum, malrotation, enteric duplication cysts).
- Patients with certain specific alarm symptoms or focal pain should be considered for diagnostic laparoscopy.

Editor's Comment

Chronic and recurrent abdominal pain is one of the more common indications for referral to a pediatric surgeon, especially the experienced laparoscopist with a known willingness to operate on these children. Many patients will have suffered for months or years with debilitating pain and are desperate for relief at any cost, but it is important to remain objective and consider surgical intervention only in those cases in which it is likely to be of benefit. In this respect, the Rome criteria are a major advance, and should help us to do a better job deciding which patients are more likely to benefit from an operation.

Until very recently, clinicians routinely assumed that abdominal pain with no proven organic basis was psychosomatic or, worse, a harbinger of psychiatric illness. Although the patient experiencing an acute attack of abdominal pain can occasionally appear restive or erratic, the enlightened physician of the twenty-first century understands that the etiology of chronic pain is much more complicated and that the patient could very well be suffering from an organic syndrome that simply eludes our detection at this point in our history. The picture is especially muddled in patients with an underlying neuropsychiatric illness such as autism, who often have a very high pain threshold and the inability to communicate effectively.

Perhaps the most common cause of recurrent abdominal pain is constipation. However, one must be careful not to assume this or casually dismiss a complaint of abdominal pain as "just constipation," which is often an insensitive oversimplification. A more tactful approach is to recommend empiric therapy for constipation while a systematic and thoughtful evaluation is being carried out. Appendiceal colic is also underappreciated as a cause of recurrent abdominal pain. This is partly due to the fact that the classic picture (postprandial right lower quadrant or periumbilical pain associated with nausea and pallor) is absent in many cases and the appendix is invariably normal by imaging studies, and partly due to the fact that many surgeons do not believe it to be a genuine phenomenon. I believe it is real and I always perform an empiric appendectomy whenever I do a diagnostic laparoscopy for abdominal pain. It is surprising how often there is pathology (fibrous obliteration of the lumen, fecalith)

and how often patients feel better after the operation. Remember also that endometriosis in young girls has a different appearance than the "powder burns" classically described in women. Instead, they often appear as tiny nondescript bumps or subtle whitish plaques on the peritoneal surface. Any questionable lesion should be excised and sent for biopsy.

Preoperative Preparation

- ☐ Proper laboratory and imaging work up, especially for retroperitoneal structures
- ☐ Pregnancy test
- ☐ Informed consent, including a frank discussion regarding the likelihood of success

Parental Preparation

- Surgery is not indicated in all cases.
- There is a significant possibility that the pain will persist after surgery.
- It is reasonable and generally safe to remove the appendix as a matter of course.
- Even if the diagnostic operation is negative and the patient continues to have pain, this does not mean that people should assume it is a psychosomatic or psychiatric illness.

Technical Points

- Patients and their families are often desperate and will sometimes be willing to consent to an operation without carefully considering the potential benefits and risks.
- The diagnostic surgical procedure of choice is a meticulous laparoscopic exploration.
- At laparoscopy, rule out adnexal pathology, endometriosis, Crohn's disease, Meckel's diverticulum, malrotation, and other anatomic abnormalities.
- Strongly consider empiric appendectomy.

Suggested Reading

Boyle JT. Abdominal pain. In: Walker WA, Goulet O, Kleinman RE, Sherman PM, Shneider BL, Sanderson IR, editors. Pediatric gastrointestinal disease – pathophysiology, diagnosis, management. 4th ed. Hamilton, ON: BC Decker; 2004. p. 225–43.

Boyle KJ, Torrealday S. Benign gynecologic conditions. Surg Clin North Am. 2008;88(2):245–64.

Di Lorenzo C, Colletti RB, Lehmann HP, et al. Chronic abdominal pain in children: a clinical report of the American Academy of Pediatrics and the North American Society for Pediatric Gastroenterology, Hepatology and Nutrition. J Pediatr Gastroenterol Nutr. 2005a;40: 245–8.

Di Lorenzo C, Colletti RB, Lehmann HP, et al. Chronic abdominal pain in children: a technical report of the American Academy of Pediatrics and the North American Society for Pediatric Gastroenterology, Hepatology and Nutrition. Pediatrics. 2005b; 115:e370–81.

Haricharan RN, Proklova LV, Aprahamian CJ, et al. Laparoscopic cholecystectomy for biliary dyskinesia in children provides durable symptom relief. J Pediatr Surg. 2008;43:1060–4.

Kolts RI, Nelson RS, Park R, et al. Exploratory laparoscopy for recurrent right lower quadrant pain in a pediatric population. J Pediatr Surg Int. 2006;22:247–9.

Levine JS. Gastrointestinal manifestations of systemic disease. In: Yamada T, Alpers DH, Kaplowitz N, Laine L, Owyang C, Powell DW, editors. Textbook of gastroenterology. 4th ed. Philadelphia, PA: Lippincott Williams & Wilkins; 2003. p. 2661–704.

Meyers RL, McCollum MO. Acute and chronic pancreatitis and exocrine pancreatic tumors. In: Mattei P, editor. Surgical directives: pediatric surgery. Philadelphia, PA: Lippincott Williams & Wilkins; 2003. p. 585–95.

Rasquin A, Di Lorenzo C, Forbes D, et al. Childhood functional gastrointestinal disorders: child/adolescent. Gastroenterology. 2006;130: 1527–37.

Teh SH, Pham TH, Lee A, et al. Pancreatic pseudocyst in children: the impact of management strategies on outcome. J Pediatr Surg. 2006;41:1889–93.

Chapter 56
Crohn's Disease

Peter Mattei

Crohn's disease is one of the two commonly seen inflammatory bowel diseases. As opposed to ulcerative colitis, which only directly affects the colon and rectum, Crohn's disease can affect any part of the intestinal tract. It can also involve the full thickness of the bowel wall, which accounts for many of the complications seen with the disease. Surgery is not curative but is reserved for the treatment of complications that are refractory to medical management. The etiology is unknown but it is increasingly clear that most patients have a genetic predisposition, though what purported environmental triggers are involved is less clear. Medical therapy has improved significantly, especially with the development of infliximab and adalimumab, but the prevalence of the disease is increasing, more patients are being identified at a younger age, and many still develop complications that require surgical intervention.

Although the disease can affect any part of the GI tract "from the mouth to the anus," nearly all patients who come to the attention of a surgeon have one of three distinct patterns of disease: ileal, colonic, or perianal disease.

Ileal Disease

Children with acute ileitis will sometimes present with right lower quadrant pain, fever, and GI symptoms, thus mimicking acute appendicitis. When findings consistent with ileitis are seen on an abdominal CT scan, the patient is usually treated medically for presumed infectious ileitis by the medical service and evaluated for the possibility of Crohn's disease as an outpatient. If a patient is brought to the operating room for presumed appendicitis and found instead to have ileitis, the surgeon has a decision to make: resect, biopsy, appendectomy, or simply close. In the setting of chronic symptoms (abdominal pain, diarrhea, poor weight gain, growth retardation) and

P. Mattei (✉)
Department of General Surgery, Children's Hospital of Philadelphia, Philadelphia, PA 19140, USA
e-mail: mattei@email.chop.edu

severe disease in the ileum that is clearly chronic (fibrosis, chronic bowel obstruction, creeping fat, or fistulae), ileocecal resection with primary anastomosis is acceptable and safe. On the other hand, if the symptoms are clearly of recent onset and the ileal disease appears to be mild, non-obstructing, and acute, then resection might be considered excessive and unnecessary. Biopsy is inadvisable because of the risk of postoperative fistula formation or abscess. Appendectomy is probably safe if the base of the appendix and the cecum are clearly normal. Regardless, it is important to document the findings in great detail in the operative note and, whenever possible, with intra-operative photographs.

More commonly, the surgeon is consulted for the patient with known Crohn's disease who has developed severe chronic symptoms or an acute complication. The most common chronic picture is that of a partial small bowel obstruction due to a fibrotic stricture or recurring bouts of complete bowel obstruction that respond to high-dose steroid therapy. Other common presenting complaints include chronic and recurrent abdominal pain, failure to thrive, short stature, and delayed sexual maturation. Some patients develop adverse reactions or intolerance of medical therapy or simply desire relief from taking too many drugs. Ileal disease can also fistulize to other loops of bowel, the colon, or the bladder. Sinus tracts that open into the peritoneum can result in free perforation or an enterocutaneous fistula but more commonly produce an intra-abdominal abscess.

Except for the exceedingly rare case of free perforation and the occasional complete bowel obstruction that does not respond to bowel rest and corticosteroids, these patients are nearly always able to be treated on a semi-elective basis. This is preferable to having to perform an operation emergently as the risks are greater, the likelihood of needing a temporary diverting ileostomy is probably slightly higher, and the need to make a large laparotomy incision is greater. While awaiting operation, patients should be given nasogastric or intravenous nutrition. Abscesses should be drained percutaneously and the drain left in place (controlled enterocutaneous fistula) while the patient is treated with antibiotics: intravenous for two weeks and oral for two to three weeks until the day of surgery. Formal bowel preparation is not necessary, but having the patient take nothing but clear liquids for 24 h prior to operation seems to help to decrease the amount of feculent material in the ileum and the diameter of the chronically obstructed bowel.

Diagnosis

The decision to operate is based principally on the patient's clinical picture and response to medication, however medical imaging can help to identify the most active site of disease and over time can reveal the rate of progression of the disease. The upper GI contrast study with small bowel follow-through helps to demonstrate the location of disease and gives some information regarding its severity (Fig. 56.1). It is very sensitive for small bowel strictures but gives little information regarding the relative contributions of inflammation and fibrosis on the origin of the stricture. This is potentially important regarding prognosis as in theory inflammation is reversible while fibrosis is not. When reviewing these images, it is important to focus not only on the more vivid luminal contrast but also to the negative space in the image, which represents the thickened wall of the affected bowel segment pushing other contrast-filled loops out of the

way. This study will also sometimes demonstrate a fistula or bowel distension due to chronic obstruction.

Computed tomography is also a very useful study in patients with Crohn's disease but tends to be less commonly used than UGI, perhaps because of the perception that it exposes the patient to more radiation. MRI is being used more frequently, but interpretation of the images can be difficult. This will improve with cumulative experience and it will likely soon become the diagnostic study of choice in these patients.

Surgical Treatment

Bowel resection is the treatment of choice for long segments of Crohn's disease of the small intestine. In the vast majority of cases, this entails ileocecectomy (Fig. 56.2). A primary anastomosis is almost always feasible as ileostomy is almost never, if ever, indicated. The operation can and should be performed through a very small lower midline, periumbilical, or transverse right lower quadrant incision, made just big enough to allow removal of the diseased bowel (typically 4–7 cm). For ileocecectomy, the right colon is easily mobilized up to and including the hepatic flexure using a laparoscopic approach, which then allows the resection and anastomosis to be performed through a very small incision created by extending one of the port sites. A small transverse right lower quadrant muscle-splitting incision is cosmetically acceptable and associated with little postoperative discomfort. A side-to-side, functional end-to-end, stapled anastomosis is preferred: it is quick, associated with a minimal risk of leak, and has been shown to have superior long-term patency rates compared to traditional hand-sewn anastomoses, particularly in patients with Crohn's disease. All incisions should be closed primarily with absorbable suture in standard fashion and the use of cyanoacrylate glue results in excellent cosmesis and a very low incidence of wound infection.

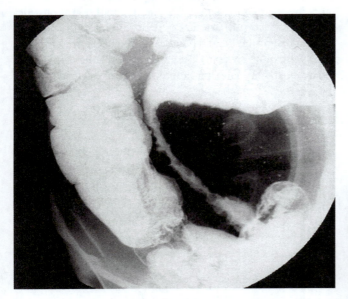

Fig. 56.1 Upper GI contrast study with small bowel follow-through in a patient with Crohn's disease of the terminal ileum. This image demonstrates a long segment of stricturing disease in the ileum. Note the "negative space" adjacent to the thin column of contrast within the strictured segment, which is the bowel wall, thickened by inflammation and fibrosis, displacing adjacent contrast-filled loops of bowel. (Reprinted from von Allmen D. Surgical management of Crohn's disease. In: Mamula P, Markowitz JE, Baldassano RN, editors. Pediatric inflammatory bowel disease. New York: Springer; 2008, p. 459.)

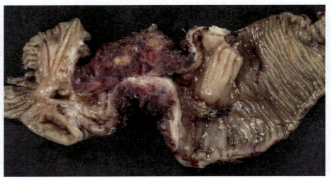

Fig. 56.2 Pathologic specimen from patient with Crohn's disease and ileal stricture. Note the thickness of the wall of the strictured segment and the large diameter of the chronically obstructed and dilated ileum proximal to the stricture (*right*)

Besides complete laparoscopic mobilization of the right colon, there are several other maneuvers that can help to minimize the size of the open incision. The cecum is usually uninvolved and can be delivered into the incision first. Divide the right colon with a stapling device just above the cecum, place a stay suture at the corner of the distal colon staple line, and drop it back into the abdomen. Next try to deliver the diseased bowel, sometimes pausing to divide the mesentery between absorbable ligatures. (The mesentery in Crohn's disease is often thick and hypervascular, making suture ligatures the safest way to control bleeding from the mesentery that is to remain.) When trying to deliver the diseased bowel, a laparotomy sponge provides a good grip on the bowel, while a gentle back-and-forth rocking motion and simultaneously sliding a short one-inch Richardson retractor around the incision to push the skin and fascia down and away will often allow the phlegmonous bowel to be delivered. The proximal bowel is divided just proximal to the diseased segment (it does not need to be histologically normal) and that end is marked with a stay suture and dropped back inside. The mesentery is then divided in the usual fashion. Prior to making an anastomosis, the small bowel should be inspected all the way to the ligament of Treitz to be sure there are no other areas of severe disease that might require resection. Mild disease is left alone while short strictures can be treated by resection or a standard Heineke–Mikulicz stricturoplasty. Every effort should be made to preserve bowel length. It is also a good idea to close the mesenteric defect before performing the anastomosis, as it is much easier to perform this way. It also allows you to rule out the presence of a twist in the bowel. Again, ileostomy is almost never indicated.

In many cases, fistulae to normal adjacent bowel or sigmoid colon can be controlled laparoscopically by application of a gastrointestinal endostapler across the fistula where it meets the normal bowel. If the involved loop is also diseased, then it should be resected as well. Dividing the fistula laparoscopically will allow both loops to be delivered sequentially through the same small incision rather than as a large, phlegmonous mass. Fistulae to the bladder usually require suture repair of the bladder with absorbable suture and Foley catheter decompression for several days. Unexpected abscesses can be evacuated and the adhesions forming the walls of the abscess lysed. Resection of the diseased bowel is still indicated if it can be freed from all adhesions.

Colitis

Crohn's disease can create colonic strictures that are resected using a laparoscopic-assisted technique as described for small bowel disease, but this is an uncommon presentation. However, when it occurs near the recto-sigmoid junction or when the disease extends into the rectum, this is one of the rare indications for colostomy, as a low anterior or rectal anastomosis is perilous under these circumstances. The diagnosis is usually confirmed by colonoscopy or contrast enema. Abdominal CT or MRI are also increasingly being used.

The more common clinical manifestation of Crohn's colitis is fulminant hemorrhagic colitis. It is often confused with ulcerative colitis and it is this difficult distinction that creates some of the uncertainty regarding the best surgical course of action. If ulcerative colitis is likely and the patient with hemorrhagic colitis fails to respond to maximal medical therapy, one should feel comfortable recommending a subtotal colectomy with ileostomy and delayed proctectomy with ileo-anal reconstruction. On the other hand, Crohn's colitis will in some cases respond to simple ileal diversion or segmental colectomy, thus allowing preservation of at least part of the colon and the entire rectum.

Diverting ileostomy is a reasonable option in some children with severe colitis and a high suspicion for Crohn's disease, but it is rarely done. The decision to reverse the ileostomy is then often delayed indefinitely and is difficult due to persistence of disease in the colon and vacillation regarding the appropriate next step. In addition, after ileostomy takedown, there is a high incidence of disease recidivism. In most cases of fulminant hemorrhagic colitis, whether the ultimate diagnosis is UC, Crohn's colitis, or indeterminate colitis, the best course of action is usually a subtotal colectomy, preferably performed laparoscopically. This allows the patient to heal, improve nutrition, and wean medications (corticosteroids) while the diagnostic conundrum is resolved with reasonable certainty. When the patient is healthy, reconstruction can be in the form of a proctectomy and J-pouch ileo-anal reconstruction or, if the patient turns out to have Crohn's disease, an ileo-sigmoid colostomy or ileorectostomy.

Laparoscopic subtotal colectomy is a safe and straightforward operation. Two 10–12-mm trocars are placed, on at the umbilicus and one in the right lower quadrant at the site marked for an ileostomy. A third 5-mm port is placed in the left lower quadrant. The lateral attachments of the colon and the omentum are mobilized using the harmonic scalpel while the mesocolon is divided up and away from the deeper structures with a bipolar electrocautery device designed to handle larger blood vessels. I prefer to start at the sigmoid colon, mobilize the splenic flexure, start taking the omentum of the left lateral transverse colon, and then begin to divide the left mesocolon down to the distal sigmoid and across to the middle colic vessels. I use a 60-mm endostapler to divide the sigmoid and then begin to take down the hepatic flexure and right colon. The colon can then be brought out through an ileostomy incision created by extending the right lower quadrant port site slightly. Hemostasis is confirmed, the abdomen is irrigated, and the port sites are closed. Finally, a Brooke ileostomy is matured in the standard fashion.

Patients with ulcerative colitis but are well-nourished and on less than 20 mg daily of oral prednisone can be considered for a one- or two-stage colectomy/ileo-anal reconstruction. Any uncertainty regarding the possibility of Crohn's colitis should be considered a contraindication to proctectomy and ileo-anal reconstruction. These patients are candidates for diverting ileostomy, parial colectomy or subtotal colectomy with ileostomy.

Perirectal Disease

Crohn's perirectal disease can range from mild and annoying to stubborn and heart-breaking. The clinical manifestations include: skin tags, anal fissures, fistula-in-ano, perirectal abscess, and anorectal stricture. The pattern of disease is usually acute-on-chronic and medical therapy is improving the plight of these patients to some degree. Nevertheless, surgical intervention is frequently required to treat symptoms, prevent worsening of disease, and avert complications. We tend to try our best to avoid fecal diversion except in the most severe cases, mostly because of the obvious significant emotional and psychological issues related to having a stoma in adolescence, but also because although the infectious complications of the disease often resolve after diversion, the inflammatory and destructive components of the disease often persist and progress. Nevertheless, colostomy is unfortunately sometimes the only practical and safe option.

Skin tags should almost never be excised as they usually grow back and the procedure is often complicated by poor wound healing. It is sometimes useful as a diagnostic maneuver since the skin tags frequently have the characteristic granulomata on histopathologic analysis. Fissures are considered a marker of the degree of active inflammatory disease and are also not treated surgically because of poor wound healing and a high recurrence rate. They are treated with local measures and systemic anti-inflammatory medications.

Fistulae-in-ano are treated surgically but conservatively. Fistulectomy should be avoided as wound complications and sphincter injury are too often the result. Simple debridement, temporary drainage, injection of fibrin sealant, or placement of collagen plugs sometimes allow the simplest of fistulae to close, but complex fistulae associated with chronic infection, severe inflammation, or rectal stricture almost never respond to such measures. Fistulae are often complex and deep-seated. They can burrow circumferentially and up to the labia or scrotum, and can form multiple external skin openings along a single long tract. The mainstay to the surgical approach is examination under anesthesia (EUA), however pelvic MRI is an excellent way to assess the true extent of disease prior to going to the OR. In the OR, the fistula should be probed gently, avoiding the creation of a false passage, but all will have an external skin opening and an internal opening in the rectum. A No. 2 silk thread should be passed through the fistula and tied to itself loosely in the form of a non-cutting seton. This is well-tolerated and can be left in place indefinitely, keeping the fistula open at both ends and preventing the formation of an abscess. The seton usually falls out on its own in 12–18 months or it can be removed painlessly in the office if medical therapy has allowed complete resolution of all signs of active inflammation and chronic infection. If better drainage is needed, a silastic vessel loop tied to itself can be placed in parallel with the silk seton and removed in two to three weeks in the office. Complex fistulae require creative combinations of drains and setons. It usually best to find a way to tie the drains to themselves to avoid premature dislodgement and obviate the need for stitches to the skin. An alternative is to secure the drain with a rapidly dissolving suture material to allow the drain to fall out on it own within a few weeks.

In patients with Crohn's disease, a perirectal abscess is always associated with a fistula and is therefore best managed in the operating room. This allows complete evacuation of the abscess, which is often quite large and complex, and control of the fistula with a silastic drain (short-term) and a seton (long-term).

Abscesses and fistulae are also strongly associated with anorectal strictures, usually as they heal. Infliximab has the reputation for "causing" strictures, but this is probably because it is so effective at getting fistulae to heal. Short and distal strictures usually respond well to anal dilatation with cervical dilators. This is always done in the OR and usually needs to be repeated periodically. Some patients, after being taught how to do so in the office, are able to use a dilator every day at home to keep the stricture from closing down.

Long, recalcitrant, or high strictures can sometimes be treated with periodic dilatation but these are the patients at risk for perforation of the distal sigmoid colon, especially if the disease extends up into the abdomen. It is therefore best in these cases to recommend empiric diversion or, if the patient refuses to consent to colostomy, perhaps a single attempt at dilatation in a controlled setting, possibly with balloon dilatation, in the operating room, with all precautions taken in case of a perforation (hospital admission, intravenous antibiotics, frequent radiographic assessment, low threshold for surgical intervention if there are any signs of a bowel injury).

Crohn's disease can also produce vulvar edema and fissures in girls. A fistula should be sought for by MRI and EUA but can be difficult to identify. Recto-vaginal fistulae are a feared complication that are often, but not always, considered an indication for fecal diversion. If the inflammatory component can be treated medically but the fistula persists, then surgical closure with tissue flap advancement should be considered. Results are certainly better when performed in the setting of a temporary colostomy. It is reasonable in most cases to start with conservative measures but to offer colostomy for those who fail to respond.

Though perianal Crohn's disease is not cured by surgical intervention, it can usually be controlled when managed attentively. This requires frequent office assessment and periodic MRI and/or EUA. Asking the adolescent with perianal disease to come for follow-up visits "as needed" is discouraged because it is important to start therapy before the disease has progressed too far. The goal should be to maintain patient comfort, prevent infectious complications, and stay ahead of strictures and complex fistulae, while all the while helping the patient cope with issues related to hygiene, peer interaction, and sexual function.

Postoperative Care

Most patients can be discharged to home after EUA and placement of a drain or seton, unless they require intravenous antibiotics, intravenous pain control, or specific observation. After small bowel resection, ileocecectomy, or subtotal colectomy, patients are admitted and can usually be treated using a fast-track protocol. This includes: no routine nasogastric tube, early oral intake of fluids, advance to regular diet as tolerated, minimizing narcotics and intravenous "maintenance" fluids, early ambulation, and administration of a rectal suppository to initiate a bowel movement on postoperative day two. Most patients can expect to be discharged on postoperative two or three after elective ileocecectomy, an on postoperative day three or four after subtotal colectomy.

Criteria for discharge include: tolerating a regular diet, ambulating without assistance, good pain control with oral analgesics, and no fever. It is also preferable that they have a bowel movement prior to discharge.

Prophylactic antibiotics should be given within 60 min of incision and, although there is no evidence to support the practice, can be continued for up to 24 h postoperatively. Corticosteroids should be weaned slowly in the postoperative period, not because of the risk of adrenal insufficiency, which is actually quite rare in children under these circumstances, but rather because of the risk of intestinal pseudo-obstruction, which occurs with surprising frequency when corticosteroids are weaned too quickly after an abdominal operation. Narcotics should be weaned quickly after the night of surgery. Ketorolac is an excellent alternative that allows most patients to avoid the use of narcotics until oral analgesia is tolerated. There is a general reluctance to use NSAIDs in patients in with Crohn's disease because of the perceived but ill-defined risk of inducing a flare. Nevertheless, we use it routinely in these patients and have had excellent results and no evidence of adverse effects.

The results of surgery for Crohn's disease are generally excellent and durable. The majority of patients have a long period of remission with near complete resolution of symptoms, significant tapering of their medical regimen, excellent weight gain and growth, and substantial improvement in their quality of life. Long-term results depend on the severity of the underlying disease and patient compliance with their medical regimen, but it is unusual for patients to require a second abdominal operation for Crohn's disease within eight to ten years of their first operation. The hope is, of course, that medical advances will eventually make this disease manageable without surgery or completely curable with drugs alone.

Summary Points

- Crohn's disease can affect any part of the GI tract, but the three common patterns of disease that come to the attention of the surgeon are ileal, colonic, and perianal disease.
- The terminal ileum is the most common site of severe disease, where it can cause strictures, fistulae, or abscesses.
- Ileocecectomy is the most common surgical procedure in patients with Crohn's disease and is well-suited to a laparoscopic-assisted approach.
- Most operations can be performed on a semi-elective basis rather than as an emergency.
- Ileostomy is rarely indicated after ileocecectomy, and only under extreme circumstances.
- Patients with severe Crohn's colitis are candidates for ileal diversion, partial colectomy, or subtotal colectomy.
- Colectomy can often be performed laparoscopically.
- It is sometimes difficult to distinguish fulminant ulcerative colitis and severe Crohn's colitis.
- Crohn's perianal disease is manifests principally as skin tags, fissures, fistulae, abscess, and/or stricture.
- Fistulae are rarely cured with surgery but are best controlled with temporary drains and non-cutting silk setons.
- Strictures may respond to periodic anal dilatation but in severe cases are an indication for colostomy.

Differential Diagnosis

- Crohn's disease
- Ulcerative colitis
- Infectious ileitis
- Behçet's disease

Preoperative Preparation

- ☐ Clear liquids only by mouth for 24 h
- ☐ Prophylactic antibiotics
- ☐ Work up to confirm diagnosis of Crohn's versus ulcerative colitis
- ☐ Informed consent

Parental Preparation

- Extremely low likelihood of needing an ileostomy or colostomy
- Chance of finding additional areas of severe disease elsewhere in the small intestine
- Potential complications are rare but include: infection (wound, anastomotic leak, intra-abdominal abscess), bleeding, injury to other structures (ureter, bladder, bowel), anastomotic stricture, recurrence
- Barring a complication, expect discharge as early as day 2–3 after ileocecectomy or day 3–4 after subtotal colectomy with ileostomy
- Small possibility of requiring a blood transfusion
- Surgery is not curative and medication will be needed but there is a high probability that the patient will enjoy a period of clinical remission and a good quality of life after surgery

Diagnostic Studies

- Upper GI contrast study w/small bowel follow through
- Abdominal CT scan
- Abdominal MRI
- Upper and lower endoscopy
- Anorectal examination under anesthesia
- Pelvic MRI

Technical Points

- The main reason to use laparoscopy for ileocecectomy is to mobilize the entire right colon and hepatic flexure to allow resection of the diseased segment and anastomosis through a small lower abdominal incision.
- The incision can be right lower quadrant transverse, extended periumbilical, or lower midline.
- The stapled side-to-side functional end-to-end anastomosis is quick, secure, and good long-term patency rates.
- Before completing the operation, run the entire small bowel to identify other severe areas that should be resected or opened by stricturoplasty.
- Patients with fulminant or hemorrhagic colitis, subtotal colectomy with ileostomy is usually the best option, though consideration can be given to diverting ileostomy or partial colectomy.
- Colectomy is an operation well suited to a laparoscopic approach.
- Patients with perianal disease can benefit from a thorough examination under anesthesia.
- Skin tags and fissures are generally not treated surgically because of poor healing and a high rate of recurrence.
- Abscesses should be drained and the associated fistula-in-ano controlled to prevent recurrence.
- Fistulectomy is associated with poor healing and complications and is usually best avoided.
- Drains and/or setons can placed through the fistula and tied to themselves loosely to avoid sutures placed in the perianal skin.

Suggested Reading

Bousvaros A, Antonioli DA, Colletti RB, et al. Differentiating ulcerative colitis from Crohn disease in children and young adults: report of a working group of the North American Society for Pediatric Gastroenterology, Hepatology, and Nutrition and the Crohn's and Colitis Foundation of America. J Pediatr Gastroenterol Nutr. 2007;44(5):653–74.

Carvalho R, Hyams JS. Diagnosis and management of inflammatory bowel disease in children. Semin Pediatr Surg. 2007;16(3):164–71.

Strong SA. Perianal Crohn's disease. Semin Pediatr Surg. 2007;16(3): 185–93.

Vogel J, da Luz Moreira A, Baker M, Hammel J, Einstein D, Stocchi L, et al. CT enterography for Crohn's disease: accurate preoperative diagnostic imaging. Dis Colon Rectum. 2007;50(11):1761–9.

Von Allmen D. Surgical management of Crohn's disease in children. Curr Treat Options Gastroenterol. 2005;8(5):405–10.

Von Allmen D, Markowitz JE, York A, Mamula P, Shepanski M, Baldassano R. Laparoscopic-assisted bowel resection offers advantages over open surgery for treatment of segmental Crohn's disease in children. J Pediatr Surg. 2003;38(6):963–5.

Chapter 57
Ileostomy and Colostomy

Oliver S. Soldes

In any age group, creation of an intestinal stoma is a significant event with major physiologic, body image, lifestyle, and psychosocial implications. Management and indications for ostomies in infants and young children are often different than in adolescents and adults. This is a consequence of the differing diagnoses, physiology, size, growth and development issues, complications, and unique patient and parental adjustment concerns.

Intestinal stomas in the pediatric population are more likely to be temporary adjuncts in the management of surgical emergencies and congenital anomalies. Permanent intestinal stomas are usually only formed for failures of management of some congenital disorders (anorectal malformations, myelomeningocele), inflammatory bowel disease, or, rarely, unresectable pelvic, abdominal or intestinal tumors (desmoid tumor, giant neurofibroma, sarcoma) and then more commonly in older children after unsuccessful reconstructive procedures. Fortunately, small bowel and colonic stomas of all types are often reversed within a few months or years, and, with rare exception, every effort is made to eventually eliminate the need for an ileostomy or colostomy. There are also several special types of ostomies rarely used outside of pediatric practice that are employed for certain conditions unique to pediatric surgical practice, examples of which include the Bishop–Koop ileostomy for meconium ileus and the divided descending/sigmoid colostomy for high imperforate anus.

Indications

The indications for an ostomy are dictated by the diagnosis and the desired function of the stoma (Table 57.1). The function of an ileostomy or colostomy is usually diversion of the fecal stream, decompression of dilated or obstructed bowel, or access for irrigation and evacuation of stool or inspissated meconium. Stomas commonly used for diversion and decompression include the end stoma, the double-barrel stoma, and the loop stoma and its variations (rodless end-loop stoma, divided loop ileostomy). Stomas for irrigation and evacuation include appendicostomies and catheterizable cecal conduits, tube cecostomy, and tube sigmoidostomy. Venting stomas with end-to-side anastomosis and distal vent (Bishop–Koop) or side-to-end anastomosis and proximal vent (Santulli) perform both diverting and irrigation functions and are still occasionally used in the management of meconium ileus.

In pediatric surgical practice, roughly three fourths of ostomies are placed in neonates and infants. In neonates, enterostomies are utilized in the management of diverse diagnoses such as necrotizing enterocolitis with perforation, complicated intestinal atresia, volvulus, Hirschsprung disease, meconium ileus, imperforate anus, or cloaca. The young child or adolescent will sometimes require an ostomy for the management of medically refractory Crohn's disease, as part of the staged operative approach to ulcerative colitis, bowel perforation with extensive peritoneal contamination or ischemia (volvulus, trauma, inflammatory bowel disease) and failure of reconstruction and management of congenital anomalies (high imperforate anus, myelomeningocele, Hirschsprung disease).

When fashioning an ileostomy or colostomy, a decision must be made as to whether to use a loop or end stoma, or a variant of these types (Fig. 57.1). The type of stoma is determined by a variety of factors, including the indication for diversion, anticipated length of time the stoma will be required, planned future procedures, underlying disease process, and anatomy. Loop ileostomy and colostomy are generally utilized when a temporary stoma is desired to protect a distal anastomosis, or to relieve distal obstruction and decompress the proximal bowel prior to definitive surgical management of the obstruction. The main advantage of a loop ostomy is ease of reversal. Loop stomas can be reversed with a localized procedure around the stoma, avoiding a full laparotomy. The marginal blood supply to the distal stoma is also more

O.S. Soldes (✉)
Department of Pediatric Surgery, Cleveland Clinic Foundation, Desk M14, 9500 Euclid Avenue, Cleveland, OH 44195, USA
e-mail: soldeso@ccf.org

P. Mattei (ed.), *Fundamentals of Pediatric Surgery*,
DOI 10.1007/978-1-4419-6643-8_57, © Springer Science+Business Media, LLC 2011

easily preserved with a loop stoma. A major disadvantage of a loop ostomy is a greater tendency to prolapse, retract or develop parastomal hernias, due to the larger fascial opening needed to bring out both ends of the bowel. A double-barrel stoma is similar to loop stoma but the bowel is completely divided.

End stomas are selected in the setting of bowel resection, when a permanent or long duration stoma is anticipated, or complete fecal diversion is desired. End stomas are often employed in the setting of an abdominal surgical

emergency, such as one involving bowel necrosis, ischemia or perforation with gross contamination. An end stoma is usually chosen when a segment of bowel is resected and there is significant concern for leakage following a primary anastomosis (necrotizing enterocolitis with perforation, tenuous blood supply, acidotic and poorly perfused patient). It might also be chosen for anatomic considerations, such as limited mesenteric length, that preclude loop ostomies.

The end stoma is generally formed at the site of resection. The distal end of the intestine must be managed as either a Hartmann's pouch or by the creation of a mucous fistula. In the absence of distal obstruction, the distal bowel segment may be closed and dropped back into the abdomen at the time of the initial operation (Hartmann's procedure). Future closure of the end stoma is usually facilitated by tacking the closed distal end of the bowel to the side of the proximal bowel or to the fascia.

If there is distal obstruction or if there is a reason to need access to the distal bowel segment, then a mucous fistula is created. The advantage of the end stoma is that it is completely diverting and less likely to prolapse. The main disadvantage of the end stoma is that it often requires a somewhat bigger operation to bring the two bowel ends together to form an anastomosis.

Table 57.1 Function and types of ileostomy and colostomy

Stomas for intestinal diversion and decompression
    End ostomy
    Loop ostomy and variants (rodless end-loop stoma)
    Double-barrel ostomy
Stomas for irrigation and evacuation
    Appendicostomy
    Catherizable cecal conduit
    Tube cecostomy or sigmoidostomy
Stomas for both diversion and irrigation/evacuation
    Distal venting ileostomy with end-to-side anastomosis
    (Bishop–Koop)
    Proximal venting ileostomy with side-to-end anastomosis (Santulli)
    Divided descending sigmoid colostomy for high imperforate anus

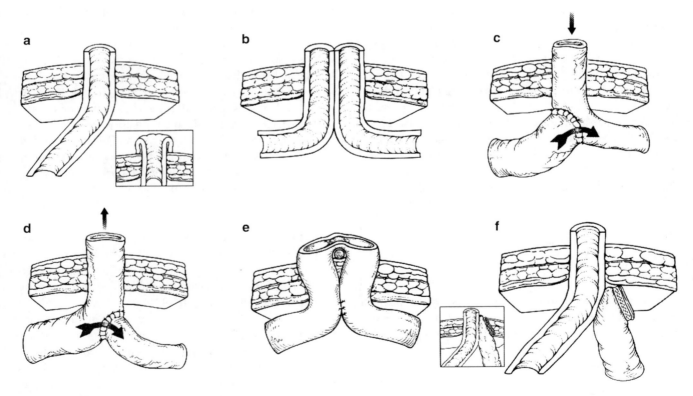

Fig. 57.1 Stoma variants. (**a**) End stoma amd Brooke maturation (inset). (**b**) Double-barrel stoma. (**c**) Bishop–Koop: distal stoma with proximal end-to-side anastomosis. (**d**) Santulli: proximal stoma with side-to-end distal anastomosis. (**e**) Loop ostomy. (**f**) End stoma with Hartmann's clo-sure and rodless end-loop variation (*inset*). (From Gauderer MWL. Stomas of the small and large intestine, Chapter 96. In: Grosfeld JL, O'Neill JA, Fonkalsrud EW, Coran AG, editors. Pediatric surgery. 6th ed. Philadelphia, PA: Mosby; 2006, with permission from Elsevier.)

Several types of permanent stomas are used for daily irrigation of the colon in patients with failed reconstruction of high imperforate anus, Hirschsprung disease, chronic constipation, and overflow incontinence. These irrigating stomas serve to improve cleanliness and the quality of life for children with chronic soiling, poor control of defecation, and leakage of stool. They include intermittently catheterizable appendicostomy and cecal conduits, tube cecostomy, and sigmoidostomy. All are intended primarily to facilitate the instillation of an antegrade enema by intermittent catheterization or indwelling tube. A large-volume (15–20 mL/kg or more) warm tap water or saline colonic enema is given daily, usually in the evening, to achieve a daily bowel movement. The colon is then emptied nightly and allowed to function as a passive reservoir for stool until the next enema. The volume is titrated to effect. The saline enema solution is usually made at home by the caregiver, mixing 1½ teaspoons of table salt in 1,000 mL of warm water. The intermittently catheterizable stomas have the advantage of enhanced body image because there is no appliance on the abdominal wall. The umbilical appendicostomy is fashioned at the base of the umbilicus by open or laparoscopic technique where it is well hidden. Continuously catheterized tube stomas, such as the cecostomy button (usually a standard gastrostomy button), endoscopically placed ("pull-type" percutaneous endoscopic gastrostomy style tube), or radiologically placed (Chait) tube, leave the patient with an external appliance that allows access to the GI tract. These types of tubes are prone to the usual gastrostomy tube complications (displacement, mechanical malfunction, infection, skin irritation and breakdown, peristomal fistula) and need to be replaced periodically. Intermittently catheterized stomas are complicated by stenosis, retraction or perforation of the intestine by the intestinal tube. With time, neurologically intact older children and adolescents are usually able to completely assume all of the care associated the enemas.

Preoperative Preparation

Intestinal stomas in the children are much more likely to be created in management of unexpected abdominal surgical emergencies and congenital anomalies. As such, the opportunity for preoperative counseling and parental preparation might be limited, but should be undertaken whenever possible. A notable exception is in patients undergoing elective or semi-elective procedures for IBD, imperforate anus, and Hirschsprung disease. In this setting, preoperative consultation with an enterostomal therapist is useful for counseling, stoma site marking, and education. Discussion of the possible need for an ostomy should be

part of the informed consent prior to any procedure likely to involve a bowel resection.

In the case of elective formation or closure of an ileostomy or colostomy, pre-operative bowel preparation is generally performed outside of the neonatal period. At minimum, an oral clear liquids diet is given for 24 h prior to surgery. We prefer a traditional bowel preparation, particularly for colon surgery, in children older than one year, who are usually admitted the day before surgery. A slender nasogastric feeding tube (6-0 Fr) is placed and polyethylene glycol (PEG) solution is administered at a rate of 25 mL/kg/h until the output is clear. Adolescents can undergo bowel preparation at home with standard regimens (sodium phosphates oral solution or PEG) used for adult surgery. Sodium phosphates oral solution is sometimes better tolerated by adolescents because a lower volume is needed than for PEG solution. Neonates and infants undergoing ileostomy and colostomy formation or closure require only preoperative clear liquids with or without retrograde distal intestinal irrigation on the floor or in the operating room prior to incision. Mechanical bowel preparation is usually not possible when there is obstruction and perforation. Three doses of oral antibiotics (erythromycin 15 mg/kg/dose and neomycin 30 mg/kg/dose or metronidazole 7 mg/kg/dose, up to adult dose) are still given by some surgeons, particularly for older children and adolescents, as is distal tap water or 1% neomycin enemas. Appropriate perioperative intravenous antibiotics are always used in every age group, prior to incision and for up to 24 h postoperatively.

Pre-operative contrast studies of the distal bowel (rectal contrast enema, ileostomy injection or colostogram) are generally indicated prior to elective closure of enterostomies, especially in the setting of previous necrotizing enterocolitis, ischemia, volvulus, and atresia. Neonates and infants with a history of necrotizing enterocolitis or ischemic volvulus can have unsuspected distal strictures that develop during recovery from their initial illness.

Ileostomy

In newborns and infants, an ileostomy is usually performed when an anastomosis is judged to be unsafe during an operation for necrotizing enterocolitis, meconium ileus, complex intestinal atresia, or volvulus with necrosis. These are most commonly end ileostomies and a mucous fistula is usually created as well. They can be brought up through the primary incision or a separate incision. Using the primary incision has the disadvantage of a higher risk of wound complications and infection. The distal end is also sometimes be tacked to the proximal end or the fascia to make later closure easier. In the setting of extensive patchy necrotizing enterocolitis or multiple atresias, multiple ostomies can be formed to salvage segments of bowel that cannot be safely anastomosed, to preserve bowel length, and to mitigate short bowel syndrome.

When the functional end of the bowel is brought through or close to the laparotomy incision and peritoneal contamination is minimal, we close the remainder of the primary incision with cyanoacrylate topical skin adhesive, which acts as an effective barrier. The bowel is secured to the fascia or skin with interrupted 4-0 polyglycolic acid sutures. In neonates, where possible, at least 1 cm of ileum should be allowed to protrude. The bowel is tacked to the skin edges with partial-thickness 4-0 polyglycolic acid sutures. Maturation of the end of the stoma and mucocutaneous sutures are avoided in small premature infants, in whom the end of the bowel is fragile and easily traumatized. Within two weeks, the end of the small bowel will spontaneously roll back to mature itself. In full-term newborns and older infants, a few fine interrupted absorbable sutures should be placed to form a Brooke ileostomy. In the situation where there is concern about additional atresias or the possibility of late strictures, exteriorization of the distal segment as a mucous fistula has the added advantage of facilitating contrast studies of the distal end segment prior to re-establishing intestinal continuity. A mucous fistula also allows refeeding of stoma effluent to improve nutrient absorption and as a trophic stimulant for bowel growth and adaptation. The intestine distal to an atresia is often diminutive and the proximal end so dilated that an anastomosis between the two, though mechanically patent, is functionally obstructed. A period of diversion with refeeding will allow for growth and salvage of the distal intestine and a better size match later.

A loop ileostomy is commonly used for postoperative diversion following total colectomy and ileal pouch-anal anastomosis for ulcerative colitis or transabdominal endo-rectal pull-through for Hirschsprung disease. It can also be used to decompress a massively dilated distal colon prior to redo endorectal pull-through procedures for Hirschsprung disease or anastomotic stenosis. The advantages of a loop ileostomy in this setting are the avoidance of the risk of compromise of the marginal colonic blood supply that could occur with the formation of a colostomy and decompression of and access to the distal segment for follow-up contrast studies. Furthermore, the loop ileostomy used to protect the distal colo-anal anastomosis will already have been formed. Another clinical situation in which a loop ileostomy is useful is when total colonic Hirschsprung disease is unexpectedly encountered.

There are several ileostomy variants employed in pediatric surgery for special situations. The Bishop–Koop or double-barrel Mikulicz stoma sre sometimes used specifically in the management of obstruction related to meconium ileus. These stomas allow irrigation of the distal intestinal segment to disimpact the inspissated meconium. In the rare situation where a feeding jejunostomy is needed in an infant (for example, multiple failed fundoplications for reflux in the setting of congenital diaphragmatic hernia or long-gap esophageal atresia), a Roux-en-Y feeding jejunostomy can be employed. In infants, application of the Witzel technique can narrow the bowel lumen significantly when the jejunostomy tube is imbricated to form the tunnel, causing obstruction. The Roux-en-Y feeding jejunostomy obviates this problem in small diameter bowel. The Roux-en-Y feeding jejunostomy also allows the use of a conventional balloon enterostomy feeding tube or button in larger children, without obstruction of the small bowel lumen by the balloon.

Colostomy

Colostomies formed in the management of necrotizing enterocolitis, volvulus or perforation in neonates require the same technical considerations as ileostomy in this age group. Colostomies for Hirschsprung disease and imperforate anus are special categories. In patient with rectosigmoid Hirschsprung disease, colostomy is now rarely performed because of the increasing popularity of single-stage transanal primary endorectal pull-through procedures with or without laparoscopic assistance. In the event that a colostomy is chosen as the initial treatment, a "leveling" colostomy is made in the normal colon just proximal to the level of the transition zone. A loop sigmoid colostomy or end-sigmoid colostomy and mucous fistula are created. The access to the distal colonic segment afforded by a loop colostomy or mucous fistula is preferred so as to allow passage of mucus or irrigation of the distal colon. The colostomy is generally performed as distal as possible within the normal bowel, taking great care to be well above the transition zone.

In patients with high imperforate anus, a divided descending colostomy is employed. This colostomy has the advantage of decompressing the congenitally obstructed bowel, completely diverting the fecal stream from the fistula to the urinary tract in males, and allowing sufficient space on the abdominal wall to apply a proper ostomy appliance. It also allows performance of a distal colostogram and drainage of any urine from the fistula, minimizing its reabsorption and subsequent metabolic acidosis. This ostomy is generally left in place following anorectal reconstruction by posterior sagittal or laparoscopic technique. Unlike the sigmoid colostomy in Hirschsprung disease, care is taken not to perform this colostomy too distally, so as avoid tethering of the rectosigmoid colon during the anorectal reconstruction.

Colostomies for fecal diversion in older children and adolescents are generally formed using the same techniques as for adults in the settings of perforation, necrosis or IBD.

Stoma Closure

Contrast studies of the distal intestine are generally performed prior to takedown of an enterostomy to detect unanticipated obstruction or stricture, particularly when a full laparotomy with inspection of the distal bowel and lysis of adhesions is not planned. In infants and young children, the ostomy closure anastomosis is generally performed with a single-layer handsewn inverting technique because of the small size of the bowel. A single-layer technique with interrupted fine polyglycolic acid sutures is preferred to avoid narrowing of the anastomosis by excessive imbrication of the bowel ends that can occur with a double layer closure. In adolescents and adults, the anastomosis may be handsewn in one or two layers, or using a surgical stapling device, according to the surgeon's preference. Loop stomas are closed after local mobilization and anastomosis of the intestinal ends without a larger laparotomy.

Postoperative Care

Parental concerns and education require substantial time and support from the surgeon and an enterostomal therapist. Successful management of an ostomy by a parent at home requires attention to their concerns. Few parents of young children will have had any experience in such home care. Failure to support these needs and provide sufficient education prior to discharge sometimes results in unnecessary readmission and frequent return visits as an outpatient. Parents and patients, when age appropriate, must be instructed in care of an ostomy appliance and recognition of ostomy complications (Table 57.2).

The most important and serious complications include high stoma output with dehydration and electrolyte disturbances, prolapse, and stenosis. Infants and young children, because of their small size can become rapidly dehydrated from gastroenteritis or overfeeding in the setting of malabsorption. Several weeks of post-operative inpatient feeding titration is required, particularly in the newborn with a very proximal stoma. Neonates with mid-level or high jejunostomies can sometimes

Table 57.2 Complications of ileostomy/jejunostomy and colostomy

Fluid and electrolyte disturbances
Prolapse
Retraction
Ischemia
Stenosis
Parastomal hernia
Peristomal skin excoriation/candidiasis
Fistula
Granulation tissue
Catheter-related perforation
Ostomy appliance complications
Intestinal volvulus
Technical errors (exteriorization of incorrect end)
Spillover of stool into mucous fistula with subsequent stool impaction (Hirschsprung, imperforate anus)

be managed successfully on home parenteral nutritional therapy but more typically require inpatient care until the ostomy is reversed. High output from a stoma is generally defined as an output of greater than 30–40 mL/kg/day. This is most likely to occur in the patient with a high jejunostomy. Postoperative advancement of feeding in patients with ileostomy or jejunostomy should be slow, especially once output approaches 30 mL/kg/day, to avoid overwhelming the absorptive capacity of the intestine. Agents to reduce ostomy output such as loperamide (0.1 mg/kg/dose 3–4 times daily) can be used with variable success. Cholestyramine can be added to the feeds of patients with a colostomy and short small intestinal length, where unresorbed bile acids in the colon produce diarrhea. The ostomy output should be checked for pH and reducing substances. Low pH (<5.5) or positive reducing substances indicates malabsorption. When output exceeds 30–40 mL/kg/day, feeds should be held completely for 12–24 h to allow non-absorbed sugars to clear. Simply slowing the feed rate will result in continued high output due to the presence of non-absorbed and osmotically active sugars within the intestinal lumen.

Permanent stomas are relatively rare in pediatric practice. Prolapse or stenosis is most often managed by closure of the temporary stoma. In the event of prolapse, retraction, parastomal hernia or stenosis of a permanent enterostomy, revision and re-siting of the stoma is sometimes necessary.

Summary Points

- The indications for pediatric stomas vary and several unique types of stomas are available.
- The function of an intestinal stoma is to divert the fecal stream, to decompress dilated or obstructed intestine, or to irrigate and evacuate stool.
- Stomas are constructed when an anastomosis is judged to be unsafe, there is a distal obstruction, or as protection of a distal anastomosis.
- Most pediatric intestinal stomas are temporary. Permanent intestinal stomas are used when attempts at reconstruction have failed.

Editor's Comment

In children, stomas should be rare and reversible. Although the decision to create a stoma is to some degree always a matter of judgment, there are some indications that are largely technical (high imperforate anus, long-segment Hirschsprung disease, ileal pouch-anal anastomosis), some that are somewhat obvious because an anastomosis would clearly be unsafe (NEC with necrotic bowel, fecal peritonitis with sepsis), and finally some that are more or less a matter of style or personal preference on the basis of experience and training. These decisions often serve to define a surgeon as "conservative" or "aggressive." Regardless, because stomas are not without complications and make life difficult for the patients and their parents, the decision to create a stoma should not be taken lightly, the surgeon should be able to justify the decision in that particular patient in that particular circumstance, and, to the extent possible, the parents' opinion should be sought ahead of time. It is clear that many of the traditional indications for creation of a stoma are historically based and, although we will likely never see a randomized trial to prove it, there are many surgeons with the courage to challenge surgical dogma and who have generated a great deal of experience that supports the informed and thoughtful decision to avoid a stoma under certain circumstances.

The Bishop–Koop ileostomy was a major advance in the surgical treatment of meconium ileus when it was first introduced several decades ago and many pediatric surgeons still routinely use it in these patients. Many surgeons, however, have found that evacuation of the inspissated meconium by irrigating through an enterotomy made in the dilated portion of the ileum that is then closed primarily works well and avoids the issues related to the care and closure of a stoma. Likewise, stomas should almost never be necessary in healthy children after ileocecal resection for intussusception, severe appendicitis, or even Crohn's disease. Leveling colostomy in healthy infants with short-segment Hirschsprung disease should rarely, if ever, be necessary as primary repair in the newborn period has proven to be safe and effective. Bowel perforations after blunt or penetrating trauma can usually be safely repaired primarily without creation of a stoma unless there are clear extenuating circumstances – significant delay in diagnosis, severe chemical peritonitis, profound sepsis. In the end, although it is clearly important to learn from historical precedent, the surgeon should be able to justify the creation of a stoma with more than "because this is how it has always been done."

Despite the historical variation in types of stomas, stomas are essentially either end-stomas, in which case they should be matured in the manner of a Brooke ileostomy, or some modification of the loop ileostomy. End-colostomies can be flush but function better and are easier to care for when they are matured somewhat. There is no need to routinely use a rod or tube to secure a loop stoma – proper suture placement and a small but adequate fascial opening should be enough to prevent retraction of the stoma. In the case of Hirschsprung disease or imperforate anus, the mucous fistula should be brought up separately so as to avoid spillover and subsequent impaction of stool. To prevent prolapse, the mucous fistula should not be matured and, in fact, is probably best made flush and rather small, perhaps by using just the corner of a stapled bowel end closure. In most other cases, a double-barrel or Turnbull stoma should be used. The latter involves "Brooking" the proximal end and leaving the distal end flush with the skin. Most of the other stomas described were designed to allow closure at the bedside because a trip to the operation room was so dangerous. There is little need to use these old-fashioned constructs today.

Complications of stomas are not uncommon but are largely preventable. Parastomal hernias are often due to an excessively large fascial opening and improper suture fixation of the bowel. The same factors predispose to prolapse, which is one of the more frustrating complications of stomas. Prolapse is more common in mucous fistulas, probably due to the effect of peristalsis in bowel that has been fixed in this way. Maturing the mucous fistula makes matter worse because the everted segment of bowel peristalses in the direction of prolapse. Prolapse of the proximal segment usually occurs in stomas created when the bowel was extremely dilated and has now decompressed to a more normal size. In these cases, it is probably best to either find a way to remove the stoma or to completely re-site it. Proximal jejunal stomas should be avoided if at all possible because of the fluid and electrolyte and skin care problems that arise from the high output. Whenever possible, all stomas should be placed in the lower abdomen at a site that has been carefully marked by an enterostomal therapist. Transverse colostomies should also be avoided as they are difficult for patients to manage and accept. Bowel obstruction frequently occurs at or near ostomies, sometimes simply due to adhesions and other times due to volvulus around the stoma. Operation should not be delayed simply because the surgeon is convinced that "the stoma is patent" based on digital exam or intubation of the stoma. Finally, an examining finger should rarely if ever be placed in a child's ileostomy due to the significant risk of circumferential injury to the bowel or its blood supply.

Diagnostic Studies

– Contrast studies of the distal intestine prior to stoma closure.

Parental Preparation

- Stoma formation has major physiologic and psychosocial effects, but most children are able to function normally with a stoma.
- We will only create a stoma if there is no safe alternative.

Preoperative Preparation

☐ Bowel preparation, if necessary
☐ Prophylactic antibiotics
☐ Informed consent to include "possible stoma"
☐ Mark the ideal stoma site prior to going back to the OR

Technical Points

- In infants, stomas may be brought out through the wound or through a separate incision.
- Multiple stomas are commonly employed in the management of patchy NEC and multiple atresias to preserve bowel length.
- Intestinal stomas in neonates do not need to be matured as they are able to auto-mature.
- Loop stomas are usually fashioned for temporary diversion and are at greater risk for prolapse and retraction than end stomas, but they are generally easier to close.
- Permanent stomas are generally end stomas.
- At stoma closure, single-layer bowel anastomosis is preferred in neonates and infants.
- Patients with proximal stomas are prone to dehydration and electrolyte imbalances – stoma output greater than 30–40 mL/kg/day is associated with the greatest risk.

Suggested Reading

Gauderer MWL. Stomas of the small and large intestine. In: Grosfeld JL, O'Neill JA, Fonkalsrud EW, Coran AG, editors. Pediatric surgery. 6th ed. Philadelphia, PA: Mosby; 2006. p. 1479–92.

Lavery IC. Techniques of colostomy construction and closure. In: Fischer JE, Bland KI, editors. Mastery of surgery. 5th ed. Philadelphia, PA: Lippincott Williams & Wilkins; 2007. p. 1439–49.

Maidl L, Ohland J. Care of stomas. In: Fischer JE, Bland KI, editors. Mastery of surgery. 5th ed. Philadelphia, PA: Lippincott Williams & Wilkins; 2007. p. 1449–64.

Rowe MI, O'Neill JA, Grosfeld JL, Fonkalsrud EW, Coran AG. Intestinal procedures. In: Rowe MI, O'Neill JA, Grosfeld JL, Fonkalsrud EW, Coran AG, editors. Essentials of pediatric surgery. 1st ed. St. Louis, MO: Mosby-Year Book; 1995. p. 129–37.

Williams JG. Intestinal Stomas. In: Souba WW, Fink MP, Jurkovich GJ, Kaiser LR, Pearce WH, Pemberton JH, Soper NJ, editors. ACS surgery: principles and practice 2006. New York, NY: WebMD Professional; 2006. p. 803–14.

Part VIII
Colon, Rectum, and Anus

Chapter 58
Constipation

Linda Nicolette

Constipation is defined as a stool frequency of less than 3 times per week. These patients will have bulky, hard, dry bowel movements that can be painful to pass. The age range for this diagnosis can obviously be from a newborn infant to an older child, though the most common age of presentation is between 1 and 5 years. The work up and management is often dependent on the age of the patient. Most children with constipation are well managed by pediatricians and pediatric gastroenterologists. The patients that are referred to the pediatric surgeon are often those who rarely or never have bowel movements without some mechanical assistance, either orally or per rectum. They may have had difficulty since birth or gradually developed worsening constipation as they transitioned off breast milk or formula and onto cow's milk. Sometimes they will have a diagnosis that might indicate the possibility of a functional disorder of the colon, such as gastroschisis, Hirschsprung disease or cystic fibrosis. Rectal sphincter disorders, such as imperforate anus, cloacal anomalies and myelomeningocele also contribute to constipation issues. There are children who have conditions such as trisomy 21 and cerebral palsy and who are more likely to be constipated. Finally, children with complex neuromuscular disorders (muscular dystrophy, spinal muscular atrophy, intestinal pseudo-obstruction), might require surgical assistance with the problems of constipation.

Encopresis is defined as the passage of normal stools in abnormal places. These children do not have stools that are difficult to pass, but rather functional, cognitive or behavioral problems that allow for stooling accidents. This group of patients is best treated by a dedicated practitioner using bowel management programs that include behavioral techniques and strict dietary management.

Initial Evaluation

A thorough history and physical exam will often give the surgeon a good indication as to the likelihood of a surgical solution to the constipation problem. The age of the patient along with the history really determines how the patient is approached. How long has the patient had difficulty passing bowel movements? Was there ever a period of normal bowel movements? Was there any change in diet or health prior to onset of the problem? Was there any change in the family situation? What is the nature of the bowel movement? This history should include the frequency of bowel movements as well as the size and hardness of the stools. In infants, color can also give a clue in that hard, green movements are often a sign of iron intake either on the part of the infant or maternal breast milk. A history of sudden onset of constipation, especially after a particularly stressful event such as potty training or family discord usually indicates a problem that can be dealt with using oral medications, sometimes rectal medications such as suppositories and enemas, dietary education, and behavioral training. These children sometimes have other historical clues such as fecal staining of the underwear though stool accidents is considered normal in children less than 5 years of age.

Diagnostic Evaluation

On physical exam, many patients with constipation have stool palpable on abdominal examination and sometimes smell of feces. As the children get older and have more problems with soiling accidents, they become more and more withdrawn, depressed and reclusive.

Contrast enema can be diagnostic and at least temporarily therapeutic. It will show the area of colon that is filled with stool, how dilated it is and also indicate the size of the rectum to evaluate for Hirschsprung disease. Especially if this is done with an agent such as diatrizoate meglumine (Gastrografin) it will also help to clean out the colon and

L. Nicolette (✉)
Department of Pediatric Surgery, Presbyterian Hospital, 201 Cedar St. SE Suite 503, Albuquerque, NM 87106, USA
e-mail: linda.nicolette@gmail.com

P. Mattei (ed.), *Fundamentals of Pediatric Surgery*,
DOI 10.1007/978-1-4419-6643-8_58, © Springer Science+Business Media, LLC 2011

relieve the child of bulky hard stool so that a bowel management program can be instituted. Surgical disimpaction is sometimes necessary.

Newborns

Any infant who fails to pass stool in the first 48 h of life, or fails to pass bowel movements at least every other day should be closely evaluated. This should include a thorough physical examination, looking specifically for anal stenosis, ectopic anus, a presacral mass or an anal fissure. Plain abdominal radiographs will sometimes suggest a particular diagnosis or simply reveal evidence of intestinal obstruction. Unless the infant has peritonitis and needs to go quickly to the operating room, a contrast enema will usually aid in the evaluation. It might reveal a suspicion for small left colon syndrome, meconium ileus, meconium plug syndrome, or Hirschsprung disease.

Infants

After the newborn period and until about 2 years of age, the most common problems with constipation will most likely be "functional." Frequently there is a family history of constipation. There is often an association with transition from maternal breast milk to formula and as new foods are added, some may be more constipating. Historically, the infant may have hard stools that are difficult to pass and the parent must help the infant pass the stool by bending the knees up over the abdomen or manually removing the stool. Often there is a report of blood in the stool from an anal fissure that has developed from passing hard stools. If there is any doubt as to the cause, then a contrast enema should be performed and a suction rectal biopsy considered.

If the workup points towards functional constipation, these children should first have more water added to their diet. Some children will also respond to the addition of juice to the diet. A formula change might be beneficial if juice and water do not improve the situation. Some children respond to just changing the brand of formula, but changing from cow's milk or soy formula to something more elemental can be very helpful. The formula should be evaluated for iron content, and if iron treatment is not indicated, a low- or no-iron formula should be used. If the mother is breast feeding and taking a vitamin with iron, this should also be eliminated. Many recommend that if the mother is breast feeding, the mother should eliminate cow's milk products from her diet, as it can be constipating for the infant.

If the child is on cereal, they should be taking oat cereal rather than rice cereal to increase fiber. The parent should also be instructed to avoid feeding the child bananas and apple sauce, two of the first foods often started in the diet after rice cereal. All these foods can be constipating. As the child transitions to finger food, some will respond to fruits and vegetables, especially raisins.

If parents are willing, I try to encourage natural remedies before prescribing laxatives. Some infants will respond very well to probiotics, others to ground flax seed or flax seed oil. Most local health food stores are more than happy to counsel parents about the best product for the digestive health of their infant. Unfortunately, the response to these products is not consistent and compliance can be a problem.

If all these measures are unsuccessful, then a laxative should be added to the regimen. I will usually start with polyethylene glycol 3350 (MiraLax) as it easy to administer (tasteless and odorless and mixes well with any fluid), easy to adjust dosages, and generally well tolerated. The most important aspect of giving any laxative is to educate the parents on how to adjust the dosage. A typical scenario is the laxative is started, then the infant has liquid stools, so the medicine is stopped, which allows for rebound constipation, and a negative cycle begins. The parents should be instructed to increase the dose until the infant has soft, easy-to-pass bowel movements at least daily. If the movements are too loose, then the dose is cut in half for a few days and in half again if necessary, but parents should not discontinue the regimen unless they have discussed this plan with their provider.

One of the exceptions to this rather drawn out treatment plan is when the child has an anal fissure. In these cases, it is prudent to be more aggressive to achieve soft bowel movements as soon as possible to allow the fissure to heal. If this is the case, in addition to starting a laxative early in the course of management, with parent education, adding a sitz bath several times a day and prescribing a steroid cream to be massaged into the inflamed area might facilitate healing.

Toddlers

A new onset of constipation in the toddler age group is most often due to factors outside colonic motility, often related to toilet training. It is still necessary to closely review the stooling history of the patient as there is a possibility of short segment Hirschsprung disease or even ectopic anus presenting in this age group. In children with cerebral palsy and other neurologic disorders, we often begin seeing more problems with gastrointestinal motility in this age group.

If physical exam and contrast enema do not reveal an anatomical reason for the constipation, then motility studies may be indicated. There are several centers in the United States that have become well known for their expertise in bowel motility but it is unfortunately often quite a burden on the family to travel to these clinics and therefore usually reserved for the most difficult cases. A sitzmark study is a crude but effective way to study colonic transit. It can be done in any radiology department as it is a study common to adults. The patient takes a capsule filled with 24 small radiopaque rings and serial x-rays are taken over the next 5 or 5 days. A child with normal motility will pass all the rings within 2–3 days. If a cluster of rings remain in the colon, then it is determined if they are in the right, left, sigmoid or entire colon and this can help pinpoint the location of the disordered motility. The results of a sitzmark study are much more reliable if the colon is first cleaned of excess stool or fecal impaction. Anal manometry, which is also becoming more widely available, should be considered if the diagnosis of short segment Hirschsprung disease or internal sphincter achalasia is suspected.

Treatment in this age group generally includes dietary modifications, teaching good toileting habits, use of laxatives and possible use of suppositories or enemas to help retrain the bowel. Probably the most difficult cases to deal with in this age group are the children with imperforate anus and poor rectal innervation who are toilet training. These children often do well with a daily regimen of suppositories or enemas but stool softeners may have the unwanted effect of allowing for increased soiling accidents. It can be a challenge to keep the stool hard enough so it doesn't leak, yet soft enough to be able to pass.

School Age Children

New onset of constipation in this age group is uncommon. It must be determined if the constipation is really a new issue or if it is a chronic one that has never been treated effectively or at all. If it is truly a new problem then one must consider the most common causes of constipation in this age group. Emotional, physical or sexual abuse should be considered as a possible cause of a sudden onset of constipation in a previously healthy child, but other things to consider are tethered spinal cord or occult spina bifida. One can also see patients in this age group with other GI motility disorders that finally decompensate and need surgical intervention. This would most commonly include children with spina bifida, imperforate anus and some patients with Hirschsprung disease who have poor rectal control. In my own practice I have seen a number of children with cerebral palsy whose upper or lower GI function decompensates during this period of their life.

If there is concern for a tethered spinal cord or occult spina bifida, the evaluation should include an MRI of the lumbarsacral region. The distal spinal cord should be no lower than L2. An MRI might also be very helpful in evaluating the patient who has had a pull-through for imperforate anus and cannot achieve bowel continence. This will show where the rectum is with respect to the sphincter muscle complex and if there is enough muscle to warrant trying to correct one that is not in the center of the complex. About 25% of patients with imperforate anus will also have tethered spinal cord.

Evaluation of children with corrected Hirschsprung disease often warrants a rectal biopsy to ensure there are ganglion cells at the anastomotic area. In this age group, a full thickness biopsy will be more reliable than a suction rectal biopsy. The diagnosis of "short segment" Hirschsprung disease should also be entertained in children with chronic constipation. This is especially important in the child who has a tunnel-like anal canal and explosive stool on digital rectal exam. Typically these are children who have a rectum full of stool but do not always soil their underwear.

Generally, the evaluation of these children should include a contrast enema. It might also be helpful to do a sitzmark study. If there is one particular area that is dilated and retains markers, especially the sigmoid colon, resection of this segment can result in complete resolution of the problem. Formal motility studies can be very helpful in these cases and the option of using adult equipment becomes more realistic if the patient is old enough and the gastroenterologist is willing. However, for those practicing away from large centers that do motility studies on children, this is when it is really worth it for the family to travel to these centers for a more formal motility work up.

Along with the work-up, the surgeon is often faced with doing a surgical disimpaction. Giving several doses of mineral oil from above, as well as mineral oil enemas several times for a day or two before the disimpaction can soften very hard stool. Many surgeons keep a long handled tablespoon on their surgical set for "scooping" the stool softened by the oil from the rectum. It is also helpful to have fluoroscopy and some dilute Gastrograffin solution ready to give as an enema in the operating room to flush above the impaction and facilitate removal of any retained stool after everything within reach has been removed.

Surgical Therapy

If a child has a diagnosis that is not amenable to a specific surgical therapy (Hirschsprung disease, poorly aligned rectum-to-sphincter complex in imperforate anus, isolated hypomotile segment), consideration of surgically creating a way to administer therapy, namely some form of a stoma, might be warranted. If it is available, the appendix is usually the first choice: the ACE (Malone antegrade continent enema) or simply ACE procedure. If there is no appendix, than using a Monti-Yang ileocecostomy (creating a tube from ileum and anastomosing it between the cecum and the anterior abdominal wall) is an option, or creating a tube from a flap of cecum and bringing it up to the anterior abdominal wall is also an option. This access, through which the child can self-administer an enema or laxative, can mean independence and a drastic improvement in quality of life.

A continent stoma brought out through the umbilicus is generally concealed and easy to access. Some children with spina bifida or other urologic problems either already have a Mitrofanoff stoma accessing the bladder for self-catheterizations at the umbilicus, or they will need one. If the child is in need of both a Mitrofanoff and an ACE, then I defer to the urologist to use their preference of stoma sites and stoma conduits and I use what is available. The urinary system is more functionally delicate and prone to complications than the bowel, which is generally more forgiving. If the patient is small and thin, the a long appendix can be divided on its mesentery and used for both conduits. The distal appendix is generally used on a mesentery to the bladder and brought out through the umbilicus, and the remaining appendiceal stump can be brought out in the right lower quadrant. If the patient is larger or even mildly obese, the conduits may not reach without compromising the blood supply, in which case two separate conduits should be considered. In obese patient, bringing a conduit on its mesentery through a thick abdominal wall is fraught with complications and needs to be carefully considered.

If the patient only requires an ACE, and there are no other contraindications, then laparoscopic assisted procedures are ideal. Bowel prep is done before surgery and a first generation cephalosporin administered prior to incision. I prefer to mobilize the right colon and bring the appendix up through a generous defect created in the umbilical fascia. Through this defect, the cecum can be pexed to the anterior abdominal wall to decrease the risk of internal hernia or volvulus. The appendix should be shortend so the cecum nearly abuts the abdominal wall to decrease the risk of volvulus. Most operative descriptions of this procedure describe imbricating cecum over the appendix to act as an anti-reflux valve. This is difficult to do in some cases without compromising the mesentery of the appendix or compromising the passage of a catheter. In these cases, I will try to intussuscept the base of the appendix into the cecum for a short distance rather than imbricating it within a tunnel. I have not seen significant problems with stool leakage, especially if the patient is compliant and has good washouts.

When using the umbilicus, it is important to generously excise the thickened skin at the base. If too much of this is left, it leads to stomal stricture, a common complication with this procedure. The thickened skin at the base of the umbilicus should be removed, which leaves a circle in the base of umbilicus without skin. A "V" is then cut on the inferior lip of the umbilical ring, with the apex of the V in the deepest part of the umbilicus. This apex is then stitched to a slit made on the anti-mesenteric side of the appendix and also fixed to the fascia so, when tied, it pulls everything down into the base of the umbilicus and creates an epithelial "slide" for the catheter to follow into the appendiceal conduit. Do not tie this fixation stitch until the rest of the stoma has been completed. It is important not to make this V too small or the slit in the appendix too short or you will be frustrated with stoma stricture or an exposed stoma with mucus leak. Ideally the broadest part of the V is about 10 mm in width and about 15 mm long. The remaining mucosa is stitched to the remaining circle of skin around the umbilicus and finally, the stitch at the tip of the V is tied. During this construction, the catheter should be passed in and out frequently to ensure that no stitch compromises access to the cecum. When it is finished, the V should be extending into the base of the umbilicus at the fascial level. Even if there is a good deal of the mucosa exposed, in a short amount of time, if the base is fixed to the fascia, the rest of the mucosa will retract and the stoma will be quite cosmetic in several weeks to months. Finally, I leave an 8–14 Fr silastic balloon catheter, taped securely away from the stoma, in place for 6 weeks. If the catheter is stitched in place, the skin is irritated, it causes more discomfort for the child and the stitch usually pulls out before the catheter is ready to be changed. The balloon catheter seems to hold well and keeps the child a lot more comfortable. I also use the largest catheter that the conduit allows without stretching the wall to the point of ischemia, as it will allow the enema administration to go more quickly. One of the frustrations for these patients is the time required for them to administer the enema and then allow it to work. Anything that can be done to shorten this time is beneficial. I have not found that a larger catheter makes the stoma more unsightly.

In the patient who is undergoing a Mitrofanoff or already has a Mitrofanoff, then the umbilical site is typically used for this and the ACE will be brought out through a stoma in the right lower quadrant. There are several descriptions of creating tubular stomas that utilize skin flaps so the mucosa is buried in the wall of the abdomen with a tube of skin being part of the tunnel. These include the VQZ, VQQ and VR techniques, all of which create a tunnel in which the first several millimeters are skin, before the mucosa begins. These are all superior to a stoma that brings mucosa to the skin surface which is fraught with mucus leakage, skin break down and stoma strictures.

If the appendix is not available, using a Monti tube (a segment of small bowel that is tubularized in a transverse fashion) or a colon flap, which can be from cecum, right, transverse or left colon can also be used. There is a higher incidence of complications in these conduits, in particular false passages created by passing the catheter through the suture line. These conduits are generally not possible in the obese patient as the mesentery is not long enough to bring the tube through the abdominal wall. Another consideration when using the Monti tube is that the mesentery can become a source for an internal hernia. These tubes also secrete much more mucus and can be less appealing because of this.

Irrigations are begun as soon as bowel function returns. Most surgeons start with small volumes of warm tap water and increase it every few days to a point where the child gets a good washout and stays clean for 24 h until the next irrigation. Eventually, a patient may be able to irrigate every other day or even 3 times a week, but for the first several months, a daily schedule is most effective. If the amount necessary is getting quite large, and certainly if it is more than 1,500 mL, modification of the recipe to avoid larger volumes and achieve a better washout is in order. This is where creativity and patience is really critical. Adding something that draws more water into the stool or stimulates peristalsis might be helpful. One of the most successful things I have used is to crush one or two Dulcolax tablets in a small volume of water and administer this 15–20 min before the irrigation. Phosphosoda solutions are often quite helpful but there is always a risk of hyperphosphatemia. Bowel management nurses, internet sites and other parents can be invaluable resources of new ideas for achieving good washouts.

The patient is brought into the office about the third postoperative week for the catheter to be changed. If all is going well and the catheter passes easily, then the child is taught to change the catheter at 6 weeks. At this point, a short mentor catheter, the same French as the balloon catheter, is easier for the patient to use as it is stiffer and easier to pass.

Mention should also be given to a "left-sided" ACE. Traditionally, the ACE was described using the appendix. However, if the problem is with sphincter relaxation and emptying the rectal vault, placing a tube or button in the sigmoid colon can allow a prompt and effective washout with less volume than a right sided irrigation that must travel through the entire colon to be effective. This is typically done with a tube or a button and not an intestinal conduit, so the patient must be willing to have permanent hardware. It is possible to transpose the appendix or create a Monti tube on the left side, but issues with the mesentery to the conduit make this more risky than is generally acceptable.

Complications

The complication rate of these procedures can be as high as 25%. The most frequent complication of the stoma is stricture, usually at the skin site, though if the conduit itself becomes ischemic a stricture can form along the tunnel. Some of these can be treated with dilation but most will require surgical revision. Stoma leakage may be treated with injection of dextranomer/hyaluronic acid copolymer, though this might also require surgical revision with imbrication of the conduit in the wall of the colon. False passages can occur in the Monti tube or the colon patch. If they can be safely re-accessed, leaving a tube in for several weeks might allow salvage of the conduit.

One of the most difficult situations is when a colon simply does not empty after irrigation. This can usually be anticipated on the basis of pre-operative motility studies showing the entire colon is hypomotile or a sitz-mark study suggesting a hypomotile segment. Generally, these patients will not evacuate the irrigation, no matter the recipe, and then over the next day or two, leak liquid stool. If it can be predicted pre-operatively, resection of most of the colon along with doing the ACE should be considered. If colonic hypomotility is recognized after the ACE, then resecting most of the colon between the ACE and the lower sigmoid can be done. Even then, some rectums will not empty easily and a permanent ileostomy should be considered.

Summary Points

- A variety of organic, functional and anatomical problems can lead to constipation. These must be thoroughly evaluated and addressed before the symptom of constipation can be treated.
- A thorough history and physical exam will help the clinician decide which studies might be helpful.
- Contrast studies are indicated in most patients for diagnosis, treatment and predictive purposes.
- Evaluation of difficult patients can be enhanced by motility studies.
- Sitzmark study often add information regarding colonic motility.
- Dietary, medical and behavioral therapy is indicated in most situations.
- The ACE procedure can be very helpful in difficult cases or those with neurological problems that cannot be addressed any other way.
- There is a relatively high minor complication rate for these procedures.
- If an ACE is performed, dealing with the complications of the surgery and dedication to finding irrigation solutions that are effective takes time and patience.
- A dedicated bowel management expert as a resource for patients with chronic constipation is invaluable.

Editor's Comment

Patients with constipation are referred to the pediatric surgeon for one of three indications: for fecal disimpaction, for consideration of an antegrade enema procedure, and for "rule out Hirshsprung's disease." Though unpleasant and sometimes tedious, fecal disimpaction is often quite rewarding. It should be performed with an aggressive but careful bimanual technique and accompanied by saline irrigation of the left colon through a red-rubber catheter. The anal dilatation that invariably occurs can be helpful for a time after the procedure but deliberate forceful dilatation of the anal sphincter is no longer recommended because of the risk of incontinence.

Antegrade continent enemas do nothing to treat the underlying disorder, but they can help patients with intractable constipation and encopresis stay clean for up to 24 h. The procedure should be done laparoscopically whenever possible and, to make it truly continent, some form of an antireflux valve must be created at the base of the conduit. This procedure is clearly undervalued and offered not nearly as often as it should be for patients who could clearly benefit. This might be due to the fact that it can be technically challenging, the postoperative care is laborious and fraught with frequent minor complications (recurrent stenosis, stool leakage), and perhaps because some are uneasy recommending a procedure that treats a symptom rather than an underlying disease.

Hirschsprung disease can generally be excluded by a careful history, but once the possibility has been raised it is often impossible to disprove without a rectal biopsy. In children older than about 4 months, this needs to be done as an open procedure under general anesthesia. A contrast enema should also be performed, but the sensitivity of this test for Hirschsprung disease is disappointingly low.

Be very careful to avoid stating or even implying that a child's symptoms are due to "just constipation," as this can provoke anger and resentment in parents, many of whom interpret this as evidence of a lack of empathy or an overt criticism of their parenting. Severe constipation can be a serious issue that causes a great deal of anxiety and physical discomfort. I am confident that most cases of "functional" constipation will someday prove to have a genuine underlying pathophysiologic mechanism that we simply have yet to appreciate. Finally, the traditional and sometimes self-righteous recommendations that clinicians frequently give (drink more water, increase dietary fiber intake, avoid "constipating" foods) are almost never enough for children with severe or symptomatic constipation; laxatives or cathartics are almost always necessary in these cases.

Differential Diagnosis

Newborns

- Imperforate anus
- Anal stenosis
- Meconium ileus
- Hirschsprung disease
- Ileal atresia
- Meconium plug syndrome

Infants

- Hirschsprung disease
- Anal stenosis
- Functional/familial

Toddlers

- Environment/psychological
- Functional constipation
- Hirschsprung disease
- Ectopic anus
- Neurologic dysmotility (cerebral palsy)

School age

- Environment/psychological
- Functional constipation
- Tethered spinal cord/occult spina bifida
- Neurologic dysmotility

Diagnostic Studies

- Abdominal radiograph
- Contrast enema
- Suction rectal biopsy or full thickness rectal biopsy
- Anal manometry
- Colonic manometry
- Sitzmark study

Parental Preparation

- Education about diet, medication, and behavior modification programs.
- Finding the right combination takes patience and a great deal of trial and error.
- If surgery is an option, the minor complication rate is high but overall patient satisfaction is high.
- Finding the right irrigation recipe can take time and creativity.

Preoperative Preparation

☐ Bowel preparation
☐ Prophylactic antibiotics

Technical Points

- All anastomoses should be tension-free.
- Always handle the mesentery carefully to avoid ischemia and subsequent stricture.
- If the umbilicus is chosen for the site of an appendicostomy, remove the thickened skin at base of umbilicus prior to creating the stoma.
- If a RLQ site is chosen, use a technique that creates a skin tunnel with generous skin flaps.

Suggested Reading

Bani-Hani AH, Cain MP, Kaefer M, et al. The Malone antegrade continence enema: single institution review. J Urol. 2008;180: 1106–10.

Barqawi A, De Valdenebro M, Furness III PD, Koyle MA. Lessons learned from stomal complications in children with cutaneous catheterizable continent stoma. BJU Int. 2004;94:1344–7.

Herndon CDA, Cain MP, Casale AJ, Rink RC. The colon flap/extension malone antegrade continence enema: an altenative to the monti-malone antigrade continence enema: an alternative to the monti-malone antegrade continence enema. J Urol. 2005;174: 299–320.

Kajbafzadeh AM, Chubak N. Simultaneous malone antegrade continent enema and mitrofanoff principle using the divided appendix: report of a new technique for prevention of stoma complications. J Urol. 2001;165:2404–9.

Ransley PG. The 'VQZ' plasty for catherizable stomas. In: Frank DJ, Gearhart JP, Snyder III HM, editors. Operative pediatric urology. 2nd ed. London: Churchill Livingstone; 2002. p. 111–4.

Rintal RJ, Pakarinen M. Other disorders of the anus and rectum, anorectal function. In: Grosfeld JL, O'Neill JA, Fonkalsrud EW, Coran AG, editors. Pediatric surgery. 6th ed. Philadelphia: Mosby; 2006. p. 1590–5.

Voskuijl W, de Lorijn F, Verwijs W, et al. PEG 3350 (Transipeg) versus lactulose in the treatment of chronic functional constipation: a double blind, randomixed, controlled trial. Gut. 2004;53(11): 1590–4.

Chapter 59
Perianal Disease

Cynthia D. Downard

Perianal problems in pediatric surgery can be a source of significant distress to patients and families, but offer an excellent opportunity for satisfying intervention. Often during medical training, management of perianal problems is relegated to junior members of the surgical team, as the issues may seem mundane and uncomplicated. In fact, correct identification and treatment of perianal problems can be challenging. It is important to know how to differentiate among the diverse perianal pathologies seen in the pediatric population as their treatments vary. One must also remember that many perianal problems are a sign of internal pathology and warrant further evaluation beyond management of the external disease. While perianal diseases are usually self-limiting and rarely life threatening, they do cause significant pain for children and angst for their parents.

Rectal Prolapse

Rectal prolapse is most often seen in children under 3 years of age. It initially presents as a protrusion of rectal mucosa through the anal canal, but if not addressed properly can progress to full thickness prolapse (procidentia). The initial instance of rectal prolapse often accompanies straining to have a bowel movement and can be quite alarming for parents. Personnel unfamiliar with the appearance of prolapsed rectum may also mistake it for something else, and may not attempt reduction in a timely manner. Most often though, by the time the patient reaches a medical facility, the prolapsed rectum has spontaneously reduced.

Anatomic factors, including the relatively straight course of the rectum, colon mobility, and the presence of little pelvic fat and fascia, combined with increased intra-abdominal pressure predisposes toddlers to rectal prolapse. Additional factors, such as cystic fibrosis or rectal polyposis, must also be considered if prolapse becomes a chronic problem. In general, rectal prolapse should be considered a symptom of an underlying pathology. It is important to identify the cause of this underlying problem, particularly making sure that constipation is treated adequately and testing for cystic fibrosis has been carried out.

Immediate therapy of rectal prolapse involves manual reduction. In children with recurrent rectal prolapse, it is important to teach their parents to do this. Steady pressure on the prolapsed rectum usually allows a successful reduction. If the rectum is significantly edematous, reduction with sedation or general anesthesia may be necessary.

Initial therapy of recurrent rectal prolapse involves identifying the underlying cause of straining to have bowel movements. This most often includes dietary changes and addition of stool softeners to facilitate regular bowel habits, but testing for cystic fibrosis or anatomic variants of pelvic anatomy including spina bifida occulta must be considered. Parents should be reassured that this is usually a self-limited problem, and most patients will outgrow it once they are past the toddler years and have developed more regular bowel habits. Patients rarely present with rectal prolapse after age four, but usually have a more difficult time with resolution of the issue. It is particularly important to consider alternate pathology such as cystic fibrosis or variants of pelvic anatomy in older children with rectal prolapse.

Patients with refractory prolapse despite adequate control of constipation with dietary alterations and laxatives for several months, operative intervention may become necessary. Several procedures have been proposed for treatment of recurrent rectal prolapse, each with its own advantages and limitations. In determining the best course of action, it is important to consider the long-term functional outcome, as permanent alterations in rectal and pelvic anatomy in youth can lead to a lifetime of stooling difficulty.

A relatively straightforward initial intervention involves perirectal injection of a sclerosing agent, such as hypertonic saline (25%), concentrated dextrose (D_{50}) or 5% phenol. This intervention is thought to allow scarring and subsequent adherence of the external surface of the rectum to the

C.D. Downard (✉)
Department of Surgery, University of Louisville, Kosair Children's Hospital, 315 East Broadway, Suite 565, Louisville, KY 40202, USA
e-mail: c0down01@louisville.edu

P. Mattei (ed.), *Fundamentals of Pediatric Surgery*,
DOI 10.1007/978-1-4419-6643-8_59, © Springer Science+Business Media, LLC 2011

surrounding tissues by creating an intense local inflammatory reaction. Injection sclerotherapy is done in the operating room and permits a thorough digital examination under anesthesia to exlude the presence of a rectal polyp or other lead point for the prolapse. Injection sclerotherapy carries a greater than 80% success rate in multiple series, though more than one injection is sometimes required.

Thiersch cerclage, in which a non-absorbable suture or wire is passed circumferentially in the submucosal plane of the rectum at the level of the anal sphincter, might be required for increased scarring of the rectum and perirectal tissues. It is important that the suture be adequately "loose" to permit bowel movements without straining. The cerclage suture is then removed several weeks to months after placement, but the scarring it causes remains. Several types of rectopexy and resections of the rectum have been reported in patients refractory to other measures, but these operations irrevocably alter the anatomy of the rectum and should be reserved for extreme cases.

It is important that after any surgical procedure for rectal prolapse, that treatment of the underlying constipation continue. Close follow up and gradual tapering of medications should permit a successful outcome most patients.

Fistula-in-Ano

While buttock abscesses occur relatively frequently in the pediatric population, a fistula-in-ano is observed much less often. Fistula-in-ano may first present as a perianal abscess, most often seen in infants under 6 months of age. The abscess from a fistula-in-ano is often closer to the anal verge than one would expect with a routine perirectal abscess. If a fistula-in-ano is identified in a child older than 1 year of age, investigation of alternate conditions such as Crohn's perianal disease should be undertaken. There is a striking male preponderance of this problem. Fistula-in-ano should be suspected with the close association of an abscess near the anus in a young infant.

An infant with a fistula-in-ano might present to the pediatric surgeon after drainage of a perianal abscess by another physician. When the abscess persists or recurs in the same site, it certainly raises concern for a fistula. Perianal abscess incision and drainage is followed approximately one third of the time by a fistula-in-ano, so close postoperative evaluation is advised.

Fistula-in-ano is thought to develop from infection in abnormally deep anal crypts just inside the dentate line. The goal in treatment of the fistula is to completely open the external fistula to the internal abnormal crypt, and excise or

cauterize the granulation tissue between the two openings. The fistula tract is usually identified by placing a lacrimal probe through the entire tract to identify the abnormal crypt, then completely opening the tract and using a curette and cautery to destroy granulation tissue along the tract. In addition, one can search for other abnormally deep crypts at the same operation and open these slightly to permit better drainage, though the likelihood of developing an additional fistula-in-ano in a new location is extremely low. The fistula tract is almost always well inside the anal sphincter complex, so performing a full fistulotomy should not affect long-term continence. It is important, however, to warn parents that the fistula will sometimes recur and that follow up is important.

Some surgeons advocate non-operative management of fistula-in-ano as this appears to be a self-limited condition. A prospective observational study found that in healthy neonates, perianal abscess and fistula-in-ano can resolve spontaneously and do not routinely require antibiotics. The patients treated in this expectant manner had symptoms for an average of 6 months and were seen frequently during that period until resolution of the problem occurred. In addition, infants in the series who had significant discomfort or systemic signs of infection underwent operative treatment. Although non-operative therapy is an option for treatment of fistula-in-ano, it should be approached cautiously, and only if familial support allows continued re-evaluation.

Anal Fissure

Anal fissure may be suspected in children with constipation, extreme pain with defecation, rectal bleeding, or blood in the stool. There is no clear cause for anal fissure, but it can be associated with constipation, difficult bowel movements, and hypertonicity of the anal sphincter. This results in a vicious cycle of pain with bowel movements, and subsequent reluctance to have bowel movements and constipation.

The diagnosis of anal fissure is made on clinical examination, with a linear disruption of the anoderm on visual inspection. Digital rectal examination is very painful if an anal fissure is present, but should be attempted if the diagnosis is not clear, to rule out other possibilities for anal pathology. If the diagnosis is clear on visual evaluation, omitting the digital examination is advisable.

The treatment for anal fissure should be aimed at interrupting the vicious cycle of painful bowel movements, subsequent reluctance to have bowel movements, and the resultant constipation. The goal of easy daily bowel movements will allow for gradual healing of the fissure. Initial therapy usually involves dietary changes including increasing fiber to add bulk to bowel movements and decrease straining with defecation. Soaking in the bathtub or sitz baths can provide some pain relief, and topical local anesthetic creams are sometimes also useful.

In the past, failure of initial medical management for anal fissures has resulted in surgical treatment such as internal anal sphincterotomy or anal dilations under anesthesia to relieve the hypertonicity of the anal sphincter and supposedly permit healing. These procedures are associated with a significant risk of incontinence. More recently in adults, nitroglycerin ointment has been used to reduce anal sphincter hypertonicity and is gradually replacing anal sphincterotomy as the preferred treatment for anal fissure. Prospective, blinded, placebo-controlled trials of treatment with 0.2% topical nitroglycerin ointment, local anesthetic cream, and placebo carried out in children have suggested that topical nitroglycerin ointment results in faster complete healing of the anal fissure and resolution of symptoms. Regardless of the treatment chosen, it will likely take several weeks for symptoms to subside, and this must be shared with the family at the outset of treatment.

Pilonidal Disease

Pilonidal sinuses are fistulous tracts that extend from the sacrum to the skin at the superior aspect of the gluteal crease. They often have hair and cutaneous debris within them. If present, pilonidal sinuses often become problematic in the adolescent years, and come to medical attention because of infection over 50% of the time.

Pain and drainage in the uppermost part of the gluteal crease are usually the first signs of pilonidal disease. An adolescent with tenderness at the top of the gluteal crease should be considered to have a pilonidal sinus until proven otherwise. There may be minimal visible external signs of significant underlying pathology. A small opening may or may not be evident on simple inspection, and if pain is the presenting symptom, a thorough examination of the upper part of the buttocks is difficult without anesthesia.

Adolescents with likely pilonidal disease and a possible pilonidal abscess benefit from examination under anesthesia and drainage in the operating room. It is important to prepare the patient and family that if an underlying infected pilonidal sinus is present, extensive resection of tissue may be necessary in order to eradicate the disease. In addition, multiple operations may be required to completely treat the process, particularly if significant inflammation is present.

Operative treatment usually requires general anesthesia, as the patient must be positioned jackknife-prone with the buttocks taped apart for optimal inspection of the area of suspected pilonidal disease. First, evaluation for draining sinuses should be carried out. Once identified, a probe is placed in the tract and the overlying skin is completely opened and all infectious material is evacuated. Most surgeons will then resect back to healthy tissue to adequately treat the pilonidal disease.

The real controversy in treatment of pilonidal disease lies in what to do with the wide-open wound after resection of all unhealthy tissue, often down to the sacrum itself. Four general options exist for treatment of the pilonidal area, and these should be discussed with the family before the operation. The option chosen is largely dependent on local practice and family cooperation: (1) One can leave the wound completely open, and allow it to heal by secondary intention. This is a difficult proposition as many adolescents with pilonidal disease are overweight, and will need significant help from family members to adequately care for a challenging open wound. Also it can take several months for the wounds to heal. (2) One can place a vacuum-type dressing over the wound, and gradually decrease the size of the packing sponge to let the wound heal in slowly. This method should yield substantial healing in 6–8 weeks, but considerable resources are expended in obtaining the vacuum device and home health assistance to facilitate use of the device. (3) Primary closure or marsupialization of the edges can be attempted. Primary closure, even if a drain is used, is often complicated by recurrent infection and repeat operations. Marsupialization of the edges of the wound (sewing the skin open) should help decrease the likelihood of recurrent infection as it allows some drainage, but subsequent deep infection may develop. (4) Reconstructive procedures, including musculocutaneous flap coverage of the defect, can be undertaken even in the face of infection. Unfortunately, this requires careful attention to optimize outcome of the flap, which can suffer pressure necrosis from sitting on the reconstructed buttocks. In addition, if infection persists, the flap may be lost, leaving an even larger resultant defect.

Currently, pilonidal disease in the face of significant infection seems to be well-treated with primary wide local excision and vacuum-type dressing application. This carries a minimal risk of recurrent infection, offers a reasonable solution to difficult dressing changes, and facilitates relatively quick closure of the wound. Primary closure can be considered if minimal infection is present, but the difficult nature of this problem must be explained to the patient and family prior to surgical creation of a large soft-tissue defect.

Summary Points

- Correct anatomic diagnosis of perianal problems, guided by the patient age and presenting history, is critical.
- Always consider the underlying internal pathology when treating the external perianal problem.
- Rectal prolapse is nearly always due to chronic constipation and normally resolves when the underlying condition is adequately treated.
- Cystic fibrosis should be ruled out by sweat chloride measurement in all children with rectal prolapse.
- There are several techniques described for the surgical repair of rectal prolapse, which is rarely necessary.
- Fistula-in-ano is common in infants and is usually self-limited with conservative management.
- Fistulectomy is offered when symptoms persist or recur over a long period of time.
- Older children with fistula-in-ano should be evaluated for possible Crohn's disease.
- Anal fissure is nearly always due to chronic constipation and normally resolves when the underlying condition is adequately treated.
- Pilonidal disease is not a true perianal problem but is often confused with one.

Editor's Comment

Rectal prolapse should rarely require surgical treatment. It is generally harmless but evokes an extreme emotional response in many parents and some children. It nearly always resolves when the underlying constipation is treated but it can take months for the child to break the habit of straining at stool and for the tissue laxity to improve. All children with rectal prolapse should have a sweat chloride test to rule out cystic fibrosis regardless of how well they appear to be. Surgical repair becomes necessary only in extreme cases. I prefer to avoid sclerotherapy because it is painful, usually needs to be repeated, and makes subsequent surgical repair very difficult. Instead, a modified Delorme procedure, in which the mucosa and submucosa layers of the rectum are mobilized and resected, is safe, straightforward to perform, and works quite well. I add a modified Thiersch stitch using a heavy braided absorbable suture to encircle the anus at the level of the sphincter to prevent early recurrence, which could disrupt the repair. Patients whose rectal prolapse recurs after a transanal procedure should undergo a laparoscopic rectopexy using an absorbable mesh or biological collagen sheet.

A rectal polyp will sometimes pass through the anus and be confused with rectal prolapse. If the stalk is narrow, it can be ligated painlessly in the office. In young children, these are nearly always juvenile polyps but a work up to rule out polyposis is recommended.

Anal fissures can be painful but are also usually due to anal trauma from passing hard stool, though rarely they can be a harbinger of Crohn's disease. They heal slowly and are reinjured by the passage of subsequent hard stools. Relief of the constipation cures the condition in the vast majority of patients. Surgical treatment is almost never necessary. The presenting symptoms can be pain or bleeding, but perhaps the most common presenting complaint is a skin tag. For reasons that are unclear, fissures frequently cause adjacent perianal skin and subcutaneous tissue to become heaped up in such a way that a broad-based polypoid skin tag is the result. These are harmless and generally "cosmetic" concerns but parents are sometimes distressed by them. To make matters worse, they can persist for months or years (for life?) even after the fissure heals. I suppose they can be excised but parental reassurance is usually all that is necessary.

Fistula-in-ano in infants can and should be treated nonoperatively. A painful abscess can be drained and cellulitis or fever should be treated with antibiotics and acetaminophen, but fistulectomy should be reserved for only the most severe cases. In reality, the usual trigger for surgical intervention is severe parental anxiety and sometimes care-giver frustration. Luckily these are nearly always superficial and respond very well to fistulectomy. Older patients with Crohn's disease and perianal fistula should not undergo fistulectomy because wound complications and poor healing are extremely common. Infliximab and other newer medical therapies for Crohn's disease have been useful in the treatment of fistulae but the risk of abscess formation in the setting of an uncontrolled fistula is high. These patients should have a #2 silk suture (non-cutting seton) placed through the fistula and tied to itself. This keeps the fistula open at both ends, reducing the risk of abscess and fistula progression. They can be left indefinitely to fall out on their own in 12–18 months or they can be removed when there is no longer any induration, drainage, or other signs of active inflammation.

Thrombosed external hemorrhoids occur infrequently in adolescents and should be treated by incision and clot extraction when they are very painful. Otherwise they should be observed. Internal hemorrhoids are actually quite rare in children but are easily treated with sclerotherapy or banding. In extremely rare cases, atypical hemorrhoidal tissue should be considered a sign of a more serious systemic disorder such as portal hypertension or lymphoma.

The mainstay of therapy for all anorectal problems in children is rectal examination under anesthesia (EUA). The patient should be in a dorsal lithotomy position with all pressure points padded. "Candy-cane" stirrups work well for these purposes. In the case of complex fistulae or Crohn's disease, this should be preceded by a pelvic MRI. Fistulae should be gently probed to avoid the creation of false passages. It is preferable to tied drains to themselves rather than stitching them to the skin. Perirectal abscesses should be thoroughly drained and debrided but never packed with gauze, as this is never necessary and always extremely painful. A passive drain is all that might be required but often simple drainage is sufficient. Skin tags can be biopsied to look for the granulomata characteristic of Crohn's disease but resection is fraught with complications and recurrence.

Anal condylomata are rarely seen but can be very distressing for patients, parents, and surgeons. In the past they were considered a definitive sign of sexual abuse but this association has been questioned. Severe carpeting disease should be treated aggressively with surgical excision and fulguration under general anesthesia. Circumferential disease should be treated in stages (2 or 3 non-contiguous quadrants at a time) to avoid a circumferential scar and subsequent anal stricture. Like most viral warts, they have been known to resolve spontaneously in patients who have stopped taking immunosuppressive drugs (corticosteroids) and in others over time for no apparent reason.

Diagnostic Procedures

- Anorectal examination under anesthesia (EUA)
- Pelvic MRI

Differential Diagnosis

- Rectal prolapse
  - Full-thickness prolapse
  - Mucosal prolapse
- Rectal polyp
- Anal fissure
- Fistula-in-ano
- Skin tag
- Perirectal or perianal abscess
- Anal condyloma
- Systemic diseases
  - Idiopathic constipation
  - Hirschsprung disease
  - Crohn's disease
  - Cystic fibrosis
  - Polyopsis
  - Anal trauma (sexual abuse)

Suggested Reading

Festen C, van Harten H. Perianal abscess and fistula-in-ano in infants. J Pediatr Surg. 1998;33:711–3.

Lee SL, Tejirian T, Abbas MA. Current management of adolescent pilonidal disease. J Pediatr Surg. 2008;43:1124–7.

Rosen NG, Gibbs DL, Soffer SZ, et al. The nonoperative management of fistula-in-ano. J Pediatr Surg. 2000;35:938–9.

Sonmez K, Demirogullari B, Ekingen G, et al. Randomized, placebo-controlled treatment of anal fissure by lidocaine, EMLA, and GTN in children. J Pediatr Surg. 2002;37:1313–6.

Chapter 60
Pilonidal Cyst Disease

Daniel P. Doody

Pilonidal sinus disease is a chronic subcutaneous inflammation in the upper part of the gluteal cleft. First described by Mayo in 1833, this "nest of hairs" was aptly named by Hodges in 1880, who first used the term pilonidal sinus (Latin *pilus* hair, *nidus* nest). For some time, the midline nature and presence of hair in the wound misled physicians, who hypothesized that pilonidal disease was an infection of a congenital cyst or pit of the sacrococcygeal area. However, over the past 60 years, it has been argued convincingly that this disease is acquired and the "cystic" nature of the abscess cavity is likely due to chronic infection and inflammation. This acquired etiology is supported by: (1) the occurrence of similar lesions in other sites of the body, occasionally associated with minor trauma (interdigital spaces of hair stylists and barbers), (2) the increased incidence associated with a sedentary occupation or lifestyle (jeep-drivers disease of World War II), and (3) the absence of typical histological features in the pilonidal "cyst" to suggest a congenital origin (absence of hair follicles and skin appendages despite the presence of hairs in the cyst wall, lack of epithelium of the internal cyst wall).

There is an increasing consensus that the pilonidal pits, which are located within the internatal cleft, originate from abnormal hair follicles in the midline. With the onset of puberty, hormones associated with sexual maturation affect the pilosebaceous glands, and a hair follicle becomes distended with keratin. If the skin surface closes over the follicle, the entrapped hair and non-hair follicular elements can become secondarily infected, initiating microabscess formation. This leads to infection of the subcutaneous tissue, creating an underlying cavity. If this local abscess also opens to the skin, a pilonidal sinus is created. With time, the walls of the sinus will epithelialize, establishing a path to the underlying subcutaneous tissue. Surrounding loose hairs, by friction and negative pressure created by normal motion (particularly sitting), may enter through the pilonidal sinus and become entrapped in the subcutaneous space. It is this entrapped hair that initiates a foreign body tissue reaction, often with secondary infection, leading to abscess formation and enlargement of the underlying subcutaneous hollow.

The typical patient with pilonidal disease is male, hirsute, and overweight. The disease is more common in Caucasians, particularly Caucasians of Mediterranean descent, and less common in Africans and Asians, possibly as a result of hair and skin characteristics. The incidence of pilonidal disease in the general population is 26/100,000 population, and while pilonidal disease can occur at any age, the greatest incidence of pilonidal sinus disease occurs between puberty and age 30. Prevalence in young adults is as high as 0.7%. In groups at extreme risk (Mediterranean males of military age), authors have found evidence of pilonidal sinuses in 9% of Turkish recruits to as high as 33% in the Greek military services. The natural history of the disease suggests that there is a decline in incidence after age 30 years, even in those previously affected.

An early article reported the incidence of pilonidal disease in college-age adults varied by sex, with an almost tenfold increase in incidence in males as compared to females (1.1 vs. 0.11%). While this incidence is high, others report a male-to-female ratio of approximately 3:1.

At initial presentation, the patient may or may not have evidence of ongoing infection. Those who present with an acute abscess are often very uncomfortable with swelling in the natal cleft, erythema, leukocytosis, and fever. They are often unable to sit directly on the sacrococcygeal area and have trouble walking. This acute presentation accounts for nearly half of the initial encounters for pilonidal sinus disease. Others present with chronic drainage and staining of underclothes. Some present with odor due to a chronic gluteal cleft infection. Infrequently, the incidental finding of a pilonidal sinus will be made, and the patient referred for surgical evaluation. In general, examination alone is sufficient to establish the diagnosis of pilonidal sinus disease. If a sinus opening is visible, hair is often seen protruding from it.

The differential diagnosis includes fistulous disease complicating inflammatory bowel disease, other infections of the

D.P. Doody (✉)
Department of Pediatric Surgery, Massachusetts General Hospital, Harvard Medical School, Boston, MA, USA
e-mail: ddoody@partners.org

P. Mattei (ed.), *Fundamentals of Pediatric Surgery*,
DOI 10.1007/978-1-4419-6643-8_60, © Springer Science+Business Media, LLC 2011

skin and subcutaneous tissue such as folliculitis, osteomyelitis involving the sacrococcygeal region, and hidradenitis suppurativa. Infrequently, a perirectal or perianal abscess is confused with pilonidal disease. A very young child with a congenital sacral pit is sometimes inappropriately given a diagnosis of pilonidal sinus.

At tertiary centers, some patients will be referred after multiple surgical attempts to address the pilonidal disease. These patients are often quite challenging, and surgical correction may require more complex flap reconstruction.

Abscess Drainage

When a young adult patient presents with acute onset of severe pain in the sacrococcygeal area, the treating clinician can reasonably assume that this is related to pilonidal sinus disease with abscess formation. While soft tissue edema associated with an acute abscess in the internatal cleft may hide the causative pilonidal sinus, the presence of an abscess in the superior central or slightly lateral sacrococcygeal position is almost invariably associated with pilonidal sinus disease.

While drainage of the abscess can be performed in the office or in an emergency department setting, the best location is in the operating room. The physician chooses a side for drainage lateral to the internatal cleft and the abscess cavity. If the abscess has a bias to one side, that side is the preferable site for incision and drainage. Even if the area of greatest fluctuance is centrally located in the cleft, the surgeon should perform drainage through a lateral approach. As recovery will depend on having an appropriate postoperative environment, the area should be shaved for a distance of 3–4 cm around the internatal cleft.

With the patient in the prone position, a field block using lidocaine or a combination of lidocaine with bupivacaine is performed. The area is then prepared and draped in a sterile fashion. At least 2 cm lateral to the internatal cleft, an incision is made on the skin of the medial buttock. The dissection continues down into the superficial subcutaneous tissue, and then a hemostat is passed medially towards the abscess cavity. The abscess cavity often has a fibrous wall, and the surgeon will need to push firmly to enter the abscess cavity, with the subsequent expression of an often malodorous purulent drainage, which should be cultured. If anesthesia is adequate, the surgeon should debride the abscess cavity using gauze or curettes. This debridement of the abscess cavity provides the best chance of recovery without the need for additional surgery.

The abscess cavity may be loosely packed with gauze. The patient should be discharged home with oral antibiotics to cover aerobic and anaerobic organisms. If the patient has extensive cellulitis or signs of systemic toxicity, hospitalization for intravenous antibiotic therapy and pain management

is appropriate. Packing is removed in 48 h and if purulent drainage persists, the wound is packed again and the patient seen in 24–48 h. Healing occurs on average in 3–5 weeks.

After the acute drainage, the patient should be seen in 7–10 days. At that time, the infectious and postsurgical edema has usually resolved, and the surgeon might be able to see an obvious pilonidal sinus. If the surgeon was unable to debride the abscess cavity with the acute presentation, the next procedure (lateral drainage and excision of pits) should be performed with anesthesia. The lateral wound is opened and the chronic abscess cavity is debrided with curettes and gauze sponges. The midline sinuses may be treated by opening the sinus tract or by excision of the sinus with primary closure using an absorbable monofilament suture. The sinus excision only should involve the sinus tract, usually a 2-mm excision around the sinus is all that is needed. If one chooses to excise several midline pits, one should try to avoid a large midline incision, as this may lead to recurrent disease.

Chronic pilonidal disease is the result of surgical or spontaneous drainage of an acute pilonidal abscess. However, a fair number of patients will first present with multiple sinuses, persistent drainage and soilage, and occasional pain without a history of past abscess formation or surgical drainage (Fig. 60.1).

As with most disease processes that have multiple procedures to address the problem, chronic pilonidal disease has no single surgical treatment that is 100% effective. Despite the seeming simplicity of the problem, surgical management of chronic pilonidal disease is often unsuccessful and can be quite frustrating.

Nonoperative Management

Conservative treatment of relatively asymptomatic chronic pilonidal sinus disease includes the establishing of a favorable environment to prevent chronic irritation in the area and entrapment of additional hairs. Personal hygiene would include washing the area at least once and preferably twice daily. Hair should be removed by shaving or application of a depilatory for a distance of 2–3 cm around the internatal cleft. Any hairs that are identified in the sinus opening should be individually removed by the surgeon or a family member. Initially, careful outpatient follow-up on a weekly to bimonthly basis is recommended.

Although less accepted in Western Europe and North America, centers in Eastern Europe have reported some success using phenol in the medical treatment for pilonidal sinus disease. After the surrounding skin is protected with paraffin jelly, an 80% phenol solution is injected into the cavity and allowed to reside there for 1 min. The phenol solution is then expressed and the sinus cavity curetted. Up to three separate

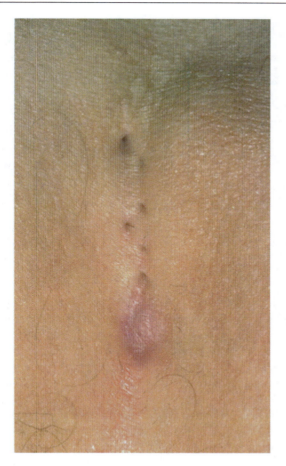

Fig. 60.1 Typical appearance of chronic pilonidal sinus disease with multiple sinuses located superior gluteal cleft over sacrococcygeal region. Hair can be seen protruding from the middle sinus. (Courtesy of Dr. Paul Shellito)

treatments are performed in a single session. The treatment is painful and sometimes require overnight admission for pain management. The therapy would then be repeated in 4–6 weeks. Recurrence is reported to be between 7 and 27%.

Definitive Surgical Therapy

Problems of addressing pilonidal disease came to the fore during World War II. Over 78,000 young adults were admitted and treated for this disease in service hospitals and they remained hospitalized for an average of 44 days. Arguments were made for open treatment of this disease although controversy existed whether wide excision of affected tissue down to the sacrococcygeal fascia or less extensive excision with marsupialization of the fibrotic abscess wall to the skin would lead to a better outcome. Both were associated with a delayed return to duty, although marsupialization seemed to have a more rapid recovery with an average time to complete healing and return to duty of 30 days. With both methods,

there were some wounds that were recalcitrant to healing and remained open for months. The controversy persisted and several military surgeons argued that primary closure in their hands resulted in a more rapid return to duty with a low recurrence rate. This controversy, excision with healing by secondary intention or primary closure, persists today.

Paraphrasing Hull and Wu, the ideal treatment for pilonidal disease should be technically simple, require minimal postoperative wound care, avoid hospitalization if possible, and have a low recurrence rate. An ideal operation would lead to rapid return to normal activity and an improved quality of life. However, the treating surgeon will often have to adjust the treatment and planned procedure to the type of presentation. The intergluteal cleft is a notoriously difficult place to heal because of moisture, bacteria, and stress created by the activities of daily living.

Wide Excision

The classic wide excision entails the surgical debridement of pilonidal sinus tracts and abscess cavity, frequently down to the sacrococcygeal fascia, and converting the multiple sinuses and abscess cavity into a large open wound to heal by secondary intention. Technically, it is the easiest method. While this procedure has the lowest recurrence of pilonidal disease, it has the significant disadvantage of prolonged wound healing, a more painful postoperative course with dressing changes, an often extended hospital stay, and a delayed return to normal activity. Frequent follow-up visits are needed in the postoperative period to remove granulation tissue and to prevent premature skin bridging. In the current era, many surgeons have moved away from wide excision because of the associated morbidities.

Marsupialization

Buie was one of the original authors to describe this technique in the 1930s and reported it as a preferred treatment of the "jeep-driver disease" of World War II. Briefly, a probe is placed in the sinus cavity and the skin superficial to the probe is opened. The surgeon removes any overhanging skin edges. The abscess cavity is identified and any hair and foreign material is removed. The internal surface of the cavity is then curetted until the fibrous base is identified. Using an absorbable monofilament suture, the skin edges are then sutured circumferentially to the edges of the abscess cavity (Fig. 60.2) The patient may shower the day after surgery and dressing changes are performed daily using a wet-to-dry technique to promote a gentle debridement and gradual epithelialization

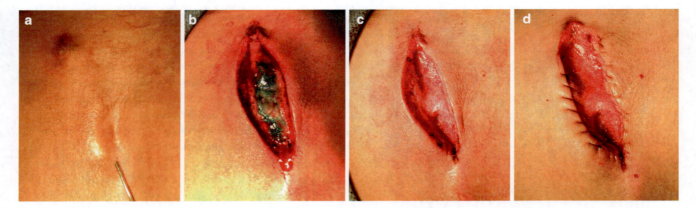

Fig. 60.2 Lay-open with marsupialization. (**a**) Identification of the direction of the abscess cavity using a probe through the pilonidal sinus. A secondary tract is appreciated superior to the chronic sinus. (**b**) Mat of hair and exudative debris in abscess despite near-normal appearance of overlying skin. (**c**) Following debridement of pilonidal abscess using curette and gauze. (**d**) Marsupialization of skin edges to the fibrous base of abscess cavity. (Courtesy of Dr. Paul Shellito)

of the raw surface. Shaving the hair around the area for 3–4 cm is important to prevent recurrence as the wound closes.

Marsupialization tends to constrict the wound while having the advantage of preventing premature wound closure. The average time to healing is 4–8 weeks. Authors have reported the use of vacuum-assisted closure dressings to treat these open wounds with the hope of diminishing time to full recovery. Like wide excision, recurrence following marsupialization is infrequent (1–2%). However, particularly for large cavities, recovery to healing following marsupialization can be prolonged, on occasion up to several months.

Excision with Primary Closure

Excision with successful primary closure results in simple postoperative care and a more rapid return to school or work. Unfortunately, primary closure following midline excision is more frequently associated with wound dehiscence, postoperative infection, other postoperative complications (seroma and hematoma), and recurrence of pilonidal sinus disease, making it less optimal than other procedures. As a result of these historically known complications associated with midline excision and closure, most experts recommend asymmetrical incisions and closures.

Karydakis Procedure (Lateral Advancement Flap)

The Karydakis procedure relies on the creation of an asymmetrical flap to avoid a midline closure and to create a more shallow depression between the buttocks. This elevation of the gluteal cleft helps to prevent the conditions that favor the creation of pilonidal disease. With the patient in the prone jackknife position, an elliptical incision is made on the left or right side. The surgeon incises close to the gluteal cleft and sinuses on one side and excises the skin and soft tissue on the opposite side at least 2 cm from the midline. The entire sinus cavity and underlying subcutaneous tissue are excised in asymmetrical fashion down to the sacrococcygeal fascia.

The medial flap is then undermined laterally at the subcutaneous-fascial junction for a distance of at least 2 cm. The subcutaneous tissue of the medial flap is then approximated to the sacrococcygeal fascia and the subcutaneous tissue of the opposite side using 2-0 polyglactin or polydioxanone sutures. A suction drain is placed in the more superficial subcutaneous tissue. Then the superficial subcutaneous tissue is approximated using polyglactin or polydioxanone sutures. The skin may be closed with a subcuticular suture or interrupted nylon sutures that will be removed. Care must be taken not to leave suture holes or drain sites closed to the midline, as these increase the risk of recurrence. The drain is removed in 2–3 days. Sutures are removed in 10–14 days.

In a modification of the Karydakis technique and in an effort to create a tension-free closure, Kitchen created a superficial and secondary flap at a depth of 1 cm from the skin edge that was anastomosed to the laterally incised wound margin.

Bascom Flap (Cleft Lift Procedure)

In 1987, Bascom described a surgical treatment for recurrent or refractory pilonidal disease based on the asymmetrical incision of the Karydakis but associated with less dissection of the underlying subcutaneous tissue. The procedure confined the surgical dissection primarily to the skin, excising only the underlying abscess cavity while leaving the surrounding normal subcutaneous tissue in place. In 2002,

Bascom modified this technique to excise skin in an asymmetrical fashion but preserve almost all of the subcutaneous tissue, including the debrided abscess cavity. After the subcutaneous granulation tissue is debrided, the fibrous tissue that remains is used to help create the soft tissue foundation on which the asymmetrical skin flap will be closed. The fibrous tissue of the abscess cavity is removed only if the surgeon is unable to achieve a tension-free mobility of the medial skin flap to cover the laterally displaced wound. This excision addresses the root cause of pilonidal sinus disease, the hair follicles in the internatal cleft, by removing the involved skin and creating a more shallow depression in the gluteal cleft (Fig. 60.3).

The patient is placed in the prone jackknife position. The buttocks are pressed together and the skin above the natal cleft is marked on the left and right side of the buttocks at the point of contact. This designates the lateral margin of the skin flap that will be raised to cover the asymmetrical excision of the midline pilonidal pits. The buttocks are then taped apart. A site is chosen that will be the recipient site of the flap. Methylene blue is not injected into the sinuses or pits as it may stain normal tissue, and this stained normal tissue, if excised, leaves a much larger soft tissue wound and may lead to a less successful outcome.

The surgeon then marks the area to be excised. This skin area will be primarily to one side of the gluteal cleft. The ends of this elliptical incision should be 2 cm below and 2 cm above the offending sinuses, but these endpoints should be 2 cm lateral to the midline cleft. This off-midline ellipse, 4 cm at its greatest diameter but including the sinuses in the gluteal cleft as the medial margin, is traced. The incision is begun at the midline approximately 1 mm lateral to the midline sinuses. Unlike the Karydakis flap, in which the underlying soft tissue is excised, the Bascom excision and subsequent flaps are skin-based. The ellipse of

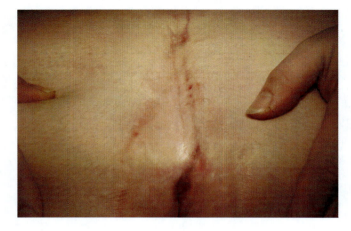

Fig. 60.3 Excision and primary closure using asymmetrical flap (Bascom). Five weeks following Bascom procedure in 17-year-old who presented with an acute abscess and recurrent disease after two previous attempts at wide excision with closure by secondary intention

skin from one buttock is excised with the midline pilonidal sinuses, preserving the underlying subcutaneous tissue. The midline abscess cavity is debrided with curettes and gauze, and the base of the cavity is preserved. If other fistulas originate from the chronic abscess but track to normal skin lateral to the gluteal cleft, these secondary openings are slightly enlarged and the fistulous tract is debrided by passing a gauze sponge through the tract. Most typically, these fistulas will not be excised but will heal by secondary intention.

On the buttock opposite the side of excision, a 7- to 10-mm thick skin and subcutaneous tissue flap is raised and will act as a donor skin flap to cover the laterally placed wound. Undermining this flap should extend to the initially marked point of contact between the buttocks. Traction on the donor skin flap, drawing it onto the recipient site, will roll the underlying subcutaneous tissue from the donor site into the gluteal cleft, creating a more shallow depression in the gluteal cleft. If the underlying scar from past pilonidal infection prevents tension-free mobilization of the donor skin flap, it should be excised.

The tape used to open the buttock cleft is released. A round suction drain is placed at the base of the wound and brought out through a separate stab incision off the midline. The soft tissue of the medial (donor) flap is then sutured to the subcutaneous tissues of the lateral (recipient) side using 3-0 or 4-0 polydioxanone sutures. A subcuticular polydioxanone suture is used to close the skin closest to the anus. However, the greater part of the length of the incision is closed with a subcuticular suture of polypropylene or monofilament nylon that will be removed in 10–14 days. Steri-strips are placed to reinforce the skin closure.

With both procedures that perform primary closure with asymmetrical flaps, the patient may be discharged home with oral antibiotics, including coverage for anaerobic bacteria, which will continue for 4–5 postoperative days. Ambulation and sitting may begin immediately. The patient may begin washing the wound after the drain is removed and the primary dressing is taken down on the second to fourth postoperative day.

Complex Flaps

More complex flaps including Z-plasties, rhomboid rotational flap (Limberg), V–Y advancement flaps, and large musculocutaneous flaps have been used in the treatment of chronic pilonidal sinus disease. These more complex flaps are typically considered when other operations have failed but are often associated with prolonged hospitalizations and may have greater morbidity. I believe that most surgeons will find that the asymmetrical flaps of Karydakis or Bascom provide excellent results, are technically simpler, and can be performed in transient surgery while requiring no, or very short, hospitalizations.

Treatment of pilonidal sinus disease can be frustrating for the patient and surgeon. Recurrence and delayed healing, are not unusual even in the most experienced hands.

Postoperative Care

The patient who presents with an acute abscess and undergoes emergent drainage will have recurrence of disease in approximately 50% of cases. Those who present with recurrence but are asymptomatic can be followed with conservative therapy that includes regular washing of the gluteal cleft and removal of hair by shaving, use of a depilatory, or laser therapy to minimize the risk of recurrent disease. Hair remains the initiating and potentiating factor in pilonidal disease. Careful and regular follow-up is needed if one chooses this conservative management.

The use of wide excision with healing by secondary intention or the lay-open technique with or without marsupialization is not only associated with a delayed recovery, but also with recurrent pilonidal disease despite the extensive resection (approximately 5%). Although the patient who has had multiple failed attempts at primary closure may be an appropriate candidate for this more radical excision, most patients will be able to avoid a prolonged postoperative recovery by use of appropriate excisions with primary closure.

Excision and primary closure using a midline incision should be avoided. While the surgeon may be able to achieve complete excision of the pilonidal disease without recurrence or wound breakdown, the risk of failure is much greater using this technique. In a large meta-analysis, McCallum compared techniques and noted a nearly 12% risk of recurrent disease with midline excision and primary closure.

As with all procedures associated with the treatment of chronic pilonidal disease, asymmetrical flaps do have postoperative infections, seroma formation, and superficial wound dehiscence. However, both in the literature and personal experience, the incidence of complications from primary closure with asymmetrical flaps is small, and these problems tend to be minor. The patients avoid the prolonged morbidity of postoperative dressings associated with the open technique and the often delayed time to full recovery that is coupled with secondary closure, particularly of the large pilonidal wound. In McCallum's meta-analysis, the recurrence rate reported for all off-midline closures (including more complex flaps) was 1.4%.

A very late and rare complication reported with the long-standing irritation associated with pilonidal sinus disease is dysplasia and carcinoma of the gluteal cleft. These patients are of middle age and had chronic pilonidal disease with a mean duration of symptoms of 22 years. The most frequent carcinoma is squamous cell, and this malignancy is much more aggressive than the more typical nonmelanoma skin cancers. It has been speculated that this malignancy is similar to those seen with chronic irritation (Marjolin ulcers) and it makes a strong argument that chronic pilonidal disease cannot be ignored.

There is no operation that meets the ideal standard and there is continued controversy regarding the best treatment of chronic pilonidal sinus disease. Whether dealing with an acute abscess or chronic pilonidal disease, the surgeon should avoid the midline as it is in the midline that persistent and recurrent problems are found. For symptomatic chronic pilonidal disease, excisional therapy with closure by secondary intention and primary closure with asymmetrical flaps result in minimal recurrence of the disease and are associated with infrequent complications. As the risk of complications appear equivalent for the two treatment plans, the more rapid return to normal activity would make primary closure with asymmetrical flaps (Karydakis or Bascom) the preferred treatment for most patients who suffer with chronic pilonidal sinus disease.

Summary Points

- Pilonidal disease is a common disease of young adults and in the 15–30 year age group may have an incidence of 0.7%.
- With an acute abscess complicating pilonidal disease, the abscess needs to be incised and drained. Even if the area of greatest fluctuance is in the midline, the incision for drainage should be at least 2 cm lateral to the midline cleft. If anesthesia is adequate, the clinician should "scrub" the abscess cavity with gauze to remove any entrapped hair.
- Chronic pilonidal sinus disease can be a difficult problem, often associated with complications following surgical treatment.

- In any surgical treatment of pilonidal disease, closure of the midline is associated with a high incidence of postoperative complications and recurrent disease.
- If wide excision is chosen, the lay-open technique with preservation of the fibrous abscess capsule and marsupialization is associated with a shorter recovery.
- Excision with primary closure using asymmetrical flaps is associated with infrequent recurrence or infection.
- For extensive pilonidal disease, complex flaps may be indicated.

Editor's Comment

I have found that most patients with pilonidal disease can avoid surgery with a combination of meticulous hygiene, hair removal, and close follow up, so that drill hairs can be removed from the pits, minor infections can be treated early, and small granulating areas can be debrided before being allowed to erode into lateral tissues. Because the morbidity is high, the recovery prolonged, and the results questionable, an operation should only be offered when conservative management has failed and there is clearly no alternative. Though the disease is clearly acquired and probably related to hairs being driven into the skin at the midline by movement while walking, there are some patients who have a true nest of subcutaneous hairs growing under the skin. These are the patients most likely to require a more aggressive surgical approach.

In most cases, incision and drainage of an excruciatingly painful, tense abscess with shiny overlying skin is easily done in the office, and provides instant relief. Local anesthetics are useless and unnecessary if the abscess is "pointing." Extensive debridement and packing of the wound are painful and also unnecessary. Cultures rarely contribute useful information and antibiotic coverage should be broad regardless of the results. The incision should be generous and the patient encouraged to allow water from the bath or shower to enter the cavity freely at least daily. A single abscess is not an indication for definitive surgical therapy, though a history of multiple recurrent abscesses should prompt discussion regarding surgical options.

The success of definitive surgical therapy depends on a tension-free closure and patient compliance, the effects of both of which are mitigated by using a flap technique with the incision off the midline and closed-suction drainage. Most techniques describe making an elliptical incision, but unless the ellipse is to include the midline pits, a crescent-shaped excision minimizes loss of healthy tissue and decreases tension of the final wound closure.

There are some patients, usually after having failed multiple procedures, who will be left with an open wound that needs to heal by secondary intention over the course of weeks or months. It is in these circumstances that the vacuum-assist closure device is most useful. It substantially shortens the time to heal these extensive wounds and, though the logistics can be daunting, this option should be explored on behalf of each of these patients, who stand to lose several months of their active and productive lives waiting for the open wound to heal by secondary intention.

Differential Diagnosis

- Folliculitis
- Osteomyelitis
- Hidradenitis suppurativa
- Fistulous disease complicating inflammatory bowel disease
- Perirectal abscess
- Congenital sacral pit

Diagnostic Studies

- Physical examination
- Medical imaging (rarely necessary)
- Ultrasound, for suspected abscess
- MRI, for complex disease

Parental Preparation

- Incision and drainage of an acute pilonidal abscess is associated with a 50% recurrence of problems related to pilonidal disease.
- Surgical treatment of pilonidal disease is associated with a relatively high risk of complications including recurrence and infection.
- Superficial dehiscence is common, but treated with local wound care.

Preoperative Preparation

☐ Prophylactic antibiotics

Technical Points

- Avoid making an incision in the midline.
- Closure of the wound off the midline (asymmetrical flaps) are associated with a lower risk of recurrence and infection.
- Preserve the underlying subcutaneous tissue to act as a foundation for the skin flaps.
- Maintain a tension-free closure.

Suggested Reading

Bascom J. Pilonidal disease: origin from follicles of hairs and results of follicle removal as treatment. Surgery. 1980;87:567–72.

Bascom J, Bascom T. Failed pilonidal surgery: new paradigm and new operation leading to cures. Arch Surg. 2002;137:1146–50; discussion 1151.

Buie LA. Jeep disease (pilonidal disease of mechanized warfare). South Med J. 1944;37:103–9.

Cintron JS, Abcarian H. Pilonidal disease. In: Cameron JL, editor. Current surgical therapy. 7th ed. St. Louis, MO: Mosby; 2001. p. 316–22.

Hull TL, Wu J. Pilonidal disease. Surg Clin North Am. 2002;82: 1169–85.

Karydakis GE. Easy and successful treatment of pilonidal sinus after explanation of its causative process. Aust N Z J Surg. 1992;62: 385–9.

Kitchen PR. Pilonidal sinus: experience with the Karydakis flap. Br J Surg. 1996;83:1452–5.

McCallum IJ, King PM, Bruce J. Healing by primary closure versus open healing after surgery for pilonidal sinus: systematic review and meta-analysis. BMJ. 2008;336:868–71.

Chapter 61
Hirschsprung Disease

Jacob C. Langer

Hirschsprung disease is a developmental disorder of the enteric nervous system that is characterized by the absence of ganglion cells in the myenteric and submucosal plexuses of the distal intestine. This results in absent peristalsis in the affected bowel and the development of a functional intestinal obstruction. In most cases, the aganglionosis involves the rectum or rectosigmoid, but it can extend for varying lengths and in 5–10% of cases can involve the entire colon or even a significant amount of the small intestine. The incidence of Hirschsprung disease is approximately one in 5,000 live born infants.

The etiology of Hirschsprung disease is incompletely understood. Ganglion cells are derived from the neural crest and are known to migrate through the gastrointestinal tract from proximal to distal. Infants with Hirschsprung disease suffer a failure of complete migration or in some cases possibly a failure of differentiation or survival of ganglion cells in the distal bowel. There is increasing evidence that mutations in a variety of genes might be the cause of Hirschsprung disease with the most commonly identified being the *Ret* proto-oncogene and the endothelin family of genes. The mechanisms by which these mutations result in aganglionosis are currently under investigation.

Hirschsprung disease tends to present in one of three ways: neonatal distal intestinal obstruction, chronic constipation, or enterocolitis. Between 50 and 90% of children with Hirschsprung disease present during the neonatal period. This percentage has increased in recent years with greater awareness of the disease. The neonate presents with a distended abdomen and feeding intolerance with bile-stained aspirates or frank emesis. Rarely, cecal perforation is

the initial event. Passage of meconium is usually, but not always, delayed. Plain radiographs usually show dilated bowel loops throughout the abdomen. The differential diagnosis of this presentation includes meconium ileus, meconium plug syndrome, intestinal atresia, or a number of other less common conditions.

Some children do not become obstructed in the neonatal period but present later with chronic constipation. This is most common among breast-fed infants, who sometimes develop constipation around the time of weaning. Although most children who present after the neonatal period have short-segment disease, this history can also be found in those with long segment or even total colonic disease, particularly if the child has been exclusively breast-fed. Because constipation is frequently seen in childhood, it is often difficult to differentiate Hirschsprung disease from more common causes of constipation. Clinical features that point to this diagnosis include failure to pass meconium in the first 48 h of life, failure to thrive, gross abdominal distention and dependence on enemas without significant encopresis.

Approximately 10% of children with Hirschsprung disease present with fever, abdominal distention and diarrhea due to Hirschsprung-associated enterocolitis (HAEC), which can be chronic or severe and life-threatening. As Hirschsprung disease is generally thought of as causing constipation, the diagnosis can easily be missed. A careful history, including the failure to pass meconium and the presence of intermittent obstructive episodes, should lead to an investigation for Hirschsprung disease. The etiology of HAEC is unclear, but it is thought that stasis and bacterial overgrowth caused by the functional obstruction of the aganglionic bowel plays a role. Particular infectious agents such as *Clostridium difficile* or rotavirus have been postulated as causative, but there is little evidence to support a specific pathogen. There is some evidence implicating alterations in intestinal mucin production and defects in the mucosal production of immunoglobulins in children with HAEC, which presumably results in loss of intestinal barrier function and allows bacterial invasion.

J.C. Langer (✉)
Hospital for Sick Children, Division of Thoracic and General Surgery, University of Toronto, 1526-555 University Avenue, Toronto, ON, M5GF 1X8, Canada
e-mail: jacob.langer@sickkids.ca

P. Mattei (ed.), *Fundamentals of Pediatric Surgery*,
DOI 10.1007/978-1-4419-6643-8_61, © Springer Science+Business Media, LLC 2011

Many children with Hirschsprung disease have other anomalies, such as malrotation, genitourinary abnormalities, congenital heart disease, limb abnormalities, cleft lip and palate, hearing loss, mental retardation and dysmorphic features. In addition, it is sometimes seen in association with certain syndromes such as trisomy 21, congenital central hypoventilation syndrome, or one of the neurocristopathies.

Diagnosis

For the neonate with a clinical picture and plain radiographs suggesting distal neonatal bowel obstruction, the first step in the diagnostic pathway should be a *water-soluble contrast enema*. The pathognomonic finding of Hirschsprung disease on contrast enema is a transition zone between normal and aganglionic bowel (Fig. 61.1). It is important to use a water-soluble material, since the enema could be the definitive

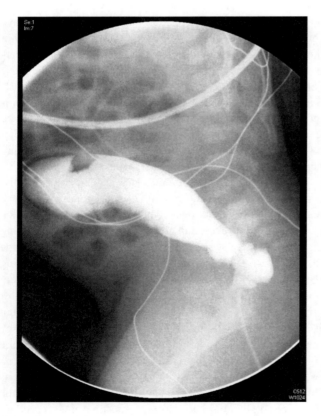

Fig. 61.1 Water soluble contrast enema demonstrating a transition zone in the rectosigmoid. The lateral view is the most important one to identify a low transition zone. Other findings on the contrast enema which suggest the diagnosis of Hirschsprung disease include a rectosigmoid index (the ratio of rectal diameter/sigmoid diameter) less than 1.0, and retention of contrast on a 24-h post-evacuation film

treatment for some of the other conditions in the differential diagnosis, such as meconium ileus and meconium plug syndrome. It is also important to remember that approximately 10% of neonates with Hirschsprung disease lack a demonstrable transition zone, so a negative contrast study does not definitively rule out the disease. In older children, an unprepped barium enema should be done rather than a water-soluble contrast study. The absence of a transition zone is less common in this age group, but can easily be missed if the aganglionic segment is very short.

The recto-anal inhibitory reflex (reflex relaxation of the internal anal sphincter in response to rectal distension) is present in normal children but absent in the vast majority of children with Hirschsprung disease. *Anorectal manometry* is not widely available for neonates and can be somewhat operator dependent. In older children, the test is technically easier but false positive results may occur due to masking of the relaxation response by contraction of the external sphincter or artifacts created by movement or crying. Anorectal manometry is most useful in the evaluation of the older child with chronic constipation, where documentation of a normal recto-anal inhibitory reflex effectively rules out Hirschsprung disease and avoids the need for a rectal biopsy.

Definitive diagnosis of Hirschsprung disease is based on histological evaluation of a *rectal biopsy*. In neonates, most surgeons use a suction biopsy technique, which is very safe, painless, and can be performed at the bedside. For children in whom the suction biopsy yields an inadequate specimen (inflammatory exudate, uncooperative patient, active stooling, technical difficulties) and in older children, punch biopsies or full-thickness open biopsies provide more tissue and deeper levels but often require sedation or general anesthesia.

The absence of ganglion cells is the hallmark of the disease and in most cases hypertrophied nerve trunks should be noted as a way to confirm the diagnosis. Because there is normally a paucity of ganglion cells in the area 0.5–1.0 cm above the dentate line, the biopsy should be taken at least 1.0–1.5 cm above it; however taking the biopsy too far proximally may miss a short aganglionic segment. The biopsy analysis can be enhanced by staining for acetylcholinesterase, which has a characteristic staining pattern in the submucosa and mucosa and is markedly increased in patients with Hirschsprung disease.

Treatment

The first priority is resuscitation, particularly in neonates with intestinal obstruction or enterocolitis. Intravenous fluids and antibiotics should be administered and a nasogastric tube should be inserted. Children with enterocolitis should undergo active colonic decompression using digital rectal stimulation and saline rectal irrigations (10–20 mL/kg every 6–8 h), and, if extremely ill, an urgent diverting ostomy. Children with associated abnormalities such as cardiac disease or congenital central hypoventilation syndrome must have these issues dealt with prior to definitive surgical repair.

Once a child has been stabilized and decompressed, surgery can usually be done semi-electively. While waiting for surgery, most children can be fed breast milk or an elemental formula, in combination with rectal stimulation and irrigations. Those that do not tolerate oral or nasogastric feeds can be nourished with parenteral nutrition. In the older child with an extremely dilated colon, weeks or months of irrigations may permit the colon to come down to a more normal size prior to definitive surgery, though some might benefit from a colostomy in order to adequately decompress the dilated colon.

The goals of surgical management for Hirschsprung disease are to remove the aganglionic bowel and reconstruct the intestinal tract by bringing the normally innervated bowel down to the anus while preserving normal sphincter function. The most commonly performed operations are the Swenson, Duhamel and Soave procedures. There is no compelling evidence that any one is best and all three are acceptable options in the hands of a well-trained and experienced surgeon. Outside of North America the Rehbein operation is still done and some surgeons also advocate simple anal myectomy for patients with short-segment disease.

The initial description of a surgical approach to Hirschsprung disease was by Swenson in the late 1940s. Swenson's initial description was a one-stage procedure, but a relatively high incidence of stricture, leak and other adverse outcomes led him and others to routinely perform a preliminary colostomy and, following a period of growth, a subsequent reconstructive operation. This approach persisted until the 1980s, when a number of surgeons reported series of single-stage pull-through procedures even in small infants. Since then, one-stage operations have become increasingly popular and many have documented the safety of the approach. A single-stage procedure avoids the known morbidity of stomas in infants and is probably more cost effective. It is important to remember, however, that a stoma may still be indicated for children with severe enterocolitis, perforation, malnutrition, or massively dilated proximal bowel. A staged approach should also be used in situations where there is inadequate pathology support to reliably identify the transition zone on frozen section from the operating room.

In the early 1990s, Georgeson described a laparoscopic approach to surgery for Hirschsprung disease. This operation involves laparoscopic biopsy to identify the transition zone and mobilization of the rectum below the peritoneal reflection, followed by a short mucosal dissection performed transanally. The rectum is then everted through the anus and the anastomosis completed from below. This approach has been associated with a shorter time in hospital and the early results appear to be equivalent to those reported for the open procedures. Excellent short-term results have also been reported for laparoscopic versions of the Duhamel and Swenson operations.

The transanal Soave procedure utilizes the same mucosal dissection from below as the Georgeson operation, but without intra-abdominal mobilization of the rectum. The mucosal incision is made 0.5–1.0 cm above the dentate line and the mucosa is stripped from the underlying muscle for a distance of several centimeters. The rectal muscle is then incised circumferentially, and the dissection is continued on the rectal wall, dividing the vessels where they enter the rectum. The entire rectum and part of the sigmoid colon can be delivered through the anus. The transition zone is identified visually and confirmed by frozen-section biopsy and the anastomosis is completed transanally (Fig. 61.2). This approach can also be used in a patient with a colostomy, by using the stoma as the end of the pull-through and performing the rest of the dissection using the transanal technique. The transanal approach has a low complication rate, requires minimal analgesia, and is associated with early feeding and discharge. Although there have been no studies published to date comparing the transanal and laparoscopic approaches, the transanal pull-through can be done by any pediatric surgeon, including those without laparoscopic skills, and by pediatric surgeons in parts of the world where access to appropriately miniaturized laparoscopic equipment is limited.

There is controversy surrounding the need to determine the level of the transition zone prior to beginning the anal dissection during the laparoscopic or transanal pull-through. Proponents of preliminary biopsy point to the inaccuracy of the contrast enema in predicting the level of aganglionosis: approximately 8% of children with an apparent rectosigmoid transition zone on contrast study turn out to have a more proximal pathological transition zone at operation. This is particularly important for the surgeon who does a different operation for long-segment disease than for rectosigmoid disease. Options include biopsy by laparoscopy or through a small umbilical incision, both of which can also be used to mobilize the splenic flexure in children with higher transition zones. The advantage of the umbilical approach is that it can be done by any surgeon, anywhere in the world, and doesn't require laparoscopic skills or equipment.

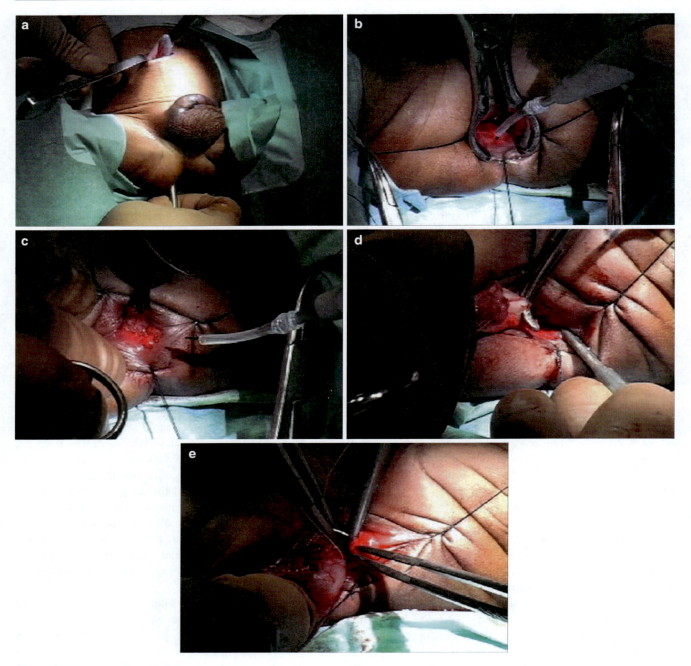

Fig. 61.2 The transanal Soave pull-through. (**a**) An umbilical incision is used for a preliminary biopsy. A Heger dilator is used to push the sigmoid into the umbilical incision. (**b**) Eversion sutures are placed, and a nasal speculum is used to provide exposure to the anal canal. A circumferential incision is made 5 mm from the dentate line. (**c**) The submucosal dissection is carried 2–3 cm. (**d**) Once the muscle cuff has been divided circumferentially, the dissection is carried proximally, staying right on the colonic wall. (**e**) The bowel is divided at least 2 cm above the biopsy showing ganglion cells, and the anastomosis is performed. Care must be taken to do the anastomosis to the rectal mucosa, not to the transitional epithelium, or normal sensation will be lost and the risk of incontinence will be increased

Postoperative Care

Postoperatively, the child is fed immediately and most can be discharged within 24–48 h. The anastomosis should be calibrated with a dilator or finger 1–2 weeks after surgery. Although many surgeons have the parents dilate the anus on a daily basis, we have found that this is unnecessary in most cases and weekly calibration is adequate for a period of 4–6 weeks. Protection of the buttocks with a barrier cream is mandatory, since at least 50% of children will have frequent stools postoperatively and are prone to perineal skin breakdown. Fortunately, this problem tends to resolve over time. The family should be educated about the signs and symptoms of enterocolitis (fever, lethargy, abdominal distension, diarrhea, passage of blood or mucus from the anus) and told to bring the child to the hospital immediately if there is any concern.

Long-term problems in children with Hirschsprung disease include ongoing obstructive symptoms, incontinence and enterocolitis. Quite often an individual child may have a combination of problems. These complications are more common than previously recognized and it is incumbent upon the surgeon to follow these children closely, at least until they are through the toilet training process.

Obstructive Symptoms

Abdominal distension, bloating, vomiting or ongoing severe constipation may be present immediately after surgery, or may develop later after an initial period of normal bowel function. The five major reasons for persistent obstructive symptoms following a pull-through are: mechanical obstruction, recurrent or acquired aganglionosis, disordered motility in the proximal colon or small bowel, internal sphincter achalasia or functional megacolon caused by stool-holding behavior. An organized approach to this problem is essential (Fig. 61.3).

Mechanical obstruction is usually the result of a stricture after a Swenson or Soave procedure, or a retained aganglionic spur from a Duhamel procedure, which can fill with stool and obstruct the pulled-through bowel. Obstruction can be identified using digital rectal examination and a contrast enema. Although some strictures can be managed using repeated dilatations, many require an operative revision of the pull-through. Duhamel spurs can be resected from above or managed by extending the staple line from below, with or without laparoscopic visualization.

Children who present with obstructive symptoms after a pull-through procedure should undergo rectal biopsy to confirm the presence of ganglion cells above the anastomosis or in the posterior aspect of the neorectum in patients who have had a Duhamel procedure. *Persistent or acquired aganglionosis* is rare and may be due to pathologist error, a transition zone pull-through or ganglion cell loss after the pull-through. The pathology from the original operation should be carefully reviewed to ensure that there was normal innervation at the proximal margin. In most cases, the best treatment for persistent or acquired aganglionosis is a repeat pull-through. This can be done using either a Soave or a Duhamel approach.

Children with Hirschsprung disease may have an associated *motility disorder*, which can be focal (usually involving the left colon) or diffuse. In some cases these abnormalities are associated with histological abnormalities such as intestinal

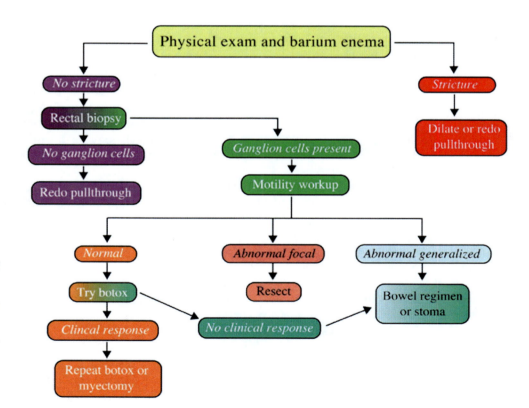

Fig. 61.3 Algorithm for the investigation and management of the child with obstructive symptoms following a pull-through. (Reprinted from Langer JC. Persistent obstructive symptoms after surgery for Hirschprung's disease: development of a diagnositc and therapeutic algorithm. J Ped Surg. 2004;39:1458–62, with permission from Elsevier)

neuronal dysplasia. In children who have been shown not to have a mechanical obstruction and who have normal ganglion cells on rectal biopsy, investigations for a motility disorder should be undertaken. This includes a radiographic shape study, radionuclide colon transit study, colonic manometry and laparoscopic biopsies looking for intestinal neuronal dysplasia. If a focal abnormality is found, consideration should be given to resection and repeat pull-through using normal bowel. If the abnormality is diffuse, the appropriate treatment is bowel management and the use of prokinetic agents.

Internal sphincter achalasia refers to the lack of a normal recto-anal inhibitory reflex that is present in all children with Hirschsprung disease but can in some can significantly impair normal defecation. This is a diagnosis of exclusion, after ruling out mechanical obstruction, aganglionosis and dysmotility. The standard treatment has been internal sphincterotomy or myectomy, but since this problem tends to resolve on its own in most children, we prefer the use of intrasphincteric botulinum toxin. In many cases, repeated injection of botulinum toxin or applications of nitroglycerine paste or topical nifedipine are necessary while waiting for resolution of the problem.

Functional megacolon refers to stool-holding behavior, which is a common cause of constipation in children without Hirschsprung disease, and is probably even more common in children with the disease. This problem is best treated using a bowel management regimen consisting of laxatives, enemas and behavior modification, including support for the child and family. In the most severe cases, the child may best be served by cecostomy for administration of antegrade enemas or even an ostomy, either of which can usually be reversed when the child reaches adolescence.

Incontinence

Incontinence after a pull-through can be caused by abnormal sphincter function, abnormal sensation or "overflow" incontinence due to severe chronic constipation. Abnormal sphincter function might be due to sphincter injury during the pull-through or to a previous myectomy or sphincterotomy. Anorectal manometry can usually identify this problem. Abnormal sensation sometimes involves lack of sensation of a full rectum (identifiable using anorectal manometry), or due to loss of the transitional epithelium if the anastomosis was made too low. If both sphincter function and sensation are intact, a common cause of incontinence after a pull-through is overflow of stool because of ongoing constipation. This should be managed with laxatives and bowel management. A final consideration is hyper-peristalsis in the pulled-through bowel, which makes it difficult for the child to control his stools despite normal sphincter function. Children

with this problem might benefit from a constipating diet along with bowel management.

Enterocolitis

Enterocolitis may be present both before and after surgical correction of the disease, and can be very severe, even life-threatening. Although the clinical features of enterocolitis are generally agreed upon (fever, abdominal distention, diarrhea), a precise definition has not been developed. Recurrent enterocolitis is more common in children with long-segment disease and those with trisomy 21.

The treatment of postoperative enterocolitis involves nasogastric drainage, intravenous fluids, broad-spectrum antibiotics and decompression of the rectum and colon using rectal stimulation and irrigations. To minimize the risk of recurrence, consider routine rectal irrigations, daily administration of metronidazole and probiotic agents, particularly in those who are thought to be at highest risk based on clinical or histological grounds. Since enterocolitis is the most common cause of death in children with Hirschsprung disease and can occur postoperatively even in children who did not have it preoperatively, it is extremely important that the surgeon educate the family about the risk of this complication and urge early return to the hospital if the child should develop any of the characteristic symptoms.

Despite the relatively common occurrence of postoperative problems, most children with Hirschsprung disease overcome these issues and do very well. Obstructive symptoms, incontinence and enterocolitis, in the absence of an ongoing source of obstruction, usually resolve after the first 5 years of life. For the vast majority of patients, sexual function, social satisfaction and quality of life all appear to be normal. Two specific subgroups have less optimistic outcomes, namely children with long-segment disease or trisomy 21. For reasons that are not entirely clear, both have a higher risk of enterocolitis, incontinence and recurrent bouts of dehydration. Finally, the prognosis is poor for children with co-morbidities, such as those with congenital central hypoventilation syndrome, congenital heart disease, and syndromes that are associated with mental retardation or other forms of disability.

Special Forms of Hirschsprung Disease

Long-Segment Hirschsprung Disease

Long-segment Hirschsprung disease is defined as a transition zone which is proximal to the mid-transverse colon. The most common form (5–10%) is total colonic aganglionosis, which usually also includes at least part of the distal ileum. In rare cases, most or all of the small bowel is also involved. Long-segment disease is more likely to be associated with a positive family history and more frequently diagnosed prenatally. Contrast enema typically reveals a shortened, relatively narrow colon, often with a transition zone in the small bowel. The rectal biopsy shows absence of ganglion cells, but in many cases there are no hypertrophic nerves or abnormalities of acetylcholinesterase staining.

Early resuscitation and management is similar to that described for standard Hirschsprung disease. Laparotomy or laparoscopy should be done and biopsies obtained for frozen section identification of the transition zone. For surgeons who choose not to use a laparoscopic approach, a small umbilical incision can be used to access all parts of the colon, and the ileostomy, if necessary, can be brought out through the umbilical incision. Although initial biopsies can be focused on an obvious area of size discrepancy, the pathological transition zone may differ from what the surgeon sees grossly. Some surgeons start with an appendectomy, assuming that lack of ganglion cells in the appendix is diagnostic of total colonic disease, however, this has resulted in a false positive diagnosis of total colonic Hirschsprung disease, since there may be a paucity of ganglion cells in the appendix even in children with shorter segment disease.

Once the level of aganglionosis has been identified, most surgeons create a stoma, wait for permanent sections, and do a definitive reconstructive procedure at several months of age. Although primary pull-through without ileostomy for total colonic disease has been reported, this approach requires a high degree of confidence in the pathologist, since it requires doing a total colectomy on the basis of frozen sections alone. In addition, many surgeons believe that the results of pull-through surgery are better once the stool has thickened, which usually occurs after the first few months of life.

The options for reconstruction of children with long-segment Hirschsprung disease can be divided into three main categories: straight pull-through, colon patch and J-pouch construction. Straight pull-through procedures can be done using any one of the standard techniques (Swenson, Duhamel, Soave), and can be done open, through a small umbilical mini-laparotomy or laparoscopically. The concept of a colon patch is to do a side-to-side anastomosis between normally innervated small bowel and aganglionic colon, using the small bowel for motility and the colon for water absorption and as a reservoir for storage of stool. Options include the Martin procedure, which consists of a long Duhamel reconstruction involving the entire left colon, or the Kimura procedure, which uses the right colon and requires a staged approach. Several authors have published modifications of Kimura's operation. Although the colon patch procedures theoretically result in decreased stool output due to better water absorption, the aganglionic colon gradually tends to dilate, and

many of these patients develop severe enterocolitis requiring removal of the patch or a permanent stoma. The J-pouch procedure is the same as that done commonly for children and adults with ulcerative colitis and familial polyposis syndrome. Although it has been used by a small number of surgeons for Hirschsprung disease, there has been little written about the results of this approach.

Near-Total Intestinal Aganglionosis

This condition is extremely rare and results in intestinal failure and the need for total parenteral nutrition from birth, a situation associated with a very high risk of mortality from liver failure. The extent of aganglionosis should be established at the time of the first laparotomy, and a stoma brought out at the most distal point that has normally innervated bowel. Some surgeons prefer to bring out a more distal stoma, but this increases the risk of chronic intestinal obstruction and bacterial overgrowth. A central venous catheter should be inserted for parenteral nutrition and a gastrostomy should be considered for continuous "trophic" feeding with breast milk or elemental formula.

There are several surgical options available for the management of near-total intestinal aganglionosis, particularly for those in whom there is not enough absorptive capacity and inadequate adaptation. For those children who develop significant proximal dilatation of the normally innervated bowel, tapering, imbrication or bowel lengthening procedures such as the Bianchi or serial transverse enteroplasty (STEP) procedure should be considered. Zeigler has popularized a technique known as "myectomy-myotomy," in which a long myectomy is created along the length of aganglionic small bowel distal to the transition zone. Although a few successful cases using this technique have been reported, most surgeons have not found it to be successful and have noted a high complication rate. For children with ongoing liver failure, small bowel or combined small bowel-liver transplantation might offer the only chance for survival.

"Variant" Hirschsprung Disease

There are a number of conditions that resemble Hirschsprung disease in presentation and clinical course, but are not characterized by absence of ganglion cells on rectal biopsy. The diagnostic criteria, clinical features and even the existence of many of these conditions remain controversial. The best known is intestinal neuronal dysplasia (IND), which in its usual form consists of dysplasia of the submucous plexus with thickened nerve fibers and giant ganglia, increased acetylcholinesterase staining, and identification of ectopic ganglion cells in the lamina propria. It is often present in children who also have Hirschsprung disease, although it occurs by itself. Hypoganglionosis is even rarer and is characterized by sparse, small ganglion cells, usually in the distal bowel. There can also be abnormalities in acetylcholinesterase distribution. It is important to differentiate hypoganglionosis from immature ganglion cells, which is seen in preterm children who present with distal intestinal obstruction due to underdeveloped colonic motility; this is self-limited and therefore should not be treated surgically. Both IND and hypoganglionosis can be either focal or diffuse. If the lesion is focal, the appropriate treatment is to resect the abnormal colon and perform a pull-through procedure, much as one would do for a child with Hirschsprung disease. If the problem is diffuse, surgery is not indicated and bowel management combined with prokinetic agents is the treatment of choice.

Virtually all children with Hirschsprung disease lack the recto-anal inhibitory reflex. However, there are some children with ganglion cells present on rectal biopsy who also lack the inhibitory reflex and may develop obstructive symptoms that resemble those of Hirschsprung disease. This condition has been termed internal sphincter achalasia or ultra-short segment Hirschsprung disease (although others reserve the latter term for children with a documented aganglionic segment of less than 3–4 cm). These children should be initially managed with a bowel management regimen. If this is unsuccessful, some surgeons advocate anal sphincter myectomy. Others have had success with temporary sphincter-relaxing measures such as botulinum toxin or nitroglycerine paste. The latter choices have some appeal due to the likelihood that the symptoms will improve significantly over time in most of these children.

Summary Points

- Hirschsprung disease must be considered in any neonate with distal intestinal obstruction, or any older child with persistent severe constipation or enterocolitis.
- Although the diagnosis can be suspected on the basis of history, physical examination, and radiology, the gold standard for diagnosis is an adequate rectal biopsy showing aganglionosis.
- Most children can be treated with a one-stage pull-through procedure, although a stoma may still be appropriate for those with severe enterocolitis, malnutrition, massive colonic distention, inadequate pathology support, or long-segment disease.
- The Swenson, Soave, and Duhamel procedures are all excellent, and the surgeon should do the operation that he/she is trained to do and does frequently. The laparoscopic and transanal approaches are associated with less pain, earlier feeding, and shorter hospital stay than the open procedures.
- When doing a laparoscopic or transanal pull-through, a preliminary biopsy should be done to identify the pathological transition zone prior to beginning the anal dissection. This can be done laparoscopically or through an umbilical incision.
- Many patients will have ongoing problems after a pull-through, including obstructive symptoms, incontinence, and enterocolitis. An organized approach to diagnosing and managing these complications is essential.
- Patients with long-segment disease, trisomy 21, and other syndromes and anomalies are at higher risk for problems and complications.

Editor's Comment

When done by experienced surgeons, the clinical outcomes of the various operations for the treatment of Hirschsprung disease are all quite similar. It is therefore important to become very familiar with one of the procedures described. I prefer the transanal Soave, with laparoscopic assistance when the transition zone is in question or if the splenic flexure needs to be taken down to mobilize the distal colon. I try to avoid colostomies whenever possible, but for infants with total colonic aganglionosis I perform an ileostomy followed by an ileal Duhamel between 6 and 12 months of age. Likewise, I will usually recommend a temporary colostomy for children who present late and have a true megacolon and most patients with trisomy 21.

It is important to realize that the operation for Hirschsprung disease is not curative, but rather palliative. Most children continue to have some degree of constipation and are at risk for enterocolitis. This is probably due to the fact that the sphincter is abnormal, the recto-anal reflex remains dysfunctional, and, as research has shown, there is more to this disease than simply a lack of ganglion cells. Nevertheless, most patients can function reasonably normally and do well in the long term. The exceptions are patients with long-segment disease and those with trisomy 21, who generally do quite poorly for a long time, though most seem to improve eventually.

When a patient fails, it is important to do a rectal biopsy to rule out recurrent aganglionosis, even though we fear that others will be critical of our initial operation. Although some few cases might appropriately be blamed on surgeon or pathologist error, in many cases there is clearly an as yet unexplained and mysterious process at work (ischemia? denervation?) that causes ganglion cells to disappear. These patients are probably best served by redoing the pull-through, which, if enough time has passed, is not always as difficult as one would expect. To avoid pulling through the transition zone, it is important to rely on the intra-operative biopsies and ignore the results of the contrast enema. Finally, when performing a Soave procedure, it is probably best to avoid excessive stretching of the anal sphincter, create only a short muscular cuff, and always perform a complete myotomy of the cuff in the midline posteriorly.

Differential Diagnosis

Neonatal presentation

- Meconium ileus
- Intestinal atresia
- Meconium plug syndrome
- Obstructing congenital band
- High anorectal malformation
- Motility disorder/intestinal pseudo-obstruction
- Systemic problem (i.e., septic ileus, hypothyroidism, electrolyte disorder)

Chronic constipation

- Colonic motility disorder
- Internal sphincter achalasia
- Intestinal neuronal dysplasia/hypoganglionosis/desmosis coli
- Functional megacolon/stool-holding behavior

Enterocolitis

- Gastroenteritis
- Malabsorption
- Necrotizing enterocolitis
- Malrotation and volvulus
- Congenital chloride diarrhea

Diagnostic Studies

- Plain abdominal radiograph
- Contrast enema
- Anorectal manometry
- Rectal biopsy

Parental Preparation

- The diagnosis of Hirschsprung disease can only be confirmed by rectal biopsy.
- A temporary colostomy is sometimes necessary to increase the likelihood of a good long-term result.
- Most children with Hirschsprung disease do well and live a full and normal life, but some have ongoing problems.

Preoperative Preparation

- ☐ Make sure the diagnosis is definitive, based on review of the rectal biopsy by an experienced pediatric pathologist
- ☐ Settle down any enterocolitis by using antibiotics and bowel irrigation
- ☐ Preoperative prophylactic antibiotics
- ☐ Informed consent

Technical Points

- Wash out rectum and distal colon in the operating room prior to beginning.
- Preliminary biopsy to determine normal ganglion cells using either laparoscopy or umbilical incision.
- Start mucosal incision 5–10 mm from dentate line, depending on the size of the child. Making the anastomosis too low will predispose to incontinence from interference with sensation, and making the anastomosis too high will predispose to persistent obstructive symptoms.
- Make a short rectal cuff, no more than 2–3 cm long. If you do make a longer cuff, make sure to divide it before completing the pull-through.
- Once in the extra-rectal space, keep dissection right on the wall of the colon.
- Divide bowel and do anastomosis at least 2 cm above the biopsy showing normal ganglion cells, to avoid a transition zone pull-through.

Suggested Reading

Amiel J, Lyonnet S. Hirschsprung disease, associated syndromes, and genetics: a review. J Med Genet. 2001;38(11):729–39.

Dasgupta R, Langer JC. Diagnosis and management of persistent problems after surgery for Hirschsprung disease in a child. J Pediatr Gastroenterol Nutr. 2008;46:13–9.

Georgeson KE, Cohen RD, Hebra A, et al. Primary laparoscopic-assisted endorectal colon pull-through for Hirschsprung disease: a new gold standard. Ann Surg. 1999;229:678–83.

Hoehner JC, Ein SH, Shandling B, Kim PCW. Long-term morbidity in total colonic aganglionosis. J Pediatr Surg. 1998;33:961–5.

Langer JC. Persistent obstructive symptoms after surgery for Hirschprung's disease: development of a diagnositc and therapeutic algorithm. J Ped Surg. 2004;39:1458–62.

Langer JC, Durrant AC, de la Torre L, et al. One-stage transanal Soave pullthrough for Hirschsprung disease: a multicenter experience with 141 children. Ann Surg. 2003;238(4):569–83; discussion 83–5.

Minkes RK, Langer JC. A prospective study of botulinum toxin for internal anal sphincter hypertonicity in children with Hirschsprung disease. J Pediatr Surg. 2000;35(12):1733–6.

Pini Prato A, Gentilino V, Giunta C, Avanzini S, Mattioli G, Parodi S, et al. Hirschsprung disease: do risk factors of poor surgical outcome exist? J Pediatr Surg. 2008;43:612–9.

Teitelbaum DH, Coran AG. Enterocolitis. Sem Pediatr Surg. 1998; 7:162–9.

Teitelbaum DH, Coran AG. Reoperative surgery for Hirschsprung disease. Sem Pediatr Surg. 2003;12:124–31.

Yanchar NL, Soucy P. Long-term outcomes of Hirschsprung disease: the patients' perspective. J Pediatr Surg. 1999;34:1152–60.

Chapter 62
Appendicitis

Shawn D. Safford

Appendicitis is the most common indication for abdominal surgery in children. Most patients present with abdominal pain and about one third of children with symptoms and signs that suggest the possibility of appendicitis require admission. The lifetime risk of developing appendicitis is approximately 9% in males and 7% in females. The peak incidence of appendicitis in children occurs in early adolescence and it is exceedingly rare in children under 2 years of age. Children less than 5 years of age typically present with nonspecific symptoms and have a much higher incidence of perforated appendicitis.

The etiology of most cases of appendicitis is thought to be obstruction of the appendiceal lumen by either lymphoid hyperplasia or a fecalith. Accumulation of secreted mucous and overgrowth of colonizing bacteria then leads to distension of the appendix, frank suppuration and, if relief of the obstruction is not provided within 24–48 h, ischemia and perforation.

Diagnosis

There are a myriad of possible signs and symptoms associated with the visceral irritation of acute appendicitis. Only approximately one third of children present with the classic clinical presentation that includes crampy periumbilical or right lower quadrant pain, nausea, vomiting, and anorexia, together with focal tenderness and guarding in the right lower quadrant on physical examination. An additional diagnostic challenge arises in children less than 5 years of age who are unable to clearly articulate their complaints. Various scoring systems have attempted to delineate which patients are clearly candidates for operative intervention without exposing them to potentially harmful radiographic studies, but these have been inconsistent and difficult to reproduce across institutions. Nevertheless, the tenets of a careful history and physical exam

are essential in aiding the clinician in confirming or excluding the diagnosis of appendicitis.

Early appendicitis usually starts with mild periumbilical pain that progresses over the first 12–24 h. The pain is usually – but not always – associated with anorexia and nausea or vomiting. The initial symptoms are due to distension of the appendix, a hollow viscus derived from the embryological midgut, and are therefore nonspecific. As the appendiceal wall becomes infected and eventually ischemic, the serosal inflammation causes a limited peritonitis, which produces more intense pain that is now localized in the right lower quadrant, as well as a low grade fever and more intense gastrointestinal symptoms (vomiting and sometimes diarrhea). The pain becomes more severe until gangrene develops and perforation occurs, at which point there might be some improvement of symptoms as the pressure within the dilated appendiceal lumen is relieved. If the appendix is retrocecal or successfully walled off by adjacent bowel and omentum, a localized abscess will form. On the other hand, if the appendix is intraperitoneal, generalized peritonitis can occur. Once perforation occurs, the child might appear toxic, sometimes progressing to a clinical picture of sepsis. On physical examination, there is usually diffuse tenderness or a rigid abdomen. Focal right lower quadrant pain should raise the suspicion for appendicitis, especially in boys (symptoms due to ovarian pathology frequently mimic appendicitis).

The importance of early diagnosis and treatment lies in the significant morbidity associated with perforated appendicitis. In children, the incidence of perforation ranges from 25 to 75%, with younger children at the highest risk. Half of children with perforated appendicitis have associated complications, compared to only 2–4% of children with nonperforated appendicitis. The significantly higher complication rate also leads to longer lengths of stay and higher costs.

Laboratory values should include a complete blood count, C-reactive protein and a urinalysis. This should also include a pregnancy test and, in girls who are sexually experienced, a pelvic exam with cultures. The white blood count usually is moderately elevated with an increase in the band count (a left shift). In the child without peritonitis or sepsis, a WBC that is extremely high without a left shift suggests the possibility of

S.D. Safford (✉)
Department of Surgery, National Naval Medical Center, Bethesda, MD, USA
e-mail: shawn.safford@med.navy.mil

P. Mattei (ed.), *Fundamentals of Pediatric Surgery*,
DOI 10.1007/978-1-4419-6643-8_62, © Springer Science+Business Media, LLC 2011

a viral syndrome rather than appendicitis. The CRP has been shown to be helpful in excluding appendicitis if less than the normal value for the institution. Finally, the urinalysis can suggest other etiologies of appendicitis including renal calculus, pyleonephritis or cystitis, though inflammation of an appendix located near the bladder or ureter can lead to white blood cells in the urine.

Most cases of acute appendicitis can be identified on the basis of the history, physical examination, and basic laboratory tests. Further work up is necessary when the history and physical exam do not correspond with laboratory values or in pubescent girls with focal lower abdominal pain. The next diagnostic studies include abdominal ultrasound or computed tomography. The study of choice depends on the availability and expertise of the ultrasound technician, the body habitus of the patient, and the ability of the child to tolerate the procedure.

In children, the sensitivity and specificity of ultrasound for appendicitis range from 45 to 95%, but is considered a good initial study because it is quick and relatively inexpensive and does not expose the patient to ionizing radiation. It is generally used in children with equivocal clinical findings and to aid in the diagnosis of other abdominal pathology that mimics appendicitis, especially adnexal pathology. Ultrasound findings consistent with appendicitis include a noncompressible, fluid-filled, tubular structure with a diameter (measured from outside wall to outside wall) greater than 6 mm. Other findings suggestive of appendicitis include the presence of an appendicolith, pericecal or periappendiceal fluid, and increased periappendiceal echogenicity. Findings of perforation include loss of the echogenic submucosal layer and presence of loculated fluid, phlegmon, or abscess.

The utility of ultrasound varies. Identification of the appendix is not always possible, especially in the obese patient and those with gaseous distension of the bowel. Some studies demonstrate no improvement in outcomes and no change in the perforation rate, complication rate, or cost. In fact, some studies have found a significantly higher negative appendectomy rate in children with suspected acute appendicitis following the introduction of ultrasound.

Helical CT has been shown to be highly sensitive and specific for appendicitis and is less dependent than US on operator expertise. The administration of rectal contrast further increases the sensitivity and specificity. The appendix usually arises from the posteromedial aspect of the cecum approximately 1–2 cm below the ileocecal junction. Findings suggestive of appendicitis include: appendix greater than 7 mm in diameter, appendiceal wall thickening and enhancement, an appendicolith, pericecal fat stranding, free intraperitoneal fluid, and intraperitoneal phlegmon or abscess. CT also helps to identify the precise location of an abscess and the extent of associated loculations, which are useful when planning a drainage procedure.

Treatment

The treatment of appendicitis is appendectomy, but the timing varies depending on the duration of symptoms and the clinical state of the child. If the onset of symptoms was more than 5 days prior to presentation, or there is evidence of an abscess on physical examination or medical imaging, then initial nonoperative management should be considered. However, for most children, prompt appendectomy is the best course of action.

At initial presentation, the child should be fluid resuscitated, given broad-spectrum antibiotics (usually a single agent is sufficient) and, once the decision to operate has been made, narcotics for pain relief. The timing of surgery has changed over the years from emergent to urgent. In fact, for patients who are admitted late in the evening or in the night, it is standard and accepted practice in many institutions to delay appendectomy until the first case of the next morning.

An appendectomy can be performed either open or laparoscopically without significant differences in cost, comesis or length of stay. Many pediatric surgeons perform an appendectomy laparoscopically and feel that visualization is better, allowing for more complete exploration of the abdomen, and that they can avoid the large incision that is sometimes necessary when the appendix is in an unusual location or intensely adherent. During exploration for presumed appendicitis, approximately 3% of patients have another surgical process that was not suspected preoperatively.

In preparation for the operating room, patients should evacuate their bladder, which avoids the risks associated with placement of a Foley catheter. The patient should be placed in a supine position with the left arm tucked and padded. The laparoscopic approach starts with an infrumbilical incision and exposure of the inifraumbilicial fascia. The base of the umbilicus is grasped with a Kocher clamp and a second clamp is applied approximately 3 cm inferior on the linea alba. Both of these are lifted as the fascia is incised using electrocautery. Once the peritoneal cavity is entered, a blunt 12-mm trocar is placed into the abdomen and is confirmed to be intraperiteoneal with the laparoscope before starting insufflation. Insufflation should begin with low flow initially with a maximal pressure of 15 mmHg. The surgeon should locate the appendix and place two 5-mm trocars: one lateral to the inferior epigastric vessels and another in the lower midline just above the level of the bladder. These sites can be adjusted depending on the location of the appendix. The lateral trocar should be placed first so that it can be used to assist the second trocar being placed in the lower midline where the peritoneum is more redundant.

The appendix can then be mobilized without grasping it to avoid causing the indurated organ to rupture (Fig. 62.1). If there is a significant phlegmon and the anatomy of the appendix cannot

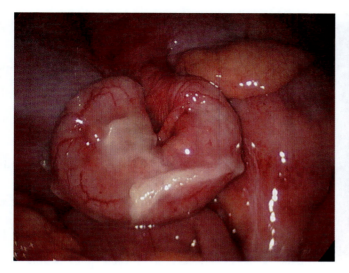

Fig. 62.1 The inflamed appendix. Note the presence of the fat pad at the ileocecal valve

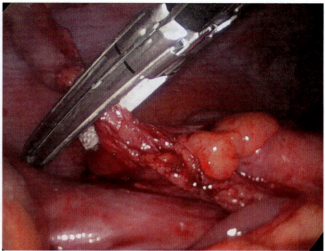

Fig. 62.3 The base of the appendix is stapled across the base using a endo-GIA

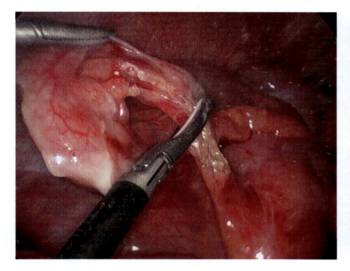

Fig. 62.2 The mesoappendix is ligated using the harmonic scalpel

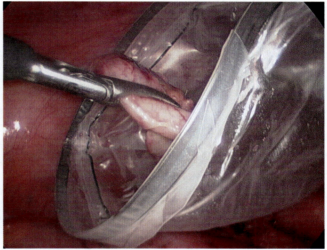

Fig. 62.4 The appendix is placed in an endo-bag and removed through the umbilical incision

be adequately visualized, the cecum and right colon should be mobilized to free the base of the appendix and allow for more precise dissection. Once the mesoappendix and the appendix are identified, the mesoappendix is ligated using the harmonic scalpel or electrocautery (Fig. 62.2). The appendix can be traced to its base where an endo-gastrointestinal stapling device or endo-loops can be used to ligate the base of the appendix (Fig. 62.3). The appendix is then placed in an endo-bag and removed through the periumbilical incision (Figs. 62.4 and 62.5). Irrigation is used sparingly with only removal of frank soilage; the liberal use of irrigation might increase the risk of a postoperative abscess. For closure, the 5 mm trocars are removed under direct visualization and then, if possible, the fascia is closed with absorbable suture. The periumbilical incision should always be closed at the level of the fascia. I use cyanoacrylate skin adhesive for the 5-mm port

site incisions but I prefer to close the umbilical skin incision loosely with interrupted sutures and steri-strips, as the umbilical incision has the highest risk for developing a superficial wound infection and the loose closure should theoretically allow spontaneous drainage of fluid.

Perforated Appendicitis with Abscess

Patients with appendicitis who present more than 5 or 6 days after the onset of symptoms are likely to have a well-defined abscess and should be considered for nonoperative therapy with intravenous antibiotics and percutaneous drainage.

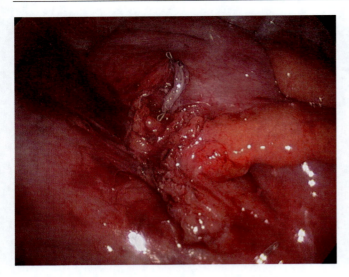

Fig. 62.5 The base of the appendix is healthy without any evidence of necrosis

Patients with a phlegmon can be treated with antibiotics alone. Failure of the nonoperative approach (persistent fevers, worsening pain, bowel obstruction) should prompt surgical intervention. A contraindication for the nonoperative approach includes the presence of a fecalith, diffuse peritonitis, or clinical instability.

Postoperative Care

Postoperatively, children with acute appendicitis without perforation should be allowed to advance their diet as tolerated. Antibiotics are continued for 24 h and the patient can usually be discharged the following day.

The treatment of perforated or gangrenous appendicitis has evolved somewhat. Our current protocol includes treatment with broad spectrum intravenous antibiotics until the child is afebrile, asymptomatic, and tolerating a regular diet. Once these criteria are met, a white blood count is checked, and if normal, the patient is discharged on oral antibiotics until a total of 14 days of antibiotics have been completed.

Some controversy exists regarding the appropriate management of the child who has been treated nonoperatively for perforated appendicitis. Most recommend an interval appendectomy 4–6 weeks after completion of the course of antibiotics. However, some have noted that the complication rate is approximately 12% after interval appendectomy, while the risk of recurrent appendicitis is only about 10%. In addition, though most surgeons recommend interval appendectomy, some recommend watchful waiting and some parents, after having reviewed the data themselves will decide to forego appendectomy unless symptoms recur.

Delay in diagnosis and treatment increases the risk of perforation, abscess formation, peritonitis, wound infection, sepsis, infertility, adhesions, bowel obstruction, and, in very late state of presentation, even death.

The risk of abscess increases significantly in the setting of gangrenous or perforated appendicitis. No specific interventions have been shown to decrease the formation of abscess. No studies have identified any significant difference in the development of abscess between open appendectomy and laparoscopic appendectomy. An abscess can form up to 4 weeks postoperatively and cannot be predicted based on any specific laboratory value. Most children present at approximately 1 week with fever, abdominal pain, or signs of obstruction including anorexia and vomiting. The child who presents with these signs should undergo a CT scan to assess for a drainable abscess. If a large abscess is identified, percutaneous drainage of the abscess should be performed.

Once drained, the abscess catheter should be flushed and monitored for output and broad-spectrum antibiotics should be administered for a 14-day course. The child's clinical condition should improve with drainage over the course of 2–3 days. Once the drainage output is minimal, the catheter can be removed. Plans should be made to send the child home with the intravenous antibiotics administered through a PICC line.

The small subset of patients who present with perforation and the presence of an appendicolith pose a special situation. These patients are less likely to respond to nonoperative management and should undergo surgery. If an appendicolith is missed and found postoperatively, the likelihood of developing a postoperative abscess is quite high and the surgeon should consider early re-exploration for retrieval of the appendicolith.

Summary Points

- Clinical judgment remains paramount to the diagnosis and treatment of appendicitis.
- Computed tomography is not without a small potential risk of future malignancy and should be used only when necessary, for example in the setting of clinical uncertainty.

Editor's Comment

Nearly every appendectomy can be safely performed laparoscopically. I prefer the laparoscopic approach because the outcomes have been shown to be the same or better than those of traditional appendectomy, and I have found it to be a superior when the appendix is retrocecal or stuck way down in the pelvis. The only shortcoming of the technique is its greater overall cost, which might someday become an important factor. I prefer to avoid instrumentation including Foley catheters and nasogastric tubes unless absolutely necessary.

The only reason to perform an appendectomy in the middle of the night is the inability to secure a guaranteed early start the next morning. The benefits of nonoperative therapy outweigh the risks only in patients who present with a well-defined abscess, usually more than 5 days after the onset of symptoms. Antibiotics use is excessive in most patients with appendicitis. All patients undergoing an appendectomy need prophylactic antibiotics, preferably given within 60 min of making an incision, but removal of a normal appendix requires no additional doses, removal of a suppurative appendix warrants perhaps one more dose and certainly no more than 24-h worth, and gangrenous or frankly perforated cases need intravenous antibiotics until afebrile and asymptomatic unless they develop an abscess, in which case a 10–14-day course of intravenous antibiotics and a PICC line are justified. I also believe that the risk of postoperative abscess is lower when patients with perforated appendicitis take oral antibiotics (trimethoprim/sulfamethoxazole and metronidazole, or ciprofloxacin and metronidazole) for 7–10 days after discharge.

If an open appendectomy is performed in a child with perforated appendicitis, it is never necessary to leave the wound open to heal by secondary intention. In fact, I use cyanoacrylate on all incisions in every patient with appendicitis and, if anything, the risk of a superficial surgical site infection appears to be much lower than with steri-strips.

Differential Diagnosis

Nonsurgical causes

- Mesenteric adenitis or gastroenteritis
- Omental torsion
- Pneumonia of the right lower lobe
- Streptococcus pharyngitis
- Nephrolithiasis/pyleonephritis
- Crohn's disease
- Henoch–Schonlein purpura
- Sickle cell disease with crisis
- Hemolytic uremic syndrome
- Pancreatitis

Surgical causes

- Meckel's diverticulitis
- Ectopic pregnancy
- Gastro-intestinal perforation of other source including gastric and intestinal ulcers
- Cholecystitis
- Pelvic inflammatory disease
- Idiopathic intussusception

Diagnostic Studies

- Complete blood count with differential
- C-reactive protein
- Ultrasound
- Computed tomography

Parental Preparation

- There is a small chance that the operation will need to be converted to an open operation.
- The postoperative course will vary depending on whether the appendix is perforated or nonperforated.
- There is a less than 5% chance that the appendix will in fact be normal, in which case we would still remove it and perform a brief exploration to rule out other causes of pain.
- Potential complications include wound infection, postoperative intra-abdominal abscess, injury to other structures, and error in diagnosis, but the overall competition rate is quite low.

Preoperative Preparation

☐ Intravenous hydration.
☐ Prophylactic antibiotics.
☐ Patient should urinate immediately before arriving to the operating room.

Suggested Reading

Adibe OO, Barnaby K, Dobies J, Comerford M, Drill A, Walker N, et al. Postoperative antibiotic therapy for children with perforated appendicitis: long course of intravenous antibiotics versus early conversion to an oral regimen. Am J Surg. 2008;195(2):141–3.

Frush DP, Donnelly LF, Rosen NS. Computed tomography and radiation risks: what pediatric health care providers should know. Pediatrics. 2003;112:951–7.

Henry MC, Walker A, Silverman BL, Gollin G, Islam S, Sylvester K, et al. Risk factors for the development of abdominal abscess following operation for perforated appendicitis in children: a multicenter case-control study. Arch Surg. 2007;142(3):236–41.

Chapter 63
Ulcerative Colitis and Familial Polyposis

Stephen E. Dolgin

Ulcerative colitis (UC) is a chronic idiopathic illness that causes cramping abdominal pain and bloody diarrhea. It is managed medically but can only be cured surgically. However, there is significant morbidity associated with the surgical remedies. For this reason, families and gastroenterologists generally utilize medical management until the affected children have suffered considerable morbidity. When finally coming to surgical therapy, it is unusual for the child to be doing well with minimal toxicity from the medical therapy.

Subtotal Colectomy

Some children experience a fulminant onset of UC that requires hospitalization. They have frequent bloody bowel movements, severe abdominal cramps, and tenderness on examination. Blood transfusions are often required. Management includes intravenous corticosteroids. Diagnosis is confirmed with flexible colonoscopy that reveals rectal involvement, no skip areas, and mucosal friability. The terminal ileum will be free of inflammation. Stool should be cultured for infectious pathogens and should be assayed for *Clostridium difficile* toxin to exclude pseudomembranous colitis.

Cyclosporine has been added in an attempt to avoid colectomy in patients with fulminant colitis. This is a common choice for so called "rescue therapy." Both fulminant colitis and extensive colitis, defined as colitis extending from the rectum proximal to the splenic flexure, are more common in children than in adults.

Toxic megacolon, a life threatening complication highlighted by colonic dilatation, demands emergency colectomy and has become rare in recent decades. Nonetheless, if a child

receiving medical therapy for virulent colitis experiences progressive tenderness, especially if associated with colonic dilatation, the threshold for emergency colectomy should be low. If bloody diarrhea and abdominal cramps are unremitting despite maximum medical management, colectomy is indicated, although a specific time limit for the non-operative approach cannot be dictated.

If after 5 days of intravenous steroids, frequent stools and nocturnal bowel movements persist with elevated inflammatory markers, such as C-reactive protein and erythrocyte sedimentation rate, rescue therapy such as cyclosporine is appropriate. About half of children with fulminant colitis for will come to colectomy during their admission to the hospital.

In this setting the simplest and safest way to stop the hemorrhage and the toxicity of the medications is a subtotal colectomy (STC). Ideally, the surgical option for fulminant colitis would be ileal pouch anal anastomosis (IPAA) with diverting ileostomy. However, when a child is acutely ill, with poor nutritional status, and receiving high-dose steroids, STC is the operation I advocate. Although the diseased rectum remains in situ, the proctitis tends to become quiescent when the fecal stream is diverted. Some blood-tinged mucus is usually passed per rectum, sometimes as often as three to four times daily. Serious ongoing bleeding from a deep rectal ulcer is a theoretical possibility but unlikely. I have not seen that occur in a single patient after performing STC in this setting in 50 children with UC. Colectomy liberates the child from the toxicity of the medications and restores him to health with good nutritional status. The early postoperative complications I have seen after STC include wound infection, small bowel obstruction and, in one child, a leak from the rectal stump. That patient did well after percutaneous drainage and antibiotics.

Even if a child with UC is managed as an outpatient, the need for infliximab (Remicade) should be a warning to the surgeon that an IPAA may not heal satisfactorily. These patients may be steroid-dependent and infliximab has been added because the colitis is refractory. Infectious complications such as fistulas from the pouch are common in this setting. This finding may not implicate infliximab per se, but

S.E. Dolgin (✉)
Albert Einstein College of Medicine, Schneider Children's Hospital, 269-01 76 Ave 1, New Hyde Park, NY 11040, USA
e-mail: sdolgin@nshs.edu

could indicate that by the time patients get that high on the therapeutic ladder, they are at increased risk for complications after a major reconstructive operation. A group at the Mayo clinic found a significant increase in infectious complications after IPAA when patients were receiving infliximab and recommend the STC as the initial operative step for these patients. I agree.

Surgical Technique

This operation is a first stage toward reconstruction. Several technical features are critical in light of future reconstruction. The best site in the abdominal wall for the ileostomy should be chosen and marked prior to the operation. The ileum should be divided at the ileocecal junction. The blood supply to the colon should be taken close to the colonic wall. There is no need to include mesentery with the specimen. The ileocolic pedicle must be preserved for the future IPAA. The rectum can be stapled above the peritoneal reflection. It is not necessary to dissect more deeply in the pelvis in order to excise more of the rectum since the fecal stream will be diverted by the ileostomy and the diseased rectum is unlikely to cause ongoing serious bleeding.

A long permanent suture in the rectal stump helps with future identification. Some surgeons advocate removing the omentum with the specimen to limit the formation of adhesions. The stoma should have adequate length above the skin so that it is easily managed. There are particular risks with a skin-level stoma in this setting. If, in the future, the child is ever faced with the need for another stoma, the memory of skin burning around the stoma may be prohibitively disturbing.

Usually children do very well after STC. I do not proceed to the reconstructive operation until good nutrition has been restored with a near normal hematocrit. Mild anemia from bloody rectal discharge is not uncommon. A few children have chosen to wait years rather than months because they are in school, doing well and are not very bothered by managing their stomas.

Ileal Pouch Anal Anastomosis

Children with UC are managed as outpatients unless their disease becomes severe. Steroids are not an acceptable maintenance therapy because of their toxicity. Some children do not do well unless they receive steroids and so steroid dependence becomes an indication for operative management.

The illness is not curable by non-operative means and the life-long risk of cancer increases as years pass. It approximates 10% per decade after the first 10 years of the illness. Gastroenterologists managing adults with UC aggressively provide a program of surveillance that includes twice yearly complete colonoscopic examinations with multiple biopsies every 10 cm for the entire length of the colon. Some gastroenterologists declare that with this program of surveillance the risk of colon cancer should not be an indication for colectomy. In my opinion, the need for life-long surveillance, the uncertainty of compliance and the threat of adenocarcinoma that may be advanced and multifocal support the application of surgical cure for childhood UC. If a child is missing school, receiving medications and suffering from chronic colitis, perhaps occasionally hospitalized, the life-long risk of cancer might help decide for the operative approach.

Extra-intestinal manifestations of UC, such as arthritis and erythema nodosum, are usually improved or cured by colectomy. Unfortunately, this claim does not hold for sclerosing cholangitis, a potentially morbid extra-intestinal manifestation that carries the risk of liver failure and hepatocellular carcinoma.

The postoperative appearance of disease lurks as a possibility for patients with UC and sometimes intimidates families from pursuing the operative treatment. Crohn's disease affects every inch of the GI tract. The prospect of recurrent inflammatory bowel disease from Crohn's disease after IPAA frightens families and gastroenterologists. The Cleveland Clinic's large series of children who underwent IPAA for UC showed that a particularly high number of patients ultimately developed Crohn's disease (15%). This is about twice the rate expected in adults. That series found correlation with Crohn's disease when children had experienced perineal disease or small bowel disease pre-operatively. My series includes half the rate of Crohn's disease as the Cleveland group, but I did not perform IPAA on any child with small bowel or perineal disease.

In frankly discussing the risks and uncertainties of the operative approach with families considering colectomy, it has been helpful to put them in touch with other families who have been through this experience. Patients are sometimes less interested in talking with other young people than their parents are in talking with other parents.

Surgical Technique

Patients undergoing elective IPAA can be admitted on the day of the operation. I limit them to clear liquids on the prior day and provide intravenous antibiotics perioperatively.

I have not used laxatives, enemas or pre-operative enteral antibiotics in these children.

Anti-inflammatory medications such as 6MP are stopped at the time of the colectomy. If they have received steroids within 3 months of the operation, they are given perioperative stress doses that are tapered after the operation. The first stress dose can be provided after induction of anesthesia. It is not necessary the day before the operation. They are usually discharged home on prednisone 10 mg daily and tapered off completely in the months after the operation.

A Foley catheter is placed after induction and not removed until the fourth postoperative day. Initially it serves to keep the bladder empty for the proctectomy. For the first few days after the operation it serves to monitor hydration and to avoid bladder distention that might put tension on the healing pouch-anal anastomosis.

The operation is begun through a midline incision, with a place marked for the ileostomy. The patient is protected in lithotomy. The operation can be done with the assistance of the laparoscope. That should be limited to surgeons with adequate experience with this technique. If the surgeon does few of these operations, the safer approach is to do it by the open technique. Some of the risks of this operation increase with the length of time the operation requires. Although compartment syndrome in the legs can occur with any type of operation in lithotomy, the risk increases after 5 h of operating time. When an operation in lithotomy takes 5 h, the patient's position should be changed and documented in an effort to avoid this serious complication. It is hard to defend a surgeon if the operation is done using the laparoscopic-assisted approach, takes a very long time, and the patient develops a compartment syndrome.

The small bowel should be examined from the ligament of Treitz to the fold of Treves to make sure there is no evidence of Crohn's disease involving the small intestine. After the small intestine has been examined, the perineal part of the operation can be done concomitantly by a second team. If a prior STC has not been done, the ileum is divided with the GIA stapler right at the ileocecal junction. The ileocolic vascular pedicle is preserved and protected.

The colorectal group at the Cleveland Clinic forcefully advocate a double stapled ileorectal anastomosis over the mucosectomy and hand-sewn ileo-anal anastomosis. Their evidence, retrospective from a large series, shows that this approach offers a lower incidence of pelvic sepsis. The double stapled ileorectal anastomosis has limited support currently for the pediatric population. It leaves a cuff of columnar mucosa that can lead to a post operative cuffitis, which represents persistent UC that usually responds to local anti-inflammatory medication. The ileorectal anastomosis also demands life-long surveillance for dysplasia of the residual columnar mucosa. The more common operation for children

with UC is the IPAA with rectal mucosectomy and a J-pouch hand sewn to the anus. The conservative approach is to include a temporary diverting ileostomy.

At the perineum, endorectal retraction is avoided. The Lone Star self-retaining retractor provides exposure. This protects sphincter tone that may be endangered by stretching. The mucosectomy is begun at the dentate line. Dissection is circumferential, visualizing and protecting the internal sphincter. Submucosal injection of epinephrine in dilute lidocaine prior to the dissection helps reduce bleeding. Pennington-type clamps can be used for retraction on the mucosal sleeve. They are adjusted as the dissection proceeds. Judicious use of the cautery provides most of the hemostasis. The dissection is complete when the mucosa has been freed just proximal to the palpable puborectalis muscle. A heavy suture ligature closes the mucosal sleeve. Then, with a large clamp, the surgeon breaks through the rectal wall above the puborectalis and below the stripped mucosa. This helps when the proctectomy is completed from the pelvis. A betadine soaked kerlex is placed in the anal canal.

The most common major risk of this operation is pelvic sepsis either from a pouch fistula or ileo-anal anastomotic separation. Several technical steps limit tension on the anastomosis. The mesentery is mobilized to the duodenum. This is done with care since portal vein thrombosis can occur after this operation. The peritoneum on each side of the mesentery can be incised with transverse cuts. Vascular branches in the ileal mesentery between arcades can be divided. A non-crushing clamp may be applied for a few minutes to help ensure that dividing a vessel will not cause ischemia to the pouch. The use of a pouch to add a reservoir and thereby reduce the frequency of bowel movements has become standard.

The J-pouch is the simplest to construct and is preferred. I choose the length of the J-pouch based on the site that provides the greatest length when pulled down to the anus. Usually the pouch in a child is about 8 cm long. It is constructed with gastrointestinal anastomosis staplers. The device can be inserted from the apex upward requiring two applications. Or, enterotomies can be made in each limb and the stapler passed upward and downward in separate applications (Fig. 63.1). The resulting septum near the apex can be divided with the same stapler after inverting the pouch through the enterotomies. The enterotomies are closed with a linear stapler. The anastomosis is hand sewn to the anus with interrupted 3-0 braided absorbable sutures. A closed-suction drain is left alongside the pouch in the pelvis and exits above the pubis (Fig. 63.2). Some utilize a rectal tube to keep the pouch decompressed, hoping to avoid distention and ileal pouch-anal disruption.

The proctectomy is completed from above. The closed suction drain is passed from the pelvis to the perineum before the pouch is passed. The pouch is passed, untwisted, from

Fig. 63.1 Steps in the construction
of a J-pouch, usually about 8 cm
long (From Bauer JJ, Gorfine SR,
eds. Colorectal surgery illustrated:
A focused approach. Philadelphia:
Mosby-Year Book; 1993. Reprinted
with permission from Elsevier)

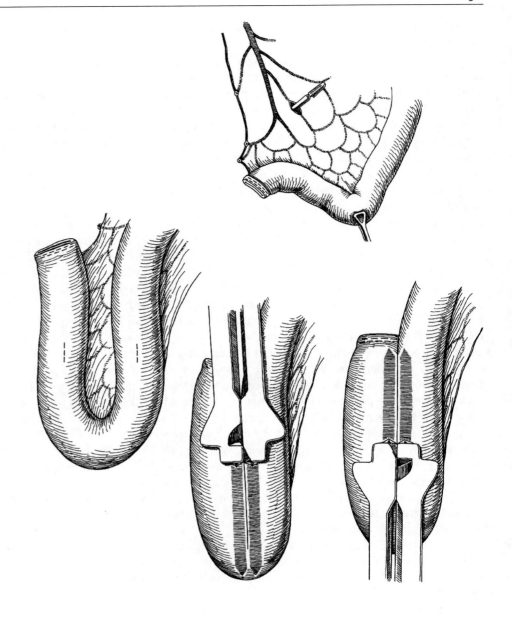

the pelvis to a surgeon at the perineum. The surgeon at the
perineum reaches through the denuded rectum with a
Babcock clamp and the surgeon at the pelvis places the apex
of the pouch into that instrument. Sometimes perirectal fat
obstructs this step and requires excision. The neoanus is
opened at the apex of the pouch. An interrupted single layer
of 3-0 braided absorbable suture is used for the ileo-anal
anastomosis. The drain is cut as the anastomosis is complete
and left just proximal to the suture line.

Some practitioners contend that a proximal diverting ileostomy should be done routinely to limit pelvic sepsis. If a
patient is in relatively good health, not cushingoid, not malnourished, not receiving infliximab, not hospitalized receiving intravenous steroids and blood transfusions, and the

operation proceeds perfectly, the surgeon can opt to forego
the ileostomy. However, an ileostomy must be fashioned
promptly if the patient suffers pelvic sepsis postoperatively.

I remove the urinary catheter on the fourth postoperative
day and the closed suction drain when the child is ready for
discharge. The ileostomy is not closed for at least 6 weeks
and then after a CT scan with intravenous contrast and contrast in the pouch injected transanally through a catheter. If
the pouch looks fine by CT, I examine the pouch under anesthesia at the time of stoma closure and proceed if no problem
is visualized. Sometimes an easily broken synechia is dilated.
The anastomosis should accept a 14 French dilator without
difficulty. If it does not, dilatation is required and ileostomy
closure should be deferred.

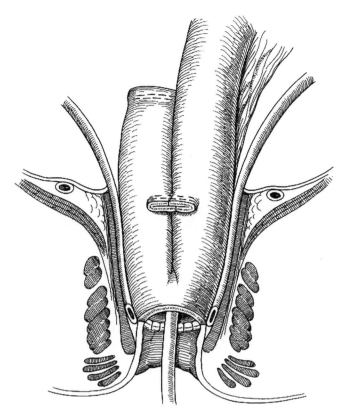

Fig. 63.2 J-pouch in place in the pelvis, the rectal tube is optional (From Bauer JJ, Gorfine SR, eds. Colorectal surgery illustrated: A focused approach. Philadelphia: Mosby-Year Book; 1993. Reprinted with permission from Elsevier)

Table 63.1 Long term problems related to ileal pouch anal anastomosis (IPAA)

Pouchitis
Crohn's disease
Irritable pouch syndrome
Cuffitis (occurs after double-stapled ileorectal anastomosis)
Stricture
Pouch fistulas

Systemic symptoms, such as weakness, aphthous ulcers or other extra-intestinal manifestations of inflammatory bowel disease, raise the specter of Crohn's disease. Blood tests reflecting inflammation such as markedly elevated ESR and CRP enhance the concern. About half the patients who develop Crohn's disease are able to keep their functioning pouches. The rest require a permanent ileostomy.

Cuffitis does not occur when all the columnar mucosa has been removed. However, it occurs after the double-stapled ileorectal anastomosis. It is managed with local anti-inflammatory medications. Irritable pouch syndrome is a pouch with physiologic dysfunction but no inflammation, analogous to irritable bowel syndrome.

Leakage at night affects about 20% of my patients. I ask the children who are old enough to exercise their perineal muscles in order to increase rectal tone. This involves squeezing perineal muscles tightly and repetitively. Loperamide can be taken before sleep. Children are discouraged from eating and drinking just before going to bed.

Ileo-anal anastomotic strictures are managed by dilatation, often requiring general anesthesia. Late-appearing fistulas and abscesses can involve the vagina and the perineal skin. They also raise the specter of Crohn's disease.

Outcome

Pelvic sepsis is the most serious acute postoperative complication, occurring in up to 10% of patients. It is the result of ileo-anal separation or pouch fistula. Pouchitis occurs in about 25% of patients. About 20% suffer nocturnal leakage. Crohn's disease occurs in about 8%. A permanent ileostomy has been required in about 5% of patients. Long term complications of the pouch are relatively uncommon (Table 63.1).

Symptoms of pouchitis include increased frequency of bowel movements, cramps, accidents, and occasionally blood in the stool and fever. Empiric treatment with oral antibiotics is commonly employed. Metronidazole is often the first choice and ciprofloxacin the second. Some benefit has been found with probiotics. If response is not prompt or symptoms recur, flexible endoscopic examination of the pouch should be done to assess the pouch and the afferent loop. Inflammation limited to the pouch and without histologic evidence of epithelioid granulomas confirms pouchitis. Inflammation of the afferent limb or the presence of epithelioid granulomas confirm Crohn's disease.

Familial Polyposis

When the phenotype of familial polyposis (FP) includes hundreds of adenomatous colonic polyps confirmed by colonoscopic appearance and biopsies, colectomy is indicated to avoid adenocarcinoma of the colon. This is an autosomal dominant disease caused by any of a variety of mutations in the adenomatous polyposis coli (APC) gene on the long arm of chromosome 5. Because of variability in gene expression, colectomy is generally not indicated unless sheets of polyps are present. I use this formulation because FP in children may be unearthed by genetic testing when a family member is affected by the disease and at present the genotype alone does not ordinarily dictate colectomy.

Symptomatic anemia is less common in childhood and suggests the possibility of malignancy. Colectomy is done because colonic cancer is inevitable. The mean age for the development of colorectal carcinoma in patients with FAP is about 39 years. Some continue to advocate ileorectal anastomosis for reconstruction, which was a more common choice before the era of IPAA. Mucosectomy and hand sewn IPAA carries the advantage of leaving no at-risk mucosa. Some advocates of the ileorectal anastomosis think that this choice can be made based on the specific genetic mutation in the APC gene, with some mutations carrying lower risk of subsequent cancer in the residual rectum.

These children are usually well. Unlike patients suffering from UC, their nutritional status is fine and they are not receiving toxic medications. If a surgeon is ever willing to perform IPAA without diverting ileostomy, that approach would apply to these children, assuming the operation goes perfectly.

Pouchitis is less common after IPAA for FP than for UC and subsequent manifestations of Crohn's disease does not occur.

Lifelong surveillance for other tumors, especially duodenal, is indicated. Depending on the genotypic variant, associated findings may include other gastrointestinal polyps, duodenal tumors, desmoids tumors, osteomas, epidermoid cysts, brain tumors, thyroid tumors, liver tumors and congenital hypertrophy of the retinal pigment epithelium (CHRPE).

Summary Points

- UC presents with bloody diarrhea and abdominal cramps. It is managed medically but only curable surgically.
- Fulminant colitis, not responding to i.v. steroids and rescue therapy, warrants urgent colectomy. STC with end ileostomy is a safe choice in this setting.
- Indications for elective operative treatment include: refractory symptoms, steroid dependence, and toxicity from therapy outweighing the therapeutic benefits.
- IPAA is the best approach, and can be done with or without a diverting ileostomy.
- A patient receiving infliximab warrants STC as a first stage to limit septic complications from IPAA.

Editor's Comment

Total colectomy, mucosal proctectomy, and J-pouch ileo-anal anastomosis with temporary ileostomy is the standard operation for children with intractable UC or polyposis. A long and often rather tedious operation, it demands patience, meticulous attention to detail, and a commitment to the patient for the foreseeable future. Experience makes one realize there is no shame in sometimes recommending the traditional "three-staged" approach, particularly when faced with the typical UC patient who is malnourished, steroid-dependent and emotionally tenuous, even though it invariably seems to every new generation of pediatric surgeons to be a hopelessly old-fashioned relic of a bygone era. I prefer to do the STC laparoscopically, and, if the proctectomy is being done the same day, I will make a Pfannenstiel incision (with the fascia opened in the midline) to use a hand-assisted approach, which saves time and minimizes blood loss. I then do the mucosal proctectomy and J-pouch procedure through the Pfannenstiel incision.

Getting the ileum to reach the anus can be quite difficult, especially in obese patients. Every surgeon should have a systematic approach, each step of which adds a few centimeters of length, including mobilizing the pedicle all the way up to the pancreas, scoring the mesentery, and dividing superfluous vessels after test clamping. This should all be done before the proctectomy is started! In the rare event that a tension-free anastomosis is impossible, it is best to abort the pull-through, create an ileostomy, and plan to try again in 6 months or so. If the proctectomy is done, placing omentum in the rectal canal will make it easier to find the lumen in the future. Then again, mobilizing too much ileum increases the risk of pouch prolapse, a vastly under-reported complication of this operation.

Pouchitis is the nemesis of the patient with a J-pouch. Interestingly, it almost never occurs in patients with polyposis, suggesting it may in fact be a forme fruste of UC. Patients with recurrent pouchitis should undergo examination under anesthesia to rule out an anastomotic stricture and Crohn's disease. Daily dietary fiber supplements, probiotics and judicious intermittent use of metronidazole are all part of a regimen that is usually effective in minimizing recurrence.

Differential Diagnosis

- Crohn's disease
- Infectious colitis

Diagnostic Studies

- Stool for pathogens and *C. difficile* toxin
- Flexible colonoscopy

Parental and Family Preparation

- Detailed discussion of short- and long-term risks and expectations
- Introduce them to other parents with similar experience
- Meet with stoma therapist before the operation for teaching and selecting the best location for stoma

Preoperative Preparation

☐ Full metabolic profile, including serum albumin, and liver function tests
☐ Complete blood count
☐ Type and cross, family designated if preferred
☐ Clear liquids for 24 h prior to operation

Technical Points

STC

- Foley catheter, leave in 48 h
- Take blood supply near colonic wall
- Divide ileum where it joins cecum
- Divide rectum above peritoneal reflection
- Create ileostomy with adequate length

IPAA

- Carefully protect patient while in modified lithotomy
- Foley catheter kept in place for 4 days
- Inspect entire small bowel to rule out Crohn's disease
- Mobilize small bowel mesentery to duodenum
- Score peritoneum of mesentery on either side
- Determine length of J-pouch by choosing a site that provides the least amount of tension for pull through
- Take a vessel if needed for length after applying a non-crushing clamp and ensuring viability of bowel
- Use the Lone Star retractor and minimize stretching of the sphincter
- Mucosectomy: inject lidocaine with epinephrine, dissect circumferentially, protect inner circular muscularis, advance proximally, stop at upper aspect of puborectalis, break through back wall of rectum below mucosal sleeve
- Pack Betadine-soaked kerlex into canal after closing the mucosal sleeve with a large ligature
- Complete the proctectomy from above
- Closed-suction drain next to pouch, leave in place until ready for discharge
- Hand sew neorectum to dentate line

Suggested Reading

Alexander F, Sarigol S, DiFiore J, et al. Fate of the pouch in 151 pediatric patients after ileal pouch anal anastomosis. J Pediatr Surg. 2003;38:78–82.

Fazio VW, Ziv Y, Church JM, et al. Ileal pouch-anal anastomoses complications and function in 1005 patients. Ann Surg. 1995;222:120–7.

Selvasekar C, Cima R, Larson D, et al. Effect of Infliximab on short-term complications in patients undergoing operation for chronic ulcerative colitis. J Am Coll Surg. 2004;204:956–62.

Shen B, Fazio VW, Remzi FH, et al. Comprehensive evaluation of inflammatory and noninflammatory sequelae of ileal pouch-anal anastomoses. Am J Gastroenterol. 2005;100:93–101.

Turner D, Walsh CM, Benchimol EI, et al. Severe paediatric ulcerative colitis: incidence, outcomes and optimal timing for second-line therapy. Gut. 2008;57:331–8.

Vasen HFA, van Duijvendijk P, Buskens E, et al. Decision analysis in the surgical treatment of patients with familial adenomatous polyposis: a Dutch-Scandinavian collaborative study including 659 patients. Gut. 2001;49:231–5.

Chapter 64
Anorectal Malformations

Marc A. Levitt and Alberto Peña

Anorectal malformations (imperforate anus) are a class of congenital anomalies that are represented by a wide spectrum of defects, some relatively mild and some quite severe. The most feared sequelae associated with the care of these defects is fecal incontinence. Nevertheless, the majority of patients do well and 75% can achieve a good degree of bowel control, provided they receive expert surgical care and adequate postoperative treatment, especially for constipation.

Current terminology is based on the location of the rectal fistula, which has both prognostic and therapeutic implications. (Table 64.1) Inaccurate terms such as *high, intermediate*, and *low* are confusing and should no longer be used.

Over 80% of male patients with imperforate anus will have a fistulous connection between the rectum and the urinary tract (*recto-bladderneck fistula, recto-prostatic urethral fistula*, or *recto-bulbar urethral fistula*) and about 15% have a *recto-perineal fistula*, in which the rectal opening is on the perineal skin. Rarer still, but more commonly found in patients with trisomy 21, is *imperforate anus without fistula*, in which the rectum ends blindly in the pelvis, almost always at the level of the bulbar urethra.

In females, there are three main types of malformations: *recto-perineal fistulas, recto-vestibular fistulas* and *cloacas*. A *perineal fistula* opens on the perineal skin, anterior to the anal dimple. In the case of a *vestibular fistula*, the opening lies within the introitus, but outside of the hymen (Fig. 64.1). A *cloaca* is a malformation in which the rectum, vagina and urethra all open into a single channel, which subsequently opens onto the perineum (Fig. 64.2). True *recto-vaginal fistulas* are extremely rare, but unfortunately this is a term that is overused and almost always inaccurate.

Diagnosis

The initial diagnosis of imperforate anus is almost always made during the first newborn physical examination. The lack of an anal opening is usually fairly obvious. Occasionally, a perineal fistula will be missed. Two important questions must be answered in the first 24 h of life: The first is whether a colostomy should be opened, deferring the repair of the defect until later in life, or whether to proceed with definitive repair during the newborn period without a protective colostomy. Physical examination, especially the perineal inspection, will provide enough clinical evidence to reach a decision about the need for a diverting colostomy in over 90% of the patients. The second question is whether the patient needs urgent treatment for an associated defect (Figs. 64.3 and 64.4).

Males

The presence of a well-developed midline groove between the buttocks, a prominent anal dimple and meconium exiting through a small orifice located anterior to the sphincter in the midline of the perineum is evidence that the patient has a perineal fistula. Occasionally one may see a prominent skin bridge over a tiny opening, giving the appearance of a bucket handle, or a midline raphe, which can appear as a white or black ribbon of subepithelial meconium. These malformations can all be repaired via a perineal approach during the newborn period without a colostomy. On the other hand, a flat bottom, with no evidence of a perineal opening and the presence of meconium in the urine are indications of a recto-urethral fistula. Most surgeons will open a colostomy in these patients.

One should not be too hasty in ruling out a fistula. Unless meconium is definitely seen on the perineum or in the urine, a conclusion as to the presence or absence of a fistula cannot be made with certainty on the basis of physical examination alone. However, it takes some time for the intraluminal pressure to force the meconium past the pelvic musculature and out through

M.A. Levitt (✉)
Colorectal Center for Children, Cincinnati Children's Hospital
Medical Center, Pediatric Surgery, 3333 Burnet Avenue, ML 2023,
Cincinnati, OH 45229, USA
e-mail: marc.levitt@cchmc.org

P. Mattei (ed.), *Fundamentals of Pediatric Surgery*,
DOI 10.1007/978-1-4419-6643-8_64, © Springer Science+Business Media, LLC 2011

Table 64.1 Classification

Males
  Cutaneous (perineal fistula)
  Rector-urethral fistula
    Bulbar
    Prostatic
  Recto-bladder neck fistula
  Imperforate anus without fistula
  Rectal atresia
Females
  Cutaneous (perineal fistula)
  Vestibular fistula
  Imperforate anus without fistula
  Rectal artesia
  Cloaca
  Complex malformations

Source: Pena A, Levitt MA. Imperforate anus and cloacal malformations. In: Pediatric surgery, 4th ed. Philadelphia, PA: Elsevier; 2005. Reprinted with permission from Elsevier

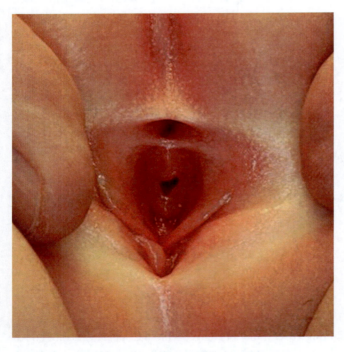

Fig. 64.1 Classic appearance of imperforate anus with recto-vestibular fistula. Note that the fistula is located within the introitus but outside of the hymenal ring

a perineal or urinary fistula. This usually does not occur until after the first 24 h of life. If the diagnosis is still in doubt after 24 h, a cross-table lateral radiograph of the abdomen and pelvis with the infant in prone position should be obtained (Fig. 64.5). A radiopaque marker should be placed at the anal dimple to allow you to estimate the size of the gap between the end of the dilated bowel and the skin. If this distance is less than one cm, a primary repair can usually be performed. If the distance is greater than one cm, we recommend that a colostomy be performed. This film is necessary in less than 10% of male patients.

Females

The presence of a single perineal orifice in a newborn female establishes the diagnosis of a cloaca. All infants with cloaca require a colostomy and some may also require a vaginostomy to drain a hydrocolpos.

In a female with a normal urethra, the presence of a rectal orifice located within the vestibule of the female genitalia but outside of the hymen confirms the diagnosis of a recto-vestibular fistula (Fig. 64.1). This malformation is by far the most common defect seen in females. In these cases, some surgeons simply dilate the fistula to allow stool to pass and alleviate abdominal distention. Other surgeons prefer to open a colostomy and perform the repair at a later date. Surgeons who are experienced in the treatment of this abnormality may choose to do a primary repair in the newborn period without a protective colostomy. This decision is made by the primary surgeon depending on his or her level of experience and comfort.

When the rectal orifice is located anterior to the center of the sphincter but posterior to the vestibule of the genitalia (in the perineal body), the diagnosis of perineal fistula is established. These babies can undergo a primary anoplasty without a protective colostomy.

The absence of any of the above findings and the lack of meconium coming out through the genitalia after 24 h of life indicates that the patient most likely has imperforate anus without a fistula (more common in patients with trisomy 21). Again, the prone cross-table lateral radiograph can be useful in this situation (Fig. 64.5).

True *recto-vaginal* fistulas are located above the hymenal ring. Occurring in less than 1% of all females with imperforate anus, they are so exceedingly rare as to be practically nonexistent. Nevertheless, it is the most common misdiagnosis given to female babies born with anorectal malformations.

The waiting period of 16–24 h can be used to answer the second question concerning associated defects, the majority of which are of the genito-urinary system. In general, the more severe the anorectal anomaly, the more likely an associated defect will be present. Patients with cloacas have up to a 90% risk of an associated defect and patients with vestibular fistulas have approximately a 40% risk. The incidence of associated defects in males with imperforate anus is 90% for patients with a recto-bladder neck fistula, 60% for those with a recto-prostatic fistula and 30% for boys with a recto-bulbar urethral. Both males and females with a perineal fistula have a less than 20% incidence of a other abnormalities. All patients must have an ultrasound study of the kidneys to rule out hydronephrosis, the most common cause of which is vesico-ureteral reflux. In newborns with cloacas, the abdominal ultrasound must include the pelvis to rule out the presence of hydrocolpos or a distended bladder.

Fig. 64.2 Cloacal malformation. The urethra, vagina and rectum meet to form a single common channel. (**a**) Short common channel. (**b**) Long common channel. (From Pena A. Atlas of surgical management of anorectal malformations. New York: Springer; 1989. Reprinted with permission from Springer Science + Business Media)

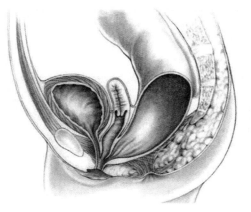
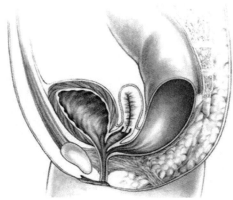

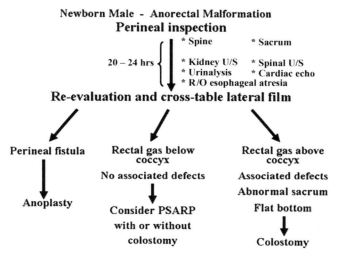

Fig. 64.3 Clinical algorithm for males with imperforate anus. (From Pena A, Levitt MA. Imperforate anus and cloacal malformations. In: Pediatric surgery, 4th ed. Philadelphia, PA; Elsevier; 2005. Reprinted with permission from Elsevier)

A nasogastric tube should be passed to rule out esophageal atresia, which occurs in about 5% of cases. It also helps to decompress the gut while waiting for clinical evidence of a recto-urethral or perineal fistula. All patients with imperforate anus should have an echocardiogram, as about 10% of patients are found to have patent ductus arteriosus or a more serious structural cardiac defect such as tetralogy of Fallot or ventricular septal defect.

An ultrasound of the spine is also important to rule out the presence of a tethered cord, which occurs in about 25% of all patients with anorectal malformations. This finding has important therapeutic and prognostic implications. A radiograph of the spine must also be obtained. The presence of hemivertebra of the spine or sacrum indicates an increased risk of associated urologic defects and has negative prognostic implications in terms of bowel control. Anterior-posterior (AP) and lateral radiographs of the sacrum allow calculation of the *sacral ratio* (Fig. 64.6). A poorly formed sacrum (ratio <0.5) is associated with more severe malformations and carries with it a poor

prognosis for bowel control. The presence of a hemisacrum might indicate the presence of a presacral mass, such as a teratoma, lipoma, anterior meningocele or a mix of all or part of these. A spinal ultrasound or magnetic resonance imaging (MRI) can confirm this suspicion.

During the diagnostic period, the infant needs intravenous fluids, intravenous antibiotics and gastric tube decompression. The decision regarding primary repair or diverting colostomy should be made within the first 48 h of life to avoid the risk of colonic perforation.

Surgical Technique

Colostomy

The ideal colostomy is created at the junction of the descending and sigmoid colon (Fig. 64.7). Creating the stoma too distal in the sigmoid is the most common error we see. Making the stoma more proximal ensures that the distal colon will be long enough to allow a tension-free pull-through later. In addition, stomas fashioned from the distal descending colon almost never prolapse because the colon is tethered by retroperitoneal attachments. To prevent prolapse of the more mobile distal stoma, the mucous fistula should be made with a very small external opening; the colon may also be fixed to the lower anterior wall for a few centimeters. The stomas should be far enough apart on the abdomen that the ostomy appliance can be placed comfortably over the functional stoma and not cover the mucous fistula.

Loop colostomies are contraindicated in patients with imperforate anus, as they are frequently incompletely diverting. The subsequent overflow of stool into the distal limb exposes the patient to fecal contamination of the genitourinary tract. Under no circumstances should the distal stoma be closed as a Hartmann pouch, as this will result in a mucocele and make it impossible to perform contrast studies of the distal rectum. A transverse colostomy is not recommended for

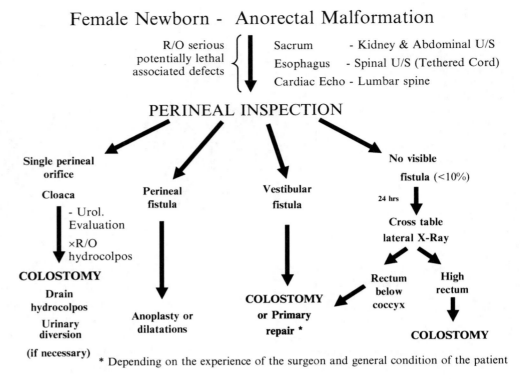

Fig. 64.4 Clinical algorithm for females with imperforate anus. (From Pena A, Levitt MA. Imperforate anus and cloacal malformations. In: Pediatric surgery, 4th ed. Philadelphia, PA: Elsevier; 2005. Reprinted with permission from Elsevier)

Female Newborn - Anorectal Malformation

R/O serious potentially lethal associated defects
- Sacrum — Kidney & Abdominal U/S
- Esophagus — Spinal U/S (Tethered Cord)
- Cardiac Echo — Lumbar spine

PERINEAL INSPECTION

Single perineal orifice
Cloaca
- Urol. Evaluation
×R/O hydrocolpos
COLOSTOMY
Drain hydrocolpos
Urinary diversion
(if necessary)

Perineal fistula
Anoplasty or dilatations

Vestibular fistula
COLOSTOMY or Primary repair *

No visible fistula (<10%)
24 hrs
Cross table lateral X-Ray
→ Rectum below coccyx
→ High rectum → **COLOSTOMY**

* Depending on the experience of the surgeon and general condition of the patient

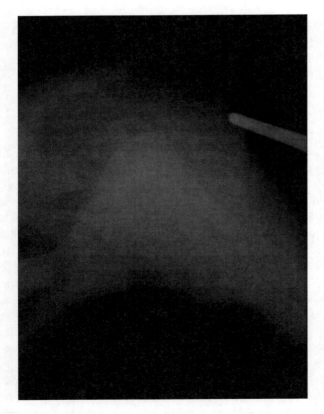

Fig. 64.5 Prone cross-table lateral radiograph. Wait 24 h after birth for air to pass distally. Infant should be prone for 15–20 min prior to shooting the film to allow gas to move above the meconium. Note the radiopaque marker at the anal dimple and the proximity of the rectum to the perineal skin. (From Levitt MA, Pena A. Management in the anorectal newborn period. In: Holschneider AM, Hutson J, eds. Malformations in children. Berlin: Springer; 2006. Reprinted with permission of Springer Science + Business Media)

several reasons: it makes it very difficult to clear inspissated meconium from the distal colon, it does not allow an adequate distal colostogram to be performed, and, in the presence of a fistula to the urinary tract, it may result in the resorption of urine, which can cause significant acidosis. At the time of the colostomy, use a soft rubber catheter to gently irrigate the distal limb with warm saline to remove all of the meconium from the lumen; this will prevent significant problems with inspissated meconium later on. A colostomy in a newborn is a delicate operation and should be done with meticulous attention to detail. Complications such as stenosis and prolapse are causes of significant morbidity and must be avoided.

Hydrocolpos

If the baby has hydrocolpos, it must be drained during the initial operation (Fig. 64.8). In the rare case of a giant hydrocolpos, in which the vagina reaches close to the diaphragm, the vagina can be exteriorized like a colostomy. At other times, a tense hydrocolpos is present but the vagina is no larger than the bladder and cannot be brought up to the abdominal wall. In such situations, the hydrocolpos can be drained by tube vaginostomy. If there is bilateral hydrocolpos, a window should be created between the hemivaginas. An undrained hydrocolpos will often cause hydronephrosis due to ureteral compression at the trigone. No treatment for the hydronephrosis should be considered until the hydrocolpos has been addressed. Once the vagina has been drained, the hydronephrosis should disappear. Even in the absence of hydronephrosis, it is important to decompress a hydrocolpos

Fig. 64.6 Sacral ratio. Line A is drawn so as to connect the uppermost aspect of the iliac crests. Line B is drawn so as to connect the lowest point of sacro-iliac joints. Line C is drawn parallel to line B at the tip of the coccyx. The ratio is calculated by dividing the distance between lines B and C by the distance between lines A and B. (From Pena A. Anorectal malformations. Semin Pediatr Surg. 1995;41(1):35–47. Reprinted with permission from Elsevier)

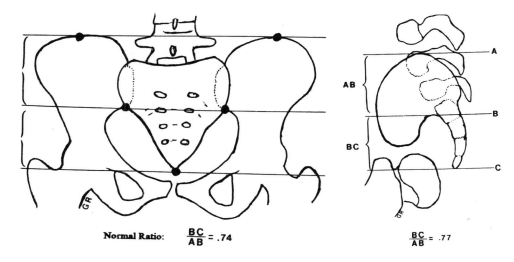

Normal Ratio: $\frac{BC}{AB} = .74$

$\frac{BC}{AB} = .77$

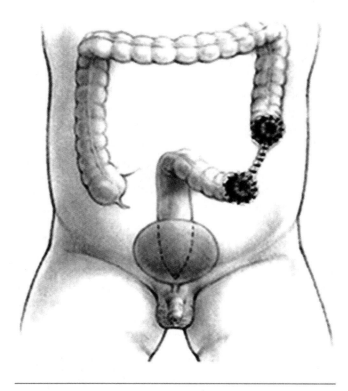

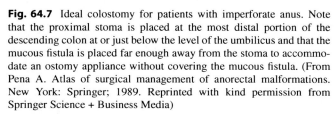

Fig. 64.7 Ideal colostomy for patients with imperforate anus. Note that the proximal stoma is placed at the most distal portion of the descending colon at or just below the level of the umbilicus and that the mucous fistula is placed far enough away from the stoma to accommodate an ostomy appliance without covering the mucous fistula. (From Pena A. Atlas of surgical management of anorectal malformations. New York: Springer; 1989. Reprinted with kind permission from Springer Science + Business Media)

as the undrained vagina can become infected (pyocolpos), which can then lead to perforation or sepsis and may result in loss of the vagina.

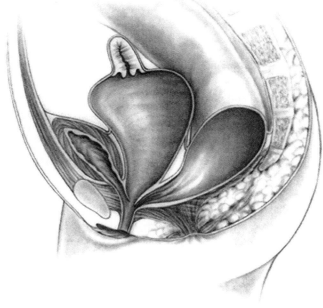

Fig. 64.8 Hydrocolpos. The vagina is hugely distended with fluid. Hydrocolpos should be decompressed by tube drainage or creation of a vaginostomy. (From Pena A. Atlas of surgical management of anorectal malformations. New York: Springer; 1989. Reprinted with kind permission from Springer Science + Business Media)

Anoplasty

In infants with a perineal fistula, a formal anoplasty can be performed during the first several days of life without the need for a protective colostomy. Older infants who are passing stool (as opposed to meconium) should have a full preoperative bowel prep. The operation utilizes a minimal posterior sagittal incision from the fistula to the anal dimple. Multiple 6-0 silk stitches are placed circumferentially around the rectal opening to facilitate uniform traction. Circumferential full-thickness dissection of the rectum is performed until enough length is gained that the rectum can be placed accurately within the limits of the sphincter. In male patients, keep in mind that the rectum and urethra are closely associated and that special care is needed to avoid urethral injury. A Foley catheter should always be placed prior to anoplasty in a male. If a baby with a perineal fistula is very sick, significantly premature or otherwise at high risk of an anesthetic complication, the fistula can be serially dilated to allow passage of meconium and the repair delayed indefinitely.

Almost all infants with a perineal fistula eventually have excellent bowel control. Fecal incontinence develops in patients who have undergone an overly aggressive operation that damages important anatomic structures necessary for bowel control and those with associated spinal anomalies.

Distal Colostogram

It is extremely important that the surgeon know the location of the distal rectum prior to the definitive repair. An augmented-pressure distal colostogram should be performed in all male patients who undergo a colostomy and all females with a cloaca, and can be done 4 weeks after the colostomy is opened. It is the most valuable diagnostic study in the treatment of these patients. It shows the location of the fistula between the rectum and the genito-urinary tract, the length of available colon from the colostomy to the fistula site, the distance between the rectum and the anal dimple and the relationship of the rectum with the sacrum. It may also demonstrate the characteristics of the urethra in males, the characteristics of the vagina in females and the presence of vesico-ureteral reflux. There is no other study that provides all this information. Eliminating this study or performing it improperly prior to definitive repair is the cause of many of the complications that occur in these patients.

The study should be performed in the fluoroscopy suite, ideally with the surgeon present. It is begun with the patient in the supine position. A #8 Foley catheter is introduced through the mucous fistula and the balloon is inflated with 1–2 mL of water. The catheter is pulled back firmly against the abdominal wall, occluding the lumen and allowing hand controlled injection of contrast material under pressure. Water-soluble contrast material should be used as barium is contraindicated in the presence of a recto-urinary tract fistula. A radiopaque marker is placed at the anal dimple. With the patient in the supine position, the surgeon can see the length of bowel available for the pull-through. The patient is then turned onto his or her side. As the injection is performed, contrast material will usually stop progressing at the pubo-coccygeal (PC) line. This line represents the upper limit of the levator muscles. It requires a significant increase in hydrostatic pressure for the contrast material to progress beyond this point. A lack of understanding of this fact will lead to early termination of the study and a conclusion that the patient has a "high imperforate anus with no fistula." It should be obvious that the abrupt flattening of the contrast column is actually due to compression of the distal rectum by the sphincteric funnel. In a male, the injection continues until the contrast material passes into the urethra. Usually the contrast goes up into the bladder rather than toward the penis and the injection should continue until the bladder is full and the baby starts to void. Films are taken during the entire sequence, particularly during voiding. The surgeon should be able to see the location of the fistula and its relationship to the bladder, bladder neck and urethra (Fig. 64.9).

A distal colostogram is not necessary in patients who have a vestibular fistula, because the diagnosis is obvious just by inspection. In patients with cloaca, this study is a bit more complex. The contrast material usually passes into the reproductive tract, defining the vagina or frequently two hemivaginas, but rarely enters the bladder. One can complement the

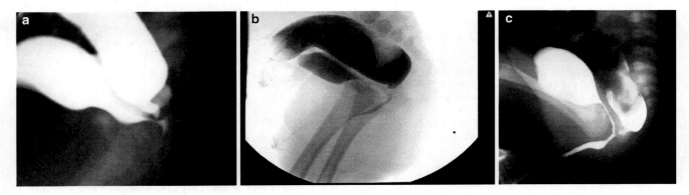

Fig. 64.9 Distal colostogram in the male with imperforate anus. (**a**) recto-bladder neck fistula; (**b**) recto-prostatic fistula; (**c**) recto-bulbar urethral fistula. Note that the bladder is filled with contrast and observed until after voiding

study by inserting a catheter into the perineal orifice and injecting contrast to delineate the bladder and vagina. If a vesicostomy, cystostomy or vaginostomy are present, these should also be injected with contrast. The goal of the study in patients with cloaca is to have images of all three crucial structures, bladder, vagina and rectum, in AP and lateral projections, and, if possible, in three dimensions.

In patients with cloaca, the information provided by the distal colostogram is extremely important. It allows the surgeon to estimate the prognosis by determining the precise nature of the defect and helps the parents avoid false expectations. It allows for planning of the primary repair, including an estimation of the length of the operation and the best technical maneuvers applicable for each case. If the study shows the presence of a bladder neck fistula, the surgeon knows that the rectum cannot be reached through a posterior sagittal incision and must be approached by laparoscopy or laparotomy. If the surgeon fails to understand this important point, the result can be a difficult and awkward search for the rectum through a posterior sagittal incision, the consequences of which are frequently urological injury and major morbidity. When the study shows a prostatic fistula, the surgeon knows to look for the rectum in the soft tissue 1–2 cm deep to the coccyx during the posterior sagittal approach or just below the peritoneal reflection at laparoscopy. The presence of a bulbar urethral fistula indicates that the rectum will easily be found just deep to the levator muscles within 3–4 cm of the perineal skin. In the case of an imperforate anus with no fistula, the surgeon will not need to spend time looking for the fistula site and knows that the distal rectum is located adjacent to the bulbar urethra. For cloacas, the study allows the surgeon to estimate the length of the common channel, predict the need for a vaginal replacement, and determine whether proper reconstruction can be performed through a perineal incision alone or require a combined abdominal-perineal approach.

Posterior Sagittal Anorectoplasty

Males

Patients with a recto-urethral fistula can be repaired using the posterior sagittal approach. It is mandatory that a Foley catheter be placed prior to commencing the operation. The patient is placed in the prone position with the pelvis elevated. The incision is made in the midline from above the coccyx to below the anal dimple. A fine needle-tip cautery is used for the entire dissection and an electrical stimulator is used to determine the location of the sphincter. One must stay exactly in the midline, leaving an equal amount of muscle on each side of the incision. The incision is continued until the posterior wall of the rectum is located. The rectum is opened in the

midline and traction sutures are placed on both sides. The incision in the rectal wall is continued distally up to the fistula site. The rectum is then separated from the urinary tract. This step is the most delicate part of the operation because injury to the urinary tract can easily occur. The anterior wall of the rectum and the posterior wall of the urinary tract are intimately attached and there is no obvious plane of separation. It is important to remember that the more inferior the rectum extends, the longer is this common wall. We place multiple 6-0 silk mucosal stitches in a semicircle just above the fistula to allow uniform traction on the rectum. The mucosa is incised between the silk stitches and the fistula. A submucosal dissection is performed for about 2 cm above the fistula until a more obvious plane of separation is reached. The fistula is then closed on the urinary tract side with fine long-term absorbable sutures. One should not attempt to open the urethra or see the Foley catheter. Likewise, maneuvers such as circumferential dissection around the rectum with a right-angled clamp should be avoided because the clamp may go around both the rectum and the urethra, resulting in urethral injury or even complete division of the urethra.

The dissection should be performed as close to the rectal wall as possible without injuring it. The rectum has a characteristic pale white fascia that defines the plane of dissection. All of the extrinsic vessels of the rectum are divided and cauterized. Keeping the rectal wall intact will ensure that the intramural blood supply of the distal rectum is preserved. The dissection continues until enough rectal length has been gained that an anastomosis between the rectum and the skin of the perineum can be created without tension. The electrical stimulator is used to determine the location of the sphincter mechanism, the anterior and posterior limits of which are marked on both sides with silk sutures. The anterior portion of the incision is closed, and the rectum is placed within the sphincter (Fig. 64.10). The rectum may occasionally be very dilated, in which case the posterior wall should be excised and the rectum tapered in order to allow it to fit more easily within the sphincter mechanism. The posterior edges of the levators are reapproximated behind the rectum. The posterior aspect of the muscle complex is also sutured together in the midline, which should include a portion of the posterior rectal wall in order to anchor the rectum. Finally, the anoplasty is performed by creating an anastomosis between the rectum and skin with interrupted long-term absorbable sutures.

Ten percent of male patients with an anorectal malformation have a bladder neck fistula. These patients have a rather poor functional prognosis and a high incidence of associated defects. This is also the only group of patients who must have a combined abdominal-perineal approach. At the time of the main repair, the colostomy is packed to avoid contamination and a total body prep from the costal margins inferiorly is performed. This allows the entire lower half of the child to be in the field and provides access to both the

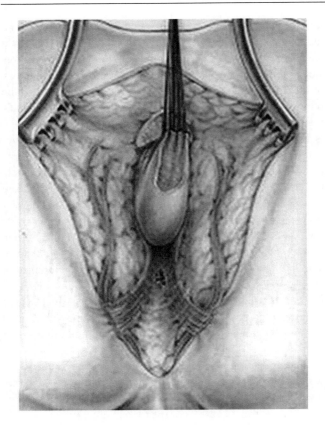

Fig. 64.10 A typical view during posterior sagittal anorectoplasty. The limits of the sphincter mechanism should be assessed both visually and by direct electrical stimulation. Note that the incision is placed exactly in the midline with the same amount of muscle left on each side. (From Pena A. Atlas of surgical management of anorectal malformations. New York: Springer; 1989. Reprinted with kind permission from Springer Science + Business Media)

perineum and abdomen. The operation begins with a laparoscopic approach, in which the distal rectum is dissected and the fistula is ligated. Further dissection is then performed to allow for the rectum to comfortably reach the perineum. This is a technically challenging step. The dissection is performed as close as possible to the rectal wall to avoid injury to nerves, reproductive structures and the ureters. If getting the distal rectum to reach is difficult because the colostomy has been placed too distal in the sigmoid, it may be necessary to take down the mucous fistula. If the distal rectum is excessively dilated and needs to be tapered, this might require conversion to laparotomy. It may also be necessary to ligate one or more branches of the inferior mesenteric vessels in order to allow complete mobilization of the rectum. Careful inspection of the vasculature is necessary to determine which vessels can be divided while still preserving the blood supply to the rectum (Fig. 64.11). Because the arcades might have been disrupted by the colostomy, one must be careful to ligate these branches close to the rectal wall, relying on its excellent intramural blood supply. Once adequate length has been achieved, the rectum is ready to be pulled through.

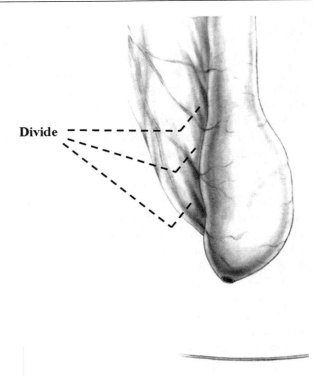

Fig. 64.11 Rectal vessel ligation to gain length when mobilizing the rectum from within the abdomen. The vessels should be divided close to the rectal wall, relying on the rich intramural blood supply of the rectum

The posterior sagittal incision is then made to create a path that goes from the presacral space down to the anal dimple. This can be done with the child in the lithotomy position. The anoplasty is then performed and the small posterior sagittal incision closed.

Females

Perineal fistulae in females are repaired as described in male patients. Vestibular fistulae are repaired using a limited posterior sagittal incision. All pediatric surgeons should become adept at this repair because this malformation is the most common defect seen in girls. When properly treated, these patients should have excellent bowel control. Technical errors and complications should be considered unacceptable as they can significantly impact functional prognosis.

With the patient in prone position, a posterior sagittal incision is made, dividing the sphincter mechanism exactly in the midline. Multiple 6-0 silk stitches are placed circumferentially in the external orifice of the fistula, as uniform traction on the rectum facilitates the creation of a dissection plane. The posterior rectal wall is identified by its characteristic whitish fascia and the dissection is continued between this fascia and the rectal wall, staying as close as possible to the rectal wall. The dissection progresses laterally on both sides, always staying in the same plane. The dissection must continue in a circumferential manner in order to finally approach the most delicate part of the operation, the separation of the distal rectum from the vagina. These two structures have a very thin common wall with no true plane of separation. A submucosal plane on the rectal side must be developed for the first 2 cm or so, until eventually a full-thickness plane can be developed. Separation of the two structures becomes relatively easy at this point and an areolar plane of separation is identified. Once the rectum has been separated from the vagina, a circumferential dissection is performed to gain enough length to allow the creation of an anastomosis of the rectum to the skin without tension. If defects were made in the posterior vagina or anterior rectum during the dissection, the rectum is mobilized further until it can be positioned such that the two suture lines are not adjacent to each other, a situation that can result in formation of a recto-vaginal fistula. The perineal body is reconstructed using interrupted long-term absorbable sutures, bringing together the anterior limits of the sphincter, and the rectum is placed within the limits of the sphincter. The levator muscle and the posterior edge of the muscle complex are sutured together in the midline, along with the posterior wall of the rectum. The wound is closed and the anoplasty is performed as previously described.

In the uncommon circumstance of a true recto-vaginal fistula, the technique used is essentially the same, except that the degree of exposure and dissection of the rectum is greater than for a vestibular fistula.

Posterior Sagittal Anorectovaginourethroplasty (PSARVUP) for the Repair of Cloacas

Cloacal malformations represent a wide spectrum of defects, the surgical repair of which represents one of the most significant technical challenges in pediatric surgery. Cloacas with a common channel shorter than 3 cm are generally straightforward and most of these can be safely repaired by general pediatric surgeons who have had adequate training in this procedure. At the other end of the spectrum are complex malformations with a long common channel, the repair of which can often be exceptionally challenging.

Vaginoscopy and cystoscopy are performed as a separate procedure after the newborn period. With the scope positioned at the urethral orifice, the length of the common channel, also known as the *urogenital sinus*, is measured from the tip of the endoscope to the perineal skin. When the common channel is shorter than 3.0 cm, it should be possible to repair the entire malformation at the perineum, without having to open the abdomen. If the common channel is longer than

3.0 cm, it is better to prepare the patient with a total body prep in order to be able to turn the patient and open the abdomen if necessary. In our experience, laparotomy is required in approximately 25% of cases.

The operation starts with a posterior sagittal incision, dividing the entire sphincter mechanism in the midline. The incision is continued anteriorly until the surgeon reaches the single perineal orifice. The common channel is then opened in the midline, which usually results in excellent visualization of the anatomy. Total urogenital mobilization can be done in the majority of cases and avoids the need to separate the vagina from the urethra, which formerly represented the most difficult portion of this operation and led to frequent complications such as urethro-vaginal fistulas, vaginal strictures and acquired vaginal atresia. About 50% of cloacas have a common channel shorter than 3.0 cm and will be amenable to repair using this approach alone. The rectum needs to be dissected off of the posterior aspect of the vagina as previous described. The vagina and urethra are then mobilized and advanced down to the perineum as a single unit, usually providing about 2–3 cm of length. The urethral orifice is sutured immediately behind the clitoris so as to create a normal anatomic arrangement. The vaginal edges are sutured to the introitus resulting in a remarkably normal appearance. If the patient has two hemivaginas, the vaginal septum should be excised. The perineal body is reconstructed with interrupted long-term absorbable sutures and the rectal component of the malformation is repaired as previously described.

When dealing with a longer common channel, total urogenital mobilization is still utilized but additional length is frequently needed. The decision-making process for these cases is complex and requires a great deal of experience in the management of these malformations. The urogenital complex can be mobilized further via laparotomy. If the length is still not adequate, then the urinary tract and vagina must be separated, which is the most difficult part of the operation. This must be done with extreme caution because both ureters usually run within the common wall that separates the vagina from the urinary tract. Prior to separating the vagina and bladder, we recommend opening the bladder and passing a catheter into each ureter to allow their identification and prevent injury.

It is important also to study the characteristics of the vagina. In the event of a small or high vagina, it is necessary to replace the vagina. We prefer to use the colon but small bowel is a reasonable alternative if colon is not available. If the patient has a very long or very dilated rectal segment, one can create a neovagina by dividing the rectum transversely or longitudinally. For very long common channels, the anterior urethral dissection can sometimes be avoided by using the common channel to replace the urethra while the vagina is pulled through separately or replaced. On the other hand, if the patient has two large hemivaginas that are located up in

Fig. 64.12 Vaginal switch operation, a good option for girls with cloaca, a long common channel and a double vagina. The right hemi-uterus has been removed, preserving the ovary. The two hemivaginas have been separated and the right hemivagina is inverted to create a single long vaginal tube. Note that the left hemivagina is not detached from the urinary tract so as to preserve its blood supply. (From Peña A, Levitt MA, Hong AR, Midulla P. Surgical management of cloacal malformations: a review of 339 patients. J Ped Surg. 2004; 19(3):470–279. Reprinted with permission from Elsevier)

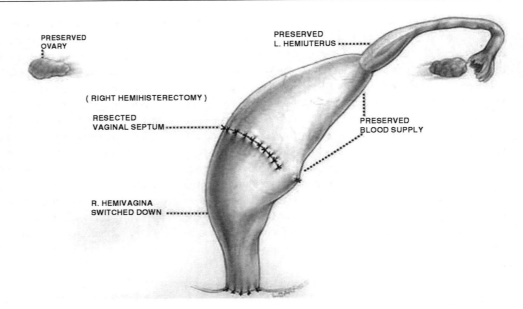

PRESERVED OVARY

PRESERVED L. HEMIUTERUS

(RIGHT HEMIHISTERECTOMY)

RESECTED VAGINAL SEPTUM

PRESERVED BLOOD SUPPLY

R. HEMIVAGINA SWITCHED DOWN

the pelvis, a vaginal switch maneuver can be used (Fig. 64.12). This involves the complete separation of one hemi-vagina from the urinary tract and mobilizing the other side only partially in order to preserve its blood supply. The hemi-uterus is resected from the mobilized vagina while preserving the ovary, the vaginal septum is resected, and the hemi-vaginas are placed end-to-end to create a single unit. The previous dome of the right hemivagina is brought down to the perineum. This maneuver may allow the creation of a single vagina without the use of bowel.

If a laparotomy is needed during the main repair or at the time of colostomy closure, the Müllerian structures must be inspected so that problems related to menses and obstetrics can be anticipated and treated. In patients with the more complex malformations described above, a suprapubic cystostomy tube is inserted and a urethral catheter left in place for 2–3 weeks. If the patient has severe vesico-ureteral reflux, a vesicostomy is sometimes required.

Postoperative Care

Complications after colostomy should be avoided and a properly performed procedure is the first step in accomplishing this goal. Once the colostomy is working, the child is allowed to feed. A stoma therapist should teach the parents how to take care of the colostomy site. The mucous fistula is usually left exposed. Prolapse occurs when the colostomy is opened in a mobile part of the colon and can usually be avoided by fixing the mobile segment to the anterior abdominal wall.

Recovery after a PSARP is usually rapid and generally straightforward. The children seem to have surprisingly little pain. Patients with a colostomy can eat the same day of

surgery. When the operation is performed in an infant who is still passing meconium, we withhold feeds for a minimum of 5 days after surgery. In babies who are already passing stool, we withhold oral nutrition for 7–10 days after surgery, during which time they are maintained on parenteral nutrition. Broad-spectrum intravenous antibiotics are continued for 48 h. The patient is discharged with the Foley catheter in place. For males, the Foley catheter can usually come out 7 days after surgery. Neurogenic bladder and urinary retention in male patients should not occur and are almost uniformly due to surgical technique. Patients with recto-bladder neck fistula may benefit from a suprapubic tube as neurogenic bladder related to associated spinal anomalies is common. If the Foley catheter is accidentally removed before the recommended time, it need not be replaced since the majority of patients will be able to void and the potential for urethral injury during recatheterization is significant.

Two weeks after surgery, the anus is calibrated in the clinic with Hegar cervical dilators. This should cause very little discomfort for the infant. The parents are then taught how to dilate the anus. The well-lubricated dilator is gently passed through the anus into the rectum, and held in place for 30 s. The dilator is removed and then passed again. The anus must be dilated twice per day. Every week the size is increased until the appropriate size for the patient's age is reached: #12 for a newborn of normal size, #15 for a 1 year old, #16 for a preschooler and #17 for older patients. The dilation process must not be interrupted, for there is a high likelihood that a stricture will develop. Once the desired size is reached, the frequency of dilations is tapered to once daily for a month, then every other day for 1 month, twice per week for 1 month, and finally once a week for 1 more month. The colostomy can be closed anytime after the desired size has been reached.

A primary anastomosis of the two stoma ends is performed when the anal dilatations have reached the desired size. After the colostomy is closed, patients often initially have very frequent bowel movements that produce a severe perianal rash. It may take some time for this to heal. A variety of creams and ointments are available that attempt to create a barrier, usually with variable success. The best treatment for the severe diaper rash is to avoid prolonged contact between stool and the skin. We instruct parents to wash the perineum with mild soap and water every time stool appears. Soon the number of bowel movements will decrease and the patients typically develop constipation. Parents should be forewarned of this change so that they are ready to treat it.

Constipation is the most common problem seen in patients with anorectal malformations. It is more severe in the benign group of malformations. The more complex malformations have a poorer prognosis in terms of bowel control, but a lower incidence of constipation. It is extremely important that constipation be treated aggressively. Complications from prolonged constipation include soiling, overflow pseudoincontinence and megarectum. Megarectum, in turn, provokes more constipation, which worsens the megarectum, creating a vicious cycle. In order to avoid this, the child should empty the rectum every day, which is best achieved with a high-fiber diet and laxatives as needed.

When properly treated, 75% of all patients with anorectal malformations will have voluntary bowel movements by the age of 3 years. However, about half still soil their underwear intermittently. This is usually due to constipation. If the soiling does not improve by the age of potty training, a bowel management and enema program should be initiated.

Surgeons who operate on patients with anorectal malformations are morally obligated to follow and care for them after their operation and to ensure that they are clean and dry. In our experience, 25% of all patients with anorectal malformations suffer from fecal incontinence. However, these patients should be able to remain clean and completely free of "accidents" without having to wear diapers. An aggressive bowel management program that includes the use of enemas allows them to achieve this goal. However, the program is much more involved than just administering an enema every day and needs to be tailored to the individual patient. For example, the volume and concentration of the enemas need to be adjusted until the colon remains clean for the entire day. Prior to initiating the program, a contrast enema will demonstrate the anatomy of the colon and allow us to estimate the ideal enema volume. Parents are taught how to give the enema without causing significant discomfort for the child and a daily abdominal X-ray is taken to evaluate the results of the previous day's enema. Changes are made in concentration and volume until the colon is clean.

A difficult concept for most surgeons to understand is that patients can be fecally incontinent and yet still have a tendency towards constipation. These patients typically still have their entire colon but have a megarectum. Most of these patients require a large volume (500–1,000 mL) saline enema. Constipation is actually somewhat helpful as the colon remains quiet (and the patient remains clean) between enemas. Other patients may have lost their distal colon, usually due to a technical mishap during the operative repair. These patients are more difficult to successfully manage, because they have a fast moving colon without the distal reservoir function normally provided by the rectum. For these patients, medications are used to slow the colon to help make the stool more solid, foods that have a laxative effect are avoided, and small volume (250–400 mL) enemas are given.

Once it is demonstrated that the bowel management has been successful, patients with severe constipation can be offered a Malone procedure, also known as a continent appendicostomy or antegrade continent enema (ACE) procedure (Fig. 64.13). An appendicostomy is created, preferably within the umbilicus. This allows the enemas to be given in an antegrade fashion. The cecum is plicated around the base of the appendix to create a valve that prevents stool from leaking back through the umbilicus. This operation is usually recommended when the patient wants to become more independent, as it allows the administration of the enema without parental assistance. The Malone procedure is essentially just another way to administer an enema; therefore it should only be performed in patients for whom bowel management has been successful. If the enema does not work through the rectum, it probably will not work through an appendicostomy.

With the exception of an occasional patient with myelomeningocele, a severe sacral abnormality or tethered cord, boys with imperforate anus nearly always have good urinary control. In the absence of a predisposing condition, we believe that most cases of urinary incontinence in male patients are due to injury during the peri-bladderneck dissection. This is also true of girls, with the exception of those with cloaca. Although the vast majority of patients with a common channel shorter than 3 cm have normal urinary control, approximately 20% may require intermittent catheterization for a flaccid bladder. With a common channel longer than 3 cm, approximately 80% will have difficulty with urinary continence requiring intermittent catheterization or some form of continent diversion.

The management of patients with anorectal malformations is complex and requires an understanding of the multiple problems that these children can have. Although it is extremely important for the surgeon to be able perform the operations without causing injury, technical mastery alone is clearly not sufficient. It is essential that the surgeon be able to manage the significant post-operative functional sequelae that many of these patients have and recognize that these are patients for life.

Fig. 64.13 Malone procedure. An appendicostomy is created at the umbilicus to allow the patient to receive an antegrade enema. The cecum is imbricated around the base of the appendix to create a valve (inserts), which prevents escape of gas or liquid through the appendix. (From Levitt MA, et al. Continent appendicostomy in bowel management. J Ped Surg 1997; 32(11)1630–3. Reprinted with permission from Elsevier)

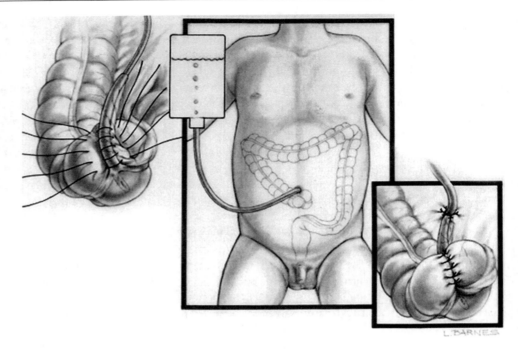

Summary Points

- Infants with a perineal fistula can usually be safely primarily repaired in the immediate newborn period without a colostomy.
- A decision regarding colostomy or primary repair should ideally be made within the first 48 h of life.
- Depending on the expertise and comfort level of the surgeon, many girls with a vestibular fistula (within the introitus but outside the hymen) can be repaired primarily in the immediate newborn period.
- Infants without a fistula or with a fistula to the urinary tract are best treated initially with a diverting colostomy and delayed repair.
- All infants with imperforate anus should undergo a comprehensive workup for associated anomalies: passage of a nasogastric tube, renal ultrasound, echocardiogram, spinal ultrasound and plain radiographs of the axial skeleton and forearms.
- Repair of cloacal anomalies can be exceptionally challenging and requires experience, meticulous planning and precise surgical technique.
- Girls with cloaca frequently have gynecologic anomalies that can result in hydrocolpos in the newborn period and obstetrical issues in the long term.
- Nearly every patient with imperforate anus will have some degree of constipation, which needs to be addressed aggressively and proactively.
- In the absence of a spinal anomaly or surgical misadventure, the majority of patients with imperforate anus should expect to have adequate fecal continence.
- Regardless of the nature of the anomaly or the adequacy of repair, keeping the child clean, without soiling or odor, is of paramount importance.
- Patients with anorectal anomalies should be considered patients for life.

Editor's Comment

Imperforate anus is one of the more common congenital anomalies requiring surgical correction and pediatric surgeons should be well versed in the correction of its more common varieties. One of these is the perineal fistula in girls, commonly referred to as the "anterior displaced anus." Some controversy exists over the best way to correct these seemingly benign lesions. Regardless of the technique used, the functional result is the same: moderate to severe constipation.

In the past, the fistula was often simply dilated, which allows meconium to pass; however patients were incontinent and needed extraneous methods to evacuate. Similarly, for a time it was popular to use the "cutback anoplasty," in which the fistula is opened in the midline posteriorly to the center of the anal sphincter and the rectal mucosa is anastomosed to the perianal skin. The result is a keyhole-shaped anal opening that is only partially surrounded by sphincter musculature. A better anatomic and functional result is achieved when the rectum is brought up through the anal sphincter with either a "mini-Peña" procedure or anal transposition.

Girls with cloaca are treated in many children's centers by a team of surgeons that includes a pediatric surgeon, a pediatric urologist, and sometimes an expert in pediatric gynecologic anomalies. Pediatric urologic consultation can also be useful when searching for a high rectum in boys, who are at risk for injury to the urethra, bladder neck, seminal vesicles and vasa deferentia during the very difficult and tedious dissection that is often required in these cases. One can also be lulled into a false sense of security by the rare male infant with an apparent perineal fistula, usually associated with a low lesion and straightforward repair, but who instead has a rectum that ends at the level of the prostate and a long, narrow fistula that opens on the perineum. These infants often need to have a laparotomy for proper mobilization of the rectum.

In boys with no apparent fistula, it might be difficult to see evidence of urethral passage of meconium as it is diluted by urine and soaks into the diaper. It is useful in these cases to place a gauze pad over the penis within the diaper. The urine passes through the gauze while the meconium is trapped in the interstices of the cotton mesh.

Finally, although it is certainly better to make a decision regarding repair or colostomy within 48 h, there are rare situations in which an infant with a severe cardiac anomaly and no apparent fistula is felt to be too unstable even for a bedside colostomy or is thought to be unlikely to survive for long with or without cardiac reconstruction. With adequate gastric decompression, these children can sometimes be maintained for a surprising length of time and, in very rare cases, will begin to pass meconium through the perineal dimple a few weeks after birth, at which point they may be amenable to dilation.

Differential Diagnosis

- Rectal atresia
- Anal stenosis
- Intersex anomalies

Diagnostic Studies

- Physical examination
- Cross-table lateral radiograph of the abdomen and pelvis, to measure gap between rectum and perineal skin
- AP radiograph of the sacrum, to calculate sacral ratio
- Plain radiograph of the spine, to rule out vertebral anomalies
- Plain radiograph of the forearms, to rule out radial limb anomalies
- Abdominal ultrasound, to rule out renal anomalies
- Echocardiogram, to rule out cardiac defects
- Spinal ultrasound, to rule out tethered cord
- Vaginoscopy, to measure common channel in patients with cloaca
- Distal colostogram

Parental Preparation

- Colostomy is unavoidable in some cases.
- After definitive repair, twice daily anal dilatations done by the parents at home are essential to achieve a good result.
- Nearly all patients will have some degree of constipation after repair.
- Some patients will have incontinence of feces, which is sometimes due to inadequately treated constipation.
- Patients with imperforate anus are patients for life.

Preoperative Preparation

- ☐ Nasogastric tube decompression
- ☐ Intravenous antibiotics
- ☐ Medical imaging to rule out associated anomalies
- ☐ Serial physical examination

Technical Points

- The colostomy should be completely diverting (not a loop) and created from the proximal sigmoid colon (to maintain adequate length for the pull-through and to avoid prolapse) while the mucous fistula should be small, separated from the stoma and adequate for proper performance of a distal colostogram.
- During a PSARP, it is important to keep the incision exactly in the midline.
- The plane of dissection should be close to the rectal wall, relying on the intramural blood supply of the rectum.
- An electrical stimulator is used to define the precise limits of the anal sphincter mechanism.
- Placement of a Foley catheter is mandatory for safe repair of anorectal anomalies in boys.
- Multiple fine silk stay sutures are useful to apply even circumferential tension on the rectum during dissection, especially near the vagina or urinary tract.
- A very dilated rectum should be trimmed posteriorly and tapered so as to fit adequately within the anal sphincter mechanism.
- Precise technique should be used when dissecting near the urinary tract or vagina to avoid injuries that can result in urinary or fecal incontinence or sexual dysfunction.
- Cloacas with a common channel shorter than 3 cm can usually be repaired by urogenital mobilization through a perineal approach.
- Cloacas with a common channel longer than 3 cm usually require a combined abdomino-perineal approach.

Suggested Reading

Levitt MA, Pena A. Management in the anorectal newborn period. In: Holschneider AM, Hutson J, editors. Malformations in children. Berlin: Springer; 2006.

Levitt MA, Soffer SZ, Peña A. Continent appendicostomy in the bowel management of fecal incontinent children. J Pediatr Surg. 1997;32(11):1630–3.

Levitt MA, Stein DM, Peña A. Gynecological concerns in the treatment of teenagers with cloaca. J Pediatr Surg. 1998;33(2):188–93.

Levitt, M, Falcone R, Pena, A. Pediatric fecal incontinence. In: Fecal incontinence: diagnosis and treatment. Milan: Springer; 2007. p. 341–50, Chapter 36.

Levitt MA, Peña A: Imperforate anus and cloacal malformations. In: Ashcraft KW, Holcomb GW, Murphy JP, editors. Pediatric surgery. 4th ed. Philadelphia: Saunders; 2010, p. 468–490

Pena A. Anorectal malformations. Semin Pediatr Surg. 1995;41(1):35–47.

Peña A. Atlas of surgical management of anorectal malformations. New York: Springer; 1989. p. 25–47.

Peña A. Total urogenital mobilization – an easier way to repair cloacas. J Pediatr Surg. 1997;32(2):263–8.

Peña A, Guardino K, Tovilla JM, Levitt MA, Rodriguez G, Torres R. Bowel management for fecal incontinence in patients with anorectal malformations. J Pediatr Surg. 1998;33(1):133–7.

Peña A, Levitt MA, Hong AR, Midulla P. Surgical management of cloacal malformations: a review of 339 patients. J Pediatr Surg. 2004;39(3):470–9.

Chapter 65
Gastroschisis

Aimen F. Shaaban

The term gastroschisis ("belly cleft") was coined in 1894 by Italian pathologist Cesare Taruffi, who used it in "Storia della Teratologia" to define a variety of congenital malformations in which the abdomen remains open at birth, though the condition had been reported sporadically since 1557. In 1887, William P. Hogue of West Virginia reported the first successful repair by reduction of the viscera and application of plaster strips. The child survived and appeared to have spontaneous closure of the defect by 5 weeks of age. This case provides the first evidence of the hardiness of the infant with gastroschisis, an observation that has been reinforced in the medical literature ever since.

Postulated etiologies of gastroschisis include: (1) failure of the differentiation of the embryonic mesenchyme due to exposure to a teratogen during the fourth week of gestation; (2) rupture of the amnionic membrane at the umbilical cord base during the time of physiologic herniation in the sixth week of gestation; (3) an abnormal involution of the right umbilical vein leading to reduced viability of the surrounding mesenchyme and a defect in the abdominal wall to the right of the umbilicus; (4) disruption of the omphalomesenteric artery leading to necrosis at the base of the cord with subsequent gut herniation; and (5) a failure of development of one or more folds responsible for abdominal wall closure. Unfortunately, none of these overlapping theories completes our understanding of this disease. Furthermore, scientific support for any hypothesis suffers greatly from the lack of a relevant animal model.

Despite disagreement regarding the pathogenesis of gastroschisis, a number of risk factors have been identified. Because large international databases report that only 1.2% of infants with gastroschisis have a chromosomal abnormality, a greater effort has been applied to the study of epigenetic factors. Various independent risk factors include, in order of decreasing certainty: young maternal age, maternal use of salicylates like aspirin, maternal genitourinary infection just before or during the first trimester, maternal cigarette smoking, and maternal alcohol and illicit drug use. The reported incidence of gastroschisis is 1 in 2,000–3,000 live births. A rising incidence of this anomaly is documented in the medical literature of every decade since the 1940s. The incidence of associated anomalies remains relatively stable at 10%, including mostly gastrointestinal and cardiac anomalies. Therefore, gastroschisis represents a majority of the congenital gastrointestinal anomalies encountered in fetal and newborn healthcare. Given the potential for the development of significant morbidity, specialty-trained pediatric surgeons should be fluent in both the prenatal counseling and the postnatal management of this disease.

Diagnosis

Most cases of gastroschisis are suspected by abnormal maternal serology and reliably confirmed by fetal ultrasound. Since several reports document a survival advantage for fetuses born in a center where both neonatal and surgical care can be provided, the utility of maternal screening in improving outcomes cannot be overstated. Ultrasound diagnosis in the late first trimester is possible as physiologic return of the intestines to the peritoneal cavity is normally complete by 11 weeks. The identifying sonographic features of gastroschisis are the findings of multiple loops of bowel floating freely in the amniotic fluid. Herniated bowel is typically seen to the right of the umbilical cord insertion. Gastroschisis is differentiated sonographically from an omphalocele by the lack of a membranous covering of the bowel and the strong association of omphalocele with cardiovascular and genitourinary anomalies. The associated anomaly rate for gastroschisis ranges from 10 to 15% and includes other GI anomalies, central nervous system, cardiovascular, musculoskeletal, and genitourinary anomalies. Although the incidence of cardiac anomalies associated with gastroschisis appears to be increasing, the limited severity of the identified disease brings to question the benefit of detailed

A.F. Shaaban (✉)
Department of Surgery, University of Iowa Carver College of Medicine, University of Iowa Hospitals and Clinics, 1500 JCP, 200 Hawkins Dr, Iowa City, IA 52242, USA
e-mail: aimen-shaaban@uiowa.edu

P. Mattei (ed.), *Fundamentals of Pediatric Surgery*,
DOI 10.1007/978-1-4419-6643-8_65, © Springer Science+Business Media, LLC 2011

prenatal diagnosis. Overall, most tertiary centers do not perform routine prenatal echocardiography in cases of gastroschisis. Because of the low incidence of chromosomal anomalies, the risks of amniocentesis are unwarranted in cases of isolated gastroschisis.

Significant and potentially irreversible injury of the herniated bowel resulting from exposure to the amniotic fluid or contracture of the umbilical ring is also characteristic of gastroschisis. Indeed the progression of injury can be tracked with serial ultrasound. Risk stratification of bowel injury in affected fetuses has been proposed based upon the ultrasound characteristics. Sonographic parameters include matting and dilatation of the bowel, loss of peristaltic activity, changes in bowel wall echogenicity, alterations in mesenteric blood flow, and changes in stomach position. Despite the ominous appearance of the anatomy, none of these parameters appear to correlate with postnatal outcomes. Furthermore, prospective studies of planned early delivery or amniotic fluid exchange have not been shown to be helpful. Nonetheless, some of these infants experience severe bowel injury during the third trimester that results in much of the long-term morbidity associated with this disease. It is hoped that future research will more accurately identify these factors so that treatment may be optimized.

The characteristic gross appearance of gastroschisis involves a defect to the right of the umbilicus that has smooth edges and is usually less than 4 cm in diameter. The defect is frequently separated from the base of the umbilical cord by a small bridge of skin (Fig. 65.1). The intestines are usually thickened and matted with no overlying membrane. A few anatomic variants have been described. The most notable of these is that of "closed" or "vanishing" gastroschisis, in which it is presumed that the umbilical defect closed antenatally, resulting in ischemic injury and necrosis of the bowel. Prenatal ultrasound

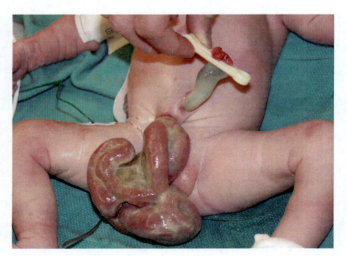

Fig. 65.1 Gross appearance of gastroschisis. Note herniation to the right of the umbilicus and lack of membranous covering associated with edema of the bowel and an exudative peel

studies have documented the pathogenesis of this anatomic deformity. The outcome of these infants relates directly to the amount of remaining viable bowel. Characteristically, long hospitalizations and repeated operations are necessary in the surviving infants. Another variant is left-sided gastroschisis in which the defect is to the left of the umbilicus. Although only small cases series exist, the incidence of associated anomalies, frequency of complications, and overall survival does not appear to be significantly different when compared to right-sided gastroschisis.

Different approaches regarding both the timing and mode of delivery for fetuses with gastroschisis have been explored. In most studies, larger infants born closer to term seem to fare better overall while premature infants or those with evidence for intrauterine growth retardation have worse outcomes. Although a few infants with complicated gastroschisis might benefit from early delivery, parameters for selecting these patients have not been well-defined. Furthermore, Cesarean section has not been shown to improve outcomes. Therefore, following a critical review of the available literature, each center should develop guidelines for planning the timing and mode of delivery of these infants. These guidelines should maintain a bias toward term vaginal delivery for the vast majority of patients and permit alternative planning for a subset of patients who develop ominous findings during prenatal surveillance.

Treatment

The various closure techniques differ to the degree in which the skin and fascia are closed with sutures or assisted by the natural process of umbilical ring contracture. Some methods preserve varying lengths of the umbilical cord for either cosmetic or functional purposes. While one or two of these approaches may seem to have a broader application, recognition that umbilical contracture is a conserved process permits consideration for non-operative closure in select infants.

The initial focus for the pediatric surgeon called to participate in the delivery of the gastroschisis newborn is the resuscitation and optimal handling of the exposed viscera. Following delivery of the infant, the need for intubation and ventilation should be determined and quickly established. An 8 or 10 French orogastric decompression tube should be passed while IV access is obtained. The umbilical cord should be clamped 6 in. or so from its insertion to the abdomen. The entire torso, abdomen, and lower extremities of the newborn should be then placed in a sterile plastic bowel bag that is loosely secured around the chest just above the nipple line. This allows direct visualization of the bowel during transport. Bowel congestion can be easily identified and any kinking in the mesentery alleviated by repositioning. The liberal administration of intravenous normal saline including at least one 20 mL/kg bolus is beneficial in nearly all cases of gastroschisis. It is also routine to administer an initial dose of ampicillin and gentamicin shortly after arrival in the nursery.

The medical literature is replete with studies of varying quality and opposite conclusions comparing early and delayed (silo-assisted) or staged closure of gastroschisis. However, an average length of dependency on parenteral nutrition (average 14–21 days) and total hospital length of stay (30–50 days) for newborns with gastroschisis suggests that multiple variables affect these outcome measures to a greater degree than the timing of repair. At a tertiary center for neonatal care, a rate of major perinatal morbidity and mortality not exceeding 5% should be the targeted goal. Given that gastroschisis newborns exhibit a varying severity of bowel injury and co-morbidity, the application of a singular approach to all patients is probably too simplistic. Both early and delayed primary closure have their advantages and a familiarity with the nuances and pitfalls of either approach will best serve these infants.

Following resuscitation and warming of the infant, an assessment of the bowel and its potential for primary closure can be made. The short-term benefits of primary closure must be weighed against the risks of ventilatory compromise or bowel ischemia. Such risks are likely to be inappropriate in the more pre-term infants or those with markedly edematous bowel. These risks are amplified when infants arrive to the operating room hypothermic and dehydrated after an incomplete resuscitation for an aggressive attempt at primary closure. Additionally, after-hours repair of gastroschisis frequently places an unnecessary strain on limited anesthesia and ICU resources. Alternatively, if the abdominal defect is quite narrow or the status of the bowel and infant favorable, an attempt at primary repair following resuscitation and warming is sensible.

In practice, these situations are infrequent; therefore, it has been our practice to place the bowel in a preformed silo in the vast majority of cases of gastroschisis. This should be performed at an opportune time in the delivery room or, more commonly, shortly after arrival in the intensive care nursery.

Application and maintenance of a silo is easier in an overhead warming bed than in an isolette. The bowel bag should be removed and sterile towels used to drape the abdomen and the bedding. An assistant wearing sterile gloves is particularly useful during this process. The bowel should be closely inspected for signs of ischemia, volvulus, or venous congestion. Any concerns for bowel viability related to a small abdominal defect or inability to assess the bowel should prompt replacement of the bowel bag and expeditious transfer to the operating room for further evaluation. The availability of better lighting and a variety of essential instrumentation in the operating room might avoid a disaster. Next, the abdominal wall defect should be closely examined. Skin adhesions to

the mesentery or the exudative peel of the bowel should be divided. Minor bleeding is easily controlled with gentle pressure. The defect diameter is usually smaller than that of the edematous eviscerated contents and may cause venous congestion. An exceptionally narrow defect is best managed by incising the umbilical ring prior to placement of a silo or an attempt at primary repair. If an index finger passes easily into the peritoneal cavity through the defect adjacent to the mesenteric pedicle, it is unlikely venous congestion will be a problem.

The spring-loaded silo (Bentec Medical, CA) should be selected for the smallest diameter that comfortably accommodates the bowel contents. The most frequent size is a 5-cm silo. The silo is removed from the packaging in sterile fashion and opened completely. It is pre-moistened with a small amount of warm saline. With the help of an assistant, the bowel is passed into the silo, carefully sliding it along the entire length of the bowel prior to insertion of the ring into the peritoneal cavity. With the bowel completely in the silo, the ring is then pinched and the corner passed into the peritoneal cavity. With gentle persistence and patience using both hands, the spring-loaded ring can be fully deployed inside the peritoneal cavity. Care should be taken to avoid trapping the intra-abdominal viscera between the ring and the abdominal wall. Once the silo has been positioned, it can be stretched above the infant by tension on the suspension hole at the top of the bag (Fig. 65.2). The impression of the spring-loaded ring can be seen externally on the abdominal wall and its full deployment confirmed at this time. The bowel should be well-perfused and free of venous congestion. Some degree of narrowing normally occurs as the silo passes through the defect into the abdomen. Excessive bottlenecking should prompt widening of the umbilical ring. Any concerns regarding bowel trapping or incomplete ring expansion should be immediately addressed.

The silo is suspended from the overhead warmer by passing tracheostomy tape through the suspension hole and over the warming apparatus. A modest degree of tension on the silo helps to lift the abdominal wall and reduce the leakage of peritoneal fluid. A one inch strip of petrolatum gauze can be applied at the junction of the silo with the abdominal wall skin to provide a moist dressing. This is typically covered with two or three loose circumferential wraps of rolled gauze. The bowel should be visible above the gauze so the bedside nurse may provide a continual assessment of bowel perfusion, which should be reviewed frequently.

Ideally, discussions regarding the tempo and timing of serial reduction were addressed at prenatal counseling sessions with the family. If not, time spent counseling the family following silo placement is imperative. Three to five days of serial reduction are needed prior to silo removal and operative repair. The goal during the initial 24–48 h of silo suspension should be to minimize trauma to the bowel and allow natural reduction of edema by gravity with a minimum of stress to the

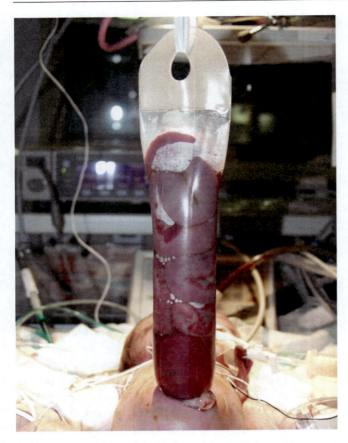

Fig. 65.2 Appropriate placement of silo. Bowel is placed in the smallest size silo that will accommodate it. Viable and well-perfused bowel visible within silo without much bottle-necking at level of defect

infant. Patients who were initially ventilated at the resuscitation can usually be extubated during this time. A PICC line may be attempted and total parental nutrition should be initiated. As the bowel becomes less edematous, it begins to settle in the base of the silo. Straw colored peritoneal fluid will accumulate alongside the bowel within the silo. Beginning on the second or third day, the bowel should be manually reduced within the silo toward the peritoneal cavity. A slow, deliberate reduction facilitates cooperation from the patient. Heavy analgesia is not particularly helpful as significant discomfort by the newborn should prompt release of tension. There is no advantage to a rapid reduction. Additionally, cases of bowel ischemia within the silo during aggressive reduction attempts have been reported. The reduction is maintained with an encircling umbilical tape applied around the silo above the level of the partially-reduced bowel. Initial efforts at reduction should be very gentle. As the bowel edema subsides, larger reduction steps may be taken. Once the bowel is reduced below the level of the umbilical ring, plans are made for definitive closure.

For repair in the operating room, a few basic preparation steps save both exposure time and unnecessary field contamination. An arterial catheter is essential for intra-operative monitoring, especially in cases of either complicated gastroschisis or anticipated tight reductions. Placement of a fresh orogastric catheter also ensures optimal decompression of the proximal gut. In anticipation of a tight reduction, anal dilatation and colonic irrigation for decompression of meconium is helpful prior to the preparation and draping of the operative field. This is best done with an assistant manipulating the bowel in a sterile manner. In most cases, simple anal dilatation with a dilator or examining finger is sufficient. The neck, chest, abdomen, and lower extremities to the knees are prepared with betadine solution. Chlorhexidine and solutions containing alcohol should never be used directly on the bowel as they are toxic at all concentrations. The silo can be held by one assistant while the area is prepared around the base of the silo and umbilical ring. A second assistant who is gowned and gloved can then hold the baby steady while the silo is removed from the abdomen and the field. Following draping of the patient, the bowel can be eviscerated. Thereafter, reducing the bowel into the abdomen is usually quite easy, and concerns regarding inability to replace the bowel are usually overstated. The exposure permits a close examination for associated anomalies. Additionally, major adhesions causing sharp kinks in the bowel can be identified and divided. This step seems sensible given that adhesive small bowel obstructions occur in up to one third of patients in the first year. Conversely, midgut volvulus is extremely rare and as such, a Ladd's procedure is not routinely added. If an atresia is encountered, the surgeon must decide whether to perform an enterostomy or simply defer repair of the atresia until a second operation 4–6 weeks later. A distal atresia is usually best managed with a diverting ileostomy while treatment of a proximal atresia is best deferred. Abdominal closure following repair of edematous atretic bowel frequently results in anastomotic leakage and is strongly discouraged. Prior to replacing the bowel within the abdomen, the foregut can be easily decompressed through the orogastric tube and the distal colon decompressed through the anus. The peritoneal cavity can be examined specifically noting the presence of a gallbladder, color and texture of the liver, and position of the spleen. With gentle pressure the bladder can be decompressed.

Once the bowel is replaced within the peritoneal cavity a limited effort to stretch the abdominal wall is usually helpful. This is best accomplished by inserting an index finger into the peritoneal cavity and pushing it against the abdominal wall with counter pressure applied by two fingers externally. With slow, steady, and migrating pressure, the abdominal wall can be noted to become more pliable in all directions due to reduction in edema and some degree of actual stretch. Next, skin and subcutaneous flaps should be circumferentially mobilized from the fascia for 2–3 cm from the edges of the umbilical ring. Great care should be taken to avoid injuring the rectus fascia. The umbilical vein should be divided between absorbable ligatures while the umbilical artery and the urachus are left undisturbed. The cord remnant should be left adherent to the fascia along the left hemi-circumference.

The fascia may be approximated by either a transverse or longitudinal closure. Using interrupted simple or Smead-Jones knots of long-term absorbable monofilament suture, the fascia edges are approximated without strangulating or tearing. Care is taken in the region of the umbilical vessels to avoid bleeding. Following placement, the sutures are then pulled up in unison to distribute the tension evenly and avoid bowel entrapment (Fig. 65.3). After securing the knots, inspect the closure can be for gaps, particularly adjacent to the umbilical cord remnant.

The skin is then approximated around the base of the cord remnant. The goal should be to provide coverage of the fascia while preserving all of the umbilical skin. The natural process of wound contracture and scar formation following auto-amputation of the cord remnant yields the most aesthetically pleasing appearance to the umbilicus and is easy to perform. The umbilical cord remnant is trimmed 1 cm from the skin edge. Using a 3-0 or 4-0 short-term monofilament absorbable suture, the umbilical skin is drawn around the base of the cord remnant in a purse-string fashion. The first pass should be through the fascia immediately to the right of the umbilical cord. The open end of the suture is clamped with a hemostat and a purse string is created through the edges of the surrounding umbilical skin. Periodic tensioning on the suture facilitates the progress of the closure and evenly distributes the tension on the skin edges. Following completion, the knot is secured beneath the level of the skin (Fig. 65.4a). Tiny gaps surrounding the cord remnant prevent serous collections from accumulating beneath the skin flaps. Eventually wound contracture will eliminate these gaps leaving a relatively normal-appearing umbilicus (Fig. 65.4b). The wound should be dressed with a dry gauze and non-occlusive tape. A single epidural application of local anesthetic helps to control pain.

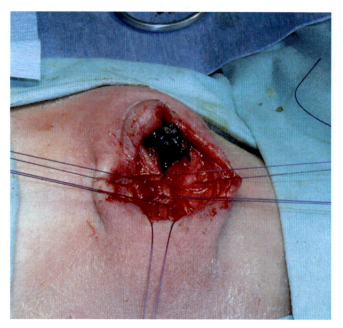

Fig. 65.3 Operative closure of defect. Skin and subcutaneous flaps have been mobilized 2 cm from the edges of the fascia. Interrupted knots of long-term absorbable mono-filament suture are used to close defect transversely while preserving cord remnant at left-lateral margin

Postoperative Care

Post-operatively, the surgeon must remain sensitive to the potentially serious complications that can result from high intra-abdominal pressures. Balanced fluid management preserves visceral perfusion and minimizes edema. Intra-abdominal pressure is monitored using the clinical parameters of abdominal exam, urine output, serum acid-base balance, ventilatory compliance, and lower extremity perfusion. The intra-abdominal pressure can also be directly measured by transduction of bladder or stomach. Pressures above 20 mmHg are excessive and

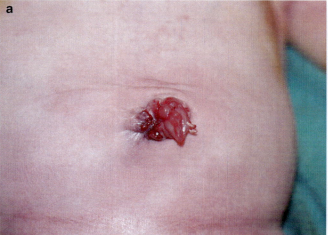
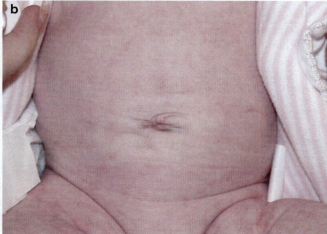

Fig. 65.4 Skin closure and long-term appearance of the umbilicus. Umbilical skin is drawn around cord remnant using purse-string of short-term absorbable monofilament suture. Wound contracture following auto-amputation of cord remnant provides aesthetically acceptable appearance of the umbilicus

should prompt opening of the abdominal wall closure and replacement of the silo at the bedside. The surgeon should be acutely attentive to this, especially in the first 24 h following closure.

Patients are usually extubated on the second or third post-operative day. Antibiotics are routinely continued for 3 days postoperatively. Although mild erythema typically develops in the region of the mobilized skin, concern for cellulitis usually wanes by the third or fourth day. Gastric decompression is maintained and parenteral nutrition is optimized until bowel function returns, usually between post-operative days 7 and 14. Suppositories are helpful around this time. Feedings are initiated with either elemental formula or breast milk with a slow initial advancement. In addition, awareness that occasional bilious emesis or aspirates are routinely observed without consequence in these patients minimizes the frequent stop-start cycles that frequently plague the management of infants with gastroschisis. Typically, full feedings are not achieved until 3 or 4 weeks post-operatively. We utilize anti-reflux medications in all patients and continue them for at least 6 months. Significant malabsorption or late onset necrotizing enterocolitis occurs in up to 10% of patients postoperatively. Line sepsis can be expected in up to one third of patients. Concerns for a missed atresia or adhesive bowel obstruction are best sorted out clinically or confirmed with radiologic contrast studies performed after the fourth or fifth postoperative week.

"Plastic" Sutureless Repair

An alternative approach has been described in which closure of the abdominal wall defect is obtained without placing a single suture. In this technique, the bowel can be reduced shortly after delivery or following silo reduction as the situation requires. An essential ingredient is preservation of a length of the umbilical cord needed to fill the defect after reduction of the bowel. Good communication with the obstetrical and neonatology teams is needed so that the cord will be clamped and cut at least six inches from its insertion. Heavy sedation and mechanical ventilation is required for early reduction and gentle anal dilatation and colonic irrigation are performed to evacuate meconium prior to reducing the bowel into the abdomen. Alternatively, silo reduction can be performed without ventilation or heavy sedation and the cord is preserved in a wrap of petrolatum gauze.

Once the bowel has been reduced, the umbilical cord is trimmed to a few inches and coiled to fill the abdominal wall defect. The skin surrounding the umbilical ring is protected with Skin Gel protective dressing wipe (Hollister Inc., Ill.). The umbilical cord and defect are then directly covered with two large occlusive dressings, which are removed on the third day and replaced with dry dressings. This allows the cord remnant to desiccate and the umbilical ring to contract leaving an approximately one centimeter area of granulation centrally. Feeding can be initiated when bowel function returns.

In a prospective study of 10 consecutive sutureless repairs, the average time to initiation of feeds (12.5 days) and total hospital length of stay (28.3 days) compared favorably with most series of either primary or silo-assisted closure. No patient experienced bowel ischemia or fistulization. Interestingly, two of the ten patients in the series underwent primary repair of an intestinal atresia prior to sutureless defect repair. Many of the infants have a small umbilical hernia, which closes spontaneously in the first few years. Although a larger experience is still being collected, sutureless repair appears to be safe and might have significant advantages over other techniques. Perhaps this is the ideal method for treatment of the occasional unstable pre-term gastroschisis patient with a tenuous ventilatory status.

Summary Points

- Most cases of gastroschisis are suspected by abnormal maternal serology and reliably diagnosed by fetal ultrasound.
- The identifying sonographic features of gastroschisis are the findings of multiple loops of bowel floating freely in the amniotic fluid without a membranous covering of the bowel.
- The associated anomaly rate for gastroschisis ranges from 10 to 15%.
- Term vaginal delivery is preferred for most patients as neither planned early delivery nor Cesarean section has been shown to improve outcomes of fetuses with gastroschisis.
- The initial focus for the pediatric surgeon called to participate in the delivery of the gastroschisis newborn is the resuscitation and optimal handling of the exposed viscera.
- Silo-assisted staged reduction is associated with fewer complications than early primary repair and should be employed in most cases of gastroschisis.
- Post-operatively, the surgeon must remain sensitive to the potential disasters that can result from high intra-abdominal pressures.
- Average time to full feedings is about 3 weeks.
- Line sepsis can occur in up to 1/3 of patients and necrotizing enterocolitis in up to 10%.

Editor's Comment

Over the past 10 years or so, three major advances have greatly improved the care of infants with gastroschisis: (1) the defect is now almost always detected antenatally, which allows for appropriate obstetrical and parental preparation; (2) the routine use of the preformed, spring-loaded silo has transformed the care of these infants from an obligatory emergency operation (nearly always in the middle of the night!) to a more relaxed, albeit still urgent, and straightforward bedside procedure; and (3) PICC lines have for the most part supplanted tunneled central venous catheters, which were associated with significantly more infectious and mechanical complications in these newborns who need intermediate- and long-term parenteral nutrition. I am confident that prospective studies will continue to show significant improvement in outcomes.

Infants with gastroschisis have a great deal of "third-space" and insensible fluid losses and therefore require large amounts of intravenous fluids, sometimes up to 80 mL/kg in the first 24 h. Unless tissue perfusion and urine output are monitored closely, there can be serious consequences if adequate replacement for fluid losses is not provided.

Silo placement requires experience, patience, and careful technique to avoid bleeding and bowel injury. If the defect is too small, the fascia (and sometimes skin) should be opened inferiorly in the midline. Fibrous bridges should be carefully lysed with electrocautery or ligated to avoid the bleeding that can result from traumatic disruption when the silo is being placed. At the time of fascial closure, it is important to avoid excessive intra-abdominal pressure and the risk of abdominal compartment syndrome. If it is too tight, it is best to apply a temporary dressing or another silo and delay the repair for a few days. Alternatively, a patch of artificial material can be used at the level of the fascia, but these almost invariably become infected and eventually need to be removed. The best intra-operative sign of excessive pressure is the peak inspiratory pressure needed to maintain adequate minute ventilation: a PIP of 25 or more is too high.

After reduction and fascial repair, return of bowel function can be very prolonged. It has always been assumed that this is due to the obvious injury sustained by the intestine, presumably caused by exposure to amniotic fluid, even though there is no correlation between the apparent degree of injury (induration, foreshortening, exudative peel) and the severity or duration of the bowel dysfunction. An alternative hypothesis posits that the bowel dysmotility is the primary lesion and is therefore the *cause* of the defect rather than the *result* (perhaps intestine that is poorly motile in early gestation cannot easily return to the abdominal cavity). Regardless, most infants with gastroschisis eventually respond to slowly advance feeds as tolerated until able to wean from parenteral nutrition, which can take many weeks or, in some cases, months. Infants with gastroschisis who do not tolerate full feeds by 4–6 weeks after fascial closure need to be evaluated for stricture. Contrast enema or upper GI contrast study might reveal a change in caliber of intestine due to an obstruction, but even in the absence of an obvious stricture on an imaging study, one should have a low threshold for empiric laparotomy, lysis of adhesions, and tapering or resection of dilated segments of bowel. Finally, retaining the umbilical stump almost always results in a better cosmetic result than a neo-umbilicus created with a purse-string suture or flap umbilicoplasty. On the other hand, it is never advisable to leave the child with no belly button as this causes anguish for children and their parents and has resulted in lawsuits.

Differential Diagnosis

- Omphalocele
- Gastroschisis
- Complicated gastroschisis

Diagnostic Studies

- Maternal serum alpha-fetoprotein level
- Level II prenatal ultrasound

Parental Preparation

- Prenatal counseling regarding challenges associated with bowel compromise and the possibility of associated anomalies is essential.
- Counseling should introduce options for treatment including early primary closure vs. staged silo-assisted reduction and repair.
- Discuss risks for short-term (bowel ischemia, necrotizing enterocolitis and line sepsis) and long-term complications (gastroesophageal reflux, gut dysmotility, adhesive small bowel obstruction and short bowel syndrome).

Preoperative Preparation

- □ Orogastric decompression.
- □ Fluid resuscitation and correction of hypothermia.
- □ Arterial catheter for intra-operative monitoring.
- □ Central venous catheter for post-operative nutrition.
- □ Anal dilatation and evacuation of meconium prior to repair.

Technical Points

- The spring-loaded silo should be selected for the smallest diameter that comfortably accommodates the herniated bowel contents.
- Once the silo has been positioned, it can be stretched above the infant by tension on the suspension hole at the top of the bag.
- Three to five days of serial reduction are needed prior to silo removal and operative repair.
- The goal of initial 24–48 h of silo suspension should be to minimize trauma to the bowel and allow natural reduction in edema.
- Beginning on the second or third day, the bowel may be manually reduced toward the peritoneal cavity with the silo in place.
- The reduction is maintained with an encircling umbilical tape applied around the silo above the level of the partially-reduced bowel.
- After the bowel is reduced below the level of the umbilical ring, plans may be made for closure.
- Once the bowel is replaced within the peritoneal cavity a limited effort to stretch the abdominal wall is usually helpful.
- The fascia may be approximated by either a transverse or longitudinal closure using interrupted simple or Smead-Jones knots of long-term absorbable mono-filament suture.
- The umbilical skin is drawn around the cord remnant using a monofilament purse-string suture.

Suggested Reading

Aina-Mumuney AJ, Fischer AC, Blakemore KJ, et al. A dilated fetal stomach predicts a complicated postnatal course in cases of prenatally diagnosed gastroschisis. Am J Obstet Gynecol. 2004;190: 1326–30.

Badillo AT, Hedrick HL, Wilson RD, et al. Prenatal ultrasonographic gastrointestinal abnormalities in fetuses with gastroschisis do not correlate with postnatal outcomes. J Pediatr Surg. 2008;43: 647–53.

Feldkamp ML, Carey JC, Sadler TW. Development of gastroschisis: review of hypotheses, a novel hypothesis, and implications for research. Am J Med Genet A. 2007;143:639–52.

Kidd Jr JN, Jackson RJ, Smith SD, Wagner CW. Evolution of staged versus primary closure of gastroschisis. Ann Surg. 2003;237:759–64. discussion 764–5.

Logghe HL, Mason GC, Thornton JG, Stringer MD. A randomized controlled trial of elective preterm delivery of fetuses with gastroschisis. J Pediatr Surg. 2005;40:1726–31.

Mastroiacovo P, Lisi A, Castilla EE, et al. Gastroschisis and associated defects: an international study. Am J Med Genet A. 2007;143: 660–71.

Midrio P, Stefanutti G, Mussap M, D'Antona D, Zolpi E, Gamba P. Amnioexchange for fetuses with gastroschisis: is it effective? J Pediatr Surg. 2007;42:777–82.

Pastor AC, Phillips JD, Fenton SJ, et al. Routine use of a SILASTIC spring-loaded silo for infants with gastroschisis: a multicenter randomized controlled trial. J Pediatr Surg. 2008;43:1807–12.

Salihu HM, Emusu D, Aliyu ZY, Pierre-Louis BJ, Druschel CM, Kirby RS. Mode of delivery and neonatal survival of infants with isolated gastroschisis. Obstet Gynecol. 2004;104:678–83.

Sandler A, Lawrence J, Meehan J, Phearman L, Soper R. A "plastic" sutureless abdominal wall closure in gastroschisis. J Pediatr Surg. 2004;39:738–41.

Vogler SA, Fenton SJ, Scaife ER, et al. Closed gastroschisis: total parenteral nutrition-free survival with aggressive attempts at bowel preservation and intestinal adaptation. J Pediatr Surg. 2008;43:1006–10.

Chapter 66
Omphalocele

Kenneth W. Liechty

Omphalocele is a common congenital abdominal wall defects. It consists of a central defect in the umbilical ring that allows herniation of the viscera into the umbilical cord, resulting in a membrane-covered defect. The mortality has been historically reported to exceed 25%, however this has been reduced by advances in prenatal diagnosis, pediatric anesthesia, mechanical ventilation, nutritional support, operative techniques, and neonatal intensive care units.

The etiology is thought to be a defect in body infolding between 3 and 4 weeks of gestation. During this period, the abdominal wall is formed by the infolding of cranial, caudal, and two lateral embryonic folds. If the deficit is primarily with the cranial fold, then the omphalocele is associated with other cranial fold defects, such as an anterior diaphragmatic hernia, cardiac anomalies, a pericardial defect, and a sternal cleft (the pentalogy of Cantrell). If the deficit is primarily with the caudal fold, then the omphalocele may be associated with bladder extrophy. The result of this error in infolding is a spectrum of defects ranging from umbilical hernias to giant omphaloceles.

The incidence is approximately 1 in 5,000 births. It is associated with advanced maternal age. In contrast to gastroschisis, patients with omphalocele have a high incidence of associated defects, ranging from 50 to 70% (Table 66.1), as well as a 30% incidence of chromosomal abnormalities. An associated syndrome is Beckwith-Wiedemann, which is marked by macroglossia, organomegaly, hypoglycemia, and an increased risk of malignancy, specifically Wilms tumor, hepatoblastoma, and neuroblastoma. Patients with omphalocele also have a high incidence of cardiac defects (50%). Interestingly, the smaller the omphalocele, the higher the incidence of chromosomal and cardiac anomalies. The survival of patients with omphalocele is generally dependent on the severity of the associated defects.

Diagnosis

The majority of omphaloceles are detected in the prenatal period, either by routine screening ultrasonography or as the result of obstetrical indications such as an elevated maternal serum alpha-fetoprotein (MSAFP). During the second trimester, MSAFP is elevated two-fold in about 80% of cases. This is less sensitive than for other abdominal wall defects, such as gastroschisis, where MSAFP is elevated two-fold in 99% of patients. This may be related to the omphalocele having a membrane covering the viscera, limiting the diffusion of fetal AFP.

On prenatal ultrasound, omphalocele appears as a central mass anterior to the abdominal wall fascia (Fig. 66.1). The mass consists of a sac or membrane containing bowel and potentially stomach and liver. The sac is comprised of an inner peritoneal layer and an outer amnion layer, with Wharton's jelly in between. The umbilical cord inserts on the sac and can be identified by Doppler ultrasound. By definition, a giant omphalocele is larger than 5 cm in diameter. It contains liver and the intrahepatic umbilical vein can be visualized within the defect. A potential diagnostic dilemma is created when the omphalocele is ruptured, which occurs in approximately 10% of cases, making it difficult to distinguish from gastroschisis. The identification of the umbilical cord insertion, the presence of liver in the defect, and the identification of the intrahepatic umbilical vein can help to distinguish a ruptured omphalocele from gastroschisis. In addition to identifying the omphalocele, ultrasonography can be helpful in identifying other associated defects.

Fetal MRI in an important diagnostic adjunct to fetal ultrasonography, providing better structural detail and aiding in the diagnosis of other associated anomalies (Fig. 66.2). Once the diagnosis of omphalocele is made, fetal echocardiography and a karyotype analysis should be performed.

There is currently no fetal intervention for omphalocele. Survival in patients with omphalocele is highly dependent on the associated anomalies and the prenatal detection of these anomalies allows appropriate prenatal counseling. If the decision is made to continue the pregnancy, serial biophysical profiling and ultrasonographic evaluation should be performed weekly after 32 weeks gestation to monitor for fetal

K.W. Liechty (✉)
Departments of General Thoracic and Fetal Surgery,
University of Pennsylvania, Children's Hospital of Philadelphia,
Philadelphia, PA, USA
e-mail: kliechty@umc.edu

P. Mattei (ed.), *Fundamentals of Pediatric Surgery*,
DOI 10.1007/978-1-4419-6643-8_66, © Springer Science+Business Media, LLC 2011

Table 66.1 Associated syndromes

Beckwith-Wiedmann syndrome
Cloacal extrophy
Fibrochondrogenesis
Lethal omphalocele-cleft palate syndrome
Marshal-Smith syndrome
Meckel-Gruber syndrome
Trisomies 13–15, 18, 21

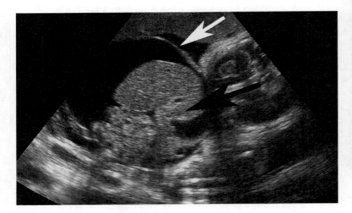

Fig. 66.1 Prenatal ultrasonography of a fetus with a giant omphalocele. The extraperitoneal liver is indicated by the *black arrow*. The membrane covering the omphalocele is indicated by the *white arrow*. Ascites is seen within the sac

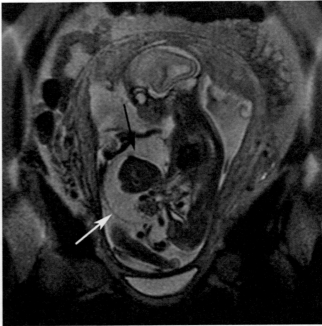

Fig. 66.2 Prenatal ultrafast high resolution MRI of a fetus with a giant omphalocele. The covering membrane is indicated by the *white arrow*. The liver contained in the sac is indicated by the *black arrow*

growth and to look for signs of fetal distress or other complications, such as intra-uterine growth retardation (6–35%), preterm labor (24–65%), and omphalocele rupture (10%).

To maximize fetal growth and lung development, the goal should be to deliver patients with omphalocele as close to term as possible. Delivery should be in a tertiary care setting with the availability of pediatric surgeons. There is no advantage to caesarean delivery over vaginal delivery, except in the case of giant omphalocele or in patients with significant liver herniation, which can result in omphalocele rupture, birth dystocia, or liver trauma.

Postnatal Care

Following delivery, the newborn is observed for respiratory insufficiency and intubated if necessary. The stomach is decompressed by oro- or nasogastric tube to prevent bowel distention, vomiting, and aspiration. Because of the association with Beckwith-Wiedemann syndrome, blood glucose is checked immediately and then frequently thereafter. The membrane covering the omphalocele is protected and dressed with non-adherent gauze to prevent injury or desiccation. If the omphalocele is ruptured, then urgent bowel coverage, either by silo or placement of a sterile mesh, is warranted.

Once the infant is stabilized, a complete physical examination is performed. If not sent prenatally, a karyotype and Genetics consultation is requested. Echocardiography must be done and a chest radiograph is obtained to evaluate for a narrow and elongated thorax ("dog chest" deformity), which is a sign of pulmonary hypoplasia (Fig. 66.3).

Operative Treatment

After the initial assessment, the surgical approach to the correction of the abdominal wall defect is decided upon. This is dictated by the size of the defect, the presence of comorbidities (prematurity, respiratory insufficiency, cardiac disease), and the presence of other congenital anomalies or syndromes. There are three principal therapeutic options: primary closure of the defect, which is used in small omphaloceles (<3 cm), delayed closure ("paint and wait"), which is used when the patient has significant comorbidities, and the amnioinversion technique, which is used in patients with large defects and no significant comorbidities.

Primary Closure

For primary closure of small omphaloceles, the skin is dissected circumferentially from the amnion and down to the

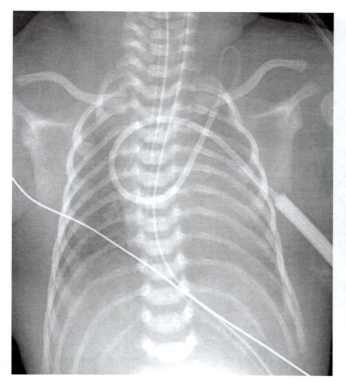

Fig. 66.3 Antero-posterior chest X-ray from a patient with a giant omphalocele. The "dog chest" deformity is clearly seen with the narrow thorax and small lung fields consistent which is consistent with pulmonary hypoplasia

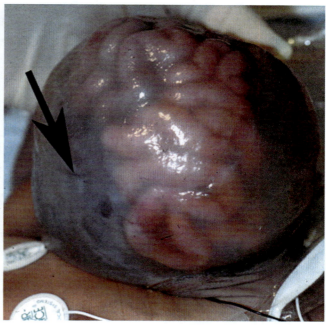

Fig. 66.5 Giant omphalocele with bowel and liver (*black arrow*) seen within the sac

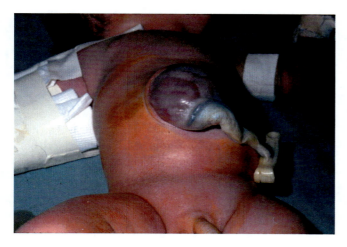

Fig. 66.4 Small omphalocele with bowel visible and the umbilical cord inserting on the sac

abdominal wall fascia (Fig. 66.4). The umbilical cord structures are dissected, isolated, and ligated. The fascial edges of the enlarged umbilical ring are approximated, in the midline or transversely, with interrupted absorbable suture. An umbilicoplasty is performed to close the skin over the repair and to fashion a neo-umbilicus.

The advantages of primary repair include a secure fascial closure, fewer procedures, and a less risk of fistula formation. In addition, earlier enteral feeding decreases other complications such as parenteral nutrition-associated cholestasis and hepatic dysfunction, line infection, and sepsis. A potential disadvantage to primary closure is the risk of abdominal compartment syndrome resulting from the closure being too tight. When abdominal compartment pressures are greater than 20 mmHg, splanchnic and renal perfusion is compromised and associated with significant morbidity and mortality. In addition, increased abdominal pressure can result in abdominal competition and respiratory insufficiency. To avoid this serious complication, selection of the proper closure technique is essential.

Delayed Closure

Delayed closure is an option for infants with giant omphalocele or comorbidities that contraindicate the use of other techniques. The cord is ligated at the junction with the amnion and the excess cord excised (Figs. 66.5 and 66.6). The amnion is then dressed daily with topical sulfasalazine, non-adherent dressing, and dry sterile gauze. Over the subsequent weeks or months, the amnion becomes epithelialized. At between 1 and 2 years of age, when comorbidities have improved and the size of the abdominal defect has decreased relative to the size of the abdominal wall, definitive closure can performed. A vertical incision is made inferior to the

Fig. 66.6 (**a**) An infant with giant omphalocele managed non-operatively with topical therapy because of comorbidities including prematurity and respiratory distress. The entire omphalocele has epithelialized. (**b**) The abdominal wall after reduction of the omphalocele and closure of the abdominal wall

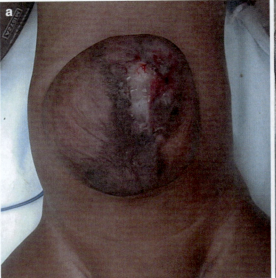
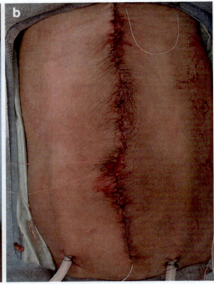

epithelialized omphalocele and dissected down to fascia. The omphalocele sack is then entered and the incision extended superiorly under direct vision and with care not to injure the liver, which is often adherent to the skin. Skin flaps are raised circumferentially and the omphalocele contents reduced into the peritoneal cavity. The fascia is the approximated in the midline with care to avoid an excessively tight closure, which can produce an abdominal compartment syndrome. Rarely, this requires the placement of lateral relaxing incisions in the external oblique fascia. The skin is then closed in the midline over closed-suction drains.

The primary advantage of delayed closure is the prevention of further exacerbation of underlying comorbidities, such as respiratory insufficiency from pulmonary hypoplasia or prematurity, or hemodynamic instability in patients with significant cardiac disease. Another advantage is the ability to provide early enteral nutrition, which is associated with fewer complications than parenteral nutrition. Disadvantages of delayed closure include the need for daily dressing changes, the requirement for subsequent fascial closure, and the risks of amnion rupture and wound infection. In addition, there are psychosocial and developmental considerations related to limitations of being able to spend time in the prone position or crawling, which may be precluded by the large anterior abdominal wall mass.

Amnioinversion

The amnioinversion technique is used for infants with large omphaloceles that preclude primary closure but who lack significant comorbidities (Fig. 66.7). All of the dissection stays extraperitoneal and the amnion is inverted. First, the skin is circumferentially dissected from the amnion and the fascia identified. Flaps of skin and subcutaneous tissue are then raised off the fascia, extending several centimeters from the edge of the defect. For the very large omphalocele, the fascia at the top and bottom of the defect is incised for 1–2 cm to aid in the reduction of the omphalocele contents and subsequent closure. Care is taken to stay extraperitoneal and to avoid injuring the hepatic veins superiorly and the bladder inferiorly. A sheet of polytetrafluoroethylene netting is then secured to the fascia on either side of the defect with a running 3-0 polypropylene suture, approximately 1–2 cm from the edge of the mesh. This mesh cuff is then placed down on the fascia and secured with a running 3-0 absorbable monofilament suture. Tissue in-growth from the fascia through the interstices of the mesh helps to further anchor it in place. Povidone ointment is applied to the mesh and the skin flaps are sutured to the mesh to prevent skin retraction. The wound is then dressed with dry gauze and an impermeable drape. The mesh is sequentially tightened every other day using horizontal mattress sutures to remove the slack, gradually reducing the omphalocele and inverting the amnion. Eventually, the abdominal contents and amnion are reduced to the level of the fascia. Once the fascial edges are touching, the fascia is closed with interrupted absorbable suture and the mesh is removed. The skin edges are trimmed of excess skin and approximated in the midline over a vessel-loop drain, which is brought out through a stab incision inferior to the wound, and an umbilicoplasty performed.

The main advantage of the amnioinversion technique is that the fascia is closed and is done so without entering the peritoneum, thereby decreasing the risk of adhesions. In addition, there is the potential for extubation with subsequent tightenings being done under sedation. These patients are also able to be prone and may progress through normal developmental

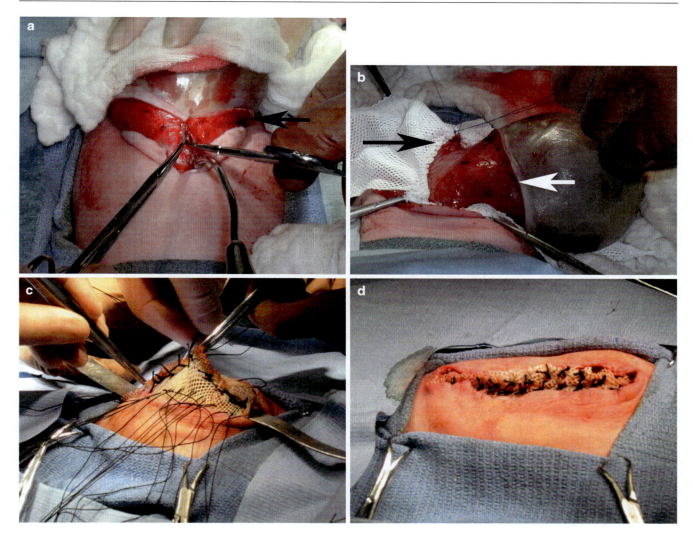

Fig. 66.7 Amnioinversion technique. (**a**) Dissection of the skin from the amnion, the identification of the fascia, and the raising of skin flaps. This is performed circumferentially around the omphalocele, extends several centimeters beyond the edge of the fascia, and keeps the amnion intact. (**b**) The suturing of artificial mesh to the fascia. This is performed 1–2 cm from the edge of the mesh using a running polypropylene suture. The cuff of mesh is secured to the anterior abdominal wall fascia with absorbable suture in an onlay fashion. Tissue in-growth from the fascia through the mesh helps to secure it in place. (**c**) Sequential tightening of the mesh using horizontal mattress silk sutures through the mesh to remove the slack and reduce the omphalocele. (**d**) After several reductions, the omphalocele is at the level of the fascia. Once the fascia is touching, the fascia is closed and the mesh removed

milestones. The disadvantages of this technique include the need for multiple procedures, a delay in enteral nutrition, and the risk of wound infection.

Complications

Complications of omphalocele can be classified into early and late (Tables 66.2 and 66.3). Some, such as pulmonary hypoplasia and subsequent chronic lung disease, are related to the disease process. As all infants with omphalocele are malrotated, there is a risk of midgut volvulus, but this occurs rarely. Other complications are related to treatment or the intensity of medical therapy, such as delayed enteral nutrition resulting in cholestasis, episodes of line sepsis, or developmental delay and hypotonia. Early complications such as the exacerbation of respiratory insufficiency or renal failure are related to the surgical closure of the abdomen being too tight, resulting in abdominal competition and decreased renal perfusion.

Late complications, such as hernia and GERD, might also be the result of increased intra-abdominal pressure. These complications highlight the need to select the appropriate treatment modality based on the size of the omphalocele and the associated comorbidities.

Survival of patients with omphalocele is largely related to associated anomalies. These infants are also at risk for chromosomal abnormalities and other comorbidities, such as pulmonary

Table 66.2 Early complications

Pulmonary hypoplasia
Respiratory insufficiency
Line sepsis
Wound infection
Dehiscence
Renal failure
TPN cholestasis
NEC
Bowel obstruction
Fistula formation
Midgut volvulus

Table 66.3 Late complications

GERD
Chronic lung disease
Hernias
Developmental delay
Hypotonia
Bowel obstruction
Midgut volvulus

hypoplasia. Associated anomalies and comorbidities dictate the postnatal management of these complex cases. The selection of the appropriate operative approach is essential to minimize reduce morbidity and mortality and optimize outcomes. Early involvement of a pediatric surgeon, preferably in the antenatal period, is an important part of the management of these patients and requires the early referral of these patients and their families to tertiary care centers where such care is available.

Summary Points

- Omphalocele occurs in approximately 1 in 5,000 births, is associated with advanced maternal age and chromosomal abnormalities in 30%.
- Infants with omphalocele are at risk for cardiovascular anomalies and should undergo a thorough cardiovascular examination including echocardiography.
- Infants with omphalocele are at risk for Beckwith-Wiedemann syndrome (hypoglycemia, macroglossia, gigantism, risk of malignancy, omphalocele) and therefore blood glucose levels should be checked urgently and then serially.
- For defects small than 5 cm in diameter, primary closure is usually possible and should be attempted if the baby is healthy and without significant associated anomalies.
- For giant defects (larger than 5 cm or containing a portion of the liver), it is best to use a staged approach (amnio-inversion technique): a mesh is sutured securely to the fascia, the amnion is preserved, and the fascia reapproximated every other day until the edges are approximated.
- For infants who are compromised due to cardiovascular or pulmonary disease, one might consider using a delayed closure approach, in which the amnion is coated with an antiseptic and allowed to epithelialize.

Editor's Comment

For all practical purposes, omphalocele and gastroschisis are the only congenital abdominal wall defects and though each is often listed in the other's differential diagnosis, they are so completely different as to never be confused with one another, except occasionally on antenatal US when the membrane has ruptured. Omphalocele is covered by a membrane, it involves the umbilical ring and the umbilical cord, the size of the defect is highly variable, it can include the liver, and, most importantly, it is frequently associated with one of several syndromes and anomalies in other organ systems, most notably cardiovascular and genitourinary. Today, the diagnosis is almost always made antenatally, which allows the parents to receive proper counseling and the infant to be transferred quickly to an appropriate neonatal care center. The only emergency steps that need to be taken are a blood glucose measurement and placement of a clean, moist dressing on the amnion.

All simple defects should be repaired primarily whenever possible or, if larger than 5 cm, with the staged approach originally described by Schuster. The delayed closure technique ("paint and wait") could still potentially be used in extreme situations but, because of the significant long-term morbidity and debilitation associated with this approach, its use in the modern era is almost never justified. Complicated defects that involve extrophy of the bladder or cardiothoracic defects (pentalogy) can be quite difficult to repair and usually require a multidisciplinary approach and a well-conceived plan. All infants with omphalocele have intestinal nonrotation, which rarely if ever needs to be corrected, as the risk of volvulus appears to be quite low.

Differential Diagnosis

- Gastroschisis
- Beckwith-Wiedemann syndrome

Preoperative Preparation

☐ Complete work up for associated anomalies
☐ Blood glucose
☐ Prophylactic antibiotics
☐ Intravenous hydration

Parental Preparation

- Babies with omphalocele sometimes have associated anomalies, which explains why we need to perform other tests.
- If the omphalocele is small, we recommend trying to place the bowel back in the abdomen and close the opening in the abdominal wall.
- If the omphalocele is large, we will need to close the opening gradually over the course of the next week or two, until we can perform the final operation to close it up completely.
- All babies with omphalocele have malrotation of the intestines but it is rarely necessary to correct it.

Diagnostic Studies

Prenatal

- Maternal serum AFP
- High resolution ultrasonography
- Fetal MRI
- Fetal ECHO
- Fetal karyotyping

Postnatal

- Serum glucose
- CXR
- Echocardiography
- Genetics evaluation and karyotyping

Technical Points

- The fascia can be closed transversely or in the midline.
- The fascia should be closed without tension and with care to avoid producing an abdominal compartment syndrome.
- For delayed closure techniques, the amnion should be preserved, which decreases the risk of sepsis and adhesions.

Suggested Reading

Biard JM, Wilson RD, Johnson MP, et al. Prenatally diagnosed giant omphaloceles:short- and long-term outcomes. Prenat Diagn. 2004;24:434–9.

How HY, Harris BJ, Pietrantoni M, et al. Is vaginal delivery preferable to elective cesarean delivery in fetuses with a known ventral wall defect. Am J Obstet Gynecol. 2000;182:1527–34.

Koivusalo A, Rintala R, Lindahl H. Gastroesophageal reflux in children with a congenital abdominal wall defect. J Peditr Surg. 1999;34:1127–9.

Ledbetter DJ. Gastroschisis and omphalocele. Surg Clin N Am. 2006;86:249–60.

Mann S, Blinman TA, Wilson RD. Prenatal and postnatal management of omphalocele. Prenat Diagn. 2008;28:626–32.

Schuster SR. A new method for the staged repair of large omphaloceles. Surg Gynecol Obstet. 1967;125(4):837–50.

Wilson RD, Johnson MP. Congenital abdominal wall defects: an update. Fetal Diagn Ther. 2004;19:385–98.

Chapter 67
Eventration of the Diaphragm

Samuel Z. Soffer

Eventration of the diaphragm constitutes an abnormal elevation of one or both hemidiaphragms and can be the result of congenital or acquired causes. Congenital eventration is less common and results from the development of a structurally intact but abnormal thin diaphragmatic muscle. The etiology of congenital eventration is unknown, though infectious causes such as rubella or cytomegalovirus have been implicated, and there is no known familial predisposition. Congenital eventration can be difficult to distinguish from a congenital diaphragmatic hernia with a sac, as both subsets of these patients present with milder pulmonary symptoms than the typical diaphragmatic hernia patient.

Acquired eventration of the diaphragm most often follows thoracic surgery or a traumatic birth (Erb's palsy), which result in injury to the phrenic nerve. In these instances the diaphragmatic muscle itself is normal but it functions poorly. In addition, eventration of the diaphragm is associated with spinal muscle atrophy (Werdnig-Hoffman syndrome), in which a generalized progressive loss of neurologic function leads to eventration.

Eventration may be associated with other congenital abnormalities including congenital heart disease, cerebral agenesis, and chromosomal anomalies. In a small number of patients, it is also associated with pulmonary hypoplasia. Physiologically, altered diaphragmatic function causes a restrictive deficit manifested by reduced lung volume, decreased tidal volume, and increased work of breathing, leading to respiratory compromise, sometimes requiring mechanical ventilation.

Many infants and children with eventration of the diaphragm are asymptomatic and the diagnosis is sometimes noted incidentally on a chest radiograph for an infectious or pulmonary manifestation. Other patients may incur respiratory embarrassment at birth or following intrathoracic surgery with injury to the phrenic nerve.

Asymptomatic patients can usually be treated conservatively with periodic follow-up, whereas most symptomatic patients require surgical correction. With severe congenital eventration, the baby may develop respiratory distress soon after birth requiring mechanical ventilation and hemodynamic resuscitation. Alternatively, the baby might have persistent or recurrent respiratory infections, wheezing, chronic bronchitis or pneumonia unresponsive to conventional treatment. The most common presentation of acquired diaphragmatic eventration is postoperative respiratory failure following an intrathoracic procedure. Gastrointestinal symptoms are most commonly seen with left-sided eventrations and include intermittent vomiting, postprandial pain, bloating, and failure to thrive.

Diagnosis

Unilateral eventration is diagnosed by chest radiograph when the right hemidiaphragm is more than two rib levels higher than the left or the left hemidiaphragm is more than one rib level higher than the right (Fig. 67.1). Rarely, bilateral eventration (usually congenital), is suspected when both hemidiaphragms are elevated. Fluoroscopic evaluation of the diaphragm ("sniff test") was used historically and will show paradoxical movement of the diaphragm, but the ease of ultrasound has supplanted fluoroscopy as the initial diagnostic test of choice. Ultrasonography provides an even better assessment of the diaphragm since dynamic function can be assessed during respiration. Absent or paradoxical diaphragmatic movements during inspiration are suggestive of eventration. In addition, both CT and MRI have been used to confirm the diagnosis. MRI provides the best resolution overall but often requires anesthesia for optimal imaging.

S.Z. Soffer (✉)
Albert Einstein College of Medicine, Division of Pediatric Surgery, Schneider Children's Hospital, 269-01 76th Avenue, New Hyde Park, NY 11598, USA
e-mail: SSoffer@nshs.edu

P. Mattei (ed.), *Fundamentals of Pediatric Surgery*,
DOI 10.1007/978-1-4419-6643-8_67, © Springer Science+Business Media, LLC 2011

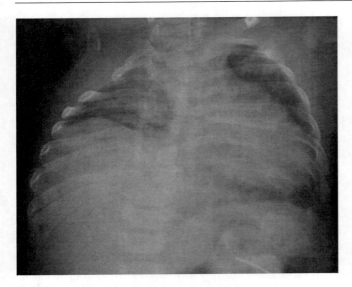

Fig. 67.1 Right sided diaphragmatic eventration in a baby with ventilator dependence and pulmonary hypoplasia

Treatment

Small eventrations with minimal respiratory symptoms may be left untreated and can safely be observed. Most large eventrations, even if asymptomatic, are repaired surgically with plication of the diaphragm, but associated anomalies such as pulmonary hypoplasia sometimes mitigate the modest improvements in respiratory function even after surgical repair. Preoperative preparation for congenital eventrations must include a thorough workup for chromosomal abnormalities and congenital cardiac defects. An echocardiogram should be performed to rule out associated structural cardiac anomalies. Children with acquired eventration following an intrathoracic procedure or even following birth should be given a period of conservative management since phrenic nerve function can improve with time, thus obviating the need for surgery. Children who do not improve will require an operation and intraoperative assessment of the diaphragm can determine the etiology of the eventration and the optimal type of repair.

Diaphragmatic eventration can be repaired with either a thoracic or abdominal approach, and can be performed laparoscopically or thoracoscopically. Unilateral eventration is most commonly approached via a seventh intercostal space thoracotomy. Thoracotomy allows for ideal visualization of the phrenic nerve and its branches as they course into the diaphragm. This offers the best chance for protecting the phrenic nerve from injury during the operation.

Transthoracic repair of a congenital eventration involves excising the thinned portion of the hemidiaphragm (usually centrally located) and approximating the edges with non-absorbable, interrupted, 2-0 sutures. The goal is to bring muscularized diaphragm together without excessive tension. Rarely, a prosthetic patch is required. Transthoracic repair of

an acquired eventration involves plicating redundant areas of diaphragm to create a taut closure. This is done by grasping the central portion of the affected hemidiaphragm with a non-crushing clamp and marking the extent of the plication with a surgical marker. The plication should be oriented in an anteromedial to posterolateral configuration. Again, non-absorbable sutures are used and care must be taken to avoid incorporating abdominal viscera in the repair with an overly aggressive bite.

Minimal access approaches are gaining in popularity. I prefer a thoracoscopic approach both for eventrations of the diaphragm as well as babies with congenital diaphragmatic hernias with minimal pulmonary hypertension. One 5-mm and two 3-mm trocars are used and it is useful to orient placement of the ports in a more anterior location on the lateral chest wall of the affected side to facilitate manipulation of the diaphragm. Intuitively, this operation seems perfect for a minimally invasive approach, but it can be technically challenging as it is difficult to place intracorporeal knots that do not fray the delicate diaphragmatic tissue. In addition, one must carefully avoid incorporating phrenic nerve branches into the repair. I find the use of 2-0 braided nylon sutures cut long with a tie-knot device, utilizing extracorporeal titanium fasteners that are brought down with perfect tension ideal for this type of repair. If the diaphragm does begin to tear, one should not hesitate to open since, if most of the sutures do not hold, a chest radiograph several days later will look as if nothing had been done. There is a tendency for the diaphragm plication to loosen over time and any compromise in operative technique will likely result in a suboptimal long-term repair. Laparoscopic repair of diaphragmatic eventration has also been described and the approach is nearly identical to laparoscopic repair of a congenital diaphragmatic hernia.

Bilateral eventration is best approached via a transverse upper abdominal incision which allows for the best exposure of the complete diaphragm. Eventrations presenting with GI symptoms or cases of suspected malrotation should also be approached abdominally. The liver, stomach and spleen are carefully retracted. Plicating sutures are oriented in the same manner as a transthoracic approach and care must be taken to avoid the phrenic nerve based on its expected location.

Postoperative Care

Outcome related to the surgery itself is usually good with improvement in respiratory function. Most children can be weaned from the ventilator within 1 week of surgery. However, a small subset of patients will continue to be require mechanical ventilation even after a technically good repair. Intrapleural drainage is maintained for several days following the transthoracic and thoracoscopic approaches.

Recurrent eventration requiring re-operation is rare. Children with bilateral eventration do not seem to do as well as unilateral eventrations due to severe pulmonary hypoplasia. In contrast, there is potential for lung growth following repair of significant unilateral diaphragmatic eventration. This may be responsible for the overall favorable prognosis in these patients if other associated anomalies, such as cardiac defects, can be adequately addressed.

Summary Points

- Eventration of the diaphragm can be congenital or acquired.
- Congenital eventration can be difficult to distinguish from a congenital diaphragmatic hernia with a sac.
- Acquired eventration most often follows thoracic surgery or trauma during birth.
- Asymptomatic patients may be treated conservatively with periodic follow-up, whereas most symptomatic patients require surgical correction.
- Unilateral eventration is diagnosed by chest radiograph when the right hemidiaphragm is more than two rib levels higher than the left or the left hemidiaphragm is at least one rib level higher than the right.
- Preoperative preparation for congenital eventrations must include a thorough workup for chromosomal abnormalities and congenital cardiac defects.
- Diaphragmatic eventration can be repaired with either a thoracic or abdominal approach, thoracoscopically or laparoscopically.
- Outcome related to the surgery itself is usually good with significant improvement in respiratory function.

Editor's Comment

Most children with unilateral eventration of the diaphragm seem to have very little if any respiratory compromise, which is the traditional indication for surgical intervention. However, over time, the diaphragm can rise quite high in the chest, restricting lung expansion and compromising growth and development of both lungs during early childhood. This, combined with the fact that the minimally invasive approach is effective and well-tolerated, favors an aggressive surgical approach for patients with severe eventration. Nevertheless, since many cases that are due to phrenic nerve injury will improve or resolve over time, a period of observation and close monitoring with serial chest radiographs is warranted.

The thoracoscopic approach is straightforward and should allow a repair that is equivalent to that performed through a thoracotomy. Excision of the redundant portion of the diaphragm is probably the best way to prevent a recurrence, especially in infants, but when breakdown of the suture line does occur, the result is a diaphragmatic hernia. It appears to be important to use nonabsorbable interrupted sutures, placed in a way that distributes the tension evenly across the entire repair. Extracorporeal knots (Roeder or square) seem to work best, but one must frequently check the status of the repair and to have a low threshold to cut and replace any and all sutures that are under too much tension.

The laparoscopic approach is especially useful when a fundoplication or gastrostomy tube is needed and can be done concomitantly. The principles of the actual repair are essentially the same as for the thoracoscopic approach, though an extra port is often needed for bowel or liver retraction.

Differential Diagnosis

- Congenital diaphragmatic hernia with a peritoneal sac.
- Pulmonary hypoplasia/pulmonary insufficiency of any etiology.

Diagnostic Studies

- Plain chest radiograph
- Ultrasound
- CT scan
- MRI
- Real time fluoroscopy

Parental Preparation

- Plication of the diaphragm in symptomatic babies is usually helpful but not always.
- Weaning of respiratory support may be a slow process.
- Thoracoscopic/laparoscopic repair may require conversion to an open procedure.
- High likelihood of postoperative chest tube.

Preoperative Preparation

□ Karyotype
□ Echocardiogram
□ Multiple attempts at weaning prior to surgical intervention, particularly for mild eventration.

Technical Points

- The diaphragm should be plicated so that it is well flattened but it need not be tense.
- Interrupted permanent sutures must be carefully placed to prevent the diaphragm from tearing.
- Do not incorporate phrenic nerve branches into the repair.
- Do not inadvertently incorporate abdominal viscera into the repair.
- For thoracoscopic approach, place ports slightly anterior.
- Extracorporeal knots can be helpful to avoid tearing of the diaphragm.
- There should be a low threshold to convert to open the diaphragm is tearing, or if the repair is in any way suboptimal.

Suggested Reading

Jawad AJ, al-Sammarai AY, al-Rabeeh A. Eventration of the diaphragm in children. J R Coll Surg Edinb. 1991;36:222–4.

Kizilcan F, Tanyel FC, Hicsonmez A. The long term results of diaphragmatic plication. J Pediatr Surg. 1993;28:42–4.

Langer JC. Phrenic nerve palsy. In: Fallis JC, Filler RM, Lemoine G, editors. Pediatric thoracic surgery. New York: Elsevier; 1991. p. 210–4.

Stolar CJH, Dillon PW. Congenital diaphragmatic hernia and eventration. In: Grosfeld JL, O'Neill JA, Fonkalsrud EW, Coran AG, editors. Pediatric surgery. 6th ed. Philadelphia: Mosby Elsevier; 2006. p. 946.

Chapter 68
Congenital Diaphragmatic Hernia

Peter Mattei

Congenital diaphragmatic hernia occurs in approximately 1 in 3,000 live births. There are two distinct anatomic forms that differ significantly in their physiologic effects. The more common and certainly more challenging type is the posterolateral (Bochdalek) hernia. Anterior defects (Morgagni) are much less common and also much less morbid, often not presenting until well beyond infancy.

Bochdalek Hernia

Congenital diaphragmatic hernia usually refers to the more common and physiologically more significant posterolateral defect. Although the etiology is unknown, it is thought in most cases to be the result of an error in mesenchymal cell differentiation between the fourth and tenth week of gestation when the pleuroperitoneal folds normally develop. The result is incomplete formation of the diaphragm and herniation of intestine and solid organs into the chest cavity. The presence of a space-occupying lesion in the chest during this critical stage in development has several serious developmental effects. Pulmonary hypoplasia occurs bilaterally, worse on the ipsilateral side, and results in a limitation of the number of branches that form in the bronchial tree, overmuscularization and a decrease in the number of pulmonary arterioles, and surfactant deficiency. There is also some degree of cardiac hypoplasia, and the severe mediastinal shift can cause hydrops fetalis.

Infants with CDH are also at risk for associated anomalies in other organ systems. Approximately 10% have chromosomal abnormalities such as trisomy 18 or 13 or other chromosomal abnormalities and in rare cases CDH can be part of a syndrome or association such as Apert, Beckwith-Wiedemann, or CHARGE. The incidence of neural tube defects and severe cardiac anomalies is much higher in infants with CDH who are stillborn. Because the bowel is in the chest and therefore not available to undergo the normal pattern of rotation and fixation within the abdomen, nearly every individual with CDH is expected to have intestinal nonrotation or malrotation. Despite the inherent risk, however, volvulus and intestinal atresia appear to be rare.

In many ways, at least from a surgical perspective, the hernia itself is a relatively straightforward anatomic problem that can usually be repaired using some combination of basic techniques, while it is the effects of pulmonary hypoplasia that have proven to be extremely difficult to manage. Respiratory insufficiency can usually be managed with supportive measures or mechanical ventilation at birth and because the lungs continue to grow (and more branches develop) until the age of approximately 8 years, this tends to be a self-limited problem. Likewise, surfactant deficiency can be corrected at birth with the administration of exogenous surfactant. Thus far, however, pulmonary hypertension remains the Achilles heel of CDH management. There are few effective vasodilators available that specifically target the pulmonary vessels. Some infants demonstrate few if any effects of pulmonary hypertension, while others demonstrate severe shunting that once triggered seems to worsen inexorably in spite of all efforts to control it. Furthermore, these infants are at risk for iatrogenic lung injury due to overzealous attempts to optimize oxygenation and ventilation, which can result in barotrauma, volutrauma, and oxygen toxicity.

Antenatal Diagnosis

CDH is increasingly identified by antenatal ultrasound. The images reveal a heterogeneous intrathoracic mass with peristalsis and the stomach bubble is sometimes seen in the chest. For left-sided lesions, which account for 85–90% of cases, the finding that liver has herniated up in the chest is associated with a poor prognosis (more complications, more likely to need ECMO, decreased survival: 40% vs. 90+%). Other clinical features that appear to correlate with a poor prognosis include early gestational age at diagnosis, polyhydramnios,

P. Mattei (✉)
Department of General Surgery, Children's Hospital of Philadelphia, 3400 Civic Center Blvd, Philadelphia, PA 19146, USA
e-mail: mattei@email.chop.edu

P. Mattei (ed.), *Fundamentals of Pediatric Surgery*,
DOI 10.1007/978-1-4419-6643-8_68, © Springer Science+Business Media, LLC 2011

cardiac hypoplasia, and diminished total lung volume. Right-sided defects are also associated with a higher morbidity and mortality. In infants with left-sided defects, lung area-to-head circumference ratio (LHR) can be used as measure of severity and is predictive of mortality; however, as treatment continues to improve, it is less predictive of morbidity than in the past. The ratio is obtained, usually at 24–26 weeks gestation, by measuring the cross-sectional area of the right lung at the level of the atria (in square millimeters) and dividing it by the head circumference (in millimeters). In general, an LHR ≤1.0 is associated with low survival while a ratio of >1.4 is associated with improved outcome. Fetal lung volumes calculated by ultrafast fetal MRI also correlate with morbidity and survival. At this time, the best predictor of poor outcome in infants with left-sided CDH is liver herniation ("liver up"). In those without liver herniation ("liver down"), LHR and lung volumes continue to have some predictive value but this is evolving as treatments improve.

There was once hope that in utero surgical repair of fetuses with CDH could help to reduce mortality, but this has not been the case. After several well-designed controlled studies, it is clear that the fetuses who do well with prepartum repair are the ones who are likely to have done well with standard therapy and the survival of high-risk fetuses is not improved by repair before birth. Another fetal intervention that holds some promise is tracheal occlusion. Occluding the trachea early in gestation leads to the accumulation of lung fluid and a dramatic increase in lung size. This has been shown in a fetal sheep model and in limited human studies to be a potentially useful technique, presumably by minimizing the herniation of bowel and allowing the lungs to grow more than they might have otherwise. The techniques available to occlude the trachea have evolved from surgical application of a metal clip that is removed at birth to a fetoscopically placed endotracheal balloon that is ruptured at birth. This technique is being studied in ongoing human trials and awaits approval for use in the US.

Although fetal surgical intervention is currently not feasible, antenatal diagnosis of CDH is a relatively common indication for referral to a fetal treatment center. Early referral is helpful for prospective parents as they can be provided counseling, prognostic information that helps them decide whether to continue the pregnancy, and help with the considerable preparation required for the safe delivery and postnatal care of these infants. Because of the small but significant risk of associated anomalies and chromosomal abnormalities, we recommend fetal echocardiography and karyotype analysis, which is most safely and accurately performed by amniocentesis. Ultrafast fetal MRI is performed to help identify associated anomalies and liver herniation, and to measure lung volumes. Genetic counseling is offered as well; specifically array comparative genomic hybridization (aCGH) is recommended under some circumstances as

a useful tool for the identification subtle chromosomal abnormalities. Fetal US is repeated at 2-week intervals to assess fetal growth and amniotic fluid volume, and to rule out complications such as bowel ischemia, ascites, hydrops, or particulate matter (meconium) in the amniotic fluid. Nonstress testing is performed twice per week starting at 33 weeks and corticosteroids are administered for preterm labor as indicated per standard protocol.

The best timing and mode of delivery of infants with CDH is not known with certainty. There is no advantage to scheduled cesarean delivery though, based on retrospective reviews, some believe that there might be an advantage to early term delivery (37–38 weeks). Nevertheless, we recommend scheduled induction of labor at 38–39 weeks, preferably at a center where proper monitoring and all aspects of advanced care, including ECMO, are available. Delivery by cesarean section is performed when indicated by standard criteria. The Special Delivery Unit of The Children's Hospital of Philadelphia is unique in that infants are delivered at a free-standing tertiary-care children's medical center, where neonatal and surgical specialists are immediately available, obviating the need for transportation to another facility.

Medical Management

Although some remain well-perfused and stable with little or no sign of respiratory compromise or cardiovascular instability, every infant with CDH is considered at risk for severe pulmonary hypertension that can easily spiral out of control, often without warning and sometimes inexplicably after a period of apparent stability. The principles of medical management of the infant with CDH include: (1) Using gentle ventilation techniques (permissive hypercapnia) to minimize iatrogenic lung injury; (2) Minimizing the onset and impact of pulmonary hypertension; (3) Performing diagnostic studies to rule out associated anomalies and to prepare the infant for the possibility of ECMO; and (4) Delaying surgical repair until hemodynamic stability has been maintained for at least 24 h. Infants who need to be transferred to a tertiary care center for definitive management should be prepared for transportation with frequent updates communicated with the accepting NICU. Every newborn nursery should have a specific evidence-based and frequently updated protocol for the stabilization and initial medical treatment of these infants.

Infants are subjected to continuous cardiac monitoring and placement of a nasogastric tube, bladder catheter, and umbilical vein and artery cannulas. Oxygen saturation (SaO$_2$) is measured continuously by pulse oximetry in a preductal (right arm, head) and postductal location. Initial studies should include a chest radiograph to confirm the diagnosis and assess the degree of lung expansion and bowel distension; echocardiography to rule out associated anomalies and to measure changes in the pulmonary artery pressure, left-to-right shunt fraction and flow across the ductus arteriosus; and a head US to rule out intraventricular hemorrhage in anticipation of the possible need for ECMO. In low-risk infants (liver down), it is best to delay the echocardiogram until the second day of life so as to avoid over-estimation of pulmonary hypertension. Surgical intervention is considered non-urgent.

Infants with a known CDH are orotracheally intubated immediately. Though some have promoted the early administration of surfactant, this has not been shown to improve outcomes. We therefore administer surfactant only in premature infants (<35 weeks gestation). A gentle ventilation strategy with permissive hypercapnia has been shown to be effective and minimizes barotrauma. The goals are to minimize ventilator-associated lung injury, prevent pressure-related complications (pulmonary interstitial emphysema, pneumothorax), and, if possible, avoid the need for ECMO. Hypercarbia ($PaCO_2$ 60–65 mmHg, or transiently up to 70) is permitted as long as pH can be maintained above 7.20 with bicarbonate therapy. Some protocols prohibit the use of muscle relaxants and call for minimization of sedation, although these are sometimes necessary to help control ventilation and reduce airway pressures. Infants who are hypoxemic, severely hypercarbic, shunting, or agitated are treated with a fentanyl infusion at 1 μg/kg/h that is titrated to effect. We use muscle relaxants for refractory hypoventilation and for surgical procedures.

Mechanical ventilation is started in conventional IMV mode at a rate of 40/min and increased as needed up to 80. Typical settings include an I:E ratio of 1:2, and a PEEP of 3–5 cmH_2O. Peak inspiratory pressure is set initially at the lowest pressure that provides adequate chest movement (TV 5–6 mL/kg), and increased to an upper limit of 25 cmH_2O, if necessary. A PIP of 28–30 is probably safe for short periods and as a bridge to ECMO. FiO_2 is initially set at 100% and weaned very slowly to avoid sudden or severe hypoxemia, which is thought to be a trigger for shunting. Oxygen is weaned in high-risk infants (LHR <1.0, liver up) after 6 h if they are stable and have a PaO_2 >150 mmHg and in low-risk infants (liver down) after 2 h if the PaO_2 is >200 and then only by 3% per hour.

Failure of low-rate conventional ventilation, as evidenced by severe retractions or paradoxical chest movement, worsening tachypnea, preductal SaO2 <80–85%, or $PaCO_2$ >60–65 mmHg, is an indication for escalation of therapy. The next step at some institutions is high-frequency conventional ventilation (IMV = 100) but we prefer gentle high-frequency oscillator ventilation (MAP <14, Hz 6–8). The goal is a $PaCO_2$ of 60–65 mmHg with pH >7.20, and a preductal SaO_2 above 85%. Failure of HFOV or any complication of barotrauma (pneumothorax, PIE) is usually an indication for consideration of ECMO.

Pulmonary hypertension is manifested by an increasing need for ventilator support and a widening gap between pre- and postductal SaO_2 ("shunting"). It can also be assessed by echocardiography. Once it starts, there is the well-founded fear that it will worsen rapidly and inexorably. But the triggers are poorly understood, leading to institutional practices that border on the superstitious. Nevertheless, it is recommended that the infant be kept warm and not be exposed to loud noises, abrupt changes or rough handling, that painful procedures and endotracheal tube suctioning be avoided, and that all ventilator changes be made incrementally. We prefer to not even weight the baby at first (the weight is estimated). We try to avoid overhydration by using small boluses of crystalloid only as needed for poor perfusion or low urine output. Blood is transfused as needed to maintain a hemoglobin of around 14 g/dL.

If needed for hypotension, dopamine is started at 5 μg/kg/min and titrated to maintain a mean systemic blood pressure equal to or above the patient's gestational age in weeks, up to a maximum of 30 μg/kg/min. Dobutamine (5–10 μg/kg/min) is used if moderate to severe cardiac dysfunction is identified by echocardiography. For infants with significant left ventricular dysfunction, milrinone (0.25 μg/kg/min) can be used as an adjunct to low-dose dopamine. Low-dose epinephrine infusion is considered only in rare instances. Infants with persistent hypotension despite increasing dopamine receive hydrocortisone (1 mg/kg IV q12h×2, then 0.5 mg/kg q12 h×2). Children with hypotension that is refractory to pressors should undergo echocardiography again to rule out a missed cardiac anomaly or severe cardiac dysfunction and are considered candidates for ECMO.

For some infants, nitric oxide is an effective pulmonary vasodilator. We use inhaled nitric oxide when pre- and postductal SaO_2 measurements differ by more than 10 points, postductal PaO_2 is less than 100 mmHg, or there is echocardiographic evidence of pulmonary hypertension. We start with a dose of 20 ppm. The infant is considered an iNO nonresponder if there is a less than 10% increase in PaO_2, a less than 10% decrease in the oxygenation index, or the OI remains 25 or greater despite adequate lung inflation. Nonresponders are considered potential candidates for ECMO.

Infants who respond to iNO can be transitioned to enteral sildenafil, which has been used safely in newborns with pulmonary hypertension. It is contraindicated in the setting of hepatic or renal dysfunction and requires off-label use consent. Because its mechanism of action is mediated in part by NO, it is not used in infants who have failed to respond to iNO. A typical dosing regimen is 0.25 mg/kg per NGT q6h and titrated up to 2 mg/kg q3h for maintenance therapy. We use it to transition patients off iNO after surgical repair of their defect.

Criteria for starting ECMO are similar to those used for other neonates with respiratory failure: preductal SaO_2 <85%

or postductal PaO_2 < 30 mmHg; oxygenation index ([FiO_2·MAP]/PaO_2) greater than 40; PIP > 28, TV > 7 mL/kg, or MAP > 15; persistent metabolic acidosis or rising serum lactic acid levels; hypotension refractory to pressors; acute deterioration after surgical repair; and failure to respond to maximal medical treatment. ECMO should be considered only if the pulmonary hypoplasia is not felt to be severe enough to preclude survival and in the absence of other life-threatening anomaly or chromosomal abnormality. Most infants with CDH should begin with VA-ECMO, unless they are hemodynamically stable, off pressors, and demonstrating good cardiac function by echocardiogram; in which case one can start with VV-ECMO and convert to VA if necessary in the event of clinical deterioration. Parents should be reminded that ECMO is not considered therapeutic but rather serves as a bridge that allows time for maturation of the lungs, transition from fetal to newborn circulation, and normalization of pulmonary arterial pressure.

Surgical Management

Surgical repair of the actual defect is often the most straightforward aspect of the care of the infant with CDH. Treatment protocols have evolved from emergency surgery as soon as possible after birth to current strategies that emphasize gentilation and stabilization, followed by elective repair. Furthermore, hernia repair is felt in most cases to provide very little immediate clinical benefit – most actually get worse before they get better. For a time, in fact, it was thought that surgical repair was entirely incidental – reduction of the herniated bowel and closure of the defect, it was argued, had little immediate therapeutic effect on the lung hypoplasia or pulmonary hypertension, which were much more important determinants of outcome. This resulted in the uncommon decision, rarely understood or accepted by parents, to forego repair in infants who have failed to demonstrate improvement after a certain number of days or weeks on ECMO and instead to withdraw support and let them expire without having been repaired. However, because some infants do seem improve after repair, most centers will offer surgical repair as a final maneuver before recognizing the futility of further therapy.

The optimal timing of surgical repair is not known with certainty. For the stable infant without significant pulmonary hypertension, surgical repair can usually safely be performed after a period of stabilization lasting more than 24–48 h. In unstable infants, repair should be delayed until their condition improves significantly. Patients on ECMO pose a challenge regarding the best time to operate. Options include: operating early in the course of the ECMO run, to allow for more time on ECMO after the operation; waiting until the infant is close to coming off, in case the patient deteriorates postoperatively or needs to come off abruptly due to bleeding; and delaying surgery until after decannulation, so that the risk of bleeding is minimized, but recognizing that a few will need to go back on ECMO. Ultimately, the decision as to when to operate is based on institutional mores and surgeons preference. We prefer to wait until the child is nearly ready to come off ECMO or has already been decannulated.

Patients who undergo surgical repair while on ECMO are at significant risk of hemorrhage. Platelets must be maintained above 100,000/mm³ and the heparin infusion should be decreased to bring the activated clotting time down to between 170 and 180 s. Some routinely use ε-aminocaproic acid (Amicar 100 mg/kg IV load followed by 20 mg/kg/h IV infusion) to decrease intra-operative bleeding, but one must consider the increased risk of thrombotic events and clotting of the ECMO circuit. Tissues should be handled gently with minimal blunt dissection and liberal use of electrocautery. The spleen is especially friable and splenectomy is sometimes necessary to stop bleeding from what would otherwise be considered a minor injury.

The operation can be performed in the operating room when the infant is perfectly stable, but it is nearly always preferable to undertake repair in the NICU. The infants is prepared by starting muscle relaxants the evening before to help minimize bowel gas, blood products are prepared and supplied in syringes at the bedside to allow rapid infusion, and adequate IV and arterial access is secured ahead of time. An open abdominal approach is standard; however options include: laparoscopy, thoracoscopy, and thoracotomy (apparently favored by Koop). We currently favor laparotomy but are starting to perform the operation using a minimally invasive approach in select patients. The infant is positioned supine with a small roll placed across the back at the level of the diaphragm. A transverse incision in the upper quadrant allows excellent exposure and typically heals nicely, though some prefer a subcostal incision. The peritoneum is entered and with gentle traction, the stomach, spleen, tail of pancreas, and small and large intestine are reduced into the abdomen. It is best to keep the bowel in the abdomen, tucked behind a moist laparotomy pad and kept in place with gentle traction. This decreases heat and insensible water loss, minimizes bowel edema, and increases the likelihood that a tension-free fascial closure will be achievable. The kidney is sometimes partially herniated into the chest, obscuring the posterior rim of diaphragm, and should be gently retracted inferiorly. A hernia sac is found in 10–15 % of cases and should be completely excised.

The edges of the defect are then carefully inspected. The posterior remnant, sometimes collapsed accordion-like in the retroperitoneum, should be sought out and unfurled. A decision needs to then be made as to whether a primary repair can be achieved without tension. If the defect is too large, most surgeons prefer to use a polytetrafluoroethylene patch. Such repairs are generally durable but increase the risk of infection, recurrent hernia, chest wall deformity, and scoliosis as the child grows. Alternatively, a latissimus dorsi flap can be used and is especially useful if the patch becomes infected and needs to be removed. Primary repair is performed with interrupted simple or figure-of-eight 3-0 polypropylene sutures. Some prefer to place a chest tube but this is usually unnecessary as the air will gradually be replaced by fluid and then eventually by lung and adjacent tissue. Alternatively, the air can be replaced with saline prior to completing the closure. Because of the high risk of postoperative bleeding in the child being repaired on ECMO, it is better to leave a chest tube (and a closed-suction peritoneal drain).

If the intestine is malrotated, a formal Ladd procedure should be undertaken. Appendectomy should be performed by inversion, especially if a patch was used. A tension-free fascial closure is sometimes difficult to achieve and occasionally requires use of a temporary silo, especially if there is respiratory embarrassment or concern about a possible abdominal compartment syndrome. Some will use an absorbable mesh or simply close the skin, leaving an incisional hernia, but these techniques are to be condemned because of the risk of complications and the extreme difficulty of the subsequent fascial repair. For all but the largest defects, a small transverse incision allows for excellent exposure, secure fascial approximation, and acceptable cosmesis.

Right-sided defects pose additional challenges – the patients are generally sicker and the defects are more difficult to repair. Exposure can be difficult, sometimes necessitating a thoraco-abdominal or primarily thoracic approach. Reduction of the liver into the abdomen can cause kinking of the hepatic veins or inferior vena cava, resulting in abrupt hemodynamic instability. This must therefore be done gradually and with continuous cardiac and blood pressure monitoring. The liver capsule is typically also friable and prone to rupture.

Outcomes

The overall survival of infants with CDH now approaches 80%. However, despite many advances and the widespread application of ECMO, the mortality remains disappointingly high. This can be attributed somewhat to comorbidities but is mostly due to the clinical effects of pulmonary hypertension, for which a specific and effective treatment has been elusive.

Some infants will require long-term ventilator support for severe pulmonary hypoplasia. There is also a higher risk of late effects of therapy including ototoxicity, neurocognitive deficits, and feeding difficulties. For optimal follow up of these complex patients, we employ a multidisciplinary approach that includes a pediatric surgeon, an experienced surgical nurse practitioner, a neonatologist, a pulmonologist, a cardiologist, a developmental pediatrician, a social worker, and a nutritionist. Others are consulted as needed: gastroenterology, speech, audiology, ophthalmology, feeding team, and orthopedics.

Gastroesophageal reflux is a common clinical problem for patients who have undergone repair of a CDH. Failure to thrive or complications such as aspiration pneumonia, reactive airways disease, or life-threatening events related to aspiration are indications for antireflux surgery. Children with concomitant feeding difficulty might also benefit from placement of a gastrostomy button.

Some patients will develop complications related to the presence of the artificial patch as they grow, including an obvious chest wall deformity or scoliosis. Elective removal of the patch might improve the cosmetic appearance but this is by no means assured.

Minimally Invasive Approaches

Minimal access surgical techniques are increasingly being applied to the repair of congenital diaphragmatic hernia. Despite the seemingly straightforward concept of suture repair or patch replacement of a simple tissue defect, many technical challenges remain. These include: how best to reduce the hernia contents and keep them from getting in the way during the repair, how to place the sutures securely and in such a way that tension is distributed evenly, and how best to place a patch in such a small space without increasing the risk of recurrent herniation. It is also usually not feasible to perform a minimally invasive operation in the NICU, making it necessary to transport a potentially labile infant a long distance to the operating room.

The thoracoscopic approach has the theoretical advantage of one not having to work around the reduced abdominal organs. It is also a larger and "cleaner" field to work in. Some believe that the positive pressure generated by CO_2 insufflation helps to push the bowel down into the abdomen, which is true at first, but once the gas fills the abdominal cavity, as it inevitably does through the hernia defect, the pressure gradient disappears. In addition, gas insufflation in the chest can compromise ventilation and venous return and if the child is positioned in a decubitus position, ventilation of the dependent "good" lung is further limited. Thoracoscopy is sometimes made more difficult in newborns due to very high end-tidal CO_2 levels, which often requires high inspiratory pressures and increased minute ventilation, options not considered safe in most infants with CDH. Nevertheless, many feel the thoracoscopic approach is superior and allows them to place multiple sutures that are brought out through the chest wall before being tied down one by one to allow an even distribution of tension. In the end, the surgeon must resist the temptation to cut corners or leave even a single stitch that is inadequate – if the operation is not being done with same attention to detail and quality as the open repair, then it should not be done.

The laparoscopic approach is feasible and especially useful for smaller defects, Morgagni hernias, and when dealing with older children. It is common to require an extra port for retraction of abdominal contents and proper exposure. A liver retractor is useful to hold the spleen and stomach down and away from the surgical field. The same principle of tension-free closure is paramount. Even with experience, good exposure, and meticulous technique, these operations can be very long and extremely tedious, making operator fatigue and exposure of a fragile infant to an excessively long operation potential patient safety concerns that need to be weighed carefully when deciding on the best approach. This is especially true for large defects that require patch closure, which should probably be an indication for conversion to open.

Morgagni Hernia

Anterior diaphragmatic hernias are due to defects in the pars sternalis of the diaphragm. They are thought to represent no more than 5% of all diaphragmatic hernias, are nearly always on the right side, and often cause no symptoms. Herniated organs usually include the transverse colon and omentum. Associated anomalies are described in up to half of cases, including congenital heart disease and chromosomal abnormalities. Although strangulation and ischemia of hernia contents has been described, many are discovered incidentally as an anterior chest mass or "pneumonia." If suspected on the basis of a chest radiograph, the diagnosis is confirmed by CT or MRI.

Asymptomatic Morgagni hernias in asymptomatic adults can sometimes be observed, but surgical repair is recommended in children. The surgical approach can be open or minimally invasive, thoracic or abdominal. Laparoscopic repair is probably the most effective and has become the standard at many centers. Nearly all have an associated hernia sac, which can often only be partially removed because it is densely adherent to the pericardium. Primary repair is usually feasible and can be performed by bringing the anterior and posterior portions of the defect together with interrupted permanent sutures, although patch repair is sometimes necessary. Insufflation of the abdomen has a tendency to enlarge the defect and create tension on the repair. It is therefore recommended that the insufflation pressure be lowered to 5 or 6 mmHg and that the repair be effected by starting at the lateral aspects of the defect and working sequentially towards the middle. Manually pushing down on the lower portion of the sternum during the operation is also sometimes helpful.

These children do not have the same physiologic derangements that are seen in those with Bochdalek hernias and usually tolerate the operation extremely well. Some are coincidentally noted to have malrotation but this is not a common feature. Results of surgical repair are generally quite good but recurrence has been described and patients should be followed for at least a year or two to check for this. If the sac is not completely excised, it frequently fills with fluid, giving the appearance of a possible recurrence. However, patients are typically asymptomatic and these "cysts" can usually be safely observed until they eventually resolve spontaneously.

Summary Points

- There are two distinct anatomic forms of congenital diaphragmatic hernia, which also differ significantly in their physiologic effects.
- The more common posterolateral defect (Bochdalek) produces clinically significant pulmonary hypoplasia and a predilection for pulmonary hypertension.
- Anterior defects (Morgagni) are rare and frequently cause few symptoms.
- The management of newborns with CDH has evolved from an emphasis on aggressive mechanical ventilation and emergency surgery to a strategy that includes gentle ventilation, ECMO when necessary, and elective surgical repair.
- The goal of gentilation with permissive hypercapnia is to avoid ventilator-associated lung injury and allow some time for the lung to mature and for pulmonary hypertension to resolve.

Differential Diagnosis

- Congenital cystic adenomatoid malformation (CCAM)
- Pulmonary sequestration

Diagnostic Studies

- Chest X-ray
- Ultrafast fetal MR
- Amniocentesis
- Echocardiogram

Parental Preparation

- The principal causes of morbidity and mortality in infants with CDH are pulmonary hypoplasia and pulmonary hypertension, not the hernia itself.
- ECMO is a bridge that allows the lungs to mature but is not a treatment.

Preoperative Preparation

- ☐ Echocardiogram
- ☐ Stabilization of cardiopulmonary status

Technical Points

- Surgical repair is best delayed until the infant is stable.
- Most surgeons use an open transabdominal approach, though repair can also be performed by thoracotomy, thoracoscopy or laparoscopy.
- If the repair is performed while the infant is on ECMO, lower the activated clotting time somewhat and consider using ε-aminocaproic acid to minimize the risk of bleeding.
- Primary repair, usually with interrupted permanent sutures, is ideal but not always possible.
- If the defect is too large to close primarily, most surgeons use a polytetrafluoroethylene patch.
- A muscle flap can also be used to repair the diaphragm, especially if the artificial patch has become infected and needs to be removed and replaced.
- A chest tube is not usually necessary unless there is an air leak from the lung or a significant risk of bleeding (on ECMO).

Suggested Reading

Al-Salem AH. Congenital hernia of Morgagni in infants and children. J Pediatr Surg. 2007;42(9):1539–43.

Arca MJ, Barnhart DC, Lelli Jr JL, Greenfeld J, Harmon CM, Hirschl RB, et al. Early experience with minimally invasive repair of congenital diaphragmatic hernias: results and lessons learned. J Pediatr Surg. 2003;38(11):1563–8.

Danzer E, Davey MG, Kreiger PA, Ruchelli ED, Johnson MP, Adzick NS, et al. Fetal tracheal occlusion for severe congenital diaphragmatic hernia in humans: a morphometric study of lung parenchyma and muscularization of pulmonary arterioles. J Pediatr Surg. 2008;43(10):1767–75.

Hedrick HL. Management of prenatally diagnosed congenital diaphragmatic hernia. Semin Fetal Neonatal Med. 2010;15(1):21–7.

Hedrick HL, Crombleholme TM, Flake AW, Nance ML, von Allmen D, Howell LJ, et al. Right congenital diaphragmatic hernia: prenatal assessment and outcome. J Pediatr Surg. 2004;39(3):319–23.

Kim AC, Bryner BS, Akay B, Geiger JD, Hirschl RB, Mychaliska GB. Thoracoscopic repair of congenital diaphragmatic hernia in neonates: lessons learned. J Laparoendosc Adv Surg Tech A. 2009;19(4):575–80.

Nasr A, Struijs MC, Ein SH, Langer JC, Chiu PP. Outcomes after muscle flap vs prosthetic patch repair for large congenital diaphragmatic hernias. J Pediatr Surg. 2010;45(1):151–4.

Ruano R, Aubry MC, Barthe B, Dumez Y, Benachi A. Three-dimensional ultrasonographic measurements of the fetal lungs for prediction of perinatal outcome in isolated congenital diaphragmatic hernia. J Obstet Gynaecol Res. 2009;35(6):1031–41.

Chapter 69
Uncommon Hernias

Shaheen J. Timmapuri and Rajeev Prasad

Hernias are among the most common conditions encountered by pediatric surgeons. Although inguinal and umbilical hernias are by far the most prevalent, rarer types of hernias are occasionally encountered in children. Because they are so rare, most of the information regarding the treatment of these conditions is anecdotal. A clear understanding of the anatomy and techniques for repair of these hernias is critical for developing an appropriate management plan. An incorrect or delayed diagnosis can lead to significant complications, including bowel obstruction, ischemia, or perforation.

Unusual Inguinal Hernias

Incarcerated hernias with unusual contents and historically named after Littre, Amyand, and Richter, can occur in any abdominal wall or inguinal defect. Although rare in any age group, *Littre's hernia*, in which the hernia sac contains a Meckel's diverticulum, are extremely uncommon in the pediatric population. Preoperative diagnosis is nearly impossible. Radiographic evaluation (US, CT) is often unhelpful, aside from confirming the presence of a hernia. The usual evaluation for a suspected incarcerated hernia should be undertaken to ensure prompt reduction and to prevent ischemic consequences. Besides bowel ischemia, other complications include pain, bleeding, and perforation. Inflammation of the Meckel's diverticulum can create dense adhesions to the hernia sac. The optimal treatment consists of hernia repair and resection of the diverticulum. If thorough inspection and proper resection are not possible through the inguinal incision, it might be necessary to make an additional incision on the abdomen. Proponents of laparoscopic hernia repair have reported cases in which the Meckel's diverticulum was identified and reduced laparoscopically, and then resected through an umbilical incision.

This approach might allow better visualization of the bowel than is possible through a standard inguinal incision.

Amyand's hernia is an inguinal hernia in which the hernia sac contains a normal or acutely inflamed appendix. As with Littre's hernias, they are nearly impossible to diagnose preoperatively. The presentation is similar to that of any incarcerated or strangulated inguinal hernia: tenderness, erythema, inability to reduce the hernia contents. There are several case reports in the literature of acute appendicitis occurring within a hernia sac mimicking a strangulated inguinal hernia or testicular torsion. The significance of acute appendicitis within the sac is unclear. Inflammation of the appendix can be incidental or perhaps a consequence of incarceration.

The treatment of Amyand's hernias consists of hernia repair and appendectomy, which can be performed using a laparoscopic-assisted approach. Postoperative management depends on the condition of the appendix at the time of surgery. Prolonged hospitalization for long-term antibiotics is sometimes necessary for perforated appendicitis and patients should be monitored for complications such as intra-abdominal abscess and sepsis.

Richter's hernia occurs when only the antimesenteric portion of a segment of bowel wall protrudes through a hernia defect. Because the entire circumference of the intestine is not involved, these hernias do not present with the usual symptoms of a bowel obstruction even in the setting of incarceration. This can lead to bowel wall ischemia and perforation if unrecognized or if an involved ischemic segment is unknowingly reduced. Therefore, surgeons should have a high index of suspicion for ischemia if a child has abdominal symptoms following hernia reduction or repair. The treatment is a standard hernia repair, with careful inspection of the involved intestinal segment, if necessary using an abdominal counter-incision.

Femoral Hernias

Femoral hernias account for approximately 1% of pediatric groin hernias. They are frequently misdiagnosed, as often as 75% in some series. The femoral hernia is often confused

S.J. Timmapuri (✉)
Department of Pediatric Surgery, Drexel University, St. Christopher's Hospital for Children, Erie Ave at Front Street, Philadelphia, PA 19134, USA
e-mail: shaheen.timmapuri@tenethealth.com

P. Mattei (ed.), *Fundamentals of Pediatric Surgery*,
DOI 10.1007/978-1-4419-6643-8_69, © Springer Science+Business Media, LLC 2011

with an indirect inguinal hernia and the correct diagnosis is usually made upon inguinal exploration. It can also be mistaken for an enlarged lymph node, lipoma, or abscess. Because these hernias are so rare in children, understanding the anatomy is critical for making a correct diagnosis and ensuring appropriate and prompt treatment.

The etiology remains unclear but an anatomic defect, such as an enlarged femoral ring, is probably the cause in most cases. Though more common in adults, acquired etiologies (increased intra-abdominal pressure, prior inguinal surgery) are in some cases thought to be contributing factors. The majority of pediatric patients with femoral hernias are less than 10 years of age, supporting a congenital rather than acquired etiology.

As the diagnosis is usually not considered preoperatively, many patients present with a recurrent groin bulge after an inguinal hernia repair. Femoral hernias are located lateral and inferior to the pubic tubercle and inferior to the inguinal ligament. The diagnosis can usually be made by thorough physical examination. Some patients complain of pain in the ipsilateral lower extremity, which is caused by pressure on the femoral nerve. The pain disappears with flexion of the thigh (Astley Cooper sign).

Many surgical techniques for the repair of femoral hernias have been described; but because these hernias are rarely reported in children, no large series exist to objectively compare them. The McVay hernia repair (approximation of Cooper's ligament to the conjoined tendon) is probably the most widely used technique. Laparoscopy has recently been described for the diagnosis and repair of femoral hernias.

The most common error made regarding femoral hernia repairs is misdiagnosis. This results in inadequate treatment at the first operation and patients being subjected to repeated procedures for a "recurrent" hernia. In patients with negative explorations for suspected indirect inguinal hernias, the diagnosis of a femoral hernia should be considered. The most significant operative complications are recurrence and intestinal compromise secondary to strangulation.

Spigelian Hernias

Fewer than fifty cases of Spigelian hernia in the pediatric age group have been reported in the literature. These hernias occur lateral to the rectus abdominus muscle along the semilunar line. In adults and older children, these hernias are thought to be the result of trauma, neoplasms, or prior abdominal operations. However, the occurrence of Spigelian hernias in neonates has raised the possibility of a congenital etiology. In these patients, associated findings of inguinal hernias and cryptorchid testes have been described.

The diagnosis of a Spigelian hernia can be made clinically when a bulge is present along the semilunar line. This is often a subtle finding because of the overlying intact external oblique muscle, which prevents complete herniation of abdominal contents. If unclear clinically, US, CT or MRI sometimes aids in confirming the diagnosis. Once diagnosed, Spigelian hernias should be repaired in order to alleviate associated discomfort and prevent incarceration. Primary repair is almost always possible in children and can be accomplished through a transverse incision directly over the fascial defect. Prosthetic material is sometimes necessary for larger defects. Laparoscopy has been found to be very useful for both diagnosis and treatment. The hernias can be repaired entirely laparoscopically or by using laparoscopy as an adjunct to identify the exact site of the hernia and guide incision placement.

Because of the often subtle nature of Spigelian hernias, the diagnosis is challenging. In patients without an obvious bulge on examination but with a good history, radiologic studies might be helpful. Recurrence after repair is rare, especially with small defects. Other complications relate to intestinal ischemia secondary to incarceration.

Lumbar Hernias

Although approximately 10% of all lumbar hernias are congenital in origin, congenital lumbar hernias (CLH) account for the majority of cases in children. In older children and adults, acquired lumbar hernias result from trauma, infection or prior surgery. The most common types are Grynfelt-Lesshaft hernias and Petit hernias. *Grynfelt-Lesshaft hernias* occur in the superior lumbar triangle, bordered by the inferior aspect of the 12th rib, the internal oblique muscle, and the quadratus lumborum. *Petit hernias* occur in the inferior lumbar triangle, whose borders are the external oblique muscle, the latissimus dorsi muscle, and the iliac crest. Combinations of both hernia types are occasionally seen and result in a large defect.

The etiology of CLH is not completely clear. Possible factors are developmental anomalies, such as aplasia of lumbar muscles, nerve entrapment, and increased pressure due to an intra-abdominal mass. Most present in the first year of life. They tend to be unilateral and have well-defined borders. The diagnosis is made on physical examination and the classification is based on the anatomic location. Associated anomalies are present in nearly two-thirds of patients with CLH. These include lumbocostovertebral syndrome, caudal regression syndrome, diaphragmatic hernia, ureteropelvic junction obstruction, cloacal exstrophy, and, rarely, lipomeningocele.

After the associated medical conditions are properly addressed, repair of CLH is recommended to prevent incarceration. As with other hernia types, primary repair is the preferred method; however, especially with combined defects, the hernia can involve the entire lateral abdominal wall, and repair with prosthetic material is often necessary. Recurrence is rare and usually occurs in patients with other significant morbidities.

Traumatic Abdominal Wall Hernias

Traumatic abdominal wall hernias (TAWH) are rare defects which result from high- or low-velocity blunt trauma. The actual injury is caused by an object projecting enough force to cause damage to muscle and fascial layers without penetrating the skin. The elastic nature of the skin allows it to remain intact while the other abdominal wall layers are disrupted. Three types of TAWH have been described: Type I hernias are small defects caused by blunt trauma (handlebar injury), Type II result from high-velocity traumas (motor vehicle accidents, falls) and tend to be larger, and Type III, which typically result from deceleration injuries and involve herniation of intra-abdominal contents. TAWH are usually seen in the lower abdomen but can occur anywhere on the abdominal wall.

Not all TAWH are evident immediately following the traumatic event but rather can present in a delayed fashion weeks or months later. To make the diagnosis of TAWH, patients should have had clear abdominal wall trauma without evidence of a hernia prior to the injury. The diagnosis is usually based on history and physical examination, however swelling or hematoma in the area of injury can obscure the bulge of the hernia, in which case radiographic studies (plain abdominal films, US, CT) can be useful for confirming the diagnosis and excluding other injuries.

Although all patients with abdominal trauma must be carefully evaluated, children with the smaller Type I defects rarely have concurrent intra-abdominal injuries. Repair is indicated whenever the diagnosis is made. Other traumatic injuries must be appropriately addressed, sometimes necessitating laparotomy. However, in the absence of other intra-abdominal pathology, a local wound exploration with primary closure of the hernia in multiple layers should be performed. Larger defects might require the use of prosthetic material for an adequate tension-free closure. Diagnostic laparoscopy is used in some patients to evaluate abdominal injuries and obviate the need for a larger laparotomy incision. This approach allows for a thorough abdominal exploration and subsequent local hernia repair in patients with no additional injuries.

Rare hernias in the pediatric population are frequently difficult to diagnose. Physical findings are vague and radiographic studies are unhelpful. Misdiagnosis of these defects can have serious consequences such as bowel ischemia, obstruction, and perforation. A clear understanding of the anatomy, along with a preoperative management plan, aid in the diagnosis and treatment of these uncommon hernias.

Summary Points

- Understanding the anatomy and repair techniques for various uncommon hernias is critical for appropriate diagnosis and management.
- Diagnosis of most hernias is based on history and physical examination.
- Misdiagnosis leads to complications, including bowel obstruction, incarceration, and perforation.

Editor's Comment

One of the rarest hernias seen in children is the direct inguinal hernia. Essentially all pediatric inguinal hernias are of the indirect variety (patent processus) and therefore high ligation is all that is necessary. It is very rare to discover that the floor of the inguinal canal is deficient either before or during an inguinal hernia repair. With the possible exception of a second recurrence or a child with a known connective tissue disorder, the use of an artificial material is not recommended for inguinal hernia repair in a child because of the uncertain long-term effects and the possibility of injury to adjacent structures. Rather, a traditional technique, such as the McVay Cooper ligament repair, is favored.

Spigelian hernias are frequently considered but rarely found. Patients will sometimes provide a history that is textbook, only to have intact fascia by physical examination, imaging studies, and even local exploration. It can be very frustrating for all involved. Although MRI and laparoscopy provide the best available techniques for confirmation of a hernia, no study or combination of studies is especially accurate.

The eponymous inguinal hernias are mostly of historical interest as they rarely cause true clinical mayhem – when performing an inguinal hernia repair, the surgeon must be prepared to deal with any number of surprises. The one exception is the Richter's hernia, which can be easily missed when one assumes that incarcerated hernia has been ruled out because of the absence of obstructive symptoms. The consequences of this error, bowel necrosis and perforation, can be dire. Imaging studies can also be deceiving, reinforcing the adage that, when in doubt, the patient should be explored.

Diastasis recti is not a true hernia and should never be operated upon, but parents often need to be repeatedly reassured. Likewise, epigastric hernias (epiploceles) should only be repaired if they become large or symptomatic. Despite being true hernias, they are almost always tiny, allowing only a small amount of properitoneal fat to herniated, and are thus generally harmless. Finally, incisional hernias can occur whenever a surgical procedure has been performed and are usually easily confirmed on physical examination. The exception is the rare trocar site hernia, which can be difficult to diagnose. The combination of pain and a lump at a trocar site should usually prompt surgical exploration to rule out a hernia.

Differential Diagnosis

- Littre's hernia (contains Meckel's diverticulum)
- Amyand's hernia (contains appendix)
- Richter's hernia (incarcerated antimesenteric portion of bowel)
- Femoral hernia
- Lymphadenopathy
- Abscess
- Spigelian hernia
- Traumatic abdominal wall hernia
- Lumbar hernia
- Traumatic abdominal wall hernia

Diagnostic Studies

- Plain radiographs
- Ultrasound
- CT
- MRI

Preoperative Preparation

- ☐ Informed consent
- ☐ Careful evaluation of preoperative studies

Parental Preparation

- Risk of infection, bleeding (hematoma), error in diagnosis, and recurrence.
- Some abdominal wall hernias are rare and difficult to confirm or exclude even with sophisticated imaging modalities.

Technical Points

- Although not always possible, accurate preoperative diagnosis allows appropriate operative planning.
- Careful evaluation of involved bowel is critical to identify an ischemic or perforated segment.
- Laparoscopy is a useful adjunct in the diagnosis and management of unusual hernias.

Suggested Reading

Chan KW, Lee KH, Mou JWC, et al. The use of laparoscopy in the management of Littre's hernia in children. Pediatr Surg Int. 2008;24:855–8.
DeCaluwe D, Chertin B, Puri P. Childhood femoral hernia: a commonly misdiagnosed condition. Pediatr Surg Int. 2003;19:608–9.
Fakhry SM, Azizkhan RG. Observations and current operative management of congenital lumbar hernias during infancy. Surg Gynecol Obstet. 1991;172:475–9.
Goliath J, Mittal V, McDonough J. Traumatic handlebar hernia: a rare abdominal wall hernia. J Pediatr Surg. 2004;39:e20–2.
Livaditi E, Mavridis G, Christopoulos G. Amyand's hernia in premature neonates: report of two cases. Hernia. 2007;11:547–9.
Losanoff JE, Richman BW, Jones JW. Spigelian hernia in a child: case report and review of the literature. Hernia. 2002;6:191–3.
Messina M, Ferrucci E, Meucci D, et al. Littre's hernia in newborn infants: report of two cases. Pediatr Surg Int. 2005;21:485–7.
Temiz A, Akcora B, Temiz M, et al. A rare and frequently unrecognized pathology in children: femoral hernia. Hernia. 2008;12:553–6.
Tycast JF, Kumpf AL, Schwartz TL, et al. Amyand's hernia: a case report describing laparoscopic repair in a pediatric patient. J Pediatr Surg. 2008;43:2112–4.
Wakhlu A, Wakhlu AK. Congenital lumbar hernia. Pediatr Surg Int. 2000;16:146–8.

Chapter 70
Umbilical Diorders and Anomalies

Adam J. Kaye and Daniel J. Ostlie

An abnormal umbilicus represents one of the most frequent indications for pediatric surgical consultation. In the newborn, the majority of umbilical abnormalities are related to the embryologic development and function of the umbilicus. The formation of the umbilical region of the abdominal wall begins in the fourth week of gestation. The embryo attaches to the primitive placenta by a stalk that will eventually house the umbilical vessels and the allantois, which together form the umbilical cord. The vitelline duct also briefly runs within this stalk connecting the yolk sac as it divides into intracoelomic and extracoelomic portions by the in-folding embryo. The intracoelomic portion forms the alimentary canal and the remaining extracoelomic yolk sac feeds the embryo through the vitelline duct. This duct normally closes between the fifth and seventh week of gestation as the placenta begins to provide nutritional support to the embryo.

The allantois is a diverticulum that forms from the posterior aspect of the yolk sac during the third gestational week and ultimately remains in the umbilical cord to serve as the extra-embryonic portion of the urachus, which connects to the urinary bladder. With normal development, the urachus obliterates into a band-like structure leaving no patent connection between the bladder and umbilicus.

Between the sixth and tenth weeks of gestation there is rapid intestinal growth and the developing midgut forms outside of the peritoneal cavity, within the base of the umbilical cord. The midgut eventually returns to the peritoneal cavity and, with intestinal rotation and fixation, comes to rest in its proper orientation. The umbilical ring then normally contracts and closes near birth. Any deviation from this normal development manifests as an umbilical anomaly. These abnormalities are commonly associated with persistent embryonic umbilical cord structures or failure of the umbilical ring to close at birth, and can be categorized as masses, infections, or drainage.

Umbilical masses make up the majority of referrals and usually involve a reducible bulge, a hard mass, or excess skin at the umbilicus. There are four major anomalies associated with these findings: umbilical granuloma, umbilical polyp, umbilical hernia and the trunk-like umbilicus.

Umbilical Granuloma

The umbilical cord separates from the umbilicus 3 days to 2 months after birth. Following separation, a small painless mass of beefy red granulation tissue usually forms at the base. These granulomas vary in size from 0.1 to 1 cm in size and produce variable amounts of drainage that can irritate the skin. Umbilical granulomas are normally treated with silver nitrate though more than one treatment is often necessary. If it does not respond to normal chemical cauterization techniques, an umbilical polyp should be suspected. If a duct remnant can be ruled out by a detailed history and careful inspection, a pedunculated umbilical granuloma can usually be safely and painlessly ligated in the office with a surgical suture. The parents are instructed to bathe the infant as per their usual routine and the granuloma should dry up and fall off within 2 weeks.

Umbilical Polyp

An umbilical polyp is most commonly a retained portion of the vitelline duct. They are generally shiny red and smooth in appearance and contain portions of small bowel mucosa. However, there are case reports of umbilical polyps containing bladder mucosa originating from the urachus. Umbilical polyps will not regress with cauterization and should be surgically excised.

Umbilical Hernia

Umbilical hernias are associated with failure of normal closure of the umbilical ring. A peritoneum-lined sac protrudes through the hernia defect and is attached to the overlying skin.

A.J. Kaye (✉)
Department of Pediatric Surgery, Children's Mercy Hospital, 2401 Gillham Road, Kansas City, MO 64108, USA
e-mail: ajkaye@cmh.edu

P. Mattei (ed.), *Fundamentals of Pediatric Surgery*,
DOI 10.1007/978-1-4419-6643-8_70, © Springer Science+Business Media, LLC 2011

Fig. 70.1 (a) The typical appearance of an umbilical hernia in a 4-year-old African American male. (b) A proboscoid umbilical hernia in a 6-year-old male. Note the beak-like extension outward and the significant redundant umbilical skin

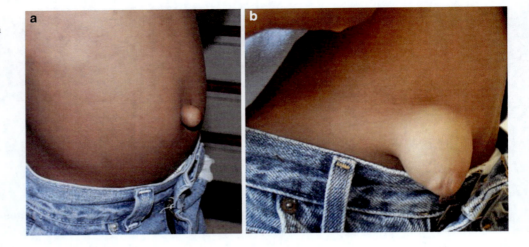

Umbilical hernias show no gender predilection, however there is a higher incidence in children of African descent. Umbilical hernias also occur very commonly in low birth weight infants but most will resolve. Umbilical hernias diagnosed within the first 6 months of life and less than 1 cm in size will generally close spontaneously by 4 years of age. Since most small hernias will close spontaneously, it is standard to delay any surgical correction until the children is at least 2 years of age. Umbilical hernias larger than 2 cm or those with a large amount of excess skin (proboscoid) are not likely to close spontaneously and should be surgically closed once the child is older than 2 years of age. (Fig. 70.1) For hernias smaller than 1 cm, it is reasonable to wait until 4 or 5 years of age. However, if the child has any signs of obstruction (abdominal pain associated with the hernia or bilious emesis) or if the hernia becomes a tender hard mass, immediate exploration and repair of the hernia is required.

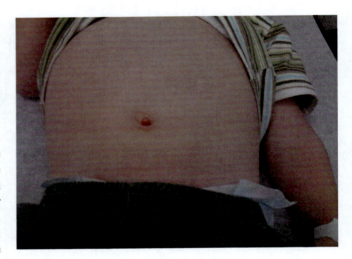

Fig. 70.2 A trunk-like umbilicus in a 1-year-old. At operative repair, there was no herniation, but rather redundant skin and subcutaneous fat

Trunk-Like Umbilicus

A trunk-like umbilicus protrudes from the abdomen in a proboscoid fashion. This finding was first described by Esch *et al.* in 2004. The umbilical skin does not house a hernia or an abdominal wall defect. Instead there is simply excess skin and fat protruding ventrally. (Fig. 70.2) The diagnosis should prompt a careful search for an anomalous association or dysmorphic syndrome. Three rare syndromes associated with a large protuberant umbilicus include Reiger's syndrome, Aarskog–Scott syndrome and Robinow's syndrome. These syndromes have other more severe findings and early diagnosis can help limit morbidity. The umbilical abnormality can be revised with simple excision or umbilicoplasty.

Infections

Omphalitis

Omphalitis is an infection of the umbilicus that is generally seen in hospitalized newborns. Modern infection control techniques, such as antibiotic ointments and alcohol preparations applied to the umbilical stump, have reduced the rate of omphalitis from 65% to less than 1%. The primary pathogens associated with omphalitis are skin flora, especially *Staphylococcus aureus* and *Streptococcus pyogenes*, though many infections are now polymicrobial and can include gram negative bacteria. Rarely, omphalitis can progress to necrotizing fasciitis.

Urachal Cyst

Although the urachus normally obliterates completely throughout its course from the bladder to the allantois, sometimes a cyst will form along its route. These cysts usually remain undiagnosed until they become infected, presenting as a tender mass, often with overlying skin erythema. The mass is usually located in the midline between the umbilicus and the pubis. An ultrasound study is usually adequate for diagnosis, however computed tomography has been used more frequently of late (Fig. 70.3). Control of the infection with antibiotics and incisions and drainage of the abscess may be required, eventually followed by surgical resection to excise the cyst entirely. Surgical excision is difficult and potentially hazardous in the presence of residual infection so waiting 4–6 weeks after treatment is often recommended.

Drainage

Patent Urachus

A patent urachus develops secondary to failure of normal obliteration of the tract between the umbilicus and bladder, leaving a draining sinus. Clear drainage from the umbilicus should raise the suspicion for a patent urachus. An erythematous or excoriated rash due to constant contact with urine may also occur. A patent urachal tract can be further defined by taking a lateral abdominal X-ray after injecting contrast into the draining umbilical sinus (Fig. 70.4). It is important to completely evaluate the urinary tract prior to repairing this anomaly, as the patent urachus may be serving as a release

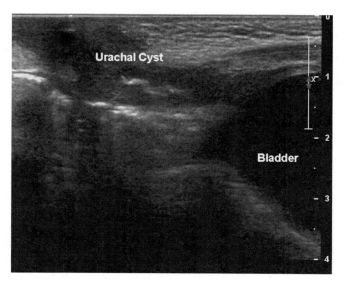

Fig. 70.3 An abdominal ultrasound scan showing an inflamed urachal cyst (UC) just above the dome of the bladder (B)

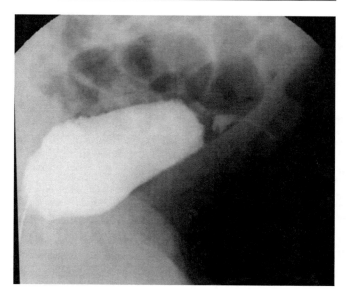

Fig. 70.4 A lateral view of contrast injected into a draining sinus from the umbilicus demonstrating a patent urachus with contrast entering the bladder

valve in the setting of a more distal obstruction such as posterior urethral valves. As such, males are three times more likely to have a patent urachus than females.

Patent Vitelline (Omphalomesenteric) Duct

The vitelline duct connects the embryonic midgut and yolk sac. A number of abnormalities can arise from incomplete obliteration of this duct. In addition to the umbilical polyp, other remnants include cysts containing intestinal or pancreatic mucosa, Meckel's diverticulum, and patent vitelline duct, the diagnosis of which is usually suggested by the drainage of succus or fecal material from the umbilicus. In some cases, the proximal or distal ileum may prolapse through the umbilicus (Fig. 70.5). Contrast studies through the draining sinus are rarely necessary for diagnosis.

Umbilical-Appendiceal Fistula

There are reports of a transected vermiform appendix being found in the umbilicus causing an umbilical-appendiceal fistula. Though some have posited that this may be a type of vitelline duct remnant that forms from the appendix rather than its usual location in the ileum, the most likely explanation is that an appendix that protrudes through the umbilical ring at birth is severed when the umbilical cord is cut. This fistula is usually mistaken for a patent vitelline duct and the true diagnosis is usually only noted at the time of the operation.

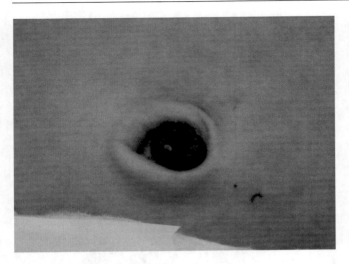

Fig. 70.5 Prolapsed intestinal mucosa from the umbilicus related to a patent vitelline (omphalomesenteric) duct

Treatment

Preoperative Preparation

Treatment for an umbilical hernia or trunk-like umbilicus is performed in an outpatient setting in an otherwise healthy child. No special preoperative preparation is necessary. Children with a patent urachus should be evaluated for the presence of a distal urinary tract obstruction, which should be repaired prior to closure of the urachus.

Surgical Technique

Umbilical herniorrhaphy has changed little since it was first described by Robert Gross in 1953. The mainstays of the surgery are a secure fascial closure and preservation of the umbilicus. The child is positioned supine and an incision is made in the inferior fold of the umbilicus. The subcutaneous tissue is divided down to the linea alba and the hernia sac is circumferentially dissected around the base of the umbilicus. The hernia sac is transected from its attachments to the posterior aspect of the umbilical skin. The fascial edges are identified and approximated transversely using interrupted absorbable sutures. To decrease the risk of intestinal injury secondary to a needle stick, as well as to ensure adequate fascial incorporation, stitches are tied only after all have been placed. The umbilicus is then inverted and the posterior aspect of the umbilical skin is sutured to the fascia with two dermal stitches, one superior and one inferior. The skin is then closed with a running subcuticular absorbable stitch.

Surgical correction for any of the draining anomalies begins with either a curvilinear incision in the inferior fold of the umbilicus, coring out the fistulous tract as it enters the abdomen, or through a midline infraumbilical incision. It is of utmost importance that one identify all of the umbilical structures for a definitive diagnosis. A patent vitelline duct can be traced back to its origin, usually the distal ileum. The duct is then resected, and the ileum is closed primarily in two layers. Rarely, because of ileal inflammation, a segmental resection of the intestine will be required.

The urachal cyst or patent urachus is identified just beneath the fascia in the preperitioneal space. When a urachal cyst is present, it can usually be removed without entering the peritoneum, however the muscular layers of the bladder will need to be closed using absorbable suture. In the case of a patent urachus, the urachus is dissected down to its origin, usually the dome of the bladder, and resected. The bladder defect is repaired in two layers with absorbable suture. The underlying fascial defect is closed and umbilicoplasty is performed to repair the umbilical defect. Laparoscopic repairs of both vitelline duct and urachal anomalies have been reported with good results. Regardless of the approach, the bladder should always be closed using absorbable suture to reduce the risk of stone formation. A standard stapled resection of the ileum is an acceptable alternative in cases of vitelline duct remnants, especially when the laparoscopic approach is utilized.

Umbilicoplasty

When repairing a hernia or trunk-like umbilicus, there can be excessive umbilical skin that prevents an optimal cosmetic result. Conversely, after removal of a patent urachus or vitelline duct, inadequate skin may remain to form a normal appearing umbilicus.

Multiple techniques for umbilicoplasty have been proposed to address these situations, but none is perfect. All umbilicoplasty techniques can be complicated by effacement of the umbilicus, infections, and chronic wounds.

When a large skin defect exists after repair of a patent urachus or vitelline duct, the Marconi technique can result in a satisfactory appearance of the umbilicus. The skin edges around the defect should be trimmed to viable edges and dissected from the underlying subcutaneous tissue. An absorbable monofilament suture is initially placed in the fascia where the center of the umbilical depression will be located. The stitch is then placed intradermally around the edges of the defect in a running purse string fashion. Once the purse string is complete, the suture is tied resulting in inversion of the skin edges.

When there is excess skin, Ikeda et al. describe a different approach that starts with an infraumbilical incision. The subcutaneous fat is removed and two fan-shaped sections of the inferior aspect of the skin are removed, resulting in an arrow head-shaped inferior portion of skin. Each side of the arrow is then sutured using 5-0 absorbable suture to the skin lateral to it, forming a cone. The cone is then inverted and secured to the fascia to make the umbilical depression and the remaining infraumbilical incision is closed with running subcuticular suture.

Postoperative Care

The umbilical hernia patient can be discharged the same day. Historically, it was common practice to place a pressure dressing over the newly repaired umbilicus for 5–7 days to prevent hematoma or seroma. A recent prospective trial showed no difference in outcome with or without such a dressing. The repair of a patent urachus or urachal cyst is also usually undertaken in an outpatient setting. Occasionally patients will experience bladder spasms after urachal resec-

tions. These spasms are best treated with oral oxybutynin. Bladder catheterization is not routinely required for removal of urachal anomalies.

Patients after repair of vitelline duct anomalies will generally require a period of overnight observation. Patients with urachal cysts and ducts that do not require a segmental resection of the intestine can be allowed an unrestricted diet postoperatively. In cases where a segmental resection of the intestine is required, the patient's diet can be advanced after the return of bowel function. Gastric decompression with a nasogastric tube is not required, even when intestinal resection is performed.

Long-term follow up for these abnormalities is not necessary as the underlying disease process is corrected by the appropriate surgical technique, and these children should not require special surgical follow up.

Summary Points

- Umbilical granulomas can be treated with several applications of silver nitrate, or simple ligation in the office if a duct remnant can be ruled out.
- Umbilical polyps contain mucosa and should be surgically excised.
- Most umbilical hernias close spontaneously and can be safely observed until age 3 or 4, while the rare symptomatic or incarcerated umbilical hernia should be repaired emergently.
- The trunk-like umbilicus can be treated with simple excision with or without umbilicoplasty but should prompt a search for signs of a congenital syndrome.
- Thanks to modern infection control techniques, omphalitis is now rarely seen but can be associated with necrotizing fasciitis.
- Umbilical cysts usually present with infection (tender infra-umbilical mass and erythema), and should be treated with antibiotics and surgical drainage before being surgically excised 4–6 weeks later.
- Patent urachus (urachal remnant) permits drainage of urine from the umbilicus that can cause skin excoriation and are occasionally associated with distal urinary obstruction. It is repaired through an infra-umbilical, extraperitoneal incision and excised close to the bladder, which should be repaired in two layers of absorbable suture.
- Vitelline (omphalomesenteric) duct remnants are usually associated with a Meckel's diverticulum, creating an ileal fistula. They are excised through a peri-umbilical incision and occasionally require bowel resection.

Editor's Comment

Most new attending pediatric surgeons are astounded by the number and variety of umbilical disorders that present almost daily in outpatient practice. Umbilical granulomas can usually be treated with silver nitrate, but the pediatrician will have tried two or three times already. Pedunculated granulomas can be ligated after application of alcohol or Betadine using a 000 braided absorbable suture, though almost any sterile suture will do. The granuloma nearly always falls off within 2 weeks. Those that are not amenable to ligation can be treated more aggressively with silver nitrate: apply Vaseline to the surrounding skin, apply the silver nitrate with firm pressure, and repeat the application (or have the parents apply it) on 3 consecutive days. Surgical excision should rarely be necessary and raises the suspicion of a duct remnant.

Parents are often disappointed when the surgeon refuses to repair their child's umbilical hernia before the age of 2 or 3. Usually, gentle reassurance is enough to dissuade them. It is probably true that infants and young children are at greater risk, have inferior long-term cosmetic results, and are more prone to recurrence than children who are repaired after age 2, but none of these statements has been proven. Most pediatric surgeons are taught to excise the sac, close the fascia transversely and use absorbable suture, but there are many experienced surgeons who simply invert the hernia sac into the abdominal cavity after separating it from the skin, close the fascia in the midline, or use permanent sutures (or even running suture) and have excellent results. It is better to decide whether the child will need an umbilicoplasty before you begin the operation, so that the proper incision can be made. There are several different ways to perform an umbilicoplasty, but regardless, it is important to leave some excess skin to prevent effacement of the umbilicus as the child grows. A simple purse-string closure (after amputating the tip of the proboscis) is usually adequate in most cases, though excising three inverted triangles of skin from the edge usually allows better dermal apposition and improved cosmesis. Meticulous hemostasis is crucial, but pressure dressings should never be necessary.

Urachal and omphalomesenteric duct remnants are interesting but relatively straightforward anomalies to repair. A peri-umbilical incision should be used in most cases as it provides the necessary exposure and is more cosmetically acceptable than a midline or large laparotomy incision. A minimal access technique can be used but in most cases is probably more invasive than a simple peri-umbilical incision. It is almost always a mistake to attempt resection of a urachal cyst that is actively infected, as this turns a simple procedure into a complicated and potentially dangerous operation.

Omphalitis can be life-threatening and usually warrants aggressive treatment with hospital admission, intravenous antibiotics, and meticulous surveillance for a necrotizing process. Necrotizing fasciitis is a devastating complication that requires aggressive surgical debridement of the abdominal wall and advanced surgical techniques for delayed reconstruction.

Differential Diagnosis

Mass

- Umbilical hernia
- Umbilical granuloma
- Umbilical polyp
- Trunk-like umbilicus

Infection

- Urachal cyst
- Omphalitis

Drainage

- Patent urachus
- Patent vitelline (omphalomesenteric) duct
- Umbilico-appendiceal fistula

Parental Preparation

- Asymptomatic umbilical hernias require surgical repair if they do not close spontaneously by age 3 or 4, though a large hernia with a great deal of excess skin is unlikely to close after age 2.
- The risks of surgery include infection, hematoma, injury to underlying bowel and recurrence, all of which are very rare.

Diagnostic Studies

Mass

- None

Infection

- Ultrasound
- Computed tomography

Drainage

- Contrast fistulogram

Preoperative Preparation

☐ Standard preoperative checklist.
☐ Antibiotic prophylaxis for urachal and vitelline duct remnant procedures.

Technical Points

- Umbilical hernia repair can be performed safely with absorbable suture. Mesh reinforcement should rarely, if ever, be used, except perhaps in the case of a multiply recurrent hernia, and in no circumstances should the umbilicus be excised or discarded.
- Umbilicoplasty should be performed when there is a great deal of excess skin after umbilical hernia repair. There are several good techniques available.
- Urachal remnants can usually be approached through an infra-umbilical incision in the extra-peritoneal space and should be excised down to the bladder, which is repaired with absorbable suture in two layers.
- Vitelline duct remnants can usually be approached through a cosmetically acceptable peri-umbilical incision and should be excised at the ileum, which can be stapled or closed in standard fashion.

Suggested Reading

McCollum MO, Macneily AE, Blair GK. Surgical implications of urachal remnants, presentation and management. J Pediatr Surg. 2003;38:798–803.

Merei JM. Umbilical hernia repair in children: is pressure dressing necessary. Pediatr Surg Int. 2006;22:446–8.

O'Neill JA, Grosfeld JL, Coran AG, Caldamone AA, editors. Disorders of the umbilicus. Principles of pediatric surgery. St Loius, MO: Mosby; 2003. p. 432–6.

Pomeranz A. Anomalies, abnormalities, and care of the umbilicus. Pediatr Clin North Am. 2004;51:819–27, xii.

Snyder CL. Current management of umbilical abnormalities and related anomalies. Semin Pediatr Surg. 2007;16:41–9.

Chapter 71
Peritoneal Dialysis

Danny Little and Monford D. Custer

The peritoneal cavity has been used in the treatment of critically ill children for the past century. Reports from Blackfan and Maxcy in 1918 demonstrated the feasibility of intraperitoneal injections of saline to resuscitate dehydrated children. The origins of continuous peritoneal lavage stem from the work of Bloxsum and Powell in 1948 and Swan and Gordon in 1949. Their early techniques used large dialysate volumes and continuous gravity dependent flow through a metal peritoneal catheter.

Today, the occasional child with renal failure will undergo pre-emptive transplantation. However, the vast majority of children with chronic renal failure, or those presenting with acute renal failure, will need dialysis access. Hemodialysis, hemofiltration, and peritoneal dialysis are acceptable alternatives to renal replacement. Continuous ambulatory peritoneal dialysis (CAPD) was first used in a child in 1978 in Toronto. Currently, more than 150,000 patients are receiving peritoneal dialysis, and approximately two thirds of children with renal failure will undergo peritoneal dialysis. A reliable catheter is the cornerstone of successful peritoneal dialysis. Implantation technique and postoperative nursing care greatly influence catheter longevity.

The peritoneum possesses several advantages that make it a natural second filter. Percent body surface area, peritoneal blood flow, and vascular permeability all contribute to the effectiveness of peritoneal dialysis (Table 71.1).

Preoperative Preparation

Indications for dialysis in pediatric patients are summarized in Table 71.2. Experience has shown that peritoneal dialysis can be successfully performed in most clinical scenarios including polycystic kidney disease, presence of a vesicostomy or colostomy, prune belly syndrome, recent abdominal surgery, ventriculoperitoneal shunt, and concurrent immunosuppressive therapy. Additionally, although renal replacement therapy can be used in newborns with early renal failure, the one-year mortality for infants is three times that of older children. Success depends on a multidisciplinary team approach that includes nephrologists, surgeons, dialysis specialty nurses, renal dietitians, social works, psychiatrists, and child life therapists.

Optimal medical management for associated fluid and electrolyte derangements should be completed before the child is taken to the operating room. Additionally, azotemic children are at risk for excessive bleeding. Correction of anemia and cessation of anticoagulation combined with the use of desmopressin acetate, conjugated estrogens, and cryoprecipitate help correct a uremic bleeding diathesis. Further, given that children have a high metabolic rate, they can generate harmful solutes more quickly than adults and thus require earlier renal replacement. These patients are characterized by impressive catabolism with rapid accumulation of potassium and phosophate. Children undergoing catheter placement should receive a single dose of a first-generation cephalosporin. Pre-incision antibiotic administration should be tailored appropriately to those known to be colonized with methicillin-resistant organisms.

Surgical Technique

Open Approach

The technique for peritoneal dialysis placement varies based on the size and clinical stability of the child, the urgency of initiating dialysis, and surgeon preference. Temporary dialysis access may be accomplished by placing a commercially available intra-abdominal catheter via the Seldinger technique. These techniques have been particularly useful in the

D. Little (✉)
Division of Pediatric Surgery, Scott and White Hospital,
615 West Garfield Avenue, Temple, TX, USA
and Department of Surgery, Texas A&M
Health Science Center, Temple, TX, USA
e-mail: dlittle@swmail.sw.org

P. Mattei (ed.), *Fundamentals of Pediatric Surgery*,
DOI 10.1007/978-1-4419-6643-8_71, © Springer Science+Business Media, LLC 2011

Table 71.1 Benefits of peritoneal dialysis

Home treatment
Self control of the therapy
No needles
Facilitates school attendance/employment
Extended travel is possible
Better preservation of remaining kidney function
Lower doses of medication needed to treat anemia
Better results after kidney transplantation
Less abrupt fluid shifts than hemodialysis
Easy to learn (3–5 days)
High level of patient satisfaction and well-being

Table 71.2 Indications for urgent dialysis (AEIOU)

Metabolic *A*cidosis
*E*lectrolyte disturbance
*I*ngestion/toxin
Fluid *O*verload
*U*remic syndrome

critical care setting. The child should be given intravenous narcotics and sedation, adding a local anesthetic with 1% lidocaine. Temporary catheters are infrequently required.

Elective procedures should be performed in the operating room with general anesthesia and muscle relaxant. A transverse incision over the rectus abdominus muscle, slightly superior to the umbilicus and semicircular line of Douglas is preferred. A small defect is created in the anterior fascia, and the rectus muscle is then gently spread, not divided. A second small defect is then established through the posterior rectus sheath. Omental adherence remains a common source of catheter failure. A partial omentectomy is therefore strongly recommended. A 3-0 monofilament suture is used in a purse-string fashion to secure the posterior rectus. It is best to use multiple short bites through the fascia, rather than large advancing bites. A curled pediatric peritoneal dialysis catheter is then straightened over a wire stylet and advanced deep into the pelvis. Intra-operative fluoroscopy is useful to confirm an appropriate location. The cuff should be positioned immediately above the peritoneum. The purse string suture is then tied. The catheter is then brought out through the second incision via a subcutaneous tunnel after it is brought out from the rectus sheath either through the anterior sheath incision or through a separate, more lateral incision. The second cuff is positioned in the subcutaneous tissue, several centimeters away from the final exit site. When possible, the exit site should be inferolateral to the skin incision. Additionally, with double-cuffed catheters, the second cuff should be at least 2 cm from the exit site in order to avoid cuff extrusion.

The catheter should be checked to ensure good flow. Infusion of 30 mL/kg of saline into the abdomen should be adequate to check for leakage and adequacy of flow. If inflow is good, the fluid is allowed to return by gravity back into the bag, which is placed on the floor of the operating room. An 80% return should be expected and constitutes an acceptable return flow. The catheter should be securely immobilized with a nonabsorbable skin suture and the primary wound closed in layers to avoid leakage of peritoneal fluid.

There are relatively few contraindications to placement of a peritoneal dialysis catheter. Naturally, the absence of an adequate peritoneal space, as can occur in children with multiple previous laparotomies or a history of peritonitis, makes it difficult to perform dialysis or even to place the catheter. Nevertheless, when necessary, an aggressive open or laparoscopic lysis of adhesions can sometimes allow the creation of enough space to perform peritoneal dialysis. The presence of an open, draining abdominal wound is a contraindication to peritoneal dialysis, but. children with urinary or intestinal diversion have successfully been treated with peritoneal dialysis. Though not uniformly agreed upon, some would consider the presence of a ventricular-peritoneal shunt or acute respiratory distress syndrome to be relative contraindications.

Laparoscopic Approach

Since the mid-1990s, laparoscopic peritoneal dialysis access techniques have become increasingly popular. The main goal of this new strategy was to reduce catheter-related complications, principally migration and subsequent outflow obstruction. Although the ideal method is still somewhat controversial, proponents of the minimally invasive approach site numerous advantages including ease of subtotal omentectomy, proper positioning of the catheter under direct vision, and ability to perform lysis of adhesions to increase peritoneal surface. Additional procedures, such as a renal biopsy, can also be performed concomitantly.

Several reports on laparoscopic techniques have been published. Authors vary on trocar placement, required incisions, tunneling techniques, and catheter security. We place the patient in the supine position and create a subumbilical fascia defect. Suction is used to deliver the omentum and a partial omentectomy is performed. A 12-mm trocar is then advanced through this umbilical incision, and an insufflation pressure of between 10 and 15 mmHg is established. A single-cuffed curled catheter is then placed through this port, followed by the laparoscope. Next, a stab incision is made in the right lateral abdomen through which endoscopic shears are advanced. A separate stab incision is made in the left lateral abdomen, and a Maryland grasper is inserted and tunneled through the abdominal wall towards the pubis. Using the right-hand endoscopic shears, a window is created for the left-hand Maryland to enter the peritoneum. The proximal end of the dialysis catheter is grasped and brought through the tract to be exteriorized.

Finally, a separate counter-incision is made lateral and inferior to the original left lateral abdomen incision to give the catheter a downward bend when exiting. Another small suprapubic incision is made extending into the subcutaneous fat only. An endoscopic fascial closure device is used to place a 2-0 absorbable monofilament suture around the catheter with two passes through the fascia. The catheter is thus secured to the abdominal wall and directed deep into the pelvis. The knot is tied anterior to the fascia and buried in the subcutaneous space. Alternatively, the catheter can be sutured to the bladder in males or uterus in females with a permanent monofilament stitch. The catheter is flushed with saline and drainage by gravity is confirmed.

At Arkansas Children's Hospital, a total of 50 patients have undergone 68 peritoneal dialysis procedures since 2001. Thirty-six procedures were approached laparoscopically while the remaining 32 were placed using a standard open approach. Focal segmental glomerulosclerosis was the most common indication. Operative times were similar between the two groups with laparoscopy averaging 47 min and open placement averaged 42 min. Exit site infections were decreased in the laparoscopic group (0.57 vs. 1.33 episodes per patient year). Although the total number of catheter migrations was similar, time to catheter failure or migration was significantly longer in the laparoscopic group (9 vs. 2.4 months).

Postoperative Care

The clinical condition will dictate when dialysis exchanges begin. There are two types of peritoneal dialysis: CAPD and automated peritoneal dialysis (APD). With CAPD, exchanges are done manually while APD uses a small machine with automatic exchanges occurring mainly at night while the child is sleeping. Thus, the child is "dialysis-free" during the day.

Catheter-care procedures vary between centers. Sterile technique, including the use of surgical masks and thorough hand scrub is recommended for those manipulating the catheter. Exchange fluid should be warmed to body temperature before use by using a heating pad or heating plate. Failure to do so can produce hypothermia, especially in infants and small children.

Dialysis will be directed by the pediatric nephrologist, however the surgeon should be familiar with the basic principles of peritoneal dialysis. The dialysate will contain glucose, amino acids, or icodextrin, or a combination thereof. Icodextrin is a starch-derived, water-soluble, glucose polymer colloid. The glucose strength (1.5, 2.5, or 4.25%) determines how much water is removed. Increased tonicity of the dialysate results in

the greater ultrafiltrate. The clinician must closely observe for the development of hyperglycemia, which can be controlled by the addition of insulin to the dialysate. The amino acids will move from the dialysate solution to the systemic circulation and thus improve a child's nutritional status. Icodextrin removes more water than dextrose solutions, creating longer intervals between exchanges. Additionally, this glucose-free regimen is advantageous both for the peritoneum and the body as a whole. Solutes are removed at different rates, as follows: urea > potassium > sodium > creatinine > phosphate > uric acid > calcium > magnesium. Thus, hyperkalemia is relatively easily controlled, usually within a few hours of initiating peritoneal dialysis.

Despite advances in catheter design and dialysis procedures, complications remain relatively common and include: bleeding, peritonitis, dialysate leakage, inguinal hernia, and soft-tissue infection. Rare complications include hydrothorax, chylous ascites, and organ or bowel perforation.

Blood-tinged dialysate or frank bleeding is commonly noted with the initiation of the first few exchanges. Attributed to bleeding from the catheter insertion site, this complication will generally resolve spontaneously. Heparin (250 units/L) should be added to the dialysate to prevent catheter obstruction from blood clots.

Infectious complications are a common source of catheter failure and subsequent morbidity. The incidence of peritonitis approaches one infection per patient per year. In most cases, bacteria enter the abdomen during a solution exchange. Traditionally, straight dialysis catheters have been used. The introduction of curved single- or double-cuffed catheters has led to a considerable reduction in peritonitis.

Classically, the diagnosis of peritonitis was noted by the presence of cloudy peritoneal dialysate effluent, fever, and abdominal pain. Increased pain and difficulty with fluid exchange are common. Dialysate fluid should be sent for complete blood count and differential. Greater than 100 WBC/mm^3 or more than 50% polymorphonuclear leukocytes is an indicator of peritonitis. Serum leukocytosis is sometimes seen but this is not a consistent finding. Occasionally, peritoneal eosinophilia is noted shortly following catheter placement. If cultures are negative, no therapy is indicated.

Most cases of peritonitis can be successfully managed with intraperitoneal antibiotic administration. This produces a high intraperitoneal concentration of antibiotics and often allows dialysis to continue. Improvement in the child's status, including a clear dialysate fluid, resolution of abdominal pain, and improving dialysate cell counts are generally seen within 48 h. Failure of therapy necessitates catheter removal and establishment of temporary hemodialysis access.

Increased intra-abdominal pressure from the instillation of dialysate contributes to fluid leakage. These leaks most often occur early, during the first few days or week of dialysis. Causes include high exchange volumes, excessive catheter manipulation, underappreciated catheter traction, or patient repositioning. Leaks occurring late may present with abdominal wall or genital edema. Whether early or late, the diagnosis may be established by detecting elevated glucose content from the expressed fluid. Confirmatory contrast or radionuclide studies may be required. Initial attempts at smaller exchange volumes or night-only cycling is sometimes successful. Prevention is preferable. Treatment of an associated exit site infection may prove beneficial. If the leak persists despite all therapeutic maneuvers, catheter revision is required.

Regardless of the source, excess intra-abdominal fluid is a factor in the development of an inguinal hernia. The development of an inguinal hernia is inversely proportional to the age of the child receiving dialysis, with children under the age of one have the highest frequency of inguinal hernia. Estimated risk of inguinal hernia ranges from 7 to 15%. These hernias should be repaired promptly followed by no or low-flow dialysis for several days.

Prevention of *exit-site infections* with meticulous sterile dressing procedures from caregivers is recommended. When exit-site or tunnel infections occur, they are commonly a result of infection with *Staphylococcus* or *Pseudomonas* species. Redness and pain will be noted. Prompt diagnosis and therapy might prevent the development of peritonitis. Empiric therapy should be instituted with antibiotic therapy directed against the susceptibilities of the cultured organism. Treatment should continue for two to four weeks. In cases of MRSA, nasal carriage status of family members should be assessed and those colonized should be treated appropriately with intranasal mupirocin.

Dialysis becomes necessary when conservative management of renal failure in children is no longer effective. Peritoneal dialysis has become the standard therapy for children with acute and chronic renal failure. Advantages include the relative simplicity of placement for the surgeon and ease of therapy for the child and caregivers. The pediatric surgeon's primary goal is to establish an intraperitoneal catheter with rapid flow rates and no fluid leaks. Additionally, a low incidence of catheter-related infections with strict adherence to sterile technique is achievable. Both open and laparoscopic techniques are acceptable.

Summary Points

- Peritoneal dialysis is an excellent way to provide dialysis for a child with end-stage renal disease while preserving quality of life and avoiding the pain and risk of hemodialysis.
- Peritoneal dialysis catheters can be placed using a traditional open technique or a laparoscopic approach, both of which are safe and associated with minimal risk.
- There are very few contraindications for peritoneal dialysis, including lack of a peritoneal space due to excessive adhesions, peritonitis, and active abdominal wall infection.
- Peritoneal dialysis can be used in patients with polycystic kidney disease, vesicostomy or colostomy, prune belly syndrome, recent abdominal surgery, or ventriculoperitoneal shunt.

Editor's Comment

Although the pediatric surgeon's role in the care of the child with end-stage renal disease is primarily technical, it is extremely important that every detail of the operation to place a peritoneal dialysis catheter be performed with the utmost care. For children with renal failure, these catheters are lifelines and any complication can have profoundly deleterious effects. This means that the catheter must work reliably, without leakage, and the risk of infection should be minimized. I find little advantage to the laparoscopic approach except for some redo operations and to troubleshoot a malpositioned or poorly functioning catheter. The critical maneuvers are to use an appropriate-length curled catheter placed carefully in the pelvis, to place a precise purse-string suture, to perform a partial omentectomy, to tunnel the catheter in such a way that it stays in the pelvis, and to close all layers with running suture to prevent leaks.

The catheter should be placed as though it were permanent: don't cut corners so that it will be easier to remove it someday. A catheter placed on the right side will usually find the right place in the pelvis more easily because the sigmoid colon is less likely to get in the way. The stylet used to place the catheter is usually very long and can easily become contaminated on the surgeons mask or an unsterile object outside the field, in which case it must be removed from the field and replaced with a new one. Place the purse string with small bites before entering the peritoneum and catch a tiny bite of cuff so that it stays snug against the posterior rectus sheath. The catheter should be brought out the lateral aspect of the rectus sheath so that the anterior sheath can be closed water-tight. A second cuff is generally superfluous. Finally, do not leave the operating room until the catheter functions perfectly and there is zero leakage; otherwise, you will be sure to return in the near future to repair or replace it. You should have the confidence to let the nephrologists use it the night of surgery, if this becomes necessary.

Inguinal hernias are probably not caused per se by the dialysis but it is more likely that a pre-existing hernia is made clinically apparent sooner due to the increased intra-abdominal pressure created by the infusion of dialysate. Given that repair of these hernias can be challenging and prone to recurrence, perhaps it makes sense to use laparoscopy to assist in the placement of the catheter (this would obviate the need for fluoroscopy) and rule out the presence of an inguinal hernia. Removal of the catheters can be difficult due to the adhesions at the cuff. It is ideal (but probably not critical) to close the peritoneum to prevent leaks and hernias. A rare but devastating complication of peritoneal dialysis is sclerosing encapsulating peritonitis (SEP), which causes recurrent bowel obstruction and chronic bowel dysfunction. The cause is unknown but it is clearly associated with the use of chlorhexidine-based antiseptics (formerly used to clean the tubing and equipment used for peritoneal dialysis) and immunosuppression. Treatment includes radical excision of the extensive fibrotic peel that envelops the bowel, but the recurrence rate and mortality are high.

Diagnostic Procedures

- Electrolytes
- Coagulation studies
- Intra-operative fluoroscopy for confirmation of proper catheter placement
- Diagnostic laparoscopy with lysis of adhesions, if needed
- Peritoneal fluid for complete blood count and culture, if peritonitis is suspected

---

Preoperative Preparation

□ Prophylactic antibiotics
□ Correction of coagulopathy
□ Correction of hyperkalemia, fluid overload, severe acidosis

---

Parental Preparation

– Peritoneal dialysis catheters usually function well and are generally safe.
– Risks include: infection at the exit site or peritonitis; catheter migration, dislodgement or obstruction due to adhesions; and inguinal hernia formation.

Technical Points

- Use an intraoperative first generation cephalosporin.
- Perform partial omentectomy to prevent outflow obstruction.
- Place exit site far from stomas.
- Direct catheter exit towards an inferolateral site.
- Use intra-operative fluoroscopy to verify a deep pelvic position for the catheter.
- Consider fibrin glue sealant at peritoneum opening if leakage is persistent.

Suggested Reading

Gajjar AH, Rhoden DH, Kathuria P, et al. Peritoneal dialysis catheters: laparoscopic versus traditional placement techniques and outcomes. Am J Surg. 2007;194(6):872–5.

Johnson DW, Wong J, Wiggins KJ. A randomized controlled trial of coiled versus straight swan-neck Tenckhoff catheters in peritoneal dialysis patients. Am J Kidney Dis. 2006;48(5):812–21.

Stringel G, McBride W, Weiss R. Laparoscopic placement of peritoneal dialysis catheters in children. J Pediatr Surg. 2008;43(5):857–60.

Strippoli GF, Tong A, Johnson A, et al. Catheter type, placement and insertion techniques for preventing peritonitis in peritoneal dialysis patients. Cochrane Database Syst Rev. 2004a;18(4):CD004680.

Strippoli GF, Tong A, Johnson A, et al. Antimicrobial agents for preventing peritonitis in peritoneal dialysis patients. Cochrane Database Syst Rev. 2004b;18(4):CD004680.

Warady BA. Peritoneal dialysis. In: Kher KK, Schnaper HW, Makker SP, editors. Clinical pediatric nephrology. 2nd ed. London: Informa Healthcare; 2007. p. 391–406.

Wiggins KJ, Craig JC, Johnson DW, et al. Treatment for peritoneal dialysis-associated peritonitis. Cochrane Database Syst Rev. 2008;23(1):CD005284.

Wright MJ, Bel'eed K, Johnson BF, et al. Randomized prospective comparison of laparoscopic and open peritoneal dialysis catheter insertion. Perit Dial Int. 1999;19(4):372–5.

Chapter 72
Neonatal Hyperbilirubinemia

Clyde J. Wright and Michael A. Posencheg

Neonatal hyperbilirubinemia, or jaundice in the newborn, is caused by deposition of bilirubin in the skin. It manifests in over 50% of newborns but relatively few require therapy. Bilirubin is a breakdown product of heme proteins, the most abundant of which is hemoglobin. The heme moiety is converted by heme oxygenase to biliverdin, which is reduced to unconjugated bilirubin by biliverdin reductase. Unconjugated bilirubin is bound to albumin in the blood and is taken up by the liver and conjugated by uridine diphosphate glucuronyl transferase (UDPGT). Conjugated bilirubin is excreted by the liver into the small intestine and eliminated in the stool. However, conjugated bilirubin can be de-conjugated in the bowel, reabsorbed into the blood, and delivered again to the liver, a process called enterohepatic circulation. Elevation of unconjugated bilirubin is the result of increased heme breakdown, decreased uptake of bilirubin by the liver, decreased bilirubin conjugation, or increased enterohepatic circulation. In contrast, elevation of conjugated bilirubin is primarily due to decreased liver excretion, bile duct abnormalities, or hepatocyte dysfunction.

Jaundice is the clinical manifestation of elevated unconjugated or conjugated bilirubin; however the skin discoloration is somewhat different when comparing the two. Unconjugated hyperbilirubinemia produces a more yellow–orange hue, while conjugated hyperbilirubinemia produces a yellow–green hue. The initial challenge to the clinician is determining which form of jaundice is present and whether or not it is pathologic. Conjugated hyperbilirubinemia is always considered pathologic and is defined as a conjugated fraction of greater than 1 mg/dL in the setting of a total serum bilirubin (TSB) less than 5 mg/dL, or more than 20% of the TSB if it is above 5 mg/dL. More than 70% of cases are due to either idiopathic neonatal hepatitis or biliary atresia. In preterm or sick term infants, the most common cause is parenteral nutrition-associated cholestasis. The complete differential diagnosis for conjugated hyperbilirubinemia contains over 100 diagnoses. We will focus on the differential diagnosis and management of the more common condition of unconjugated hyperbilirubinemia.

Hyperbilirubinemia presents a challenge to the clinician due to the acute and chronic neurological sequelae than can occur in infants with markedly elevated levels. When unconjugated bilirubin concentrations exceed the infant's capacity to bind with albumin, either because of an exceedingly high bilirubin level or a low albumin level, there is an increased concentration of unbound bilirubin. This bilirubin freely crosses the blood-brain barrier and is toxic to neurons of the basal ganglia and brainstem nuclei. The clinical manifestation is termed acute bilirubin encephalopathy or bilirubin-induced neurological dysfunction (BIND). These symptoms are often confused with those of sepsis or asphyxia and initially include lethargy, poor feeding, and hypotonia. This can progress to stupor, irritability, fever, high-pitched cry, seizures, and hypertonia. The hypertonia associated with hyperbilirubinemia has been classically described as backward flexion of the neck (retrocollis) and trunk (opisthotonos). Lastly, if unchecked, acute bilirubin encephalopathy can progress to a shrill cry, loss of ability to feed orally, apnea, coma, and death. The long-term sequelae of this brain injury is kernicterus, which can include choreoathetosis, sensorineural hearing loss, dental enamel dysplasia, paralysis of upward gaze, hypotonia, and delay in acquisition of motor skills. The goal in treating hyperbilirubinemia is to prevent both the acute and chronic sequelae.

Diagnosis

The differential diagnosis of unconjugated hyperbilirubinemia in the newborn is extensive and includes physiologic jaundice, which is part of the normal transition from fetal to neonatal life. In utero, bilirubin produced by the breakdown of heme proteins easily crosses the placenta and is conjugated and excreted by the mother's liver and intestinal tract. Many factors make the newborn infant ill-equipped to deal with the loss of this route of excretion. Newborns have a larger mass

C.J. Wright (✉)
Department of Pediatrics, Children's Hospital of Philadelphia, 34th Street and Civic Center Boulevard, Philadelphia, PA 19104, USA
e-mail: wrightcl@email.chop.edu

of red blood cells, and therefore a higher hemoglobin load. Additionally, these cells have a shorter life span when compared to older children and adults. Furthermore, the newborn liver exhibits reduced UPDGT activity (<1% of adult activity in the first few days of life), and delayed passage of meconium with a prolonged intestinal transit time increases enterohepatic circulation. The combination of these factors results in a physiologic hyperbilirubinemia that occurs in more than half of newborns, peaking around the fourth day of life. Average peak TSB is 5–6 mg/dL in formula-fed term newborns and approaches 9 mg/dL in breast-fed infants. While classically it has been taught that a TSB of 5 mg/dL approximates the minimum serum level required to detect clinical jaundice, it is important to remember that estimating bilirubin levels by clinical exam is unreliable. Any jaundice detected clinically, especially when detected in the first 24 h, requires prompt laboratory evaluation.

When the bilirubin level is elevated in the first 24 h of life, rapidly rising, or above 17 mg/dL, further work-up is necessary. Any one of these conditions is likely to represent a process other than physiologic jaundice. The evaluation of such an infant begins with a review of the pertinent maternal and neonatal history. Maternal factors such as blood type, Rh status, and antibody profile might contribute to an increased risk of hyperbilirubinemia. Isoimmune hemolytic disease can manifest when maternal antibodies cross the placenta and bind to antigens present on newborn red blood cells including major blood group antigens (A, B), minor blood group antigens (Kell, Kidd, Duffy), or Rh factor.

Regarding ABO incompatibility, only infants born to mothers with type O blood are at risk for major blood group incompatibility, as their anti-A and anti-B antibodies are more likely to be IgG and cross the placenta. Mothers with type A or type B blood develop anti-B and anti-A IgM antibodies, which cannot cross the placenta and therefore pose no risk to the newborn. Rhesus isoimmunization occurs in Rh positive infants born to Rh negative mothers who have developed anti-Rh IgG antibodies from previous exposure to Rh positive blood. While Rh isoimmunization requires prior sensitization and therefore does not occur in first pregnancies, ABO incompatibility can occur in the first child. This is an important history to establish as immune-mediated hemolysis can cause significantly elevated bilirubin levels and requires specific therapeutic interventions.

Other important maternal factors include TORCH infection, maternal diabetes, intra-uterine growth restriction, and the use of medications such as sulfonamides, nitrofurantoin, anti-malarials or oxytocin. All of these can contribute to an increase in unconjugated bilirubin by different mechanisms.

Delivery and neonatal history are also important. Evidence of birth trauma such as ecchymosis and cephalohematomas increase the amount of hemoglobin that must be degraded. It is important to know the infant's gestational and postnatal age as this determines treatment thresholds. The infant's ethnicity increases the risk of certain disease processes. For example, G6PD deficiency is more common in infants of African, Mediterranean, Middle Eastern, or Southeast Asian descent. Some states test for this condition as part of the newborn screen. Breast-feeding is associated with higher bilirubin levels than formula feeding. Additionally, the infant's voiding and stooling pattern must be investigated as these represent the major routes of elimination.

Along with a thorough history, the physical exam can provide clues that impact the aggressiveness with which one evaluates the infant's hyperbilirubinemia. Jaundice becomes clinically apparent as yellow–orange skin discoloration at levels above 5 mg/dL. Furthermore, it progresses in a cephalocaudal manner, from the face to the chest, trunk and lower extremities. However, multiple studies have shown the clinicians' ability to predict bilirubin values on the basis of this progression to be poor. Jaundice is best evaluated by assessing the color of skin that has been blanched with light pressure in natural light.

Other physical exam findings are important to note and are sometimes associated with higher bilirubin levels. The infant with polycythemia often appears ruddy, in contrast to the pale infant undergoing hemolysis. Infants with long standing hemolysis in utero may have evidence of hydrops fetalis, such as pleural effusions or ascites. Microcephaly, petechiae, and hepatosplenomegaly suggest the possibility of a TORCH infection. Lastly, jaundiced infants should be monitored closely for signs and symptoms of acute bilirubin encephalopathy or BIND.

The laboratory evaluation of an infant with clinical jaundice should always include a fractionated bilirubin level, with total serum, unconjugated, and conjugated levels determined. These individual fractions must be determined as the diagnosis and subsequent therapeutic interventions depend on this information. A blood type, Coombs' test, and complete blood count with reticulocyte count can determine whether ongoing hemolysis is occurring. A G6PD level can be helpful in establishing the diagnosis in infants with the appropriate ethnic background. Serum albumin, the primary protein transporter for bilirubin in the blood, should be measured as low serum levels of albumin increase the risk of developing neurological sequelae due to the increased amount of free bilirubin crossing the blood-brain barrier. The newborn screen provides information regarding rarer conditions associated with increased total and conjugated bilirubin such as galactosemia, tyrosinemia and hypothyroidism. Lastly, if an infant demonstrates signs or symptoms of sepsis, the appropriate tests should be sent to establish this diagnosis, including a urine culture. Urinary tract infections have been associated with late-onset as well as conjugated hyperbilirubinemia.

Treatment

The primary reason to evaluate infants with hyperbilirubinemia is to prevent the neurological sequelae of markedly elevated bilirubin levels by instituting the appropriate therapies aimed at decreasing serum bilirubin levels. Phototherapy is the mainstay of treatment for the majority of infants with *un*conjugated hyperbilirubinemia. In 2004, the American Academy of Pediatrics published updated clinical practice guidelines for the management of hyperbilirubinemia, which provide clear guidelines regarding the prevention and evaluation of hyperbilirubinemia, as well as follow-up of infants with this condition. Also provided are new nomograms with gestational age and postnatal age-specific recommendation for the use of phototherapy and, in more severe cases, double-volume exchange transfusion (DVET).

Unconjugated bilirubin absorbs light maximally in the blue portion of the visible spectrum (approximately 450 nm). Phototherapy with a light source that approximates this wavelength results in the photoisomerization of unconjugated bilirubin into a polar, water-soluble, and more readily-excreted form. Both configurational and structural isomers are formed, the most common of which is lumirubin. The efficacy of phototherapy is related to the wavelength and irradiance of the light, the surface area of exposed skin, and the distance between the light source and the skin. To ensure maximal effectiveness of phototherapy, the clinician should request maximal skin exposure of the infant including removal of any head covering, use of a fiberoptic pad (or bili blanket) under the infant, and use of an irradiance of >30 μW/cm^2/nm (in infants ≥35 weeks gestational age). Irradiance can be measured with a radiometer at the bedside.

The level of TSB that warrants the use of phototherapy in infants with a gestational age of 35 weeks or greater can be determined using the standard age-specific nomogram. Several items of clinical data must be applied when using this chart. The primary determinants include gestational age, actual age, and TSB concentration. Furthermore, a review of the infant's clinical condition will reveal if there are any risk factors for acute bilirubin encephalopathy. Increased hemolysis, increased permeability of the blood-brain barrier, and decreased binding to albumin are further risk factors that can be due to isoimmune hemolytic disease, G6PD deficiency, asphyxia, lethargy, sepsis, temperature instability, acidosis, or albumin <3.0 g/dL.

The guidelines for use of phototherapy in infants less than 35 weeks gestation are not well established. Studies have not determined a safe level of bilirubin for these infants. Some experts suggest starting phototherapy based on the infant's birth weight. One method to approximate the level to start phototherapy involves dividing the first two digits of the infant's birth weight by two. For example, for a 1,500 g infant,

consider starting phototherapy at a total serum bilirubin of 7.5 mg/dL.

In some instances, the total serum bilirubin continues to rise despite the appropriate use of phototherapy, in which case hemolysis should be strongly considered as a cause. In the setting of antibody-mediated isoimmune hemolytic disease, the use of intravenous γ-globulin (IVIG) has been shown to decrease the need for a DVET with less risk to the infant. The current recommendation from AAP is to administer IVIG 0.5–1 g/kg over 2 h if the TSB is rising despite phototherapy, or the TSB is within 2–3 mg/dL of the exchange transfusion level. This dose can be repeated in 12 h.

For some infants, the use of phototherapy and IVIG is not sufficient to control the rising bilirubin level. Alternatively, some infants may have neurological sequelae of bilirubin toxicity despite bilirubin levels below suggested therapeutic levels. In these instances, a DVET is indicated. This process is labor intensive and must be anticipated far in advance. Preparatory steps include acquiring a sufficient volume of blood, establishing adequate vascular access, and setting up the equipment, including a blood warmer. This often takes hours to complete. A DVET involves removing twice the infant's blood volume with simultaneous isovolemic replacement of reconstituted whole blood. This process achieves two separate but related goals: it removes bilirubin and, in the setting of isoimmune hemolytic disease, it removes the offending maternal antibodies. Some experts suggest performing a DVET at even lower levels than recommended in the guidelines when significant antibody-mediated hemolysis is occurring.

To calculate the amount of blood to order and exchange, estimate the infants blood volume (between 80 and 100 mL/kg based on level of prematurity and amount of perinatal blood loss) and multiply the result by two. Blood is ordered as reconstituted whole blood, using O-negative red blood cells and AB-positive plasma. Blood should be withdrawn at a rate of 1–2 mL/kg/min and simultaneously replaced at the same rate. Exchange of twice the infants blood volume in this manner replaces approximately 86% of the infant's own blood (a single volume exchange replaces approximately 63%). The distribution of bilirubin in both the intravascular and extravascular spaces does not allow for the removal of an equivalent percentage. One can expect a bilirubin level of approximately 45% of pre-exchange levels at the conclusion of the procedure and the eventual rebound to at least 60% of pre-exchange levels. Some infants require more than one DVET.

The optimal method for performing a DVET involves two operators, one responsible for blood removal and the other for infusion. This continuous process is best done using an umbilical arterial catheter for withdrawal and umbilical venous catheter with the tip above the diaphragm for infusion. Other combinations are possible and include variations of umbilical and peripheral catheters. If only one line can be inserted, a push-pull technique can be employed to remove and then infuse blood in small aliquots. This technique is more time consuming and more prone to both error and complications.

There are many potential complications associated with the DVET. These include electrolyte disturbances, arrhythmias, cardiac arrest, thrombotic or embolic sequelae, metabolic acidosis, thrombocytopenia, DIC, infection, necrotizing enterocolitis, temperature instability, and blood-borne infection. Before, during, and after the procedure,

attention should be paid to the following blood tests: serum electrolytes (especially calcium), blood glucose, bilirubin, CBC, and reticulocyte count. Some experts utilize a calcium infusion during the procedure, especially if the blood products contain citrate, which chelates calcium. Serial bilirubin levels should be followed after the procedure to ensure the rebound is not significant enough to warrant repeat DVET.

Summary Points

- Clinical jaundice is a result of elevated bilirubin concentrations in the blood, called hyperbilirubinemia.
- Elevations in both the unconjugated and conjugated fraction of bilirubin can be seen and have a very different differential diagnosis and therapeutic options.
- Over 50% of newborn infants will become jaundiced in the first few days of life; breast-fed infants are more likely than formula-fed ones to demonstrate jaundice.
- Jaundice appears in cephalocaudal manner, however prediction of bilirubin levels based on this progression is unreliable.
- Most jaundice is physiological and may not require therapy.
- The challenge to the clinician is to identify infants at risk of neurological sequelae from hyperbilirubinemia and initiate therapy accordingly, thus preventing kernicterus.
- Phototherapy is the mainstay of therapy and converts unconjugated bilirubin in a non-enzymatic fashion into a polar, water-soluble form that is more readily excretable.
- Hemolysis is strongly suggested in an infant receiving intensive phototherapy when the total serum bilirubin continues to rise or fails to decrease significantly.
- Rh incompatibility requires prior sensitization and therefore does not happen in a first pregnancy. ABO incompatibility can occur in a first-born infant.
- IVIG is indicated in infants with isoimmune hemolytic disease resulting in hyperbilirubinemia that is approaching levels at which a DVET is suggested.
- A low albumin level decreased the infants' ability to bind unconjugated bilirubin, increasing the fraction of free, unbound bilirubin, which increases an infants' risk for neurological toxicity. The bilirubin/albumin ratio can be used as an adjunct in determining the need for DVET, emphasizing the risk of a low serum albumin.
- A DVET is reserved for infants who fail phototherapy and IVIG (if indicated) and removes approximately 86% of the infant's own blood.
- Close monitoring of serum electrolytes, CBC, and bilirubin levels after a DVET should be performed to evaluate the infant for complications or need to repeat the procedure.

Editor's Comment

Depending on the admission standards at a given institution, infants in the neonatal intensive care unit who need surgery are often admitted to the Surgery service. Regardless of the arrangement, surgeons need to monitor their newborn patients for hyperbilirubinemia for several important reasons. The first is that even surgical newborns can develop hyperbilirubinemia of infancy and might be at higher risk for brain injury due to their exposure to other potential neurotoxins in the form of drugs and anesthetics. Second, elevated levels of conjugated bilirubin can be a sign of parenteral nutrition-associated cholestasis and impending liver

dysfunction, in which case measures must be taken to prevent progression of this disease process including cycling of the parenteral nutrition, advancing enteral feeds as tolerated, and considering supplements such as omega-3 fatty acids. Finally, infants with a persistent elevation of conjugated bilirubin must be considered to have biliary atresia until proven otherwise. The success rate of establishing biliary drainage and avoiding liver transplantation diminishes significantly the later infants with biliary atresia undergo Kasai portoenterostomy. It therefore becomes critical that the rare infant with biliary atresia undergo the proper diagnostic evaluation without delay. It is often surprisingly difficult to distinguish the infant with biliary atresia from the more common case of parenteral nutrition-induced cholestasis. It is reasonable to start with an ultrasound to confirm the presence of a gallbladder and then proceed with HIDA scan if there is still some question. It is not uncommon for there to remain some concern about the differential diagnosis even after these two studies have been performed. Some recommend liver biopsy at this point, though even experienced pathologists can have difficulty distinguishing the two entities. It is occasionally necessary to proceed with an intra-operative cholangiogram to confirm the presence of patent bile ducts. The one consolation in the case of a negative study is that infants with cholestasis often appear to benefit from having their biliary tree flushed and cleared of inspissated bile. Many are also at risk for gallstones and therefore benefit from what becomes a prophylactic cholecystectomy.

Differential Diagnosis

Unconjugated Hyperbilirubinemia

Increased bilirubin production

- Isoimmune hemolytic disease – ABO, Rh, minor blood antigens
- Red blood cell enzyme defects – glucose-6-phosphate dehydrogenase deficiency, pyruvate kinase deficiency, hexokinase deficiency
- Red blood cell membrane defects – hereditary spherocytosis, elliptocytosis, pyknocytosis.
- Hemoglobinopathies – alpha-thalassemia
- Increased red blood cell load – ecchymosis, polycythemia, cephalohematoma

Decreased bilirubin uptake or conjugation

- Hypothyroidism / hypopituitarism
- Gilbert syndrome
- Crigler–Najjar (type I and II)
- Lucy-Driscoll syndrome
- Sepsis – bacterial, viral, fungal

Increased enterohepatic circulation

- Breastfeeding jaundice
- Breast milk jaundice
- Bowel obstruction or ileus
- Pyloric stenosis

Conjugated Hyperbilirubinemia (Limited Differential Diagnosis)

- Biliary Atresia
- Idiopathic neonatal hepatitis
- Choledochal cyst
- Infection – UTI, TORCH, bacterial sepsis, HSV, enterovirus, etc.
- Metabolic disorders – Galactosemia, tyrosinemia, alpha-1-antitrypsin deficiency, Alagille syndrome, etc.
- Neonatal hemochromatosis
- Total parental nutrition (TPN)-related cholestasis

Diagnostic Studies

- Total serum, unconjugated and conjugated bilirubin
- Infant blood type and Coombs' test
- Complete blood count with reticulocyte count
- G6PD level
- Albumin level
- Urine culture
- Newborn screen
- Abdominal ultrasound
- Serum electrolytes, including calcium, pre-DVET

Parental Preparation

- Most infants with hyperbilirubinemia either do not require therapy or require phototherapy only. Therefore, the common challenge is parental anxiety regarding the discoloration or separation for phototherapy. If a DVET is required, parental consent should be obtained and include a discussion of potential complications of the procedure which rarely results in death.

Preoperative Preparation

Double-Volume Exchange Transfusion

- □ Obtaining vascular access – preferably umbilical arterial and venous catheters.
- □ Order reconstituted whole blood – approximately 160 mL/kg body weight plus additional small volume for the tubing.
- □ Obtain DVET infusion kit including blood warmer.

Technical Points

Double-Volume Exchange Transfusion

- Preferred access is umbilical arterial catheter for withdrawal and umbilical venous catheter for replacement.
- Withdraw blood at 1–2 mL/kg/min and infuse at the same rate.
- Monitor serum electrolytes and glucose during procedure.
- Monitor CBC and bilirubin levels at beginning and end of procedure.

Suggested Reading

American Academy of Pediatrics, Subcommittee on Hyperbilirubinemia. Management of hyperbilirubinemia in the newborn infant 35 or more weeks of gestation. Pediatrics. 2004;114(1):297–316.

Bhutani VK, Johnson L, Sivieri EM. Predictive ability of a predischarge hour-specific serum bilirubin for subsequent significant hyperbilirubinemia in healthy term and near-term neonates. Pediatrics. 1999;103:6–14.

Dennery PA, Seidman DS, Stevenson DK. Neonatal hyperbilirubinemia. N Engl J Med. 2001;344(8):581–90.

Johnson LH, Bhutani VK, Brown AK. System-based approach to management of neonatal jaundice and prevention of kernicterus. J Pediatr. 2002;140:396–403.

Maisels MJ, McDonagh AF. Phototherapy for neonatal jaundice. N Engl J Med. 2008;358(9):920–8.

Moyer V, Freese DK, Whitington PF, Olson AD, Brewer F, Colletti RB, et al. Guideline for the evaluation of cholestatic jaundice in infants: recommendations of the North American Society for Pediatric Gastroenterology, Hepatology and Nutrition. J Pediatr Gastroenterol Nutr. 2004;39(2):115–28.

Watchko J, Claassen D. Kernicterus in premature infants: current prevalence and relationship to NICHD phototherapy study exchange criteria. Pediatrics. 1994;93(6 Pt 1):996–9.

Watchko JF, Oski FA. Kernicterus in preterm newborns: past, present, and future. Pediatrics. 1992;90:707–15.

Wong RJ, Stevenson DK, Ahlfors CE, Vreman HJ. Neonatal jaundice: bilirubin physiology and clinical chemistry. Neoreviews. 2007;8(2):e58–67.

Chapter 73
Biliary Atresia

Peter C. Minneci and Alan W. Flake

Biliary atresia is an uncommon disorder of the newborn, occurring in 1 in 10,000 to 1 in 15,000 live births worldwide. It is a cholangiopathy characterized by inflammation of the bile ducts leading to progressive fibroproliferative obliteration of the extrahepatic biliary tree and, to a variable extent, the intrahepatic bile ducts. The progressive destruction of the bile ducts leads to cholestasis, liver fibrosis, and cirrhosis. The etiology of biliary atresia remains unknown, but it is likely a multi-factorial process involving environmental, genetic, and immunologic factors.

Both anatomic and clinical classification systems have been developed to characterize different types of biliary atresia. The anatomic systems are based on the degree of patency of the extra-hepatic biliary tree. One commonly used schema describes three types of biliary atresia: Type I involves the common bile duct, Type II includes involvement of the hepatic duct, and Type III, the most common, describes atresia at the porta hepatis. Types I and II have historically been referred to as "correctable" biliary atresia because it was once felt that when a patent extra-hepatic bile duct exists it could be used for reconstruction. It is now recognized that even the "correctable" types of biliary atresia should be treated by portoenterostomy. Type I or II biliary atresia account for 10–15% of all cases, while the remainder are type III.

The clinical classification system divides biliary atresia into two forms, of which *acquired* or *perinatal* biliary atresia is the more common, accounting for up to 90% of cases. These patients are usually well-appearing newborns who develop or have progression of bile duct inflammation and obliteration after birth. They will typically have a jaundice-free period after birth and present with cholestasis between four and 6 weeks of age. *Syndromic*, also referred to as *embryonal* or *fetal*, biliary atresia is the less common form. These patients have associated congenital anomalies (Table 73.1)

and usually do not have a jaundice-free period after birth. In a recent series from the NIH-sponsored Biliary Atresia Research Consortium (BARC), 25% of cases of biliary atresia from 1997 to 2000 (26/104 cases) were syndromic, with half of the patients having one anomaly and half having more than one. The most common anomalies were: splenic malformation (12), interrupted IVC (11), cardiac malformation (9) and malrotation (9). Of the 13 patients with more than one anomaly, 11 had biliary atresia splenic malformation (BASM) syndrome.

Both the anatomic and clinical classification systems have prognostic significance with higher rates of liver transplantation and higher mortality rates reported in patients with Type III biliary atresia and in patients with syndromic biliary atresia.

Diagnosis

The typical patient with biliary atresia is a full-term, healthy-appearing infant with normal birth weight, who develops jaundice that persists at 4–6 weeks and is associated with acholic stools, dark urine, and hepatomegaly. There is often a delay in the diagnosis because nearly two thirds of all newborns develop jaundice, the overwhelming majority of which are due to physiologic jaundice (usually lasts only 2–3 days) or breast milk jaundice (can last up to 4 weeks). Only a minority of cases are due to neonatal cholestasis (1/500 cases of jaundice in infants between 2–4 weeks old). Nevertheless, biliary atresia should be suspected in any infant who remains jaundiced for more than 2 weeks (3 weeks if breastfed) because early diagnosis and surgical intervention are associated with improved outcomes. The American Academy of Pediatrics recommends that total and direct bilirubin levels be checked in any infant that is jaundiced at 3 weeks. Physiologic and breast milk jaundice are related to liver immaturity, increased bilirubin production, decreased bilirubin clearance or excretion, and excessive enterohepatic recirculation. Therefore, the total bilirubin level will be elevated but the conjugated (direct) level account for less than 20% of

P.C. Minneci (✉)
Department of Surgery, Children's Hospital of Philadelphia,
34th Street & Civic Center Boulevard, Wood 5,
Philadelphia, PA 19104, USA
e-mail: minneci@email.chop.edu

P. Mattei (ed.), *Fundamentals of Pediatric Surgery*,
DOI 10.1007/978-1-4419-6643-8_73, © Springer Science+Business Media, LLC 2011

Table 73.1 Anomalies associated with syndromic biliary atresia

Splenic malformation (asplenia, polysplenia)

Interrupted IVC (suprarenal) with azygous continuation

Cardiac malformations

Gut malrotation

Aberrant hepatic arterial supply (left hepatic from left gastric or SMA)

Situs inversus

Preduodenal portal vein

Annular pancreas

Duodenal, esophageal or jejunal atresia

the total. Neonatal cholestasis is due to intrinsic liver disease or dysfunction, and therefore the total bilirubin will be elevated with more than 20% being conjugated bilirubin. In biliary atresia specifically, the conjugated bilirubin levels might represent 50–80% of the total bilirubin level.

An infant with evidence of cholestasis (elevated total bilirubin with greater than 20% conjugated) must undergo a complete workup to rule out both extrahepatic and intrahepatic causes. As surgeons, we are most often involved in the search for extrahepatic causes of neonatal cholestasis, however this should be part of a more comprehensive medical work up to exclude infectious, metabolic, genetic, and toxic causes of cholestasis.

The evaluation of extrahepatic causes of neonatal jaundice starts with laboratory tests demonstrating increased serum alanine aminotransferase (ALT), aspartate aminotransferase (AST), alkaline phosphatase, and especially gamma-glutamyl transpeptidase (GGT), which is usually disproportionately elevated in infants with biliary atresia. The ensuing diagnostic workup varies from center to center. A fasting abdominal ultrasound should be obtained and will often demonstrate an enlarged liver and either a contracted or absent gallbladder. Other findings that have been reported with a focused and detailed ultrasound include abnormal gallbladder wall configuration, shape or contractility, nonvisualization of the common bile duct, enlarged hepatic artery diameter, and a focal area of increased echogenicity anterior to the bifurcation of the portal vein (the triangular cord sign), which represents the fibrotic remnant of the extrahepatic biliary tree. The results of the ultrasound are both technician- and center-dependent and therefore highly variable in their diagnostic value. Ultrasound does not allow us to confirm the diagnosis of biliary atresia but it can support the diagnosis, and is useful to exclude other extrahepatic causes of neonatal cholestasis, such as a choledochal cyst.

Hepatobiliary scintigraphy is often obtained to assess the patency of the extrahepatic bile ducts. It can exclude the diagnosis of biliary atresia when bile flow into the duodenum is demonstrated. In the case of biliary atresia, hepatobiliary scintigraphy usually demonstrates good hepatic uptake with absent or reduced excretion at 24 h. The diagnostic value of hepatobiliary

scintigraphy can be improved by using [99]technetium-labeled disopropyliminoacetic acid (DISIDA scan) after administration of phenobarbital (a choleretic). In reported series, the sensitivity of hepatobiliary scintigraphy approaches 100%, but specificity ranges from 40 to 100%. The findings of hepatobiliary scintigraphy remain nonspecific and additional workup is required.

Percutaneous liver biopsy is often the next step in the diagnostic workup. In infants with biliary atresia, there will be expanded fibrous portal tracts with edema, fibrosis, and inflammation, bile ductule proliferation, and canalicular and bile duct plugs. These histologic findings are diagnostic of neonatal cholestasis, they are nonspecific. The differential diagnosis still includes choledochal cyst, bile duct stricture or stone, and other toxic, metabolic or genetic causes. The final step and still the gold standard for the diagnosis of biliary atresia is to demonstrate an atretic biliary tree by abdominal exploration and intra-operative cholangiogram.

Newer modalities being used to evaluate patients with suspected biliary atresia include ERCP and MRCP. These modalities are not routinely used because of limited availability and experience with these procedures in neonates. Both have theoretical value in the diagnostic workup of biliary atresia and are likely to play a more prominent role in the future.

It is critical that the diagnostic evaluation be not only thorough but also rapid, as earlier age at treatment has been consistently shown to improve survival and decrease the need for liver transplantation. Adequate nutrition has been shown to improve outcomes. Fasting should be minimized and calories and fat-soluble vitamins should be supplemented. Finally, family education about biliary atresia is important and should include detailed discussions regarding the risk of perioperative complications, the potential for inadequate biliary drainage after portoenterostomy, the possibility of liver transplantation within the first year of life, and the fact that some patients have progressive disease despite maximal medical and surgical therapy and can go on to develop cirrhosis and need a liver transplantation. In addition, families of patients with BASM or syndromic biliary atresia should be made aware of the worse outcomes in this patient subgroup.

Treatment

The treatment of biliary atresia is surgical, starting with portoenterostomy and, if necessary, liver transplantation. Without definitive surgical therapy, the natural history invariably includes progressive liver fibrosis, cirrhosis, end stage liver disease, and death, usually within 2 years. Most patients with biliary atresia should be offered portoenterostomy.

Exceptions include patients who present after the first 120 days of life and those with cirrhosis or portal hypertension. These patients should instead be considered for primary liver transplantation.

The goal of the portoenterostomy (the Kasai operation, Fig. 73.1) is to establish bile flow from still-patent bile ductules below the fibrous plate of the liver capsule. We perform portoenterostomy under general endotracheal anesthesia supplemented with epidural analgesia. A nasogastric tube and Foley catheter should be placed and prophylactic antibiotics administered prior to making incision. We begin with a 2-cm subcostal incision and expose the undersurface of the liver and gallbladder fossa. If the gallbladder is a fibrotic remnant without a lumen, then the cholangiogram can be omitted. Otherwise, the gallbladder is dissected out of its fossa and a cholangiogram is performed by placing a purse-string suture in the dome of the gallbladder, excising the tip of the gallbladder, and inserting a 24-gauge intravenous cannula. With the catheter secured in place, contrast material is injected under fluoroscopic guidance. Extravasation of the contrast material around the catheter without flow into the duodenum or liver confirms the diagnosis of biliary atresia. The catheter is removed and the incision extended to a full right subcostal incision.

The liver is mobilized by taking down the falciform and triangular ligaments, allowing the entire liver to be mobilized up through the incision, providing excellent exposure of the portal structures. We then proceed with a meticulous dissection of the hilum and preparation of the fibrous plate for portoenterostomy. The hepatic artery and its branches are identified and dissected. The portal vein is identified and dissected free at its bifurcation, clearing its upper margin away from the underlying liver capsule (the location of the fibrous plate). Tiny portal venous branches to the capsule are ligated and divided, if necessary, to gain enough exposure around the fibrous plate and to accommodate the portoenterostomy sutures. This portal dissection is carried out to the first branches of the hepatic arteries bilaterally. The cystic artery is ligated, the gallbladder is taken down off of the hepatic bed, and any common bile duct remnant is dissected and divided, leaving the extrahepatic ductal remnants attached only at the fibrous plate. Next, fine monofilament traction sutures are placed circumferentially around the fibrous plate to the depth of the liver capsule. The fibrous plate is then placed on maximal traction and sharply divided at the depth of the liver capsule. A smooth, glistening cut surface should be the result. Hemostasis is achieved by placing an epinephrine-soaked gauze and gentle pressure (never use electrocautery!). The specimen should be oriented and sent to pathology.

The liver is then placed back into the abdominal cavity and a Roux-en-Y limb created. The proximal jejunum is divided 10–20 cm distal to the ligament of Treitz and a 20–30 cm Roux limb is created by performing an end-to-side jejuno-jejunostomy with a single layer of interrupted absorbable sutures. The mesenteric defect is closed and the Roux

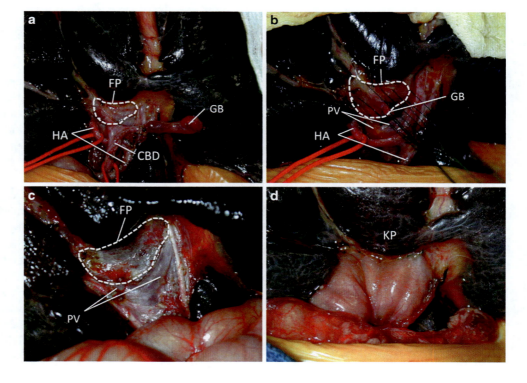

Fig. 73.1 The Kasai portoenterostomy (KP). (**a**) Exposure of the area of the fibrous plate (FP – *dotted line*) prior to division of the common bile duct (CBD) remnant. The hepatic arteries (HA) have been dissected to their first hepatic branch and the gall bladder (GB) dissected off the liver. (**b**) The portal vein (PV) bifurcation has been dissected away from the FP and traction sutures placed around the margins of the plate. (**c**) The transected fibrous plate. Note the glistening fibrotic surface and the bile staining around the periphery of the plate. (**d**) The completed portoenterostomy

limb is passed through a defect created in the transverse mesocolon so as to lie in a retrocolic position. The liver is then brought up and out again and the fibrous plate is examined for hemostasis. When adequate hemostasis has been achieved, an enterotomy is made in the antimesenteric border of the Roux limb to approximate the size of the fibrous plate. The portoenterostomy is then performed using interrupted fine absorbable monofilament sutures. The posterior rim of the anastomosis, between the portal vein and the fibrous plate, is performed with horizontal mattress sutures add the knots tied internally. The anterior half of the anastomosis is then completed with the knots tied externally. The viscera are returned to the abdominal cavity, hemostasis is confirmed, and the incision is closed in layers with absorbable suture.

Postoperative Care

After portoenterostomy, it is important to determine if bile flow has been established and to maintain adequate nutrition. Patients are usually maintained on bowel rest, with or without a nasogastric tube in place, until return of bowel function. The clinical hallmark of a functioning portoenterostomy is the production of pigmented stools. Stools should be green, tawny or brown. Persistently acholic stools, even when intermittent, are concerning for inadequate bile drainage and should be investigated. An ultrasound might reveal a fluid collection, which is concerning for a bile leak or Roux limb obstruction, but a nuclear medicine biliary scintigraphy scan should be performed if there is any question about the adequacy of bile drainage.

Early postoperative complications like bleeding and anastomotic leak should always be considered in neonates who do poorly after portoenterostomy. In addition, ascites might initially worsen in the immediate postoperative period, particularly in patients with cirrhosis, and requires careful fluid management. Prophylactic antibiotics should be continued throughout the peri-operative period. These infants are especially prone to cholangitis, which occurs in 45–60% of patients overall: more than half occur within 6 months, 90% within the first year. The incidence of cholangitis is inversely correlated with bile flow. Many centers administer prophylactic antibiotics orally for 3–12 months postoperatively in an effort to prevent cholangitis. No strong evidence is available to support this practice. Patients who initially achieve good drainage after a Kasai procedure and then develop an acute rise in bilirubin levels should be considered for revision of the portoenterostomy. This is an uncommon scenario and some surgeons discourage reoperative revision of the portoenterostomy.

In addition to monitoring for complications such as bleeding, obstruction, and cholangitis, it is common to administer medical therapies intended to stimulate bile flow. Corticosteroids are thought to stimulate bile flow by inducing cannalicular electrolyte transport. Some believe they might also limit the progression of bile duct injury and fibrosis and prevent the closure of microscopic bile ducts through their anti-inflammatory and immunosuppressive effects. There is a lack of consensus on the benefit of steroids in biliary atresia. Retrospective studies suggest improved outcome. Reports from Japan suggest marked benefit with an aggressive regimen that includes prednisolone 10 mg intravenous twice daily for 7 days, then 20 mg orally every day for 4 days, gradual tapering of subsequent doses, and stopping when the total bilirubin level is below 2 mg/dL for 3 months. Researchers there claim that this leads to clearance of jaundice in greater than 80% of patients and a 10-year survival without transplantation of 60%. However, in a study from Europe, high-dose steroids did not lead to improved outcomes compared to historical controls. Furthermore, a recent small randomized controlled trial from the United Kingdom that used prednisolone 2 mg/kg orally on postoperative days 7–28 demonstrated that steroids were well tolerated and led to decreased bilirubin levels at 1 and 3 months, but no difference at 6 and 12 months. The need for liver transplantation was also the same. The use of corticosteroids remains controversial and therefore larger clinical trials are underway.

Ursodeoxycholic acid (Ursodiol, Actigall) is another therapy used frequently at many centers to encourage bile flow and decrease the toxicity of circulating bile acids. Despite a lack of strong evidence to support its use, it is more widely accepted and administered because it is well tolerated and has few side effects.

Most patients with biliary atresia have ongoing issues with malnutrition, mainly due to increased caloric needs in the setting of fat malabsorption and fat-soluble vitamin deficiencies. They require life-long nutritional support with oral fat-soluble vitamin supplementation and a high-calorie, high-protein diet with at least 125% of recommended caloric intake. In some patients, supplemental nocturnal feedings with semi-elemental formulas and medium chain triglycerides are necessary to meet nutritional goals.

Several factors that influence the success rates of portoenterostomy have been identified. (Table 73.2) Age at treatment has been consistently associated with better long-term survival with native liver, with the best outcomes reported when portoenterostomy is performed before 60 days. This relationship might be explained by age serving as a proxy for the extent of liver damage present at the time of the procedure. Histologic features of the excised biliary remnants, including fewer and a smaller cross-sectional area of residual biliary

Table 73.2 Factors influencing outcomes after portoenterostomy

Age at treatment
Histologic characteristics of residual biliary ductules
Surgeon and center expertise
Syndromic biliary atresia or BASM
Anatomic pattern of biliary atresia
Episodes of cholangitis
Presence of cirrhosis at the time of surgery

ductules indicates lower probability of successful restoration of bile flow with portoenterostomy. In addition, some studies suggest that the experience of the medical center and expertise of the surgeon play a role, with centralization of care of patients with biliary atresia leading to improved 5-year survival with native liver (pre-centralization: 40%; after centralization: 60%), but these findings have not been reported in all centers. The presence of syndromic biliary atresia or BASM has been associated with lower survival (32% vs. 77%) and survival with native liver (47% vs. 91%). Many attribute these poorer outcomes to the prevalence of associated cardiac anomalies in these patients. The anatomy of the extrahepatic biliary remnant also affects outcome, with "correctable" forms of biliary atresia, types I or II, having better outcomes. Ten-year survival with native liver in patients with no patent ducts is 21%; with patent gallbladder, cystic duct and common bile duct it is 36%; with a cyst at the liver hilum and communicating dystrophic intrahepatic ducts it is 56%; and with atresia of common bile duct only it is 83%. As expected, the presence of cirrhosis or liver fibrosis at time of portoenterostomy is associated with a higher risk of developing advanced liver disease and requiring liver transplantation in the future. The occurrence of postoperative cholangitis is also considered a risk factor for progressive liver fibrosis and cirrhosis and a marker of poor bile drainage.

Markers predictive of outcome have also been reported. Postoperative total bilirubin levels at 3 months strongly correlate with outcome of portoenterostomy. A bilirubin level under 2 mg/dL is predictive of a good outcome, while a level over 6 mg/dL is predictive of a poor outcome at 2 years. In another series, 60% of patients with total bilirubin levels under 2 mg/dL at 3 months survived with native liver at 2 years, compared to 15% with levels over 2 mg/dL. In addition, hepatobiliary scans demonstrating bile flow at either 6 weeks or 6 months after portoenterostomy are predictive of long-term survival with native liver.

Portoenterostomy adequately restores bile flow in 40–60% of patients. Subsequently, the course of the disease is highly variable, with many patients developing cirrhosis and complications of portal hypertension due to ongoing intrahepatic biliary injury. Overall, 20–30% of patients have long-term stability of their disease with reported 10- and 20-year survival rates with native liver of 30–35% and 14–23%.

Transplantation

Biliary atresia is the leading indication for pediatric liver transplantation, accounting for more than 40% of all pediatric liver transplants and more than 75% of liver transplants in children under 2 years of age. Despite an adequately draining portoenterostomy, progressive fibro-proliferative obliteration of the intrahepatic biliary ducts leads to fibrosis, cirrhosis, and liver failure in many patients, 70–80% of whom eventually need liver transplantation. Common indications for liver transplantation in biliary atresia patients include: (1) poor early response to portoenterostomy with persistently acholic stools, bilirubin greater than 6 mg/dL at 3 months, and failure to thrive, ascites or variceal hemorrhage; (2) late-onset (adolescence) cholestasis with hepatic dysfunction and cirrhosis; (3) primary treatment for neonates who present late (more than 120 days old) or have significant ascites or portal hypertension; (4) recurrent cholangitis; (5) variceal hemorrhage in the setting of jaundice or if refractory to endoscopic management; and (6) refractory ascites with advanced liver disease.

Outcome after liver transplantation is excellent, with 1-, 5- and 10-year patient survival of 95, 90, and 88%, and graft survival rates of 87, 82, and 81%. Furthermore, patients demonstrate a period of catch-up growth and normal development after liver transplantation. Malnutrition adversely affects both waiting-list and post-transplantation mortality; therefore, aggressive use of fat-soluble vitamin supplementation, supplemental enteral feedings and medium-chain triglyceride enteral nutrition formulas should be considered in patients with progression of biliary atresia. Overall long-term patient survival rates greater than 90% are now being achieved with portoenterostomy and liver transplantation options.

Future Directions

Ongoing efforts to characterize the etiology of the disease should lead to the development of novel treatments. In the meantime, international multi-institution initiatives have been formed to facilitate studying the clinical aspects of this disease and to perform definitive clinical trials of treatments. These include the NIH-sponsored Biliary Atresia Research Consortium (BARC) in the United States, the Japanese Biliary Atresia Registry, and the European Federation for Biliary Atresia Research.

In addition to these research initiatives, new screening methods and better physician education should improve outcomes in biliary atresia by leading to earlier diagnosis and treatment. One promising screening tool is the use of stool color cards. In a study from Taiwan, stool color cards given to parents prior to discharge from the hospital led to an earlier diagnosis of biliary atresia with 23 of 30 cases (79%) of biliary atresia diagnosed before 30 days of age and 26 of 30 (90%) diagnosed before 60 days of age. The sensitivity, specificity, and positive and negative predictive values in this study were 90, 99, 29, and 99%. Larger studies investigating the impact of stool cards are ongoing. Other screening modalities being investigated include measuring direct bilirubin levels in blood spots and blood specimens. Beyond screening, physician education and awareness might play a role in improving outcomes. This includes educational initiatives to increase awareness that infants with jaundice persisting into the second and third weeks of life need to be evaluated for neonatal cholestasis, and considering a change in the routine visit schedule for newborns. In the United States, follow-up visits are typically at 2 and 8 weeks of age while the peak presentation of biliary atresia occurs at between 4 and 6 weeks of age. Finally, from a surgical perspective, advances in liver transplantation and immunosuppression continue to lead to improved outcomes in patients with biliary atresia.

Summary Points

- Biliary atresia is characterized by inflammation of the bile ducts leading to progressive fibro-proliferative obliteration of the extrahepatic biliary tree and, to a variable extent, the intrahepatic bile ducts.
- Acquired biliary atresia is more common (75–90%) and presents in well-appearing newborns with no other associated anomalies; Syndromic biliary atresia is less common (10–25% of cases) and is associated with other congenital anomalies.
- The typical patient with biliary atresia is a full-term, healthy, well appearing, normal birth weight infant that develops persistent jaundice by weeks for to six of life with icteric sclera, jaundice, acholic stools, dark urine, and hepatomegaly.
- Neonatal cholestasis, characterized by an elevated total bilirubin and greater than 20% direct bilirubin, must undergo a complete workup to rule out both extrahepatic and intrahepatic causes.
- The gold standard for the diagnosis of biliary atresia is abdominal exploration with cholangiogram that demonstrates an atretic biliary tree.
- Treatment of biliary atresia is surgical with portoenterostomy and liver transplantation, when necessary.
- Commonly used postoperative medical therapies include antibiotics, corticosteroids, ursodeoxycholic acid, and nutritional supplementation.
- Factors that might influence the success of portoenterostomy include: earlier age at surgery (preferably less than 60 days), favorable histology, degree of surgical expertise, biliary anatomy, presence of syndromic biliary atresia, and occurrence of postoperative cholangitis.
- Postoperative total bilirubin levels at 3 months strongly correlate with outcome of portoenterostomy with total bilirubin levels less than 2 mg/dL predictive of a good outcome.
- Portoenterostomy adequately restores bile flow in 40–60% of patients; overall, 20–30% of patients have long-term stability of their disease.
- Outcome after liver transplantation is excellent and overall patient survival rates greater than 90% are being achieved with portoenterostomy and liver transplantation options.

Editor's Comment

Children with biliary atresia clearly do best when a meticulous portoenterostomy is performed early in the course of the disease by a surgeon with a great deal of experience. They should also be treated at tertiary-care centers where there-is expertise in Gastroenterology/Hepatology, Nutrition, Pathology, Radiology and Nursing. Less clear are the benefits of postoperative prophylactic antibiotics, corticosteroids, and choleretics like ursodeoxycholic acid.

The standard diagnostic approach (ultrasound, DISIDA scan, percutaneous liver biopsy, and ultimately intra-operative cholangiogram, in that order) is certainly invasive but highly accurate. I suspect a minimal access or percutaneous approach will someday become standard, though it is uncommon for a child to undergo a cholangiogram and not have biliary atresia. Furthermore, even when biliary atresia has been ruled out, the diagnosis is usually cholestasis, in which case clearing the extrahepatic biliary tree of inspissated bile and sludge by performing a cholangiogram is often therapeutic.

The Kasai portoenterostomy works by allowing bile (in the form of lymph?) to escape from the liver through tiny canaliculi located just below the fibrous plate at the convergence of the hepatic ducts. The critical maneuver is the proper excision of the fibrous plate to expose these microscopic ducts, after painstakingly exposing as much of the fibrous plate as possible at the bifurcation of the portal vein. The cut should be neither too superficial nor too deep, as though shaving a thin slice of thickened capsule, and should be made with a fresh blade or very sharp tenotomy scissors. The cut surface should weep a clear yellow fluid. Bleeding should be controlled with pressure and very warm saline- or epinephrine-soaked gauze sponges. Cautery and hemostatic agents should never be used.

Postoperative cholangitis and technical complications (bile leak, bleeding, roux limb obstruction) should be treated promptly and aggressively, with reoperation if necessary. The traditional approach is to revise the portoenterostomy if the child drains initially and then stops draining, and proceed directly to liver transplantation if adequate drainage is never achieved. Routine surgical revision is unlikely to salvage a large percentage of livers that fail to drain but, used selectively, it is a reasonable option for some patients.

Differential Diagnosis

Extrahepatic Causes

- Biliary atresia
- Choledochal cyst
- Inspissated bile plug (cystic fibrosis)
- Gallstones
- Bile duct stricture or stenosis
- Spontaneous perforation of the common bile duct
- Tumor
- Intrahepatic causes:
- Toxic:
- Parenteral nutrition
- Medications

Infectious

- Viral (Hepatitis, Herpes, Adenovirus, Enterovirus, HIV)
- Bacterial sepsis
- Metabolic/Genetic disease:
- Alagille Syndrome
- Mitochondrial disorders
- Cirhin deficiency
- Alpha-1 antitrypsin deficiency
- Cystic fibrosis
- Hemochromatosis
- Disorders of glucose, amino acid, lipid or bile acid metabolism
- Idiopathic neonatal hepatitis

Diagnostic Studies

- Liver function
- Ultrasound
- Hepatobiliary scintigraphy
- Liver biopsy
- MRCP
- ERCP

Parental Preparation

- There are several possible immediate and long-term complications, including infection, bleeding, anastomotic leak, cholangitis, and inadequate bile flow.
- Children with inadequate bile flow or progressive liver dysfunction might eventually need liver transplantation.

Preoperative Preparation

- ☐ Informed consent
- ☐ Hydration
- ☐ Supplemental nutrition
- ☐ Vitamin supplementation (including Vitamin K)
- ☐ Type and screen
- ☐ Prophylactic antibiotics

Technical Points

- Surgical exploration and intraoperative cholangiogram are the gold-standard diagnostic study for biliary atresia.
- Once the diagnosis is confirmed, one should perform a meticulous dissection of hepatic artery, portal vein, and the remnant hepatic ducts.
- The gallbladder and biliary remnant should be carefully excised, exposing the fibrous plate.
- A widely patent portoenterostomy should be created between the fibrous plate and a jejunal Roux limb.

Suggested Reading

Bassett MD, Murray KF. Biliary atresia: recent progress. J Clin Gastroenterol. 2008;42(6):720–9.

Chen SM, Chang MH, Du JC, et al. Screening for biliary atresia by infant stool color card in Taiwan. Pediatrics. 2006;117(4): 1147–54.

Davenport M, De Ville de Goyet J, Stringer MD, et al. Seamless management of biliary atresia in England and Wales (1999-2002). Lancet. 2004;363(9418):1354–7.

Davenport M, Stringer MD, Tizzard SA, McClean P, Mieli-Vergani G, Hadzic N. Randomized, double-blind, placebo-controlled trial of corticosteroids after Kasai portoenterostomy for biliary atresia. Hepatology. 2007;46(6):1821–7.

Humphrey TM, Stringer MD. Biliary atresia: US diagnosis. Radiology. 2007;244(3):845–51.

Kelly DA, Davenport M. Current management of biliary atresia. Arch Dis Child. 2007;92(12):1132–5.

Muraji T, Nio M, Ohhama Y, et al. Postoperative corticosteroid therapy for bile drainage in biliary atresia–a nationwide survey. J Pediatr Surg. 2004;39(12):1803–5.

Nio M, Ohi R, Miyano T, Saeki M, Shiraki K, Tanaka K. Five- and 10-year survival rates after surgery for biliary atresia: a report from the Japanese Biliary Atresia Registry. J Pediatr Surg. 2003;38(7): 997–1000.

Petersen C. Pathogenesis and treatment opportunities for biliary atresia. Clin Liver Dis. 2006;10(1):73–88. vi.

Petersen C, Harder D, Melter M, et al. Postoperative high-dose steroids do not improve mid-term survival with native liver in biliary atresia. Am J Gastroenterol. 2008;103(3):712–9.

Roach JP, Bruny JL. Advances in the understanding and treatment of biliary atresia. Curr Opin Pediatr. 2008;20(3):315–9.

Shneider BL, Brown MB, Haber B, et al. A multicenter study of the outcome of biliary atresia in the United States, 1997 to 2000. J Pediatr. 2006;148(4):467–74.

Shneider BL, Mazariegos GV. Biliary atresia: a transplant perspective. Liver Transpl. 2007;13(11):1482–95.

Sokol RJ, Shepherd RW, Superina R, Bezerra JA, Robuck P, Hoofnagle JH. Screening and outcomes in biliary atresia: summary of a National Institutes of Health workshop. Hepatology. 2007;46(2): 566–81.

Wadhwani SI, Turmelle YP, Nagy R, Lowell J, Dillon P, Shepherd RW. Prolonged neonatal jaundice and the diagnosis of biliary atresia: a single-center analysis of trends in age at diagnosis and outcomes. Pediatrics. 2008;121(5):e1438–40.

Chapter 74
Surgical Therapy of Disorders of Intrahepatic Cholestasis

Peter Mattei

Medical management of patients with certain disorders of intrahepatic cholestasis, including progressive familial intrahepatic cholestasis (PFIC) and Alagille disease, can often delay the need for liver transplantation for many years. Some of these patients, however, develop severe and intractable pruritus, apparently due to excessive serum levels of bile salts. The pruritus can be debilitating, driving some patients to consider suicide.

Liver transplantation is curative for both PFIC and Alagille disease and was formerly the only option for patients with intractable pruritus. However, there are now available several operations that are designed to lower the serum concentration of bile salts and can provide substantial relief of pruritus in these patients. The two most commonly used operations are partial external biliary diversion (PEBD) and ileal bypass.

Disorders of Intrahepatic Cholestasis

Alagille disease is a genetic disorder (autosomal dominant) characterized by conjugated hyperbilirubinemia, congenital heart disease (usually tetrology of Fallot), vertebral abnormalities, and a characteristic facies. In addition, some develop multiple subcutaneous xanthomas and a characteristic thickening of the skin on the palms and soles, both of which can be painful and quite bothersome to the patient. The diagnosis is confirmed by liver biopsy, which classically demonstrates a paucity of bile ducts. Some develop rapidly progressive liver failure and require life-saving liver transplantation. Others are managed symptomatically and with choleretics

and do reasonably well, surviving well into adulthood. However, patients for whom the pruritus and skin changes are debilitating should be considered for a biliary drainage procedure.

PFIC is a group of autosomal recessive genetic disorders that results from a mutation in one of several genes involved in the transport or metabolism of bile salts. Three distinct types have been described, each characterized by cholestasis and progressive liver dysfunction, although the clinical patterns and timing of onset differ. PFIC-1 (Byler disease) is caused by a mutation in the gene that codes for FIC-1, an ATPase involved in phospholipid translocation. PFIC-2 often presents in infancy and is caused by a bile salt export pump (BSEP) protein deficiency. PFIC-3 is caused by a mutation in the multidrug resistance protein-3 (MDR-3) and is associated with elevated serum GGT and a later onset. This form of the disease is not usually associated with severe pruritus and is not effectively treated with non-transplant surgery. Children with PFIC-1 or -2 develop high serum concentrations of bile acids, causing severe pruritus. Surgical therapy is indicated for severe pruritus but, because surgery also appears to ameliorate liver damage in these patients, it is now recommended as primary therapy.

Surgical Technique

There are several operations described for the treatment of intrahepatic cholestasis. PEBD and ileal bypass have a reasonably good track record of success and are the standard of care at some centers. Cholecysto-appendicostomy and cholecysto-jejuno-colostomy (partial internal biliary diversion) are relatively new, are rarely performed, and await further studies before they can be recommended.

PEBD involves the creation of a jejunal conduit between the gallbladder and a skin-level ostomy, where the bile empties into an ostomy appliance and is discarded by the patient. Only some of the bile is diverted but it is enough to

P. Mattei (✉)
General, Thoracic and Fetal Surgery, The Children's Hospital
of Philadelphia, 34th Street and Civic Center Boulevard,
Philadelphia, PA 10104, USA
e-mail: mattei@email.chop.edu

P. Mattei (ed.), *Fundamentals of Pediatric Surgery*,
DOI 10.1007/978-1-4419-6643-8_74, © Springer Science+Business Media, LLC 2011

cause a decrease in the total amount of bile salts available for enterohepatic circulation. The operation itself is very straightforward. Through a small transverse right upper quadrant incision, a 15- to 20-cm segment of proximal jejunum is isolated on a generous mesenteric pedicle and intestinal continuity is reestablished by primary anastomosis. The proximal end of the jejunal conduit is anastomosed end-to-side to the gallbladder using absorbable sutures. This must be done in a way that anticipates the final position of the gallbladder when the liver retractors are removed, otherwise the conduit will become kinked. This usually means dividing the jejunum at an angle, longer on the mesenteric side and shorter on the antimesentery. The distal end is brought out through a separate incision, made below the primary incision to encourage dependent drainage, and matured in the manner of a Brooke ileostomy. The operation can also be performed using a laparoscopic-assisted approach.

Ileal diversion is simply an ileocolostomy that bypasses the distal 15% of the length of the small intestine. The goal is to prevent the resorption of bile salts, which normally occurs in the terminal ileum. Through a small transverse right lower quadrant incision, the bowel is measured twice and a gastrointestinal stapling device is used to divide the bowel at a point 85% of the distance between the ligament of Treitz and the ileocecal valve. The proximal end is then anastomosed end-to-side to the right colon just above the cecum. The mesenteric defect is obliterated to prevent an internal hernia.

Postoperative Care

The postoperative care of the patient who has undergone PEBD or ileal bypass is the same as for any bowel procedure, with the notable exception that vitamin K should be administered, especially in patients with PFIC. Without intravenous supplementation for at least three days or until the patient is able to tolerate a regular diet, there is a significant risk of postoperative bleeding. Even with a proximal jejunal anastomosis, a fast-track protocol may be used (no routine nasogastric tube, advance diet as tolerated from postoperative day one, minimize narcotics). For patients who have undergone ileal bypass, especially in infancy, providing adequate nutrition is a real concern, even though it is rare to encounter malabsorption or malnutrition when only 15% of the bowel length is bypassed. Absorption of the fat soluble vitamins (A, D, E, K) is diminished and supplementation becomes more important than ever in this susceptible population. Likewise, there is the potential for vitamin B12 deficiency, which should be supplemented intravenously.

Results

The results of PEBD are generally quite good, with most patients experiencing complete or near-complete relief of pruritus. Patients with Alagille disease also frequently note improvement in the hyperkeratosis of their hands and feet and a substantial decrease in the size and number of painful subcutaneous xanthomas. In addition to relief of symptoms, most patients with PFIC also experience improved growth and a slowing in the progression of liver dysfunction – for these patients, it is therapeutic, not just palliative. Many have even documented an improvement in the histological appearance of subsequent liver biopsies. PEBD is now recommended as primary therapy of PFIC.

The results of ileal diversion appear to be less consistent, less dramatic, and probably less durable. Some recent series tout excellent early results, however the immediate and long-term results tend to be worse, presumably because of bowel adaptation and a gradual increase in the ileal absorption of bile salts.

The results of cholecysto-appendicostomy are difficult to assess as there are few reports. We have one patient who had it done and had a great deal of technical difficulty because of the small size of the conduit and required intermittent catheterization to maintain patency. The idea of partial internal biliary diversion is appealing in that it avoids an external ostomy and theoretically should accomplish the same degree of relief. The biggest concern, of course, is the risk of ascending infection when the colon is used as the drainage site. In addition, it is likely that patients will experience increased frequency and urgency of defecation when bile is allowed to dump directly into the colon. We have tried to create a reservoir using the jejunum in which a gastrostomy tube is placed, with the idea that the patient could intermittently empty the bile without having to wear an external appliance. This has not worked as planned, perhaps because the pouch was created in a dependent area (RLQ), but more likely because of the viscosity and rheological properties of bile – it is slippery and tends to leak around the gastrostomy, ultimately necessitating the use of an ostomy appliance.

Although the PEBD operation works much better than the ileal bypass procedure, patients generally hate to have to wear an ostomy appliance. This is especially true in adolescents, who often forget how miserable they before the procedure. These patients frequently request to be converted to some form of an internal drainage procedure. This is technically straightforward but generally involves cholecystectomy and thus removes the ability to be converted back to PEBD should the ileal bypass fail. We have preserved the jejunal conduit by creating an end-to-side anastomosis to the proximal jejunum, which has worked well and should allow us to perform PEBD again in the future should the patient change her mind again.

Complications

Patients are at risk for small bowel obstruction due to adhesions and entrapment within an internal hernia. Many also require revision of the stoma due to retraction, prolapse or parastomal hernia. Revision of the conduit is sometimes necessary because of kinking or excessive length. Cholangitis appears to be extremely rare. Postoperative bleeding can occur due to vitamin K deficiency, thus the recommendation that it be administered intravenously in the postoperative period.

Summary Points

- Some patients with Alagille disease or PFIC develop severe and intractable pruritus and are candidates for non-transplant surgical therapy.
- The two most common operations designed to lower serum concentrations of bile salts are PEBD and ileal bypass.
- For most patients with PFIC, PEBD provides effective relief of pruritus and also improves growth and liver function.
- For most patients with Alagille disease, PEBD provides effective relief of pruritus, lessens palmar hyperkeratosis, and decreases the size and number of soft tissue xanthomas.

Differential Diagnosis

- Alagille disease
- PFIC-1, -2, and -3
- Cholestasis of other etiology
- Biliary atresia
- Choledochal cyst
- Cholangitis

Diagnostic Studies

- Ultrasound
- HIDA scan
- Cholangiography
- MRCP
- Liver biopsy

Preoperative Preparation

☐ Prophylactic antibiotics
☐ Improvement in nutritional parameters
☐ Vitamin K supplementation

Parental Preparation

- Risks include infection, bleeding, injury to adjacent structures, need to revise the ostomy, conduit or anastomosis, small bowel obstruction, and failure to relieve pruritus.
- PEBD is more consistently effective in relieving pruritus and, in patients with PFIC, in improving liver function, but it involves the creation of an ostomy.
- The ileal bypass avoids the ostomy but the results are less predictable and less durable.

Technical Points

- For PEBD, the jejunal conduit should be long enough to prevent ascending infection and to comfortably allow creation of an ostomy, but short enough to provide little resistance to drainage and to avoid the potential for kinks – 15–20 cm.
- Ileal diversion is an ileocolostomy that bypasses the distal 15% of the length of the small intestine (measure twice, cut once).
- Patients should be given intravenous vitamin K postoperatively to avoid bleeding complications.

Suggested Reading

Davis AR, Rosenthal P, Newman TB. Nontransplant surgical interventions in progressive familial intrahepatic cholestasis. J Pediatr Surg. 2009;44(4):821–7.

Mattei P, von Allmen D, Piccoli D, Rand E. Relief of intractable pruritus in Alagille syndrome by partial external biliary diversion. J Pediatr Surg. 2006;41(1):104–7.

Modi BP, Suh MY, Jonas MM, Lillehei C, Kim HB. Ileal exclusion for refractory symptomatic cholestasis in Alagille syndrome. J Pediatr Surg. 2007;42(5):800–5.

Whitington PF, Whitington GL. Partial external diversion of bile for the treatment of intractable pruritus associated with intrahepatic cholestasis. Gastroenterology. 1988;95(1):130–6.

Yang H, Porte RJ, Verkade HJ, et al. Partial external biliary diversion in children with progressive familial intrahepatic cholestasis and Alagille disease. J Pediatr Gastroenterol Nutr. 2009;49(2):216–21.

Chapter 75
Cholecystitis

Andrè Hebra and Aaron Lesher

Introduction

Cholecystitis and cholelithiasis are occurring with increasing frequency in children. Cholecystectomy for symptomatic cholelithiasis, cholecystitis, and biliary dyskinesia now comprise approximately 4% of all cholecystectomies performed in this age group. Although younger boys and girls have similar rates of gallstone disease, girls are more commonly affected as age increases, with a female-to-male predominance of between 10 and 20–1. Once thought to be isolated to patients with hemolytic disease, gallstone formation is also associated with prolonged parenteral nutrition, trauma, sepsis, pregnancy, and obesity. Non-hemolytic cholelithiasis is more prevalent than hemolytic cholelithiasis. In our experience, the incidence of cholesterol gallstones as an indication for laparoscopic cholecystectomy far exceeds that of pigmented stones. Pediatricians and pediatric surgeons should consider the possibility of gallbladder pathology in every child presenting with abdominal pain.

Gallstones are usually classified into one of three types: cholesterol stones, pigment stones, or mixed-type. Cholesterol stones usually result from cholesterol saturation of bile and stasis and are found in children and adolescents without hemolytic disease (Fig. 75.1). These stones are radiolucent and form within the gallbladder, sometimes migrating into the ductal system. Obesity, Western diet, pregnancy, and advancing age are risk factors for cholesterol stones. Pigmented stones are radiopaque and associated with supersaturation of bile with calcium bilirubinate, usually due to hemolytic disease. Brown stones are associated with bacterial cholangitis and can form within the ductal system.

Cholecystitis is inflammation of the gallbladder wall, often due to irritation by retained stones or sludge within the gallbladder. In children, acute and chronic calculous cholecystitis may represent two different points in the same disease process, as many gallbladders removed for acute cholecystitis have signs of chronic inflammation and fibrosis. Acute or chronic acalculous cholecystitis can also occur in children without gallstones. Acute acalculous cholecystitis is not uncommon in children and is often associated with serious chronic illness. Although the etiology is poorly understood, risk factors include hyperalimentation, mechanical-assisted ventilation, ileus, and prolonged fasting. Biliary dyskinesia, or chronic acalculous cholecystitis, is a distinct clinical entity that is characterized by decreased gallbladder contractility and signs of chronic cholecystitis on histologic study after cholecystectomy. This condition is now more commonly seen in adolescents with chronic or recurrent right upper quadrant pain. Cholelithiasis in infancy is often related to hyperalimentation and is associated with a variety of risk factors, including congenital biliary tract abnormalities, parental nutrition, hemolytic disease, and prolonged fasting. Obstruction of the common bile duct may occur due to gallbladder sludge and stasis.

Diagnosis

Cholelithiasis and cholecystitis should be included in the differential diagnosis of any patient who presents with right upper quadrant or epigastric abdominal pain with or without jaundice, especially in children with risk factors. The patient with biliary colic typically complains of intermittent right upper quadrant pain of variable intensity. Symptoms of biliary colic due to gallstones often precede those of acute cholecystitis, although the child may have acute cholecystitis at the first presentation. The pain may be diffuse or it can radiate around to the scapula or to the epigastrium. Younger children may have nonspecific abdominal pain, irritability, jaundice or acholic stools. The clinical presentation depends on the location and degree of obstruction caused by the offending stone, which dictates the nature of medical and surgical treatment. The differential diagnosis includes acute hepatitis, gastroesophageal reflux, pancreatitis, appendicitis, colitis, irritable bowel syndrome, pneumonia, and bowel obstruction, including intussusception.

A. Hebra (✉)
Department of Surgery, Medical University of South Carolina,
Children's Hospital, 96 Jonathan Lucas Street,
Charleston, SC 29425, USA
e-mail: hebra@musc.edu

P. Mattei (ed.), *Fundamentals of Pediatric Surgery*,
DOI 10.1007/978-1-4419-6643-8_75, © Springer Science+Business Media, LLC 2011

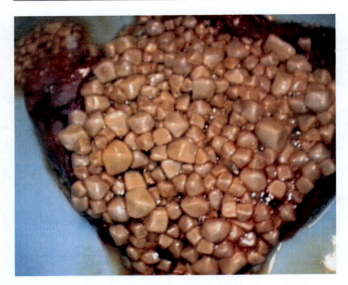

Fig. 75.1 Gallbladder of a 13-year old with morbid obesity and multiple cholesterol stones

While the physical examination of a child with biliary colic is sometimes unremarkable, right upper quadrant tenderness suggests the presence of cholecystitis. Acute calculous cholecystitis, an increasingly common disease process in children, usually presents with the recent onset of unremitting right upper quadrant pain that persists for hours. Most patients have a low-grade fever, nausea, and anorexia. Vomiting occurs in about one third of patients. Laboratory tests usually reveal a mild leukocytosis ($12,000–15,000/mm^3$) and, if there is common bile duct obstruction from stones or edema, elevated conjugated bilirubin. In younger children, the pain is often more generalized. Patients sometimes have a positive Murphy's sign, which is classically described as arrest of deep inspiration and pain during palpation of the gallbladder. Charcot's triad (fever, right upper quadrant pain, jaundice) suggests ascending cholangitis. Jaundice is seen more frequently in the pediatric population than in adults and, because it implies biliary tract obstruction, necessitates a more extensive workup. Chronic cholecystitis and asymptomatic cholelithiasis are more common than acute cholecystitis in the pediatric population. Chronic cholecystitis presents with recurrent episodes of abdominal pain. The diagnosis can be differentiated from biliary colic by the presence of right upper tenderness. However, most children with gallstones have some measure of chronic gallbladder wall inflammation, so differentiating biliary colic from chronic cholecystitis might be purely academic.

While plain abdominal films can demonstrate the 15% of gallstones that are radiopaque, ultrasound is relatively inexpensive to perform, 95% accurate in identifying gallstones, and might reveal evidence of cholecystitis. With ultrasonography, gallstones are seen as discrete echodensities with acoustic shadowing. Ultrasound findings of cholecystitis include gallbladder wall thickening (greater than 3.5 mm), pericholecystic fluid, and gallbladder sludge. Ultrasound can also provide information about the common bile duct, revealing stones or duct dilation. If the ultrasound findings are equivocal, the diagnosis of acute cholecystitis can also be made by cholescintigraphy. Hepatoiminodiacetic acid (HIDA) scanning involves intravenous injection of a radiolabeled tracer that is taken up and excreted by the liver. Nonvisualization of the gallbladder despite passage of tracer into the duodenum is diagnostic of acute cholecystitis, but false positive results can occur in fasting patients or those receiving parenteral nutrition. Using morphine to cause sphincter of Oddi spasm can improve the sensitivity of the test.

Acute acalculous cholecystitis is often diagnosed in association with another systemic disease state and is rarely seen. Patients are typically in critical condition with sepsis, massive burn, prior surgery or other widespread illness, particularly Kawasaki's disease. Symptoms include fever and right upper quadrant pain. Laboratory studies reveal a leukocytosis with left shift, hyperbilirubinemia, and elevated serum amylase.

Biliary dyskinesia is essentially biliary colic without evidence of gallstones. Patients, often females in their early teenage years, present with colicky right upper quadrant pain with nausea after ingesting of a fatty meal. Another cohort of patients presents with nonspecific abdominal pain. The work-up for other sources of abdominal pain, including abdominal radiographs, ultrasound and laboratory studies, is usually negative. The diagnosis is suggested by a HIDA scan that shows poor gallbladder emptying and an ejection fraction of less than 35%. With the increasing availability and use of HIDA scanning, the diagnosis of biliary dyskinesia seems to be increasing in frequency. Numerous reports have documented the efficacy of elective cholecystectomy for biliary dyskinesia, but most have short follow-up. We typically counsel patients about the risks of surgery and offer elective laparoscopic cholecystectomy if the patient and family wish to proceed.

Treatment

The management of patients with acute cholecystitis begins with stabilization of the patient and preparation for the operating room if the patient is a suitable candidate. Fluid resuscitation and a broad-spectrum antibiotic, such as cefazolin, are administered. Nasogastric tube decompression of the stomach is rarely necessary. The timing of operation varies between institutions and even within groups. We typically schedule the patient with acute cholecystitis for laparoscopic cholecystectomy within one to 2 days of presentation.

We prefer to delay surgery for 6 weeks if the patient has been symptomatic for more than 3 days.

Removal of the gallbladder is indicated for patients with symptomatic gallstone disease. Laparoscopic or open cholecystectomy can be performed safely with minimal morbidity and mortality. The laparoscopic approach has become the standard of care and now comprises more than 98% of our cholecystectomy cases. The technique for laparoscopic cholecystectomy in pediatric patients is very similar to that described for adult patients, but a few variations must be taken into account. First, the trocar placement is determined by patient size and position of the gallbladder and the liver. We usually start by placing a 10–12 mm trocar in the umbilical position. Typically the peritoneal cavity is insufflated with CO_2 using the following pressure limits: (1) obese teenage patients: 16 mmHg; (2) normal teenage patients: 14 mmHg; (3) patients 8–12 years of age: 12 mmHg; (4) patients less than 7 years of age: 10 mmHg. If the patient had any previous abdominal surgery or is significantly obese, we prefer to utilize an open technique for the initial trocar placement. In such cases, it is important to create an opening on the inferior aspect of the umbilicus until the muscle fascia and the linea alba can be visualized. Stay sutures of 2-0 braided absorbable suture are placed on each side of the muscle fascia which is then opened under direct visualization. It is not infrequent that additional braided absorbable sutures must be placed in order to elevate the fascia until the peritoneal membrane can be visualized and entered. Once the peritoneum is open, a 12-mm trocar can be inserted under direct visualization and the peritoneal cavity is insufflated.

We perform most of our laparoscopic cholecystectomies with a 5-mm, 30° laparoscope. However, in very obese patients, it is best to have a 10-mm trocar available to perform the cystic duct dissection. This is primarily due to the fact that the 5-mm laparoscope will not generate enough light inside the large abdominal cavity of an obese patient and may compromise the surgeon's ability to clearly visualize all vital structures surrounding the cystic duct. Considering that most complications related to laparoscopic gallbladder surgery occur during the dissection and exposure of the cystic duct, one should never work with poor lighting and inadequate visualization at that point of the operation. It is fairly simple to begin the procedure with the 10 mm laparoscope in place via the 12-mm trocar and to change it to a 5 mm laparoscope once the dissection and exposure of the cystic duct and artery are completed.

Subsequent trocar placement in children must be determined individually once the gallbladder fundus is visualized with the laparoscope. A 5-mm trocar is typically placed in the sub-xyphoid region. Another 5-mm trocar should be placed in the mid-right upper quadrant of the abdomen (at the level of the mid-clavicular line) in such a way to allow the introduction of a laparoscopic instrument that will be utilized to manipulate the neck of the gallbladder. This trocar is usually placed about 2 cm below the costal margin. However, in small children it must be placed closer to the costal margin. The last trocar should be a 5-mm trocar placed lateral in the right upper quadrant. This trocar will be utilized for placement of a grasping instrument such as a McKernan grasping-locking forceps that will be placed on the fundus of the gallbladder for retraction. For that reason, the trocar should not be placed too far from the costal margin. Once the gallbladder fundus is grasped, it must be displaced towards the patient's right shoulder, above the right lobe of the liver. This maneuver will allow for exposure of the neck of the gallbladder. One assistant should keep the fundus of the gallbladder pushed towards the patient's shoulder region at all times. This will elevate the neck of the gallbladder together with the cystic duct and artery, facilitating dissection and exposure.

The third important step is the exposure and dissection of the neck of the gallbladder. If significant inflammatory changes are identified, we prefer to perform an intra-operative cholangiogram to help define the anatomy of the cystic duct and its relationship to the gallbladder and common bile duct. We prefer to perform a cholangiogram through the gallbladder (Fig. 75.2), which can be easily performed by placing an intravenous catheter in the gallbladder under laparoscopic visualization. The gallbladder is filled with water-soluble dye and radiographic images are obtained with live fluoroscopy.

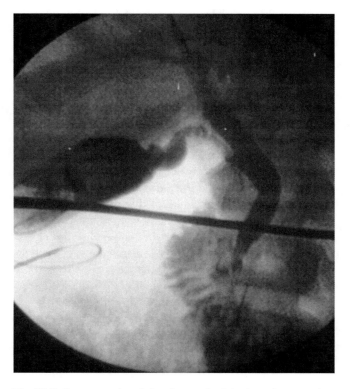

Fig. 75.2 Intra-operative cholangiogram by injection of contrast into the gallbladder demonstrating a long cystic duct, dilated common bile duct, but no evidence of biliary obstruction in a 12-year-old with acute cholecystitis

Not only does this help to identify an obstruction or stones in the common bile duct, but it can provide valuable information about the length and relative location of the cystic duct, facilitating dissection and minimizing the risk of injury to the ducts. The dissection for exposure of the cystic duct and artery is started at the neck of the gallbladder. It is important to first mobilize the visceral peritoneum and any inflammatory adhesions away from the gallbladder. This can be easily performed by using hook electrocautery. We usually have the surgeon manipulate the laparoscopic camera and use a hook or Maryland dissector in the right hand placed via the sub-xyphoid trocar. The assistant should be retracting the fundus of the gallbladder towards the right shoulder at all times and should also have a blunt grasper in the right hand to manipulate the neck of the gallbladder. This manipulation involves moving the neck towards the right or left side, providing dynamic exposure for the surgeon. The assistant should never keep the neck of the gallbladder in a fixed position.

Using careful dissection, the surgeon must achieve the so-called "critical view." This refers to the visualization of the cystic duct and artery as they enter the gallbladder. It is not necessary to expose the common bile duct. Once the point of entry of the cystic duct is clearly visualized on the gallbladder, the duct can be clipped and divided. We prefer to place one 5-mm clip on the cystic duct next to the gallbladder and two clips towards the common bile duct. The cystic artery can be clipped simultaneously with the cystic duct or separately, depending on how close it is to the duct. It is not necessary to completely dissect the artery and fully expose it, since this may lead to bleeding from small branches. In young children, it is possible to cauterize the artery or to divide it with the ultrasonic dissector. Once the cystic duct is divided with scissors, its lumen should be inspected to make sure that there is a single lumen visible and therefore no evidence of injury to the common bile duct. At this point, the surgeon should utilize the hook cautery to divide the visceral peritoneum at the plane between the gallbladder and the liver. Again, the assistant will move the gallbladder back and forth, providing continuous exposure of that plane until the gallbladder is completely free. If a hole is accidentally made in the gallbladder wall, leakage of bile and gallstones can be controlled by placing the grasping instrument over the hole. Lost stones should be removed using the suction-irrigator.

If the gallbladder is partially intrahepatic, it is usually necessary to remove a wedge of liver tissue with the gallbladder. Electrocautery dissection at high settings should be enough for hemostasis. Once the gallbladder is completely separated from the liver, we move the laparoscope to the subxyphoid port and insert a 10-mm endo-pouch through the umbilical port. The gallbladder is placed inside the bag and brought into the trocar. In most cases the gallbladder is too big to be removed through the 12 mm port. We prefer to enlarge the umbilical incision and expose the muscle fascia, which is

than divided with electrocautery. This will allow extraction of the pouch containing the gallbladder. The fascia can then be re-approximated with absorbable sutures. After the gallbladder is removed, we prefer to re-inspect the liver bed to make sure that there is no evidence of bleeding or bile leak. Any residual bile is suctioned. At this point all trocars are removed under direct laparoscopic visualization and the operation is completed. Unless the patient is less than 5 years old, the fascia at the 5-mm trocar sites does not need to be closed.

Recent experience has demonstrated the feasibility of mini-laparoscopic technique for removal of the gallbladder in pediatric patients. The laparoscopic operation can be achieved using 3-mm instruments and minimal use of ports. A three-port mini approach has been reported. However, it is important to remember that patient selection is essential when trying to perform this operation with miniature instruments. One should not sacrifice good visualization and optimal exposure of the vital structures. The risk of iatrogenic injury to the common bile duct would outweigh any benefit that can be achieved with miniature scopes and instruments. Inflammation and adhesions, frequently seen in symptomatic patients, may limit the use of the mini-laparoscopic approach.

The open approach is reserved for patients with dense adhesions whose gall bladder cannot be visualized with the laparoscope. If at the time of laparoscopy, there is evidence of gangrene, empyema, emphysematous cholecystitis, or perforation, we advocate a low threshold for conversion to open cholecystectomy. This approach is performed through either a right subcostal incision (Kocher incision), or an upper midline incision. An intra-operative cholangiogram is indicated if there is clinical evidence of obstruction prior to going to the operating room, if there is suspicion of duct injury, or if the anatomy is unclear.

Nonoperative therapies aimed at treating gallstone disease have been studied. Extracorporeal shockwave lithotripsy in combination with oral dissolution agents, such as ursodiol, has shown promise in adults. Neither of these modalities has been studied in children. In our opinion, for children and teenagers with a normal life expectancy, laparoscopic cholecystectomy as definitive treatment should be the standard of care for symptomatic gallstone disease as the risk of recurrence with all forms of nonoperative therapy is generally high.

Although uncommon in children, stones are sometimes present in the common bile duct. Every child suspected of biliary tract obstruction should undergo preoperative ultrasound and intra-operative cholangiogram. Choledocholithiasis is seen in all age groups and children with hemolysis are disproportionately affected. Jaundice is present and laboratory values are usually suggestive of elevated serum concentrations of conjugated bilirubin, alkaline phosphatase, and serum amylase. Perioperative endoscopic retrograde pancreatography can aid in the diagnosis of common bile duct stones as well as clear the common bile duct. The success of

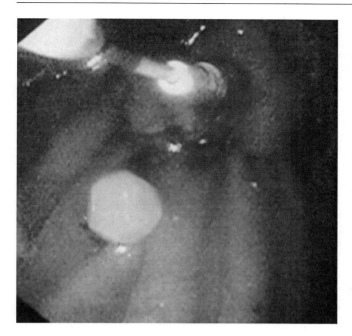

Fig. 75.3 Endoscopic view during ERCP with trans-ampullary extraction of an obstructing cholesterol gallstone in an 8-year-old with obstructive jaundice after laparoscopic cholecystectomy

therapeutic ERCP has increased significantly over the last decade and should be considered the intervention of choice for the initial management of pediatric patients with biliary obstruction (Fig. 75.3). If ERCP is unsuccessful in clearing the common bile duct, a laparoscopic or open procedure with irrigation of the biliary tree via the cystic duct or transduodenal sphincterotomy can be performed. Laparoscopic common bile duct exploration at the time of cholecystectomy has been employed in pediatric patients with excellent results.

Approximately 20% of cholelithiasis in children is related to hemolysis. Hemolytic diseases, including sickle-cell disease, thalassemia major, and hereditary spherocytosis, cause black pigmented stones with subsequent symptomatic gallbladder disease in a significant fraction of patients. These patients present with a similar picture as those patients without hemolysis. If symptomatic gallstone disease is identified, then patients are recommended for elective laparoscopic cholecystectomy. Our protocol for such patients includes hospital admission 1 day prior to cholecystectomy and PRBC transfusion to a hemoglobin of 10 mg/dL to increase the ratio of Hemoglobin A to Hemoglobin S to greater than 2:1. These patients are also aggressively hydrated for 24 h prior to surgery. For children with sickle cell anemia, the presenting symptoms of abdominal pain, jaundice, fever, and nausea may be either abdominal pain or biliary colic. For this reason, we routinely screen all sickle cell children over 10 years of age with ultrasound to rule out gallstone disease. In the absence of gallstones but continued high suspicion, a HIDA scan is appropriate. Non-visualization of the gallbladder suggests cholecystitis and

elective cholecystectomy is indicated. Patients with hereditary spherocytosis requiring splenectomy should undergo gallbladder ultrasound prior to going to surgery. If gallstones are found, we always recommend concurrent laparoscopic cholecystectomy with laparoscopic splenectomy.

Patients who are critically ill with acalculous cholecystitis are treated expectantly if the patient cannot tolerate anesthesia or the stress of operation. Mild cases are treated with nasogastric suction, fluid resuscitation, antibiotics, and expedient treatment of the underlying disease. The patient's clinical course is followed by serial abdominal ultrasounds. Increasing gallbladder distension or worsening clinical status may necessitate percutaneous placement of a cholecystostomy tube, usually performed by interventional radiology. Complications of cholecystitis, such as gallbladder wall gangrene or infarction, emphysematous cholecystitis, or empyema may require emergent open cholecystectomy. This is rarely necessary in pediatric patients.

Neonates and infants treated with prolonged total parenteral nutrition can develop cholestasis with gallstone formation or biliary sludge. We recommend observation with judicious hydration in these patients as these gallstones usually resolve with maturation of the hepatobiliary system. Ursodeoxycholic acid has been employed for dissolution of stones, but strong evidence is lacking. If jaundice persists, we advocate a laparoscopic gallbladder washout procedure.

Postoperative Care

Children who have undergone elective laparoscopic cholecystectomy are typically admitted for overnight observation. Patients are initially advanced from clear liquids to a regular diet as tolerated. Ambulation is encouraged and subsequent activity is only limited by pain. Patients treated with open cholecystectomy generally have a longer hospital course and more postoperative pain.

Children with hemolytic anemias are observed until tolerating a diet with good pain control. Intravenous narcotic needs are typically higher in this group. In patients with sickle cell disease, splenic sequestration crisis and acute chest syndrome can be precipitated by surgery. These children should be monitored closely, since the symptoms of hypoxemia and tachypnea in acute chest syndrome and abdominal pain and anemia in the case of splenic sequestration can begin suddenly with rapid clinical deterioration. Treatment is largely supportive and involved close consultation with specialists in pulmonary, critical care, and hematology medicine. Our experience has demonstrated that the use of laparoscopic technique in children with sickle cell disease does not decrease the risk of post-surgical acute crisis.

Children and adolescents with non-hemolytic gallstone disease usually do extremely well after cholecystectomy. Most modern series of cholecystectomy in children demonstrate minimal morbidity and no mortality. At discharge, parents are told to monitor for unremitting right upper quadrant pain, jaundice, or feeding intolerance, which may suggest a postoperative complication. They are seen in clinic once after 2 weeks to monitor progress and to evaluate for any possible postoperative problems.

Short-term complications include hemorrhage, wound infection, ileus, pancreatitis, cystic duct stump leakage, and common bile duct injury. Ileus and pancreatitis are treated supportively in an inpatient setting. Cystic duct stump leak and common bile duct injuries may present with bile perito-nitis or bilious drainage from the wound. Ultrasound can help to identify a fluid collection amenable to percutaneous drainage. ERCP must be performed to demonstrate the leak and it will often allow for an effective therapeutic intervention such as sphincterotomy or placement of a decompressive stent.

Long-term complications are rare and include small bowel obstruction and bile duct stricture. Small bowel obstruction should be treated according to acuity, with judicious use of laparotomy for lysis of adhesions. The incidence of postoperative bile duct strictures in children is unknown. These patients may present with ascending cholangitis or painless jaundice. Bile duct strictures should be evaluated and treated expeditiously to relieve the obstruction of bile flow.

Summary Points

- Approximately 80% of gallstones are nonhemolytic in origin.
- Diagnosis of gallbladder disease is best made by real-time ultrasonography.
- Ultrasound findings of gallbladder wall thickening, pericholecystic fluid, and echogenic stones with acoustic shadowing are diagnostic for acute cholecystitis.
- Laparoscopic cholecystectomy is the procedure of choice for symptomatic cholelithiasis or acute cholecystitis.
- Chronic acalculous cholecystitis (biliary dyskinesia) is associated with typical symptoms of biliary colic without the presence of gallstones and a HIDA scan gallbladder ejection fraction of <35%.

Editor's Comment

Indications for cholecystectomy in children include pigmented gallstones, symptomatic cholesterol stones, or biliary dyskinesia. Acalculous acute cholecystitis is also seen occasionally, especially in immunocompromised or critically ill patients. It is usually best to treat these children with percutaneous cholecystostomy tube placement, rather than a heroic attempt to remove the gallbladder. Children with incidental asymptomatic gallstones are usually recommended for cholecystectomy, though some are observed for months or years, and sometimes prescribed ursodiol, in the hope that the stones might resolve. They rarely, if ever, disappear.

The prevalence of biliary dyskinesia seems to be increasing. The diagnosis can be elusive but if the patient has: (1) intermittent RUQ or epigastric pain precipitated by meals, (2) associated nausea, and (3) a positive CCK-HIDA scan (gallbladder ejection fraction <35%), then cholecystectomy can be expected to relieve the pain in 85–90% of the cases. With only two of three of these findings, the likelihood of success is probably closer to 60 or 70%, and with only one, cholecystectomy should only be considered if the patient is truly debilitated, all other likely causes have been excluded, and the patient understands that there is a less-than-50% chance that the operation will be a success. Patients should also understand that removal of the gallbladder is not entirely without risk and that it can result in the unpleasant and often intractable problem of fecal urgency and loose bowel movements.

In general, intra-operative cholangiogram is rarely indicated and really only necessary in the rare case of anatomic confusion. Most children with one of the traditional indications for intra-operative cholangiogram (jaundice, pancreatitis, dilated CBD) and whose symptoms have resolved can safely undergo cholecystectomy without intra-operative cholangiogram. If the clinical impression is that they might actually have a stone in the CBD, they should undergo ERCP (or at least an MRCP) before undergoing cholecystectomy. Common duct exploration in children is technically difficult and potentially hazardous; it should almost never be necessary when the expertise to perform a therapeutic ERCP is available. Likewise, open cholecystectomy should rarely be necessary in children. The severe inflammation or fibrosis commonly seen in adults occurs rarely in children and the anatomy is rarely confusing.

Three-trocar cholecystectomy is certainly feasible but because it affords no significant advantage (it eliminates one 5-mm port) and the risks are almost certainly higher, it is difficult to justify its routine application. The single-port operation is being developed but whether it can be done with consistent safety remains to be seen. The operator should always control both the dissector and the assistant's grasper (rather than the camera). This is how all other operations are performed and is certainly more natural. The dissection of the cystic duct should begin at the infundibulum of the gallbladder so that there is no question that it is the cystic duct that is being isolated and divided. The cautery hook should be used more like a spatula, dividing tissue that has been placed under tension by gentle traction, rather than using it as a hook every time. There is increasing evidence that, except in the case of true acute cholecystitis or cholangitis, laparoscopic cholecystectomy can be considered a "clean" case, making prophylactic antibiotics unnecessary.

As a complication of cholecystectomy in children, common bile duct injury appears to be exceedingly rare. Reconstruction is usually best accomplished with Roux-en-Y choledochojejunostomy, which can be prone to strictures due to the small caliber of the duct in most children. Bile leaks are also quite rare but are treated in the standard fashion (percutaneous drainage, ERCP, sphincterotomy, stent). Every attempt should be made to retrieve spilled stones, although retained intraperitoneal stones discovered incidentally months or years later are rarely cause for concern. In some cases, the cystic duct can be quite large and therefore not properly controlled with even the longest endoscopic hemoclip. In these situations, it is usually best to use an endoscopic linear stapling device to come across the duct, though this can be technically challenging.

Differential Diagnosis

- Biliary colic
- Gastroesophageal reflux
- Viral hepatitis
- Irritable bowel syndrome
- Cholangitis
- Small bowel obstruction
- Pancreatitis and pancreatic pseudocyst
- Pneumonia

Diagnostic Studies

- Abdominal radiograph
- CBC, serum bilirubin
- Abdominal ultrasound
- Biliary scintigraphy (HIDA scan)
- MRCP
- ERCP

Parental Preparation

- Possible conversion to open procedure
- Possible injury to common bile duct or pancreatitis
- For patients with biliary dyskinesia, there is the possibility that abdominal pain will not be relieved by cholecystectomy

Preoperative Preparation

☐ IV hydration
☐ RBC transfusion if warranted for hemolytic disease
☐ Preoperative antibiotics
☐ Informed consent

Technical Points

- Laparoscopic trocar placement varies with patient size and body habitus
- Double clip proximal cystic duct stump
- Selective use of intra-operative cholangiogram
- Convert to open if gallbladder is gangrenous or perforated, inadequate visualization, or excessive adhesions and inflammation
- Minilaparoscopic technique employs 3-mm instruments, but visualization of vital structures must not be compromised

Suggested Reading

Balaguer EJ, Price MR, Burd RS. National trends in the utilization of cholecystectomy in children. J Surg Res. 2006;134:68–73.

Bonnard A et al. Laparoscopic approach as primary treatment of common bile duct stones in children. J Pediatr Surg. 2005;40:1459–63.

Holcomb III GW, Andrews WS. Gallbladder disease and hepatic infections. In: Grosfeld JL, O'Neill JA, Fonkalsrud EW, et al., editors. Pediatric surgery, vol. 2. 6th ed. Philadelphia, PA: Mosby Elsevier Health Science; 2006. p. 1635–50.

Holcomb Jr GW, Holcomb III GW. Cholelithiasis in infants, children, and adolescents. Pediatr Rev. 1990;11:268–74.

Nakeer A, Ahrendt SA, Pitt HA. Calculous biliary disease. In: Mulholland MW, Lillemope KD, et al., editors. Greenfield's surgery scientific principles and practice. 4th ed. Philadelphia, PA: Lipincott Williams & Wilkins; 2006. p. 978–99.

Tagge EP, Tarnasky PR, Chandler J, et al. Multidiscoplinary approach to the treatment of pediatric pancreaticobiliary disorders. J Pediatr Surg. 1997;32:158–65.

Tarnasky PR, Tagge EP, Hebra A, et al. Minimally invasive therapy for children. Gastrointest Endosc. 1008;47:189–92.

Chapter 76
Choledochal Cysts

Greg M. Tiao

A choledochal cyst is an uncommon but correctable cause of biliary obstruction that, if left untreated, can cause recurrent episodes of cholangitis and biliary cirrhosis. In the long term, chronic inflammation within the biliary epithelium may result in the development of a cholangiocarcinoma. Operative intervention is therefore warranted in all patients with a choledochal cyst.

The anatomic variations of the choledochal cyst were first classified by Alonso-Lej et al. and subsequently modified by Todani et al. into five subtypes (Fig. 76.1). The most common forms are a type I and type IV. In the case of a type I choledochal cyst, the dilatation is confined to the common bile duct. In contrast, the dilatation in patients with a type IV choledochal cyst either extends in continuity into the intrahepatic biliary tree or there is a short portion of normal-caliber common hepatic duct with isolated or multi-focal intrahepatic duct dilatation. In both type I and IV cysts, the dilated duct tapers to a normal diameter before it is joined by the pancreatic duct in the head of the pancreas.

The most widely accepted theory as to the pathogenesis of types I and IV choledochal cyst is pancreatico-biliary malunion, in which the pancreatic duct joins the bile duct proximal to the sphincter complex, allowing reflux of pancreatic enzymes into the common bile duct (Fig. 76.2). This is thought to damage the bile duct in two ways: direct enzymatic injury to the biliary epithelium and damage caused by increased intraluminal pressure.

Types II, III and V choledochal cyst are rare variants, comprising less than 2% of the cysts identified in large series. A type II choledochal cyst is a diverticulum arising from the wall of the bile duct, thought to occur because of a localized weakness in a segment of the common bile duct. A type III choledochal cyst, also known as a choledochocele, consists of a dilatation at the distal end of the common bile duct that protrudes into the lumen of the duodenum. Type V choledochal cyst, also known as Caroli's disease, consists of multiple cystic dilatations of the intrahepatic biliary tree, often with strictures between the cysts. The cysts can be confined to one lobe of the liver or found throughout the intra-hepatic biliary tree.

Diagnosis

In clinical practice, the classic triad of abdominal pain, jaundice, and right upper quadrant mass occurs rarely. Young children frequently present with one or two of these symptoms while adolescents and adults typically present only with epigastric pain. Some patients are diagnosed after an episode of cholangitis when they present with jaundice, fever, and right upper quadrant pain (Charcot's triad). When a choledochal cyst has been present for a long time, recurrent bouts of cholangitis may result in a thickened and inflamed cyst wall. The biliary epithelium can be significantly damaged, resulting in marked metaplasia or have progressed to a cholangiocarcinoma. In severe cases, the epithelium is replaced by granulation tissue and fibrosis. A giant choledochal cyst can spontaneously perforate such that a patient presents with biliary ascites. These patients have chemical peritonitis and require urgent care.

Due to the widespread application of ultrasound, the diagnosis of a cystic anomaly of the biliary tract is commonly made antenatally. The differential diagnosis for a cystic lesion arising in the hilum of the liver detected in utero includes choledochal cyst and a cystic variant of biliary atresia. These patients require assessment of the patency of the extrahepatic biliary tract soon after birth. Patency can be established based on clinical criteria (pigmented stool) or by nuclear medicine scan. If the biliary tract is obstructed, biliary atresia is likely. If the biliary tract is patent, the cystic lesion is more likely a choledochal cyst. These are ideal patients as operative repair can be performed prior to the onset of inflammatory changes that can make the dissection more difficult and dangerous.

Laboratory studies performed in patients with a choledochal cyst are usually unremarkable. Serum conjugated and

G.M. Tiao (✉)
Department of Pediatric and Thoracic Surgery, Cincinnati Children's Hospital Medical Center, Cincinnati, OH, USA
e-mail: greg.tiao@cchmc.org

P. Mattei (ed.), *Fundamentals of Pediatric Surgery*,
DOI 10.1007/978-1-4419-6643-8_76, © Springer Science+Business Media, LLC 2011

Fig. 76.1 Classification of
choledochal cysts, according to
Todani et al. (Modified with
permission from Fischer JE,
Bland KI, Callery MP, Clagett
GP, Jones DB, editors. Mastery
of surgery. 5th ed. Philadelphia,
PA: Lippincott, Williams &
Wilkins; 2006.)

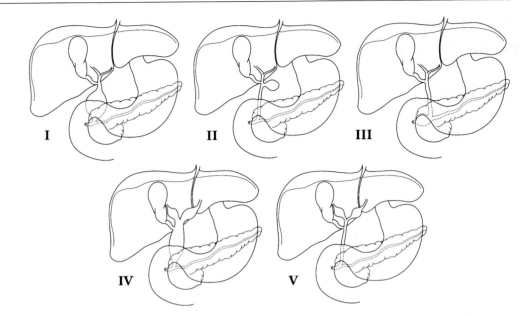

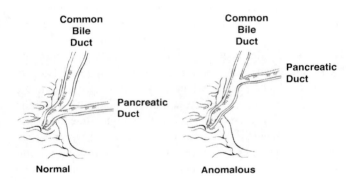

Fig. 76.2 Pancreatico-biliary malunion (PBMU): thought to be the
pathologic basis for the development of a type I and IV choledochal
cyst. (Modified with permission from Fischer JE, Bland KI, Callery
MP, Clagett GP, Jones DB, editors. Mastery of surgery. 5th ed.
Philadelphia, PA: Lippincott, Williams & Wilkins; 2006.)

unconjugated bilirubin and hepatocellular transaminase levels
are normal unless the patient has active cholangitis or has
developed cirrhosis. In patients who present with recurrent
episodes of pancreatitis, serum amylase levels are sometimes
elevated.

Three-dimensional imaging of the abdomen is necessary
to define the anatomic configuration of a choledochal cyst.
Ultrasonography is usually the first study performed and will
identify the abnormality in the bile duct, but CT or MRI
should be employed to define the anatomic extent of disease
for surgical planning purposes. On occasion, MRCP or
ERCP can be helpful to better define anatomy, especially if
the cyst is very small.

Surgical Therapy

The treatment of a patient with a choledochal cyst depends on
the subtype. For most patients, we perform definitive correction soon after diagnosis, however patients with cholangitis
should be treated with a course of intravenous antibiotics
before definitive repair is undertaken. Patients who present
with acute pancreatitis should also be treated to allow for resolution of pancreatic inflammation prior to definitive resection.

All patients receive preoperative intravenous vitamin K as
some are deficient due to underlying cholestasis. Perioperative
antibiotics are administered before incision and continued
for 24 h.

The goal of surgical intervention should always be complete excision. For patients with a type I or IV cyst, we perform excision of the cyst and a retrocolic, isoperistaltic,
Roux-en-Y hepaticojejunostomy. We use a right subcostal
incision to enter the peritoneal cavity and, if necessary, extend
the incision across the midline. In most instances, the choledochal cyst is readily apparent. Mobilization of the gallbladder will aid in the delineation of the anatomy. An intra-operative
cholangiogram performed through the gallbladder is helpful
to determine where the proper hepatic duct is of normal caliber and where the pancreatic duct joins the biliary tract.
If possible, the common duct is circumferentially mobilized,
allowing the application of traction to the choledochal cyst
and a safer dissection of the hepatic artery and portal vein. In
cases in which the size of the choledochal cyst distorts the
hilar anatomy, decompression of the cyst will facilitate safer
dissection.

Fig. 76.3 Mucosectomy of the lining of a choledochal cyst. Recurrent bouts of cholangitis within a choledochal cyst will cause extensive inflammation and fibrosis within the hilum. The choledochal cyst can be opened longitudinally and the mucosa excised leaving the residual fibrous capsule. (Modified with permission from Fischer JE, Bland KI, Callery MP, Clagett GP, Jones DB, editors. Mastery of surgery. 5th ed. Philadelphia, PA: Lippincott, Williams & Wilkins; 2006.)

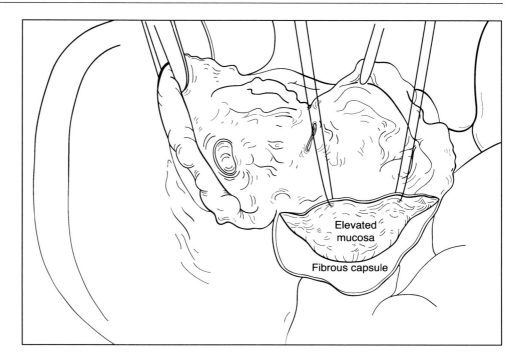

Dissection should proceed distally until the duct narrows to normal caliber, which is where the cyst should be divided. The choledochal cyst will often extend behind the first portion of the duodenum into the head of the pancreas. Although it is rare for the choledochal cyst to extend to the junction of the pancreatic duct, care must be taken to avoid injury to the pancreatic duct. Superiorly applied traction to the cyst and close adherence to the wall of the choledochal cyst allows for safer dissection. Complete resection of the cyst is important. Division at the superior edge of the duodenum may leave residual cyst wall in the head of the pancreas, which could lead to a recurrence or a future malignancy. Once the neck of the cyst is defined, it is ligated at its base using a non-absorbable suture.

In patients with a long-standing choledochal cyst, recurrent bouts of cholangitis may have resulted in significant inflammation throughout the hilum, making dissection around the choledochal cyst quite difficult and creating the potential for injury to the hepatic artery or the portal vein. In this circumstance, the choledochal cyst may be opened longitudinally and the mucosa of the cyst excised from within (Fig. 76.3). The posterior fibrous remnant of the cyst wall is left in place, minimizing the likelihood of injury to adjacent hilar structures. Here again, it is important to excise all of the cyst mucosa as there is a risk of developing cholangiocarcinoma in the abnormal biliary epithelium left behind. Dissection is carried distally until the cyst narrows to normal caliber where it is oversewn.

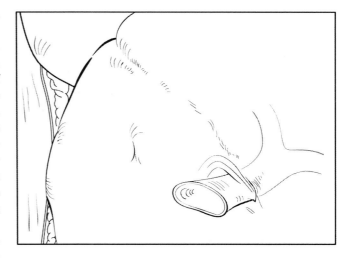

Fig. 76.4 Choledochal cyst divided. The proximal extent of dilation is identified and the choledochal cyst is divided. If the mucosa appears intact, a hepaticojejunostomy is performed to this level. If the mucosa is abnormal either at the gross or microscopic level, more proximal dissection must be performed. (Modified with permission from Fischer JE, Bland KI, Callery MP, Clagett GP, Jones DB, editors. Mastery of surgery. 5th ed. Philadelphia, PA: Lippincott, Williams & Wilkins; 2006.)

For a type I cyst, the proximal dissection in carried up the common hepatic duct to where its caliber appears normal and can be divided (Fig. 76.4). For a type IV cyst, we have found that the intra-hepatic duct dilatation usually resolves after the abnormal common bile duct has been removed. Because of this, we divide a type IV cyst just distal to the confluence of the right and left proper hepatic ducts. If the mucosa appears abnormal, we perform a frozen section biopsy at the line of division to ensure that the biliary epithelium is intact. If the mucosa appears histologically normal, hepaticojejunostomy is performed at this level. If the mucosa is abnormal, more proximal dissection must be undertaken.

We re-establish biliary drainage by end-to-side hepaticojejunostomy into a 40-cm limb of a Roux-en-Y brought to the hilum in a retro-colic position, using a single-layer interrupted anastomosis with absorbable suture. A proper anastomosis with precise mucosal apposition is important, as this minimizes the likelihood of subsequent leak or stricture. Sutures are placed such that all the knots are outside the lumen, reducing the likelihood of choledocholithiasis. Anchoring sutures from the Roux limb to tissue around the bile duct are placed to decrease tension on the anastomosis. For the cyst that extends up to the confluence of the right and left hepatic duct, we spatulate the lateral wall of both ducts to create a larger opening and a wider anastomosis.

In patients who present with a perforated choledochal cyst, the first step is to control the biliary ascites. Suitable drainage can be achieved through operative placement or by interventional radiology. Percutaneous trans-hepatic biliary drainage assists in controlling the leak and defines the cyst anatomy. Only after suitable control of the biliary leak and the treatment of accompanying sepsis have been achieved should operative resection and reconstruction be undertaken.

Recently, minimally invasive surgical techniques have been applied to the treatment of choledochal cysts. Multiple reports have demonstrated successful excision with reconstruction using a laparoscopic approach. Complete cyst excision must still be achieved when using the laparoscopic approach, otherwise residual cyst epithelium left within the head of the pancreas could lead to cyst recurrence or cholangiocarcinoma. In our experience, the dissection of the choledochal cyst into the head of the pancreas has been the most challenging aspect of the procedure.

For patients with a type II choledochal cyst, excision of the diverticulum and the extra-hepatic biliary tract with a Roux-en-Y hepaticojejunostomy is our procedure of choice. Although simple excision of the diverticulum with ligation at its base can be performed, excision of the extra-hepatic biliary tract is recommended because of the risk of the development of a cholangiocarcinoma in the remaining extra-hepatic biliary tract. We have treated one patient in which it

was difficult to define where the diverticulum arose from the biliary tract. In that case, we opened the cyst, excised all of its mucosa and fulgurated the residual cyst wall.

For patients with a type III choledochal cyst, the recommendations for treatment vary according to the type of epithelium found within the choledochal cyst. An ERCP should be performed prior to surgical intervention. At the time of ERCP, biopsy of the mucosa lining the cyst should be performed. If the biopsy reveals mucosa of duodenal origin, the lesion can be treated by a sphincterotomy or meatotomy to enlarge the opening and relieve the obstruction. This can be done endoscopically or with open surgery. In those cases where the epithelium lining the lesion appears to be of biliary tract origin, excision of the cyst with re-implantation of both the bile duct and the pancreatic duct has been recommended. Here again, it is essential to excise all of the biliary epithelium so as to minimize the likelihood of the development of a cholangiocarcinoma.

In patients with Caroli's disease (type V choledochal cyst), the extent of disease dictates the type of surgical procedure performed. In patients with disease confined to one lobe of the liver, formal lobectomy is recommended. If a patient has bi-lobar disease, liver transplantation will usually be necessary. The timing for transplantation has not been established but transplantation must take place prior to the development of a cholangiocarcinoma. These patients require close long-term surveillance.

Postoperative Care

Cholangitis is a common and potentially serious postoperative complication and therefore patients are maintained on peri-operative intravenous antibiotics until they can tolerate enteral feeds, at which time suppressive antibiotics are started and maintained for at least 6 months. If no episodes of cholangitis occur during the 6-month period, antibiotics are discontinued. The use of ursodeoxycholic acid (Actigall) might be beneficial in the peri-operative period but can be discontinued if no complications arise.

Established complications following repair of a choledochal cyst include stenosis at the hepaticojejunosotomy, intrahepatic lithiasis, and cholangiocarcinoma, any of which can occur years later. Patients who undergo excision of a choledochal cyst require long-term follow up. We obtain an ultrasound every year for the first 2 years and thereafter if symptoms arise.

Summary Points

- Choledochal cyst is a rare but correctable cause of jaundice.
- They are classified into five types, with type I and IV most common.
- The clinical presentation varies according to the age of the child, but the classic triad of pain, jaundice, and a right upper quadrant mass is rarely seen.
- Antenatal diagnosis of choledochal cyst is becoming more common and needs to be distinguished from cystic forms of biliary atresia.
- Cross-sectional imaging (CT or MRI/MRCP) is important for surgical planning.
- Surgical resection always necessary but the approach varies depending on the type of choledochal cyst and whether there is associated infection, inflammation, or fibrosis.
- Long-term follow-up important even if the entire cyst has been completely excised.

Editor's Comment

It is becoming increasingly clear that excision of the most common varieties of choledochal cyst can often be safely performed laparoscopically and that this will become the preferred approach in the very near future. It is obviously a very advanced minimally invasive technique that will not be available at every center but parents should be made aware that it is an option, even if it means transferring the child to another institution.

The critical points are that the mucosa of the cyst must be completely excised and the mucosa must be carefully approximated at the hepaticojejunostomy. It is also important to trace the distal common bile duct into the pancreas while avoiding injury to the pancreatic dust. Stents and drains are not routinely necessary but patients should be closely monitored for signs of a bile leak, which usually resolves with percutaneous drainage and one to 2 weeks of parenteral nutrition. As with most anastomoses involving the GI tract, leaks are often followed by strictures, which sometimes respond to percutaneous balloon dilation or stent placement but more often require surgical revision of the anastomosis. Cholangitis is thought to be minimized by creating a relatively long Roux limb (30–45 cm) but always suggests the possibility of an obstruction, either in the biliary tree or the Roux limb (an argument for avoiding excessive length). Stones that form within the biliary tree can also cause obstruction and cholangitis.

Differential Diagnosis

- Cystic variant of biliary atresia
- Choledocholithiasis
- Distal biliary stricture
- Other causes of cholangitis

Parental Preparation

- Resection is always necessary.
- Early postoperative complications include: leak and/or stricture.
- Long-term complications include: hepaticolithiasis, biliary cirrhosis (if stenosis is present), and, in very rare cases, cholangiocarcinoma.

Preoperative Preparation

- ☐ Type and screen
- ☐ Preoperative vitamin K
- ☐ Prophylactic antibiotics

Technical Points

- Complete resection of the cyst is essential.
- Intra-operative cholangiogram, which can be done through the gall bladder, can be extremely helpful in delineating complex anatomy, especially at the level of the hepatic ducts.
- If the anatomy is distorted or unclear, the cyst may be decompressed or simply opened.
- If the choledochal cyst is densely adherent to the hepatic artery or portal vein, it should be opened longitudinally and the mucosa completely excised, leaving the fibrous wall.
- Biliary drainage should be re-established using a 45 cm retrocolic, isoperistaltic Roux-en-Y hepaticojejunostomy with meticulous mucosal apposition.

Suggested Reading

Todani T, Watanabe Y, Narusue M, Tabuchi K, Okajima K. Congenital bile duct cysts: classification, operative procedures, and review of thirty-seven cases including cancer arising from choledochal cyst. Am J Surg. 1977;134:263–9.

Iwai N, Yanagihara J, Kazuaki T, Shimotake T, Nakamura K. Congenital choledochal dilatation with emphasis on pathophysiology of biliary tract. Ann Surg. 1992;215(1):27–30.

Akira O, Hasegawa T, Oguchi Y, Nakamura T. Recent advances in pathophysiology and surgical treatment of congenital dilatation of the bile duct. J Hepatobiliary Pancreat Surg. 2002;9:342–51.

O'Neill JA, Templeton JM, Schnaufer L, Bishop HC, Ziegler MM, Ross III AJ. Recent experience with choledochal cyst. Ann Surg. 1987;205(5):533–40.

Stain SC, Guthrie CR, Yellin AE, Donovan AJ. Choledochal cyst in the adult. Ann Surg. 1995;222(2):128–33.

MacKenzie TC, Howell LJ, Flake AW, Adzick NS. The management of prenatally diagnosed choledochal cysts. J Pediatr Surg. 2001;36(8): 1241–3.

Okada T, Sasaki F, Ueki S, Hirokata G, Okuyama K, Cho K, et al. Postnatal management for prenatally diagnosed choledochal cysts. J Pediatr Surg. 2004;39(7):1055–8.

Jun YY, Chen HM, Chen MF. Malignancy in choledochal cysts. Hepatogastroenterology. 2002;49:100–3.

Lee H, Hirose S, Bratton B, Farmer D. Initial experience with complex laparoscopic biliary surgery in children: Biliary atresia and choledochal cyst. J Pediatr Surg. 2004;39(6):804–7.

Coyle KA, Bradley III EL. Cholangiocarcinoma developing after simple excision of a type II choledochal cyst. South Med J. 1992;85(5):540–4.

Schimpl H, Sauer H, Goriupp U, Becker H. Choledochocele: importance of histological evaluation. J Pediatr Surg. 1993;28(12): 1562–5.

Todani T, Watanabe Y, Toki A, Urushihara N, Sato Y. Reoperation of congenital choledochal cyst. Ann Surg. 1988;207(2):142–7.

Chapter 77
Hepatic Resection

Heung Bae Kim

The indications for hepatic resection in children include a wide variety of both benign and malignant conditions. Benign conditions include mesenchymal hamartoma, adenomas, focal nodular hyperplasia (FNH), vascular malformations, and biliary tract cystic disease. Malignant lesions most commonly include hepatoblastoma and hepatocellular carcinoma, but other rare lesions are occasionally found including angiosarcoma, rhabdomyosarcoma, and cholangiocarcinoma. Some lesions such as inflammatory myofibroblastic tumor are considered benign but have a propensity for locally invasive disease.

Not all benign liver lesions require resection and in these cases. Expectant observation, especially when the diagnosis is not confirmed by biopsy, can often be more anxiety provoking to both the parents and the surgeon than a definitive operation but, obviously, unnecessary surgery should be avoided. Indications for resection of benign lesions include symptoms resulting from mass effect, a known risk of rupture and hemorrhage, or a well-defined natural history that includes growth of the lesion. Typically, mesenchymal hamartoma, adenoma, and biliary cysts require resection, whereas FNH and simple liver cysts that are not large or symptomatic can be safely observed.

Surgical resection is an important part of the therapy for most malignant lesions of the liver. Hepatoblastoma is the most common malignancy of the liver in young children and therapy consists of a combination of chemotherapy and complete gross surgical resection. In adolescents, hepatocellular carcinoma replaces hepatoblastoma as the most common primary malignancy of the liver. The fibrolamellar variant is most commonly encountered in this age group, but regardless of the type, surgical resection remains the mainstay of therapy for children with HCC as chemotherapy and radiation are largely ineffective. While most HCC in adults is found in the setting of cirrhosis, the majority of cases in children arise from an otherwise normal liver. In the presence of cirrhosis, even children with small otherwise resectable lesions will require liver transplantation given the significant risks associated with hepatectomy and the likelihood of disease recurrence in the remaining liver. However, as the risk of postoperative liver failure is much lower and the risk of recurrent disease is small, even very large HCC in an otherwise normal liver can usually be resected.

Diagnosis

The initial presentation of primary liver lesions is variable and depends on the type of lesion. Most malignant tumors are discovered on palpation of a large abdominal mass. Given the well-protected position of the liver behind the lower ribs, only a very large liver tumor is palpable, unless it is primarily growing inferiorly from the anterior inferior portion of the liver. In rare cases, a patient may present with tumor rupture and hemorrhage, which can be a life threatening event.

Initial radiographic evaluation is usually with ultrasound but detailed assessment of anatomy for planning surgical resection requires cross-sectional imaging with either CT or MRI. I find MRI to be most useful for determining the etiology of a lesion, especially when it is thought to be benign. An MRI is useful for differentiating cystic from solid lesions and, in some cases, for differentiating FNH from adenoma. In addition, as it is very sensitive for even small tumors and does not involve ionizing radiation, MRI is a good way to follow patients postoperatively for recurrence of malignant tumor. Despite the advantages of MRI, I believe that a CT-angiogram with arterial and venous phases provides a much higher resolution image to assist in the determination of resectability.

Physical examination must include a careful assessment for associated signs of liver disease. Jaundice is an uncommon finding, but when present indicates a lesion that is obstructing the common hepatic duct or the common bile duct. This is most commonly found in cases of biliary rhabdomyosarcoma, but can be caused by any lesion arising near the biliary bifurcation. Segmental biliary obstruction does

H.B. Kim (✉)
Department of Surgery, Pediatric Transplant Center, Harvard Medical Center, Children's Hospital Boston, Boston, MA, USA
e-mail: heung.kim@childrens.harvard.edu

P. Mattei (ed.), *Fundamentals of Pediatric Surgery*,
DOI 10.1007/978-1-4419-6643-8_77, © Springer Science+Business Media, LLC 2011

not usually cause jaundice. Splenomegaly, caput medusae, spider hemangiomata, or ascites usually suggests portal hypertension, either from portal vein thrombosis and obstruction or, less commonly, from cirrhosis. Obstruction of only one branch of the portal vein will not result in signs of portal hypertension. Ascites can also be a sign of either partial or complete hepatic vein obstruction (Budd–Chiari syndrome), or can be a sign of tumor rupture.

Laboratory assessment for patients found to have a liver mass should include a complete blood count, electrolytes, and a liver function panel including transaminases, alkaline phosphatase, GGT, albumin, fractionated bilirubin, and coagulation studies. The only true "liver function tests" among these laboratory tests are the INR and albumin. If the INR is elevated, especially in the setting of jaundice, the patient should be given a dose of vitamin K. Coagulopathy unresponsive to vitamin K usually signifies diminished functional liver mass. If there is a significant amount of uninvolved liver on imaging, then one should suspect that the remaining liver is cirrhotic. In these cases, one can expect marginal liver function following resection and so consideration should be made for preoperative biopsy of the uninvolved liver. These are the cases that might require liver transplantation, not for anatomic reasons, but for functional reasons.

Preoperative Preparation

Once it is determined that a liver lesion should be resected, the most important next step should be to determine if it can be resected safely. An easy way to think about this is in terms of anatomic resectability and functional resectability. Anatomic determination of resectability is primarily based on the vascular relationships of the tumor. In other words, liver surgery is really vascular surgery of the liver and this requires a detailed understanding of both extrahepatic and intrahepatic vascular anatomy (Fig. 77.1). Functional resectability is determined by a number of factors including the size of the potential remnant liver as well as the condition of the remnant liver (degree of fibrosis). Ultimately, all liver tumors are resectable if adequate replacement therapy is available and appropriate including, if necessary, liver transplantation.

The most common anatomic liver resections are left lateral segmentectomy, left lobectomy, right lobectomy, left trisegmentectomy, and right trisegmentectomy (Table 77.1). In the presence of a normal liver, children can generally tolerate a remnant liver volume of 25% and so all of these anatomic resections can be performed safely. However, preexisting liver disease must be accounted for to avoid leaving a patient with too little functional liver mass. On the contrary, in many cases of large liver masses, the involved liver segments may atrophy resulting in compensatory growth of

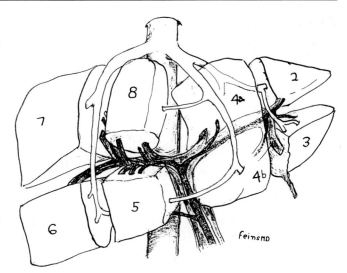

Fig. 77.1 Segmental anatomy of the liver (Courtesy of Neil Feins, MD)

uninvolved liver and more than the average expected remnant liver. This type of compensatory growth is most helpful when considering a left or right trisegmentectomy.

Of the three hepatic blood vessel systems, the hepatic veins are the most important determinants of anatomic resectability, followed by the portal vein. The reason for this is that the hepatic veins are almost entirely intrahepatic and so are difficult to "peel away" from an adjacent tumor without risking significant hemorrhage or incomplete resection. In addition, the hepatic veins are much more fragile and control of bleeding is more difficult than with the portal vein or heaptic arteries. The portal vein is extrahepatic well beyond the bifurcation, and so in many cases where the bifurcation seems involved, the vein can be dissected free of the tumor. In addition, the portal plate containing the bile ducts often separates the portal vein bifurcation from the liver parenchyma and offers a natural plane of dissection from the tumor. The left portal vein remains extrahepatic through almost its entire course and ends at the obliterated umbilical vein (Rex recessus). Branches supplying segments 1–4 can be dissected free along the course of the left vein without entering the liver parenchyma. The right portal vein can usually be dissected to the level of its first bifurcation into anterior and posterior sectors (segments 5, 8, and 6, 7, respectively), although the branching pattern can be quite variable.

The hepatic artery is usually the least important vascular determinant of resectability. Biliary structures should never determine resectability, as Roux-en-Y biliary reconstruction of even individual segmental ducts can always be performed even in small infants.

Involvement of the inferior vena cava poses its own challenges, depending on the level of involvement. Intravascular invasion via the hepatic veins can lead to tumor extension

Table 77.1 Anatomic liver resections

Common terminology	Anatomic segments resected	Hepatic vein resected	Approximate remnant liver volume (%)
Left lateral segmentectomy	2, 3	Left	75
Left lobectomy	2–4 ± 1 (caudate)	Left, middle	60
Right lobectomy	5–8	Right	40
Left trisegmentectomy	1–4 (left lobe) + 5, 8	Left, middle, anterior right	30
Right trisegmentectomy	5–8 (right lobe) + 1, 4	Middle, right	25

into the right atrium. An intrapericardial approach may be necessary to allow a clamp to be placed above the tumor and, in some cases, cardiopulmonary bypass may be necessary to complete the resection. More commonly, a tumor may appear to be compressing the IVC below the level of the hepatic veins. Often, a dissection plane can be found to resect the tumor while leaving the IVC intact, although IVC replacement with a PTFE graft is necessary in some cases. When complete or near complete IVC obstruction is present, the majority of blood flow may already be shunted through azygous vein collaterals that can be seen on CT-angiogram, and in these cases, the IVC may be resected without significant adverse outcomes.

In order to accurately assess the liver vasculature, I prefer a combination of Doppler ultrasound and CT-angiogram. Ultrasound is useful to examine direction of flow as well as to obtain baseline portal venous, hepatic venous, and hepatic arterial waveforms. CT-angiogram with arterial and venous phases gives the best assessment of the tumor relative to the vasculature and provides a roadmap for the operative procedure. While MRI is useful for assessment of the etiology of the tumor, I generally find that the resolution is not sufficient in difficult cases to accurately determine anatomic resectability.

Surgical Technique

The techniques of liver resection are quite variable, but have been significantly influenced in recent years by a growing experience with living donor and split liver transplantation. This experience has helped to define the limits of what is possible both from an anatomic and physiologic standpoint.

All liver resections can be performed through a generous bilateral subcostal incision. A midline extension up to the xiphoid is sometimes necessary to gain better exposure of the suprahepatic cava, especially in cases where intrapericardial IVC clamping is necessary to extract tumor thrombus. Initial exploration for malignant disease should include a careful inspection of the peritoneal surfaces and liver hilum for evidence of metastatic disease. In all but the most superficial wedge resections, complete mobilization of the liver is essential to provide easy exposure of the hepatic hilum and

retrohepatic IVC. The falciform ligament is completely divided up the level of the IVC and the left and right triangular ligaments are divided. Elevation of the hepatic hilum into the operative field can be achieved by placement of one or two laparotomy pads behind the right lobe of the liver. I prefer to use the Thompson retractor system as gentle retraction of the liver and bowel can be achieved without risk of injury to these structures. The porta hepatis should be skeletonized and care should be taken to completely define the hepatic arterial anatomy, which can be quite variable. Replaced arteries should be ruled out by inspection of the gastrohepatic ligament and the nodal tissue behind the portal vein.

Determination of resectability should be made after assessment of the portal vein, hepatic arteries, and the hepatic vein origins from the suprahepatic IVC. Intraoperative ultrasound may be very useful to identify the location of the hepatic veins as well as any major branches. Once resectability is confirmed, inflow to the liver segments to be resected can be temporarily clamped to demarcate a line of parenchymal transection and this should be marked with the cautery or argon beam coagulator on the surface of the liver. In most cases, the portal vein and hepatic artery branches supplying the segments to be resected should be divided prior to parenchymal transection to minimize bleeding. I generally do not take the outflow until the majority of the parenchymal transection is complete as there may be some collateral inflow to that segment of the liver and if the outflow is obstructed during parenchymal transection, this can lead to increased hemorrhage during the transection. The bile duct bifurcation should be preserved if possible, but if there is involvement with tumor, the bifurcation can easily be taken and a Roux-en-Y biliary reconstruction can be performed.

There are many methods of parenchymal transection and all of them work, so the most important thing is to find a method that is consistently available in your institution and that you are comfortable with. My personal preference is to simply use electrocautery with the coagulation level turned up sufficiently to allow for easy arcing of the current to the tissue, and to identify and ligate larger branches as they are encountered within the parenchyma using a "clamp fracture" technique. The argon beam coagulator is used for diffuse oozing of the surface of the liver after transection but should not be used as the primary dissecting instrument. Bile ducts should be sharply transected with a knife or scissors to maximize preservation of the vasculature, particularly when reconstruction will be necessary. In cases where the bile duct bifurcation must be resected, I prefer to construct a 45-cm Roux-en-Y that is brought up in a retrocolic position. I perform a mucosa-to-mucosa choledochojejunostomy and routinely use an external biliary stent to assist in evaluation should biliary complications arise. At the completion of the procedure, I routinely leave a closed-suction drain along the cut edge of liver for several days to monitor for bleeding and bile leak.

In cases of right trisegmentectomy, care must be taken at the completion of the procedure to ensure that the remnant liver is not prone to rotation, which can cause outflow obstruction of the left hepatic vein. The liver will tend to rotate into the right upper quadrant to fill the empty space, but this space should be filled by the colon and small bowel to prevent the remnant liver from rotating 180° and obstructing the left hepatic vein. Should this occur, the patient will develop ascites, a sudden rise in transaminases, and sometimes bleeding. This is an acute surgical emergency and operative intervention will be necessary to relieve the acute Budd–Chiari syndrome. In some cases, I will tack the falciform ligament to the anterior abdominal wall or the left triangular ligament back to the diaphragm to help avoid this complication.

Postoperative Care

Most patients should be monitored in the surgical intensive care unit following a major liver resection. Extubation should be performed in the operating room or as soon as possible in the ICU to prevent elevations of central venous pressure, which promotes bleeding from the IVC and the cut edge of the liver. The CVP should be maintained in the low-normal range and high pressures should be avoided for the first several days. Blood products should be given as needed, but plasma replacement should be avoided, if possible, so that the INR can be followed as a reflection of liver function. I use the INR as the primary method to determine the adequacy of

functional liver tissue following major liver resection. This is usually a major concern only in the case of left or right trisegmentectomy. Formal right or left lobectomy should almost never cause concern for inadequate liver function postoperatively. Transaminases can be monitored daily and any sudden elevations should prompt an emergency ultrasound to assess for a vascular complication. A routine ultrasound should be performed on the first postoperative day if there is any concern for vascular compromise from the surgery.

When more extensive resections are performed, the INR may not remain normal postoperatively, and a rising INR is an indication of insufficient liver volume. In mild cases, supportive care is all that is necessary to maintain the patient while the liver regenerates. This may require intermittent or continuous plasma replacement to maintain an INR less than 2.0, or lower if there is ongoing bleeding. Parenteral nutrition should be started in these cases and particular attention paid to adequate repletion of phosphorus during liver regeneration.

In more severe cases of insufficient liver volume, the "small for size syndrome" may occur. This has been defined for split-liver transplantation and consists of progressive jaundice, coagulopathy, and ascites. This can be partially due to portal hyperperfusion to a small remnant liver resulting in hepatocyte injury. If it progresses faster than liver regeneration can occur, this can eventually result in encephalopathy, liver failure, and death if liver replacement therapy is not immediately available. However, if a patient can be supported through this time period with plasma replacement and nutritional support, liver regeneration will eventually result in resolution of symptoms and normal liver function. Complete resolution can take months.

Following discharge, I routinely obtain blood tests and perform an ultrasound at three months following surgery, and then, depending on the clinical situation, only as needed. Obviously, patients with malignant disease will require lifelong follow up for tumor recurrence. I utilize CT angiography if there are any concerns for postoperative vascular compromise. If AFP levels were elevated preoperatively, they should be followed carefully following surgery to detect any residual or recurrent tumor.

Summary Points

- Malignant liver lesions almost always require complete resection as part of therapy.
- Benign liver lesions may require resection if they are symptomatic or have a known natural history of significant growth or risk of rupture.
- Initial diagnosis of liver lesions is often by ultrasound.
- MRI is better for characterizing liver lesions but CT angiography is better for surgical planning and determination of resectability.
- Resectability is determined by two factors: anatomic resectability and functional resectability.

- Anatomic resectability depends primarily on the vascular relationships of the tumor. Hepatic veins are the most important determinants of anatomic resectability followed by the portal veins and hepatic artery branches. Bile ducts should never determine resectability.
- Functional resectability is determined by the size of the remnant liver as well as the overall condition of the remnant liver.
- Ultimately, all liver tumors are resectable with the use of liver transplantation.

Editor's Comment

In many pediatric centers, major hepatic resections are increasingly being performed by transplant surgeons or surgeons who care for adults. This undoubtedly results in fewer pediatric surgeons having the experience and training to perform the operations, which in turn results in more referrals to the transplant surgeons. Though obviously one should always take the path that is safest for the child given the resources available at one's institution, the best way for pediatric surgeons to maintain their preeminence in this field is to continue to demonstrate that we can perform these operations safely and achieve excellent outcomes. This demands careful preoperative planning, meticulous technique, and attention to every detail of the operation and postoperative care.

Modern three-dimensional imaging allows us to define the vascular anatomy of the liver with a great deal of precision, and for any segmental or nonanatomic liver resection (anything more than a simple wedge biopsy) the surgeon should insist on having a CTA or MRA before going to the operating room. This is especially important when the indication for resection is a tumor, for which a well-done major resection can be for naught if the margin is inadequate or a second nodule is left behind. It is also important to understand whether the liver is healthy or cirrhotic to be sure that what remains will be able to regenerate.

Intraoperatively, the child should be carefully monitored, preferably with an indwelling arterial line and a central venous catheter. There is still no safe way to perform a liver resection through a tiny incision and a generous bilateral subcostal incision can mean the difference between a safely performed operation and an intraoperative disaster. The entire liver should be mobilized and all vessels, including the suprahepatic and infrahepatic IVC, the portal vein, and the hepatic artery should all be dissected and controlled with vessel loops or ties. For most major resections, the extrahepatic biliary anatomy should be defined as well, often starting with a cholecystectomy as a point of reference. Blood loss is minimized by ligating all vessels supplying or draining the segment to be removed, which sometimes entails dissecting out second-order branches of the portal vein and hepatic artery within the liver parenchyma. Control of the major hepatic branches can be difficult and whether it is safe to pursue this in a given operation is a matter of judgment. How to come across the liver parenchyma is a matter of preference and experience. The harmonic scalpel works well, though bile duct branches and larger vessels need to be recognized early and ligated individually. The parenchyma just beneath the liver capsule is usually more compact and less vascular for a depth of about a centimeter or two and this "rind" can be incised first with the electrocautery, exposing the deeper "pulp" of the liver where the larger vessels reside. After resection, bleeding from the raw surface of the liver is controlled with the argon beam coagulator and precise placement of absorbable figure-of-eight sutures as needed. Application of fibrin sealant is now customary, while the routine placement of drains is no longer considered obligatory.

Initial postoperative care should take place in the PICU, though most healthy children recover uneventfully. Much is made of the need to have plenty of phosphate substrate available to the regenerating liver, but this is rarely a significant issue if the child is provided adequate nutrition before and after the operation. Complete regeneration of the liver in a child with healthy liver parenchyma can occur within a few weeks of a major hepatic resection.

Differential Diagnosis

Malignant

- Hepatoblastoma
- Hepatocellular carcinoma
- Rhabdomyosarcoma
- Angiosarcoma
- Cholangiocarcinoma
- Metastatic lesions

Benign

- Mesenchymal hamartoma
- Adenoma
- Focal nodular hyperplasia
- Hemangioma
- Vascular malformations
- Cystic lesions

Diagnostic Studies

- Ultrasound
- Magnetic resonance imaging (MRI)
- Computed tomography angiography (CTA)
- Alpha-fetoprotein (AFP)

Preoperative Preparation

- ☐ CTA to determine resectability
- ☐ CBC, Chem10, LFT's, INR
- ☐ Type and cross (need to have PRBC and FFP available for any anatomic resection)
- ☐ Informed consent
- ☐ ICU bed postoperatively

Parental Preparation

- Major operation likely to require blood transfusions.
- Potential for poor liver function postoperatively.
- Potential complications including bile leak, portal vein thrombosis, injury to blood flow to the remnant liver, and inability to completely resect tumor.
- Recurrence of malignant tumors.

Technical Points

- Use CT angiography as roadmap for resection
- A generous bilateral subcostal incision can be used for almost all resections
- Extent of resection is primarily determined by vascular involvement of the tumor
- Intraoperative ultrasound may be useful to locate the hepatic veins
- If bile ducts are involved, they can be resected and a Roux-en-Y hepaticojejunostomy can be performed
- Use the method of parenchymal transection that you are most comfortable with
- Be sure the remnant liver segments are well positioned without signs of twisting and kinking of the hepatic vein prior to closure
- Avoid plasma transfusions postoperatively so that the INR can be used as the primary indication of liver function

Suggested Reading

Blumgart LH, Fong Y, editors. Surgery of the liver and biliary tract. Philadelphia, PA: WB Saunders; 2000.

Busuttil RW, Klintmalm GB, editors. Transplantation of the liver. Philadelphia, PA: Elsevier; 2005.

Clavien P-A, Petrowsky H, DeOliveira ML, Graf R. Strategies for safer liver surgery and partial liver transplantation. N Engl J Med. 2007; 356(15):1545–59.

Orkin SH, Fisher DE, Look AT, Lux SMD, Ginsburg D, Nathan DG. Oncology of infancy and childhood. Philadelphia, PA: Elsevier; 2009.

Chapter 78
Portal Hypertension

Jaimie D. Nathan, Kathleen M. Campbell, Greg M. Tiao, Maria H. Alonso, and Frederick C. Ryckman

The management of children with portal hypertension has evolved significantly over the past two decades. Improved survival in these patients has resulted from: (a) progress in the pharmacologic control of acute portal hypertensive hemorrhage; (b) improved efficacy and safety of endoscopic methods to treat acute esophageal variceal hemorrhage, which also reduce the risk of rebleeding; (c) recognition of the role for advanced surgical therapy (portocaval shunts); and (d) improved outcomes following pediatric liver transplantation as a definitive treatment for children with end-stage liver disease or life-threatening complications of portal hypertension.

Portal hypertension is defined as an elevation of the portal pressure above 10–12 mmHg. In healthy children, portal pressure rarely exceeds 7 mmHg. Elevation of the portal pressure is most commonly secondary to obstruction of portal venous flow due to pre-hepatic, intra-hepatic, or post-hepatic block, although increased splanchnic blood flow might contribute in some cases. Increased pressure within the portal circulation leads to the formation of collateral circulatory pathways connecting the high-pressure portal vasculature to the low-pressure systemic venous system. The most common and potentially dangerous communications occur within the esophageal wall, connecting the coronary and short gastric veins to the esophageal venous plexus. Esophageal varices developing within this plexus become the site with the highest risk for massive gastrointestinal hemorrhage. Less threatening collateral communications can develop between the recanalized umbilical vein and abdominal wall systemic veins (*caput medusa*), the inferior rectal veins (hemorrhoids), and in the retroperitoneum. In addition, any surgically created interface between the portal and systemic venous circulations, such as occurs with intestinal stomas, is a potential site

of often problematic variceal development. Spontaneous natural splenorenal shunts sometimes develop in the form of favorable collateral vessels within the tissues surrounding the pancreas, duodenum, and left kidney.

The progressive development of porto-systemic collaterals has the beneficial effect of decreasing portal pressure. However, this benefit is countered by the concurrent development of a hyperdynamic circulatory state. Portal hypertension has been associated with the presence of autonomic nervous system dysfunction, as well as an excess of circulating cytokines leading to tachycardia, decreased systemic and splanchnic vascular resistance secondary to vasodilatation, plasma volume expansion, increased cardiac output, and increased portal inflow.

The combination of portal venous outflow obstruction, increased portal inflow, and extensive collateral circulation account for many of the complications associated with portal hypertension. Superficial submucosal collateral vessels, especially those in the esophagus, stomach, and, to a lesser extent, the duodenum, colon, or rectum, are prone to rupture and bleed. In addition, submucosal arteriovenous communications between the muscularis mucosa and dilated precapillaries and veins within the stomach result in vascular ectasia, or congestive hypertensive gastropathy, contributing significantly to the risk of hemorrhage from the stomach.

Each of the causes of elevated portal pressure shares the common mechanism of increased resistance to blood flow from the splanchnic portal circulation to the right atrium (Table 78.1). In children, the location of this increased vascular resistance can be: (a) pre-hepatic, usually within the portal vein and its primary feeding branches; (b) intra-hepatic, most commonly related to intrinsic liver disease, but may be secondary to pre-sinusoidal obstruction (congenital hepatic fibrosis or schistosomiasis); or, (c) post-hepatic, secondary to hepatic vein outflow obstruction.

The primary factor influencing the prognosis and treatment is the intrinsic functional status of the liver. Pre-hepatic obstruction does not result in impaired hepatic synthetic function, and, therefore, coagulopathy is absent. Treatment should be directed toward the prevention of hemorrhage through

J.D. Nathan (✉)
Division of Transplantation, Division of Pediatric and Thoracic Surgery, University of Cincinnati, Cincinnati Children's Hospital Medical Center, Cincinnati, OH, USA
e-mail: Jaimie.Nathan@cchmc.org

P. Mattei (ed.), *Fundamentals of Pediatric Surgery*,
DOI 10.1007/978-1-4419-6643-8_78, © Springer Science+Business Media, LLC 2011

Table 78.1 Pediatric diseases associated with portal hypertension

Pre-hepatic causes
Extrahepatic portal vein thrombosis
Cavernous transformation of the portal vein
Splenic vein thrombosis
Congenital portal vein malformation (web or diaphragm)
Extrinsic portal vein compression

Intra-hepatic causes
Hepatocellular disease
   Autoimmune hepatitis
   Hepatitis B, C
   Wilson's disease
   Alpha-1-antitrypsin deficiency
   Glycogen storage disease – type IV
   Toxins and Drugs
   Histiocytosis X
   Gaucher's disease
Biliary tract disease
   Biliary atresia
   Cystic fibrosis
   Intrahepatic cholestasis syndromes
   Sclerosing cholangitis
Congenital hepatic fibrosis
Schistosomiasis
Sinusoidal veno-occlusive disease

Post-hepatic causes
Budd-Chiari syndrome
Inferior vena cava obstructions (web)
Chronic congestive heart failure
Veno-occlusive disease (s/p bone marrow transplantation)
Postoperative hepatic vein stenosis
Prothrombotic disease

Hyperkinetic causes (high flow)
Arteriovenous fistula (congenital or acquired)

palliative interventional procedures while spontaneous collateral venous channels develop. However, in some children who are at higher risk of re-bleeding, portal decompression via surgical shunting may be necessary. In patients with intrinsic liver disease, routine endoscopic surveillance, selective surgical shunting, transjugular intrahepatic portosystemic shunting, and liver transplantation each play a role, depending on the degree of cirrhosis and extent of hepatic synthetic dysfunction. Post-hepatic obstruction is characterized by hepatic synthetic compromise, coagulopathy, and progressive hepatic failure. Although interventions to prevent or treat potentially fatal complications might be necessary, definitive correction with liver transplantation is often required.

Pre-Hepatic Portal Hypertension

The most common type of pre-hepatic obstruction is extrahepatic portal vein obstruction (EPVO). Risk factors for EPVO include umbilical vein infection in infants, and severe intra-abdominal infections (perforated appendicitis, primary peritonitis, inflammatory bowel disease) in older children. It can also develop secondary to primary biliary tract infection or cholangitis, or in the setting of inherited disorders associated with hypercoagulability, such as factor V Leiden mutation, or protein C, protein S, or antithrombin III deficiency. Hyperviscosity/polycythemia in infancy or umbilical vein catheterization can all lead to secondary thrombosis, especially when accompanied by neonatal dehydration or systemic infection and phlebitis. Embryological malformations resulting in tortuous, poorly developed portal veins, webs, or diaphragms can also be a primary cause for EPVO or predispose to an increased risk of thrombosis. The development of periportal collateral vessels ("cavernous transformation of the portal vein") may result from either a disordered embryologic process or from long-standing portal vein thrombosis.

Children with EPVO frequently appear completely healthy prior to an episode of hematemesis or hematochezia. Because their hepatic synthetic function is normal, they are able to recover from their variceal hemorrhage more readily than children with pre-existing liver disease. Despite thorough evaluation, over 50% of reported EPVO cases have no identifiable cause.

Intra-Hepatic Portal Hypertension

Portal hypertension in children is commonly related to progressive hepatocellular injury and fibrosis in the setting of intrinsic liver disease, broadly characterized as hepatocellular disorders and biliary tract disorders (Table 78.1). The common final pathway of increased intra-hepatic vascular resistance due to hepatic fibrosis and alterations in hepatic microcirculation is the basis for the development of portal hypertension and its associated complications in cirrhosis. The etiologies of chronic liver disease in children are myriad and include recognized disorders such as extrahepatic biliary atresia, metabolic liver diseases such as alpha-1-antitrypsin deficiency, Wilson's disease, glycogen storage disease type IV, and cystic fibrosis. When hepatic synthetic failure is not present or only slowly progressive, direct treatment of portal hypertension or its complications is indicated. However, because many of these conditions are associated with progressive liver failure, the primary treatment in most cases is liver transplantation. Other rarer intra-hepatic causes of portal hypertension include schistosomiasis, in which small intra-hepatic portal venules are destroyed, and congenital hepatic fibrosis, a hereditary disorder of portal bile duct proliferation and fibrosis.

Post-Hepatic Portal Hypertension

Post-hepatic portal hypertension is caused by obstruction of hepatic venous outflow. Hepatic vein obstruction (Budd-Chiari syndrome) can occur secondary to obstruction of the hepatic veins at any point from the sinusoids to the entry of the hepatic veins into the right atrium/inferior vena cava. Although a specific etiology is often not found, thrombosis can complicate neoplasms, collagen vascular disease, infection, trauma, or hypercoagulable states. Veno-occlusive disease, microvascular non-thrombotic occlusion of hepatic venules, also has emerged as one of the most frequent causes of hepatic vein obstruction in children. Most cases occur after total body irradiation, with or without cytotoxic drug therapy, associated with bone marrow transplantation. This condition also occurs after the ingestion of herbal remedies containing the pyrrolizidine alkaloids, which are sometimes taken as medicinal teas.

Diagnosis

Clinical history and physical examination should concentrate on identifying factors that predispose to the development of cirrhosis, including a family history of inherited metabolic disease and possible exposure to viral or toxic pathogens. Clinical examination findings suggesting underlying liver disease (ascites, liver size/contour, nutritional status), hypersplenism (splenomegaly, bruising), or hepatopulmonary syndrome (spider angiomas, clubbing, cyanosis) contribute to diagnostic evaluation and therapeutic planning. Hypercoagulability and its complications should be evaluated in both the patient and family members due to the inherited basis for these protein abnormalities.

Imaging tests are essential to confirm the presence of portal hypertension, define the portal venous anatomy, and formulate options for therapy. Initial screening with ultrasonography can suggest the presence of chronic liver disease and should determine portal venous patency. Doppler examination can demonstrate both the direction of portal venous flow and the degree of hepatopetal flow, which correlates with the risk of variceal hemorrhage. The branches of the portal venous system are examined to exclude splenic vein thrombosis or widespread portal system thrombosis. Magnetic resonance venography or contrast-enhanced computed tomography has replaced mesenteric angiography when further definition of portal anatomy is necessary, such as when liver transplantation or portosystemic shunt procedures are planned.

Upper gastrointestinal endoscopy is the most accurate and reliable method for detecting esophageal varices and for detecting the source of acute gastrointestinal hemorrhage. This modality is especially valuable in the presence of acute hemorrhage, where up to one-third of patients with known varices may have bleeding from other sources such as portal hypertensive gastropathy or gastric/duodenal ulcerations. In addition, upper endoscopy can identify features associated with an increased risk for hemorrhage, such as large varices, "cherry-red spots" apparent over varices, representing fragile telangiectasias within the shallow submucosa, and portal hypertensive gastropathy. Endoscopy is also used to intervene therapeutically when acute bleeding varices are identified and when prophylactic endoscopic treatment of varices is warranted.

Liver biopsy may be helpful in determining the etiology of intrinsic liver disease and in defining further therapy or the need for transplantation. A percutaneous approach may be utilized, unless significant coagulopathy is present, in which case liver biopsy should be performed using an open technique under general anesthesia.

Nonoperative Treatment

The decision to undertake pharmacologic, endoscopic, or surgical treatment for portal hypertension must be based on the natural history of the disease and the possibility of life-threatening complications. The prognosis is related to the primary etiology of the portal hypertension. In patients with intrinsic liver disease, prognosis is also dependent on the degree of hepatic functional reserve. It has been generally accepted in patients with portal hypertension due to EPVO that the risk of acute variceal bleeding decreases with age, concurrent with the development of spontaneous portosystemic collateral vessels. This postulated natural history has been the primary argument supporting conservative management of hemorrhage in these patients, using endoscopic therapy to obliterate esophageal varices while awaiting the development of favorable retroperitoneal and peripancreatic collateral vessels. However, children who have experienced bleeding complications prior to age 12 and those with grade II or III varices remain at significantly higher risk for further upper gastrointestinal hemorrhage at a later age. These high-risk populations should be identified and considered for preemptive aggressive intervention.

In patients with intrinsic liver disease, therapeutic choices are influenced by the probability of progression of their disease and the potential need for liver transplantation in the future. A significant number of these patients require temporizing endoscopic treatment or surgical portosystemic shunt therapy to treat complications or maintain stability prior to undergoing liver replacement.

The most common portal hypertensive complication is gastrointestinal bleeding. Regardless of the site and mechanism of bleeding, initial therapy is directed toward fluid resuscitation and, when necessary, blood replacement. A nasogastric tube should be placed to confirm the upper gastrointestinal source of bleeding and for evacuation of blood from the stomach. A proton pump inhibitor should be administered to decrease the risk of bleeding from gastric erosions, and antibiotics should be instituted as prophylaxis for bacterial infections or spontaneous bacterial peritonitis. In patients with hepatic synthetic dysfunction and coagulopathy, administration of vitamin K, fresh frozen plasma or cryoprecipitate, and platelets when thrombocytopenia is present also may be necessary. Adequate volume resuscitation is essential; however, volume overload from excessive transfusion or crystalloid administration is counterproductive because this leads to further increase in portal pressure and continued hemorrhage.

Pharmacologic Treatment

Pharmacologic intervention to decrease portal pressure is essential in patients with continued bleeding, as cessation of hemorrhage is the most critical therapeutic challenge. A variety of pharmacologic options are available when intervention is required.

Vasopressin decreases portal venous pressure by increasing splanchnic vascular tone and by decreasing splanchnic arterial inflow. It is administered as an initial bolus of 0.3 units/kg over 20 min followed by a continuous infusion of 0.002–0.005 units/kg/min. Intra-arterial infusion into the superior mesenteric artery has no advantage over intravenous routes. Vasopressin infusion has been associated with control of variceal hemorrhage in 53–85% of cases in children. However, its clinical utility is limited by its significant side effects, which are related to its potent systemic vasoconstrictive properties. Vasopressin can impair cardiac function, as well as induce peripheral ischemia, hypertension, and intestinal ischemia. Nitroglycerin has been used to augment the decrease in portal pressure and ameliorate the untoward systemic effects, but is inappropriate in the setting of low or unstable systemic blood pressure.

Somatostatin is a 14-amino acid peptide that reduces splanchnic blood flow by selective mesenteric vascular smooth muscle constriction. Its effects on variceal hemorrhage are similar to those of vasopressin, but it carries a lower risk of adverse systemic side effects. Because the short half-life of somatostatin complicates the management of patients with acute variceal hemorrhage, octreotide, an 8-amino acid synthetic somatostatin analogue, was developed. Octreotide can be administered subcutaneously, but is best used as a continuous intravenous infusion (25–50 $\mu g/m^2/h$, or 1.0–3.0 $\mu g/kg/hr$).

In adult studies, both somatostatin and octreotide have achieved excellent results in controlling acute variceal hemorrhage. Recent retrospective studies have demonstrated that octreotide is associated with a high rate of bleeding control in children with portal hypertension without significant adverse events. However, controlled studies in children are necessary to confirm this success.

While beta blockers have no role in the treatment of acute variceal hemorrhage, they have been used in an effort to prevent first variceal hemorrhage in high-risk patients, and as an option for secondary prophylaxis. The goal of therapy is a reduction in heart rate by 25%, thereby decreasing cardiac output, portal inflow, and perhaps blocking β receptor-mediated vasodilatation, allowing unopposed α stimulation within the mesenteric arterioles. Efficacy has been evaluated in two groups: (a) patients with documented varices who underwent beta-blocker treatment in an attempt to prevent the first episode of bleeding (primary prophylaxis); and (b) patients treated following the initial hemorrhage in an attempt to prevent recurrent bleeding (secondary prophylaxis). The efficacy of therapy differs based on the indication.

In adult patients treated for primary prophylaxis, betablockers were associated with significantly lower rates of bleeding and death from bleeding. Combined treatment using nadolol and isosorbide mononitrate further decreased the risk for first variceal hemorrhage by more than half in comparison with nadolol alone. The results of β blockade for secondary prevention of recurrent variceal hemorrhage are more controversial. In 11 randomized controlled trials including 755 adult patients, re-bleeding was reduced in all trials and the death rate was reduced. In low-risk patients (Child's class A), the risk of rebleeding has been reported to be as low as 3%. This advantage seems to be lost in Child's class B and C patients, where the risk for recurrent bleeding is reported to be 46–72%.

Fewer studies have been performed in children. Because of the presence of extrahepatic portal hypertension in up to half of all children who are candidates for treatment, pediatric results may not correlate directly with adult patients, nearly all of whom have intrinsic liver disease. Several investigators have confirmed that propranolol is well-tolerated with minimal side effects in children with portal hypertension, although heart block and asthma exacerbation have been reported. Similar to the adult experience, dosage must be adjusted to achieve a reduction of 25% in resting heart rate to achieve a therapeutic result; however, this guideline is complicated in the pediatric population by the frequent difficulty in assessing baseline measures. Because of these issues and the paucity of prospective data in children, betablocker treatment is not routinely recommended for primary prophylaxis in the pediatric population. While beta-blockers may be used for secondary prophylaxis in school-age and adolescent children based on individual assessment, controlled studies of this intervention are necessary.

Mechanical Tamponade

Mechanical tamponade using balloon catheter tubes (Sengstaken-Blakemore or Minnesota tubes) provides mechanical compression of esophageal and gastric fundal varices. Although balloon tamponade is usually successful in stopping refractory hemorrhage, the effect is often transient, and recurrence following removal is common. The significant number of complications and high incidence of rebleeding have limited their use to severe uncontrollable hemorrhage as a temporizing measure until a definitive intervention or surgical procedure can be performed.

Endoscopic Intervention for Esophageal Varices

In most cases, variceal hemorrhage can be controlled with fluid resuscitation, correction of coagulopathy, and pharmacologic support. However, the risk of recurrent hemorrhage and the need for accurate diagnosis of the site of hemorrhage often mandate upper endoscopy during the early posthemorrhage period. When variceal hemorrhage is confirmed or strongly suspected, variceal sclerotherapy or band ligation can be used to eradicate the present or future sites of bleeding.

The use of endoscopic methods to control acute variceal hemorrhage is well established. Endoscopic sclerotherapy (EST) has been widely used as the primary treatment for refractory variceal bleeding due to its high success rate (>90%) and the ability to institute initial treatment at the time of diagnostic endoscopy. The procedure is successful using both intra-variceal and peri-variceal injection techniques. In children, 5% ethanolamine, 1–1.5% tetradecyl sulfate, or 5% sodium morrhuate have all been used successfully. Most patients require three to six sessions at intervals of 2–4 weeks to eradicate esophageal varices. Minor early complications, which occur in almost all patients, include retrosternal pain, fever, and transient dysphagia. Esophageal ulceration at the site of injection, a direct consequence of the procedure, is seen in 70–80% of patients and can be the source of recurrent bleeding. Serious complications such as esophageal stricture, esophageal perforation, or mediastinitis occur in 10–20% of patients.

In an attempt to overcome these complications but preserve the treatment success of EST, esophageal band ligation (EBL) of varices has been developed, using techniques similar to those for banding internal hemorrhoids. Band ligation has the advantage of ligating only the submucosal venous varices, without harming the submucosal lining. Initial variceal obliteration was achieved by EBL in 73–100% of children, and rebleeding prior to completion of obliteration occurred less commonly than with EST management; however, recurrence of varices was seen in 75% of patients with intrahepatic disease. In addition, the small size of the child's esophagus limits the number of bands that can be placed at one treatment session. Size limitations associated with the commercially available EBL equipment, as well as the thinner esophageal wall of small children, which makes full-thickness ligation a risk, preclude the use of EBL in children who weigh less than 10–12 kg.

Both EST and EBL have been used for the primary prophylaxis of variceal hemorrhage. Prophylactic EST decreased the incidence of bleeding in children from 42 to 6%, but 16% developed congestive hypertensive gastropathy and 38% bled from this lesion. This was in contrast to the control group, in which only 6% had congestive hypertensive gastropathy, with no gastropathy-associated bleeding episodes. Prophylactic EST did not alter patient survival compared to the control group. We feel that EST or EBL is an acceptable and occasionally life-saving intervention when esophageal variceal hemorrhage is refractory to octreotide infusion therapy. The risk of accelerated formation of gastric varices and complications of sclerotherapy outweigh the potential benefits for EST. EBL is also not routinely recommended as primary prophylaxis in pediatric patients, although it might be a safer alternative in certain high-risk pediatric populations.

Portosystemic Shunt Operations

Numerous surgical procedures have been devised to divert portal blood into the low-pressure systemic venous circulation, thereby decreasing the portal venous pressure. Enthusiasm for the use of portosystemic shunting in children was limited by early reports suggesting that children less than 8 years of age and those with available vessels less than 8–10 mm would be unsuitable candidates due to the high risk of shunt thrombosis. In addition, Voorhees et al. suggested a high incidence of neuropsychiatric disturbances following nonselective shunts in children. More recent experience in centers skilled in pediatric vascular reconstruction has established that a high rate of success can be achieved with a minimal complication rate, even in small pediatric patients. To achieve these goals, we have found that the following principles should be followed: (a) an anastomosis constructed using fine (6-0, 7-0) monofilament sutures with a provision for growth; (b) sufficient mobilization and modification of the vessels to prevent kinking or twisting of the shunt after the viscera are returned to their normal location; (c) post-reconstructive venography to ensure division of all collateral vessels, anastomotic quality, and adequate shunt flow; (d) selective postoperative intravenous anticoagulation in high-risk patients; (e) anti-platelet

Fig. 78.1 Interposition "H"-type mesocaval shunt – a non-selective shunt involving anastomosis of internal jugular vein conduit between the superior mesenteric vein and the infrarenal inferior vena cava (modified from Zollinger RM, Zollinger RM, Atlas of surgical operations. 7th ed. New York: McGraw-Hill; 1993; with permission from McGraw-Hill Companies, Inc.)

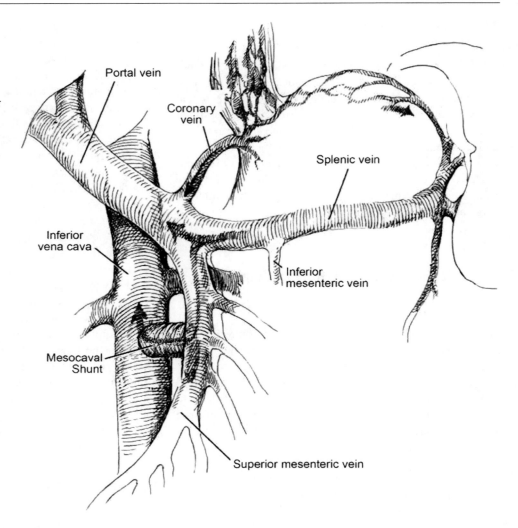

drugs in all patients for up to 90 postoperative days; and (f) a surgical team experienced and highly skilled at pediatric vascular reconstruction.

In general, portosystemic shunts can be classified into three groups: non-selective shunts, selective shunts, and direct reconstructions of the portal circulation using a vascular graft (Rex shunt).

Non-selective shunts are constructed to communicate with the entire portal venous system and therefore have the potential to divert blood from the normal antegrade perfusion to the liver. Historically, the most commonly used shunt in children was the *Clatworthy shunt*, a mesocaval shunt in which the distal IVC is ligated and divided and its proximal end is anastomosed to the side of the superior mesenteric vein. This is often complicated by the development of transient lower extremity edema, but has the advantage of using a large-caliber vein for the shunt anastomosis.

This shunt has largely been replaced by the *H-type mesocaval shunt*, which is constructed using a short segment of internal jugular vein to connect the SMV and the IVC (Fig. 78.1). This shunt retains the advantage of a larger vessel for the anastomosis and avoids ligation of the IVC.

Excellent patency (93%) and no significant episodes of encephalopathy support its use in pediatric patients. The limited intra-abdominal dissection required to construct this shunt contributes to its technical ease and if liver transplantation is necessary, the shunt can be easily occluded at that time. Other non-selective shunts have significant disadvantages in children due to the need for splenectomy (proximal splenorenal shunt), or dissection of the main portal vein (end-to-side and side-to-side portocaval shunts), which can compromise subsequent liver transplantation.

Selective shunts are constructed to divert the "gastrosplenic" portion of the portal venous flow into a systemic vein, most frequently the left renal vein or the immediately adjacent IVC. Communication between the "central" mesentericoportal circulation which perfuses the liver and the gastrosplenic portal circulation is severed by dividing the gastroepiploic veins, the coronary vein, and the retroperitoneal pancreatic collateral vessels. The most common and successful selective shunt, the *distal splenorenal shunt* (DSRS) or *Warren shunt*, preserves antegrade perfusion to the liver within the mesenteric portion of the portal circulation, while decompressing the esophageal venous plexus through

Fig. 78.2 Distal splenorenal shunt – a selective shunt allowing communication between the distal splenic vein and the left renal vein. The esophagogastric venous complex communicates via the short gastric veins, decompressing esophageal varices without decreasing perfusion through the mesenteric portal system to the liver (modified from Zollinger RM, Zollinger RM, Atlas of surgical operations. 7th ed. New York: McGraw-Hill, 1993; with permission from McGraw-Hill Companies, Inc.)

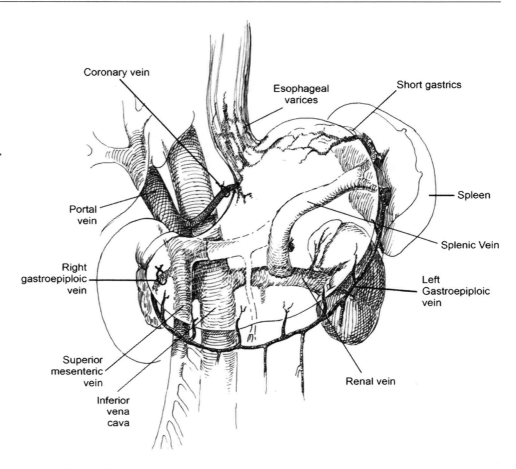

Coronary vein

Esophageal varices

Short gastrics

Portal vein

Spleen

Splenic Vein

Right gastroepiploic vein

Left Gastroepiploic vein

Superior mesenteric vein

Renal vein

Inferior vena cava

the short gastric veins and splenic vein (Fig. 78.2). We use this shunt as our primary option in children where direct reconstruction of the portal system (Rex shunt) is not possible. When the left adrenal vein is appropriately located and dilated, it serves as an alternative anastomotic site to access the left renal vein. When performed in centers experienced in complex vascular reconstruction of the portal system, as is necessary in pediatric liver transplantation, shunt patency has ranged from 83 to 100%. When shunt patency is maintained, recurrent variceal bleeding is uncommon, although decompressed varices can sometimes still be identified by upper endoscopy. Encephalopathy is uncommon following successful portosystemic shunting, even in children with intrinsic liver disease.

Direct reconstruction of the portal circulation in children with extrahepatic portal vein obstruction into the left branch of the portal vein represents the ideal solution. This mesentericoportal shunt (*Rex shunt*) re-establishes normal physiologic portal inflow into the intrahepatic portal vein, using either an interposition jugular venous graft or by transposition of the dilated coronary vein (Fig. 78.3). Candidates for this procedure should satisfy four conditions: (a) the liver parenchyma must be normal; (b) they must not have a hypercoagulable state; (c) the umbilical portion of the left portal vein must be accessible and patent; and, (d) there must be a suitable vein in the mestentericosplenic venous system to serve as

the inflow vessel. The Rex shunt is unique in that it restores hepatopetal portal perfusion and the inflow of hepatotrophic substances to the liver, and therefore patients with diffuse intrahepatic portal vein thrombosis are not candidates for this reconstruction.

Doppler ultrasonography is performed preoperatively to assess the intrahepatic portal veins, and to confirm patency of both internal jugular veins, as the left internal jugular vein is most commonly utilized as conduit for the Rex shunt. Magnetic resonance angiography is utilized to assess the intrahepatic left portal vein in cases where Doppler ultrasonography is unable to confirm its patency. If the status of the intrahepatic left portal vein still remains unclear, preoperative transjugular retrograde portal venography (Fig. 78.4) can be helpful in defining left portal vein patency. Noninvasive preoperative imaging would suggest that approximately two-thirds of children with EPVO have sufficient left portal vein patency to undergo this procedure, and of the remaining third of children, two-thirds are found at exploration to have a patent left portal vein to allow for a Rex shunt to be constructed.

Following abdominal exploration and intra-operative mesentericoportal venography under fluoroscopy, the recanalized umbilical vein is dissected down to the Rex recess between hepatic segments III and IV (Fig. 78.5). Tiny terminal branches of the left portal vein may be ligated and divided to allow for

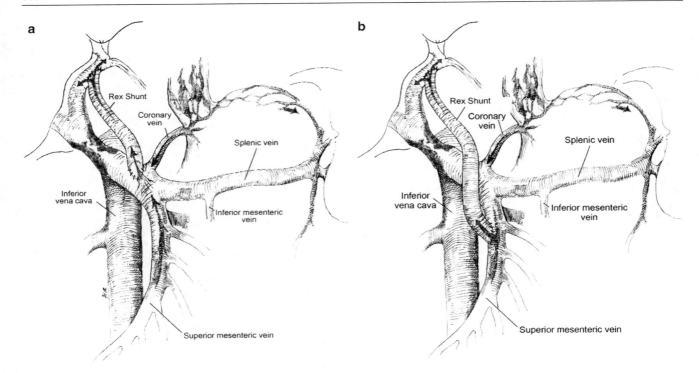

Fig. 78.3 Mesentericoportal shunt (Rex shunt) – this shunt returns portal blood flow directly to the hepatic portal circulation via the left branch of the intrahepatic portal vein, and is useful only in patients with extrahepatic portal vein obstruction and a patent intrahepatic portal venous system. Rex shunt construction usually consists of an interposition internal jugular vein conduit from either the (**a**) superior mesenteric vein (SMV), splenic vein, or (**b**) SMV-splenic vein junction to the intrahepatic left portal vein branch

adequate mobilization; however, it is important to preserve the majority of such branches, as these will serve as outflow for blood shunted via the Rex conduit. After accessing the left portal vein branch, dissection is performed to mobilize an inflow vessel, usually either the central splenic vein or the superior mesenteric vein (Fig. 78.3). Autologous vein graft is utilized as conduit. We prefer to use the internal jugular vein for this purpose. Alternatively, if the coronary vein is dilated and of appropriate length to reach the Rex recess, this vein may be mobilized, transposed, and anastomosed to the left portal vein branch. Following completion of the inflow anastomosis and left portal vein anastomosis (Fig. 78.6), completion venography and portal pressure measurements are obtained to ensure shunt patency and portal decompression.

Although experience with Rex shunt construction remains limited, recent studies have documented excellent short-term shunt patency and resolution of episodes of variceal bleeding. In a recent retrospective review of 34 children with EPVO, over 90% of those who underwent exploration had successful construction of a Rex shunt. All Rex conduits remained patent over a follow-up period of up to 7 years, with complete resolution of variceal bleeding and symptoms of hypersplenism. Thus, in appropriately selected patients with EPVO, we feel that the Rex shunt represents the optimal solution to provide adequate portal venous decompression, which also re-establishes hepatopetal portal perfusion.

The indications for portosystemic shunting have been altered by the growing success of endoscopic methods to control variceal bleeding and the improvements in pediatric liver transplantation. We now consider the following children to be candidates for portosystemic shunting: (a) children with documented variceal hemorrhage who have progressive or continued esophageal variceal bleeding despite endoscopic intervention and who have preserved hepatic synthetic function; (b) children who fail endoscopic treatment and have intrinsic liver disease, but have adequate liver synthetic function to predict that liver transplantation will not be needed for several years (selective shunt only); (c) severe portal hypertension in patients with cystic fibrosis and variceal hemorrhage whose microbiologic flora compromise liver transplant survival; (d) children with severe portal hypertension who reside a great distance from emergency medical care, endangering their survival should significant hemorrhage occur; and (e) children with EPVO and uncontrolled hypersplenism. Surgical options for shunt procedures are based on the primary etiology of portal hypertension (Table 78.2). Routine interval post-operative shunt surveillance is performed using Doppler ultrasonography or computed tomography angiography. Formal angiography is necessary if shunt patency cannot be confirmed by non-invasive imaging, or when shunt thrombosis or stenosis is identified and requires intervention.

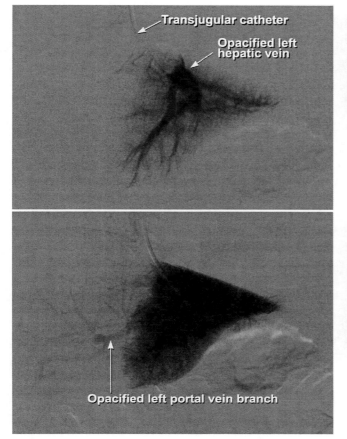

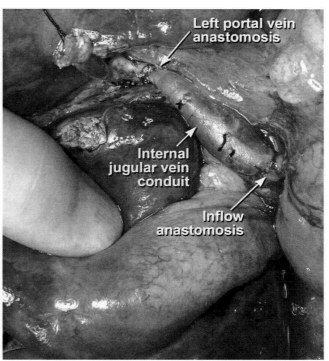

Fig. 78.6 Rex shunt construction – inflow anastomosis is typically to the splenic vein or superior mesenteric vein, and outflow anastomosis is to the left branch of the intrahepatic portal vein in the Rex recess. We prefer to use internal jugular vein as the autologous venous conduit

Fig. 78.4 Transjugular retrograde portal venography – prior to Rex shunt construction, transjugular retrograde portal venography may be used to evaluate the patency of the intrahepatic left portal vein in cases in which Doppler ultrasonography and MR angiography are unable to confirm its patency

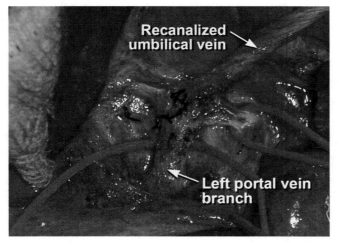

Fig. 78.5 Dissection of the Rex recess – during Rex shunt construction, initial dissection of the recanalized umbilical vein is performed down to the Rex recess between hepatic segments III and IV. Although tiny terminal branches of the left portal vein may be ligated and divided to allow for adequate mobilization, it is critical to preserve the majority of such branches, as these will serve as outflow for blood shunted via the Rex conduit

Table 78.2 Portal hypertension surgical options

Primary etiology	Preferred surgical therapies
Pre-hepatic obstruction	Rex shunt construction
Extrahepatic portal vein thrombosis	Direct venous repair
Cavernous transformation of the portal vein	
Congenital portal vein malformation	
Extrinsic portal vein compression	
Intrinsic hepatic disease	Distal splenorenal shunt
Cirrhosis	H-type mesocaval shunt
Congenital hepatic fibrosis	TIPS
Post-hepatic obstruction	H-type mesocaval shunt
Budd-Chiari syndrome	Cavo-atrial shunt
Veno-occlusive disease	TIPS
Postoperative hepatic vein stenosis	
Hyperkinetic causes (high flow)	Resection of involved liver
Arteriovenous fistula (congenital or acquired)	

Transjugular Intrahepatic Portosystemic Shunt

The introduction of transjugular intrahepatic portosystemic shunt (TIPS) has added another therapeutic option for children with complex portal hypertension. This procedure uses interventional radiologic techniques to place an intrahepatic expandable metallic stent between a portal vein branch and the hepatic vein, forming a central, transhepatic, nonselective portocaval shunt. Percutaneous access is obtained through the right internal jugular vein. The hepatic veins are identified, and a fluoroscopic/ultrasonographic-guided puncture from the hepatic vein branch into an intrahepatic portion of the portal vein is performed. This tract is then dilated, and an expandable mesh stent is placed, forming a communication between the intrahepatic portal vein and the hepatic vein branch. In infants, it is technical difficult to establishing a large enough tract for sufficient shunt flow that is safe. In children with biliary atresia, the close proximity of the biliary Roux-en-Y limb to the portal vein and the often diminutive size of the portal vein increase the risk of stent malposition and perforation. This procedure provides great benefit in the control of refractory portal hypertensive bleeding unresponsive to pharmacologic intervention and in patients needing temporary portal decompression prior to liver transplantation. The ability to embolize bleeding varices from the coronary vein at the time of TIPS placement assists in achieving primary control of bleeding sites.

The two principal long-term complications of TIPS are encephalopathy and shunt occlusion. Because it is a central non-selective shunt, the TIPS procedure can precipitate hepatic encephalopathy, especially when used in patients with severe intrinsic liver disease. The overall risk of encephalopathy ranges from 5 to 35% in adult patients, a rate similar to that seen with side-to-side surgical shunts. Most episodes of encephalopathy can be controlled with dietary protein restriction and lactulose administration. Selection of a shunt size to allow sufficient portal decompression without shunting excessive amounts of blood from the liver is also a theoretical solution. Shunt stenosis and thrombosis remain major complications following TIPS. Stenosis occurs in 25–75% of cases, with patency decreasing over time. Stenosis most commonly results from intimal hyperplasia or incorrect shunt placement. Regular monitoring for shunt patency and periodic shunt dilation or restenting is necessary.

Pediatric experience with TIPS remains limited, primarily due to a lack of appropriate candidates for the procedure. The majority of children with biliary atresia and ineffective Kasai portoenterostomy procedure develop end-stage liver disease within their first 2 years of life. These patients are poor TIPS candidates both by virtue of their size and the frequency of portal vein abnormalities within this population. The majority of experience is in children over 5 years of age. Success rates appear to approximate the adult experience, with 75–90% initial success following TIPS placement. The smaller size of the liver and its venous structures requires special skill and equipment. Shorter stent lengths and smaller diameter stents have been constructed for pediatric applications; however, the risks of hepatic perforation and stent malposition are greater in small patients.

Postprocedural encephalopathy seems to be less common in children, although limited clinical experience and the difficulties in diagnosing subtle encephalopathy in children

makes this observation tentative. The complications of shunt stenosis are equally problematic, and patient growth over time may cause the initial shunt to be too short, requiring revision or restenting to maintain access to both the portal and hepatic venous circulation. These limitations and risks make TIPS a reasonable and suitable treatment for acute unresponsive variceal hemorrhage in children with established intrinsic liver disease, as a bridge to stabilize patients awaiting liver transplantation. At the present time, long-term decompression is better achieved through surgical shunts. TIPS is not indicated in patients with extrahepatic portal vein obstruction.

Non-Shunt Procedures for Portal Hypertension

The use of non-shunt surgical procedures for the management of portal hypertension does not offer the same success as shunt surgery. Historically, these operations have included both direct variceal ligation through a transthoracic or abdominal approach, gastroesophageal devascularization procedures (Sugiura Procedure), or rarely, translocation of the spleen into the thorax (splenopneumopexy). In general, these procedures have been abandoned except in cases where widespread thrombosis of the mesenteric venous vasculature makes shunt therapy or transplantation poor alternatives.

The Sugiura procedure has been used with the most success in children. This procedure includes devascularization of the upper two-thirds of the greater and lesser curvatures of the stomach, and ligation of the left gastroepiploic, short gastric, and left gastric vessels. Ligation of all retrogastric collateral vessels, transhiatal devascularization of the lower esophagus, and esophageal transection with fundoplication and pyloroplasty if the vagus nerves are damaged complete the operative procedure. Splenectomy was advocated in the original descriptions of this procedure as well, but splenectomy has been associated with a greater risk of intraoperative bleeding, need for intraoperative blood transfusions, and postoperative portal vein thrombosis. Because of these risks and the known increased potential for postoperative infectious complications following splenectomy, we do not routinely perform splenectomy in children. Specific indications for splenectomy during non-shunt operations are severe hypersplenism, massive splenomegaly, and splenic vein thrombosis. Following extensive devascularization to achieve portoazygos disconnection, rebleeding rates of 5–10% can be achieved during long-term follow-up. Survival has been reported to be 88% at 5 years and 80% at 10 years. This is a safe alternative for variceal control in patients with anatomy unsuitable for shunting, or when the expertise for emergency portocaval shunt or liver transplantation is not available.

Liver Transplantation

The progressive improvement in both the operative techniques and the immunosuppression management of children who have undergone liver transplant has led to 1-year survival rates approaching 90% in many centers, with 5-year survival rates of 85%. Regardless of the primary etiology of portal hypertension, liver transplantation successfully resolves the portal flow obstruction and allows the resolution of hypersplenism and hypertensive portal gastropathy. The introduction of innovative surgical procedures to allow transplantation of liver segments and reduced-size grafts has increased donor availability and donor access for children of all ages. However, the use of primary transplantation as a treatment modality for portal hypertension is limited by the availability of suitable donor organs and the long-term risks of immunosuppression, opportunistic infections, and lymphoproliferative disease. When children have progressive intrinsic hepatic disease, the course of their progression and the amount of hepatic functional reserve should determine the use of primary transplantation compared with temporizing treatments, such as sclerotherapy or surgical shunts. At present, primary transplantation is recommended for children who have significant portal hypertensive complications such as bleeding, hypersplenism, or hepatopulmonary syndrome, and those who have progressive hepatic synthetic failure. Children with intrinsic liver disease but preserved hepatic synthetic function, who may not require transplantation for several years, will achieve excellent palliation with selective DSRS. TIPS is reserved for patients who have unresponsive variceal bleeding as a therapeutic bridge to transplantation, allowing them to achieve suitable stability while awaiting transplant donor organ availability.

Therapeutic options for children with portal hypertension now include a broad range of pharmacologic, endoscopic, and surgical procedures. Thoughtful application of all of these options can improve quality of life by decreasing the complications of portal hypertension, and decrease mortality by preventing the consequences of variceal hemorrhage. The development of portal hypertensive gastropathy following palliative procedures such as endoscopic sclerotherapy and band ligation may limit their long-term success in children. The excellent results now obtained with selective portosystemic shunts and liver transplantation assure that definitive surgical treatments will continue to be a critical component in the treatment of children with portal hypertensive complications or progressive liver disease. Evolving procedures, such as TIPS, represent excellent short-term life-preserving techniques to stabilize critically ill patients while awaiting liver transplantation.

Summary Points

- Etiology of portal hypertension is classified as pre-hepatic, intra-hepatic, or post-hepatic.
- Extrahepatic portal vein obstruction (EPVO) is most common type of pre-hepatic obstruction.
- Most cases of acute variceal bleeding can be controlled with fluid resuscitation, correction of coagulopathy, and pharmacologic support.
- Octreotide is most commonly used pharmacologic intervention in management of acute variceal bleeding.
- Upper endoscopy is important intervention for both diagnostic and therapeutic purposes in acute variceal bleeding.
- Endoscopic sclerotherapy or band ligation can be used to control refractory variceal bleeding.
- Classification of portosystemic shunts: non-selective shunt, selective shunt, direct reconstruction of portal circulation.
- H-type mesocaval shunt is most commonly used non-selective shunt.
- Most common selective shunt is distal splenorenal shunt.
- Extrahepatic portal vein obstruction is optimally managed by mesentericoportal shunt (Rex shunt).
- Transjugular intrahepatic portosystemic shunt (TIPS) may be used as a bridge to liver transplantation in patients with intrinsic liver disease who have acute unresponsive variceal bleeding.
- If significant portal hypertensive complications are accompanied by progressive hepatic synthetic failure, liver transplantation may be considered.
- Due to progressive liver failure in the setting of intrinsic liver disease, most cases of intra-hepatic portal hypertension are definitively managed by liver transplantation.

Editor's Comment

Regardless of the etiology, children with advanced cirrhosis should be considered for liver transplantation, although a surgical portosystemic shunt or TIPS is sometimes used as a bridge to transplant. Surgical shunts are associated with excellent outcomes when performed by experienced surgeons in high-volume centers. In general, selective shunts (distal splenorenal) are preferred over nonselective shunts (central splenorenal, mesocaval) because they result in less postoperative encephalopathy. Direct reconstruction (Rex shunt) is preferred for patients with extrahepatic portal venous obstruction, patent intrahepatic veins, and no significant hypercoagulability. It is important to choose a shunt that will not make subsequent liver transplant operation more difficult or dangerous.

In the past it was common for patients with hypersplenism due to portal hypertension to be referred for splenectomy, usually in combination with a nonselective shunt (central splenorenal) or devascularization procedure. However, except in the rare case of splenic vein thrombosis, this practice is currently frowned upon, especially since a well-constructed shunt improves venous drainage of the spleen and will almost always reverse the hypersplenism. Combined with the increased risk of bleeding and subsequent sepsis, the spleen should be preserved whenever possible.

Diagnostic Studies

- Upper endoscopy
- Doppler ultrasonography of liver
- Magnetic resonance angiography
- Transjugular retrograde portal venography (if necessary, prior to Rex shunt)

Parental Preparation

- Major operation
- Large abdominal incision.
- Decision regarding type of shunt required is usually made at time of abdominal exploration and intraoperative venography.
- Possible need for postoperative intravenous anticoagulation.
- Postoperative anti-platelet therapy.
- Postoperative shunt surveillance with Doppler ultrasonography, computed tomography angiography, or formal angiography.
- Potential complications: bleeding, shunt thrombosis, shunt stenosis.

Preoperative Preparation

☐ Evaluate presence and degree of intrinsic liver disease
☐ Upper endoscopy to evaluate degree of varices
☐ Evaluate for hypercoagulable state
☐ Doppler ultrasonography, magnetic resonance angiography
☐ Transjugular retrograde portal venography (if necessary)
☐ Complete blood count, coagulation parameters, type & cross
☐ Informed consent

Technical Points

- Intraoperative mesentericoportal venography and measurement of portal pressures
- Use of autologous venous conduit (internal jugular vein), if conduit necessary
- Adequate mobilization of inflow and outflow vessels
- Fine monofilament suture for anastomoses
- Post-reconstructive venography is critical
- Selective postoperative intravenous anticoagulation in high-risk patients
- Anti-platelet therapy for 30–90 postoperative days
- Criteria to consider Rex shunt construction in EPVO patients:
- Normal liver parenchyma
- No hypercoagulable state
- Patent and accessible umbilical portion of left portal vein
- Suitable inflow vessel

Suggested Reading

Botha JF, Campos BD, Grant WJ, et al. Portosystemic shunts in children: a 15-year experience. J Am Coll Surg. 2004;199:179–85.

Garcia-Tsao G, Sanyal AJ, Grace ND, et al. Prevention and management of gastroesophageal varices and variceal hemorrhage in cirrhosis. Hepatology. 2007;46:922–38.

Laleman W, Van Landeghem L, Wilmer A, et al. Portal hypertension: from pathophysiology to clinical practice. Liver Int. 2005;25:1079–90.

Ochs A. Transjugular intrahepatic portosystemic shunt. Dig Dis. 2005;23:56–64.

Shneider B, Emre S, Groszmann R, et al. Expert pediatric opinion on the report of the Baveno IV consensus workshop on methodology of diagnosis and therapy in portal hypertension. Pediatr Transplant. 2006;10:893–907.

Superina RA, Alonso EM. Medical and surgical management of portal hypertension in children. Curr Treat Options Gastroenterol. 2006;9:432–43.

Superina R, Shneider B, Emre S, et al. Surgical guidelines for the management of extra-hepatic portal vein obstruction. Pediatr Transplant. 2006a;10:908–13.

Superina R, Bambini DA, Lokar J, et al. Correction of extrahepatic portal vein thrombosis by the mesenteric to left portal vein bypass. Ann Surg. 2006b;243:515–21.

Tiao GM, Alonso MH, Ryckman FC. Pediatric liver transplantation. Semin Pediatr Surg. 2006;15:218–27.

Zollinger RM, Zollinger RM. Atlas of surgical operations. New York: Macmillan; 1975.

Chapter 79
Congenital Hyperinsulinism

N. Scott Adzick

Congenital hyperinsulinism (HI) is a rare derangement of glucose metabolism that occurs with an estimated incidence of 1–1.4 in 50,000 live births, accounting for about 80–120 new cases in the United States each year. Higher rates of 1 in 2,500 live births have been reported in areas of high consanguinity, such as the Arabian Peninsula. Inappropriate over secretion of insulin is the hallmark of HI. The old term "nesidioblastosis" should be discarded. HI is the most common cause of persistent hypoglycemia in neonates and can lead to seizures and irreversible brain damage. Pancreatectomy for management of persistent infantile hypoglycemia was first performed at The Children's Hospital of Philadelphia (CHOP) in 1950.

Diagnosis

Molecular biological studies have shown that abnormalities of the K_{ATP} channel, which are encoded by the sulfonylurea receptor 1 (SUR1) and Kir6.2 genes, are responsible for altered control of insulin secretion. In response to elevated glucose levels, the K_{ATP} channel closes, depolarizing the beta-cell membrane and initiating a calcium-dependent release of insulin from the beta-cell storage granules. Uncontrolled insulin secretion may occur if either the SUR1 or Kir6.2 proteins is defective. The SUR1/Kir6.2 form of HI may not be controlled with medical therapy such as diazoxide, which acts on SUR1 to suppress insulin secretion, and thus pancreatectomy is often necessary. In contrast, patients with other genetic forms of HI that result from mutations of glucokinase or glutamate dehydrogenase genes are usually responsive to diazoxide and do not require surgical intervention.

Neonates with HI may have either diffuse involvement of the pancreatic beta-cells or focal adenomatous islet cell hyperplasia. Mutations of the SUR1/Kir6.2 complex appear to be involved in both types. Recessive mutations cause diffuse HI, whereas loss of heterozygosity (LOH) and inheritance of a paternal mutation cause focal adenomatous HI: patients with recessively inherited mutations of the SUR1/Kir6.2 complex have all abnormal beta cells and therefore develop diffuse disease and patients with LOH in combination with a paternal mutation have normal beta-cells as well as one or more focal clones of abnormal beta-cells that are homozygous for the SUR1/Kir6.2 mutation. The focal lesions arise as a result of a two-hit loss-of-heterozygosity mechanism. First, there is a specific loss of maternal alleles of the imprinted chromosome region 11p15 in cells from the focal lesion but not in the surrounding normal pancreatic cells. Second, there is a transmission of a mutation of SUR1/Kir6.2 in the paternal chromosome 11p. Focal lesions have been linked to non-Mendelian expression of paternally-transmitted SUR1 mutation in which there is duplication and reduction of homozygosity of the mutant paternal allele. In the future, molecular biology testing of peripheral leukocytes may help differentiate focal from diffuse disease. However, the search for mutations is currently of limited use in clinical practice because the process takes many weeks and not all mutations are known.

One of the big challenges in diagnosis has been that the diffuse and focal forms of HI are clinically identical. Patients with either form of the disease are unusually large for gestational age, reflecting the effects of hyperinsulinemia on fetal growth. We have found that approximately 55% of our patients have focal disease and about 45% have diffuse disease. Distinguishing focal from diffuse disease is of importance in guiding the extent of surgical resection. Patients with diffuse disease often require near-total pancreatectomy, which has the long-term risk of diabetes mellitus. Conversely, babies with focal disease can be cured with a selective partial pancreatectomy with little risk of subsequent diabetes.

At the Congenital Hyperinsulinism Center at CHOP, we use a multidisciplinary approach (pediatric endocrinology,

N.S. Adzick (✉)
Department of Surgery, Children's Hospital of Philadelphia,
University of Pennsylvania School of Medicine,
Philadelphia, PA, USA
e-mail: adzick@email.chop.edu

radiology, pathology and surgery) for patients with HI to distinguish focal from diffuse disease, localize focal lesions, treat focal disease with partial pancreatectomy and treat medically-refractory diffuse disease with near-total pancreatectomy. During the past 10 years, more than 200 patients (median age 10 weeks) with HI have been treated with pancreatectomy at CHOP. We have crafted an educational DVD regarding the management of congenital hyperinsulinism that is available at the CHOP web site (www.chop.edu).

Diagnosis and Medical Management by Pediatric Endocrinology

Babies with HI present with severe and persistent hypoglycemia manifested by seizures, lethargy, apnea and other symptoms resulting from neuroglucopenia. The diagnosis of congenital HI is established if fasting hypoglycemia (glucose <50 mg/dL) occurs simultaneously with inappropriately elevated plasma insulin (>2.0 μU/mL), low plasma beta-hydroxybutyrate (<2.0 mmol/L) and free fatty acids (<1.5 mmol/L) and an inappropriate glycemic response to intravenous glucagon (>30 mg/dL rise in serum glucose level). Standard medical therapy to maintain euglycemia involves a high continuous intravenous infusion of glucose, frequent oral feedings and administration of diazoxide, glucagon and/or octreotide. In the past, efforts to distinguish focal from diffuse disease involved the injection of intravenous calcium and tolbutamide (a sulfonylurea) to elicit different types of insulin responses by focal and diffuse disease, but the results were not predictive enough to be clinically useful.

Preoperative assessment of babies with HI reveals that they are large, often fluid overloaded due to high intravenous glucose requirements, have hepatic enlargement due to steatosis, may be anemic due to frequent blood sampling and have oral aversion. They are predisposed to central venous line sepsis both pre- and postoperatively.

Localization Procedures Performed by Radiology

We have tried diagnostic radiology tests such as ultrasound (both preoperative and intraoperative), magnetic resonance imaging, computerized tomography, contrast angiography, and radio-labeled octreotide scans, but all have been unsuccessful in identifying focal lesions. For insulinoma localization in adults, intraoperative saline injection into the pancreas followed by tissue aspiration with rapid insulin measurements has been helpful, but I have found that this localization technique is untenable in the fragile neonatal pancreas.

Two interventional radiology tests have been used in an attempt to differentiate focal from diffuse disease. The arterial stimulation with venous sampling (ASVS) technique involves selective pancreatic angiographic stimulation with intra-arterial calcium, which stimulates abnormal islet cells to release insulin, followed by venous sampling. An immediate rise in insulin from stimulation in only one artery suggests focal HI in the corresponding area of the pancreas (gastroduodenal artery – pancreatic head; superior mesenteric artery – uncinate process and neck; splenic artery – pancreatic body or tail), whereas an insulin rise in all three areas suggests diffuse HI. We have also used transhepatic portal venous catheterization and selective sampling of the pancreatic veins (THPVS). Both techniques require that the patient be off all glycemic medications (5 days for diazoxide, 1–2 days for octreotide) before catheterization under general anesthesia. THPVS requires that glucose levels be maintained at 50 mg/dL during the procedure as compared to 60–80 mg/dL for ASVS. For THPVS, the pancreatic venous insulin levels are compared to simultaneously drawn plasma levels of insulin and glucose. Both ASVS and THPVS are technically very demanding and have limited specificity and sensitivity for distinguishing focal and diffuse disease. These techniques have been replaced by a new PET-CT scan technique using [18F]fluoro-L-DOPA.

Neuroendocrine cells have an affinity for amino acid precursors such as L-dihydroxyphenylalanine (L-DOPA), which are taken up and decarboxylated to form dopamine. We can therefore use radiolabeled [18F]fluoro-L-DOPA and positron emission tomography (PET) to identify focal lesions. Because of its very short half-life, the isotope is manufactured by the Cyclotron Facility at the University of Pennsylvania on the day of the PET scan and is administered to patients under an Investigational New Drug (IND) application approved by the Food and Drug Administration. The results are dramatic and visually spectacular (Fig. 79.1).

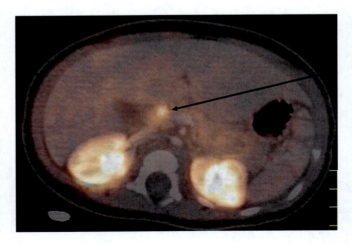

Fig. 79.1 PET scan is co-registered with a CT scan which shows a focal lesion in the head of the pancreas. Note that the kidneys excrete the [18F]-fluoro-L-DOPA and also light up

We have found that PET-CT scans read as showing a focal lesion are 100% accurate in localizing a lesion. However, about 20% of patients whose scans were interpreted as showing diffuse disease are proven during operative exploration to have a focal lesion. This false negative rate should decrease with greater clinical experience.

appear normal. Patients with diffuse disease have abnormal islets containing 5–10% of cells with enlarged nuclei present throughout the pancreas. After the operation, all samples are processed for routine histology with confirmation of frozen-section findings on the basis of paraffin-embedded sections and insulin immunohistochemistry.

Histopathology

A focal lesion is characterized by a tumor-like proliferation of islet cells that push exocrine elements aside or haphazardly incorporate them (Fig. 79.2). Unlike insulinomas, the focal lesion retains the lobular architecture of the normal pancreas and exocrine elements usually remain within the lesion. The lesions often have irregular borders and the endocrine cells frequently have enlarged nuclei. Islets outside the lesion

Surgical Technique

Open operations are approached through a transverse supra-umbilical laparotomy. The pancreas is exposed by an extended Kocher maneuver, entry into the lesser sac and mobilization of the inferior border of the pancreas. It is rarely necessary to mobilize the spleen. The pancreas is carefully palpated and inspected under 3.5× loupe magnification in an attempt to visualize a focal lesion. If no focal lesion is seen,

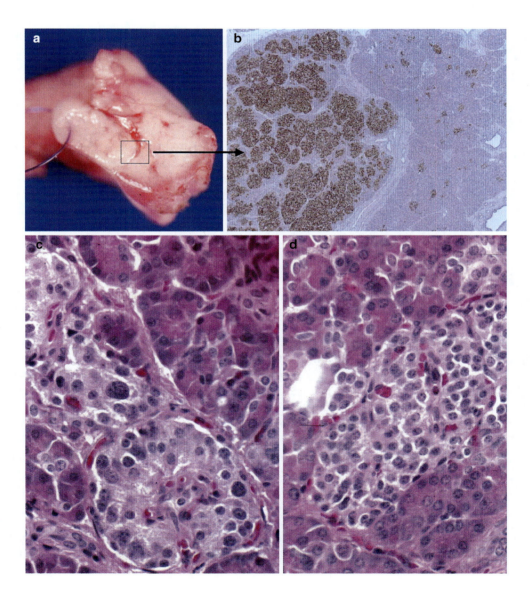

Fig. 79.2 (**a**) Cut surface of pancreatectomy specimen through a focal lesion (marked by *suture*). (**b**) Chromogranin A immunolabelling highlights the architecture of the focal lesion (*left*) and adjacent normal pancreas (*right*). (**c**, **d**) Comparison of cytologic features of the endocrine tissue in the focal lesion (**c**) and normal pancreas (**d**). Note enlarged islet cell nuclei in (**c**)

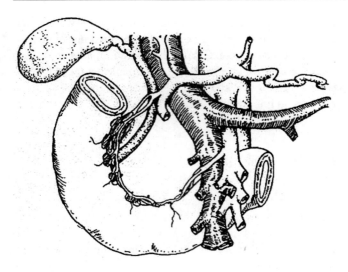

Fig. 79.3 Near-total pancreatectomy. Note that the entire common bile duct is skeletonized, and the blood supply to the duodenum is preserved

then separate 2–3 mm diameter biopsies are taken from the pancreatic head, body and tail. Patients with suspected diffuse HI have intraoperative biopsies to confirm the diagnosis and then undergo near-total pancreatectomy (Fig. 79.3). Near-total pancreatectomy (95–98%) involves resection of the entire pancreas leaving only a tiny residual portion between the common bile duct and the duodenum. The intrapancreatic course of the common bile duct should be completely dissected for an adequate near-total pancreatectomy to be performed. For children with diffuse disease treated by near-total pancreatectomy, we also place a gastrostomy tube in the event that supplemental glucose or night-time feedings become necessary in the postoperative period.

When the biopsies demonstrate normal pancreatic histology, a further search for the focal lesion using the preoperative localization data is conducted. Additional biopsies of suspicious areas are obtained until the focal lesion is confirmed by frozen section analysis. Expert pediatric pathologic interpretation is vitally important. Focal lesions tend to be less than 10 mm in size (although they can be much larger) and frequently are irregularly shaped. Some lesions have octopus-like "tentacles" that make imperative the intraoperative confirmation of clear margins by frozen section. Although focal lesions may maintain a lobular structure similar to that of the normal pancreas, subtle visual clues, ranging from a slightly reddish color to a marble-like appearance, may permit visual detection of the lesion intraoperatively. Accurate preoperative localization studies also greatly facilitate the visual search for a focal lesion. In some cases the lesion will feel firmer than the surrounding normal pancreas, however a tiny focal lesion can be buried within the pancreas and may be impossible to see or feel. Certainly,

I have learned that greater operative experience has led to more frequent intra-operative visualization or palpation of a focal lesion. Insulinomas differ from focal lesions because they are usually straightforward to identify intraoperatively and occur in older children.

Once a focal lesion is identified, partial pancreatectomy is performed and frozen section analysis of the margins is used to ensure a complete resection. For periductal lesions in the body and tail, a distal pancreatectomy is performed. With pancreatic head lesions close to the common bile duct or pancreatic duct, it can be tricky to excise the entire lesion, particularly if there are tentacles of diseased tissue that emanate from the lesion. To ensure complete lesion resection in these challenging cases, I now have a low threshold to remove most or all of the pancreatic head followed by Roux-en-Y pancreaticojejunostomy to drain the remaining pancreatic body and tail. In this way, the endocrine and exocrine function of the remaining normal pancreas is preserved. Early in my experience, I was reluctant to use this approach in neonates and infants, but this led to inadequate resection in a few cases, which necessitated either another resection or continued medical therapy. In babies, the pancreatic duct on the cut surface of the transected pancreatic body is not visible, so a meticulous anastomosis is created between the end of the Roux-en-Y jejunal limb and the capsule of the pancreatic body with fine interrupted 6-0 monofilament suture to effectively dunk the cut end of the pancreas into the small bowel lumen. Rarely, a focal lesion in the head will extend into the duodenal wall, in which case a Whipple procedure may need to be performed.

Since more than 50% of focal lesions involve the pancreatic head, subtotal pancreatectomy is inadequate therapy in many of these cases. Our experience with several referrals who underwent subtotal pancreatectomy elsewhere with the focal lesion remaining within the residual pancreas are good examples of this potential pitfall.

There are several technical tricks that can facilitate pancreatectomy in a baby. First, placing a vessel loop around the extrahepatic common bile duct and then bringing that vessel loop within the duodenal C-loop can help with dissection of the tiny common bile duct buried in the pancreatic head. Second, electrocautery (monopolar or bipolar) can be used to take the tiny pancreatic venous branches that drain into the splenic vein and the splenic arterial branches to the pancreas. Third, for pancreatic head resections, it is important to preserve the gastroduodenal artery proximally as well as the vessels supplying the third and fourth portion of the duodenum distally in order to prevent duodenal devascularization. Finally, I use fibrin glue on any remaining cut pancreatic edge after pancreatectomy instead of placing a closed suction drain.

Because PET scan localization of focal lesions has proven to be so accurate, focal lesions in the body and tail can now be resected using laparoscopic techniques. To facilitate pancreatic body and tail exposure during laparoscopy, it is useful to sew the stomach up to the anterior abdominal wall using two or three transabdominal sutures to the anterior gastric wall close to the greater curvature. The carbon dioxide pneumoperitoneum then suspends the stomach anteriorly and makes it easy to expose and dissect the pancreatic body and tail. The laparoscopic procedure is performed using four 3–5 mm ports; this permits biopsies, complete resection of a visible peripherally located focal lesion or, if necessary, distal pancreatectomy. The drawback to the laparoscopic approach is that there is little tactile feedback to help locate a non-visible focal lesion.

Postoperative Care

Postoperative management has been standardized by a clinical care pathway including the use of the Glucose Infusion Rate (GIR) to quantitate the patient's glucose requirement. The GIR is calculated as: [dextrose concentration (g/dL) × IV rate (mL/h)]/[6 × patient weight (kg)]. For the initial postoperative period, blood glucose values are determined hourly. The GIR begins at 2 mg/kg/min immediately postoperatively, is increased to 5 mg/kg/min on the morning of the first postoperative day and then usually advanced to 8 mg/kg/min by the evening of the first postoperative day. It is not unusual for an intravenous insulin infusion to be needed for the first few postoperative days. After hospital discharge, a complete response at follow-up is defined as: no requirement for glycemic medications, no need for continuous tube feedings, no evidence of diabetes mellitus and the ability to tolerate an 18-h fast without hypoglycemia.

In our entire experience, 95% of babies with the focal form of HI are cured after limited pancreatectomy. The vast majority had a less than 50% pancreatectomy. For babies with diffuse HI treated with near-total pancreatectomy, about one-third require no glycemic medications, one-third require a glycemic medication (usually octreotide) and one-third require insulin to treat diabetes. Long-term follow-up is needed for all of these children particularly with regard to neurodevelopmental issues.

Summary Points

- The diagnosis of congenital HI should be considered in any large newborn with hypoglycemia.
- The diagnosis is established by: fasting glucose of <50 mg/dL with concomitant insulin level of >2.0 µU/mL, plasma beta-hydroxybutyrate <2.0 mmol/L and free fatty acids <1.5 mmol/L, and confirmed by an inappropriate glycemic response to intravenous glucagon (>30 mg/dL rise in serum glucose level after glucagon 1 mg IV).
- There are two forms of HI: *diffuse disease*, an autosomal recessive disease, and *focal nodular disease*, which is the result of inheritance of a paternal mutation and loss of heterozygosity for the maternal allele.
- Children with congenital HI are best managed with a multidisciplinary approach that includes experienced clinicians from pediatric endocrinology, radiology, pathology, neonatology and surgery.
- Patients with focal nodular disease are treated by complete resection of the tumor with negative margins.
- Patients with diffuse disease are treated by near-total (95–98%) pancreatectomy.
- The most accurate preoperative diagnostic test is [18F]fluoro-L-DOPA PET CT scan, which is currently available at very few centers.
- Postoperative care after partial pancreatectomy almost always initially involves a continuous intravenous glucose infusion and sometimes a temporary insulin infusion.
- Postoperative care after near-total pancreatectomy may require insulin (1/3), glycemic medications (1/3), or no medication (1/3).

Editor's Comment

Congenital hyperinsulinism is such a rare condition that few pediatric surgical centers can accumulate a large number of cases. Dr. Adzick outlines an approach that is state-of-the-art and clearly based on experience with a large number of patients over many years. There are several insightful conclusions to be drawn from this nice summary: (1) Case volume and experience are necessary to generate consistently good results and a very low complication rate. (2) PET-CT scanning with [18F]fluoro-L-DOPA is clearly the most accurate and clinically useful study for preoperative diagnosis and localization of focal lesions. Although currently limited in its availability, I expect that it will soon be the gold standard test for this condition. (3) Laparoscopic techniques are clearly feasible in the treatment of patients with HI and will likely become standard for initial biopsy and diagnosis and probably for the resection of focal lesions. (4) As we learn more about the genetics and molecular biology of congenital HI, we will soon have many more options for diagnosis, classification and treatment, perhaps in some cases obviating the need for surgical intervention. (5) Infants with hyperinsulinism should always be managed very aggressively with high-dose intravenous glucose infusion (via central venous catheter, if necessary), a trial of available glycemic medications and the frequent monitoring of blood glucose levels in an intensive care setting, as the long-term neurodevelopmental sequelae of hypoglycemia can be profound, devastating and irreversible.

Differential Diagnosis

- Infant of mother with poorly controlled diabetes mellitus (usually transient)
- Beckwith-Wiedemann syndrome (gigantism, macroglossia, omphalocele)
- Inborn error of metabolism (gluconeogenesis, glycogen metabolism, others)
- Birth asphyxia
- Hypopituitarism
- Factitious hyperinsulinemia (Münchhausen syndrome by proxy)

Diagnostic Studies

- Laboratory studies: fasting glucose; insulin, betahydroxybutyrate, and free fatty acids levels.
- Provocative test: glucose level in response to intravenous glucagon injection.
- Interventional radiology studies: arterial stimulation with venous sampling (ASVS) or hepatic portal venous catheterization and selective sampling of the pancreatic veins (THPVS).
- Preoperative localization: [18F]fluoro-L-DOPA PET-CT scan (most accurate test available at this time).

Parental Preparation

- Preoperative localization studies have limitations and are not entirely accurate.
- Intra-operative localization techniques have limitations also.
- There is the possibility that a near-total pancreatectomy will be necessary and that there is a risk of recurrence and diabetes.

Preoperative Preparation

- ☐ IV Hydration
- ☐ Aggressive glucose control
- ☐ Type and screen
- ☐ Informed consent

Technical Points

- A transverse supraumbilical incision provides excellent exposure.
- The surgeon should perform a systematic and meticulous search for a suspected focal lesion using palpation and 3.5× magnification.
- If no focal lesion is found, biopsy the head, body and tail for frozen section analysis.
- If biopsies confirm diffuse disease, perform a neartotal pancreatectomy.
- Carefully dissect and preserve the intrapancreatic portion of the common bile duct.
- If a focal lesion is found, perform a partial pancreatectomy, use frozen section confirmation of negative margins, and be wary of tentacle-like extensions of tumor.

Suggested Reading

Adzick NS, Thornton PS, Stanley CA, et al. A multidisciplinary approach to the focal form of congenital hyperinsulinism leads to successful treatment by partial pancreatectomy. J Pediatr Surg. 2004;39:270–5.

De Lonlay P, Poggi-Travert F, Founet JC, et al. Clinical features of 52 neonates with hyperinsulinism. N Engl J Med. 1999;340: 1169–75.

DeLeon DD, Stanley CA. Mechanisms of disease: advances in diagnosis and treatment of hyperinsulinism in neonates. Nat Clin Prac. 2007;3:57–68.

Hardy OT, Hernandez-Pampaloni M, Saffer JR, et al. Accuracy of [18F] fluorodopa positron emission tomography for diagnosing and localizing focal congenital hyperinsulinism. J Clin Endocrinol Metab. 2007;92:4706–11.

Chapter 80
Disorders of the Pancreas

Marshall Z. Schwartz and Michael S. Katz

The pancreas is a complex retroperitoneal organ that has both major digestive and endocrine functions. In fact, the totality of the role of the pancreas has not been fully defined. Disorders of the pancreas can result from a congenital anatomic abnormality or dysfunction of either the digestive or endocrine components. The endocrine function of the pancreas is centered in the cells of the islets of Langerhans. Although the islet cells make up only approximately 2% of the pancreatic mass, they play a much larger physiologic role. There are four major types of cells within the islets, each secreting one or more specific peptides. Disorders related to each cell type or peptide can occur. The most common of these disorders is related to the Beta cells, which regulate insulin secretion. This significant topic will be covered separately. We will cover the anatomic, non-insulin endocrine, and inflammatory disorders of the pancreas.

Anatomic Abnormalities

Embryologically, the pancreas forms as a larger dorsal and smaller ventral bud. During the sixth week of gestation, intestinal rotation causes the ventral bud to come to the right and posteriorly around the duodenum where it fuses with the dorsal bud. The smaller duct of Santorini in the dorsal bud will fuse to the larger duct of Wirsung in the ventral bud, and drain into the duodenum through the bile duct at the major duodenal papilla. Variations of this rotation and fusion can lead to anatomic disorders including annular pancreas, pancreas divisum, and pancreatic cysts.

M.Z. Schwartz (✉)
Department of Surgery, Drexel University College of Medicine, St. Christopher's Hospital for Children, Philadelphia, PA, USA
e-mail: mzschwartz@msn.com

Annular Pancreas

Annular pancreas occurs when the ventral bud fails to rotate around the duodenum and instead the two buds fuse together encircling the duodenum. Fetal ultrasonography will typically show findings consistent with obstruction at the second portion of the duodenum. In the absence of previous fetal imaging, these patients usually present in the newborn period with symptoms of proximal intestinal obstruction, which is most often associated with duodenal atresia or stenosis. However, the degree of obstruction caused by the annular pancreas can vary and the patient can present later in infancy if the obstruction is less severe. The diagnosis is usually made by the presence of a double bubble of air (stomach and dilated first portion of the duodenum) on plain abdominal radiograph, but it can be confirmed by upper gastrointestinal contrast study showing obstruction at the second portion of the duodenum. It is almost always associated with duodenal atresia but whether it the cause or the result of the duodenal obstruction is not known. These patients should be admitted to the neonatal intensive care unit. They may have electrolyte derangements due to vomiting, and should receive supportive treatment including intravenous fluid hydration and placement of a nasogastric or orogastric tube.

Once the electrolytes are corrected and any other medical issues have been addressed (these infants are at risk for trisomy 21 and congenital heart defects), the patient can be taken to the operating room. With the patient in the supine position, a limited right upper quadrant transverse incision is made. After entering the peritoneal cavity the diagnosis of annular pancreas or simple duodenal atresia can be definitively made. However, from a management standpoint it makes no difference, as the surgical therapy is the same, namely duodenoduodenostomy. The pancreas should not be divided or otherwise disturbed. We prefer the diamond technique originally described by Kimura. Using electrocautery a 1–1.3-cm duodenotomy is made on the anterior surface of the duodenum proximal to the annular pancreas transversely, making sure not to enter the bile duct or major duodenal papilla. A longitudinal incision of similar length is made on the anterior aspect of the duodenum distal to the site of obstruction. It is important to evaluate the entire small bowel to exclude the possibility of a more distal atresia. This can be done by gently injecting saline through a 10 Fr catheter placed in the distal duodenum until the fluid can be seen flowing into the colon. The anastomosis is then performed with interrupted 5-0 silk sutures, taking care not to injure the major duodenal papilla.

Postoperatively, these patients are treated with parenteral nutrition and gastric drainage until bowel function returns. Gastric decompression will be continued longer than necessary if it is based on the persistence of bilious gastric drainage. It has been our practice to obtain an abdominal radiograph starting around the fifth postoperative day. If there is a considerable amount of air in the small bowel, the gastric tube can be removed. Pedialyte feedings can then be started and once tolerated, advanced to full strength breast milk or formula feeds.

Pancreas Divisum

Pancreas divisum occurs in approximately 10% of the population and is thought to occur when the buds of the pancreas rotate normally but the ducts do not fuse. This results in the main portion of the pancreas draining through the smaller duct (Santorini) and the minor papilla. The smaller inferior pancreatic head and uncinate process drain through the major duodenal papilla. In some patients, the minor papilla may be inadequate for drainage, which is thought to cause stasis in the pancreatic duct and recurrent bouts of pancreatitis. Pancreas divisum occurs in 5–10% of children with pancreatitis and as many as 25% of children with chronic pancreatitis.

The diagnosis of is best made by either magnetic resonance cholangiopancreatogram (MRCP) or endoscopic retrograde cholangiopancreatogram (ERCP). An MRCP will visualize the duct of Santorini draining the full length of the pancreas as well as an absent or atretic duct of Wirsung. An ERCP might only demonstrate one duct, depending on which papilla is being injected. The advantage of ERCP is that it can be both diagnostic and therapeutic. If the minor papilla is identified, a sphincterotomy with or without placement of a stent can be performed to alleviate the high pressure in the duct. If the patient is in the early stages of chronic pancreatitis, this might be adequate. However, if the process has been chronic, some patients will have developed multiple dilated segments of the pancreatic duct ("chain of lakes"), which can benefit from a side-to-side pancreatico-jejunostomy (Puestow procedure, Fig. 80.1).

Patients requiring a Puestow procedure should not have active pancreatitis. A left upper quadrant transverse incision is made and can be extended to the right side as needed. Palpation of the anterior surface of the pancreas helps to elucidate the location of the dilated pancreatic duct. If this is

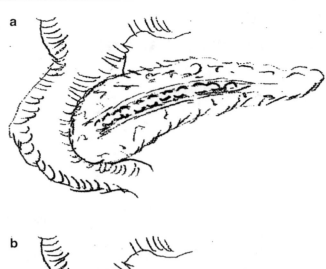

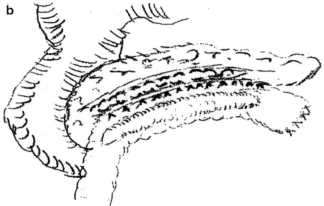

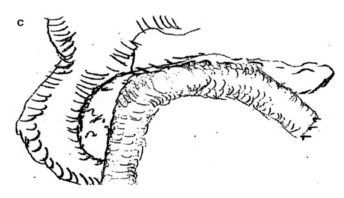

Fig. 80.1 Puestow procedure

unsuccessful, intra-operative ultrasound can be used. Once the pancreatic duct is identified, it should be opened along its length using a scalpel, giving special care not to enter the papilla or injure the bile duct. The jejunum is divided 20–30 cm distal to the ligament of Treitz. The distal end is oversewn and passed through an opening in the transverse mesocolon. An enterotomy is made with electrocautery on the anti-mesenteric border of the jejunum to match the length of the opening in the pancreatic duct. Anastomosis of the jejunum and pancreatic duct is done in a duct-to-mucosa fashion using interrupted 4-0 or 5-0 absorbable sutures. An appropriately sized closed-suction drain should be placed adjacent to the anastomosis. After completion of a standard end-to-side Roux-Y anastomosis, the abdomen is closed.

Parenteral nutrition should be continued in the postoperative period and the patient kept NPO with gastric decompression until return of bowel function, at which point a clear liquid diet can be started and advanced as tolerated. The drain should be left in place until the patient is tolerating a regular diet and there is minimal output. If the patient has a large output from the drain, the fluid should be sent for amylase and lipase. Levels of amylase or lipase greater than 20,000 U/mL confirms the presence of an anastomotic leak. These patients will need to continue to be NPO and on parenteral nutrition until the leak resolves and the drain output is minimal.

Pancreatic Cysts

Congenital cysts of the pancreas are rare. In contrast to pseudocysts, they have an epithelial wall and contain non-enzymatic fluid. They are usually found in the distal pancreas and their symptoms relate to compression on surrounding structures such as the stomach or bile duct, manifesting as feeding intolerance or jaundice. They can also be part of von Hippel-Lindau syndrome.

Surgical treatment is warranted in the symptomatic patient, as these congenital cysts will not regress spontaneously and are likely to continue to grow. Depending on the location and size of the cyst, the surgical options include marsupialization, enucleation, distal pancreatectomy, or internal drainage. Preoperative localization of the cyst is best performed by ultrasonography or abdominal CT scan. Percutaneous drainage of these cysts is not recommended because they always recur. Some patients have concomitant pancreatitis due to either congenital duct anomalies or due to compression of the duct by the cyst. In the setting of acute pancreatitis, surgical intervention should be delayed.

Surgical management can be either by a laparoscopic or open technique. Preservation of pancreatic mass by cyst removal or marsupialization is optimal. However, if the cyst is large and located in the body or tail of the pancreas, distal pancreatectomy is the optimal procedure, especially if the patient has other smaller cysts in the area or has developed a chronically dilated pancreatic duct due to the pressure exerted by the cyst.

Endocrine Disorders

Pediatric patients can develop a number of endocrine disorders of the pancreas. The most common abnormality is hyperinsulinism. The islets of Langerhans also contain alpha cells, which secret glucagon, gamma cells, which that secrete somatostatin, and G cells, which secrete gastrin. Each of these cells can be the source of a benign or malignant tumor secreting their respective peptide. A tumor of the G cells (gastrinoma) is the only non-beta cell pancreatic tumor that can present in the neonatal period. The presentation is that of gastric acid hypersecretion and subsequent peptic ulceration. The excessive gastric hypersecretion also causes diarrhea, this symptomatology being known as the Zollinger-Ellison syndrome. The diagnosis is made by determination of serum gastrin levels in the fasting state. Once a diagnosis is made, the difficult problem is identifying the site of the gastrinoma. Frequently, these tumors are within the pancreas. However, they can also occur in the wall of the duodenum or jejunum, or in the mesentery or omentum. Because these tumors are frequently quite small (<1 cm), they can be difficult to visualize by MRI or CT.

The optimal treatment is resection of the tumor, which cures the hypersecretion (Fig. 80.2). Prior to the availability of agents that can significantly block acid secretion (histamine blockers, proton pump inhibitors) the next step in management was subtotal or total gastrectomy to remove the source of gastric hypersecretion. Because medical management can be effective in the absence of identifying the primary tumor, it is currently the treatment of choice. Major gastric resection should be avoided. A treatment algorithm that applies to the common endocrine tumors of the pancreas is depicted in Fig. 80.3.

Although abnormalities of the endocrine portion of the pancreas are rare, they can be life threatening. The diagnosis can be made by identification of the hormone or peptide that is being hypersecreted. Prompt diagnosis and treatment are critical to a successful outcome.

If the tumor has been localized, surgical treatment is warranted. Resection of the tumor is considered to be the best treatment, either by enucleation or pancreatic resection. These tumors are known to sometimes metastasize, in which case medical therapy or gastrectomy are the only viable options.

Patients should be prepared for the operating room by controlling the symptoms of their underlying disorder. Often this can be done with a somatostatin analogue. The patients should receive intravenous fluid and electrolyte abnormalities should be corrected. If they have had weight loss, consider a course of parenteral nutrition to increase the albumin level above 2.5 g/dL.

The operative plan will depend on the location of the tumor. If the tumor is in the head, neck, or proximal body of the pancreas, enucleation should be performed. If the tumor is in the distal body or tail of the pancreas and enucleation is not an option, then distal pancreatectomy should be performed. It is not always possible to localize the tumor prior to surgery. This is a common issue for patients with insulinoma or gastrinoma. Since most VIPomas in children are

Fig. 80.2 Optimal treatment of
endocrine tumors (reprinted with
permission from Schwartz MZ.
Unusual peptide-secreting tumors
in adolescents and children. Semin
Pediatr Surg. 1997;6:141–6;
Copyright 1997 Elsevier)

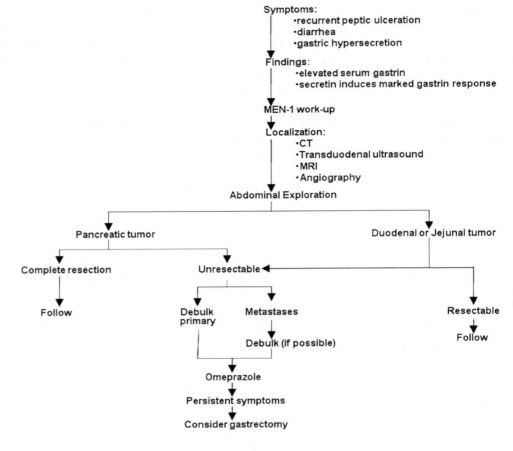

extra-pancreatic in location, a search for the tumor in other parts of the abdomen should be done. Special attention should be given to the adrenal glands and retroperitoneum. The majority of VIPomas, glucagonomas, and somatostatinomas are malignant and are usually several centimeters in diameter. When dealing with any type of islet cell tumor, aggressive attempts to localize the tumor intra-operatively should be made. The best imaging procedure is probably intra-operative ultrasonography. This allows for identification of 95–97% of tumors and can be done laparoscopically. The mass is usually seen as homogeneous, hypoechoic, and with smooth margins.

The search for a pancreatic mass should be systematic and thorough. The spleen and the body and tail of the pancreas should be mobilized medially. This allows bimanual palpation of the pancreas, which is essential. These tumors are sometimes multifocal and the localization of one tumor does not rule out other foci of disease or metastasis. Once all foci of tumor have been localized as well as any metastasis, the decision must be made whether to proceed with enucleation or to perform a distal pancreatectomy. To aid in localization and to confirm completeness of tumor resection, intraoperative hormone measurements can be performed. Serum hormone or peptide levels should be measured peripherally at

the beginning of the procedure. Twenty minutes after all identified tumor has been resected, a second serum level should be rechecked. The time interval allows for the half life of the hormone or peptide to be cleared. If the level has returned to normal, resection may be considered complete with 94% accuracy. However, if the serum level is still elevated, there is residual tumor and further exploration or resection must be considered. In a small percentage of patients who have a normal serum hormone or peptide level at the beginning of surgery, intra-operative serum levels will not be useful.

Pancreatitis

Inflammation is one of the most common diseases of the pancreas in children. There are several etiologies for pancreatitis in children (Table 80.1). In contrast to adults, cholelithiasis and alcohol are not major etiological factors for pancreatitis in children, with the exception of those with hemolytic diseases who develop gallstones. Most patients with pancreatitis will be treated by correction of the cause and supportive management. However, a small percentage

Fig. 80.3 Treatment algorithm for common endocrine tumors of the pancreas (reprinted with permission from Schwartz MZ. Unusual peptide-secreting tumors in adolescents and children. Semin Pediatr Surg. 1997;6:141–6; Copyright 1997 Elsevier)

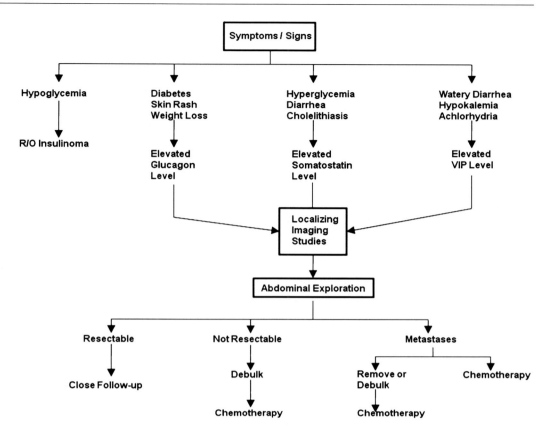

Table 80.1 Common causes of pancreatitis in children

Trauma to the head of the pancreas or adjacent duodenum
Disorders of the biliary tract or pancreatic duct
Pancreas divisum
Choledochal cyst
Cholelithiasis (hemolytic disorders)
Pancreatic cysts
Drug Induced
Immunosuppressive agents
Steroid medications
Valproate
Azathioprine
Genetic disorders
Cystic fibrosis
Hyperlipidemia
Schwachman-Diamond Syndrome
Iatrogenic
ERCP
Injury to the biliary tree or pancreas during abdominal surgery

will develop necrotizing or hemorrhagic pancreatitis and require extensive surgical debridement.

Children with pancreatitis can present with a spectrum of symptoms ranging from mild upper abdominal pain, nausea, and vomiting to multisystem organ failure and shock. When a patient presents with suspicion of pancreatitis, the first step is intravenous fluid hydration while confirming the diagnosis and assessing its severity. A complete history and physical examination should be performed with special attention to upper abdominal tenderness. Serum white blood cell count and chemistries should be done, paying specific attention to amylase and lipase levels. Though elevation of one or both of these enzyme levels suggests that the patient has developed pancreatitis, the levels do not reflect the severity of the disease. Severity is still estimated by using Ranson's criteria. Specifically, on admission, age > 55 years, serum white blood cell count >16,000/mm^3, serum lactate dehydrogenase level >350 mg/dL, serum aspartate aminotransferase level >250 IU/L, and serum glucose >200 mg/dL. While age criteria does not apply to the pediatric population, patients with three or more of these criteria should be considered to have severe pancreatitis. At 48 h, a >10% decrease in hematocrit, fluid sequestration >6 L, serum calcium <8 mg/dL, arterial pO$_2$ <60 mmHg, albumin<3.2 g/dL, and an increase in serum blood urea nitrogen >50 mg/dL would be considered to be severe. Severe cases should receive prophylactic antibiotics as they are at risk for necrotizing pancreatitis and subsequent infection. Both ultrasonography and CT are useful imaging studies for pancreatitis. A CT scan should be performed with intravenous contrast as the presence of an unenhanced area of the pancreas on contrast CT indicates pancreatic necrosis. Alone this is not an indication for surgery as many patients with sterile pancreatic necrosis will improve without surgical intervention. However, if the patient's condition continues to deteriorate or if air is present in the necrotic area of the pancreas, the diagnosis of necrotizing pancreatitis must be considered and prompt surgical treatment is warranted.

Resuscitation with large volumes of intravenous fluid is usually required due to severe third space losses and hemodynamic instability. These patients often require ventilator support and pressor agents as their disease warrants. Once the patient has been stabilized, they should be taken to the operating room for resection of the infected necrotic pancreas. This is a damage-control operation with the goal being to debride as much of the necrotic tissue as possible. The pancreas will be severely inflamed and often liquid in consistency. Depending on the severity, much of the pancreas may be removed. The abdomen should then be irrigated with several liters of warm saline as the pancreatic enzymes could now have spread throughout the abdominal cavity. All saline should be suctioned from the abdomen. Large sump drains should be placed in the pancreatic bed and brought out laterally. Depending on the severity and the amount of swelling of the bowel, the abdomen may either be closed in a normal fashion or left open with a vacuum-sponge dressing placed over it. Do not attempt to close the abdomen under pressure as these patients are at high risk for acute abdominal compartment syndrome. It is often necessary to do a second-look operation for further resection of necrotic tissue.

Central venous and arterial line placement should be placed as these are often highly unstable patients. Ventilator support and nasogastric suction should be continued. Electrolytes should be checked on a serial basis as large fluid shifts should be expected. Parenteral narcotics should be used as the pain can be significant. Meperidine or hydromorphone is preferred over morphine due to the possible effect of sphincter of Oddi spasm. Parenteral nutrition should be provided as oral feeds will stimulate pancreatic secretions. Antibiotics should be continued and tailored to the cultures that are taken in the operating room.

Sump drains should not be removed unless the fluid output is minimal and there is no evidence of a pancreatic fistula. Parenteral nutrition should be continued until the patient has a return of bowel function and normalization of pancreatic enzyme levels, at which point a clear liquid diet can be started. However, keep in mind that if a large amount of the pancreas has been removed, these patients might not be able to elevate their amylase and lipase levels despite having pancreatic inflammation.

Pancreatic Pseudocyst

Regardless of the severity of the pancreatitis or its cause, patients can develop pancreatic pseudocysts. Pseudocysts are formed when the inflammation of the pancreas causes pancreatic secretions to leak from the pancreatic duct and begin to digest the surrounding tissue. The inflammatory response walls off the pancreatic leak forming the pseudocyst. The diagnosis should be suspected in any post-pancreatitis patient with persistent abdominal pain or nausea and vomiting. Diagnosis is often made by ultrasonography or CT.

Treatment depends on the degree of symptoms. Patients are often dehydrated and should be resuscitated with intravenous fluids. Some will benefit from nasogastric decompression and parenteral nutrition. The majority of pseudocysts will resolve with conservative management. Patients with identified pseudocysts should be re-imaged at around 4 weeks. If the pseudocyst is smaller, conservative management should be continued. However, pseudocysts unchanged in size or enlarged should be considered for surgical management. Percutaneous drainage is not an effective option due to the high incidence of recurrence and pancreatic fistula formation.

There are three surgical management options for a pseudocyst. Those that are in contact with the posterior wall of the stomach should be drained by cyst-gastrostomy, while those in contact with the duodenum can be treated with cyst-duodenostomy. The technique for each of these is similar. The anterior wall of the stomach or duodenum opened, at which point a bulge from the pseudocyst will be noted in the posterior wall. A large-bore needle should be passed through the posterior wall of the organ into the pseudocyst and contents aspirated to confirm both location of the pseudocyst and its adhesion to the wall of the organ. The common wall of the stomach or duodenum and the pseudocyst can then be opened using electrocautery. A gastrointestinal stapling device can be used to extend the opening at least 4–5 cm. Necrotic material should be evacuated and the cavity gently irrigated. Once this is complete, the anterior wall of the stomach is closed by using a stapling device. This procedure can also be performed laparoscopically.

Some patients will require cyst-jejunostomy. These include infected pseudocysts, immature pseudocysts, pseudocysts found to not be connected to the stomach or duodenum, and pseudocysts iatrogenically disconnected from the stomach or duodenum. In these cases, a cystjejunostomy should be performed using a Roux-en-Y limb. The jejunum is divided approximately 40 cm distal to the ligament of Treitz. The pseudocyst is opened and the distal end of the bowel is anastomosed to the pseudocyst after necrotic material is suctioned from the cavity. If this is being done for infected or immature pseudocysts, then large closed-suction drains should be left in the area of the cyst and brought out through the lateral abdominal wall.

Pancreatic pseudocyst patients will often do very well postoperatively. The relief of pressure or obstruction will allow them to be started on a diet and advanced once their bowel function returns. Drains may be removed when the output is nearly zero.

Summary Points

- Tumors arising from cells in the islets of Langerhans can produce symptoms by oversecretion of peptides normally produced by these cells: insulinoma, gastrinoma, glucagonoma, VIPoma.
- Hyperinsulinsm is the most common endocrine disorder of the pancreas in children.
- Gastrinoma causes peptic ulcer disease and diarrhea (Zollinger-Ellison syndrome) due to hypergastrinemia.
- Gastrinomas are often very small, can arise within the pancreas or the wall of the small bowel, and may be multiple or malignant with metastases.
- Single islet-cell tumors can be enucleated or removed by partial pancreatectomy, while multifocal or metastatic disease is treated medically or, for gastrinoma, near-total gastrectomy.
- Acute pancreatitis in children can be caused by gallstones, anatomic abnormalities such as pancreas divisum, or idiopathic.
- Acute pancreatitis is managed with supportive measures and attempts to treat the underlying cause.
- Pancreatic pseudocysts are the result of a contained pancreatic fistula and usually resolve spontaneously.
- Surgical therapy of pancreatic pseudocyst is by establishing drainage into the stomach, duodenum, or jejunum.

Editor's Comment

The pancreas is an organ that is treated with a great deal of respect by surgeons. Most of the pancreatic disorders commonly seen in adults are much less prevalent in children but are much better tolerated by children. Annular pancreas is probably not a cause of duodenal obstruction but rather an anatomic variant that occurs in the setting of duodenal atresia. Although previous concerns about the risks of dividing the pancreas are probably exaggerated, there is no reason to disturb it while creating a duodenoduodenostomy for repair of the duodenal atresia. Pancreas divisum is probably a normal anatomic variant and not a frequent cause of acute pancreatitis. Nevertheless, some patients with recurrent or chronic pancreatitis appear to benefit from endoscopic sphincterotomy.

Most cases of acute pancreatitis in children are idiopathic though the workup should include a search for gallstones, severe hyperlipidemia, toxins (L-asparaginase chemotherapy), anatomic abnormalities, cysts, and a positive family history. Treatment is supportive and individualized but Ranson's criteria are relatively useless and imaging does not correlate with severity. Pancreatic necrosis is uncommon and infected pancreatic necrosis requiring intervention is exceedingly rare. If the patient is relatively stable, percutaneous drainage or laparoscopic debridement might be reasonable before embarking on a morbid and protracted course of serial surgical resections.

Given enough time, pancreatic pseudocysts almost always eventually resolve spontaneously. Indications for intervention include persistent symptoms or a cyst that persists for more than 6 weeks. Radiology-guided percutaneous drainage and placement of internal stents is gaining in popularity and seems to work in many cases. When indicated, surgical therapy should be performed using a minimally invasive approach whenever possible. Chronic pancreatitis with a dilated pancreatic duct responds well to Roux-en-Y pancreatico-jejunostomy (Puestow procedure) but the drainage should be extended to include the head of the pancreas (Frey procedure).

Pancreatic tumors include not only endocrine tumors such as insulinoma and gastrinoma but also pancreatoblastoma, solid-cystic papillary tumor, inflammatory myofibroblastic tumor, and sarcoma. The treatment is primarily surgical but should be coordinated with an experienced pediatric oncologist. The operations are the same as those used in adults, namely distal pancreatectomy for lesions in the body or tail and Whipple procedure for lesions in the head of the pancreas. These are very rarely performed but very well tolerated in children. Aggressive attempts to balance negative margins and normal function of adjacent organs should be made. Nevertheless, depending on the tumor type, recurrence and a poor prognosis are relatively common.

Preoperative Preparation

- ☐ Intravenous fluid resuscitation
- ☐ Parenteral nutrition
- ☐ Resolution of acute pancreatitis

Diagnostic Studies

- – Abdominal MRI
- – Abdominal CT scan
- – Ultrasonography
- – MRCP
- – ERCP

Technical Points

- It is unnecessary and potentially dangerous to disturb the pancreas in the case of duodenal atresia with annular pancreas.
- A Puestow procedure is for chronic pancreatitis and allows drainage of an enlarged and chronically obstructed pancreatic duct by way of a Roux-en-Y panreatico-jejunostomy.
- Pancreatic pseudocysts that do not resolve spontaneously should be drained by creating an anastomosis between the wall of the pseudocyst and an adjacent hollow viscus, namely stomach, duodenum, or jejunum, depending on which organ the cyst has adhered to.
- Intra-operative exploration for an islet cell tumor should be systematic and thorough, with mobilization of the spleen and body of the pancreas to allow for bimanual palpation.
- Intra-operative ultrasound is useful for the localization of islet-cell tumors.
- Pancreatic necrosis can be treated non-operatively except when they become infected, in which case surgical debridement and drainage are required.
- Large closed-suction drains should be used in all procedures in which the pancreatic duct is entered.

Suggested Reading

Callender GG, Rich TA, Perrier ND. Multiple endocrine neoplasia syndromes. Surg Clin North Am. 2008;88(4):863–95.

Johnson PR, Spitz L. Cyst and tumors of the pancreas. Semin Pediatr Surg. 2000;9(4):209–15.

Miyano T. The pancreas. In: Grosfeld JL, O'Neill JA, Fonkalsrud EW, Coran AG, editors. Pediatric surgery. 6th ed. Philadelphia: Elsevier; 2006.

Nijs E, Callahan MJ, Taylor GA. Disorders of the pediatric pancreas: imaging features. Pediatr Radiol. 2005;35(4):358–73.

Schwartz MZ. Unusual peptide-secreting tumors in adolescents and children. Semin Pediatr Surg. 1997;6(3):141–6.

Stringer MD. Pancreatitis and pancreatic trauma. Semin Pediatr Surg. 2005;14(4):239–46.

Chapter 81
Disorders of the Spleen

Melissa E. Danko and Henry E. Rice

Knowledge of the unique splenic anatomy is essential to guide surgical therapy. The spleen develops within the dorsal mesogastrium during the fifth week of gestation and is located in the left upper quadrant of the abdomen. It abuts the diaphragm superiorly, posteriorly, and laterally. The visceral relationships of the spleen include the left kidney, splenic flexure of the colon, stomach, and tail of the pancreas. The splenic capsule is covered by parietal peritoneum, except at the splenic hilum, and the peritoneum forms its suspensory ligaments.

The main arterial supply of the spleen is from the splenic artery, with accessory flow from both the gastroepiploic and short gastric arcades. Before entering the splenic hilum, the splenic artery divides into numerous branches within the splenorenal ligament. Two variations of splenic vasculature have been described that are important to recognize during splenectomy. In the *magistral pattern*, the artery and vein form a single pedicle that enters the hilum. In the *distributed pattern*, multiple arterial branches arise from the main trunk about 2–3 cm before reaching the hilum.

As small arteriolar branches divide in the spleen, their adventitial layer is replaced by a sheath of lymphatic tissue composed of T cells with embedded B cell germinal centers (white pulp). The marginal zone is between the white and red pulp and is rich in dendritic cells. When arterioles lose their sheath of lymphatic tissue, they cross the marginal zone and enter the red pulp, which is a skeleton of reticular cells, macrophages, endothelial passages and splenic sinuses. Venous sinusoids drain into veins which travel along trabecular veins that empty into major tributaries that join to form the splenic vein. The splenic vein lies inferior to the artery and posterior to the pancreatic tail in the splenorenal ligament. Behind the neck of the pancreas, the splenic vein joins the superior mesenteric vein to form the portal vein.

The spleen's unique circulatory system enables it to perform several critical filtering functions. The majority of the blood flow enters the macrophage-lined reticular network of the red pulp and flows back into the venous circulation via venous sinuses, labeled the "open" system. In this pathway, formed blood elements are required to pass through small slits in the lining of the venous sinuses or they become entrapped and are engulfed by phagocytes. This mechanical filtration is one of the most important functions of the spleen, allowing it to clear circulating pathogens and remove damaged or abnormal cells. The spleen processes immature red blood cells and destroys deformed and aging RBCs. Functional or anatomical asplenia can be recognized by the presence of Howell-Jolly bodies (micronuclei or nuclear remnants).

Splenic Function and Considerations for Splenectomy

The spleen performs a range of varied immunologic functions which must be taken into account prior to consideration of any splenic surgery. Overwhelming post-splenectomy infection (OPSI) is the most significant complication following total splenectomy. Various hypotheses have been proposed to account for the increased infection risk in asplenic individuals, including lack of opsonins or marginal zone macrophages, altered T-cell function, impaired clearance by the reticuloendothelial system and loss of the mechanical filtration function of pathogens by the spleen. The spleen also plays a role in the antibody response to immunizations and is required for early antibody production after exposure to intravenous antigens. Asplenic patients do not have optimal response to new antigen exposure and may have decreased levels of IgM.

The most commonly used methods for assessing splenic immune function include the quantification of immunoglobulin levels and observing specific antibody response to pneumococcal or other immunizations. These tests give a broad and relatively non-specific measure of an intact immune response. The gold standard for determining splenic phagocytic function is the liver-spleen radionucleotide scan. This study evaluates the ability of splenic macrophages to phagocytize [99m]technetium sulfur colloid. Uptake of radionuclide

M.E. Danko (✉)
Department of Surgery, Duke University Medical Center,
Durham, NC, USA
e-mail: danko004@mc.duke.edu

P. Mattei (ed.), *Fundamentals of Pediatric Surgery*,
DOI 10.1007/978-1-4419-6643-8_81, © Springer Science+Business Media, LLC 2011

is interpreted as a demonstration of intact splenic phagocytic function. Use of this test in children is limited by concerns of radioactive exposure. Other measures of splenic phagocytic function are the observation of clearance of Howell-Jolly bodies (micronuclei) or the quantification of circulating erythrocytic vesicles (pit count). Both of these tests are labor intensive and require special equipment. A newer technique of enumerating micronuclei has been described using flow cytometry. This method appears to correlate with splenic functional status and might offer a more sensitive measure of preserved splenic phagocytic function.

Recently a population of $IgM^{bright}IgD^{dull}CD22^+CD27^+$ human peripheral B cells or "IgM memory B cells" has been described that might offer a novel measure of splenic-specific immune function. Memory B cells are similar to the murine B-1a B cell subset producing both natural antibodies as well as antibodies against T-independent antigens such as pneumococcal polysaccharides. Memory B cells correspond to circulating splenic marginal zone B cells and are lacking in patients without a spleen. The absence of IgM memory B cells correlates with diminished serum anti-pneumococcal polysaccharide IgM antibody responses in splenectomized children.

The ability of memory B cells to protect against common childhood infections has been supported by the study of children with common variable immunodeficiency (CVID), a heterogeneous group of immune disorders characterized by the inability to mount protective antibody responses. Memory B cells are lacking in children with CVID, and this lack of memory B cells is associated with recurrent childhood infections from encapsulated bacteria. This model disease suggests that splenic preservation may have far-ranging implications not only for reducing the incidence of postsplenectomy sepsis but also for controlling many common childhood infections.

The removal of the spleen is required for many conditions, but total splenectomy places a patient at risk for a host of immune and other complications. In addition to concerns of OPSI, other potential risks of splenectomy include thrombosis and increased intravascular hemolysis, which may lead to long-term risks of hypertension, pulmonary hypertension and cardiovascular disease. All the risks of splenectomy must always be taken into account prior to surgery. Over the past decade, partial splenectomy has been increasingly used as an alternative to total splenectomy for children with many diseases, including various hemolytic anemias, trauma, and other conditions.

Hereditary Spherocytosis

Hereditary spherocytosis (HS) is a group of RBC membrane structure disorders and with an incidence of 1 in 5,000 is the most common cause of hemolytic anemia in North America. HS involves a defect or deficiency of one of the components of the erythrocyte cytoskeleton, such as alpha- or beta-spectrin, ankyrin, protein 3, or protein 4.2. The clinical features of HS include anemia, jaundice, and splenomegaly. Most children are either asymptomatic or minimally symptomatic. A peripheral blood smear will contain spherocytes with occasional nucleated RBCs and there will usually be signs of ongoing hemolysis, such as an elevated reticulocyte count and conjugated bilirubin. The definitive diagnostic test is the RBC osmotic fragility test.

For severely affected children with HS, the traditional surgical treatment has been total splenectomy. Splenectomy markedly decreases the rate of hemolysis, improves the hemoglobin levels, and has generally been considered curative for most children. Classic indications for total splenectomy include severe anemia and the need for multiple transfusions. In general, delay of the operation until after the fifth year of life has been recommended in the past, as young children are at the highest risk for postsplenectomy sepsis. Nevertheless, the use of partial splenectomy as a treatment for children with HS has become increasingly advocated by many surgeons and may allow surgical intervention at a younger age.

Other conditions associated with abnormal erythrocyte cell membrane include hereditary elliptocytosis, hereditary pyropoikilocytosis, and hereditary hydrocytosis. Splenectomy is indicated for most of these conditions if patients are affected by severe anemia. For all children with RBC membrane disorders, any consideration of splenectomy should be decided on a case-by-case basis, carefully weighing all risks and benefits.

Thalassemia

The thalassemias are caused by a defect in hemoglobin synthesis leading to accelerated hemolysis and splenic sequestration. Splenomegaly, transfusion requirements and splenic infarcts are the results of progressive splenic sequestration. The most common types of thalassemias are decreased or absent production of the beta-globin chains or alpha-globin polypeptides. Classic indications for total splenectomy in children with thalassemia are severe transfusion requirements or splenomegaly. We recommend careful consideration of individual symptoms and severity of disease, making the decision for surgical resection on a case-by-case basis in light of complications of splenectomy. In particular, splenectomy in children with thalassemia appears to be associated with complications associated with a hypercoagulable state, including portal vein and pulmonary vein thrombosis. This appears to be due to abnormal phospholipid endothelial cell membranes.

Sickle Cell Anemia

The sickle cell anemias are a group of disorders of abnormal hemoglobin synthesis. Seventy percent of the sickle cell anemia cases in the United States are homozygous sickle cell disease (HgbSS). A smaller number of children have HgbSC disease, which generally carries a less severe phenotype. Sickle cell disease is characterized by varying degrees of chronic hemolysis and vascular occlusion. The slow microcirculation of RBCs through the spleen permits polymerization of the sickle hemoglobin and leads to splenic infarction, which can occur as early as the first 3–6 months of life. Progressive splenic sequestration may eventually lead to functional asplenia. The early development of splenic dysfunction is especially critical, as bacterial infection is the leading cause of death in children with sickle cell disease.

The disease pattern for children with sickle cells disease is quite variable, and total splenectomy is indicated for children who have repeated or severe episodes of splenic sequestration, anemic crises or severe chronic hemolysis. Total splenectomy results in elimination of splenic sequestration and decreases transfusion requirements. Many children with sickle cell disease will also have gallstones, and consideration should be given to concomitant cholecystectomy performed at the time of splenectomy.

Erythrocyte Enzyme Deficiencies

The most common RBC enzyme disorders include pyruvate kinase (PK) deficiency and glucose-6-phosphatase dehydrogenase (G6PD) deficiency, both of which cause abnormal glucose metabolism and can result in hemolytic anemia. PK deficiency is an autosomal recessive disease that causes a decrease in RBC deformability. Severely affected children with PK deficiency may require total splenectomy. G6PD deficiency is an X-linked disease in individuals of Mediterranean, Middle Eastern and African descent that results in hemolytic anemia, particularly following exposure to specific drugs or chemicals. Splenectomy is rarely indicated in these patients.

Immune Thrombocytopenic Purpura

Immune thrombocytopenic purpura (ITP) is one of the most common bleeding disorders in childhood. For unclear reasons, these children acutely develop antibodies against a variety of platelet membrane receptors. These antibody-coated platelets become sequestered in the spleen and engulfed by phagocytes. Most cases of acute ITP have a limited course with appropriate medical therapy, including glucocorticoids, gamma-globin,

anti-D immunoglobin and newer agents like rituximab. Splenectomy is rarely required for children with acute ITP.

In contrast to acute ITP, chronic ITP is defined as a persistently low platelet count 6 months after initial diagnosis and occurs in about 15–20% of cases. Management depends on the severity of thrombocytopenia. Splenectomy is often recommended for patients with severe symptoms or a platelet count below 10,000–20,000. Total splenectomy results in a normal platelet count in about 70–80% of cases of severe chronic ITP, particularly in patients who have shown a previous response to medical therapy. Partial splenectomy is not an option for ITP or other immune-mediated conditions.

Splenic Abscess

Abscesses of the spleen are unusual and are often associated with previous trauma, systemic or local infections, immunosuppression or hemoglobinopathies. Patients often have fever and fatigue, as well as vomiting and left upper quadrant pain. Imaging with CT scan or ultrasound is often necessary to make the diagnosis. The most common pathogens isolated from a splenic abscess are *Staphylococcus* and *Streptococcus* species. Failure of medical treatment should lead to prompt total splenectomy, which is usually followed by rapid clinical improvement. Other options include partial splenectomy or percutaneous drainage, particularly in the case of a solitary thick-walled abscess.

Splenic Cyst

Splenic cysts are categorized into true cysts and pseudocysts. True cysts have an epithelial lining and are either parasitic or nonparasitic. The presence of symptoms is often related to size. Symptoms may include early satiety, upper abdominal fullness, left shoulder or chest pain or renal symptoms. Rarely, splenic cysts present with rupture, hemorrhage or infection. The diagnosis is confirmed by ultrasonography or CT scan. Parasitic cysts are found in areas with endemic hydatid disease, and cyst wall calcifications and daughter cysts are often seen on imaging. Although rare, it is prudent to exclude the possibility of hydatid disease before surgical treatment, due to risk of spillage of cyst contents. Pseudocysts comprise 70–80% of the nonparasitic cysts of the spleen, and a history of prior trauma is usually elicited from these patients. These cysts are unilocular, smooth, and thick-walled.

Operative intervention is indicated for symptomatic cysts or for cysts greater than 5 cm in diameter, as these cysts have an increased risk of rupture or hemorrhage. Surgical options include total or partial splenectomy as well as cyst wall resection. Parasitic cysts can be sterilized with 3% sodium chloride solution, alcohol, or 0.5% silver nitrate. We advocate partial splenectomy whenever technically feasible to allow for preservation of splenic function, but total splenectomy should be performed if the operation is technically difficult. Some surgeons suggest treatment with percutaneous drainage, although there is minimal data supporting the long-term efficacy of this approach.

Malignancy

Splenectomy as part of staging laparotomy for Hodgkin's disease was historically performed to evaluate the extent of disease below the diaphragm. The use of imaging such as CT and PET scan has virtually eliminated the need for staging laparotomy. This procedure is still indicated in the select patients with low clinical stages of disease (IA or IIA) with unclear radiographic staging, in whom pathologic staging would significantly influence treatment decisions. Staging laparotomy should include a thorough abdominal exploration, bilateral liver biopsies, splenectomy with hilar lymphadenectomy, retroperitoneal lymphadenectomy, iliac crest bone marrow biopsies and oophoropexy in premenopausal females.

Non-Hodgkin's lymphoma (NHL) is the most common primary splenic neoplasm, and NHL can develop as a secondary cancer after treatment for a primary neoplasm. Splenectomy can be important in the diagnosis and staging of older children and adults, but its role remains unclear in younger children. Patients with NHL isolated to the spleen may present with symptomatic hypersplenism and can be successfully treated by splenectomy. Splenectomy is indicated in patients with NHL if they experience symptoms of hypersplenism.

Vascular tumors, such as benign hemangiomas and malignant angiosarcomas, are the most common primary splenic neoplasms of childhood. Children often present with splenomegaly, hemolytic anemia, ascites, pleural effusions or splenic rupture. If malignant, these vascular tumors can be highly aggressive. Splenectomy can be performed as treatment or palliation.

Preoperative Preparation

Prior to elective total or partial splenectomy, children should be immunized against *Streptococcus pneumoniae*, *Haemophilus influenzae* type b, and *Neisseria meningitides*. If possible, vaccinations should be completed at least 2 weeks prior to surgery. Ideally, all children should receive an age-appropriate course of conjugated pneumococcal and meningococcal vaccine followed by their polysaccharide counterparts.

Children with sickle cell disease should receive preoperative intravenous fluid hydration to minimize the risk of perioperative sickling complications and some also require blood

transfusion. Preoperative hemoglobin is ideally 10–12 g/dL with a low Hgb S level. Patients with chronic ITP may require platelet transfusion prior to surgery, although platelet transfusions are much more effective following control of the splenic artery.

Partial Splenectomy

Given the risks of total splenectomy for many diseases, including congenital hemolytic anemias, trauma and splenic cysts, a partial splenectomy is increasingly considered a reasonable alternative. For children with congenital hemolytic anemias, the intent is to remove enough spleen to gain a desired hematological effect while preserving splenic function. For partial splenectomy, our goal is to remove 80–90% of splenic tissue. These practices are based on animal models that suggest that 20% of normal splenic mass will preserve the phagocytic response to *S. pneumoniae*.

The option of partial splenectomy is being used with increasing frequency, particularly in children with hereditary spherocytosis, for whom we and others have shown that partial splenectomy increases hemoglobin levels, prolongs red cell life-span, and preserves splenic function (Fig. 81.1). One concern cited for a partial splenectomy is that of regrowth of the splenic remnant and the potential for recurrent symptoms. In our experience, there is variable splenic regrowth after partial splenectomy as noted by sonographic measurement of splenic volume. However, splenic regrowth does not appear to be associated with recurrent hemolysis in children with hereditary spherocytosis.

Currently several centers throughout North American are enthusiastic supporters of partial splenectomy with HS, while others have not adopted this option at all, citing a lack of comparative clinical studies. These divergent opinions are based

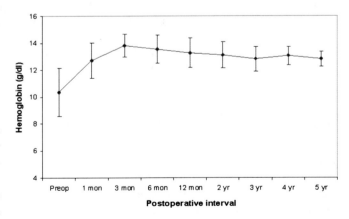

Fig. 81.1 Mean hemoglobin levels after partial splenectomy for most recent 12 children with hereditary spherocytosis undergoing partial splenectomy at Duke. Hemoglobin levels increased compared to preoperative values throughout 4–6 years of follow-up (*P* < 0.05 by paired Student *t* test). *Error bars* show standard deviation

on a decided lack of clinical information, suggesting that it is time for a critical analysis of partial splenectomy in children with HS. Our group is leading the development of the first multicenter prospective clinical study to compare total splenectomy with partial splenectomy for children with HS.

Surgical Technique

Whether total splenectomy is performed using an open or a minimal access technique is dependent on many factors, including surgeon experience and preference, the size of the spleen and underlying patient medical condition. For the patient with a normal or only mildly enlarged spleen, laparoscopic splenectomy is preferred by most pediatric surgeons. In cases of massive splenomegaly or severe splenic inflammation, open splenectomy via a left subcostal or midline abdominal incision is generally reliable and well-tolerated.

Laparoscopic Splenectomy

In experienced hands, laparoscopic splenectomy can be performed safely and effectively in almost all children. Laparoscopy results in a rapid postoperative recovery and shorter hospital stay than laparotomy, but it may entail longer operative time and increased costs. Relative contraindications for laparoscopic splenectomy include massive splenomegaly as well as significant medical comorbidity.

Our preference is to position the patient in a supine position, although others prefer a slight right lateral decubitus position. The patient is placed in slight reverse Trendelenburg position to allow gravity to assist the retraction of the viscera away from the left upper quadrant. A nasogastric tube is inserted and a urinary catheter should be considered for longer cases. Pneumatic compression stockings are applied. Both the surgeon and first assistant position themselves on the right of the patient. Pneumoperitoneum is established using either an open Hasson cannula or Veress needle, with carbon dioxide pressure maintained at 10–15 mmHg. We use four or five 5-mm ports and a 30° telescope, with one umbilical port, two upper midline ports, and a left upper quadrant port. The port placements are chosen carefully, as low insertion of the ports makes visualization of the splenic hilum during dissection more difficult. The left upper quadrant and umbilical ports are used as working access, and the upper midline and subxiphoid ports used for the camera lens and for retraction.

Meticulous exploration of the abdomen is performed, identifying any accessory spleens in the gastrosplenic ligament, splenocolic ligament, greater omentum, and splenophrenic ligament. Upon opening the gastrosplenic ligament, the splenic pedicle is inspected behind the tail of the pancreas. The dissection proceeds in five stages: (1) division of the splenocolic ligament, (2) ligation of the inferior polar vessels, (3) division of the short gastric vessels, (4) hilar control, and (5) division of the phrenic attachments of the spleen. We prefer using endoscopic bipolar electrocautery shears for the majority of the dissection. Gentle retraction of the inferior pole exposes the hilar groove, and the vascular distribution of the hilum is evaluated.

We ligate the splenic hilum with an endoscopic stapler in most cases. Once the hilum is controlled, the remaining short gastric vessels and the phrenic attachments are divided. The specimen is placed on its convex surface. The umbilical port is removed, and the spleen placed within a puncture-resistant large retrieval bag. The spleen can be removed *in toto* by extending the umbilical incision or can be morcellated with ring forceps and removed in large fragments. During all manipulations, caution is employed to avoid spillage of splenic fragments. The abdomen is inspected and all port sites are closed at the level of the fascia.

Partial Splenectomy

For use of partial splenectomy, preoperative work-up includes measurement of splenic size by ultrasonography. Splenic volume can be calculated using a formula for the volume of a prolate ellipsoid: volume (mL) = length (cm) × width (cm) × height (cm) × 0.52.

For immunoprophylaxis, children are prepared with appropriate immunizations to reduce the risk of postsplenectomy sepsis. In the absence of definitive data in regards to the preservation of splenic immune function following partial splenectomy, we encourage preparation as if each child is going to be functionally asplenic. In addition, intraoperative conversion from a partial splenectomy to total splenectomy may be required, and therefore preparation for total splenectomy is recommended.

For postoperative chemoprophylaxis, children receive oral penicillin or an appropriate alternative. In the absence of definitive data documenting the preservation of splenic immune function following partial splenectomy, we encourage treatment of all subjects with chemoprophylaxis following surgery. The duration of treatment will depend on the age and clinical status of the child.

Either laparoscopy or laparotomy is feasible for most cases of partial splenectomy, and the choice of approach is based on surgeon preference. For either approach, we partially devascularize the spleen to maintain flow either from the short gastric arcades to the upper pole or from the left gastroepiploic artery to the lower pole. The ischemic portion of the spleen is allowed to demarcate. Prior to splenic transection, the devascularized tissue can be compressed to essentially autotransfuse the blood back into the circulation. We transect the splenic parenchyma using a combination of an endoscopic stapling device and the bipolar electrocautery shears. Bleeding from the splenic bed

can be controlled with an argon-beam coagulator, suture ligation of vessels, or topical hemostatic agents. Children receive
standard postoperative care, and the length of postoperative
stay is generally 2–3 days. We restrict activities for 6 weeks to
minimize the risk of bleeding.

Splenic Cystectomy

A laparoscopic or open approach can be employed for resection of a splenic cyst. Once the splenic cyst is exposed, it can
be decompressed with drainage of the fluid via puncture and
introduction of a suction device. Epithelial and traumatic
cysts are excised using bipolar electrocautery shears or harmonic scalpel. A small margin of normal spleen must be
taken with the edge of the cyst. The raw splenic surface that
remains is treated with cautery and topical hemostatic agents.
Inadequate excision permits the edges to oppose and can
lead to recurrence.

Postoperative Complications

Overwhelming postsplenectomy sepsis is the most significant complication following total splenectomy. Concern for
this devastating event restricts the use of total splenectomy in
young children. The risk of OPSI is increased in children
compared to adults and might be as high as 20% for children
who undergo splenectomy before the age of five. Although
the risk of OPSI is reduced by appropriate immunizations
and long-term postoperative antibiotic prophylaxis, its risk is
never eliminated. Although young children are at highest
risk, it should be noted that older children and adults are at
increased risk of infection for life, especially given ongoing
concerns of incomplete protection by vaccinations, antibiotic
resistance, and poor compliance.

Physicians must be vigilant to recognize signs and symptoms of infection in patients with asplenia, as progression of
sepsis can be extremely rapid. OPSI usually begins with a
prodromal phase characterized by fever, chills, vomiting,
sore throat, myalgias, malaise, and diarrhea. Any suspicion
of sepsis should prompt hospital admission, blood cultures,
and immediate empiric treatment with intravenous antibiotics.
Rapid progression can lead to hypotension, respiratory distress, disseminated intravascular coagulation and death within
hours. Despite the use of broad-spectrum antibiotics and
intensive care, the mortality rate remains as high as 70%.
Complications from OPSI include osteomyelitis, deafness,
extremity gangrene, and bacterial endocarditis.

Following splenectomy, postoperative antibiotic chemoprophylaxis is recommended for all young children. We generally prescribe oral penicillin for at least 1 year for children
undergoing total or partial splenectomy, although concerns

persist with low compliance and breakthrough infections.
The appropriate duration of antibiotic prophylaxis is unclear.
Most young children continue chemoprophylaxis for several
years after splenectomy, with older children and teenagers
able to wean off prophylaxis therapy more quickly. The
greatest risk is in the immediate postoperative period, but
there have been reports of sepsis occurring many years after
splenectomy. In addition to vigilant surveillance, the physician should provide thorough patient and family education
including advocating wearing a medical bracelet.

In addition to decreased immune competence, splenectomy
may result in a number of other problems, including vascular
derangements. Following removal of the spleen, the main site
of extravascular hemolysis, there is an increase in intravascular hemolysis and free hemoglobin. This triggers deleterious
effects on vascular homeostasis mediated by nitric oxide (NO),
as endothelium-derived NO is scavenged by free hemoglobin
and incapable of diffusing into vascular smooth muscle. In
most conditions, the ability of hemoglobin to block NO is limited by compartmentalization of hemoglobin inside the erythrocyte. However, with increased intravascular free hemoglobin,
these homeostatic mechanisms are compromised.

An increase in intravascular hemolysis may contribute to
the development of hypertension, vascular thrombosis, pulmonary hypertension and cardiovascular disease. Hemoglobin
also exerts direct cytotoxic, inflammatory and pro-oxidant
effects that adversely affect endothelial function. Understanding the biology of increased intravascular hemolysis
following splenectomy is important from the broad perspective of public health and requires further study.

One increasingly recognized complication of total splenectomy is the development of thromboembolic events,
including portal vein thrombosis and deep vein thrombosis.
Clinically evident thrombosis may occur in up to 10% of
adults and children following total splenectomy, although
the true incidence of thrombosis may be much higher than is
clinically appreciated. Given the increasing recognition of
the risks of thrombosis following total splenectomy, the
option of partial splenectomy may be increasing employed
for children with various conditions.

Splenectomy is not an operation that should be entered into
lightly in the pediatric population. The spleen plays an important role in the filtering of erythrocytes and contributes to host
defenses. Patients with functional or surgical asplenia are at
risk for a variety of complications, including OPSI, increased
hemolysis, and arterial and venous thrombosis. However, for
severely affected children with various congenital anemias,
splenectomy can be curative and may be quite helpful. Total
splenectomy can be performed via laparotomy or laparoscopy;
the minimally invasive approach has been shown to have
decreased recovery time and shorter hospital stay. Some
groups advocate the use of partial splenectomy as an alternative for select patients, although the long-term efficacy of this
approach remains unclear and will require further study.

Summary Points

- The spleen plays an important role in mechanical filtration as well as the maintenance of host defenses.
- IgM memory cells in the peripheral blood may be a novel measure of splenic-specific immune function, and seem to be essential for the prevention of common childhood infections.
- Splenic phagocytic function can be measured using the liver-spleen radionucleotide scan, pit cell measurement, or micronuclei enumeration studies.
- Total splenectomy places patients at risk for overwhelming post-splenectomy sepsis (OPSI), increased rates of thrombosis, and increased intravascular hemolysis.
- Children should be prepared for elective splenectomy with immunizations against *Streptococcus pneumoniae*, *Haemophilus influenzae* type b, and *Neisseria meningitides*.
- Partial splenectomy is increasingly used as an alternative surgical option in children with congenital hemolytic anemias.
- Laparoscopic splenectomy has become the preferred approach for most pediatric surgeons, with faster postoperative recovery and shorter hospital stay.
- Children should receive postoperative antibiotic prophylaxis with oral penicillin for at least 1 year following splenectomy.

Editor's Comment

There is in this day and age almost never a valid excuse for performing an open splenectomy in a child as a planned procedure. The open incision is invariably large, painful, and potentially morbid, whereas the instrumentation and expertise to perform the procedure safely using the laparoscopic approach are widely available. The patient can be supine or slightly tilted with a bump. A line should be drawn where an open incision would be made should it become necessary to do so in a hurry. For reasons of exposure, postoperative comfort, and cosmesis, this incision should be transverse or oblique, rather than subcostal. Three or four ports are used, all 5 mm except for the umbilical port which should be a 10/12-mm port. For total splenectomy, I prefer to completely mobilize the spleen, leaving the hilum for last. The hilar vessels can be easily controlled with an endoscopic stapling device maneuvered through the umbilical incision, being careful not to transect the tail of the pancreas (which is actually generally well-tolerated). A 15-mm endo-bag device will fit through the periumbilical incision after removal of the port and slight enlargement by stretching with a large hemostat. A safe, effective, and inexpensive morcellator has yet to be developed; however morcellation by hand using curved sponge clamps and a large plastic Yankhauer suction tip works quite well.

Partial splenectomy can also be performed laparoscopically, but parents should be warned about the slightly higher risk of conversion to open. The upper-most short gastric vessels should be preserved until it is clear that suitable branches of the hilar vessels can been preserved. Division of the appropriate hilar vessels causes the spleen to demarcate. Transection of the splenic parenchyma is challenging and often rather daunting. The devascularized portion of the spleen is a reservoir for a large amount of blood and release of this blood while coming across the spleen can be difficult to distinguish from active bleeding.

Also, although the harmonic scalpel is probably the best energy source to use to come across the spleen, it is not perfect, and adjuncts, such as clips, electrocautery, fibrin sealants, or stapling devices, are often needed. The argon-beam coagulator can be used on the raw surface of the cut spleen with good effect.

The clearest and perhaps most common indication for partial splenectomy is the splenic cyst. Some surgeons have advocated partial excision of the cyst, using the argon-beam coagulator to "destroy the remaining epithelium" on the back wall that remains. This is impossible, of course, especially since the epithelial surface of the splenic cyst is usually trabeculated. The recurrence rate for cysts managed in this fashion approaches 100%. Partial splenectomy for hematologic conditions makes sense and certainly should be studied in a formal way to be certain that the recurrence rate is low and that splenic function can indeed be adequately preserved.

There are sometimes requests for splenectomy for unusual indications. The wandering spleen syndrome is presumably due to intermittent volvulus of the spleen because of inadequate peritoneal attachments. The diagnosis is suggested in patients with intermittent abdominal pain or by imaging studies that reveal a spleen with an unusual lie or tilted axis of orientation. The diagnosis is confirmed at laparoscopy and best treated by creating a peritoneal pocket within which the spleen can be placed and secured. Rarely, the pediatric surgeon will be asked to remove a spleen simply because it is too big, due to a perceived risk of traumatic or "spontaneous" rupture. This is a difficult predicament as there are no accepted parameters whereby the risk of rupture can be predicted simply on the basis of size of the spleen. Unless the spleen is truly massive, reassurance and the use of a spleen guard are probably the best recommendations. Pediatric surgeons are still sometimes asked to remove the spleen in the child with portal hypertension and secondary hypersplenism. The preferred management of these children is treatment directed at the underlying cause, namely portosystemic shunt or liver transplantation. Finally, we are occasionally asked to biopsy the spleen, which is not as difficult or dangerous as it sounds. It can be done safely as a core-needle biopsy under image guidance and with surgery "on standby," or laparoscopically with electrocautery or sutures used on the capsule to stop the bleeding after tru-cut needle biopsy.

Differential Diagnosis

Hematologic

- Hereditary spherocytosis
- Hereditary elliptocytosis
- Hereditary pyropoikilocytosis
- Hereditary hydrocytosis
- Thalassemia
- Sickle cell anemia
- Pyruvate kinase deficiency
- Glucose-6-phophatase dehydrogenase deficiency
- Immune thrombocytopenic purpura

Infection/trauma

- Splenic abscess
- Splenic cyst

Malignancy

- Hodgkin's disease
- Non-Hodgkin's lymphoma
- Vascular tumors

Diagnostic Studies

- Liver-spleen radionucleotide scan
- Pitted cell measurement
- Micronuclei enumeration
- Immunoglobulin levels and subtypes
- Lymphocyte subsets
- Peripheral blood smear
- Hgb, MCV, reticulocyte count
- Abdominal ultrasound
- CT scan

Preoperative Preparation

- ☐ Immunizations against *Streptococcus pneumoniae*, *Haemophilus influenzae* type b, and *Neisseria meningitides*.
- ☐ If patient has sickle cell disease, IV fluid hydration and blood transfusion to Hgb > 10–12 g/dL.
- ☐ If patient has chronic ITP, platelet transfusion to count >50,000 (although more effective when performed in the OR).

Parental Preparation

- – Major operation, risk of bleeding, sepsis, thrombosis, conversion to open, recurrence, asplenia.
- – Need for preoperative immunizations against *Streptococcus pneumoniae*, *Haemophilus influenzae* type b, and *Neisseria meningitides*.
- – Potential complications: bleeding, overwhelming post-splenectomy infection (OPSI), thrombosis, increased hemolysis.
- – Need for postoperative antibiotic prophylaxis for at least 1 year.
- – Following partial splenectomy, splenic regrowth is possible.

Technical Points

- Laparoscopic splenectomy is preferred in most cases with normal spleen size.
- Open splenectomy used in cases of massive splenomegaly or severe splenic inflammation.
- For partial splenectomy, we aim to remove 80–90% of splenic tissue.
- In a partial splenectomy, either the upper or lower pole of the spleen is devascularized, the ischemic portion demarcates, and is then removed following splenic transection.

Suggested Reading

American Academy of Pediatrics Committee on Infectious Diseases. Policy statement: recommendations for the prevention of pneumococcal infections, including the use of pneumococcal conjugate vaccine (Prevnar), pneumococcal polysaccharide vaccine, and antibiotic prophylaxis. Pediatrics. 2000;106:362–6.

Farah RA, Rogers ZR, Thompson WR, et al. Comparison of laparoscopic and open splenectomy in children with hematologic disorders. J Pediatr. 1997;131:41–6.

Price VE, Blanchette VS, Ford-Jones EL. The prevention and management of infections in children with asplenia or hyposplenia. Infect Dis Clin North Am. 2007;21:697–710.

Rescorla FJ, West KW, Engum SA, et al. Laparoscopic splenic procedures in children: experience in 231 children. Ann Surg. 2007;246:683–8.

Rice HE, Oldham KT, Hillery CA, Skinner MA, O'Hara SD, Ware RE. Clinical and hematological benefits of partial splenectomy for congenital hemolytic anemias in children. Ann Surg. 2003;237:281–8.

Chapter 82
Vesicoureteral Reflux

Pasquale Casale

Vesicoureteral reflux, the retrograde flow of urine from the bladder to the collecting system, is one of the most common indications for referral to a pediatric urologist. Most children can be managed expectantly; however some require an operation for disease that is severe or intractable. Reflux per se is thought to be harmless; however it can have serious sequelae, mostly related to recurrent urinary tract infections and permanent renal parenchymal injury. The goal of therapy is to mitigate the effects of UTI and prevent end-organ injury.

Reflux is prevented in the normal ureter by several factors that combine to achieve a functional one-way valve at the level of the ureterovesicular junction (UVJ). The ureter itself is a muscular structure that propels urine towards the bladder, generating up to 40 cmH_2O of pressure. The ureter also inserts into the bladder wall obliquely, such that a relatively long length of distal ureter is surrounded by detrusor muscle. Bladder distension and increased pressure thus effectively prevents flow from the bladder into the ureter. The ratio between this length of intramural ureter and its diameter, normally approximately 5–1, appears to be critical. Primary reflux occurs when the ureter has a large caliber or the intramural segment is short. Ureteral orifices that cannot coapt due to scarring from recurrent UTI can also allow reflux.

Secondary reflux occurs when bladder pressure is chronically or persistently elevated such that the ureter cannot empty properly. When bladder pressure exceeds 40 cmH_2O, the ureter cannot empty and becomes dilated, eventually causing the valve mechanism to fail. This is a common scenario in patients with bladder dysfunction (neurogenic bladder, spina bifida) but can also be due to anatomic abnormalities such as posterior ureteral valves in boys or ureteroceles in girls.

The incidence of reflux in healthy children is probably on the order of 1%, with girls out-numbering boys by about 5–1. The etiology is multifactorial and in many cases there is clearly a genetic predisposition. The incidence is higher in children with imperforate anus, some anomaly associations (VACTERL, CHARGE), and certain urologic anomalies, such as ureteral duplication, bladder diverticula, renal agenesis, and multicystic dysplastic kidneys.

Diagnosis

The diagnosis is usually suspected in the patient who presents with signs and symptoms of a urinary tract infection, one third to one half of whom will demonstrate reflux. The diagnosis is also increasingly recognized by prenatal ultrasound. Voiding cystourethrogram (VCUG) is the definitive test for reflux but some use renal US as a noninvasive screening study in susceptible individuals. Nuclear cystography is another noninvasive study that is increasingly accepted as a screening tool. It is especially useful for following patients with known reflux over time. A complete work up is indicated in children less than 5 years old with a documented UTI (sterile collection, >100,000 colony-forming units), any child with a febrile UTI, girls with recurrent UTIs, and boys with a UTI who are not sexually active and have no urologic history. Cystoscopy is still used by some in the evaluation of reflux but, except as part of a preoperative evaluation, its role is limited.

The severity of reflux is graded from I to V based on the degree of hydronephrosis on VCUG (Fig. 82.1): *grade I* – reflux of contrast into a non-dilated ureter only; *grade II* – reflux into the ureter, renal pelvis and calyces without dilation; *grade III* – reflux with mild–moderate dilation but minimal blunting of the calyceal fornices; *grade IV* – moderate dilation with tortuosity of the ureter; *grade V* – severe dilation of renal pelvis and calyces with loss of renal papillary impressions and gross ureteral tortuosity. In the past, VCUG was often delayed until after the UTI was fully treated for fear of worsening the infection or causing undue discomfort. These concerns are probably overstated and a delayed VCUG can occasionally miss the mild case of reflux that is worsened by a UTI.

P. Casale (✉)
Department of Urology, Children's Hospital of Philadelphia,
Philadelphia, PA 19104, USA
e-mail: casale@email.chop.edu

P. Mattei (ed.), *Fundamentals of Pediatric Surgery*,
DOI 10.1007/978-1-4419-6643-8_82, © Springer Science+Business Media, LLC 2011

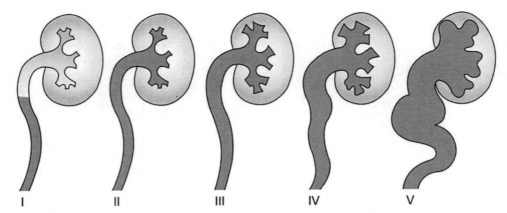

Fig. 82.1 International grading system of hydronephrosis based on VCUG results. *Grade I*: urine refluxes into the ureter. *Grade II*: urine refluxes into the ureter, renal pelvis and calyces, but the renal calyces are intact. *Grade III*: urine refluxes into the collecting system, the ureter and renal pelvis are mildly dilated, and the calyces are mildly blunted. *Grade IV*: urine backs up into the collecting system, the ureter and pelvis are moderately dilated, and the calyces are moderately blunted. *Grade V*: there is reflux into the ureter and collecting system, the pelvis is severely dilated, the ureter appears tortuous, and the calyces are severely blunted (from Gargollo PC, Diamond DA. Therapy Insight: what nephrologists need to know about primary vesicoureteral reflux. Nat Clin Pract Nephrol. 2007; 3:551–63. Reprinted with permission from MacMillan Publishers Ltd)

Treatment

With the possible exception of chronic and severe high pressure, sterile reflux is not thought to be harmful. Recurrent ascending infection, however, can cause renal scarring, progressive nephropathy, and eventually even hypertension or renal insufficiency. The incidence of nephropathy correlates with grade of reflux (I – 5%, V – 50%). Therefore, children with documented reflux are treated with low-dose antibiotic prophylaxis, usually with amoxicillin, trimethoprim-sulfamethoxazole or nitrofurantoin, and monitored with urine cultures every 3 months. Treating patient only when symptomatic or when a UTI has already developed is not effective in preventing renal scarring. Those with bladder dysfunction are treated with anticholinergics. It is also important to improve toilet hygiene and aggressively treat constipation.

Most reflux improves over time, especially in infants and young children, but the likelihood of spontaneous resolution depends on severity: approximately 85% in grades I, II or III, 25% in grade IV, and 10% in grade V. Medical management is initially recommended for asymptomatic children with low-grade (I–III) reflux. Many patients with grade IV – and even some infants with grade V – can be safely managed medically, at least until it is clear that spontaneous resolution is unlikely to occur. Repeat nuclear cystogram or VCUG is performed every 12–18 months. Antibiotic therapy can be stopped after the reflux has resolved.

Surgical Therapy

Indications for surgical intervention include: (1) children with severe reflux and evidence of nephropathy, (2) reflux that fails to resolve as the child approaches puberty, and (3) most adolescents with reflux. Parents should understand that UTIs might still occur even after successful operative repair but that the ultimate goal of the operation is to prevent pyelonephritis and nephropathy.

There are many operations described for the surgical treatment of reflux. All share the common goal of creating an effective on-way valve by increasing the intramural length of the distal ureter. Recurrent reflux is usually the result of an inadequate length-to-diameter ratio or unrecognized bladder dysfunction. It is also important to avoid excessive skeletonization of the ureter, preserving its blood supply, minimizing tissue handling, and creating gentle curves in the course of the ureter to prevent kinks and angulations. Fine, absorbable sutures are used and in most cases a ureteral stent is not necessary. The ureter that is significantly dilated should be surgically tapered so as to achieve the proper the length-to-diameter ratio.

The cross-trigonal (Cohen) technique is an intravesical approach that involves creation of a long submucosal tunnel and a new ureteral orifice situated across the posterior midline of the bladder. The ureteral advancement (Glenn-Anderson) technique is similar in that a submucosal tunnel is created, but the original hiatus is preserved. A very popular technique in the past, the Politano-Leadbetter technique involves blind creation of submucosal tunnel and a new hiatus positioned medial and inferior to the native hiatus. The extravesical (Lich-Gregoir) technique leaves the bladder intact, thus minimizing the incidence of postoperative bladder spasms and hematuria, but the more extensive dissection of the posterior aspect of the bladder raises concerns about the possibility of nerve injury and subsequent bladder dysfunction. The detrusor trough is created by incising the bladder wall, being careful to avoid mucosal tears, and preserving the native ureteral orifice.

Reflux can also be treated by cystoscopic injection of an inert material (silicone, collagen, autologous cartilage) behind the ureter, providing the backing necessary to cause coaptation when the bladder fills. The short-term results with this technique have been encouraging but long-term results are not known.

When surgery is indicated, there are two approaches: open and laparoscopic, involving either an extravesical or intravesical approach. For an open approach, a low transverse (Pfannenstiel) incision is typically utilized. With the laparoscopic approach using a transvesicle cross-trigonal ureteral reimplantation for VUR, the patient is placed in the dorsolithotomy position and the trocars are placed under cystoscopic guidance directly into the bladder. Ureteral catheters are placed during cystoscopic evaluation at the beginning of the case. Two 3-mm trocars are used for the working ports and a 5-mm trocar is used for the midline camera port housing a 5-mm/zero-degree laparoscope. Typical insufflation pressures are between 7 and 8 mmHg with flow rates between 12 and 15 mL/min to avoid bladder contractions. After the trocars are in place, the 8F pediatric feeding tube is left in place through the urethra and connected to a suction device. When suction is needed, the suction tubing is unclamped and manipulated with an instrument. The ureters are anchored with 4-0 absorbable sutures. Whether open or laparoscopic, bladder defects are closed with 3-0 absorbable sutures.

For a laparoscopic extravesical approach, a transperitoneal route is used with a 5-mm umbilical trocar for the camera and two 5-mm working ports, each lateral to the rectus sheath at the level of the anterior superior iliac spine. The peritoneal reflection is incised and the posterior aspect of the bladder visualized. Ureteral dissection should be kept distal to the uterine arteries. Care must be taken in each case to identify the pelvic plexus to avoiding injury in this area and allowing ureteral mobilization at the hiatus. A 3–4-cm long detrusor through is made on the posterior aspect of the bladder by incising the outer layers of the bladder wall, circumnavigating the ureter and leaving the mucosa intact. The detrusor muscle is then approximated over the distal ureter with 3-0 absorbable sutures.

Uretero-Pelvic Junction Obstruction

Open pyeloplasty remains the gold standard for ureteropelvic junction (UPJ) obstruction in the pediatric population. Historically, open pyeloplasty has been the standard treatment for congenital or acquired ureteropelvic junction obstruction in adults and children, with overall success rates of 90–100%. Although endopyelotomy and retrograde dilation are alternative methods of managing ureteropelvic junction obstruction in children, the success of these two procedures is inferior to that reported for conventional dismembered pyeloplasty. Laparoscopic pyeloplasty was introduced in adults in 1993 with initial reports having operative times ranging from 3 to 7 h, but the procedure has gradually gained acceptance with a current reported success rate of over 95%, equal to that achieved with the open approach. The indications for repair include: increasing hydronephrosis, progressive deterioration of renal function, recurrent urinary tract infection, and persistent pain.

Initial cystoscopy and ureteric stenting is left to the discretion of the surgeon. An indwelling Foley catheter is placed to gravity drainage. Positioning of the patient is crucial as it facilitates optimal ergonomics for the surgeon and increased access to the operative space. A flank incision between the tenth and eleventh ribs or an anterior muscle-splitting approach off the tenth rib is utilized for the open approach. For both the transperitoneal and retroperitoneal laparoscopic approach, the patient is placed in a lateral or semi-lateral decubitus position in close proximity to the posterior edge of the table, the table is flexed, the kidney rest is elevated, appropriate padding is applied, and the patient is secured with 2-in. adhesive tape and a safety belt.

An option for the retroperitoneal approach is a modified semi-prone position with the left flank up or a 45° right lateral decubitus position (for right-sided obstruction), to allow the subsequent ureteropelvic anastomosis using the right hand (for a right-handed surgeon). Another option utilized for the transperitoneal approach is to place the patient supine with a slight 30° table rotation of the ipsilateral side. The patient is then secured to the table with 2-in. tape. The table can then be rotated as needed after visualization of the intraperitoneal field. This approach can be utilized on the left side, allowing the colon to stay lateral to the left kidney so a transmesenteric window is unobstructed.

Trocar placement for the retroperitoneal approach is decided after a working space is created by gas insufflation dissection, and the first trocar fixed with a purse-string suture applied around the deep fascia to ensure an air-tight seal. A 5-mm trocar is inserted posteriorly near the costovertebral angle, while another 5-mm trocar is inserted 10 mm above the top of the iliac crest at the anterior axillary line. For the transperitoneal approach, the first 5-mm trocar is placed at the umbilicus, either trough a small open technique or after insufflation with a Veress needle. Another 5-mm trocar is inserted subcostally, lateral to the ipsilateral rectus muscle, while the last 5-mm trocar is inserted 10 mm above the top of the iliac crest lateral to the ipsilateral rectus muscle. A transmesenteric window is created if the UPJ obstruction is on the left kidney. If the UPJ obstruction is on the right, the colon is mobilized for optimal exposure. A fourth 3- or 5-mm port might be utilized, but since sutures and suction devices can be passed through one of the working ports, it is not always necessary.

The UPJ anastomosis begins with 6-0 absorbable sutures and a tapered 3/8 circular needle. The first suture is placed from the most dependent portion of the pelvis to the most inferior point or vertex of the ureteric spatulation. To facilitate laparoscopic suturing, two 6-0 undyed polydioxanone sutures, 6 cm in length, can be tied together; one is dyed using a surgical marker, thus eliminating a cumbersome step of tying intracorporeally. Once the ureter is approximated to the pelvis, the UPJ is maintained on traction and the suture line stabilized. All pyeloplasties performed for crossing vessel pathology involve transposing the UPJ anterior to the vessels. Once half of the anastomosis is accomplished, a 4.7 F polyurethane ureteral stent is inserted through the suture line to the bladder at the end of the anterior layer reconstruction. The preferred method for this in a laparoscopic approach is by percutaneous placement of a 16-gauge peripheral IV cannula; however the stent can also be inserted through the costovertebral trocar.

Postoperative Care

Immediate postoperative care is similar to that of other abdominal operations, with advancement of oral intake and activity levels when appropriate. Perivesical drains are removed when the drainage is minimal and a urine leak is excluded. Transient bladder dysfunction is common and usually due to trigonal edema and bladder spasms. The Foley catheter and externalized stents are removed on the fifth to seventh postoperative day. Renal US is performed 6–8 weeks after surgery to rule out hydronephrosis and a VCUG is obtained in 6 months to assess the quality of the repair. Prophylactic oral antibiotics are continued until the repair is deemed adequate. Patients are then followed clinically if the studies are satisfactory. Recurrent UTIs or new hydronephrosis should prompt a complete reevaluation.

The success rate for anti-reflux surgery in experienced hands should be greater than 95%. Persistent postoperative reflux is usually low grade and will resolve spontaneously over the course of a year. Reflux that persists or worsens is usually due to an inadequate submucosal length, failure to taper the dilated ureter, or unrecognized underlying bladder dysfunction. Reoperation should be considered when medical management fails.

Summary Points

- Most children with vesicoureteral reflux can be managed expectantly; however some require an operation for disease that is severe or intractable.
- Reflux per se is harmless; however it can have serious sequelae, mostly related to recurrent urinary tract infections and permanent renal parenchymal injury.
- The goal of therapy is to mitigate the effects of UTI and prevent end-organ injury.
- The incidence of reflux in healthy children is probably on the order of 1%, with girls out-numbering boys about 5–1.
- The etiology is multifactorial and in most cases there is clearly a genetic predisposition.

Editor's Comment

Vesicoureteral reflux is relatively common in otherwise healthy children. Unrecognized VUR is still a significant cause of hypertension, chronic renal insufficiency, and complications in adulthood, especially during pregnancy. Current screening practices are not systematic and rely mostly on the chance diagnosis of a UTI in childhood that prompts further evaluation. There remains controversy as to when a complete work up in a child with a UTI is necessary and even what constitutes a true UTI. Furthermore, the work up for VUR remains somewhat invasive, usually involving placement of a Foley catheter and a VCUG. These procedures are traumatic for children distressing for their parents. As a result, the diagnosis of UTI is often made on the basis of a clean-catch urine specimen, which of course is only useful if it is negative (a positive result could be due to contamination and must therefore be confirmed), and the extent of the work up in a child with a UTI is often simply a renal ultrasound, which is useful only in the rare case of high-grade reflux and some rare renal anomalies. The refinement of nuclear cystography has offers some hope of an accurate noninvasive test but the results thus far have been disappointing.

Most children with mild reflux can be observed as spontaneous resolution is common as they grow. Most practitioners recommend prophylactic low-dose antibiotics and systematic surveillance for UTI. The goal is prevention of ascending infection and this must be strongly emphasized to the child and the parents. There are several reasons for the high rate of loss to follow up in this population: the children are typically asymptomatic, which makes parents question the need for treatment; there is a growing and pervasive societal paranoia about the risks associated with taking antibiotics; and many parents mistakenly assume that simply treating a UTI when it becomes symptomatic is adequate to prevent complications of the disease.

Children who have received a renal transplant are at risk for reflux at the neoureterovesiculostomy. Most transplant surgeons use an extravesical approach to create a submucosal tunnel, which generally works quite well. A nipple-valve technique that involves eversion of the intravesical portion of the ureter has also been described but might be associated with a higher risk of distal ureteral ischemia and subsequent stenosis.

The surgical approach to refractory reflux has historically been associated with a huge incision and a vesicotomy. The extravesical approach might therefore be more appealing, however some feel that the results are inferior, the incision in the detrusor muscle causes excessive scarring, and the sometimes extensive dissection of the bladder increases the risk of nerve injury and bladder dysfunction. The development of an effective laparoscopic approach has therefore been a welcome advancement in the field. It is likely that a minimally invasive approach that combines minimal scarring, faster recovery, and excellent results will soon become the standard of care.

Differential Diagnosis

- Idiopathic primary VUR
- Neurogenic bladder
- Ureteral duplication
- Bladder diverticula
- Uretero-pelvic junction (UPJ) obstruction

Diagnostic Studies

- Renal ultrasound
- Voiding cystourethrogram (VCUG)
- Nuclear cystography
- Cystoscopy

Preoperative Preparation

- ☐ Antibiotic prophylaxis
- ☐ Assessment of bladder function
- ☐ Cystoscopic examination
- ☐ Informed consent

Parental Preparation

- The success of surgery for children with primary reflux is greater than 95%.
- There are risks of infection, bleeding, nerve injury, bladder spasms, and recurrent reflux.
- Urinary tract infections might still occur but the goal of the operation is to prevent ascending infection and kidney injury.

Technical Points

- The ratio between this length of intramural ureter and its diameter, normally approximately 5–1, is critical for creating an effective one-way valve.
- Indications for surgical intervention include: (1) children with severe reflux and evidence of nephropathy, (2) reflux that fails to resolve as the child approaches puberty, and (3) most adolescents with reflux.
- There are intravesical or extravesical and open or laparoscopic approaches available.
- The ureter must be mobilized carefully and handled gently to preserve its blood supply and prevent scarring and subsequent stricturing.

Suggested Reading

Bell LE, Mattoo TK. Update on childhood urinary tract infection and vesicoureteral reflux. Semin Nephrol. 2009;29(4):349–59.

Casale P, Patel RP, Kolon TF. Nerve sparing robotic extravesical ureteral reimplantation. J Urol. 2008;179(5):1987–90.

Kutikov A, Resnick M, Casale P. Laparoscopic pyeloplasty in the infant younger than 6 months – is it technically possible? J Urol. 2006; 175(4):1477–9.

Onen A. An alternative grading system to refine the criteria for severity of hydronephrosis and optimal treatment guidelines in neonates with primary UPJ-type hydronephrosis. J Pediatr Urol. 2007;3(3): 200–5.

Peters CA. Urinary tract obstruction in children. J Urol. 1995;154: 1874–84.

Wein AJ, Kavoussi LR, Novick AC, Partin AW, Peters CA, editors. Ectopic ureter, ureterocele, and other anomalies of the ureter. In: Campbell's Urology, 9th ed. Philadelphia, PA: Saunders; 2006. pp. 3397–413.

Chapter 83
Renal Abnormalities

Pierluigi Lelli-Chiesa and Gabriele Lisi

The urogenital tract is the most common site of congenital abnormalities. Ultrasonographic screening programs estimate that 3.2% of infants have a genito-urinary tract anomaly, and nearby half of these will require surgical procedures.

A basic knowledge of the normal embryological development of involved organs is essential to the understanding of these anomalies, their evaluation and treatment. The urinary tract develops from two segments: the nephric system and the vesico-urethral system. The nephric system passes through two major stages: the pronephros, which completely disappears, and the mesonephros. The latter undergoes degeneration, but its persisting ducts extend caudally to communicate with the anterior cloaca. At 4–5 weeks of gestational age, the ureteral bud develops from the distal end of the mesonephric duct, at its junction with the cloaca, to elongate cranially and to meet the nephrogenic cord of the metanephros. At this point, the ureteral bud begins to form the future renal pelvis, calyces and part of the collecting ducts, passing through several levels of branching. At the same time, the metanephrogenic cap begins to differentiate, while the kidney ascends cranially. The ascent is complete at the end of the eighth week. During its ascent, the kidney will rotate medially 90° (seventh to eighth weeks), and will receive blood supply from the neighboring vessels (initially the middle sacral artery, then the common iliac and inferior mesenteric arteries, then the aorta).

A spectrum of renal abnormalities derives from errors in the induction of the metanephric blastema from the ureteral bud: (1) *renal agenesis*; (2) *renal hypoplasia*; (3) *renal dysplasia* (containing undifferentiated tissue) and (4) *multicystic dysplastic kidney* (MCDK, dysplastic organ containing massive nonfunctioning cysts) (Table 83.1).

P. Lelli-Chiesa (✉)
Department of Pediatric Surgery, Gabriele d'Annunzio of Chieti-Pescara, Santo Spirito Hospital, Via Fonte Romana, 8, Pescara, 65124, Italy
e-mail: lelli@unich.it

Unilateral Renal Agenesis

Renal agenesis is the consequence of a failed induction of the metanephric blastema by the urethral bud. A number of mutations involved in induction of the renal mesenchyme (WT1), ureteric bud outgrowth from the mesonephric duct (RET, PAX2) or deletion of genes involved in nephrogenesis (HOX, retinoic acid receptor families) have been described in animal models of renal agenesis, but the genetics of human renal agenesis has not been entirely clarified.

The incidence of unilateral renal agenesis (URA) is reportedly between 1 in 1,000–1,500, with a slight male and left side predominance. The real incidence of URA is probably underestimated since isolated, non syndromic URA is usually asymptomatic. With the advent of fetal ultrasound screening, it is clear that a portion of congenital solitary kidneys are the result of a prenatal or postnatal regression of a MCDK rather than true renal agenesis.

Diagnosis

Screening ultrasound has become the most common diagnostic tool to suspect URA, but it can fail to detect a poorly functioning dysplastic kidney, ectopic organs or hypertrophied adrenal gland as alternative diagnosis to an aplastic kidney. Radionuclide scanning (DMSA or MAG-3) is the most sensitive study for identifying small, poorly functioning kidneys and those ectopically located, and is at present the method of choice to confirm the ultrasonographic suspicion of URA.

Unilateral renal agenesis is associated with ipsilateral ureteral and hemitrigonal absence in 50–87% of cases and partial ureteral development in the remaining. Abnormalities of the contralateral kidney are reported in half of cases (vesico-ureteral reflux, pelviureteric junction obstruction, megaureter, ureterovesical junction obstruction, malrotation, ectopia) and it is therefore mandatory to investigate their co-existence, in order to preserve renal function. We suggest

Table 83.1 Renal anomalies

Anomalies in number
  Supernumerary kidney (extremely rare)
  Unilateral renal agenesis
  Bilateral renal agenesis
Anomalies of rotation
  Incomplete (non rotation)
  Hyperrotation (hilus faces dorsal or lateral)
  Reverse rotation
Anomalies of ascent (renal ectopy)
  Sacral/pelvic
  Lumbar/iliac
  Thoracic
Anomalies of fusion
  Horseshoe kidney
  Crossed renal ectopia (with or without fusion, solitary, bilateral)
Multicystic dysplastic kidney

Renal cysts
Congenital
  Polycystic kidney disease
    Autosomic recessive or infantile type (ARPKD)
    Autosomic dominant or adult type (ADPKD)
  Syndromes associated with renal cysts
    von Hippel–Lindau disease
    Tuberous sclerosis
  Medullary cystic kidney disease-nephronophthisis complex
    Juvenile nephronophthisis
    Medullary sponge kidney
Acquired
  Simple cyst
  Multilocular cyst or cystic nephroma
  Acquired cystic kidney disease

routine VCUG in all new cases of URA, to rule out VUR. Alternatively, one can perform cystosonography (ultrasonographic voiding cystographic study), which, in experienced hands, is as sensitive and specific as VCUG, with the added benefit of avoiding unnecessary radiation exposure. Patients with VUR and normal renal function can be treated with UTI prophylaxis and monthly urinalysis and culture while awaiting for the reflux to spontaneously resolve. In the case of VUR with impaired renal function, we prefer a more aggressive approach including subureteral endoscopic injection of bulking agents or an antireflux operation.

Ipsilateral adrenal gland is absent in 8% of patients. Genital abnormalities are reported in 20–40% of patients, in both sexes. In female patients, unicornuate or bicornuate uterus are common, often with rudimentary or absent ipsilateral horn and fallopian tube. Duplex uterus associated with duplicated or septate vagina has been also reported. Not uncommon is vaginal agenesis or hypoplasia (Mayer-Rokitansky-Kuster-Hauser syndrome), necessitating vaginal reconstruction to achieve normal sexual function and associated in many cases with infertility. Most of these abnormalities are asymptomatic, but hydro-emetrocolpos can occur in the case of lower genital tract obstruction and the patient can

present with pelvic mass, pain or failure to menstruate at puberty. The high incidence of genital anomalies in girls warrants routine pelvic ultrasound or MRI in all girls with URA.

If imaging studies are not conclusive, we perform vaginoscopy to evaluate the size and anatomy of the vagina and cervix. In male patients with true URA, genitalia anomalies (absence of the ipsilateral vas deferens, seminal vesicle and ejaculatory duct, cyst of the seminal vesicle) approach an incidence of 50%, while agenesis of the testis is reported in up to 7% of cases. Conversely, in males with absence of the vas deferens the incidence of URA is low. Other congenital abnormalities associated with URA include those of the cardiovascular (30%), gastrointestinal (25%) and musculoskeletal (14%) systems. URA may also be associated with malformation of the anorectum and of the lower spine (caudal regression syndrome). This association and the higher incidence of wolffian duct anomalies in males and müllerian duct anomalies in females, suggests a possible regional defect to the posterior portion of the cloaca in some cases of RA.

Renal agenesis (unilateral or bilateral) is a feature of numerous syndromes, for example branchio-oto-renal syndrome, X-linked Kallmann's syndrome (olfactory bulb agenesis and infertility) and the Fraser syndrome (cryptophthalmos and syndactyly).

After nephrectomy, the remaining kidney hypertrophies (increased cells size) and the glomerular filtration rate approaches the level of normal excretory renal function (hyperfiltration). Interestingly, hypertrophic response has been demonstrated before birth. In term of functional prognosis, the patient with URA has been classically considered not at risk for future renal problems. However, recent animal models of prenatal unilateral nephrectomy showed the potentially adverse effect of the hyperfiltration of the remaining kidney on renal function (glomerulosclerosis and progressive renal damage). Case reports regarding children or adults with URA and proteinuria, hypertension and renal impairment have been described, but the relevance of these observations are far from conclusive and it is still unclear whether individuals with URA should be treated, either with drugs or dietary restriction.

Bilateral Renal Agenesis

Bilateral renal agenesis (BRA) is not compatible with extra-uterine life. Its incidence is reported to be 0.1–0.3 per 1,000 births. A familial tendency has been reported with a risk of recurrence in subsequent pregnancies of 2–5%. The total absence of intrauterine renal function accounts for the characteristics of Potter's sequence: severe oligohydramnios causing fetal compression, typical facies (prominent epicanthal fold extended onto the cheek, broad flattened nose, low set ears), bowed legs, and clubbed feet. The most significant consequence of oligohydramnios is severe pulmonary hypoplasia, manifest as a bell-shaped thorax (narrow at the top, broad at the bottom). Forty percent of infants with BRA are stillborn, the remainder die soon after birth as a consequence of respiratory failure. The poor prognosis of BRA is an indication for early termination of pregnancy. Prenatal ultrasonographic suspicion of BRA is based on severe oligohydramnios, absence of kidneys and non visualization of the bladder, the latter confirmed with serial ultrasound at a 2-h intervals and after administration of 10 mg of furosemide to the mother. As in URA, ureters are absent in 90%. In males, concomitant testicular absence is reported in 10%, not associated with vas agenesis: this finding suggests that BRA is not related to wolffian duct abnormalities. In females, the most commonly associated genital abnormalities are related to müllerian structures. Similar to URA, BRA is associated with gastrointestinal malformations (imperforate anus, malrotation) and increased incidence of spina bifida, thus suggesting a possible regional defect to the posterior portion of the cloaca as basis for BRA.

Multicystic Dysplastic Kidney

MCDK represents the most common renal cystic disease and a common renal anomaly but its management is still controversial, due to the lack of definitive long-term data on the natural history.

Macroscopically, the MCDK was first described by Schwartz in 1936. He reported that normal renal parenchyma was totally replaced by multiple fluid-filled noncommunicating cysts, varying in size, held together like a bunch of grapes, by loose connective tissue (classic type), with an atretic proximal ureter. Analysis of fluid showed a large amount of urea, indicating previous renal function. The blood supply was in the form of a typical renal pedicle but with small vessels or was totally absent. A rarer second type (hydronephrotic type), characterized by small peripheral cysts communicating with a large central cyst, not distinguishable from a massively dilated pelvis, was described by Felson and Cussen in 1975. These two variants seem to represent a spectrum of altered renal development. Microscopically, MCDK is characterized by architectural disorganization, with cysts lined by squamous or cuboidal epithelium. Cysts are separated by dysplastic renal tissue containing immature glomeruli, primitive tubules and metaplastic cartilage, but mature renal parenchyma may be found.

MCDK is commonly believed to share a common etiology with hydronephrosis. As evidenced by classical experimental model on fetal lambs, an early ureteral ligation would determine renal dysplasia, while a late obstruction would cause hydronephrosis in a morphologically normal kidney. An alternative hypothesis recently proposed is that there is an interruption of the induction of the metanephric blastema by the ascending ureteral bud. Altered induction would occur in a non-uniform manner, creating islands of dysplastic tissue amid normal developing renal tubules. Cyst expansion at a later fetal stage would cause compression of the normal surrounding renal tissue, resulting in loss of renal function at birth.

Diagnosis

In the past, the classical presentation of MCDK was a palpable mass in an asymptomatic newborns (1/3), a vomiting or anorexic child (1/3) or as an incidental finding during work-up for urinary tract infections or at autopsy (1/3). In adolescents or adults, MCDK has been associated with abdominal pain, mass, hematuria, UTI, and hypertension. Nowadays, routine prenatal US has made it possible to detect this anomaly earlier and to clarify its natural history. It represents the second most common renal abnormality detected antenatally, after hydronephrosis. Its incidence in prenatal screening programs varies from 1 in 4,300 to 1 in 2,400, depending on the gestational age. The cysts do not enlarge prenatally until the few functioning tubules produce urine and the 16th to 18th week of gestation is the earliest period to detect it. According to European and North American multicystic kidney registries, prenatal diagnosis is reported in 72–77% of cases. At ultrasound, the MCDK appears as multiple fluid-filled cysts of varying size, randomly arranged and not communicating, non-medial localization of larger cysts, and echodense stroma between adjacent cysts. It is important to differentiate MCDK from hydronephrosis, which is characterized by a reniform shape, a visible parenchyma surrounding a central cyst, and a glove-like pattern with calyces extending from a large central renal pelvis. Prenatal cyst shrinkage has been described.

The left side is more commonly affected and the anomaly has been described more frequently in males (56–73%). Postnatally, ultrasound is the most valid instrument to confirm the diagnosis and to differentiate MCDK from hydronephrosis. Intravenous pyelography (IVP) shows absent function of the kidney. Radionuclide scan is essential to evaluate renal function, with better results than intravenous pyelography and it is now the method of choice. In order to accurately differentiate MCDK from hydronephrosis, the [^{99}Tc]MAG-3 is preferred over the [^{99}Tc]DMSA because the tracer is only detectable in the presence of glomerular and/or tubular function and because it provides washout data.

MCDK is frequently associated with contralateral renal anomalies, particularly VUR (15–28%) of which 90% are low grade, UPJ obstruction, UVJ obstruction, ureteral ectopia, ureterocele and renal dysplasia. With only one functioning kidney, associated renal abnormalities are crucial for the prognosis. Large recent series of patients with MCDK and contralateral VUR found that spontaneous resolution in a relatively short period can be anticipated for most children. Furthermore, VUR is not considered a significant threat to the growth of the solitary renal unit in the first few years of life. Ipsilateral genital anomalies have been also reported. Other major associated anomalies involve cardiac, respiratory and gastrointestinal systems.

In absence of associated contralateral renal anomalies, the functional prognosis of unilateral MCDK is excellent. The contralateral anomalies must be sought and aggressively treated to preserve renal function. The available data from the US National MCDK Registry, have clarified its natural history: 50% decreased in size or were no longer detectable by ultrasound within 5 years (18% within the first 12 months of life), 35% showed no change in size, 15% grew in size. The size at presentation did not correlate with the likelihood of involution.

It remains unclear whether MCDK could be a source of UTI or pain in infancy. None of the patients in the US National Registry needed nephrectomy for abscess. The risk of UTI appears to be more associated with contralateral VUR. In practice, those complications are reported anecdotally and only in adults.

The role of MCDK in developing hypertension is controversial. The US National MCDK Registry reports very few cases of hypertension and a recent meta-analysis showed no greater risk of hypertension. The mechanism of hypertension in MCDK is not understood. Some have found increased renin expression, while others have shown a decrease in renin expression but pronounced local renin expression within arterioles and interstitial macrophages. Controversial is also the role of surgery in resolving hypertension. A recent meta-analysis found 31 cases of which half improved after nephrectomy, particularly under 12 years of age. Older patients are at risk for irreversible arteriolar changes secondary to long-standing hypertension.

The absence of renal tissue at functional radioisotopic evaluation does not preclude the presence of dysplastic tissue, increasing the risk of malignant degeneration. Neoplastic changes have been reported both in children (Wilms tumor, all reported cases under the age of 4 years) and in adults (renal cell carcinoma, transitional cell carcinoma), but none of the 660 children reported in the US national registry developed malignancies. Nodular renal blastema develops in 2–5%, compared to around 1% in normal kidneys, but the significance of this histological finding is unclear. It has been estimated that the progression rate of nodular blastema into Wilms tumor is about 1 in 100 cases, indicating that nearly 2,000 nephrectomies in MCDK would be needed to prevent one case of Wilms tumor. On the basis of the available literature, the incidence of renal tumors in MCDK is so sporadic that nephrectomy to extirpate dysplastic tissue is not indicated and it should be balanced against the risk of morbidity for nephrectomy or the risk of dying from anesthetic or surgical complications.

Nonoperative Treatment

On the basis of our incomplete understanding of the natural history of MCDK and of the real incidence of the above mentioned possible complications or malignant degeneration, the optimal therapeutic approach to this anomaly is still debated. Data from US and European registries are the basis for a rational therapeutic program (Fig. 83.1). Once confirmed postnatally, the first step is to identify contralateral abnormalities. Patients with hydronephrosis are given UTI prophylaxis and evaluated for vesico-ureteral reflux. We perform voiding cystosonography in all patients to rule out subclinical VUR. With regard to the MCDK, a nonoperative approach with periodic renal US is applicable in most cases. Particular attention must be paid to blood pressure monitoring, considered the poor understanding of the development of hypertension in MCDK.

Surgical Therapy

Few patients with MCDK will require nephrectomy, usually indicated for uncertain diagnosis, complications, a size increase that suggests the possibility of malignancy, or poor parental compliance with the medical regimen. The nephrectomy technique is also a matter of debate. Traditionally, the MCDK has been removed trough an extraperitoneal approach by an anterior muscle-splitting technique or a dorsal lumbotomy technique. Recently, minimally invasive approaches (transperitoneal, retroperitoneal) have been reported and are now the method of choice to remove a MCDK. The retroperitoneal approach has been proposed as alternative to laparoscopy, despite being technically more challenging in infants and children, mostly because it avoids violation of the peritoneal cavity and the risk of adhesions.

For the retroperitoneal approach (open or minimally invasive), no specific bowel preparation is necessary. For laparoscopic nephrectomy, an enema is given preoperatively.

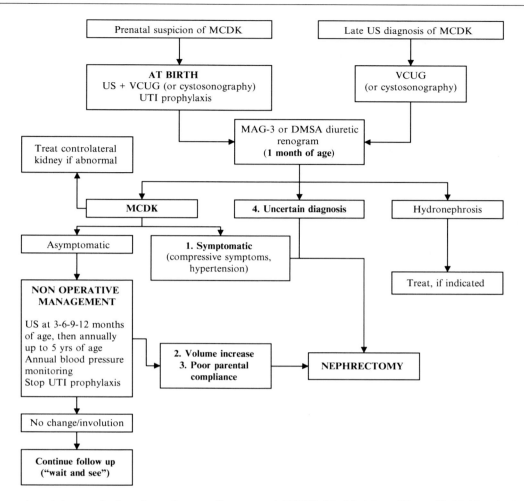

Fig. 83.1 Diagnostic and therapeutic flow-chart of antenatally suspected MCDK (Modified from Wiener JS. Multicystic dysplastic kidney. In Belman AB, King LR, Kramer SA, editors. Clinical pediatric urology. 4th ed. London: Taylor and Francis; 2002. p. 633–645)

Lateral Retroperitoneoscopic Nephrectomy

The patient is positioned laterally with a sand bag underneath the lumbar region in order to obtain a lumbar hyperflexion (wide space between the 12th rib and the iliac crest). The surgeon stands behind the patient, while the assistant stands at the left (renal phase) or at the right (ureteric phase) of the operating surgeon. The necessary instruments are: a cannula with a balloon to be inflated in order to avoid dislodgement during the procedures, a suction-irrigation device, harmonic scalpel, bipolar electrocautery device or clip applicator for the vascular pedicle. After palpating the anatomical landmarks (11th and 12th ribs, iliac crest, sacrospinal muscle), a small skin incision is made just below the 12th rib tip at the posterior axillary line (length of incision according to age, size, thickness of abdominal wall) and the first trocar is inserted with open technique.

With a muscle-splitting dissection (dissecting forceps, retractors, Metzenbaum scissors) the surgeon gains access to the retroperitoneal space, dividing the external oblique and internal oblique muscle. The dissection is concluded when the perirenal fat becomes visible. At this point, a gauze sponge is inserted into the retroperitoneum and manipulate carefully to create adequate working space, avoiding peritoneal perforation. The primary trocar (5 or 10 mm) is then secured to create retro-pneumoperitoneum (CO_2 insufflation, 8–10 mmHg for infants, 12–15 mmHg for children). After inserting the camera (0° or 30°), more space is created by moving the tip of the instrument. At the end of this phase, the anatomical landmarks (quadratus lumborum, psoas muscle, posterior aspect of kidney) must be clearly visible to the surgeon. Two additional ports (3 or 5 mm) are inserted under direct vision: a port is inserted posteriorly, in the costospinal angle, the second above the iliac crest (not too close to it, in order to avoid limited instrument mobility).

With atraumatic instruments, the Gerota's fascia is then widely opened, along the renal posterior aspect. At this point the anterior dissection of the kidney must be limited to avoid its ventral dropping and possible peritoneal injuries. Normally, during this phase, the insufflation is sufficient to push anteriorly the organ and to expose a posterior access to the hilum. Artery and vein appear as vertical in the inferior part of the operative field, but sometimes the surgeon can have difficulties in identifying the target. In this case the ureter, easy to discover in the retroperitoneal space may serve as a lead point to be followed upward up to the hilum. Once the vessels are controlled individually, hemostasis is controlled with the use of monopolar coagulation with hook for tiny vessels, while bipolar coagulation or harmonic scalpel is used for middle-sized vessels, and clips or extracorporeal ligature for large-size vessels. The artery is approached first. The remainder of the procedure involves the dissection of the renal poles, from cranial to caudal, then the anterior aspect of the organ is approach to completely free the kidney. Ureterectomy can be limited to the lumbar part and ligature is not necessary. The extraction of the specimen is preceded by the puncture of all or most of the cysts, and a retrieval bag is not necessary, unless the indication for nephrectomy is based on a possible malignant degeneration.

Polycystic Kidney

Polycystic kidney disease is bilateral, causing end stage renal disease in childhood. Two forms of polycystic kidney disease are described: *autosomic recessive* (ARPKD), which occurs with an incidence of 1:6,000–40,000, is associated with PKHD1 gene (6p21) mutation, usually becomes apparent in infancy, is characterized by small cysts (<2 cm) arising from the renal tubules tubule; and *autosomic dominant* (ADPKD), which occurs with an incidence of 1:200–1,000, is associated with PKD1, PKD2, or PKD3 mutations, usually becomes apparent in young adults, and is characterized by large cysts that involve the entire nephron. ADPKD represents the most common inherited kidney disease. Because of variability in age of presentation, the terms ARPKD and ADPKD are more precise than "infantile polycystic kidney disease" and "adult type polycystic kidney disease."

Both forms can be associated with extrarenal manifestations. ARPKD is a fibrocystic disease, characterized by nonobstructive fusiform dilatations of the renal collecting ducts resulting in enlarged spongiform kidneys and ductal plate malformation of the liver leading to congenital hepatic fibrosis/Caroli syndrome, evolving towards portal hypertension. ADPKD is a multi-organ system disease characterized by cysts in the kidneys, liver, pancreas, and ovaries, cerebral aneurysms, cardiovascular abnormalities and gastrointestinal diverticula.

Despite its rarity, ARPKD represents among the most important hereditary renal diseases. The gene PKHD1 codes for the protein fibrocystin, a hepatocyte growth factor receptor-like protein that functions on the primary cilia of renal and biliary epithelial cells. The most severe form of ARPKD/CHF involves two protein-truncating mutations, while milder forms of the disease typically have one or more missense mutations. Dysfunction of fibrocystin leads to abnormal ciliary signaling, which is normally required for regulation of proliferation and differentiation of renal and biliary epithelial cells.

The diagnosis of ARPKD can be made antenatally by ultrasound: enlarged, echogenic kidneys can be visualized beginning from the 13th weeks of gestation, oligohydramnios and absence of fetal bladder filling after the 20th week. Amniocentesis and direct genetic testing cannot yet offer an ARPKD diagnosis. The enlarged kidneys can complicate vaginal delivery. At birth, severely affected newborns can present the typical Potter facies or Potter syndrome. Ninety percent of cases are diagnosed at birth or infancy, with a mortality rate of 30–50%. Prognosis for those children who survive mechanical ventilation in the neonatal period is improving, with a 5-year survival rate of more than 80%. Individuals who survive often eventually develop portal hypertension and chronic renal failure. Although most infants presenting in the perinatal period ultimately require renal transplantation, the age at transplantation is very variable and can be occasionally delayed until adulthood. Severe systemic hypertension, often diagnosed at birth, is present in approximately 80% of patients. Children with ARPKD produce large amount of dilute urine, leading to the polyuria and polydipsia. Bed-wetting in school-aged children is not uncommon.

Simple Renal Cysts

A solitary simple renal cyst is not uncommonly identified by fetal ultrasonography, but the majority of lesions disappear before delivery. After birth, 0.3% of children have a residual cyst, while the percentage increases in adolescents and adults. A true simple cyst is a spherical lesion lined by a single-layer epithelium, with a content similar to urine. At ultrasound the cyst appears as anechoic mass with regular wall, usually located in the cortex of the upper pole of an asymptomatic patient with normal renal function. Cysts are usually stable in size (0.5–1 cm) and have a benign natural history. However, even in the case of a single cyst, a family history of ADPKD should be sought. Because of its typical location, the differential diagnosis includes a duplex collecting system with obstructed ureterocele or ectopic ureter and upper pole hydronephrosis. Large cysts (>4 cm) can cause infection, hypertension, or pain, in which case surgical therapy might be considered. Symptomatic cases or patients with atypical cysts (suggestive of malignancy) are candidates for a minimally invasive cyst marsupialisation or upper pole nephrectomy. Cyst aspiration is not indicated because of the high risk of recurrence, however sclerotherapy has been used with variable success.

Ectopic Kidney

The incidence of renal ectopy varies from 1 in 500 (autopsy studies) to 1 in 1,300 (clinical series), but the real incidence is probably underestimated. It is more common on the left. The ectopic kidney can be located in every station of the normal ascent: *sacral* or *pelvic* (opposite the sacrum and below the aortic bifurcation), *lumbar* or *iliac* (above the iliac crest but below the level of L2–3). Ectopic kidneys are usually also malrotated. In less than 5% of cases, an ectopic kidney can be found in a subdiaphragmatic position (*superior ectopic kidney*) or above the diaphragm (*thoracic kidney*), presumably due to an accelerated renal ascent prior to diaphragmatic closure or a delay in diaphragmatic development.

Renal ectopy is usually asymptomatic and is sometimes identified in children with a urinary tract infection. Symptomatic children present with vague abdominal pain related to compression of intestinal loops, renal colic (UPJ obstruction or stone formation) or palpable mass. Half also have contralateral kidney abnormalities (VUR 70%, renal agenesis 10%). Renal malrotation can cause UPJ obstruction or facilitate stone formation. Attention must be paid to the possible ultrasonographic evidence of dilatation of calyces, not related to UPJ obstruction but simply secondary to the associated malrotation. Genital anomalies are also common both in males (15%: hypospadias, undescended testis) and females (75%: vaginal duplication, bicornuate uterus, vaginal or uterine hypoplasia or agenesis).

Ultrasound is the initial imaging modality to identify and characterize an ectopic kidney. Radionuclide scan (DMSA) can more clearly show the abnormal renal position. Voiding cystourethrogram or voiding cystosonography should be performed routinely.

Renal ectopy can create problems when an operation is necessary to treat UPJ obstruction or stones because of malrotation and anomalous blood supply. The approach must be individualized. An open transabdominal approach to the UPJ might be necessary to relieve obstruction and ureterocalycostomy has been used as an alternative to pyeloplasty. Extracorporeal shock lithotripsy and endourological techniques have been described to treat stones.

Anomalies of Fusion

Two type of anomalies of fusion are described: *horseshoe kidney* and *crossed renal ectopia with fusion*. The first could result from an aberrant position of umbilical arteries during the kidney ascent from the pelvis to the lumbar region. Two different mechanisms have been proposed to explain the second type of fusion anomaly. According to the first theory, one kidney would advance slightly ahead of the contralateral organ and its lower pole would fuse together with the contralateral upper pole. Alternatively, a single nephrogenic blastema induced from the two ureteral buds, would determine both ureters crossing the midline. The fusion process occurs early in embryogenesis and is regularly accompanied by malrotation.

Horseshoe kidney is characterized by the two renal masses fused together in the midline. In 90% of cases, the lower poles are joined together with an isthmus crossing the midline consisting of fibrous tissue or renal parenchyma. The horseshoe kidney usually lies below the origin of inferior mesenteric artery, which limits renal ascent in utero. The incidence of horseshoe kidney varies from 1 in 400 to 1 in 1,800 and it is more common in males.

Patients with horseshoe kidney frequently have associated anomalies (78%) of the central nervous system, GI tract, bony skeleton, or cardiovascular system. The urinary system is also a frequent site of associated anomalies, particularly VUR, reported in up to 70% of cases. Other less frequent anomalies are ureteral duplication, MCDK, and ADPCK. Hypospadias and undescended testis are present in 4% of males; bicornuate uterus and septate vagina occur in 7% of females. Horseshoe kidney has also been described in association with trisomy 18 and Turner's syndrome.

Horseshoe kidney remain undiagnosed in nearly a third of cases throughout life and is asymptomatic in a large part of the remainders. When symptoms occur (vague abdominal pain), they are frequently related to hydronephrosis or renal stones. As in renal ectopy, hydronephrosis is related to UPJ obstruction from a high insertion of the ureter or aberrant crossing vessels.

Horseshoe kidney is also associated with an increased risk of renal malignancies, particularly hypernephromas arising from the isthmus and nephroblastoma. It is estimated that there is a sevenfold increased risk of Wilms tumor in patients with horseshoe kidney.

The main therapeutic problem in children with horseshoe kidney is related to the surgical approach in case of UPJ obstruction or stone formation, considering the associated malrotation and the anomalous blood supply. With regard to the treatment of hydronephrosis, an extraperitoneal flank approach is advisable for unilateral disease, an open transabdominal or laparoscopic approach for bilateral conditions. Standard pyeloplasty can be difficult, making ureterocalycostomy an excellent alternative. Isthmus division is not useful for relief of obstruction. Extracorporeal shock lithotripsy or endourological technique have been described to treat stones.

Summary Points

Renal agenesis

- Usually identified prenatally, but can be an incidental finding in older children.
- US is the initial imaging study but it can fail to differentiate agenesis from renal ectopia or dysplasia.
- DMSA scan is the definitive exam to confirm the diagnosis.
- Frequent association with contralateral renal anomalies and genitourinary malformations, particularly in females (perform routine VCUG, pelvic US, pelvic MRI, vaginoscopy).
- Good renal functional prognosis due to compensatory hypertrophy, unless severe contralateral disease.

MCDK

- Most common cystic renal disease.
- Prenatal diagnosis possible starting from the 16th to 18th week of gestation, but needs to be differentiated from hydronephrosis.
- Frequent association with anomalies of the contralateral kidney (VUR, hydronephrosis): perform routine US, VCUG, DMSA scan.
- Possible post-natal involution: some cases of suspected unilateral renal agenesis represents actually a former MCDK.
- MCDK usually asymptomatic, close US monitoring up to involution or stabilization, annual blood pressure monitoring lifelong.
- Possible symptoms (rare): respiratory or intestinal compression at birth, hypertension or UTI later in life.
- Possible malignant degeneration (exceptionally rare).
- Consider nephrectomy in: symptomatic patients, increasing size by serial US, poor compliance with conservative management.

PCK disease

Autosomic recessive (ARPKD)

- 1:6,000–40,000
- PKHD1 gene (6p21) mutation
- Diagnosed in infancy
- Characterized by small cysts (<2 cm) arising from the renal tubules
- Neonatal death in 50% of cases (pulmonary hypoplasia secondary to oligohydramnios)
- For survivors beyond the neonatal period: progressive development of renal hypertension and chronic renal failure and hepatic fibrosis leading to portal hypertension

Autosomic dominant (ADPKD)

- 1:200–1,000
- PKD1 (16p), PKD2 (4q), or PKD3 mutation
- Diagnosed in young adults
- Characterized by large cysts that involve the entire nephron

Editor's Comment

Renal anomalies are not uncommon and beyond their obvious significance in terms of renal function, they are important to understand when incidental to other conditions. Ectopic and horseshoe kidneys are susceptible to injury and need to be identified early in the course of a trauma evaluation. Tumors that arise within an ectopic kidney are generally straightforward to deal with while those that arise within a horseshoe kidney require careful planning and meticulous technique to avoid injury to the remaining renal parenchyma at the time of resection. Pelvic kidneys have been confused for tumors and impacted feces, rarely with deleterious results. When in doubt, abdominal ultrasound should be the first imaging study and usually settles the question easily and noninvasively.

Unilateral renal agenesis has obvious implications to the health of the patient and those at risk should be identified whenever possible. Boys with absence of the vas deferens and girls with unilateral vaginal anomalies should be screened for ipsilateral renal agenesis. As the vast majority of individuals with a solitary kidney are identified antenatally by ultrasound, it is becoming increasingly rare to encounter one incidentally in the course of another workup. Nevertheless, it is surprising how frequently patients and their families forget this important fact about their anatomy, placing the onus on the physician to be astute to this possibility.

Diagnostic Studies

- US of contralateral kidney and lower urinary tract
- Renal scan (DMSA or MAG-3)
- VCUG or cystosonography
- Pelvic US, ± pelvic MRI, ± vaginoscopy
- Serum creatinine, creatinine clearance, serum cystatin C
- Blood pressure monitoring lifelong

Preoperative Preparation

- ☐ Assess renal function
- ☐ Evaluate contralateral kidney

Parental Preparation

- No indication to termination of pregnancy (except in bilateral renal agenesis)
- Possible association with congenital anomalies of the remaining kidney
- Potential complications include compression of adjacent organs, hypertension, UTI
- US follow up to 5 years of life, blood monitoring lifelong

Technical Points (Retroperitoneoscopy)

- Size of incision adequate to patient's age, size, thickness of abdominal wall
- Create adequate working space in the retroperitoneum
- Look for anatomical landmarks while pushing the kidney upward
- Approach the vessels individually, starting with artery
- Mobilize the kidney, then extract the organ

Suggested Reading

Cambio AJ, Evans CP, Kurzrock EA. Non-surgical management of multicystic dysplastic kidney. BJU Int. 2008;101:804–8.

Corrao AM, Lisi G, Di Pasqua G, Guizzardi M, Marino N, Ballone E, et al. Serum cystatin C as a reliable marker of changes in glomerular filtration rate in children with urinary tract malformations. J Urol. 2006;175(1):303–9.

Felson B, Cussen LJ. The hydronephrotic type of unilateral congenital multicystic disease of the kidney. Semin Roentgenol. 1975;10(2): 113–23.

Merrot T, Lumenta DB, Tercier S, Morisson-Lacombes G, Guys JM, Alessandrini P. Multicystic dysplastic kidney with ipsilateral abnormalities of genitourinary tract: experience in children. Urology. 2006;67:603–7.

Miller DC, Rumohr JA, Dunn RL, Bloom DA, Park JM. What is the fate of the refluxing contralateral kidney in children with multicystic dysplastic kidney? J Urol. 2004;172:1630–4.

Miyazaki Y, Ichikawa I. Ontogeny of congenital anomalies of the kidney and urinary tract, CAKUT. Pediatr Int. 2003;45:598–604.

Narchi H. Risk of hypertension with multicystic kidney disease: a systematic review. Arch Dis Child. 2005;90:921–4.

Parrott TS, Skandalakis JE, Gray SW. The kidney and ureter. In: Skandalakis JE, Gray SW, editors. Embriology for surgeon. The embryological basis for the treatment of congenital anomalies. 2nd ed. Baltimore: Williams and Wilkins; 1994. p. 594–670.

Rabelo EA, Oliveira EA, Diniz JS, Silva JM, Filgueiras MT, Pezzuti IL, et al. Natural history of multicystic kidney conservatively managed: a prospective study. Pediatr Nephrol. 2004;19:1102–7.

Turkbey B, Ocak I, Daryanani K, et al. Autosomal recessive polycystic kidney disease and congenital hepatic fibrosis (ARPKD/CHF). Pediatr Radiol. 2009;39:100–11.

Chapter 84
Penile Anomalies and Circumcision

Douglas A. Canning

In the male, the genital tubercle gives rise to the two corporal bodies that elongate in the early part of gestation. As the genital tubercle elongates, the urethral groove forms that terminates in the urethral plate at the level of the glans. Urethral folds close between nine and 13 weeks of gestation and an in-growth of glandular surface epithelium occurs to complete the process. The process is completed by approximately 14 weeks gestational age.

Under the influence of fetal testosterone from the fetal testis, the penis elongates for the rest of gestation. The foreskin arises from paired genital folds, analogous to the labia minora in the female, that fuse to create a complete circumferential foreskin, the inner surface of which is adherent to the glans penis at the time of birth and remains that way in normal development. This close adherence of the prepuce to the glans gradually separates but can be associated with persistent filmy adhesions to adolescence in some boys.

Hidden Penis

Although subtly different, we consider the inconspicuous, concealed, hidden or webbed penis as minor variations of the same entity. All occur due to minor anomalies of the preputial ring. Specifically, the webbed penis represents an encroachment of the scrotal tissue onto the ventral portion of the penis. This condition results in considerable shortening of the ventral penile shaft skin compared with the dorsal skin. This can occur in two forms: (1) narrowing of the preputial ring proximal to the glans, resulting in a concealed penis, or (2) in the absence of preputial narrowing, resulting in a greater proportion of the penile shaft skin provided by

the inner preputial skin than the external preputial skin ("megaprepuce"). Both of these become important when considering circumcision. In these cases, circumcision performed with a Plastibell or a Gomco clamp results in excessive removal of penile shaft skin. If the circumcising incision is made along the narrow portion of the prepuce, a cicatrix will form that will "trap" the penis. This condition (trapped penis) results in a tight, firm preputial ring that requires surgical release with a rotational flap of the dorsal inner preputial skin to the ventrum of the penis.

These conditions are all relatively common. A number of successful surgical approaches address these conditions. Our preference is to harvest a flap of inner preputial skin on its vascular pedicle, transfer that pedicle to the ventrum of the penis, and suture it in place. In this way, the natural narrowing of the preputial ring is opened and the appropriate amount of residual shaft skin and inner preputial skin can then be removed to provide for good cosmesis (Fig. 84.1).

When any of these conditions are noted, it is important to refrain from newborn circumcision. Circumcision will not address the fundamental problem of proximal narrowing of the prepuce that all of these boys share.

Hypospadias

Hypospadias occurs in about 7 in 1,000 male births and may be associated with cryptorchidism and vesicoureteral reflux. Cryptorchidism occurs in up to 30% of patients with hypospadias and, when present, the surgeon needs to be wary of a coexistence of a disorder of sexual differentiation. Most hypospadias results from incomplete fusion of the paired urogenital folds. Incomplete fusion results in hypospadias with the meatus present anywhere along the ventral shaft from the perineum to the corona. More distal hypospadias results from abnormalities from the ingrowth of the glanular epithelium to meet the closing urogenital folds. Incomplete development of the penile shaft skin or corpora spongiosum results in variable ventral penile curvature, which in older textbooks is referred to as chordee.

D.A. Canning (✉)
Department of Surgery, Division of Urology, University of
Pennsylvania School of Medicine, Children's Hospital of Philadelphia,
34th Street and Civic Center Boulevard, 3rd Floor. Wood Center,
Philadelphia, PA 19104-4399, USA
e-mail: canning@email.chop.edu

P. Mattei (ed.), *Fundamentals of Pediatric Surgery*,
DOI 10.1007/978-1-4419-6643-8_84, © Springer Science+Business Media, LLC 2011

Fig. 84.1 Repair of concealed and trapped Penis. (**a**) preop AP view. (**b**) preop side view. (**c**) Preputial island flap mobilized from the dorsum of the penis. Vascular pedicle is button-holed and penile shaft brought through the hole to transfer pedicle to the ventrum. (**d**) Pedicle in place. (**e**) AP Postop appearance. (**f**) Side view of completed repair

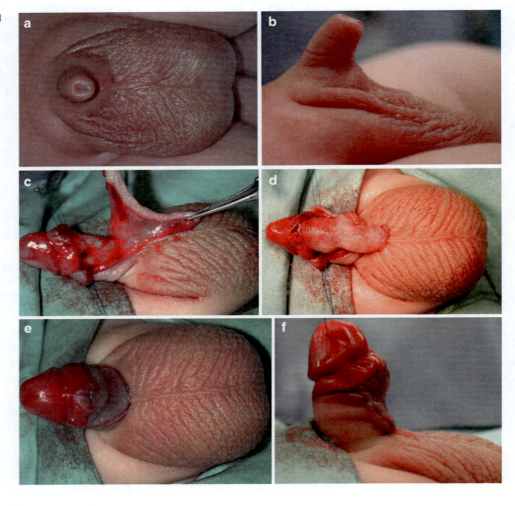

Most of the challenge in hypospadias occurs with the more proximal repairs. Of the distal repairs (distal shaft and coronal), our complication rate is about 15%. The complication rate for mid-shaft and more proximal hypospadias can be as high as 50%. Many of these repairs are associated with significant curvature, resulting in two-stage repairs at some institutions. A common distal hypospadias repairs is the tubularized incised plate (TIP) or Snodgrass repair (Fig. 84.2). More severe hypospadias repairs can be performed with a staged approach incorporating preputial or buccal mucosa grafts into the penile shaft after straightening the penis. Alternatively, a transverse island flap repair using an onlay technique (Fig. 84.3) or a rolled tube may be used (Fig. 84.4).

Surgical Technique

We operate on boys with hypospadias between age 3 months and 6 months, reserving the early surgeries for boys with severe hypospadias (Fig. 84.5). The technique varies with the severity of the defect. In general, we think of the procedure as three parts: (1) deglove the penis to assess the urethra and penile shaft, (2) straighten the penis and reconstruct the urethra, and (3) cover the penis with skin, usually rotated from the dorsal prepuce.

The first part of the operation involves placement of a holding suture into the glans penis. A circumcising incision is made skirting the urethral meatus on each side. The skin is then mobilized to the penoscrotal junction ventrally and to the penopubic junction dorsally. At this point, the spongiosal tissue and the condition of the urethra are evaluated. If the urethra appears thin with very little overlying spongiosal tissue, we cut the urethra back to the point where the spongiosal tissue becomes more normal in appearance. We then perform an artificial erection performed by placing a tourniquet at the base of the penis and injecting normal saline into one of the corpora. This helps us assess the curvature.

We then proceed to straighten the penis and reconstruct the urethra. If the ventrum of the penis is supple, we correct the curvature with a pair of longitudinal incisions on the dorsum of the penis that we close horizontally (Heineke-Mikulicz

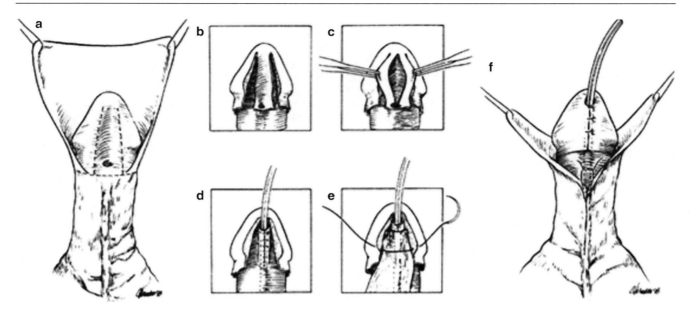

Fig. 84.2 Tubularized incised plate hypospadias repair. (**a**) Horizontal dotted line indicating circumscribing incision approximately 2 mm proximal to the meatus. *Vertical dotted lines* indicate the junction of the urethral plate to the glans wings. (**b**) Urethral plate is separated from the glans wings, which are then mobilized laterally. (**c**) The key step of the operation is a deep, midline incision into the urethral plate extending from within the meatus to its distal margin, but not continuing into the glans apex. (**d**) The plate is tubularized over a small stent leaving a generous, oval meatus. (**e**) The neourethra is covered by a dartos flap, and then glansplasty begins at the coronal margin. (**f**) Glans wings, mucosal collar, and ventral shaft skin are closed. (From Snodgrass W. Tubularized incised plate hypospadias repair: indications, technique, and complications. Urology 1999;54:6)

incisions). We place the sutures on either side of the midline or in the midline. We then repeat the artificial erection to see the effect of the plicating sutures. If there is residual ventral curvature, we incise the urethral plate and free it from the corporal bodies on the ventrum. This allows for near complete straightening and reduces the resistance to straightening when the plicating sutures are placed distally. In rare cases, we open the corpora horizontally to provide additional ventral length. Patches of dermal tissue or commercially available acellular collagen matrix can be used to provide additional lengthening. In cases where the urethral plate is supple enough to maintain as a template, we use the TIP repair or the onlay island flap repair. If the urethral plate needs to be removed, the repair can be staged by mobilizing dartos tissue and skin along the dorsum of the penis. We rotate these flaps to the ventrum of the penis and suture them in place. Alternatively, we have taken an island pedicle of dorsal preputial tissue and brought it to the ventrum by button-holing the pedicle to provide the template for the urethra to be closed at a second stage. If there is very little penile shaft skin present, a segment of buccal mucosa taken from the lip or the cheek and transferred as a free graft can be substituted for the urethra. A final option is a one-stage reconstruction using the preputial tissue that we roll in situ into a tube along the ventrum of the penis (Fig. 84.4).

Finally, we take advantage of the fact that most parents of boys born in North America prefer the boy to look circumcised

following hypospadias repair. In all but very few boys, there is ample dorsal prepuce available to cover the ventral penile shaft. The redundant dorsal skin is opened in the midline, transferred to the ventral penile shaft, and trimmed appropriately to provide for a pleasing appearance. In some cases, Z-plasties can be used to provide additional ventral penile shaft coverage (Fig. 84.6).

A myriad of dressings have been used following hypospadias repair. Dressings and stents are left for variable amounts of time depending on the severity of the defect and the type of repair selected.

In some cases, there is obvious penile curvature but the urethral meatus is at the tip of the penis and the urethra appears to be normal with relatively good spongiosal covering. In this case, rotation of the skin from the dorsum to the ventrum of the penis may be all that is required to straighten it. In other cases, rotation of skin with Heineke-Mikulicz incisions is necessary. In rare cases, curvature cannot be adequated corrected without release and repair of the urethra.

Complications

Most complications from hypospadias repair stem from one of two problems: inadequate blood supply to the reconstructed

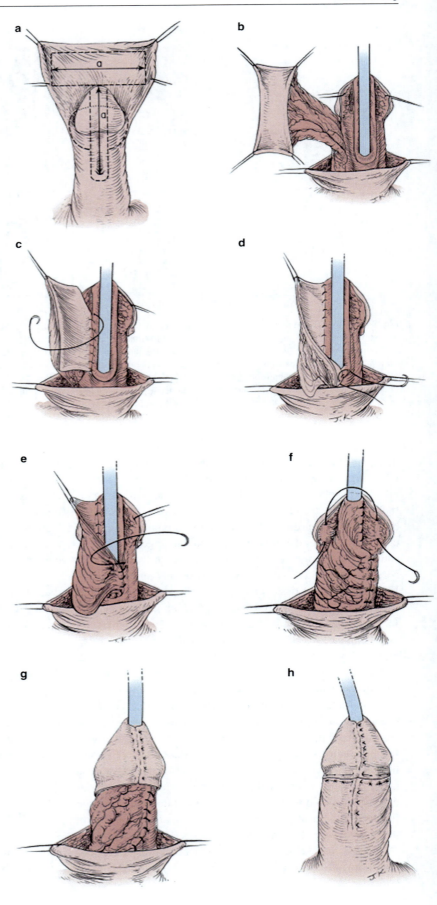

Fig. 84.3 Onlay island flap repair. (**a**) Proposed incisions for urethral plate and preputial skin onlay. (**b**) Pedicled preputial skin onlay with stay sutures. (**c**) Initial full-thickness suture approximation of onlay flap and urethral plate. (**d**) Approximation at proximal extent. (**e**) Completion of anastomosis with running subcuticular technique. (**f**) Inferolateral border of onlay pedicle has been advanced as a second layer coverage of proximal and longitudinal suture lines. (**g**) Approximated glans. (**h**) Completed repair. (Reprinted with permission from Atala A, Retik AB. Hypospadias. In: Libertino JA, editor. Reconstructive urologic surgery, 3rd ed. St. Louis: Mosby-Year Book; 1998, p. 467 Copyright 2007 by Saunders, an imprint of Elsevier, Inc.)

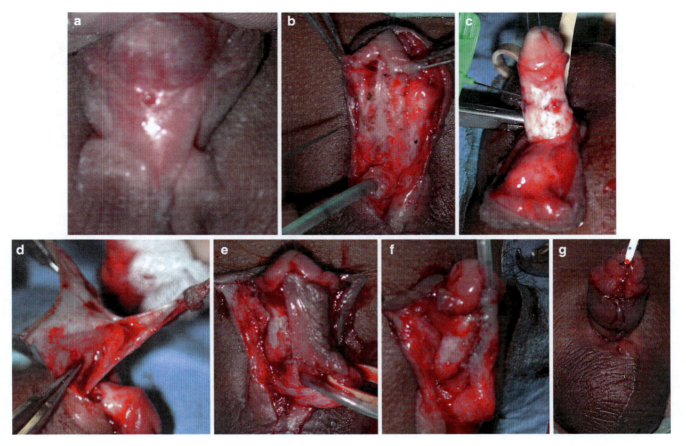

Fig. 84.4 Island tube hypospadias repair. (**a**) Preoperative appearance. Note shiny ventral tissue. This appearance suggests thinning of the ventral spongiosum and likely curvature. (**b**) Release of urethral plate with urethral meatus cannulated with feeding tube. (**c**) Artificial erection following placating sutures dorsally documents penile straightening after correction of curvature. (**d**) Dissection of dorsal preputial island flap from dorsal penile skin. (**e**) One suture line completed on midline. (**f**) Second suture line. (**g**) Completed repair

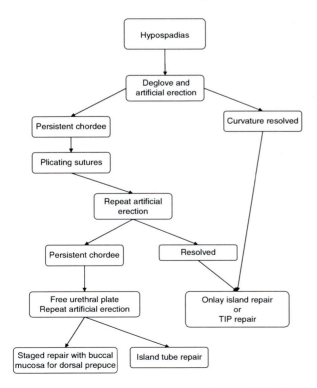

Fig. 84.5 The CHOP approach to hypospadias repair. We find this algorithm useful for intra-operative decision making

tissue, resulting in stricture or fistula, or irregularities of the circumference of the reconstructed urethra, resulting in strictures (Fig. 84.7) that subsequently result in disruption of the normal laminar flow of the voiding stream. The turbulent flow tends to create diverticula. Meatal stenosis is a narrowing of the urethral outlet at the meatus and is relatively common following hypospadias repair. Meatal stenosis often results in sprayed or diverted urinary stream with a flattened voiding curve. Nearly all of these conditions require repeat surgery. The concepts of redo surgery are similar to those of the original surgery, but extreme care must be taken to preserve the blood supply of the already compromised tissues.

We have tried to treat boys who have developed meatal stenosis the immediate postoperative period with urethral dilation. Our experience, however, is that dilation is poorly tolerated and rarely results in a good long-term outcome. In most cases, new tissue must be imported to the area of the narrowing. This tissue can come in the form of a dorsal preputial flap that we have harvested even if the first repair included a dorsal flap. Alternatively, we have taken an adjacent tissue flap taken from redundant ventral skin or an advancement of adequate tissue from the distal urethra into the glans. The postoperative care is essentially the same although sometimes we omit the use of a catheter or use it for a shorter period.

Fig. 84.6 Z-plasty closure to
provide ventral penile length.
(**a**) Penile shaft with compromised
skin fit. (**b**) Closed shaft with
Z-plasty to provide ventral length

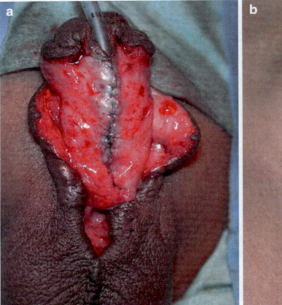
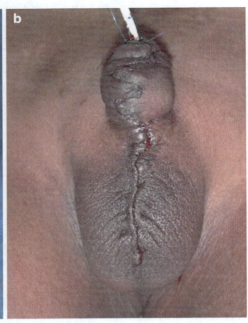

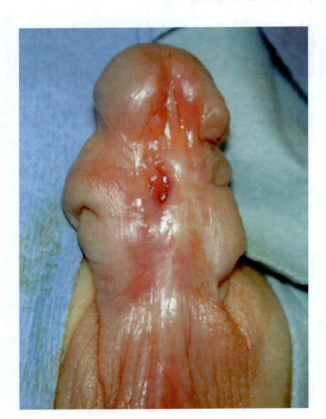

Fig. 84.7 Stricture following hypospadias repair. Distal urethra is
completely closed with obvious proximal fistula

Fistulas following hypospadias repair occur anywhere
along the path of the neourethra. They can be large, resulting
in almost complete loss of the flap, or nearly microscopic.
Tiny fistulae can present many years following repair and are

sometimes intermittent due to clogging of the fistula tract
with cellular debris. As with all fistulas, the keys to successful correction are wide exposure, mobilization of the wound
edges, debridement back to normal-appearing tissue with
good blood supply, and closure in multiple layers. Urinary
diversion is usually used but is not always essential.

Diverticula of the urethra are also relatively common following proximal hypospadias repair, particularly when we
have used segments of the prepuce for reconstruction. These
require attention since they tend to enlarge as the child continues to void. Ultimately, there develops a fairly pronounced
ventral bulge that requires mobilization and reduction.
In many cases, a relatively narrowed area is present just proximal to the diverticulum. Distal narrowing can also be present, resulting in increased pressure during voiding. Surgical
correction includes exposing the diverticula, trimming it, and
correcting any narrowing.

Hypospadias repairs are among the most difficult challenges for reconstructive urologists and there are few things
more distressing than recurrent failure. Unfortunately, each
year a number of boys present who have had multiple hypospadias repairs without success. These children will often
require aggressive straightening of the penis and urethral
replacement with buccal grafts. The goals are to straighten
the penis for adequate sexual function later, reconstruction
of the urethra, and providing adequate skin coverage. The
buccal harvest generally works well for reconstruction of
the urethra, but even in cases where the buccal tissue has
been placed along the entire length of the penis, the skin can
be short, scarred or otherwise unsuitable for coverage. In
these cases, a number of techniques have been used, including tissue expansion or rotation of the ventral reconstructed

tissue into the scrotum. A second repair after the urethra has healed to bring the penis out of the scrotum can be helpful.

Megameatus Intact Prepuce

Although megameatus intact prepuce is commonly confused with hypospadias, this defect does not present with curvature (Fig. 84.8). Because the foreskin is intact, the lesion is not always obvious. The spongiosum is also normal and so a primary closure can frequently be completed with a simple second layer of adjacent dartos tissue. The urethra, usually wide open to the level of the corona, is easily closed and the blood supply is generally excellent.

Congenital Penile Curvature

Boys with congenital penile curvature usually have relatively normal or even larger than normal penile length. The curvature is sometimes ventral but can be lateral, dorsal or even in the form of a spiral. This curvature is addressed with Heineke-Mikulicz incisions on the convex aspect, which usually provides excellent straightening. There is generally no problem with coverage since the penile skin is otherwise normal.

Preputial Glanular Adhesions

The glans penis is naturally covered with preputial tissue in uncircumcised boys, which often persists into adolescence.

However, more than 90% of foreskins can be retracted by age 3 years and only a very few patients have persistent phimosis into adolescence. We do not recommend separation of the preputial glanular adhesions if they are filmy, since many times they simply recur and it is particularly uncomfortable to pull the foreskin back.

In rare cases, however, infection occurs beneath the foreskin, which we treat with an antibiotic ointment. Oral antibiotics are only rarely required. In these cases, the inflammatory process will sometimes hasten separation. In contradistinction to physiologic or filmy adhesions, bridging adhesions can occur following penile surgery. When these occur after circumcision or hypospadias repair, the raw cut edge of the prepuce grafts to the glans penis and forms a band of varying widths that requires incision (Fig. 84.9). These are easily addressed in the operating room, sometimes in conjunction with a repeat circumcision. If the bridging adhesion is narrow, resection can be performed in the clinic if the boy and his parents are accepting. In this case, we apply an anesthetic cream, which will provide enough topical anesthesia to allow for an injection of lidocaine, which in turn will allow for a painless transection of the band following crushing of the skin with a hemostat.

Phimosis

In addition to the normal physiologic preputial glanular adhesions, scarring of the foreskin can occur from recurrent episodes of infection. When this occurs, the preputial ring itself becomes narrowed, sometimes resulting in recurrent infection and urinary spraying or ballooning of the foreskin during micturition. If this continues, resulting in true balanitis,

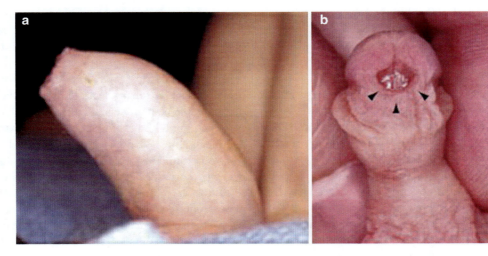

Fig. 84.8 Megameatus intact prepuce (MIP) variant of hypospadias. (**a**) Normal appearance of foreskin on lateral view. (**b**) Typical appearance of meatus *(arrowheads)* after newborn circumcision in a patient with the MIP variant. (From Borer JG, Retik AB. In: Wein AJ, Kavoussi LR, Novick AC, Partin AW, Peters CA, editors. Campbell-Walsh Urology. 9th ed. Philadelphia: Saunders; 2007; p. 3704, reprinted with permission.)

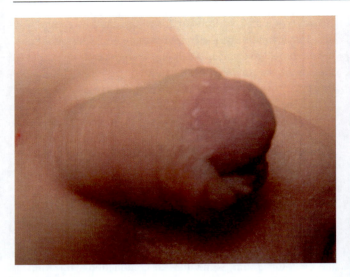

Fig. 84.9 Bridging preputial adhesions following circumcision. These adhesions along the dorsum of the glans can be incised and separated. Smegma frequently builds up beneath the adhesion in the space between the glans and the skin bridge

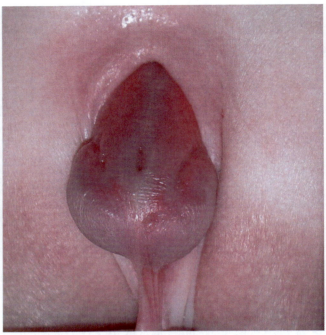

Fig. 84.10 Penopubic (complete) Epispadias. Note flattened glans with dimpling on dorsal urethral plate. Epispadias is usually associated with dorsal curvature

preputioplasty by circumcision or a ventral incision with a horizontal closure of the preputial ring may be required. In some cases, application of a corticosteroid cream three times a day for 2–3 weeks can be effective in thinning the preputial ring, resulting in resolution of the phimosis.

Epispadias

Epispadias presents most commonly as part of the classic bladder exstrophy complex that includes cloacal exstrophy, classic bladder exstrophy, and epispadias (Fig. 84.10). Epispadias is less common than classic bladder exstrophy, occurring in about 1 in 100,000 births. Boys with epispadias commonly present with the urethral plate exposed from the penopubic junction, pubic diastasis (less severe than that seen with classic bladder exstrophy), incontinence, dorsal penile curvature, and an open bladder neck.

We approach epispadias in a similar way to classic bladder exstrophy. We have a dedicated team of pediatric urologists, pediatric orthopedists, psychologists, and nurses who work together to ensure that these children optimize urinary and sexual function as they age. Because of the bladder neck defect that follows the pubic diastasis, all of these boys are incontinent. The degree of stress incontinence depends on the appearance of the bladder neck. Some degree of incontinence is present in nearly all boys and girls since the bladder neck is not completely formed even in children with distal epispadias. Along with the dorsal curvature that stems from the incomplete formation of the ventral urethral, there is

almost always vesicoureteral reflux present since the ureters enter the bladder from a relatively deep position in the pelvis. The bladder is usually a bit smaller than the age matched normal boys in part, we believe, because of the relatively open bladder neck that fails to stimulate growth and the resistance required for a combination in the bladder as it grows. As a result, boys with epispadias should have the epispadias corrected early, as early as the first few weeks of life, to assure that the bladder grows appropriately.

Epispadias repair requires mobilization of the bladder neck away from the pelvic diaphragm to enable replacement of the bladder neck within the pelvic diaphragm to provide for a more efficient sphincter complex. In the complete repair of bladder exstrophy, as described by Mitchell, the initial epispadias repair creates a hypospadias from an epispadias as the penis is separated into three components, two paired corporal bodies, the associated corpora spongiosum, and the urethra. The urethra is then dissected off of the anterior corporal bodies to the level of the prostate. In this process, the corporal bodies are separated, and the urethra is re-rolled and placed between the corporal bodies to the penoscrotal junction or partway up to the reconfigured corpora. This assures that the bladder neck is placed deep within the pelvic diaphragm. If necessary, the results in hypospadias can be corrected in a second stage 6–12 months later after the bladder is cycling appropriately. In some cases, pelvic osteotomy is required to affect further closure of the bladder neck. Continence rates following the complete repair may be as high as 70% but this remains a major challenge for these children.

Urethral Duplication

Urethral duplication can take many forms. In practice, urethral duplications are so rare that even busy pediatric urologists see only a few of these in their career. Urethral duplication usually presents with a hypoplastic, orthotopic urethra with a functional urethra that is ventral and drains to a hypospadiac position or even to the anus. Occasionally urethral duplications can be epispadiac and associated with dorsal penile curvature. The urethral duplication can be complete or partial. Treatment is individualized, usually selecting the better of the two urethras to build from with obliteration of the diminutive urethra.

Micropenis

Boys born with a penis less than 2.5 standard deviations from the normal stretched penile length are said to have micropenis. In the newborn, this means that the penis should be at least 1.9 cm long. These defects must be distinguished from the inconspicuous penis in which a normal sized penis is buried beneath layers of prepubic fat or penile shaft skin.

If fetal testosterone is abnormal prior to 12 weeks of gestation, hypospadias is often present. However, a complete microphallus in the absence of hypospadias is due to incomplete or absent testosterone after 14 weeks of gestation. Microphallus is most commonly associated with hypothalamic anomalies resulting in hypogonadotropic hypogonadism, but can also be due to deficient testosterone secretion, defects in testosterone action, or development anomalies. Occasionally the primary testicular failure from bilateral antenatal torsion can also result in microphallus. Workup for microphallus includes a karyotype and an evaluation for disorders of sexual differentiation, particularly if the microphallus is associated with cryptorchidism. Additional workup for hypogonadotropic hypogonadism is also important.

In the past, sex reassignment was often considered. However, because many of these boys have brain imprinting due to early testosterone exposure and have subsequently been found to have male sexual identity, most clinicians today avoid reassignment of the sex of rearing.

Androgen in therapy in the form of testosterone alendronate (25 mg per month for 3 months) can stimulate the penis to grow. This stimulus may be effective in predicting growth in adolescence. We recommend avoiding circumcision in boys with micropenis because it seems to draw attention to the defect rather than improve appearance.

Aphallia

Aphallia is fortunately quite rare, occurring in one in about 30,000,000 boys. This defect results from aberrant development of the genital tubercle. Associated anomalies are common, including imperforate anus, cryptorchidism, vesicoureteral reflux, horseshoe kidney, renal agenesis, and congenital musculoskeletal and pulmonary anomalies. Historically, gender reassignment was considered but virtually all of these children have normal testes and therefore adopt a male sexual identity based on early brain imprinting.

Circumcision

Although the advantages and disadvantages are widely debated, families generally feel very strongly about the decision to proceed with circumcision or not. I have had little success talking families into or out of circumcision. The risk of febrile urinary tract infection in boys who have undergone circumcision is less than age-matched uncircumcised boys up to about age 6 months. After a year of age, boys with and without circumcision have about equal risk of infection. Virtually all men who develop penile carcinoma are uncircumcised. On the other hand, in developed countries, the risk of penile carcinoma is very low even in uncircumcised males. This fact suggests that hygiene might be more of a factor in reducing the inflammatory component of the retained foreskin. Despite the relatively clear advantages and the disadvantages that come with circumcision such as complications (bleeding, meatal stenosis, injuries to the glans or penile shaft), most parents have a strong bias for or against circumcision by the time their baby boy is born. Most have made their decision regardless of whatever coaching we provide.

There are a number of different techniques used to perform a circumcision. These techniques are influenced by the age of the boy and, to a lesser extent, the presence of associated anomalies. In the newborn, local anesthesia with anesthetic cream is important. In addition, we frequently augment the injection with a penile block, which seems to provide excellent analgesia. The block aims to anesthetize the paired dorsal penile nerves that run along the dorsum of the penis and branch at the penopubic junction. An injection at the penopubic junction that favors first the left and then the right

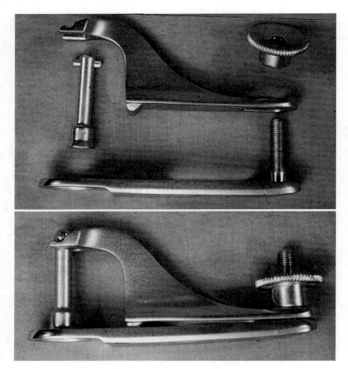

Fig. 84.11 Gomco clamp. The bell is placed within the prepuce

side and an additional circumferential block at the base of the penis provides excellent anesthesia and is relatively easy to perform even in the small newborn. The most common approach to circumcision in the newborn unit today employs a clamp or a bell. We use the Gomco clamp (Allied Healthcare Products, Inc., St. Louis, Missouri, Fig. 84.11) but the Plastibell (Hollister, Inc., Kirksville, Missouri) is equally effective. The reason we favor the clamp is that all of the hardware is removed at the conclusion of the procedure, which we believe might lessen some of the complications that occasionally occur with displacement of the Plastibell.

After the anesthetic is applied, the preputial glanular adhesions are taken down. Great care is taken to completely obliterate the preputial glanular adhesions in preparation for placing the bell over the glans. Once the bell is on, the base of the bell is fed through the orifice in the clamp and the foreskin is brought into the clamp in a symmetric fashion to provide for approximately 1 cm of penile shaft skin to be exposed. The clamp is then placed, applied, and the foreskin trimmed sharply. I like to leave the clamp for 8–10 min to provide hemostasis. Next the clamp is removed and the bell

is gently eased off the glans penis. We apply a non-stick gauze and clear plastic dressing in which a small opening is made to allow voiding. In some cases, we are now using cyanoacrylate skin adhesive along the cut edge of the penis, which obviates the use of the dressing.

The clamps come in three newborn sizes: 1.1, 1.3 and 1.45. The bell that fits the best is applied. If the child is in between clamp sizes, a relatively larger segment of inner preputial skin may be left behind. The inner preputial skin is thin and mobile. When too much inner prepuce remains, the penile shaft skin slides over the corona. The inner prepuce then attaches to the glans with easily separated filmy adhesions or forms a bridging adhesion if the separated raw edge of glans is left in contact with the cut edge of the penile shaft skin. We normally ignore filmy adhesions as they resolve spontaneously. We distinguish bridging adhesions (Fig. 84.9) from filmy adhesions by carefully looking for the circumferential penile scar that results from circumcising incision. Boys with filmy adhesions have a visible penile circumcision scar that surrounds the penis. Bridging adhesions are usually obvious because the penile shaft skin scar encroaches on the glans.

Catastrophic accidents have occurred during circumcision, including degloving injuries, significant bleeding and, worse of all, necrosis of the glans from the deployment of an electric cautery unit while the Gomco clamp is in place. However, circumcisions are relatively safe with the risk of injury under 3%. Most complications fall into three categories: meatal stenosis, glanular preputial bridging or scarring resulting in a trapped penis, or penile inclusion cysts.

Meatal stenosis results from transection of the frenular artery with resultant ischemia to the ventral portion of the urethral meatus, in combination with rotation of the urethral meatus with contact with the diaper, resulting in a web-like closure of the ventrum of the meatus. This usually results in either sprayed stream or an upwardly directed stream. We correct meatal stenosis following circumcision in the office with anesthetic cream augmented with local anesthetic. A small wedge of tissue can be removed from the ventrum of the urethral meatus it is crushed with a hemostat. If we perform this procedure in the operating room due to the parents or child's preference, we excise the same wedge but advance some of the urethral mucosal epithelium into the closure.

Penile inclusion cysts develop when a small segment of epithelial tissue becomes buried beneath the suture line. Over time this transplanted buried skin continues to slough epithelial cells, forming a cyst. These can be incised sharply but it is important to remove all of the epithelial tissue.

Summary Points

- When hidden or webbed penis is noted, it is important to refrain from newborn circumcision.
- More severe hypospadias repairs can be addressed with a staged repair incorporating preputial or buccal mucosa grafts into the penile shaft after straightening the penis.
- Separation of filmy preputial glanular adhesions is not recommend, since many times they simply recur and it becomes uncomfortable to pull the foreskin back.
- Epispadias presents most commonly as part of the classic bladder exstrophy complex that includes cloacal exstrophy, classic bladder exstrophy, and epispadias.
- Microphallus is most commonly associated with hypothalamic anomalies resulting in hypogonadotropic hypogonadism and must be distinguished from a hidden or webbed penis.
- The risk of febrile urinary tract infection in boys who have undergone circumcision is less than age-matched uncircumcised boys up to about age 6 months, but after a year of age, both groups have about equal risk of infection.
- Meatal stenosis results from transection of the frenular artery with resultant ischemia to the ventral portion of the urethral meatus combined with irritation from diaper rubbing.

Editor's Comment

Congenital anomalies of the penis are rare and should only be managed by experienced pediatric urologists. Although penile tissue is forgiving, meticulous planning and precise technique are required to achieve normal urologic and future sexual function and an acceptable appearance. Hypospadias must be recognized when performing a circumcision as any abnormality of the meatus is a contraindication – the foreskin might be needed for the reconstruction. Likewise, webbed penis, in which the scrotal skin encroaches onto the ventral shaft, is a contraindication to circumcision. Except during a circumcision, filmy foreskin adhesions should be left alone as they always recur and tend to become more painful. Repeated lysis can lead to skin bridges, which require incision under anesthesia.

There are very few medical indications for circumcision. The purported benefits are minimal, it is painful even in newborns, and the procedure is associated with a small but significant risk of major complications. Parents are nearly always motivated by misplaced cosmetic or cultural concerns. Some feel that the procedure should be more broadly condemned by society as a form of genital mutilation and only be performed when there is a clear medical indication. Nevertheless, if we can ethically justify performing the procedure at all, it is our obligation as surgeons to at least do it well and with an absolute minimum of complications. Anesthesia and antiseptic should always be used. The free-hand technique provides a nice result but it is important to avoid taking too much skin. It is far better to take too little than to take too much. It is best to place the penis on maximal stretch before deciding how much should be removed and then err on the side of leaving a little bit extra. Parents should be gently reassured that the boy is likely to need the extra skin in the future. A common complication is bleeding, which can be profuse and usually requires a trip back to the OR.

The clamp techniques all involve crushing the skin rather than incising it. Many use the Mogen clamp, variations of which have been around for centuries. The foreskin is stretched beyond the glans and then pinched transversely in the hinged metal clamp. There is a small risk of amputation of the glans. The Gomco clamp uses a metal bell placed within the foreskin. The skin is pinched against the heavy outer part of clamp by tightening a screw. Although safe in experienced hands, some find the heavy metal clamp unwieldy and the fact that the glans seems to disappear into the machinery disconcerting. The Plastibell technique is increasingly popular and comes in six sizes between 1.1 and 1.7 cm. After performing a dorsal slit and, if necessary, dividing the frenulum, the bell is placed within the foreskin and a linen cord is tied very tightly around, crushing the skin against the bell. The excess skin is trimmed and the bell is allowed to fall off in 7–10 days. The bell sometimes falls off prematurely, but this is rarely an issue, even if there is a short distance between the skin edges. After the bell detaches, the foreskin should be pulled back behind the corona at frequent intervals to prevent "recurrent" phimosis. If the bell is too large, the glans can become trapped and strangulated in the opening. When performing a dorsal slit, it is important to avoid inadvertently placing a jaw of the clamp inside the urethra. Dividing the frenular artery can result in meatal stenosis, which usually presents in toddlers as a narrow urine stream that is directed at an upward angle.

As circumcisions become less common, we should expect to see an increase in foreskin complications. Phimosis is the inability to retract the foreskin and is one of the rare indications for at least a partial circumcision. Paraphimosis is when the foreskin retracts but gets stuck, strangulating the glans. This can usually be relieved with firm manual compression of the glans to make it smaller, allowing the prepuce to be reduced. Ice does not help and risks frostbite. Usually the result of rigorous sexual activity, frenular artery tears can bleed profusely. It can sometimes be treated at the bedside with direct pressure but sometimes requires ligation under anesthesia. Balanitis is a painful skin infection that is slightly more common in the uncircumcised. It is usually treated with frequent retraction of the foreskin, gentle cleansing, and topical antibiotics. Systemic antibiotics are indicated for invasive infection.

Parental Preparation

- The more proximal the hypospadias, the more likely a complication or need for revision becomes.
- There are very few true "medical" indications for circumcision.
- Circumcision carries a risk of bleeding, injury to the penis, meatal stenosis, and the need for revision.

Technical Points

- In general, hypospadias repair has three parts: degloving the penis to assess the urethra and penile shaft, straightening the penis and reconstructing the urethra, and covering the penis with skin, usually rotated from the dorsal prepuce.
- For circumcision in the newborn, local anesthesia with anesthetic cream is important.
- Despite a risk of bleeding, injury to the penis, trapped penis, and meatal stenosis, circumcision is relatively safe, with the risk of injury under 3%.

Suggested Reading

Borer JG, Retik A. Hypospadias. In: Wein AJ, Kavoussi LR, Novic AC, Partin AM, Peters CA, editors. Campbell-Walsh urology. 9th ed. Philadelphia: Saunders; 2007. p. 3703. Chapter 125.

Elder JS. Abnormalities of the genitalia in boys and their surgical management. In: Wein AJ, Kavoussi LR, Novic AC, Partin AM, Peters CA, editors. Campbell-Walsh urology. 9th ed. Philadelphia: Saunders; 2007. p. 3745. Chapter 126.

Park JM. Normal development of the urogenital system. In: Wein AJ, Kavoussi LR, Novic AC, Partin AM, Peters CA, editors. Campbell-Walsh urology. 9th ed. Philadelphia: Saunders; 2007. p. 3121. Chapter 106.

Skoog SJ, Belman AB. Aphallia: its classification and management. J Urol. 1989;141:589–92.

Chapter 85
Inguinal Hernia and Hydrocele

André Hebra and Joshua B. Glenn

Approximately 400 years ago, Ambroise Pare described the reduction of an incarcerated pediatric hernia and the application of trusses. He recognized that inguinal hernias in children were probably congenital and that they could be cured. Despite the many historical descriptions of conservative medical management of inguinal hernias, no effective non-surgical means of treatment exists. Essentially all pediatric inguinal hernias require operative treatment to prevent the development of complications, such as incarceration or strangulation.

Inguinal hernia repair is one of the most common operations performed in children. It is a type of abdominal wall defect in which an intra-abdominal organ, such as bowel, ovary or omentum, protrudes through an opening in the inguinal region. Most hernias diagnosed in childhood are indirect inguinal hernias, caused by a patent processus vaginalis. True direct inguinal hernias are quite rare in children.

Embryology

The processus vaginalis is an outpouching of the peritoneum that is attached to the testicle and trails behind as the retroperitoneal testis descends into the scrotum. An indirect inguinal hernia results when the normal obliteration of the processus vaginalis fails to occur. The peritoneum of the coelomic cavity forms an evagination on each side of the midline into the ventral abdominal wall, which follows the path of the gubernaculum testis into the scrotal swellings and forms, along with the muscle and fascia, the inguinal canal. As the testis descends, each layer of the abdominal wall contributes a distinct layer of the spermatic cord. The internal spermatic fascia is derived from the transversalis fascia, the cremaster muscle from internal oblique muscle, the external spermatic fascia from the external oblique aponeurosis. In addition, a reflected fold of the processus vaginalis surrounds each testis (tunica vaginalis).

In the female, the ovaries descend into the pelvis but do not leave the abdominal cavity. The upper portion of the gubernaculum becomes the ovarian ligament and the lower portion becomes the round ligament, which travels through the inguinal ring into the labium majus. If the processus vaginalis remains patent, it extends into the labium majus and is known as the canal of Nuck.

Before birth, the layers of the processus vaginalis normally fuse, closing off the entrance into the inguinal canal from the abdominal cavity. The precise cause of the obliteration of the processus vaginalis is unknown, but some recent studies indicate that calcitonin gene-related peptide (CGRP), released from the genitofemoral nerve, might play a role.

When luminal obliteration fails to occur, a sac is present through which abdominal contents can herniate through the inguinal canal. Even when the processus vaginalis is patent, the entrance may be adequately covered by the internal oblique and transverse abdominal muscles, preventing escape of abdominal contents for many years. When the opening is only large enough to allow fluid to pass through, the result is a communicating hydrocele. When closure occurs proximally but fluid remains trapped within the tunica distally, a non-communicating hydrocele is the result.

Typically, hernia sacs are composed of fibrous and connective tissue. Embryonal müllerian remnants are recognized in up to 6% of surgical specimens; therefore, the finding of vas- or epididymis-type tissue in the hernia sac does not necessarily imply injury. Specific histologic features of the remnant include a smaller diameter and failure to show a prominent muscular wall with Masson trichrome staining.

Presentation

Although the exact incidence of indirect inguinal hernia in infants and children is unknown, the reported incidence ranges from 1 to 5%. Sixty percent of hernias occur on the

A. Hebra (✉)
Department of Surgery, Medical University of South Carolina, Children's Hospital, 96 Jonathan Lucas Street, Charleston, SC 29425, USA
e-mail: hebra@musc.edu

P. Mattei (ed.), *Fundamentals of Pediatric Surgery*,
DOI 10.1007/978-1-4419-6643-8_85, © Springer Science+Business Media, LLC 2011

right side. Premature infants are at increased risk for inguinal hernia, with an incidence of 2% in females and up to 30% in males. Moreover, the associated risk of incarceration is more than 60% in this high-risk population of patients. Inguinal hernias are much more common in males than in females. The male-to-female ratio is estimated to be 6:1, and approximately 5% of all males develop a hernia during their lifetime. Inguinal hernia appears to occur equally among races.

The child with an inguinal hernia generally presents with an obvious bulge at the external inguinal ring or within the scrotum (Fig. 85.1). The parents typically provide the history of a visible swelling or bulge, commonly intermittent, in the inguino-scrotal region in boys and inguino-labial region in girls. The swelling may or may not be associated with any pain or discomfort. More commonly, no pain is associated with a simple inguinal hernia in an infant. The parents may perceive the bulge as being painful when, in truth, it causes no discomfort to the patient. The bulge commonly occurs after crying or straining and usually resolves during the night while the baby is sleeping or feeding.

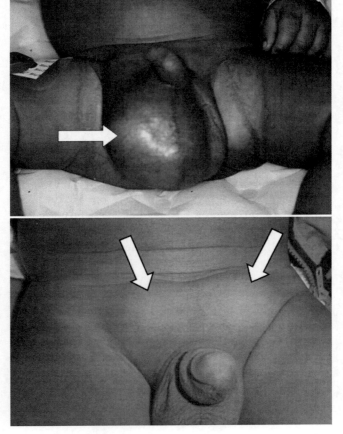

Fig. 85.1 Typical appearance of an infant with a large right indirect inguinal hernia. The right scrotal sac is enlarged and contains palpable loops of bowel and fluid

If there is a history of a painful bulge, one must suspect the presence of an incarcerated inguinal hernia. Patients with an incarcerated hernia generally present with a tender firm mass in the inguinal canal or scrotum. The child may be fussy, unwilling to feed, and crying inconsolably. The skin overlying the bulge may be edematous, erythematous, and discolored.

The physical examination of a child with an inguinal hernia typically reveals a smooth mass originating from the external ring lateral to the pubic tubercle. The mass may only be noticeable after coughing or performing a Valsalva maneuver (which can be difficult to perform in an infant), and the mass should be easily reducible. Occasionally, the examining physician may feel the loops of intestine within the hernia sac. In girls, feeling the ovary in the hernia sac is not unusual and is sometimes mistaken for a lymph node. In boys, palpation of both testicles is important to rule out an undescended or retractile testicle, which can be associated with an inguinal hernia.

When the hernia sac is palpated over the cord structures, the sensation may be similar to that of rubbing two layers of silk together. This finding is known as the "silk sign" or "silk glove sign" and is highly suggestive of an inguinal hernia. This sign is particularly important in young children and infants, in whom palpation of the external inguinal ring and inguinal canal is difficult because of their small size.

Not infrequently an inguinal hernia is noticed by the parents but eludes detection by the examining physician. In such cases, maneuvers to increase the intra-abdominal pressure may be attempted. Lifting an infant's arms above the head may provoke crying or a struggle to get free and thus increased intra-abdominal pressure. Older children can be asked to cough or to inflate a balloon or examining glove.

Direct hernias, due to muscular disruption of the so-called floor of the inguinal canal are extremely rare in children. Though classically described as occurring medial to the inferior epigastric vessels, the distinction is nearly impossible to appreciate in small children. Given the rarity of a direct hernia and the fact that direct hernias do not have elongated sacs that extend into the inguinal canal or scrotum the way indirect inguinal hernias do, the clinician can safely assume that an inguinal hernia in a child is of the indirect variety.

A femoral hernia can be very difficult to differentiate from an indirect inguinal hernia. Its location is below the inguinal canal, through the femoral canal. The differentiation is often made only at the time of operative repair, once the anatomy and relationship to the inguinal ligament is clearly visualized. The signs and symptoms for femoral hernias are essentially the same as those described for indirect inguinal hernias.

Inguinal hernia incarceration refers to the presence of a non-reducible inguinal hernia. In such cases, the herniated viscera (usually loops of intestines) become engorged, edematous, and trapped inside the inguinal canal. Incarceration is the most common cause of bowel obstruction in infants and children and the second most common cause of intestinal obstruction overall, second only to intra-abdominal adhesions from a previous operation. If the vascular supply is compromised, strangulation and ischemic necrosis develops and intestinal perforation may result, representing a true surgical emergency. When an incarceration is encountered, an attempt should be made to reduce it manually if the patient has no signs of systemic toxicity (leukocytosis, severe tachycardia, abdominal distention, bilious vomiting, discoloration of the skin over the entrapped viscera). If the patient appears toxic, emergent surgical exploration after appropriate resuscitation is indicated. It must be noted that, in experienced hands, the great majority of incarcerated inguinal hernias can be successfully reduced without surgical intervention.

In boys, differentiating between a hernia and a hydrocele is not always easy. Trans-illumination has been advocated as a means of distinguishing between the presence of a sac filled with fluid in the scrotum and the presence of bowel in the scrotal sac. However, in cases of inguinal hernia incarceration, trans-illumination may be equivocal, because any viscera that is distended and fluid-filled in the scrotum of a young infant may also trans-illuminate. A rectal examination in young children may be helpful if intestine can be felt descending through the internal ring, confirming the diagnosis of incarceration. Finally, the selective use of ultrasound can be helpful in such difficult cases, particularly because the ultrasound may be able to differentiate between hydrocele, incarcerated hernia, and testicular torsion. When in doubt, inguinal exploration is advisable.

Treatment

Inguinal hernias do not heal spontaneously and must be surgically repaired because of the ever-present risk of incarceration. Parents may be instructed on the application of gentle pressure on the bulge of an inguinal hernia to prevent incarceration until the elective operative repair is performed.

Hydrocele without hernia in neonates is the only exception in which surgical treatment may be delayed. Repair of hydroceles in neonates without the presence of hernia is typically delayed for 12–18 months because the connection with the peritoneal cavity (via the processus vaginalis) may be very small and may have already closed or be in the process of closing. Fluid in the hydrocele comes from the peritoneal cavity and is gradually absorbed if the communication has closed. If the hydrocele persists after this observation period, operative repair is usually indicated.

General endotracheal anesthesia is safe for most surgical repairs of inguinal hernia in infants and children. In addition, either a caudal anesthetic or intra-operative injection of a local anesthetic in the inguinal region is used for postoperative analgesia and to minimize the need for intravenous use of narcotics, depending on the parents' wishes and anesthetic expertise. Hernia repair is usually an outpatient procedure in the otherwise healthy full-term infant or child. Surgery should be postponed in the event of upper respiratory tract infection, otitis media, or significant rash in the groin. Very rarely, operative repair can be performed under strict local or regional anesthesia, particularly in high risk premature babies. Pre-operative antibiotics are not necessary unless the operation is being performed for treatment of an incarcerated or strangulated hernia.

Although adult surgical procedures for correction of inguinal hernias are numerous and varied, only three basic variations of the surgical techniques for repair of pediatric inguinal hernias have been described: (1) high ligation and excision of the patent sac with anatomic closure, (2) high ligation of the sac with plication of the floor of the inguinal canal (the transversalis fascia), and (3) high ligation of the sac combined with reconstruction of the inguinal floor. The most common techniques applied require open surgery. However, new developments in minimal access surgery have allowed for the use of laparoscopic techniques in the repair of pediatric inguinal hernias.

The common basic principle is high ligation and excision of the hernia sac with anatomic closure of the internal inguinal ring. Repair of the inguinal floor may be necessary if the hernia is large and has repeatedly passed through the internal ring causing enlargement of the ring and weakening of the inguinal floor. Very rarely is artificial mesh needed for repair of the inguinal floor in a child.

The steps involved in the open surgical repair of a pediatric indirect inguinal hernia include: (1) The patient is placed on the operating table in a supine position with his or her legs slightly abducted. The lower abdomen and inguino-scrotal or inguino-labial area and upper thighs must be included in the operative field. The hernia contents should be completely reduced into the peritoneal cavity before incision. (2) Incision is made in the skin of the inguinal crease just lateral and superior to the pubic tubercle. The skin incision is typically small (1–2 cm). Electrocautery may be used to control bleeding. (3) Scarpa's fascia is identified and opened. In young infants, the Scarpa's fascia may be easily confused with the aponeurosis of the external oblique. (4) One should not raise skin flaps. Dissection is started through the external oblique at the lateral aspect of the incision and extended to the inguinal ligament (it is important to clearly identify the inguinal ligament as an anatomical landmark). (5) The external ring is identified by dissecting medially along the inguinal ligament. The ring is incised and the fascia is opened, taking care to avoid injury to the ilioinguinal nerve. This incision reveals the cremasteric muscle fibers covering the cord structures. The muscle fibers are separated by blunt dissection to allow full exposure of the cord structures together with the hernia sac. (6) The hernia sac can be identified in the anteromedial aspect of the cord, and medial retraction of the sac reveals the underlying testicular vessels and vas deferens. Fine tissue forceps are used to tease these structures away from the hernia sac. An Allis clamp may be placed around the vas and the testicular vessels to keep them away and to facilitate further dissection of the sac, separating it from the cord structures. (7) When the surgeon is absolutely certain that the vas deferens has been identified and protected, the hernia sac can then be clamped and divided. The proximal sac is mobilized to the level of the internal ring, which is often identified by the presence of retroperitoneal fat. (8) Once the sac is confirmed to be empty, it is twisted on itself and doubly suture-ligated, usually with an absorbable suture. (9) If the ring is not enlarged, the distal sac is opened to drain any residual fluid and the sac is partially excised. Complete excision of the distal sac is not necessary. (10) Closure is accomplished in layers with absorbable sutures.

If the internal ring is enlarged, the cord should be elevated from its bed with a soft silastic drain. Repair of the inguinal floor is performed by placing sutures between the transversalis fascia (with or without the conjoined tendon) and the inguinal ligament in order to tighten the ring. Alternatively, a modified Bassini type of repair can be used to reinforce the entire inguinal floor. If frank disruption of the canal floor is present, a reconstructive procedure, such as that of Bassini or McVay, is necessary and mesh may be necessary. The McVay repair sometimes necessitates a relaxing incision in the rectus sheath that allows the conjoined tendon to be pulled down to the reflected edge of the inguinal ligament and the femoral sheath.

In patients with a long-standing history of inguinal hernia, the repeated protrusion of abdominal contents through the inguinal canal enlarges the internal and external rings, reducing the risk of incarceration and strangulation but increasing the likelihood of damage to the posterior inguinal wall. This makes repair more difficult and recurrence more likely (Fig. 85.2) In addition to high ligation of the hernia sac, repair of the inguinal floor is usually necessary.

In the event of surgery for an incarcerated hernia in which the peritoneal fluid is found to be bloody or turbid, material should be sent for gram stain and culture. One must consider enlarging the inguinal incision or creating a counter-incision to verify that necrotic intestine was not reduced into the abdomen.

In girls, a sliding hernia may contain the ovary or a portion of the fallopian tube. These structures should be carefully dissected from the internal wall of the sac before suture ligation. An alternate procedure involves incising the sac along the ovary and tube on either side and folding the flap into the peritoneum. A purse-string suture can then be used to close the sac. In the female, the sac can be sutured closed after division of the round ligament because no important structures pass through the round ligament and inguinal ring.

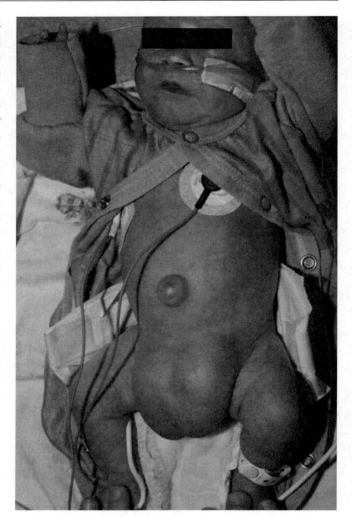

Fig. 85.2 A premature baby boy with bilateral giant inguino-scrotal hernias. Because of the large size of the hernias, operative repair sometimes requires repair of the inguinal floor in addition to the high ligation of the indirect hernia sac

An undescended testis discovered during herniorrhaphy should be fixed in the scrotum, even if the infant is younger than 12 months old. This avoids the complications of incarceration, strangulation, and testicular infarction, while possibly increasing fertility. If surgery reveals an absent vas deferens, cystic fibrosis or ipsilateral renal agenesis must be suspected. The second condition results because of the origin of the ureteral bud from the mesonephric duct, the precursor of the vas deferens.

Contralateral Exploration

The question of when the contralateral side needs to be explored is much debated. Advantages of exploration include avoidance of a second anesthetic and the risks of an incarcerated contralateral hernia. Disadvantages include the possibility

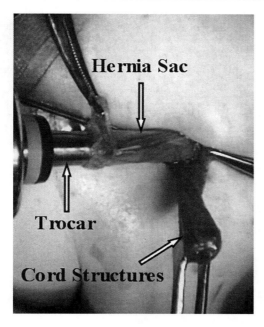

Fig. 85.3 Illustration of the technique for intra-operative diagnostic laparoscopy to evaluate for the presence of an asymptomatic contralateral inguinal hernia at the time of elective repair of an indirect inguinal hernia

of injury to the vas or testicular vessels during surgical exploration, increased operating time, and the fact that it will prove to be unnecessary in as many as 70% of patients. Unfortunately, neither age nor sex predicts whether a child has a contralateral hernia and no diagnostic test can effectively determine the presence of an asymptomatic inguinal hernia.

Peritoneoscopy offers the most accurate means of determining whether a child has a contralateral patent processus vaginalis. Diagnostic laparoscopy can be performed through the hernia sac of an indirect inguinal hernia to determine if a contralateral patent processus vaginalis is present with a false negative rate of less than 1%. Diagnostic peritoneoscopy can be accomplished through the umbilicus or the upper abdomen, using a separate incision. However, the preferred method is to perform peritoneoscopy using the ipsilateral hernia sac. The sac is opened and a 3- to 5-mm reusable laparoscopic cannula is introduced through the hernia sac. (Fig. 85.3) The peritoneal cavity is then insufflated with carbon dioxide to a pressure of 6–8 mmHg and the patient is placed in the Trendelenburg position. With a 3-mm 70° laparoscope, the contralateral internal inguinal ring can be seen, and the presence or absence of a patent processus vaginalis can be documented.

Laparoscopic Repair

As more pediatric surgeons have gained expertise in laparoscopy, the benefits have become widely recognized. Tekehara et al. were the first to describe the laparoscopic needle-assisted

repair (LNAR) that we currently use. The cosmetic results are superior to traditional open herniorraphy, recurrence rates are similar, and a lower risk of injury to the spermatic vessel and vas has been reported (Fig. 85.4–85.7).

The procedure is performed under general anesthesia with muscle relaxation. A gentle Credè maneuver is used to empty the bladder. Access to the peritoneal cavity is accomplished through the umbilicus with a Veress needle. The peritoneal cavity is insufflated with carbon dioxide to a pressure of 6–8 mmHg. A 3- or 5-mm trocar is placed through the infra-umbilical incision and a 2.7- or 5-mm 30° angled laparoscope is utilized. The diagnosis of unilateral or bilateral inguinal hernias is confirmed. A small incision is made on the lateral abdominal wall at the level of the umbilicus (lateral to the rectus muscle), opposite to the side of the hernia, to allow insertion of a 3-mm laparoscopic Maryland forceps under direct visualization. This instrument is used to move and manipulate the spermatic vessels and vas during placement of the needle for repair of the hernia. The first step is to clearly visualize the lateral and medial border of the open internal inguinal ring. A 22-gauge Tuhoi spinal needle with a 2-0 polypropylene suture threaded inside the barrel is inserted and passed underneath the peritoneum and the inguinal ligament, lateral to the internal inguinal ring, away from the spermatic vessels and vas. All needle movements are performed by the operating surgeon from outside the body cavity under laparoscopic control so that the position of the tip of the needle can be placed precisely at the desired location inside the peritoneal cavity. The Maryland dissector is used to move the cord structures and peritoneum during placement of the needle and suture. The second step is to place a suture around the internal inguinal ring: The thread is pushed through the needle into the abdominal cavity creating an internal loop. The needle is pulled out, leaving the polypropylene loop of the thread inside the abdomen. From outside the patient's body, one of the threaded ends is introduced again into the barrel of the spinal needle and the needle is than passed through the same skin puncture point, through the medial aspect of the internal inguinal ring, under the peritoneum. Again the vas and vessels are mobilized to stay away from the needle in order to prevent injury. Once the tip of the needle is in the desired position next to the loop of polypropylene (inside the abdomen), the thread is pushed in so that it passes through the loop. At this point the thread-loop is pulled out of the abdomen with the thread end caught by the loop. In this way, the suture thread of polypropylene is placed around the internal inguinal ring under the peritoneum, creating a complete purse-string suture with the ends of the suture coming out of the same skin needle hole in the groin region. The knot is tied to allow for complete closure of the internal inguinal ring and hernia opening. With this technique the knot is buried in the subcutaneous tissue. The small skin needle hole is closed with steri-strips.

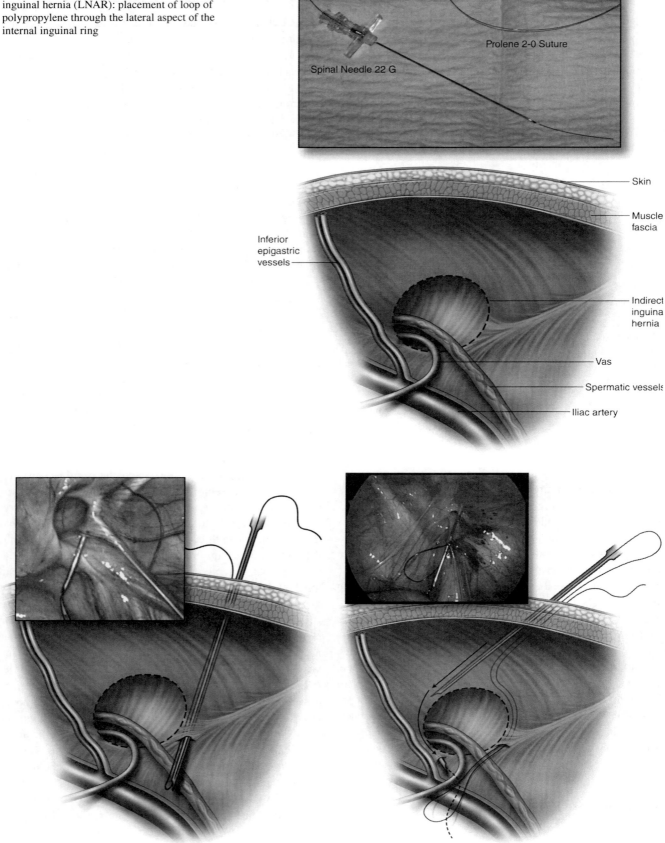

Fig. 85.4 Laparoscopic needle-assisted repair of inguinal hernia (LNAR): placement of loop of polypropylene through the lateral aspect of the internal inguinal ring

Spinal Needle 22 G

Prolene 2-0 Suture

Skin

Muscle fascia

Inferior epigastric vessels

Indirect inguinal hernia

Vas

Spermatic vessels

Iliac artery

Fig. 85.5 LNAR: placement of the spinal needle and polypropylene suture through the medial aspect of the internal inguinal ring

Fig. 85.6 LNAR: completion of the loop of polypropylene around the internal inguinal ring

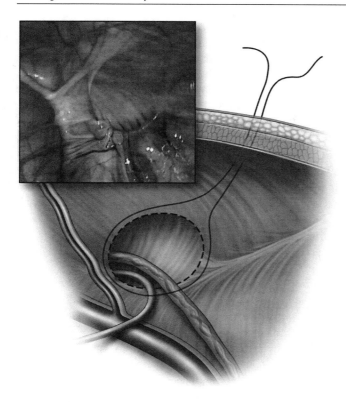

Fig. 85.7 LNAR: complete closure of the internal ring after tying the knot (extra-corporeal) of the polypropylene suture (buried in the subcutaneous tissue and not visible here)

Incarcerated Hernia

When an incarceration is encountered, manual reduction should be attempted if the patient has no signs of systemic toxicity, leukocytosis, severe tachycardia, abdominal distention, bilious vomiting, or skin discoloration. If the patient appears toxic, emergent surgical exploration is usually necessary.

Some authors have proposed the use of relaxation maneuvers to relieve the pressure on the neck of the hernia sac and to allow for the incarceration to resolve spontaneously. This involves placement of the sedated patient in a 30–40° Trendelenburg position to allow gravity to facilitate reduction. If the hernia has not reduced spontaneously within a few minutes, forceful manual reduction by an experienced physician must be attempted.

Unless the clinician suspects the possibility of inguinal hernia strangulation, manual reduction is recommended in all cases of incarcerated hernia. Such attempts are successful in more than 90% of cases and pose minimal risk to the entrapped structure. Successful reduction of an incarcerated inguinal hernia results in immediate patient comfort, relief of obstruction, and prevention of strangulation. Semi-elective operation is usually scheduled within 24–72 h after reduction primarily because recurrent incarceration is quite common. If reduction is unsuccessful, immediate surgery is performed.

Manual reduction of an incarcerated inguinal hernia is a skill that is learned by experience. The parents should be informed that reduction of the hernia will be attempted. The patient is placed in the supine position and the pelvis is grasped gently but firmly by an assistant to prevent lateral movement of the buttocks. Depending on the side of the hernia, the ipsilateral leg is then externally rotated and completely flexed into a frog-leg position. This position causes the external ring to ascend so that it more nearly overrides the internal inguinal ring. The first two fingers of the guiding hand are placed over the hernia bulge, overriding the upper margin of the external inguinal ring in such a fashion as to prevent the hernia contents from subluxating upwards and over the margin of the ring. The apex of the hernia (usually in the scrotum) is grasped between the first two fingers and thumb of the reducing hand, and steady, firm, and sometimes prolonged pressure is applied. This last point is crucial as the reducing hand must not be withdrawn after only a few seconds. One indication of the correct application of this technique is the onset of stiffness in the fingers and an ache in the thenar eminence. After several minutes, a sudden reduction of the hernia typically occurs with an almost audible thud, accompanied by complete relief in the patient.

Using this method of reduction, open operation of incarcerated inguinal hernia is rarely necessary. By successfully reducing an incarcerated inguinal hernia, the open (or laparoscopic) operation can be accomplished semi-electively and with decreased morbidity.

Once an incarcerated hernia becomes strangulated, reduction without operative intervention is not possible. Because of significant swelling from the compromised bowel, the presence of intestinal ischemia secondary to incarceration precludes the possibility of reducing the hernia back into the peritoneal cavity. In such cases, immediate operative intervention is indicated, and the viability of the intestine must be carefully assessed at the time of surgery. If necrosis has developed, one must resect the affected segment of bowel. The incidence of recurrence after emergent surgery for incarceration or strangulation is typically much higher than that reported for elective hernia repair. Moreover, other complications that are more commonly seen after surgery for incarcerated or strangulated inguinal hernia include injury to the vas and vessels, testicular ischemia and atrophy, hernia recurrence, and wound infection.

Postoperative Care

Most patients who undergo elective repair of an inguinal hernia are discharged from the hospital shortly after surgery. Overnight observation is indicated only in small premature babies (less than 60 weeks post-conception) who are at risk for postoperative apnea. Such patients are usually admitted for 24-h observation and monitoring in the hospital.

Routine follow-up care after operative repair of an inguinal hernia typically requires only one office visit or telephone consultation if the parents have reported no problems or complications. Scrotal swelling and bruising after surgery are very common and may last for 1–3 weeks. Such signs represent normal postoperative changes and do not indicate a complication. A residual postoperative hydrocele (non-communicating) is not unusual, particularly after LNAR, and does not require any operative repair since it will reabsorb spontaneously in more than 90% of the cases.

Most patients are treated with acetaminophen for 24–48 h after surgery. Codeine or other narcotics are occasionally added for pain management in children older than 1 year of age. Physical activity limitations are usually not indicated in children diagnosed with an inguinal hernia. However, following operative repair, avoidance of major physical activity for 1–2 weeks is recommended. After that time, the patient is allowed to participate in any physical activities (sports, play, swimming, biking, running). Children younger than 5 years are likely to recover extremely quickly from surgery, they are typically capable of returning to their normal level of activities within 48 h without significant limitations.

Complications following surgical repair of inguinal hernias are uncommon. Decreased testicular size (<20% of patients), testicular atrophy (1–2%), vas injury (<1%), and development of sperm-agglutinating antibodies can occur. The risk of gonadal injury in females is low. Fortunately, in the hands of experienced pediatric surgeons, such complications are quite rare. The incidence of wound infection is reported to be between 1 and 2%. Hernia recurrence rates are less than 1% when experienced pediatric surgeons perform the operation. Factors associated with recurrence include an unrecognized tear in the sac, failure to repair an enlarged inguinal ring, damage to the canal and inguinal floor, infection, history of incarceration, and conditions producing increased intra-abdominal pressure, such as chronic respiratory problems. The reported recurrence rate after laparoscopic repair of inguinal hernia has ranged from 1 to 5%. However, the few reports in the surgical literature have included the surgeon's learning curve. In the author's personal experience with LNAR of inguinal hernias in children less than 10 years of age, the recurrence rate is 1%. The vas deferens and ilioinguinal nerve are occasionally injured and should be repaired with 7-0 or 8-0 Maxon sutures. This may be technically difficult because of the extremely small vas lumen in small children. Some infertility experts advise marking the ends of the vas with permanent suture and performing vaso-vasotomy after puberty with a two-layer anastomosis. It is also important to remember that the finding of vas or epididymis on the surgical pathology report does not necessarily imply injury because, embryonal müllerian remnants have been recognized in 1–6% of surgical specimens. Specific histologic features of the remnant include a smaller diameter and failure to show a prominent muscular wall with Masson trichrome staining.

Summary Points

- Inguinal hernia repair is one of the most common surgical procedures performed in the pediatric age group.
- Nearly all inguinal hernias in children are indirect hernias.
- Incarcerated hernias occur when a portion of the intestine becomes edematous and cannot return to the abdominal cavity.
- Incarcerated hernia is an emergency because of a risk of bowel necrosis and testicular atrophy.
- Inguinal hernias present with an intermittent bulge that is usually brought out by actions that generate a Valsalva maneuver, like crying or straining.
- Hernias in children are usually painless, except when they become incarcerated.

Editor's Comment

Essentially all inguinal hernias in children are congenital and indirect. Rarely, a child with a connective tissue disorder like Ehlers–Danlos will present with a true direct hernia. A second recurrence in any child should probably be repaired with reconstruction of the floor of the inguinal canal, such as a Cooper's ligament repair. Children with a connective tissue disorder might be best served with a mesh repair; otherwise its use in children should be avoided because of uncertainty about long-term effects. The hernia "defect" is actually a normal hiatus that allows passage of the cord structures or round ligament and should therefore not require repair per se. In fact, cinching the internal ring in boys risks entrapment of the cord structures. Instead, simple ligation and division of the hernia sac should allow the hiatus to close down to a normal and more functional size.

The standard repair has withstood the test of time: it is extremely safe, well-tolerated, associated with a recurrence rate of a fraction of 1%, takes less than 10–15 min per side, and leaves a scar that is small and nearly invisible. At the risk of seeming old-fashioned, I will suggest that laparoscopic repair is unlikely to ever replace the traditional operation because of an unacceptable recurrence rate and the fact that parents will not happily accept the hydrocele that results from failing to excise the distal portion of the sac. Nevertheless, I hope to someday be proven incorrect. On the other hand, laparoscopy (2.7 mm 70° scope placed through the hernia sac) is very useful as a diagnostic maneuver to rule out a contralateral patent processus and should be used in all prepubescent children who are having an inguinal hernia repair.

The risk of incarceration is higher than once thought, especially in neonates and prematures. Though in this day and age the risk of bowel injury is extremely low, there is a significant risk of testicular atrophy and a higher complication rate of the subsequent repair, including recurrence. Therefore, repair should be undertaken soon after diagnosis, within 1–2 months, if possible, and on the same admission for those who present with incarceration. Incarcerated ovaries are rarely reducible and these hernias should be repaired within 1–2 weeks to avoid ischemia or injury to the ovary.

Reduction of an incarcerated hernia is a skill that is learned by experience. Tricks include using sedation whenever possible, which increases the success rate and minimizes discomfort; applying constant pressure over a long period of time (2–3 min straight) rather than ever-increasing pressure over a short period of time; and maintaining patience despite the resistance of the patient and the anxiety of the parents. Often, the fact that the hernia will eventually be able to be reduced is signaled by the frictional sensation of two edematous surfaces being rubbed together (similar to that of two pickles). It is useful to take a very short break between 2–3 min sessions and to try again several times before giving up. When there is doubt regarding the distinction between an incarcerated hernia and a tense hydrocele, the patient should undergo urgent surgical exploration rather than an ultrasound regardless of how asymptomatic they appear.

Ligation of the sac should be performed with absorbable suture, as there is no advantage to using silk and it can occasionally create a foreign body reaction or a cutaneous fistula. There is no need for routine pathologic analysis of the sac. The distal sac should be partially excised, but to avoid injury to the vas deferens, the portion of the sac that is adherent to the spermatic cord should be left intact. Sliding hernias can pose a challenge and should be repaired using a purse-string suture placed at the level of the internal ring

with care to avoid the vas. The fallopian tube in a sliding hernia usually has an avascular "mesentery" medially that can be divided longitudinally up into the peritoneum. The first two bites of the purse-string suture should then be placed so as to effectively close the resultant slit in the hernia sac at the internal ring.

Postoperatively, since repair does not involve muscular reconstruction, most children need no activity restrictions, with the possible exception of avoiding competitive sports for 1 week. They should also be allowed to bathe the next day and seen in routine follow up in 3–4 weeks. Infection is exceedingly rare and recurrence should occur in less than one in about 200–300 repairs. Recurrence is most common in very young premature boys, sometimes becoming evident by the morning after surgery.

Diagnostic Studies

- History
- Physical examination

Preoperative Preparation

☐ Informed consent

Parental Preparation

- Hernias in children are congenital and not due to excessive straining or muscular disruption.
- Hernias never resolve spontaneously and therefore should always be surgically repaired.
- There is as yet no imaging study that will accurately confirm or exclude the presence of an inguinal hernia.
- Incarceration is usually obvious, causing pain and vomiting, however anytime the bulge fails to resolve spontaneously the child should be urgently evaluated.
- Hernia repair in children requires general anesthesia but is very safe and has a high success rate.
- Hernia repair in children is different from that in adults: the muscles are not stitched, placement of a mesh is not required, and recovery is very rapid, typically within one or two days.

Technical Points

- Repair should include high ligation and division of the hernia sac, with repair of the floor of the inguinal canal being rarely necessary.
- Sliding hernias should be repaired with a purse-string suture at the level of the internal ring, with careful attention to avoiding injury to the vas or fallopian tube.
- At the time of repair, if the testicle is undescended or freely retractile, it should be fixed in the scrotum (orchidopexy).
- Children with a connective tissue disorder or who have had two recurrences after surgical repair should undergo repair of the floor of the inguinal canal, such as a Cooper ligament repair.
- The ilioinguinal nerve and vas deferens should be identified and protected throughout the procedure.
- Boys with absence of the vas deferens should be evaluated for cystic fibrosis and ipsilateral renal agenesis.

Suggested Reading

Given JP, Rubin SZ. Occurrence of contralateral inguinal hernia following unilateral repair in a pediatric hospital. J Pediatr Surg. 1989; 24(10):963–5.

Gonzalez Santacruz M. Low prevalence of complications of delayed herniotomy in the extremely premature infant. Acta Paediatr. 2004; 93:94–8.

Han BK. Uncommon causes of scrotal and inguinal swelling in children: sonographic appearance. J Clin Ultrasound. 1986;14(6):421–7.

Matsuda T, Muguruma K, Horii Y, et al. Serum antisperm antibodies in men with vas deferens obstruction caused by childhood inguinal herniorrhaphy. Fertil Steril. 1993;59(5):1095–7.

Miltenburg DM, Nuchtern JG, Jaksic T, et al. Laparoscopic evaluation of the pediatric inguinal hernia–a meta-analysis. J Pediatr Surg. 1998;33(6):874–9.

Myers JB, Lovell MA, Lee RS, et al. Torsion of an indirect hernia sac causing acute scrotum. J Pediatr Surg. 2004;39(1):122–3.

Othersen Jr HB. The pediatric inguinal hernia. Surg Clin North Am. 1993;73(4):853–9.

Rescorla FJ, West KW, Engum SA, et al. The "other side" of pediatric hernias: the role of laparoscopy. Am Surg. 1997;63(8):690–3.

Scherer III LR, Grosfeld JL. Inguinal hernia and umbilical anomalies. Pediatr Clin North Am. 1993;40(6):1121–31.

Skinner MA, Grosfeld JL. Inguinal and umbilical hernia repair in infants and children. Surg Clin North Am. 1993;73(3):439–49.

Stoppa R. About biomaterials and how they work in groin hernia repairs. Hernia. 2003;7:57–60.

Takehara H, Yakabe S, Kameoka K. Laparoscopic percutaneous extraperitoneal closure for inguinal hernia in children: clinical outcome of 972 repairs done in 3 pediatric surgical institutions. J Pediatr Surg. 2006;41:1999–2003.

Chapter 86
Undescended Testis

Pasquale Casale and Sarah M. Lambert

The undescended testis represents one of the more common referrals to a pediatric urologist but the presentation varies considerably. As a result, management varies widely depending on the age of the child and the location of the testis. At the extremes, a testis may be high in the retroperitoneum or retractile, migrating into and out of the scrotum. In addition, the clinician should be aware of the absent or vanishing testis and must be proficient in performing an abdominal exploration to confirm an absent testis.

An undescended testis is found in 3–5% of full-term male newborns and bilateral in nearly 2%. In premature neonates, the incidence of undescended testes is reported to be 30%, reflecting the continued descent of the testes throughout the third trimester. More recent studies demonstrate that birth weight rather than gestational age is the primary determinant of undescended testes. Postnatal testicular descent is possible and usually occurs prior to 6 months of age. This is reflected in the 1% prevalence of undescended testes at 1 year of age.

Testicular descent begins in the retroperitoneum and usually continues until the testis reaches a dependent position in the scrotum. The testis can be found in any location along this path of descent or in an ectopic location. Classification of the undescended testis includes all of these locations, though most commonly they are described as either palpable or nonpalpable. A palpable testis has descended to the level of the external ring whereas a nonpalpable testis remains intra-abdominal. This description is inherently subjective and depends solely on the clinician's examination. Accepting this degree of inconsistency, approximately 80% of undescended testes are palpable. A testis might be nonpalpable due to testicular agenesis or atrophy, or a difficult physical examination. Surgical exploration can clarify a difficult physical examination and further categorize testes into an absent, intra-abdominal, canalicular, extracanalicular, or

ectopic. At the time of surgical exploration for a nonpalpable testis, a surgeon can anticipate approximately 40% of nonpalpable testes to be distal to the external inguinal ring, another 40% to be atrophic or absent, and 20% to be truly intra-abdominal.

Most ectopic testes are found in a superficial pouch between the external oblique fascia and Scarpa's fascia. A retractile testis is one that migrates in and out of the scrotum with movement of the cremasteric muscles and poses a different challenge to clinicians. The vast majority of retractile testes do not require intervention, though a small minority can become "ascending testes," which do eventually require surgical intervention. Therefore, surveillance of these testes until they are no longer retractile is mandatory. In addition, because of the higher risk of malignant degeneration in undescended testes regardless of whether or not they have been surgically corrected, boys with undescended testes should be counseled to perform systematic testicular examination after puberty.

The undescended testis results from abnormal testicular development and descent. Many theories exist regarding the etiology of testicular maldescent. Normal spermatogenesis requires a temperature that is 2–3° cooler than normal intra-abdominal temperature. Therefore, testes remaining in the intra-abdominal cavity are at continued risk for abnormal spermatogenesis. Regulation of normal testicular descent into the protected environment of the scrotum is likely multifactorial and may be affected by androgen stimulation, somatic fetal growth, gubernacular development and intra-abdominal pressure. In addition, abnormal testicular development can result in abnormal testicular descent.

Sexual differentiation begins at the end of the sixth week of gestation. Testicular development begins early in the seventh week and requires chromosomal integrity and normal hypothalamic-pituitary-gonadal endocrine function. Abnormal testicular development can be manifested by abnormal testicular descent, infertility, or tumorigenesis. Undescended testes have abnormal germ cell morphology, varying degrees of gonadal dysgenesis, and are exposed to elevated intra-abdominal temperatures. Abnormal spermatogonia and the absence of germ cells can be demonstrated on testicular biopsy in children as

P. Casale (✉)
Department of Urology, Children's Hospital of Philadelphia,
Philadelphia, PA 19104, USA
e-mail: casale@email.chop.edu

P. Mattei (ed.), *Fundamentals of Pediatric Surgery*,
DOI 10.1007/978-1-4419-6643-8_86, © Springer Science+Business Media, LLC 2011

young as 18 months of age. This abnormal development can progress to fibrosis, basement membrane degeneration, and deposition of myelin and lipids. The relative risk of testicular cancer in patients with a clinical history of an undescended testis is up to 14 times higher than for boys with normal testicular descent and no definitive data exist to demonstrate that early orchidopexy decreases the risk of testicular cancer.

Testicular maldescent also often adversely affects fertility. Boys with bilateral undescended testes are at much greater risk of low sperm concentration and abnormal morphology than boys with a unilateral undescended testis. Men with a history of bilateral undescended testes have uniformly poor semen parameters and have a significantly decreased paternity rate when compared with men with unilateral undescended testis and the general population. On the other hand, 43% of men with a unilateral undescended testis have a sperm density of greater than 20 million/mL and paternity rates that do not differ from that of the general population. It is important to recognize that many of the studies performed demonstrating abnormalities included a large number of boys who underwent surgical repair after 2 years of age.

Diagnosis

Evaluation of the child with undescended testes begins with a comprehensive history, which should include a maternal and gestational history with clear documentation of the neonatal physical examination, medical and surgical history, and a family history to assess a potential genetic predisposition. The physical examination is of great importance and directs further interventions. A complete examination should include the penis, scrotum, perineum, inguinal canal, and potential sites of testicular ectopia. Detection of a nonpalpable testis can be improved by placing the child supine, allowing the clinician to palpate along the expected path of testicular descent using a sweeping movement after wetting his/her hands with water. During the history and physical examination, signs and symptoms of an inguinal hernia or hydrocele should also be documented. Over 90% of children with undescended testes have a patent processus vaginalis that must be ligated at the time of orchidopexy. The clinician must also be attuned to potential characteristics of congenital syndromes that are associated with undescended testes, including disorders of sexual differentiation, prune belly syndrome, and Prader-Willi syndrome.

Although radiographic studies are often an excellent adjunct to physical examination findings, in the evaluation of the undescended testis, radiographic testing is hindered by a significant rate of false-negative results. Hrebinko and Bellinger reported that ultrasonography, computerized tomography, and magnetic resonance imaging for undescended testes correlated with operative findings in 58, 33, and 0%

respectively, with an overall accuracy of 44%. Given this high false negative rate, radiographic imaging is not routinely performed in the evaluation of undescended testes.

Laboratory evaluation is utilized in the evaluation of bilateral undescended testes. Determination of the levels of follicle stimulating hormone (FSH), luteinizing hormone (LH), and testosterone can verify the presence or absence of testicular tissue. Elevated FSH in a prepubertal boy indicates anorchia. A child with bilateral undescended testes and normal gonadotropin levels can be further assessed with a human chorionic gonadotropin stimulation test prior to operative exploration. It is also critically important to promptly rule out the diagnosis of congenital adrenal hyperplasia, the work up of which should include an electrolyte panel, 17-hydroxyprogesterone level, testosterone level, pelvic ultrasound and karyotype. Diagnostic laparoscopy is often utilized in the child with a nonpalpable undescended testis and can be performed at the time of definitive surgical treatment.

Treatment

The goal of surgical repair is to remove the testis from the abdomine or inguinal canal and place it in the scrotum. Placing the testis in the scrotum allows for proper examination of suspected neoplasia or torsion, and potentially prevents further deterioration of spermatogenesis. Definitive surgical therapy is recommended between 6 months and one year of age. Operative planning depends primarily on the preoperative location of the testis. Examination of the inguinal and scrotal region after induction of general anesthesia sometimes allows for palpation of a previously nonpalpable testis and thus avoidance of an abdominal exploration.

The standard orchidopexy begins with a transverse skin incision in an ipsilateral inguinal skin crease along Langer's lines. The essential steps of this procedure include: (1) adequate mobilization of the spermatic cord and testis, (2) division of the gubernaculum, (3) high ligation of the patent processus vaginalis, (4) dissection of the internal spermatic fascial layers, and (5) fixation of the testis in a superficial sub-dartos pouch in the ipsilateral hemiscrotum. The testis should rest in the dependent portion of the scrotum without tension and care should be taken to preserve proper orientation of the spermatic vessels and vas deferens. The testis can be secured in a sutureless sub-dartos pouch, sutured at the tunica vaginalis, or sutured at the tunica albuginea. The sutures can be absorbable or nonabsorbable depending on the surgeon's preference.

In the 1980s, a prescrotal approach to the palpable testis was described by Bianchi et al. This technique is especially useful for the testis that can be brought into the scrotum by caudal traction. With the testis secured in the ipsilateral hemiscrotum by the surgeon, a scrotal incision is created to form a sub-dartos pouch. After formation of the sub-dartos pouch, the incision is deepened to the level of the tunica vaginalis and the testis is delivered into the field. As in a standard inguinal orchidopexy, the spermatic cord and testis are mobilized. In contrast to the standard approach, the gubernaculum does not need to be divided. If a patent processus vaginalis is present it is ligated near the level of the internal ring with narrow Deaver or small hernia retractors to aid in visualization. The testis is then secured in the sub-dartos pouch. After completion of the repair, the testis should rest in the dependent portion of the scrotum without tension.

High undescended testes often require further mobilization to achieve adequate length for tension-free placement into the scrotum. There are many techniques described to provide additional mobilization and length. The Prentiss maneuver involves division of the inferior epigastric vessels and opening of the transversalis fascia to allow the testis to reach the ipsilateral hemiscrotum via the most direct course. As a modification, the testis and spermatic cord can be passed under the inferior epigastric vessels thereby removing the need for ligation while still providing a direct route of descent into the scrotum.

The spermatic vessels are often the limiting factor in obtaining additional length. The Fowler–Stephens orchidopexy describes the division of the internal spermatic artery to provide additional length. After this procedure, the testis is entirely dependent upon blood supply from the deferential artery and the cremasteric attachments. Therefore, division of the internal spermatic artery may only be used prior to extensive dissection of the vas deferens and spermatic cord. The Fowler–Stephens orchidopexy, although initially described as a one-stage procedure, can be performed in two stages. Proponents of the two-stage repair suggest that the delay in complete testicular descent allows for the development of collateral blood supply and ultimately greater mobility. As an alternative to a Fowler–Stephens procedure, testicular autotransplantation via microvascular anastomosis of the testis to the ipsilateral inferior epigastric artery and vein may be used. Although this technique has been reported to have success rates of 95%, the dependence upon microvascular surgical techniques has limited its general applicability.

More recently, laparoscopic techniques have been development for the diagnosis and treatment of the nonpalpable and intra-abdominal testis. Diagnostic laparoscopy for assessment of the nonpalpable testis allows for easy distinction between a vanishing testis with blind-ending vessels above the level of the internal ring, the intracanalicular nonpalpable testis, and the intra-abdominal testis. The patient is placed supine in a slight Trendelenburg position and a Foley catheter is placed to decompress the bladder prior to entry into the peritoneum. Access to the peritoneal cavity is obtained via a semilunar supraumbilical incision that is continued though

the fascia and peritoneum under direct visualization. A blunt 5-mm trocar is then placed into the peritoneal cavity, which is insufflated with carbon dioxide. In infants who need orchidopexy or orchiectomy, one or two 5-mm working ports can be placed. The ipsilateral internal ring, spermatic vessels, and vas deferens are evaluated. The improved visualization and ease of dissection allows the surgeon to readily ascertain whether there is an intra-abdominal testis and, if necessary, perform a standard orchidopexy or Fowler–Stephens procedure. A testicular remnant ("nubbin") can usually be distinguished by its reddish-brown discoloration due to hemosiderin deposition. If a blind-ending vas deferens is visualized first, the spermatic vessels must be located prior to completion of the exploration. If blind-ending vessels are identified, no further surgical exploration is indicated but a contralateral septopexy should be considered.

Postoperative Care

Although orchidopexy represents a very common surgical procedure in the pediatric population, complications do occasionally occur. These complications include damage to the ilioinguinal nerve, injury to the vas deferens, hematoma formation, wound infection, testicular retraction, and testicular atrophy. Testicular atrophy can result from cautery injury, severe retraction upon the spermatic vessels, skeletonization of the cord, torsion of the spermatic vessels, or division of the spermatic vessels during a Fowler–Stephens repair.

The success rate of orchidopexy is affected by the preoperative testicular location and the type of repair performed. A successful orchidopexy can be defined as scrotal position and lack of testicular atrophy. A literature review including 8,425 undescended testes revealed that success rates based upon preoperative position were 74% for abdominal, 87% for canalicular, and 92% for testes located distal to the external ring. Evaluation by type of orchidopexy performed revealed a success rate of 89% for inguinal, 67% for Fowler–Stephens, 77% for staged Fowler–Stephens, 81% for transabdominal, 73% for two-staged, and 84% for microvascular orchidopexy. Although success rates for orchidopexy clearly depend on the preoperative testicular location, advances in operative techniques may increase the success rates while minimizing the risk of adverse outcomes.

In the immediate postoperative period, boys should be assessed for testicular location and the absence of complications. In 6–12 months, the patient should return for a reassessment of testicular location. As the patient continues to grow and develop through puberty, routine testicular exams should be performed. Upon transition into adulthood, all boys must be counseled regarding the performance of testicular self-examination.

Summary Points

- An undescended testis is found in 3–5% of full-term male newborns.
- The incidence of undescended testis is about 30% in premature neonates, but it appears that birth weight rather than gestational age is the primary determinant of testicular descent.
- At surgical exploration, approximately 40% of nonpalpable testes will be distal to the external inguinal ring, 40% will be atrophic or absent, and 20% will be truly intra-abdominal.
- Undescended testes are at higher risk for malignancy and impaired spermatogenesis.
- Over 90% of children with undescended testes have a patent processus vaginalis that must be ligated at the time of orchidopexy.
- Orchidopexy allows for examination of suspected neoplasia or torsion and potentially prevents further deterioration of spermatogenesis.

Editor's Comment

Bilateral undescended testes are quite rare and, when associated with a penile anomaly, can be a sign of a disorder of sexual development or an endocrinologic disorder. In the absence of an associated disorder, they are candidates for a trial of HCG therapy, which in some cases will allow the testes to descend. Unilateral undescended testis is far more common. An undescended testis puts the patient at increased risk for cancer and sterility. Orchidopexy, even when done early, probably does very little to improve either of these situations. The only reason to perform an orchidopexy is to allow surveillance for the presence of a tumor by physical examination. It is usually best to recommend orchidopexy after waiting until the child is 6 months to a year of age, as there is no urgency, the risks of general anesthesia are minimized, and, in some cases, the testis will descend, thereby obviating surgery.

A palpable testis can usually be made to reach the lower scrotum after high ligation of the patent processus and mobilization of the spermatic cord, though this occasionally requires some dissection into the retroperitoneum. The hernia sac is almost always extremely thin and difficult to separate from the spermatic cord structures. Though rarely clinically evident preoperatively, these are among the most challenging hernia repairs that we encounter, demanding patience and meticulous technique.

Nonpalable testes, on the other hand, are rarely able to reach the scrotum using standard techniques and almost always require laparoscopy to confirm the presence of a viable testis and, if a viable testis is found, a more sophisticated surgical approach, such as the Stephens–Fowler operation or microvascular revascularization. The testicular salvage rate is clearly highest when these procedures are performed by those with a great deal of experience in a high-volume pediatric urologic practice.

Boys with retractile testes can usually be safely observed, but they need to be followed closely as they approach adolescence to be sure that the testis continues to descend. Some will need an orchidopexy as they grow older if the testis remains in the upper scrotum or inguinal canal and can no longer be brought down into the lower part of the scrotum. When repairing an inguinal hernia in a child with a retractile testis, it is important to assess the adequacy of the gubernaculum and the length of the spermatic cord before closing the incision because some of these patients are at risk of the testis becoming tethered in the upper scrotum or inguinal canal by scarring in the area of the repair and along the spermatic cord and therefore benefit from having an orchidopexy done at the time of the herniorrhaphy.

Differential Diagnosis

- Undescended testis
- Ectopic testis
- Retractile testis
- Anorchia
- Disorder of sexual differentiation

Diagnostic Studies

- Physical examination
- Laboratory studies
- FSH
- LH
- Testosterone
- Medical imaging
- Ultrasound
- CT
- MRI
- Diagnostic laparoscopy

Preoperative Preparation

☐ Informed consent
☐ Trial of HCG stimulation (for bilateral undescended testes)

Parental Preparation

– An undescended testis can descend normally during the first 6 months or so of life.
– The goal of orchidopexy is to allow proper examination for tumor or torsion in the future.
– When a testis is not palpable, there is a possibility that it is no longer salvageable.
– Making an intra-abdominal testis reach the scrotum requires specialized techniques, which generally have success rate of less than 90%.

Technical Points

• The essential steps of a standard orhiopexy include: mobilization of the spermatic cord and testis, division of the gubernaculum, high ligation of the hernia sac, dissection of the internal spermatic fascial layers, and fixation of the testis in a sub-dartos pouch.
• The spermatic vessels are often the limiting factor in obtaining additional length.
• Fowler–Stephens orchidopexy can be done in one or two stages and involves division of the internal spermatic artery to provide additional length, such that the testis is entirely dependent on blood supply from the deferential artery and cremasteric attachments.
• Testicular autotransplantation with microvascular anastomosis to the ipsilateral inferior epigastric artery and vein is an option for the intra-abdominal testis.
• Laparoscopic techniques are increasingly being used in the diagnosis and treatment of the nonpalpable testis.

Suggested Reading

Bianchi A, Squire BR. Trans-scrotal orchidopexy: orchidopexy revised. Pediatr Surg Int. 1989;4:189.

Bukowski TP, Wacksman J, Billmire DA, Sheldon CA. Testicular autotransplantation for the intra-abdominal testis. Microsurgery. 1995;16(5):290–5.

Cortes D, Thorup JM, Visfeldt J. Cryptorchidism: aspects of fertility and neoplasms. A study including data of 1, 335 consecutive boys who underwent testicular biopsy simultaneously with surgery for cryptorchidism. Horm Res. 2001;55(1):21–7.

Docimo SG. The results of surgical therapy for cryptorchidism: a literature review and analysis. J Urol. 1995;154:1148–52.

Elder JS. Two-stage Fowler–Stephens orchiopexy in the management of intra-abdominal testes. J Urol. 1992;148(4):1239–41.

Hrebinko RL, Bellinger MF. The limited role of imaging techniques in managing chidren with undescended testes. J Urol. 1993;150 (2 Pt 1):458–60.

Kirsch AJ, Escala J, Duckett JW, Smith GHH, Zderic SA, Canning DA, et al. Surgical management of the nonpalpable testis: the Children's Hospital of Philadelphia experience. J Urol. 1998;159: 1340–3.

Lee PA, Coughlin MT. Fertility after bilateral cryptorchidism. Evaluation by paternity, hormone, and semen data. Horm Res. 2001; 55(1):28–32.

Lee PA, Coughlin MT. The single testis: paternity after presentation as unilateral cryptorchidism. J Urol. 2002;168(4 Pt 2):1680–2.

Mayr JM, Lawrenz K, Berghold A. Undescended testicles: an epidemiological review. Acta Paediatr. 1999;88:1089–93.

Prentiss RJ, Weickgenant CJ, Moses JJ, Frazier DB. Undescended testis: surgical anatomy of spermatic vessels, spermatic surgical triangles and lateral spermatic ligament. J Urol. 1960;83: 686–92.

Rusnack SL, Wu HY, Huff DS, Snyder HM 3rd, Carr MC, Bellah RD, Zderic SA, Canning DA. Testis histopathology in boys with cryptorchidism correlates with future fertility potential. *J Urol* Feb;169(2):659-62, 2003.

Wenzler DL, Bloom DA, Park JM. What is the rate of spontaneous testicular descent in infants with cryptorchidism? J Urol. 2004;171 (2 Pt 1): 849–51.

Chapter 87
The Diagnosis and Management of Scrotal Pain

Stephen A. Zderic

Being called upon to evaluate a young man with scrotal pain may not at first seem to represent a glamorous request for consultation. Yet its evaluation, diagnosis, and correct management represent an increasingly rare opportunity in modern medicine: one has the chance of making a diagnosis and managing a patient on the basis of nothing more than a well taken history and a careful physical examination. For the patient who presents with scrotal pain of less than 8–12 h duration, an experienced clinician can make a correct diagnosis based on the history, physical examination, and a urinalysis. However if the pain persists beyond 12 h, the findings on physical examination become less clear and, in this setting, it has proven useful to use Doppler sonography. Even experienced clinicians must exercise caution in the evaluation of these patients because if the diagnosis of testicular torsion cannot be excluded with confidence, emergent scrotal exploration is warranted. Torsion of the testis with infarction and parenchymal loss remains a leading source of litigation in pediatric surgical practices.

Diagnosis

Multiple etiologies for acute scrotal pain have been described, however torsion of the testicle, torsion of the appendix testis, and epididymitis will account for more than 90% of cases. Less common sources of scrotal pain include trauma, testicular tumor (usually on the basis of an infarction within the tumor with stretching of the tunica albuginea), orchitis (mumps orchitis is now exceedingly rare, but it can present with unilateral pain), testicular infarction, and a thrombosed varicocele. On occasion, a patient who is passing a ureteral calculus will present with referred scrotal pain.

S.A. Zderic (✉)
Department of Pediatric Urology, Children's Hospital of Philadelphia, Philadelphia, PA 19104, USA
e-mail: zderic@email.chop.edu

A careful history is essential to sorting out the various etiologies. Among the questions to be explored are the nature of the pain, the timing of its onset, whether there is radiation of the pain, and whether associated symptoms such as dysuria, nausea or vomiting are present. The pain associated with infectious epididymitis will develop slowly over a period of several hours or even days. These patients may also report dysuria or a urethral discharge, which raises the possibility of chlamydia or gonococcal epididymitis in the sexually active patient. In younger patients, dysuria may be due to a urinary tract infection associated with an obstructive uropathy as seen with posterior urethral valves, a urethral stricture, or voiding dysfunction.

In contrast, the pain associated with testicular torsion comes on suddenly; these patients can often tell you the exact time it appeared. Likewise, the pain might awaken the patient from sleep. These patients will report that they cannot find any position of comfort. Emesis is often seen with testicular torsion but is rarely seen in the other conditions. These aspects of the history become less apparent if the patient presents more than 2 days after the onset of pain.

The most striking feature of the patient who presents with a torsed appendix testis is their abnormal gait. Families will often comment on the patient's wide-based gait. These patients will also note that the pain increases whenever they move, and hence their preference is to lie as still as possible. Their appetite is unaffected.

While there is merit to the concept that the history is a powerful tool, it is equally important to keep in mind the perils of relying too much on a history. Many boys present with acute scrotal pain after sports related trauma, and in this setting it is important to remember that the trauma history may in fact represent a distracter. While rare, pain following sports injury can be due to torsion, or a rupture of the tunica albuginea. In either instance, these represent surgical emergencies. In such a setting, if operative exploration is to be avoided, a high quality Doppler sonogram is indicated and it must be unequivocally normal.

A carefully performed physical examination will often serve to confirm the impression conveyed by the history

P. Mattei (ed.), *Fundamentals of Pediatric Surgery*,
DOI 10.1007/978-1-4419-6643-8_87, © Springer Science+Business Media, LLC 2011

Table 87.1 A summary of the clinical features seen in the three main conditions that account for most episodes of scrotal pain

	Testicular torsion	Torsed appendix testis	Epididymitis
Onset	Sudden	Sudden, slowly worsens	Slow
Patient movement	Writhing	Still	Still
Emesis	Often	Rare	Rare
High riding testicle	Present	Absent	Absent
Cremasteric reflex	Absent	Present/absent	Present/absent
Point tenderness	Absent	Localized over upper outer pole	Localized to the epididymis

(Table 87.1). Upon entering the exam room, a valuable clue is offered by whether the patient is writhing about to find a comfortable position (testicular torsion) or lying still in a position of comfort (torsion of the appendix testis). While these patients should be fasted if seen in the emergency room setting, a patient who enters the ambulatory office setting while eating would suggest that the more likely diagnosis is a torsed appendix testis. Conversely, emesis during the course of the evaluation should arouse concern for testicular torsion.

Having assimilated these general observations of the patient, one should examine the abdomen and genitalia with the patient in the supine position. Palpation of the abdomen and flanks will help to rule out other possible causes of pain, such as the hydronephrosis that can occur while passing a ureteral calculus. The penis should be examined, and in older boys, it is important to check for any urethral discharge. The yellow creamy discharge characteristic of *Neisseria gonorrhoeae* contrasts with the clear discharge seen with *Chlamydia*. Such findings should be followed up with a gram stain and culture. In a pediatric population, however, such infectious etiologies are rare. The scrotum must be observed for position of the testes. A torsed testicle will be high riding within the scrotal sac because of the multiple twists of the spermatic cord. It is not uncommon to see a testis that has undergone two or even three complete rotations, and the result is a shortening of the spermatic cord.

This is also the best time to see if there is a brisk cremasteric reflex. Spiral cremasteric muscle fibers originate from the transversalis muscle and are wrapped around the spermatic cord; if the inner thigh is lightly touched or scratched, the cremasteric reflex results in a shortening of these muscle fibers, and the testes moves upwards and out of the scrotum briskly. As one might expect, if there are twists within the spermatic cord, the cremasteric reflex will be absent. Conversely the presence of a brisk cremasteric reflex will make a diagnosis of testicular torsion less likely. There are several points to bear in mind about the utility of the cremasteric reflex in this setting. The first is that the examiner must clearly distinguish between a true upward deflection of the testes. It must be a brisk movement of 2–4 cm and should be unequivocal. One may observe a slight contraction of the dartos muscle which results in changes of the scrotal ruggae, but this is not indicative of the true cremasteric reflex. The

cremasteric reflex is positive only when there is a true upward movement of the testes. The second point to remember is that the cremasteric reflex becomes less brisk or is absent in healthy teenagers making it less useful in this age group. To summarize, eliciting a brisk cremasteric reflex is helpful as it makes the diagnosis of testicular torsion unlikely in the setting of acute scrotal pain. However the absence of a cremasteric reflex is not diagnostic of testicular torsion.

At this point direct manual examination of the scrotal contents should be undertaken. It is best to begin with the asymptomatic side, palpating the testis and epididymal structures to help establish a baseline for the patient during the examination. Attention is then turned to the symptomatic side. Global testicular tenderness is a hallmark of testicular torsion. Pressing on any part of the testes will elicit severe pain. In contrast with torsion of the appendix testis, focal inflammation is seen most often on the upper outer pole of the testes. In this setting, with a careful exam, one can often elicit exquisite point tenderness localized to this area alone. One way to demonstrate this is to use a cotton-tipped applicator to gently push on the testis in various positions along its lower borders, and then end with a final push over the upper outer pole.

Ancillary Studies

The only essential ancillary study needed in the evaluation of acute scrotal pain is a urinalysis, which can be performed rapidly using dipstick testing. The presence of a urinary tract infection in the presence of acute scrotal pain raises the likelihood of epididymitis as the etiology. In the case of the patient who presents with a urethral discharge, rapid testing should be initiated to rule out chlamydia, and a culture sent for evaluation of *N. gonorrhoeae*.

When the pain has lasted longer than about 8 h, the findings on physical examination will be more difficult to interpret due to swelling and edema. Radiographic imaging is useful in this setting. Traditionally this was done with a nuclear medicine examination measuring testicular blood flow. This technique is rarely used today because it does not offer enough anatomic resolution, takes longer to complete, and is dependent upon isotope availability. Today, Doppler ultrasonography offers the opportunity to quickly visualize blood flow to the testes and avoid unnecessary surgical exploration. It is essential for the surgeon who orders this study to review it and make certain that good Doppler waveforms are actually visualized within the testicular parenchyma. The experience of the team performing such an exam might vary and it is critical to make sure that the report of "flow" to the testes actually localizes to the parenchyma and does not represent increased inflammatory blood flow to the scrotal wall. Anything short of normal testicular blood flow represents an indication for emergent scrotal exploration.

Manual Detorsion

If a patient presents early in the course of testicular torsion (less than 12 h), manual detorsion should be attempted as it offers several benefits: it confirms the diagnosis, instantly relieves the patient's pain, and minimizes the ischemic time to the testis. It should be attempted only if the examiner is convinced that the etiology of the pain is testicular torsion. The detorsion is achieved by gently rotating the affected testes outward to the lateral position. This is because 90% of the time, the testicular torsion will occur in a medial direction. Manual detorsion rarely works in patients who have been symptomatic for more than 24 h.

While manual detorsion should be used in order to gain time if an operating room is already occupied or if there is a need to transfer a patient some distance to an operative facility, it should not be used to defer exploration for any prolonged period of time. This is because though the testis that is detorsed is no longer painful, it might still have a 180° twist in the cord, which still produces venous congestion. Furthermore, the testes are still at risk for further torsion. Thus there is everything to gain by getting these patients into the operating room as soon as the diagnosis is made even if there has been a successful manual detorsion.

Surgical Management

Scrotal exploration should be undertaken with the symptomatic side to be explored first. My preference is to use a single midline incision via the midline raphè, then dissect laterally to enter the affected tunica vaginalis. Upon confirming the diagnosis of torsion, the affected testes is detorsed, wrapped in a warm saline soaked sponge, and allowed time to reperfuse. During this time, the opposite tunica vaginalis is opened and explored. My preference is to fix each testis to the midline scrotal septum using three anchoring sutures of 5-0 polypropylene sutures. While there is support in the literature for the use of a subdartos pouch and some concern regarding the reactivity of sutures within the scrotum, it is also true that retorsion after scrotal exploration has been described when non-permanent sutures were used. The use of a less reactive monofilament suture such as polypropylene should offer long-term fixation with minimal risk of a complication. Once the contralateral testis is fixed, the symptomatic side should be inspected to assess its reperfusion prior to fixing it. If after 45 min there is still no sign of reperfusion, a small incision should be made in the tunica albuginea to see if there is any evidence of arterial bleeding. Failure to see any bleeding in this setting offers support in favor of performing an orchiectomy. While all of us will share an inclination to save organs whenever possible, it is important to note that leaving a dying testicle in place will prolong the patient's pain, lengthen the recovery period, and increase the potential for abscess formation.

Torsion in the Neonate

Testicular torsion in the neonate is rare, and its management algorithm has evolved over the past 10 years. The pathophysiology differs in that neonatal torsion is caused by a twist of the spermatic cord and the entire tunica vaginalis (extravaginal torsion). In contrast, torsion in older boys takes place as the testes twists around its vascular pedicle inside the tunica vaginalis. But the most alarming feature of neonatal torsion is that it may on rare occasion occur bilaterally in either a synchronous or asynchronous manner. As these case reports of asynchronous contralateral neonatal torsion have accumulated over the years, there is a growing trend towards recommending urgent surgical exploration for the neonate, with the goal of carrying out an orchiopexy on the contralateral side. It is rare that one can salvage the torsed neonatal testes, but those in favor of urgent exploration make the valid argument that the primary goal is to save the contralateral testis from a similar fate. While contralateral torsion is a rare event, its long-term consequences of infertility and a lifelong need for androgen replacement therapy justify the more aggressive approach advocated today. This can also be justified given the major advances in anesthesia that allow for neonatal surgery in situations other than life-threatening circumstances.

Postoperative Care

After orhiopexy, most boys recover uneventfully. Postoperative edema and mild discomfort are to be expected and are usually self-limited. Provided they sought medical attention soon after the pain developed, the long-term prognosis for these patients is good. The testicular salvage rate is generally lower for adolescents, who often seek to work through or ignore their pain. This need to seek medical attention for pain should be emphasized in school health education classes along with the need to perform monthly self examination to look for scrotal masses. While several series have reported a diminished semen quality in older men with a history of testicular torsion, these reports are difficult to interpret given that semen analyses are not obtained on all patients with a history of torsion. This is an area where more long-term data with a larger cohort of patients are needed.

Summary Points

- When evaluating a boy with an acute scrotum, history and physical examination are the most important initial diagnostic steps and are sometimes sufficient to make a diagnosis.
- A positive urinalysis supports the diagnosis of epididymitis.
- A torsed testicle will often be a high-riding testicle on examination.
- The pain of testicular torsion is often of sudden onset and accompanied by nausea and vomiting.
- After about 12 h of symptoms, an exact diagnosis can be difficult to make by physical examination, in which case an ultrasound and/or surgical exploration may be indicated.
- Testicular torsion in the neonate differs in that it is caused by a twist of the spermatic cord and the entire tunica vaginalis (extravaginal torsion).
- Over the past 10–15 years, a more aggressive approach (contralateral orchidopexy) has been advocated for neonates with testicular torsion.

Editor's Comment

Although in many parts of the world boys presenting with an acute scrotum will be referred to a pediatric urologist, it is important for the pediatric general surgeon to be able to evaluate and treat this condition appropriately. As a general rule, it is better to perform a careful surgical exploration, even if the true diagnosis turns out to be epididymitis or torsion of the appendix testis, than to allow a testis to infarct while trying to establish the right diagnosis with certainty. Unfortunately, most cases will present beyond 12 h' duration, in which case the subtleties of the differential diagnosis are blurred.

When examining the boy with scrotal pain, several points bear emphasis: The history almost always includes some form of trauma, which is more often than not a red herring. The boys are invariably painfully embarrassed and it is important to approach them with compassionate patience; it is okay to acknowledge their anxiety but our demeanor needs to be measured, confident, and professional. Warm your hands and know that for some boys, even a normal examination can be painful. The examination should be systematic and precise, looking for point tenderness, masses, and the "blue-dot" sign often seen with a torsed appendix testis, but also more global secondary signs such as redness, edema, or ecchymosis.

We were taught that an ischemic testicle induces the production of antibodies that can cause infertility. Though there are still a few scattered case reports that support this concept, I do not believe it is still a widely held belief. Nevertheless, a testis that is clearly ischemic should always be removed as it causes pain and can become infected.

Finally, an incarcerated inguinal hernia usually compromises testicular blood flow to some degree, and, even might present as an acute scrotum regardless even in the absence of testicular ischemia. When in doubt, prompt exploration through an inguinal incision will confirm the diagnosis and allow reduction of the bowel. An ultrasound is almost always unnecessary and only serves to delay appropriate treatment.

Differential Diagnosis

- Testicular torsion
- Torsion of the appendix testis
- Epididymitis
- Tumor
- Trauma
- Hematoma
- Rupture of tunica albuginea

Diagnstoic Studies

- Careful physical examination
- Urinalysis
- Culture for *Chlamydia* or *N. gonorrhoeae*
- Ultrasound with Doppler

Preoperative Preparation

□ Informed consent
□ Intravenous access

Parental Preparation

- Occasionally, urgent surgical exploration is the only way to make a definitive diagnosis and offers the best chance to save an ischemic testicle.
- We will do everything we can to save the testicle, but if it is clearly dead, it will be best to remove it in order to prevent the formation of antibodies that could damage the remaining testicle.
- Silicone prostheses are available and can be placed during adolescence to achieve a more normal appearance of the scrotum.

Technical Points

- Manual detorsion can sometimes be performed early in the course of testicular torsion: the testicle is gently rotated outward at least one complete turn.
- Even after a successful manual detorsion, the patient needs to have an operation to complete the detorsion and to fix the testicles.
- A single incision in the midline raphè provides access to each hemiscrotum.
- The testicle is detorsed and observed for viability.
- The testicle can be fixed to the midline scrotal septum with three nonabsorbable sutures.
- Both testicles need to be fixed to prevent a recurrence.

Suggested Reading

Anderson MJ, Dunn JK, Lipshultz LI, Coburn M. Semen quality and endocrine parameters after acute testicular torsion. J Urol. 1992; 147:1545–50.

Arap MA, Vincentini FC, Cocuzza M, Hallak J, Athayde K, Lucon AM, et al. Late hormonal levels, semen parameters, and presence of antisperm antibodies in patients treated for testicular torsion. J Androl. 2007;28(4):528–32.

Cronin KM, Doric SA. Manual detorsion of the testes. In: King C, Heretic FM, editors. Textbook of pediatric emergency medicine procedures. 2nd ed. Philadelphia: Lippincott, Williams & Wilkins; 2008. p. 895–9.

Rupp TJ, Zwanger M. Testicular torsion. In: Emedicine http://emedicine.medscape.com/article/778086-overview.

Varghese A. Culture shock – patient as icon, icon as patient. N Engl J Med. 2008;359:2748–51.

Chapter 88
Cloacal Exstrophy

Michael C. Carr

Cloacal exstrophy represents a complex congenital anomaly that involves the gastrointestinal, genitourinary, and central nervous systems. The omphalocele-exstrophy-imperforate anus-spinal defects (OEIS) complex is believed to arise from a single localized defect in the early development of the mesoderm that ultimately contributes to the infra-umbilical mesenchyme, cloacal septum, and caudal vertebrae. The incidence of OEIS complex has been reported to be approximately 1 in 250,000 live births and is known by a number of other terms, including ectopia cloacae, vesico-intestinal fissure, exstrophia splanchnica, and cloacal exstrophy. First described by Litré in 1709, this multi-system malformation represents the most severe form of the exstrophy-epispadias sequence ranging from phallic separation with epispadias, pubic diastasis, exstrophy of the bladder, cloacal exstrophy, and OEIS complex.

In 1960, Rickham described four patients in which the vesico-intestinal fissure was preserved and this segment of bowel incorporated in continuity with the cecum and hindgut. This critical concept of refunctionalization of the hindgut prevented the short gut physiology that had occurred in previous attempts at surgical reconstruction in which this segment was used for genitourinary reconstruction. Following this early description, mortality remained at nearly 50% mostly due to malnutrition and sepsis. Refinement in parenteral nutrition and neonatal management has accounted for continued improvement in outcomes such that the mortality is now well under 10%. Increasingly important are quality of life issues for patients who are advancing through adolescence and into adulthood.

With the continued widespread use of prenatal ultrasonography, antenatal diagnosis of cloacal exstrophy is increasingly common. Early descriptions emphasized the most telling features, namely the combination of omphalocele and meningomyelocele in the setting of an elevated amniotic fluid alpha-fetoprotein. Early detection would then allow the option of early termination or appropriate counseling of the parents by a comprehensive team. Ultrasonography has been further refined and there is increasing reliance on the use of MRI to confirm the ultrasound findings.

Embryology

Prior to the fifth week of embryonic development, the urinary, genital and gastrointestinal tracts empty into the cloaca. At the caudal end of the cloaca, ectoderm lies directly over endoderm forming the cloacal membrane, which by the fourth week of development constitutes the ventral wall of the urogenital sinus. During the sixth week of development, mesoderm grows towards the midline, forming the infra-umbilical abdominal wall. Simultaneously, the urorectal septum extends caudally towards the cloacal membrane and lateral tissue folds extend from the lateral aspects of the hindgut and meet in the midline. By the seventh week of gestation, the cloaca has been divided into anterior and posterior chambers: the primitive urogenital sinus and the rectum. The cloacal membrane normally ruptures at the end of the eighth week of gestation.

Abnormal mesodermal migration between the ectoderm and endodermal layers of the cloacal membrane will cause premature rupture of the cloacal membrane. Some authors believe that the severity of the defect – cloacal exstrophy, bladder exstrophy or isolated epispadias – is determined by the stage of development when the abnormality occurs. Early damage would affect the mesenchyme that contributes to the infra-umbilical mesoderm, the urorectal septum and the lumbosacral somites and result in: (1) failure of cloacal septation, which leads to persistent cloaca and rudimentary hindgut with imperforate anus; (2) breakdown of the cloacal membrane, which causes exstrophy of the cloaca, failure of fusion of the genital tubercles and (occasionally) omphalocele; and (3) incomplete development of the lumbosacral vertebrae with hydromelia. This constitutes what has been classically recognized as cloacal exstrophy.

M.C. Carr (✉)
Division of Urology, Children's Hospital of Philadelphia, Philadelphia, PA 19104-4399, USA
e-mail: carr@email.chop.edu

P. Mattei (ed.), *Fundamentals of Pediatric Surgery,*
DOI 10.1007/978-1-4419-6643-8_88, © Springer Science+Business Media, LLC 2011

Failure in migration of the infra-umbilical mesoderm that occurs after the caudal movement of the urorectal septum has been completed by the seventh week of embryonic development will result in exstrophy of the bladder. Under normal circumstances this infra-umbilical mesoderm gives rise to the lower abdominal wall, genital tubercles and rami of the pubis. Its defective migration causes a premature breakdown of the cloacal membrane, leaving the posterior wall of the bladder exposed and also resulting in abnormalities in the other structures it normally forms, as evidenced by the epispadias and the separation of the rami of the pubis, which are frequently encountered in patients with bladder exstrophy.

Some authors consider cloacal exstrophy and bladder exstrophy as two distinct disorders, while others consider them part of a continuum. The use the acronym OEIS, although valuable as a mnemonic, has not helped to elucidate the phenotype, pathogenesis or causation of this disorder because it includes both cloacal exstrophy and bladder exstrophy without distinction. Furthermore, publications differ in the definition of the OEIS complex, with some authors including bladder exstrophy and others only cloacal exstrophy.

Bladder exstrophy is more common, occurring in approximately 1 in 50,000 live births. The male to female ratio of bladder exstrophy is 2.3 to 1 although two series have reported a 5-6 to 1 ratio. The Spanish Collaborate Study of Congenital Malformations found cloacal exstrophy to be more common in females (M:F = 0.5) and bladder exstrophy was more common in males (male:female = 1.32). They also observed that the proportion of infants with disorders of sexual differentiation or absence of the external genitalia was much higher in infants with cloacal exstrophy (46%).

Associated malformations in cloacal exstrophy sometimes involve the central nervous system, skeletal system, and the reproductive, gastrointestinal, and upper urinary tracts. Among central nervous system anomalies, the most serious are those involving spinal dysraphism. The incidence of spina bifida in various series ranges from 29 to 100% but these figures include patients with myelocystoceles, meningoceles, lipomeningoceles, hydromelia, and tethered cord. The level of myelomeningocele ranges from lumbar in 70% of cases, sacral in 15%, and thoracic in another 15%. Omphaloceles are commonly associated with cloacal exstrophy complex. Most series report an incidence of over 85%. Other serious anomalies of the gastrointestinal tract include intestinal malrotation, bowel duplication, duodenal atresia and Meckel's diverticulum. The short gut syndrome was identified in 25–50% of patients. A single umbilical artery has also been reported in association with cloacal abnormalities.

The etiology of cloacal exstrophy has not been elucidated, but appears to be heterogeneous. The higher inci-

dence of the OEIS complex in monozygotic twins suggests that these defects might have a blastogenic origin. The observation that twinning is significantly more frequent in cloacal exstrophy than bladder exstrophy also lends further support to the hypothesis that cloacal exstrophy represents an earlier origin of the defect.

Surgical Treatment

Whether cloacal exstrophy is diagnosed in utero so that a team of specialists can be involved with the prenatal counseling, the postnatal management, and surgical correction, or an infant is diagnosed postnatally, the ultimate care of such an individual should be performed at large tertiary referral centers where the expertise exists to deal with such a patient throughout life. The incidence has decreased somewhat due to prenatal detection and termination. Even in a large tertiary referral center such as ours, there are generally no more than one or two seen every several years. The surgical expertise and management of such a patient then becomes even more difficult due to unfamiliarity. Thus we have felt that it is critical to have a consistent comprehensive team of perinatologists, neonatologists, pediatric surgeons, pediatric urologists, and pediatric orthopedic surgeons.

After the patient is stabilized, a thorough evaluation can be performed. The use of saran film or Vigilon to cover the exstrophic bladder and vesico-intestinal fissure will prevent desquamation of the mucosa. The team can then assess the infant and make plans for early intervention to deal with the gastrointestinal tract first. Identification of gender is critically important as it is now clear that sex reassignment for those born with a diminutive phallic structure, as was commonly done in the past, can lead to significant psychological issues and should therefore be avoided.

Once the infant has been deemed clinically stable, the initial surgery entails closure of the omphalocele, separation of the gastrointestinal tract from the bladder halves, and closure of the vesico-intestinal fissure (Fig. 88.1). This allows creation of an end colostomy, which can be brought out in the left mid-quadrant, allowing the two bladder halves to be united. This essentially creates a bladder exstrophy anatomy. The decision then to be made is whether a one-stage closure can be performed or if a staged reconstruction is more appropriate. Some have advocated a different approach in which the cecal segment of the cloacal plate is maintained with the bladder halves to provide a natural augmentation of the bladder, however all of these patients require early parenteral nutrition. The larger exstrophy is then easier to close and more amenable to bladder neck reconstruction and ureteral reimplantation. These authors have opted for early closure of the omphalocele and creation of an ileostomy. At the same

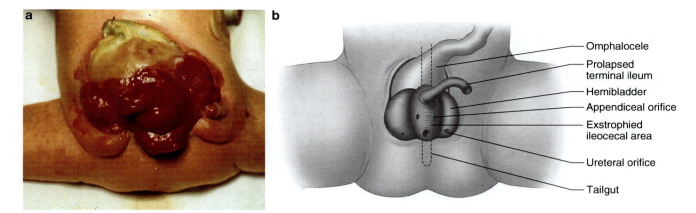

Fig. 88.1 Classic cloacal exstrophy with midline vesico-intestinal fissure dividing the bladder halves. A large omphalocele is found cephalad to this structure and many times the prolapsed terminal ileum is noted as well. The key is identifying the hindgut or tailgut which tends to be a diminutive structure and yet can be refunctionalized following closure of the vesico-intestinal fissure

time a tissue expander is placed to expand the anterior abdominal wall with subsequent closure of the bladder and creation of a thoracoepigastric flap to be used to cover the lower abdominal wall defect.

The early refunctionalization of the hindgut with preservation of the vesico-intestinal fissure into the GI tract is our recommended approach. We have also increasingly adopted the staged reconstruction due to the fact that aggressive early single-stage reconstruction with closure of the bladder can result in a postoperative abdominal compartment syndrome. The conversion of an infant from cloacal exstrophy to bladder exstrophy allows the exstrophic bladder plate to serve as an intra-abdominal pressure-relief mechanism, particularly if there is a large omphalocele. We have demonstrated that the bladder plate can easily be managed for several months by simply covering it with occlusive film. This allows the infant to gain weight and achieve positive nitrogen balance before embarking upon the next phase of reconstruction.

Following the initial procedure, thorough evaluation of the upper urinary tracts is conducted with ultrasonography. Renal anomalies are common and include pelvic kidney, unilateral renal agenesis, multicystic dysplastic kidney, ureteral duplication, or crossed-fused ectopia. Ultrasound evaluation of the spine is necessary to exclude myelomeningocele, meningocele, lipomeningocele or tethering of cord. Lower extremity anomalies include dislocated hips, talipes equinovarus or even agenesis of the lower limbs. In consultation with neurosurgical and orthopedic colleagues, an appropriate surgical plan can be outlined and priorities established.

Reconstruction of the urinary tract becomes the most challenging aspect of the management of infants with cloacal exstrophy. Magnetic resonance imaging of the pelvis provides further insight into the anatomy and allows for appropriate planning before surgery. We strongly advocate that vaginal reconstruction be performed at the same time the bladder is being created since delayed surgery will necessitate dissection in an area where prior surgery has been performed on at least two occasions. Given the likelihood of duplication of the uterus and vagina it is oftentimes better to excise one vagina and maintain the larger one.

With such a high incidence of spinal dysraphism, the likelihood of volitional voiding is low. Utilizing the principles of the complete anatomic repair for bladder exstrophy these patients can be approached in a similar fashion. Deep pelvic diaphragm dissection with division of the intersymphyseal band is crucial to allow for the appropriate positioning of the bladder and urethra. Anatomic closure of the bladder and urethra is conducted. The sphincter complex, which is identified with the aid of a Peña muscle stimulator, is closed around the bladder neck. Generally, the urethral plate will only allow the urethra to exit in a penoscrotal position. At the same time, closure of the epispadic or bifid penis can be performed to achieve "normal" anatomy. It is equally important at this time to deal with any upper urinary tract anomalies that would impede the appropriate drainage from the kidneys. Ureteral catheters can be brought through the newly reconstructed urethra and a suprapubic catheter inserted into the bladder to allow for postoperative drainage. This surgery has been successfully undertaken in infants between 3 and 6 months of age after allowing for appropriate healing from their initial closure as well as their neurosurgical procedures. With the successful second-stage closure, the infant will have a functioning colostomy and ultimately urine can drain through the urethra into a diaper (Fig. 88.2).

Infants with cloacal exstrophy usually have significant pubic diastasis and therefore require osteotomies assist in the

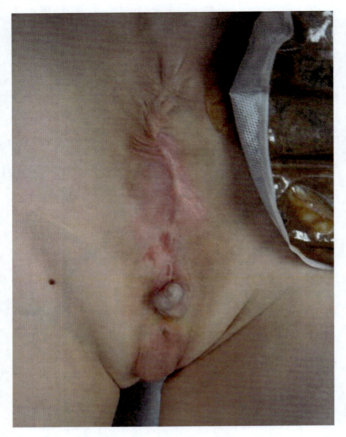

Fig. 88.2 Male cloacal exstrophy with colostomy present. Urethral meatus is present in the penoscrotal location. Second-stage reconstruction will involve creation of penile urethra and revision of midline scar

closure and posterior positioning of the urinary tract. Our orthopedic surgery colleagues perform the osteotomies prior to our attempts at bladder closure so that tension can be taken off the midline closure in addition to the bladder, pubis and the anterior abdominal wall. Our group has preferred iliac osteotomies whereas others have performed bilateral combined anterior innominate and vertical iliac osteotomies with gradual approximation of the bones over 1–2 weeks by external fixture and inter-fragmentary pins. Postoperatively, our patients are maintained in modified Bryant's traction for 3–4 weeks. The ureteral catheters are removed 10–14 days following bladder closure. An early cystogram can be performed 3 weeks following closure to document that the bladder has healed adequately and the suprapubic catheter can then be clamped to determine whether spontaneous voiding will occur. Once it has been determined that the post-void residuals are low, the suprapubic catheter can be removed. It is best to maintain infants on a low dose of antibiotic prophylaxis until an ultrasound is performed 6–8 weeks following discharge from the hospital. This excludes hydronephrosis and

allows assessment of bladder emptying. If no abnormalities are noted at the first assessment, periodic surveillance of the upper urinary tracts is performed at 3–6 months. The goal is to ensure appropriate growth and development of the individual while preserving normal renal function. This will require the expertise of a pediatrician who is able to work closely with the team and can carefully monitor the nutritional needs of the patient. We have found that these patients also benefit from the multidisciplinary experience of a spina bifida clinic.

It is important to mention at this point that there is a case report and it has been my personal observation of a small phallus being located within the urinary bladder of a patient with cloacal exstrophy. In both situations, the phallus was surgically separated from the bladder and mobilized to a more normal position. The case report describes creating a neo-urethra from tubularized bladder urothelium. Our patient has yet to have refunctionalization of his bladder and therefore no further attempts at phallic reconstruction have been attempted (Fig. 88.3).

Over the course of several years after initial reconstruction, issues include the quest for urinary continence, consideration of pull-through procedures with take-down of the colostomy, and ultimately phallic reconstruction. There are rare reports of performing the pull-through procedure in the newborn period, which can be done if sufficient hindgut is present and there is evidence of normal innervation of the perineal musculature to ensure rectal continence. Peña *et al.* have published a series of 27 patients with typical cloacal exstrophy along with 16 with covered variant, and 10 patients with complex anorectal malformations with short colon. Of these patients, 30 were deemed candidates for a pull-through procedure, 27 underwent colonic pull-through, and 20 were available for follow-up. Seventeen of these patients are clean with bowel management, two have voluntary bowel movements with occasional soiling, and one is incontinent but noncompliant. Thus the indication for pull-through depends on successful bowel management through the stoma, which depends on the ability to form solid stool. To maximize this potential, it seems important to use all available hindgut for the initial colostomy.

In most situations, achieving urinary continence necessitates augmentation of the bladder, reconstruction of the bladder neck, and creation of a catheterizable channel to allow for intermittent catheterization. Ileum can be used to augment the bladder but it is incumbent not to upset the already delicate physiology of the GI tract. Stomach has been utilized in patients with cloacal exstrophy, often with good results. There are also descriptions of creation of a composite reservoir utilizing both stomach and a portion of intestine. To date though there is no ideal tissue that can be used for augmentation. It remains to be seen whether tissue-

Fig. 88.3 (**a**) 46XY infant with cloacal exstrophy and omphalocele with wide separation of pubic symphysis and scrotum. (**b**) Postoperative appearance of patient with exteriorization of phallic structure that was located at base of bladder. Patient has a vesicostomy with some prolapse of bladder mucosa and a left-sided colostomy. Further reconstruction will involve closure of the vesicostomy, creation of a catheterizable channel, and ultimately a plastic surgical procedure to unify the scrotum

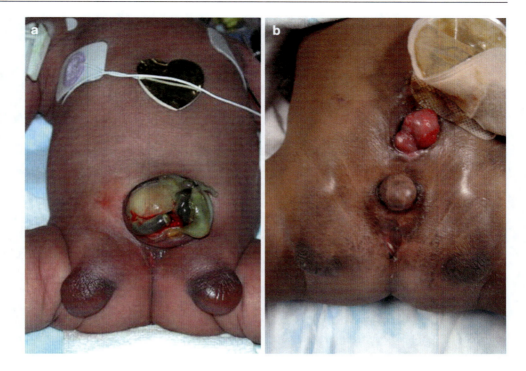

engineered bladder substitute will be a viable option. Bladder neck reconstruction involves either narrowing of the bladder neck, creation of an ileal nipple, or the novel use of a redundant portion of ureter that is tunneled submucosally and brought out to the perineum in a female patient. Closure of the bladder neck with reliance on an abdominal catheterizable channel can also be performed.

Six patients with cloacal exstrophy who underwent complete primary repair at Children's Hospital and Regional Medical Center were reported to have dry intervals and spontaneous voiding. Two patients with stress urinary incontinence have undergone bladder neck injections with Deflux. Another has undergone bladder neck reconstruction and construction of a non-orthotopic channel for clean intermittent catheterization. One patient has achieved complete dryness after toilet training and one additional patient has subsequently undergone augmentation. To date, we have one male patient who has successfully potty trained but has stress incontinence and a small bladder capacity; one girl who has successfully potty trained with 2 h dry intervals; two girls who are toddlers and leak at very low pressure into their diapers; and a patient who was left with a vesicostomy due to the complete absence of any bladder neck or urethra and who will ultimately need to undergo reconstruction.

Phallic reconstruction is accomplished according to the newest techniques with epispadias repair. This involves first-stage repair including release of the dorsal chordee and separation of any existing urethral plate with penile lengthening being accomplished due to partial detachment of the crura from their insertion on the ischial pubic rami. The crura are then advanced and approximated in the midline with dorsal skin coverage provided by reverse Byars' flaps. A second stage urethroplasty can be accomplished with tubularization of the urethral strip and mobilization of abdominal flaps with lengthening of the dorsal incision using a series of Z-plasties.

Reiner and Gearhart reported on male cloacal exstrophy patients who were given the assignment to female sex due to the issue of phallus inadequacy. Eight of 14 subjects assigned to female sex declared themselves male during the follow-up interval whereas the two raised as males remained male. In a follow-up evaluation, males with severe phallic inadequacy reared male and those reared female but converting to male have functional psychosocial developmental trajectories. Those reared female have a realistic likelihood of recognizing male sexual identity and converting to male. Those not converting to male appear to have less successful psychosocial developmental trajectories. Equally important is the experience from Children's Hospital in Seattle of patients with cloacal exstrophy. Significant differences between reassigned and non-assigned participants were found in the area of depression. All participants though had a stable gender identity whereas XY females showed more male typical gender roles. Although being born with cloacal exstrophy puts patients at risk for psychopathology and psychosocial problems, it does not necessarily mean that these problems will develop. With the appropriate support, these patients can be remarkably well-adjusted. This underscores the need to have a clinical psychologist involved in the ongoing care of these patients and in establishing a relationship with the families even in the neonatal period. This allows for appropriate counseling throughout the child's life so that the entire family can attempt to meet the needs of these unique children.

The care of the infant with cloacal exstrophy involves a tremendous commitment on the part of the practitioners who are involved in their care. A multidisciplinary approach is critical and a comprehensive, stable team is of paramount importance. The reconstructive aspects of the surgery are challenging but it is often the psychosocial issues that must be recognized and effectively dealt with that ensures the successful management of such an individual. It would make sense that regional centers of excellence should be formed to advance the care of these patients.

Summary Points

- Cloacal exstrophy represents a complex congenital anomaly that involves the gastrointestinal, genitourinary, and central nervous systems.
- Associated malformations involve the skeletal system and the reproductive and upper urinary tracts.
- It is best to have a consistent and comprehensive team of perinatologists, neonatologists, pediatric surgeons, pediatric urologists, and pediatric orthopedic surgeons involved in the care of the child with cloacal extrophy.
- Identification of gender is critically important as it is now clear that sex reassignment for those born with a diminutive phallic structure can lead to significant psychological issues and should be avoided.

Editor's Comment

Cloacal extrophy can be an extremely challenging combination of anomalies to manage and having an experienced multidisciplinary team to take care of these children is crucial. Although in some cases a primary reconstruction is feasible, many patients benefit from a staged approach. An over-aggressive attempt to incorporate all structures and close the abdomen can result in the abdominal compartment syndrome. The idea of a colonic pull-through in the newborn period is appealing, although clearly the infant needs to be stable and have well-developed pelvic anatomy. Likewise, if vaginal reconstruction can be performed early, the results are usually better. Phallic reconstruction can be most difficult, especially since the native tissue can be quite diminutive and the two halves can be quite separate. Finally, in cases of sexual ambiguity, karyotyping is extremely important because proper sex assignment needs to be established early and with certainty.

Preoperative Preparation

- ☐ Diagnostic studies to assess upper urinary tracts and associated anomalies
- ☐ Karyotyping
- ☐ Consultation with various consultants (general surgery, urology, orthopedics, neonatology) as a team to formulate a management strategy
- ☐ Frank and detailed discussions with the family regarding treatment plan, psychological issues, and long-term prognosis

Parental Preparation

- – This is a complex defect that will require extensive reconstructive surgery in multiple stages.
- – There is the potential for significant long-term psychosexual issues that will need to be addressed early on.
- – Nutrition is an important issue that will also need to be addressed.
- – There are many possible associated anomalies that will need to be identified and treated.

Differential Diagnosis

- Cloacal extrophy
- Bladder extrophy
- Ruptured omphalocele

Diagnostic Studies

- Karyotype
- Plain radiographs
- MRI of abdomen, pelvis, and spine

Technical Points

- Once the infant is stable, the initial surgery entails closure of the omphalocele, separation of the gastrointestinal tract from the bladder halves, and closure of the vesico-intestinal fissure.
- Reconstruction of the urinary tract is the most challenging aspect of the management of infants with cloacal exstrophy.
- The use of saran film or Vigilon to cover the exstrophic bladder and vesico-intestinal fissure prevents desquamation of the mucosa.
- The bladder plate can be managed for several months by simply covering it with occlusive film.
- These is usually significant pubic diastasis and osteotomies are required to assist in the closure and posterior positioning of the urinary tract.
- Achieving urinary continence usually necessitates augmentation of the bladder, reconstruction of the bladder neck, and creation of a catheterizable channel.

Suggested Reading

Carey JC, Greenbaum B, Hall BD. The OEIS complex (omphalocele, exstrophy, imperforate anus, spinal defects). Birth Defects Orig Artic Ser. 1978;14(6b):253–63.

Cromie SJ. Implications of antenatal ultrasound screening in the incidence of major genitourinary malformations. Semin Pediatr Surg. 2001;10(4):204–11.

Davidoff AM, Hebra A, Balmer D, et al. Management of the gastrointestinal tract and nutrition in patients with cloacal exstrophy. J Pediatr Surg. 1996;31(6):771–3.

Diamond DA, Jeffs RD. Cloacal exstrophy: a 22 year experience. J Urol. 1985;133:779–82.

Gearhart JP, Jeffs RD. Techniques to create urinary continence in the cloacal exstrophy patient. J Urol. 1991;146:616–8.

Hendren WH. Cloaca, the most severe degree of imperforate anus: experience with 195 cases. Ann Surg. 1998;228:331–46.

Howell C, Caldamone A, Snyder H, et al. Optimal management of cloacal exstrophy. J Pediatr Surg. 1983;18:365–9.

Hurwitz RS, Mansoni GAM, Ransley PG, et al. Cloacal exstrophy: a report of 34 cases. J Urol. 1987;138:1060–4.

Husmann DA, McLorie GA, Churchill BM. Phallic reconstruction in cloacal exstrophy. J Urol. 1989;142:563–4.

Levitt MA, Mak GZ, Falcone Jr RA, Peña A. Cloacal exstrophy – pull-through or permanent stoma? A review of 53 patients. J Pediatr Surg. 2008;43(1):164–8.

Martinez-Frias ML, Bermejo E, Rodriguez-Pinilla E, et al. Exstrophy of the cloaca and exstrophy of the bladder: two different expressions of a primary developmental field defect. Am J Med Genet. 2001;99:261–9.

Mitchell ME, Brito CG, Rink RC. Cloacal exstrophy reconstruction for urinary continence. J Urol. 1990;144:554–8.

Reiner WG, Gearhart JP. Discordant sexual identity in some genetic males with cloacal exstrophy assigned to female sex at birth. New Engl J Med. 2004;350:333–41.

Rickham PP. Vesico-intestinal fissure. Arch Dis Child. 1960;35:97–102.

Stolar JH, Randolph JG, Flanigan LP. Cloacal exstrophy; individualized management through a staged surgical approach. J Pediatr Surg. 1990;25:505–7.

Chapter 89
Disorders of Sex Development

Thomas F. Kolon

Phenotypic sex results from the differentiation of internal ducts and external genitalia under the influence of hormones and other factors. When discordance occurs among three processes (chromosomal, gonadal, phenotypic sex determination), a disorder of sex development (DSD) is the result. This has previously been identified as "intersex" or "intersexuality" but new nomenclature has replaced the use of the term intersex and now refers to it as DSD. The diagnosis and management of DSD conditions can be confusing because of the wide spectrum in physical appearance often observed. An important issue with any DSD evaluation is not to get overwhelmed by the enormity of the differential diagnosis possibilities. Instead, by working systematically through the differential diagnosis pathway based on the physical exam and laboratory findings, many possible diagnoses can be discarded along the way.

A newborn with bilateral impalpable testes or a unilateral impalpable testis and severe hypospadias should be regarded as having a DSD until proven otherwise, whether or not the genitalia grossly appear ambiguous. The reported incidence of DSD in individuals with hypospadias and cryptorchidism ranges between 17 and 50%. A complete patient history should include the gestational age at birth, ingestion of exogenous maternal hormones (such as those used in assisted reproductive techniques), and maternal use of oral contraceptives or soy products during pregnancy. It is also useful to take a careful family history of urologic abnormalities, neonatal deaths, precocious puberty, amenorrhea, infertility or consanguinity. The patient's mother should also be observed for virilization or a cushingoid appearance. An early clue to possible DSD is discordance between the fetal karyotype and the genitalia visible by antenatal sonogram.

For the purposes of diagnosis and treatment, the most important physical finding is the presence of one or two gonads. If no gonads are palpable, four main categories are possible: 46XX DSD, 46XY DSD, gonadal dysgenesis (GD), or ovotesticular DSD. Of these, 46XX DSD is most commonly seen, followed by mixed GD. A palpable gonad is highly suggestive of a testis, or rarely, an ovotestis (with primarily testis histology), since ovaries and streak gonads do not descend. If one gonad is palpable, 46XX DSD and pure GD are ruled out, while mixed GD, ovotesticular DSD and 46XY DSD remain possibilities. If two gonads are palpable, 46XY DSD or, rarely, ovotesticular DSD, is most likely (Fig. 89.1).

The child should be examined in a warm room, supine in the frog leg position with both legs free. It is important to check the size, location and texture of both gonads, if palpable. The undescended testis may be found in the inguinal canal, the superficial inguinal pouch, at the upper scrotum or, rarely, in the ectopic femoral, perineal, or contralateral scrotal regions. One should also note the development and pigmentation of the labioscrotal folds along with any other congenital anomalies of other body systems. An abnormal phallic size should be documented by width and stretched length measurements. Included is a description of the position of the urethral meatus, the amount of penile curvature, and the number of orifices.

Another critical finding on physical examination is the presence of a uterus that is palpable by digital rectal exam as an anterior midline cord-like structure. A thorough general physical examination should make note of any dysmorphic features indicating syndromic manifestations (short broad neck, widely spaced nipples, aniridia).

In the immediate newborn period, all patients require a karyotype and laboratory evaluation: serum electrolytes, 17-hydroxyprogesterone (17OHP), testosterone (T), dihydrotestosterone (DHT), luteinizing hormone (LH) and follicle stimulation hormone (FSH) levels. Once the karyotype is determined, theses levels will assist in narrowing the differential diagnosis. If the serum 17OHP level is very elevated, a diagnosis of congenital adrenal hyperplasia (CAH) can be made. Testing should be performed in the early morning as there is diurnal variation of serum 17OHP concentration.

T.F. Kolon (✉)
Department of Pediatric Urology, University of Pennsylvania School of Medicine, Children's Hospital of Philadelphia, Philadelphia, PA 19104, USA
e-mail: kolon@email.chop.edu

P. Mattei (ed.), *Fundamentals of Pediatric Surgery*,
DOI 10.1007/978-1-4419-6643-8_89, © Springer Science+Business Media, LLC 2011

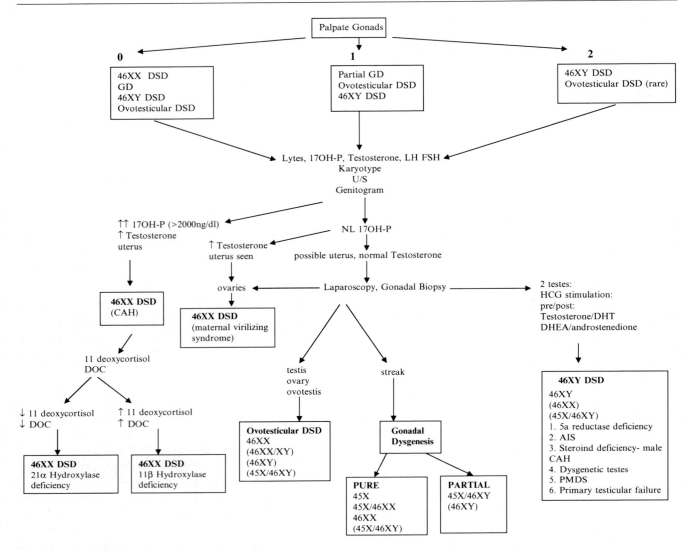

Fig. 89.1 Diagnostic algorithm for patients with DSD

Determining the serum levels of 11-deoxycortisol and deoxycorticosterone (DOC) levels will help differentiate between 21-hydroxylase and 11β-hydroxylase deficiencies. If the levels are elevated, then a diagnosis of 11β-hydroxylase deficiency can be made; low levels confirm 21-hydroxylase deficiency. If the 17OHP level is normal, a T:DHT ratio along with androgen precursors before and after hCG stimulation will help elucidate the 46XY DSD etiology. A failure to respond to hCG in combination with elevated LH and FSH and low müllerian inhibiting substance (MIS) levels is consistent with anorchia. It is important to remember that in the first 60–90 days of life, a normal gonadotropin surge occurs with a resultant increase in the testosterone level and its precursors. During this time, exogenous hCG stimulation for androgen evaluation can be postponed, allowing for the body's maternal hormonal changes to help in the evaluation.

An ultrasound should be the first radiologic exam obtained; it is noninvasive, quick, and relatively inexpensive.

Although it is only 50% accurate in detecting intra-abdominal testes, ultrasound can detect gonads in the inguinal region and can help assess Müllerian anatomy. Although more expensive, CT and MRI can also further delineate the anatomy. A genitogram can be performed to evaluate a urogenital sinus including the entry of the urethra in the vagina as well as highlighting a cervical impression.

Infants with intra-abdominal or nonpalpable testes in whom ovotesticular, mixed GD or 46XY DSD is considered will require an open or laparoscopic exploration with bilateral deep longitudinal gonadal biopsies for histologic evaluation. This will aid in determining the presence of ovotestes, streak gonads or dysgenetic testes and confirming the diagnosis. It is important to note that this procedure is a diagnostic maneuver. Therefore, removal of gonads or reproductive organs should be deferred until the final pathology report is available, a diagnosis is confirmed, and a discussion has occurred between the family and all consultants regarding a gender decision.

46XX DSD (Formerly Female Pseudohermaphroditism)

The most common DSD is 46XX DSD. The patient has a 46XX genotype with normal ovaries and Müllerian derivatives. Sexual ambiguity is limited to masculinization of the external genitalia from in utero exposure to androgens. Maternal sources of elevated androgens during pregnancy include ovarian tumors (arrhenoblastoma, luteoma of pregnancy, Krukenberg tumors) and ingestion of androgens. Congenital adrenal hyperplasia, which accounts for the majority of 46XX DSD patients, describes a group of autosomal recessive disorders that arise from a deficiency in one of five genes required for the biosynthesis of cortisol from cholesterol (Fig. 89.2). While all five of these biochemical defects are characterized by impaired cortisol secretion, only deficiencies in 21-hydroxylase (21-OH) and 11β-hydroxylase (11β-OH) activity are predominantly masculinizing disorders, with 3β–hydroxysteroid dehydrogenase (3βHSD) deficiency to a lesser extent. Females are masculinized by the excess androgens, while most male fetuses have normal genitalia.

A deficiency in activity of 21-hydroxylase accounts for approximately 90% of CAH cases. The enzyme is encoded by the *CYP21* gene and *CYP21P* pseudogene, both located on chromosome 6 between HLA-B and HLA-DR (Table 89.1). Recombination between *CYP21* and the homologous but inactive *CYP21P* account for approximately 95% of 21-OH deficiency mutations. The result is excessive androgen levels in addition to cortisol and mineralocorticoid deficiencies. Characteristic lab abnormalities include a markedly elevated level of 17OHP (as much as 50-fold above normal).

In 75% of patients with classic 21-OH CAH, an associated salt loss crisis is observed in the first week of life. Electrolyte disturbances in these patients include low serum sodium, elevated potassium, and very elevated renin levels. Because most male CAH patients have normal external genitalia, the diagnosis of the 21-OH salt-wasting type is often unsuspected and thus delayed. Patients with simple masculinizing 21-OH deficiency have been identified with a conversion mutation causing severely decreased enzyme activity, but sufficient aldosterone production to prevent salt wasting. Postnatal treatment is based on replacement of glucocorticoid and mineralocorticoid needs, typically hydrocortisone (ideally 10–15 mg/m²/day) and fludrocortisol (30–75 µg/day) in 2 or 3 daily doses. Salt supplementation (2–3 g/day) in infants is recommended for those with the salt-losing type.

In 5% of patients with CAH, a deficiency can be identified in 11β-OH, which is the last step in production of cortisol. Two 11β-OH genes, both located on chromosome 8q, have been identified in the adrenal cortex. Like 21-OH deficiencies, defects in *11β-OH* will result in androgen excess leading to varying degrees of fetal masculinization. In addition *11β-OH*

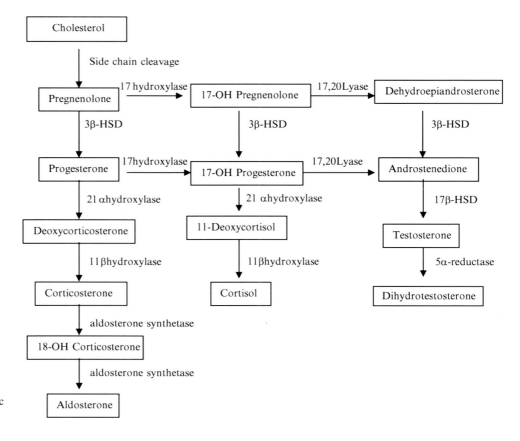

Fig. 89.2 The steroid biosynthetic pathway

Table 89.1 Genetic etiologies of DSD

Syndrome	Karyotype	Genital phenotype	Gene	Locus
21-Hydroxylase deficiency	XX	Masculinized	CYP21B	6p21.3
11-Hydroxylase deficiency	XX	Masculinized	CYP11 (B1,B2)	8q21-22
3βHSD deficiency	XX	Ambiguous	HSD3B2	1p13.1
17α-Hydroxylase or 17,20 Lyase deficiency	XX XY	Ambiguous	CYP17	10q24-25
17βHSD deficiency	XY	Ambiguous	17BHSD3	9q22
Lipoid adrenal hyperplasia	XX XY	Female, Ovarian failure (XX)	StAR	8p11.2
Leydig cell failure	XY	Ambiguous	hCG/LH receptor	2p21
Androgen insensitivity	XY	Ambiguous(female- AIS 7)	AR	Xq11-12
5α-reductase deficiency	XY	Ambiguous, pubertal virilization	SRD5A2	2p23
Persistent mullerian duct	XY	Male	AMH	19q13.3
			AMH II receptor	12q13
Complete gonadal dysgenesis	XX	Female, sexual infantilism	FSH receptor	2p16-21
	45X, 45X/46XX		X monosomy	Paternal X loss
	XY		SRY	Yp53.3
			DSS (DAX-1)	Xp 21-22
			SOX9	17q24.3-25.1
			WT-1	11p13
Partial gonadal dysgenesis	45X/46XY XY	Ambiguous	Unknown	Unknown
XY dysgenesis	XY	Ambiguous	SRY	Yp53.3
	45X/46XY		DSS (DAX-1)	Xp 21-22
			XH-2	Xq13.3
			WT-1	11p13
			SOX9	17q24.3-25.1
			SF-1	9q33
Ovotesticular DSD	XX	Ambiguous	SRY	Yp53.3
	XX/XY		Testis cascade	Unknown
	XY		Downstream genes	
Klinefelter	47XXY	Variable androgen deficiency	XY	Sex chromosome
	46XY/47XXY			Nondisjunction
XX testicular DSD	XX	Ambiguous to normal	SRY	Y translocation to X

defects also results in an accumulation of deoxycorticosterone, a potent mineralocorticoid, resulting in arterial hypertension in about two thirds of patients. Salt loss is not commonly seen; rather, patients will typically have an expanded fluid volume, low potassium, high sodium serum levels, and low renin activity. Therapy is directed towards glucocorticoid replacement. The diagnosis is made by elevated serum concentrations of DOC and 11-deoxycortisol while plasma renin levels remain suppressed.

Pregnenolone conversion to progesterone and dehydroepiandrosterone (DHEA) into androstenedione are catalyzed by 3βHSD. Two isoforms have been described, each encoded by a specific gene, HSD3B1 and HSD3B2. Complete deficiency of 3βHSD is a rare form of CAH, resulting in impaired synthesis of adrenal aldosterone and cortisol and gonadal testosterone and estradiol. These newborns have severe CAH

and exhibit signs of mineralocorticoid and glucocorticoid deficiency in the first week of life. Mild masculinization occurs as a result of DHEA conversion to testosterone in fetal placenta and peripheral tissues by the type 1 isoform. Affected females have mild to moderate clitorimegaly and males exhibit incomplete masculinization of the external genitalia.

Other more rare defects in the biosynthesis of cortisol can also lead to CAH conditions. These include defects in the enzyme CYP17 (P450) which catalyzes two reactions: (1) 17 α–hydroxylation of pregnenolone and (2) 17,20 lyase (side chain cleavage) of 17 hydroxypregnenolone and 17 hydroxyprogesterone. Steroidogenic acute regulatory (StAR) deficiency, also called *lipoid adrenal hyperplasia*, is a rare form of CAH and is the most severe genetic defect in steroidogenesis, resulting in death in days to weeks as a result of adrenocortical hormone deficiency. It is associated with severe glucocorticoid and mineralocorticoid deficiency due to failure to convert cholesterol to pregnenolone. The adrenal glands of affected children are large, containing very high levels of cholesterol and cholesterol esters.

Gonadal Dysgenesis

Mixed GD is the next most common DSD disorder. In general, GD disorders comprise a spectrum of anomalies ranging from complete absence of gonadal development to delayed gonadal failure. Gonadal dysgenesis involves a gonad that has not properly developed into a testis or an ovary such as a dysgenetic testis or a streak gonad.

Pure GD describes a 46XX child with streak gonads or, more commonly, a child with Turner syndrome (45XX or 45XX/46XX). An uncommon form of pure GD is called Swyer syndrome, characterized by a female phenotype, normal to tall stature, bilateral dysgenetic gonads, sexual infantilism with primary amenorrhea, and a 46XY genotype. Mutations in the *SRY* gene are reported in approximately 10–15% of XY sex reversal cases. Gonadectomy of both streak gonads is recommended in these patients due to the high risk of tumor formation..

Partial GD refers to disorders with partial testicular development including mixed GD, dysgenetic male pseudohermaphroditism and some forms of testicular or ovarian regression. Mixed or partial gonadal dysgenesis (45XX/46XY or 46XY) involves a streak gonad on one side and a testis, often dysgenetic, on the other side. A patient with a Y chromosome in the karyotype is at a higher risk than the general population to develop a tumor in a streak or dysgenetic gonad. Because of the 20–25% age-related risk of malignant transformation into a dysgerminoma, surgical removal of the gonad is recommended. The patient with a 45XX/46XY karyotype and normal testis biopsy could retain his testis if it is descended or can be placed in the scrotum. This child would then need a very close follow-up of the testis by monthly self exams for tumor formation.

46XY DSD (Formerly Male Pseudohermaphroditism)

46XY DSD is a heterogeneous disorder in which testes are present but the internal ducts system and/or external genitalia are incompletely masculinized. The phenotype is variable, ranging from completely female external genitalia to the mild male phenotype of isolated hypospadias or cryptorchidism. 46XY DSD can be classified into eight basic etiologic categories: (1) Leydig cell failure, (2) testosterone biosynthesis defects, (3) androgen insensitivity syndrome, (4) 5α-reductase deficiency, (5) persistent Müllerian duct syndrome, (6) testicular dysgenesis, (7) primary testicular failure (vanishing testes syndrome), and (8) exogenous hormone effects.

46XY DSD can result from Leydig cell unresponsiveness to human chorionic gonadotropin hormone (hCG) and LH. The phenotypes of these patients vary from normal female to hypoplastic external male genitalia.

Described earlier for 46XX DSD, defects in four of the steps of the steroid biosynthetic pathway from cholesterol to testosterone may also produce genital ambiguity in the male. These include the less common forms of CAH: 3βHSD deficiency, CYP17 deficiency, StAR protein deficiency, and 17βHSD deficiency. While DHEA conversion into testosterone results in masculinization in females, this same process insufficiently masculinizes affected males. Thus, male infants exhibit ambiguous genitalia with variable degrees of hypospadias, cryptorchidism, penoscrotal transposition, and a blind vaginal pouch. Males with CYP17 deficiency display a developmental spectrum from the normal female phenotype to the ambiguous hypospadiac male. The magnitude of incomplete male masculinization correlates with the severity of the block in 17α-hydroxylation. Affected males with StAR deficiency have severe testosterone deficiencies and exhibit female external genitalia with a blind vaginal pouch. No surviving 46XY patient has demonstrated testis function at puberty. The affected 46XY males with 17βHSD deficiency have external female genitalia, inguinal testes, internal male ducts, and a blind vaginal pouch. At puberty, these patients demonstrate an increase in their levels of gonadotropins, androstenedione, estrone, and testosterone. Delayed virilization occurs if testosterone levels approach the normal range.

The spectrum of androgen insensitivity syndrome (AIS) ranges from 46XY patients with complete androgen insensitivity syndrome (CAIS) to partial AIS. This syndrome is the result of mutations mainly of the steroid-binding domain of the androgen receptor resulting in receptors unable to bind androgens or receptors that bind androgens but do not function properly. This disorder occurs in approximately 1 in 40,000 live male births. The external genitalia of a child with CAIS resemble a normal female although the karyotype is XY and testes are located internally. Historically, these children have been raised as girls and most are diagnosed during surgical repair of an inguinal hernia or at puberty during an evaluation for primary amenorrhea. Management focuses on hormonal replacement, gonadectomy due to the high risk of malignancy, and possible treatment of vaginal hypoplasia. From a cross-sectional study using a self-administered validated sexual function assessment questionnaire, 90% of women with CAIS had sexual difficulties when compared with the general female population, most commonly sexual infrequency and vaginal penetration difficulty. The timing of gonadectomy (pre- vs. post-puberty) is controversial and endocrine, oncologic, and psychological issues should be taken into account. The incidence of malignancy associated with CAIS is 0.8% and usually occurs after puberty, though there has been a case report of a malignant abdominal yolk sac tumor in a 17-month-old child and several reports of benign abdominal masses. The incidence of tumor formation in PAIS is much higher and early gonadectomy is recommended.

Patients born with the autosomal recessive condition, 5α-reductase deficiency, have a defect in the conversion of testosterone to DHT causing a form of male pseudohermaphroditism. Numerous gene mutations, mainly missense mutations, have been reported. These patients are 46XY and usually have male wolffian structures but female urogenital sinus and external genitalia. In some cohorts, they are generally assigned a female sex at birth and raised as females. However, at puberty, virilization occurs as testosterone levels increase into the adult male range while DHT remains disproportionately low.

Antimüllerian hormone (AMH), or Müllerian inhibitory substance (MIS), is secreted by the Sertoli cells causing apoptosis and regression of the Müllerian duct. Since the diagnosis of persistent Müllerian duct syndrome (PMDS) is often made at the time of inguinal hernia repair or orchiopexy, this syndrome is commonly referred to as hernia uteri inguinali. PMDS can occur from a failure of the testes to synthesize or secrete MIS or from a failure in the MIS receptor. It is associated with cryptorchidism and cases of seminomas and intra-abdominal testicular torsion have been reported.

Patients with dysgenetic 46XY exhibit ambiguous development of the internal genital ducts, the urogenital sinus, and the external genitalia. Dysgenetic testes can result from mutations or deletions of any of the genes involved in the testis determination cascade, namely *SRY, DAX, WT1* and *SOX9*. Male patients with Denys-Drash syndrome have ambiguous genitalia with streak or dysgenetic gonads, progressive nephropathy, and a predisposition to develop Wilms tumor.

Ovotesticular DSD (Formerly True Hermaphroditism)

Ovotestictular DSD requires expression of both ovarian and testicular tissue that is a result from sex chromosome mosaicism, chimerism or a Y-chromosome translocation. The most common karyotype in the United States is 46XX, although 46XY or mosaicism or chimerism (46XX/46XY) can occur. Some patients with 46XX true hermaphroditism have the *SRY* gene translocated from the Y to the X chromosome. In these patients, genital ambiguity is thought to result from extensive inactivation of the *SRY*-carrying X chromosome. The gonads can be a testis on one side an ovary on the contralateral side, an ovotestis bilaterally, or an ovotestis and either a testis or ovary on the contralateral side. The external genitalia are ambiguous with hypospadias and incomplete fusion of the labioscrotal folds. The genital duct differentiation in these patients generally follows that of the ipsilateral gonad on that side, such as a fallopian tube with an ovary and a vas deferens with a testis due to local paracrine effect of hormones.

Gender Assignment

Gender assignment in the patient with DSD can often be a difficult decision, with strongly differing viewpoints regarding the timing of gender assignment. The first is to assign and complete genital reconstruction shortly after birth, which might avoid internal conflicts with the patient or external societal conflicts as the child develops. Opponents argue that gender reassignment should be a decision of the affected individual during puberty. They maintain that neither the physician nor the family can predict future gender identity and sexual orientation for the individual. Nevertheless, the decision regarding assignment of sex for rearing should be guided by three equally important factors: the functional and anatomic abilities of the genitalia (size of phallus or vagina, fertility potential), the cause of the DSD, and the values and desires of the family.

One factor in the decision making process that is becoming clearer is the large body of evidence to support the notion that the prenatal and postnatal hormonal milieu has an important role in predicting gender and sexual identity. Genetically female rats given testosterone shortly after birth do not exhibit typical female behavior during adulthood. One study showed that CAH girls with excessive prenatal androgen exposure, many have tomboyish personalities and are more likely to have bisexual or homosexual interests than women without CAH. Among women affected by CAH from 21-OH deficiencies, there appears to be outcome differences between the more severe salt-losing form and simple virilizing forms. Women with simple masculinizing CAH (when the deficiency is partial) reported greater satisfaction and fewer concerns with regard to their psychosexual outcomes compared to women with the more severe salt-losing form.

In general, newborns with ambiguous genitalia from CAH have a normal uterus and ovaries and should be raised as females. In cases of bilateral testicular dysgenesis where a vagina and uterus are present, female assignment may be desirable. Likewise, in cases of complete androgen insensitivity syndrome, a female orientation is correct. For most other instances of partial resistance, it is desirable to opt for male rearing. Male rearing is also appropriate when a deficit in 5α-reductase is identified since further virilization occurs during puberty. In cases where ovarian function can be preserved, female assignment is preferable for these cases of ovotesticular DSD. When a decision for female rearing is made in 46XY DSD, removal of testicular tissue is performed. If raised as males, careful follow-up is important due to the increased risk of gonadal tumors.

Newer research identifying the genetic and molecular etiologies of DSD has helped further our understanding of these complex conditions. In children born with a DSD condition, a methodical and thorough understanding of the physical exam, hormonal, radiographic, genetic, and psychological investigations is required for the proper diagnosis and management. Regardless, the decision regarding gender assignment has life-long implications and requires an open dialogue between the family and the child's caregivers.

Summary Points

- The term "intersex" has been replaced by disorder of sexual development (DSD).
- The differential diagnosis is often quite overwhelming at first, so a systematic multidisciplinary approach is important.
- Up to one half of boys with hypospadias and cryptorchidism will have a DSD.
- The most important initial physical finding is the presence and number of gonads.
- A uterus may be palpable on digital rectal examination.
- In the immediate newborn period, all patients require a karyotype and laboratory evaluation.
- An ultrasound should be the first radiologic exam obtained.

Editor's Comment

Few diagnoses generate more profoundly difficult ethical, emotional, psychological, and physical issues for patients and their parents than that of a disorder of sexual development. For parents, the most immediate problem is sex assignment. They need to be able to answer the question that is invariably the first one to be asked of them: "Is it a boy or girl?" The work up needs to be quick but thorough, before a rash and potentially regrettable decision is made. Sex assignment was traditionally made by the medical professionals involved (predominantly men) often in a paternalistic and categorical fashion, without input from the parents and without regard for issues related to sexual identity or psychosocial development. For the most part, if the child had a phallus, the assignment was male, and if there was no phallus (or an inadequate phallus), the assignment was female. Many of these patients eventually suffered greatly as they entered adolescence and adulthood because of inescapable feelings of having been erroneously assigned. Today, though the decision is still very difficult, more is known about the physiology of the disorders, parents are given much more of a say in the decision-making process, and, most importantly, patients are treated with considerably more compassion and acceptance than they were in the past.

Care of the child with a DSD should involve a multidisciplinary team that includes pediatric urology, endocrinology, genetics, psychology/psychiatry, and social work. Families need a great deal of emotional support and it is always best to include them as integral members of the team. The work up should be evidence-based and systematic, such that the initially overwhelming differential diagnosis can be pared down quickly and appropriately and the parents can best decide how to proceed. It cannot be overemphasized that these situations need to be handled tactfully and with the utmost empathy. Every word overheard by the parents will be scrutinized and if misinterpreted can lead to deep resentment and anger.

Differential Diagnosis

- (See Table 89.1 and Fig. 89.1)

Diagnostic Studies

- Karyotype
- Laboratory studies:
  - Serum electrolytes
  - 17-Hydroxyprogesterone (17OHP)
  - Testosterone
  - Dihydrotestosterone (DHT)
  - Luteinizing hormone (LH)
  - Follicle stimulation hormone (FSH)
- Medical imaging:
  - Ultrasound
  - CT
  - MRI
- Examination under anesthesia
- Diagnostic laparoscopy

Parental Preparation

- The list of possible diagnoses is long and we will need to perform several tests to identify the specific disorder.
- There is a great deal of support available to you from parents and patients who have had to deal with a similar situation.
- Though we recognize it is not ideal, the sex assignment might change over time, depending on information about the diagnosis and the sexual identity of the child.

Suggested Reading

Handa N, Nagasaki A, Tsunoda M, et al. Yolk sac tumor in a case of testicular feminization syndrome. J Ped Surg. 1995;30:1366.

Houk CP, Hughes IA, Ahmed SF, Lee PA, Writing Committee for the International Intersex Consensus Conference Participants. Summary of consensus statement on intersex disorders and their management. Pediatrics. 2006;118:753.

Minto CL, Liao KLM, Conway GS, Creighton SM. Sexual function in women with complete androgen insensitivity syndrome. Fertil Steril. 2003;80:157.

White PC, Speiser PW. Congenital adrenal hyperplasia due to 21-hydroxylase deficiency. Endocr Rev. 2000;21:245.

Wisniewski AB, Migeon CJ, Malouf MA, Gearhart JP. Psychosexual outcome in women affected by congenital adrenal hyperplasia due to 21-hydroxylase deficiency. J Urol. 2004;171:2497.

Chapter 90
Vagina: Diseases and Treatment

Edward J. Doolin

The diseases and anomalies of the vagina are varied and have widespread and long-lasting implications. Early in life much attention is given to the function of the urinary tract while later in life menstruation, sexual function, and fertility become more significant issues. As such, developing approaches to these diseases must take into account both the urinary and reproductive concerns as well as the two disparate time frames. The surgeon has to perform reconstructions and orchestrate therapies that will be feasible in infancy and create a reasonable lifestyle as a functional adult.

A review of the development and anatomy of the vagina is helpful in understanding the diseases and planning therapy (Fig. 90.1). In the undifferentiated stage two parallel systems, the mesonephric duct and the mullerian duct exist. As differentiation progresses, the mullerian ducts advance caudally. The proximal ducts become the fallopian tubes and, as they fuse, the distal ducts become the uterus. Most caudally the fused ducts advance as the proximal part of the vagina. This continues to descend and acquires the epithelium of the urogenital sinus (the residua of the mesonephric duct, Fig. 90.2). The distal part of this fusion is Müller's tubercle. A transverse diaphragm forms at Müller's tubercle called the hymen. This is a perforate protector of the vagina. The distal vagina arises from the urogenital sinus. The urogenital sinus also meets the external genitalia, forming the vagina. The hymen separates the external vaginal orifice from the internal vagina.

The external examination of the genitalia and vaginal orifice can be very important. This is difficult in infancy and the small size and variability of appearance in children require careful scrutiny. However, thoughtful evaluation can supply a great deal of information. The hymen will be the first part of the vaginal exam. It can be quite varied in appearance. Despite this the location of the hymen, whether or not it is patent and the presence of a vaginal orifice can be easily assessed.

E.J. Doolin (✉)
Department of Pediatric General and Thoracic Surgery,
Children's Hospital of Philadelphia, Philadelphia, PA, USA
e-mail: doolin@email.chop.edu

Vaginal Atresia

Inadequate vaginal development can present in many forms and at any age. These anomalies can exist in isolation or coexist with associated anomalies of the urinary system, hindgut or the reproductive system. Several approaches to classification have been proposed. Many of these are formed from the disease category that is being studied. Vaginal anomalies can be a part of a complex of urogenital anomalies, persistent cloaca, disorders of sexual differentiation, or anal atresia. However, to understand the development of pure vaginal anomalies the Mullerian classification system of Rock is probably the most useful. Vaginal maldevelopment can present as a completely absent vagina (1:10,000 births). Usually this is suspected early because of the abnormal hymen; however it might not present until later as primary amenorrhea and abdominal pain. The Mayer-Rokitansky-Kuster-Houser syndrome refers to an absent vagina and rudimentary upper reproductive elements. Chromosomes are usually normal, as are the ovaries; however gonadal dysgenesis has been reported.

Surgical treatment is largely focused on restoring a functional vagina. Three basic approaches include: progressive dilatations, skin grafts, and autograft substitutes. The initial anatomy, surgeon preference, and the internal reproductive structures will all contribute factors dictating the best choice. Since most of these patients have a vestigial external vagina, there is a beginning dimple that lends itself to progressive dilatations. This has a remarkable success rate and can be considered the best option in a motivated patient without another anomaly that requires surgery.

The surgical creation of a cavity in the prerectal space and ultimate grafting of skin has the advantage of a rapid result although frequent dilatations are still required (Fig. 90.3). However, skin grafts are not optimal. A donor sight is required, which is unsightly and painful. The epithelium lacks some of the elements of a normal vagina such as elasticity and mucus production. Also, the donor site might limit the size and shape of the neovagina. Ideally these reconstructions will be created with cells that are similar to vaginal

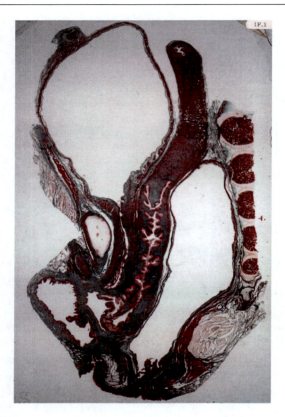

Fig. 90.1 A rare whole-mount image of the vaginal anatomy. Of particular importance are the space between the vagina (V) and rectum (R), making this an easy area to operate, and the lack of such a plane between the vagina and urethra (U). B – bladder (Stephens FD, Photographic album of anorectal anomalies and sphincter muscles prepared by Kascot Media Chicago Illinois 1987. This is the property of the Department of General Surgery, Children's Memorial Hospital 2400 Fullerton Ave, Chicago IL 60614. Reprinted courtesy of Dr. Stephens)

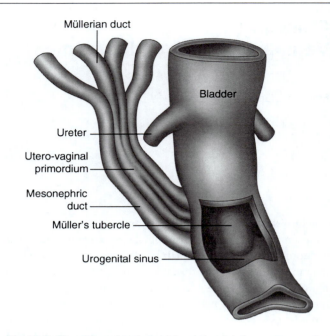

Fig. 90.2 The early embryology of the vagina. It is important to realize that the walls of the vagina come from Mullerian mesoderm but the mucosa is from urinary epithelium (reprinted with permission from Arey LB. Developmental anatomy: a textbook and laboratory manual of embryology. Philadelphia: WB Saunders; 1974)

cells. Graft engineering offers such a possibility. Even in complete vaginal atresia the perineal plate provides a good source of such epithelial cells. The size and shape of the graft can be prefabricated and tailored to the individual.

Finally, in many situations the use of adjacent organ grafts such as bladder and sigmoid colon can be considered as pedicle grafts (Fig. 90.4).

Transverse vaginal obstructions are less common. It is probably an incomplete fusion of the mullerian duct component and the urogenital sinus component of the distal vagina. These are largely found between the upper and middle third of the vaginal canal (Fig. 90.5). These are rarely associated with other urinary or pelvic anomalies. In the neonate, maternal hormonal stimulation can result in hydrometrocolpos. This causes an abdominal mass which can impact the respiration of the child. This mass can also have a secondary effect on the ureters and upper urinary system. In other patients the symptoms may present at puberty with primary amenorrhea and cyclic pain. Ultrasound and other studies are diagnostic. The treatment of transverse vaginal septae is perineal incision of the septum.

The most common and mild of these transverse obstructions is an imperforate hymen. Although this might be detected early, due to the varied appearance of the introitus in infants, it often presents as primary amenorrhea and abdominal pain. Examination demonstrates a bulging hymen. Ultrasound is confirmatory. Although this is easily diagnosed on exam, the use of ultrasound is valuable to rule out a partial vaginal atresia, caudal regression, or mullerian anomaly, any one of which can complicate treatment. Once this has been studied, hymenotomy is curative.

The distal third of the vagina obtains its epithelium from the urogenital sinus. When this development fails the proximal vagina terminates into the persistent urogenital sinus or urethra. This results in a common channel, which leads to the urethra and the superior vagina.

Tumors

Sarcoma botryoides is one of the most common solid tumors of childhood. Sarcoma botryoides is a subtype of embryonal rhabdomyosarcoma. This is the most common tumor of the lower urogenital tract in girls. It presents as a vaginal mass, usually in children less than 3 years of age. There is a second spike in incidence in adolescence. At this age it can arise from either the vagina or occasionally the cervix. This is one of five histologic types which is a polypoid form. Myxoid changes

Fig. 90.3 The use of a free skin graft and stent. The form used is a foam block or other expandable device to allow for secure placement of the graft (reprinted from Rock JA. Surgery for anomalies of the Mullerian ducts. In: Rock JA, Thompson JD, editors. TeLinde's operative gynecology. 8th ed. Philadelphia: Lippincott-Raven; 1997. p. 687–729, with permission)

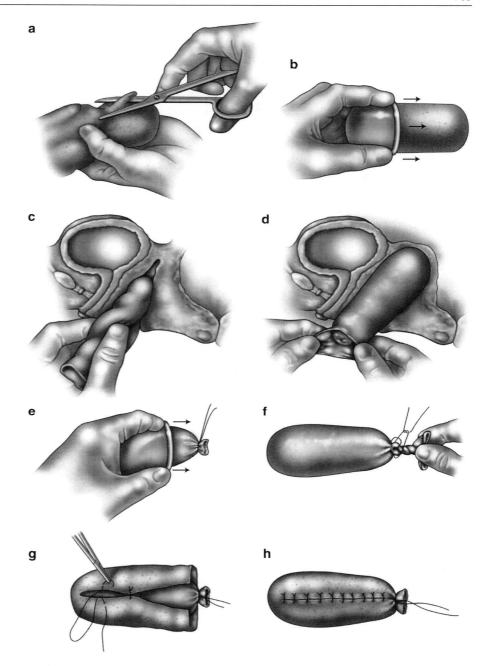

are seen and mitoses are moderate. It is a characteristic of these tumors to have a relatively acellular myxoid center and a highly cellular subepithelial area protruding against the mucosa of the vaginal.

This tumor presents as an obvious or bleeding lesion because of its superficial location. The site of origin is usually the urogenital sinus being anterior and distal. Endoscopy and biopsy are the means of diagnosis. Pan-endoscopy including the urethra and rectum will help in establishing the extent.

Treatment uses multiple modalities. Initial chemotherapy is with vincristine, adriamycin, and cyclophosphamide (VAC), which usually results in a dramatic reduction in the size of the

tumor and allows for less radical surgery. If there is no response to chemotherapy then radiation can be attempted.

Endodermal sinus tumor is usually considered a tumor of the ovary. Yolk sac in origin, the tumor would be expected to appear in a gonad; however, it can rarely be found in the vagina during infancy. Biopsy is needed for diagnosis to avoid confusion with sarcoma botryoides and other causes of vaginal bleeding or mass. The histology is marked by a reticular pattern of spaces, papillae formation, and hyaline globules. Surgery is the initial treatment; however because of the difficulty of the location and effectiveness of chemotherapy, surgery should be conservative and the vaginal structure preserved.

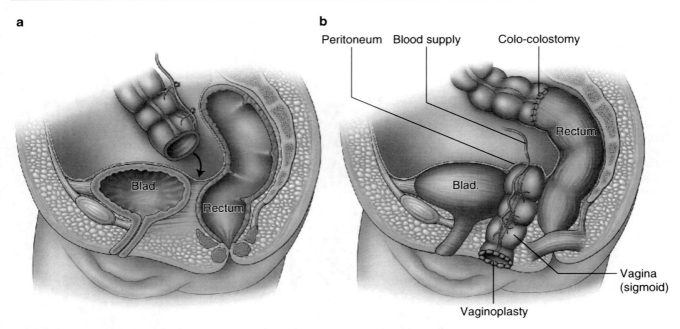

Fig. 90.4 The use of a sigmoid colon pedicle graft for the development of a vagina (reprinted from Parsons JK, Gearhart SL, Gearhart JP. Vaginal reconstruction using sigmoid colon: complications and long term results. J Pediatr Surg. 2002;37(4):630, with permission)

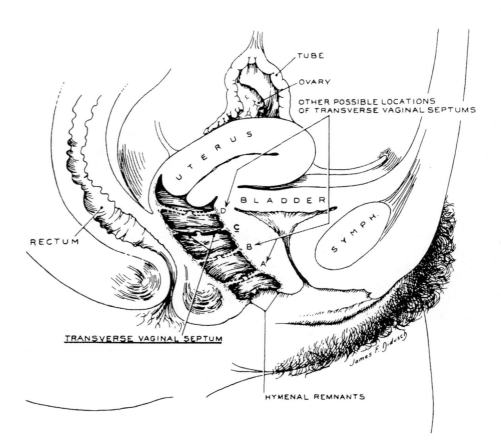

Fig. 90.5 Location of transverse vaginal septations (reprinted from Bowmen JA, Scott RB. Transverse vaginal septum, report of four cases. Obstet Gynecol. 1954:3444, with permission)

Trauma

Accidental injuries of the vagina arise from either blunt impact or penetration. The severity of these injuries has been graded by the American Association for the Surgery of Trauma: Grade I is a contusion or hematoma; Grade II is a superficial laceration (skin only); Grade III is a deep laceration into the adjacent fat and muscle; Grade IV is an avulsion injury; and Grade V includes injury of adjacent organs (urethra, rectum).

The most common circumstance that causes injury to the vaginal and vulvar area is straddle injuries. This causes compression of the vulva and vaginal orifice against the symphisis pubis and rami. One result is a vulvar hematoma. These rarely require treatment and will often resolve. Care to assure good urination and absence of urethral injury is needed. Linear lacerations of the perineum are the other result. These can extend into the vagina. Often assessment needs to be performed under anesthesia. Lacerations rarely involve critical structures. However, if surgery can be performed without delay, primary repair can shorten the time of healing and reduce pain. If the object straddled has a projection, then an impalement injury may result. This increases the risk of significant intravaginal injury and therefore evaluation under anesthesia is needed. In addition, careful assessment of the urinary and rectal area is needed.

Sexual Abuse

The second most common cause of injury is physical abuse. This can be in the form of a sexual aggression or as a component of general physical abuse. The majority of children who have suffered this type of trauma have minimal physical findings. Often the symptoms of bleeding or infection or the history of the child is what brings such injury to the attention of a physician. It is often difficult to make the differentiation between accidental injury and abuse, especially in the very young. Detailed examination under anesthesia is a large component of the evaluation. Colposcopy has played a large role in accurate assessment in the prepubertal child.

Foreign Body

In children with a vaginal foreign body, symptoms are often nondescript: pain, bleeding or discharge. The history is difficult to obtain with a positive recollection of the event in less than half of the cases. This statistic is improved after the foreign body is identified. With such challenges a diagnosis can often be elusive. In a population such as this, the presence of a foreign body must always be considered and often explains the unexplainable. In general this occurs in children ages 2 years to adult with the majority occurring before age seven. Work up includes physical exam, including the genitalia in a cooperative patient, plain radiographs, MRI, and exam under anesthesia in the younger patient when the other studies are not productive. In the older patient, self-induced foreign bodies, especially tissue paper, are common. In the younger patient a friend or sibling is usually involved and objects such as toys are often found.

Summary Points

- When managing vaginal anomalies, much attention is given early in life to the function of the urinary tract, while later in life menstruation, sexual function, and fertility become more significant issues.
- Vaginal anomalies can be a part of a complex of urogenital anomalies, persistent cloaca, disorders of sexual differentiation, or anal atresia.
- Three basic approaches to vaginal agenesis include: progressive dilatations, skin grafts, and autograft substitutes.
- Sarcoma botryoides is a subtype of embryonal rhabdomyosarcoma and is the most common tumor of the lower urogenital tract in girls.
- The most common circumstance that causes injury to the vaginal and vulvar area is straddle injuries, which cause compression of the vulva and vaginal orifice against the symphisis pubis and rami.
- In children with a vaginal foreign body, symptoms are often nondescript: pain, bleeding or discharge.

Editor's Comment

Pediatric general surgeons and urologists are frequently called upon to evaluate the young girl with a vaginal abnormality, including congenital anomalies, tumors, injuries, and foreign bodies. Imperforate hymen presents as hydrocolpos in young girls or hydrometrocolpos in pubescent females. The vagina can become quite large, sometimes palpable above the pubis as a mass. The diagnosis should be suspected in girls with abdominal pain and amenorrhea and is confirmed with a simple bedside examination in which the hymen is seen to be bulging and tense. Ultrasound is also frequently performed. The treatment is a cruciate incision (or excision) of the hymen in the operating room, in which case a large amount of dark brown fluid is often evacuated. The vagina will usually return to a normal size over time. After opening the hymen, one should examine the vagina carefully, as it is not uncommon to find a double vagina in which one hymen is patent and the other is imperforate. The longitudinal septum should be excised and the subsequent incisions on the anterior and posterior walls oversewn with absorbable suture. Most also have a duplicated uterus (two cervices) and eventually need to have an MRI or diagnostic laparoscopy to characterize their internal anatomy for fertility counseling purposes.

Sarcoma botryoides of the vagina presents as a fungating polypoid lesion and if stage I generally has a very good prognosis with chemotherapy alone. The surgeon's role is limited to biopsy to confirm the diagnosis and to exclude the rare endodermal sinus tumor. Further surgery is rarely indicated. Urethral prolapse is sometimes confused for a tumor and though there are numerous reports recommending surgical excision, as long as urinary flow is not obstructed, most can be treated with topical application of estrogen cream. Sarcoma of the uterus or cervix is also sometimes seen but is extremely rare. Vaginal foreign bodies usually consist of tissue paper or toys. It should be suspected in girls with vaginal bleeding, discharge, or itching. The history is almost never helpful. The mass can sometimes be identified on rectal examination but examination under anesthesia is usually warranted. MRI has also proven useful but if the child needs general anesthesia for the study, EAU might be more practical. In the operating room, examination of a prepubescent girl with a standard speculum is impossible. One can sometimes adequately assess the entire vagina using a nasal speculum and good lighting, but the best approach is to perform vaginoscopy using a small bronchoscope. This provides an excellent view and allows the hymen to remain intact, which is enormously important to some parents.

Perineal lacerations after straddling injuries are quite common. Most will heal without intervention. Indications for surgical repair under general anesthesia include bleeding, pain, urinary retention, obvious severe injury, or inability to fully assess the extent of injury in the office or ED. A careful examination under moderate sedation might save everyone a trip to the OR. Even moderate to severe injuries that involve the perineal body or rectal sphincter can usually be repaired primarily in layers with absorbable sutures. Colostomy should never be considered except perhaps in the rare case of severe rectal injury with devitalized tissue, gross fecal contamination, or delayed presentation. If there is any question of sexual abuse, a rape kit should be employed and the injuries should be carefully documented and photos taken.

Crohn's disease can sometimes affect the vulva and vagina with a spectrum of lesions from ulcers to fistulae or frank tissue destruction. Treatment is with anti-inflammatory drugs although fecal diversion is sometimes necessary. Severe acute herpetic lesions are sometimes seen and the possibility of sexual abuse must be investigated. Likewise, perivulvar condylomata acuminata often require surgical excision and certainly warrant investigation of inappropriate sexual contact.

Diagnostic Studies

- Pelvic ultrasound
- Magnetic resonance imaging
- Examination under anesthesia
- Vaginoscopy
- Diagnostic laparoscopy

Parental Preparation

- Vaginal anomalies are often associated with anomalies of the uterus, fallopian tubes and ovaries, which will need to be evaluated with US, MRI, or diagnostic laparoscopy.
- Examination of the vagina in a child is a delicate but safe procedure and injury to the vagina or hymen is very rare.
- In the vast majority of cases, repair of a perineal laceration should allow proper healing with minimal, if any, deleterious effect on future sexual and obstetrical function.

Suggested Reading

Adams JA, Kaplan RA, Starling SP, Mehta NH, Finkel MA, Botash AS, et al. Guidelines for medical care of children who may have been sexually abused. J Pediatr Adolesc Gynecol. 2007;20:163–72.

Berenson AB, Heger AH, Hayes JM, Bailey RK, Emans SJ. Appearance of the hymen in prepubertal girls. Pediatrics. 1992;89(3):387–94.

Borkowski A, Czaplicki M, Dobronski P. Twenty years of experience with Krzeski's cystovaginoplasty for vaginal agenesis in Mayer-Rokitansky-Kuster-Hauser syndrome: anatomical, histological, cytological and functional results. BJU Int. 2008;101:1433–40.

Deligeoroglou E, Deliveliotou A, Laggari V, Tsimaris P, Creatsas G. Vaginal foreign body in childhood: a multidisciplinary approach. J Paediatr Child Health. 2006;42:649–51.

Kihara M, Sato N, Kimura H, Kamiyama M, Sekiya S, Takano H. Magnetic resonance imaging in the evaluation of vaginal foreign bodies in a young girl. Arch Gynecol Obstet. 2001;265:221–2.

Moore EF, Jurjovich GJ, Knudson MM, et al. Organ injury scaling, VI extrahepatic. J Trauma. 1995;39:1069.

Naharaj NR, Nimako D, Hadley GP. Multimodal therapy for the initial management of genital embryonal rhabdomyosarcoma in childhood. Int J Gynecol Cancer. 2008;18:190–2.

Thomas J, Brock JW. Vaginal substitution: attempts to create the ideal replacement. J Urol. 2007;178:1855–9.

Part XII
Surgical Oncology

Chapter 91
Neuroblastoma

Natasha E. Kelly and Michael P. La Quaglia

Neuroblastoma accounts for 8–10% of all pediatric cancers and 15% of all pediatric cancer-related deaths. Seven hundred new cases are diagnosed in the United States each year. Two-thirds of the cases are diagnosed in children less than 5 years of age, and approximately one-third are in children younger than 1 year old. Neuroblastoma is more common in boys than girls (ratio 0.3:0.2) and is the most common neoplasm in infants and most common extracranial intra-abdominal solid tumor in childhood. Neuroblastoma is a solid tumor that begins in cells that are derived from the neural crest and are part of the sympathetic nervous system. It can arise in the neck, chest, abdomen, or pelvis, but most often in the abdomen (70%), with 40% arising from the adrenal medulla.

Neuroblasts are progenitor nerve cells derived from the neural crest cells found in the fetus that normally differentiate into nerve cells or adrenal medulla cells. However, neuroblasts that do not mature and continue to grow ultimately form tumors. Neuroblastoma rarely can be detected antenatally by ultrasonography. However, 70% of neuroblastomas are detected only after they have spread to lymph nodes, liver, lungs, bones, or bone marrow. Conversely, it can regress in certain patients with disseminated disease with favorable biological prognostic factors (stage 4S). The overall 5-year survival is around 69%.

Clinical Presentation

The clinical features of neuroblastoma are highly variable and depend on the primary tumor site, the degree of metastatic disease, or paraneoplastic syndromes. Approximately 40% of patients present with localized disease ranging from an incidentally discovered adrenal mass on prenatal ultrasonography to large locally invasive tumors along the sympathetic chain. Consequently, the most common presentation of neuroblastoma is an abdominal mass. Abdominal distention with respiratory compromise can sometimes occur secondary to massive liver metastasis in infants. In rare cases, some patients initially present with a varicocele, due to obstruction of the spermatic vein, and pelvic tumors can present with constipation or urinary tract symptoms. Massive abdominal tumors can present with neurological symptoms, such as extremity weakness, as a result of pressure or actual invasion of lumbosacral nerve plexuses.

The posterior mediastinum is the second most common site of origin, in which patients might present with respiratory symptoms of wheezing, cough, shortness of breath, or tachypnea. Respiratory symptoms precipitated by a pleural effusion require thoracentesis. The most common symptoms in high-risk patients are caused by tumor mass effect or bone pain due to metastasis. Proptosis and periorbital ecchymosis, also known as raccoon eyes or panda eyes, are common in this cohort of patients and are due to retrobulbar metastasis. Extensive bone marrow metastasis can cause pancytopenia, fever, and anemia. Metastatic skin nodules sometimes appear blue or purple (blueberry muffin appearance).

Since they originate in paraspinal ganglia, neuroblastomas in the thoracic, abdominal, or pelvic regions can invade the neural foramina and cause extradural compression of the spinal cord, resulting in lower extremity paralysis. Only 5% of newly diagnosed neuroblastoma patients will have neurological signs related to cord impingement such as motor weakness, pain, or sensory loss. Horner's syndrome can result from neuroblastoma in the stellate ganglion and, in the absence of an obvious cause, neuroblastoma should be ruled out in children with ptosis, miosis, enophthalmos, and anhidrosis.

Because it is one of the few cancers in children that secretes hormones, neuroblastoma can manifest as one of several paraneoplastic syndromes. Some neuroblastomas secrete catecholamines, resulting in hypertension. Tumors that secrete vasoactive intestinal peptide produce severe watery diarrhea and failure to thrive, which normally resolves after tumor excision. Opsoclonus-myoclonus-ataxia syndrome occurs in 2–4% of patients with neuroblastoma and appears to be due to an autoimmune disorder triggered by the tumor. These patients has a favorable outcome but 80% have

N.E. Kelly (✉)
Department of Pediatric Surgery, Memorial Sloan Kettering Cancer Center, New York, NY 10065, USA
e-mail: nkellymd@charter.net

long-term neurological deficits despite treatment with immunomodulating drugs and apheresis.

Diagnosis

The history and physical examination are critical to the diagnosis of patients suspected to have neuroblastoma. Initial workup includes a complete blood count to evaluate for anemia, as well as hepatic and renal function studies. Urine catecholamine metabolites including homovanillic acid (HVA) and vanillylmandelic acid (VMA) are also assessed. Serum catecholamine can also be evaluated but are not usually measured. Serum lactic dehydrogenase (LDH), neuron specific enolase (NSE), and ferritin are important prognostic indicators.

According to the International Neuroblastoma Staging System (INSS) Committee protocol, a definitive diagnosis of neuroblastoma requires either a positive bone marrow biopsy and elevated concentrations of urinary catecholamine metabolites, or a biopsy of the tumor itself. The type of biopsy performed will depend on the tumor location, and can be accomplished by CT-guided core biopsy, incisional biopsy, or excisional biopsy. A bone marrow biopsy is almost always performed for staging purposes.

Initial imaging workup usually begins with ultrasonography, which is often used to confirm the presence of a palpable abdominal or pelvic mass. Ultrasonography does not provide any characteristic radiologic information about neuroblastoma or the anatomic extent of the tumor, and does not usually allow the detection of distant metastasis. Computed tomography is the preferred imaging modality for tumors in the abdomen, pelvis, or mediastinum. When dealing with a paraspinous tumor, MRI is better for assessing invasion of the neural foramina and impingement of the spinal canal. Meta-iodobenzylguanidine (MIBG) is a particularly sensitive tool for evaluating the primary tumor and metastatic disease, as it is selectively concentrated in 90% of neuroblastomas. ^{123}I-MIBG provides better resolution than the ^{131}I isotope. Tc-diphosphonate bone scan is used to identify metastases to cortical bone. MIBG is also recommended for reassessment of high-risk patients with MIBG-avid disease during treatment and for long-term follow up. The sensitivity and specificity of PET with ^{18}fluorodeoxyglucose for detection and follow-up of metastatic disease is currently being evaluated.

Histopathology

In 1984, Shimada and colleagues developed a classification system that correlates histopathological features of the tumor to clinical behavior. These features, considered in the context of the age of the patient at diagnosis, are used to classify neuroblastomas based on the degree of neuroblast differentiation, Schwannian stroma content, and mitosis-karyorrhexis index (MKI). In general, tumors that are well-differentiated and have abundant stroma are more likely to be considered favorable.

Staging and Risk Stratification

The International Neuroblastoma Staging System is currently the standard and should be used to evaluate all new patients. The core of clinical staging is based on three factors: the extent of the primary tumor, loco-regional lymph node status, and the presence of distant metastases, but the extent of surgical resection of the primary and assessment of lymph node status are also considered important. Stage 1 tumors are generally localized to the organ of origin, completely resected with grossly negative margins, and with negative ipsilateral lymph node involvement (though the presence of positive lymph nodes that are adherent to and removed with the primary does not upstage the tumor). Stage 2 tumors are localized tumors that are either incompletely excised (2A) or associated with positive ipsilateral and unattached lymph nodes regardless of degree of resection (2B). Stage 3 tumors are unresectable tumors that cross the midline (opposite border of the vertebral column) *or* are associated with positive contralateral lymph nodes. Midline tumors with negative lymph nodes that are completely resected are usually considered stage 1. Stage 4 tumors are associated with dissemination to distant lymph nodes or other organs, most commonly bone marrow, bone, liver, skin or other organs. A special designation (4S) is given to infants with stage 1 or 2 primary tumors and metastases to the bone marrow (<10% replacement), liver and/or skin.

Even when age is considered, tumor stage alone does not predict prognosis in individual patients. To account for wide variations in tumor biology and to aid in the individualization of therapy (greatest benefit, least morbidity), the Children's Oncology Group currently uses the following characteristics to separate low-risk, intermediate-risk and high-risk tumors: (1) stage according to the INSS system, (2) age at diagnosis, (3) *MYCN* amplification status, and (4) tumor ploidy (DNA content) in children younger than 2 years old. Molecular genetics plays an important role and is a key component in risk stratification. *MYCN* amplification (more than 10 copies) is associated with a more aggressive cancer and poor outcome. This occurs in roughly 20% of primary tumors and is strongly correlated with advanced-stage disease and treatment failure. Other genetic findings that have been associated with more aggressive disease include the allelic loss of chromosome 1p and 11q and gain of chromosome 17q. DNA content (ploidy) is also a prognostic marker for patients less than

2 years of age with disseminated disease. DNA content has two categories: near diploid or hyperploid (near triploid). Near triploidy seems to be more favorable with genetic models, suggesting less aggressive tumors. On the other hand, near-diploid DNA content indicates a more aggressive variant of disease. Immunohistochemical staining for Trk A or CD44 expression may also assist in ascertaining tumor behavior, in that expression appears to confer an improved prognosis.

Neuroblastoma patients are thus classified as being low-risk, intermediate-risk, or high-risk based on these factors. Treatment is then tailored according to risk stratification. Low-risk patients are treated with surgery alone. Intermediate-risk patients are treated with surgery and chemotherapy. Within the intermediate-risk group, the duration of treatment also depends on the occurrence of the allelic loss of heterozygozity of chromosomes 1p and 11q. Several types of treatment modalities are used to treat patients with high-risk neuroblastoma due to the aggressiveness of the tumor in this subset of patients, but a typical regimen includes surgery, chemotherapy, radiation therapy, stem cell transplantation, and retinoids.

Treatment

There are four treatment strategies for neuroblastomas: surgery, chemotherapy, radiation therapy, and bone marrow/stem cell transplantation. The treatment is tailored according to the risk group to which the child's tumor has been assigned.

Surgery

Neuroblastomas can arise anywhere along the sympathetic chain, often posteriorly in the body and in close proximity to the spinal column or the great vessels. They often surround the aorta, vena cava, and major vascular branches. Complete surgical resection with negative microscopic margins is almost impossible because of the proximity of the tumor to these very important structures. Resection of all grossly visible and palpable tumor (gross total resection) is therefore the goal. Several studies have reported that gross total resection improved local tumor control and increased overall survival in patients with stage 3 or 4 disease.

Chemotherapy

Chemotherapy is used as one of the primary treatment modalities for neuroblastoma, both prior to surgery, to minimize tumor burden and make the resection more amenable to

gross total resection, and after surgery, to destroy any residual malignant cells. For patients with intermediate-risk neuroblastoma, the drugs most commonly used include combinations of cisplatin, cyclophosphamide, doxorubicin, and etoposide. For patients with high-risk neuroblastoma, combinations of cyclophosphamide, ifosfamide, cisplatin, vincristine, doxorubicin, melphalan, etoposide , teniposide, and topotecan are used more commonly.

Radiation Therapy

The most common type of radiation treatment is external-beam radiation therapy. However at some centers, intra-operative therapy is used to administer higher doses of radiation directly to the tumor bed in patients with high-risk or recurrent disease.

Bone Marrow/Stem Cell Transplantation

For most children with high-risk neuroblastoma, a more aggressive chemo- and radiation therapy regimen is used, followed by bone marrow rescue with peripheral stem cells harvested from the patient early in the course of their therapy.

Retinoid Therapy

To treat chemotherapy-resistant tumor cells, 13-*cis*-retinoic acid has been used to induce differentiation of high-risk neuroblastoma following completion of consolidation therapy.

Immunotherapy

GD2 is a disialoganglioside compound that is highly expressed on the cell membrane of most neuroblastomas. Ongoing clinical trials are currently assessing tumor-targeted immunotherapy with anti-GD2 monoclonal antibodies that are coupled with cytotoxic cytokines in patients with unresectable neuroblastoma.

Radionuclides Therapy

Recent research demonstrated a response with ^{131}I-MIBG therapy when neuroblastoma recurs. Therefore, a new clinical trial is ongoing within the COG to evaluate ^{131}I-MIBG with high-dose chemotherapy and subsequent stem cell transplant in patients with high-risk neuroblastoma.

Recurrent Neuroblastoma

Treatment of patients with recurrent neuroblastoma remains a clinical challenge and depends primarily on location of tumor recurrence and the aggressiveness of the new tumor. Despite treatment, neuroblastoma recurs in more than 50% of patients with high-risk disease. The following new therapies show promise for treating these patients:

For early neuroblastoma recurrence, cytotoxic agents such as the topoisomerase 1 inhibitors topotecan and irinotecan are used. Low-dose cyclophosphamide synergistically enhances the efficacy of topotecan. The concurrent use of irinotecan and temozolomide is currently being studied in Phase III clinical trials.

Also under evaluation for patients with recurrent neuroblastoma are immunotherapeutic agents such as G_{D2}-Interleukin 2 fusion molecule, ^{131}I-anti-G_{D2} antibody, and several other monoclonal antibodies directed against the G_{D2} antigen. Several other immunologic modulators such as DNA, cellular, anti-idiotypic vaccines and cytolytic T lymphocytes for cellular immunotherapy are currently being studied in Phase I and II clinical trials.

Ongoing additional Phase I and II clinical trials include the use of vascular endothelial growth factor (VEGF) inhibitors, CEP-701 (an inhibitor of Trk tyrosine kinase), inhibitors of the epidermal growth factor receptor (EGFR), demethylating agents such as decitabine, and histone deacetylase inhibitors.

International consensus now exists to use a unified international risk stratification schema in neuroblastoma. This new stratification system is being developed by the International Neuroblastoma Risk Group, which is defining more cogent and cohesive patient groups that will ultimately allow clinicians to better tailor treatment of their patients. A complete history and physical exam, serologic studies, and relevant radiologic imaging are instrumental in assessing risk stratification. Molecular genetic evaluation is also essential and requires an appropriate amount of tissue on initial biopsy.

Summary Points

- Neuroblastoma accounts for 8–10% of all pediatric cancers and 15% of all the cancer-related deaths in children. Neuroblasotma's clinical features are highly variable and depend on the primary tumor site, the degree of metastatic disease, or paraneoplastic syndromes.
- Forty percent of patients present with localized disease ranging from an incidentally discovered adrenal mass on prenatal ultrasonography to large locally invasive tumors along the sympathetic chain.
- The most common presentation of neuroblastoma is an abdominal mass.
- Diagnosis depends on history and physical exam, biochemical tests, urinary catecholamines, tissue biopsy or bone marrow biopsy with aspirate.
- Imaging modalities include CT scan, MRI, MIBG scan, Bone scan and PET scan for further workup.
- Treatment involves combination regimens of surgery, chemotherapy, radiotherapy, immunotherapy and stem cell transplant.
- Overall 5 year survival is 69%, but stage 4 disease 5 year survival remains less than 50%, range 10–40%.

Editor's Comment

Surgical management of neuroblastoma depends a great deal on anatomic location and stage. Cervical tumors that encase major vessels, compress the trachea, or encroach on the base of the skull are considered unresectable and a neoadjuvant approach is recommended. Likewise, tumors that extend into the chest are rarely initially resectable. At exploration for resectability, nerve stimulation should be used and muscle relaxants withheld. A transverse cervical incision placed in a skin crease usually provides the best exposure. Every effort should be made to preserve the carotid artery, internal jugular vein, and major nerves, including the brachial plexus and vagus nerve. Resection of low cervical lesions are likely to produce a Horner's syndrome and this should be discussed preoperatively with the family. Tumors that straddle the thoracic inlet sometimes require a trap-door incision and place the patient at significant risk of major vessel and nerve injury.

Most thoracic paraspinous tumors are low risk and therefore aggressive attempts at initial resection are not necessary unless the tumor can be resected easily without injury to adjacent structures. Nevertheless, an attempt should be made to remove between 50 and 90% of the mass, usually through a posterolateral thoracotomy. In some cases, a thoracoscopic approach is acceptable. The rare high-risk tumor should be more aggressively resected, including rib resection, if necessary. The phrenic, vagus, and recurrent laryngeal nerves and major vascular structures must be spared. There is high risk of Horner's syndrome when resecting apical tumors and thoracic duct injuries when the tumor infiltrates the mediastinum.

Abdominal neuroblastomas arise from the adrenal gland, the sympathetic ganglia (paraspinous), or the root of the mesentery. Small resectable tumors can be resected using a standard approach or laparoscopically. Lymph node status must be assessed properly. Most are unresectable and either intermediate or high risk, making a neoadjuvant approach the only option. They frequently encase the major branches of the aorta and sometimes penetrate into the spinal canal through the neural foramina. Spinal involvement should be assessed preoperatively with MRI and neurosurgical consultation obtained in the event laminectomy is needed for spinal decompression or tumor resection. Major vessels should be preserved and normal organs should not be removed.

Tumors that arise in the pelvis are usually located near the aortic bifurcation (organ of Zuckerkandl) or pelvic sidewall (sympathetic ganglia), where aggressive attempts at resection can be morbid. These tumors are usually associated with an excellent prognosis regardless of the extent of resection, which makes it preferable to leave residual tumor rather than risk injury to the bowel, bladder, ureters, major blood vessels or any of the numerous adjacent nerves and plexuses. Consideration should be given to using nerve monitoring for tumors near the pelvic side wall. Depending on the location of the tumor, a lower midline or low transverse incision may be used to provide adequate exposure.

Resection of the primary tumor in patients with 4S disease is usually not required. Biopsy of metastases in the liver or skin can provide enough tissue to confirm the diagnosis and conduct biological studies for proper risk grouping. Operative decompression of the abdomen is occasionally required for patients with massive hepatomegaly due to tumor infiltration and severe respiratory compromise who do not respond to emergent administration of chemotherapeutic agents.

Tumors that invade the spinal canal can cause paraplegia or paraparesis by either direct compression or intraspinal hemorrhage, the latter a risk when aggressive attempts are made to remove tumor from the neural foramina anteriorly. Patients who present with signs of spinal infiltration and who do not respond to emergent chemotherapy are candidates for urgent laminectomy and removal of tumor from the epidural space by a neurosurgeon. It is not necessary to attempt concomitant resection of the anterior portion of the mass, which is treated neoadjuvantly. In the rare circumstance in which gross total resection is felt to be necessary, putting the patient at risk for intraspinal hemorrhage, prophylactic decompressive laminectomy should be considered. Monitoring of somatosensory evoked potentials (SSEP) might also be prudent.

Inadvertent injuries to major vascular structures should be repaired. If primary repair is not feasible, the vessel should be repaired with a patch graft using autologous material or bypassed. Basic principles of vascular surgical repair should be practiced. Ureteral injuries should be repaired over a stent. Transected major nerves should be repaired primarily with the aid of magnification. Irreparable injuries of the renal artery pose a significant problem. Obvious renal ischemia can be due to vasospasm, which is temporary, but might also be due to thrombosis or emboli, in which case it is not likely to improve with time and can cause intractable severe hypertension and eventual cardiac failure. When in doubt, it is probably best to leave the kidney, though the possibility of having to return to perform a nephrectomy needs to be discussed with the parents.

Differential Diagnosis

- Wilms Tumor
- Ganglioneuroma
- Rhabdomyosarcoma
- Lymphoma

Diagnostic Studies

- CT for mediastinum, abdomen and pelvis
- MRI for paraspinal lesions
- Meta-iodobenzylguanidine (MIBG)
- Bone scan (for MIBG-negative patient)
- Position emission tomography (PET)

Parental Preparation

- Thoracoabdominal incision with potential for massive hemorrhage secondary to tumor proximity to aorta, vena cava.
- Complications include hemorrhage, diarrhea, delayed peritonitis, chylous ascites.
- Intensive care unit monitoring.

Preoperative Preparation

☐ CBC, hepatic and renal function tests, urinary catecholamine metabolites

☐ CT scan, MRI, MIBG or bone scan

☐ Tissue biopsy or bone marrow biopsy with aspirate and urinary catecholamines

☐ Histopathology

☐ Molecular genetic; MYCN, DNA ploidy, allelic loss chromosome 1p and 11q

☐ Chemotherapy, radiotherapy, stem cell transplant or immunotherapy

Technical Points

• Stage 1 and 2 disease attempt gross total resection

• Stage 2b, 3 or 4 disease combination regimen of chemotherapy, immunotherapy, radiation then surgery

Suggested Reading

Adkins ES, Sawin R, Gerbing RB, London WB, Matthay KK, Haase GM. Efficacy of complete resection for high-risk neuroblastoma: a Children's Cancer Group study. J Pediatr Surg. 2004;39(6):931–6.

Bagatell R, Rumcheva P, London WB, et al. Outcomes of children with intermediate-risk neuroblastoma after treatment stratified by MYCN status and tumor cell ploidy. J Clin Oncol. 2005;23(34):8819–27.

Brodeur GM. Neuroblastoma: biological insights into a clinical enigma. Nat Rev Cancer. 2003;3(3):203–16.

Brodeur GM, Seeger RC, Schwab M, Varmus HE, Bishop JM. Amplification of N-myc in untreated human neuroblastomas correlates with advanced disease stage. Science. 1984;224(4653):1121–4.

Castel V, Tovar JA, Costa E, et al. The role of surgery in stage IV neuroblastoma. J Pediatr Surg. 2002;37(11):1574–8.

DeCou JM, Bowman LC, Rao BN, et al. Infants with metastatic neuroblastoma have improved survival with resection of the primary tumor. J Pediatr Surg. 1995;30(7):937–40.

Evans AE, Albo V, D'Angio GJ, et al. Factors influencing survival of children with nonmetastatic neuroblastoma. Cancer. 1976;38(2):661–6.

Haase GM, O'Leary MC, Ramsay NK, et al. Aggressive surgery combined with intensive chemotherapy improves survival in poor-risk neuroblastoma. J Pediatr Surg. 1991;26(9):1119–23.

La Quaglia MP. Surgical management of neuroblastoma. Semin Pediatr Surg. 2001;10(3):132–9.

La Quaglia MP, Kushner BH, Heller G, Bonilla MA, Lindsley KL, Cheung NK. Stage 4 neuroblastoma diagnosed at more than 1 year of age: gross total resection and clinical outcome. J Pediatr Surg. 1994;29(8):1162–5.

La Quaglia MP, Kushner BH, Su W, et al. The impact of gross total resection on local control and survival in high-risk neuroblastoma. J Pediatr Surg. 2004;39(3):412–7.

Maris JM, Hogarty MD, Bagatell R, Cohn SL. Neuroblastoma. Lancet. 2007;369(9579):2106–20.

Matthay KK, Blaes F, Hero B, et al. Opsoclonus myoclonus syndrome in neuroblastoma a report from a workshop on the dancing eyes syndrome at the advances in neuroblastoma meeting in Genoa, Italy, 2004. Cancer Lett. 2005;228(1–2):275–82.

Seeger RC, Brodeur GM, Sather H, et al. Association of multiple copies of the N-myc oncogene with rapid progression of neuroblastomas. N Engl J Med. 1985;313(18):1111–6.

Shimada H, Chatten J, Newton Jr WA, et al. Histopathologic prognostic factors in neuroblastic tumors: definition of subtypes of ganglioneuroblastoma and an age-linked classification of neuroblastomas. J Natl Cancer Inst. 1984;73(2):405–16.

Chapter 92
Wilms Tumor

Peter F. Ehrlich

Wilms tumor (WT), or nephroblastoma, is the most common primary malignant renal tumor of childhood. It is the second most common solid organ abdominal tumor encountered in childhood, accounting for 6% of all pediatric tumors. The annual incidence is 8.1 per million children. This results in 600–700 new cases each year in North America. Outcomes for children with WT have improved dramatically over the last 50 years, with long-term survival in both North America and European trials approaching 85%. Moreover, many of the low-stage tumors have survival rates between 95 and 99%. The treatment strategy for children with WT has also evolved. It is currently based on traditional risk factors, such as stage and histology, as well as genetic markers, response to therapy and consideration of the risk of late effects. The goal of "risk-based management" is to maintain excellent outcomes but to spare children with low-risk tumors the long-term side effects of intensive chemo- and radiation therapy and to use more intense therapy for high-risk tumors to minimize recurrence rates (Table 92.1). Risk-based therapy requires a multidisciplinary team that includes oncologists, radiologists, surgeons, radiation oncologists, pathologists, social workers and nurses. Surgeons play a critical role in diagnosis, staging and treatment, and their technical skill and judgment have a direct impact on therapeutic decision-making and patient outcome. The current outcome data for children with WT from the National Wilms Tumor Study are shown in Table 92.2.

A child with a Wilms tumor will most often come to medical attention because of a palpable abdominal mass. The differential diagnosis of an abdominal mass is extensive and includes neoplastic and non-neoplastic lesions. WT is the most frequent tumor of renal origin but other renal tumors encountered include clear cell sarcoma, rhabdoid tumors, renal cell carcinoma and mesoblastic nephroma.

The mean age at diagnosis is 3 years with most children presenting between the ages of one and four. WT rarely occurs in children under 6 months of age or over the age of ten. The mass is usually discovered by either a parent when dressing or bathing the child or by a pediatrician during a routine office visit. Twenty percent of children with WT have microscopic hematuria, 10% have a coagulopathy (acquired von Willebrand syndrome) and 20–25% present with hypertension due to activation of the renin-angiotensin system. Fever, anorexia and weight loss occur in approximately 10% of cases. In rare instances, a child may present with an acute abdomen due to tumor rupture and bleeding, often precipitated by seemingly minor trauma. Between 5 and 10% of tumors are bilateral and can be synchronous or metachronous. Bilateral tumors are more commonly found in children with a genetic predisposition to WT, for example Beckwith-Wiedemann and WAGR syndromes.

While children with neuroblastoma may appear ill and emaciated due to the release of vasoactive tumor peptides and catecholamines, the typical child with WT is an otherwise healthy-appearing child with an abdominal mass on examination. In 13–28% of cases, congenital anomalies (aniridia, genitourinary malformations, hemihypertrophy, or signs of overgrowth) are reported. The syndromes associated with the highest risk of developing WT include: WAGR syndrome (Wilms tumor, aniridia, genitourinary malformation, mental retardation), Beckwith-Wiedemann syndrome (gigantism, macroglossia, omphalocele), and Denys-Drash syndrome (nephropathy, gonadal dysgenesis, Wilms tumor). Other maladies that are associated with a higher risk of developing WT include hemihypertrophy, Klippel-Trénaunay-Weber, Perlman syndrome and genitourinary malformations.

Diagnosis

For the child with an abdominal mass, medical imaging allows us to narrow the differential diagnosis and provides valuable information regarding local extent and staging of the tumor (Fig. 92.1). Ultrasound (US) is an excellent screening examination as it is painless, requires little patient

P.F. Ehrlich(✉)
Department of Pediatric Surgery, University of Michigan, CS Mott Children's Hospital, Ann Arbor, MI 48104, USA
e-mail: pehrlich@med.umich.edu

Table 92.1 Wilms tumor: conceptual framework for risk based therapy

| Relapse-free survival (NWTS-5) | Potential for late effects | |
	Low	Moderate to high
Excellent (≥85%)	Stage I/II FHWT, LOH-	Stage I/II CCSK
		Stage III FHWT, LOH–
Good (75–84%)		Stage IV FHWT, LOH–
		Stage II AHWT
		Stage III CCSK
Unsatisfactory (<75%)	Stage I/II FHWT, LOH+	Stage III/IV FHWT, LOH+
	Stage I AHWT	Stage III/IV AHWT
	Stage I–IV RCC	Stage V WT
		Stage IV CCSK
		Stage I–IV MRT
		Relapsed FHWT

This table represents current outcomes from the National Wilms Tumor Study 5 to the potential for late effects by stage and histology of the tumors

NWTS National Wilms Tumor Study; *FHWT* familial histology Wilms tumor; *AHWT* anaplastic histology Wilms tumor; *LOH* loss of heterozygosity; *CCSK* clear cell sarcoma of the kidney; *MRT* malignant rhabdoid tumor

Table 92.2 Four year overall survival from NWTS-5 by stage and histology

Stage	FHWT (%)	AHWT (%)	CCSK (%)	MRT (%)
I	98.3	82.5	100	50
II	97.4	82.6	88.9	33.3
III	93.9	64.7	94.8	33.3
IV	85.6	33.3	47.7	21.4
V	80.8	43.8	N/A	0

NWTS National Wilms Tumor Study; *FHWT* familial histology Wilms tumor; *AHWT* anaplastic histology Wilms tumor; *CCSK* clear cell sarcoma of the kidney; *MRT* malignant rhabdoid tumor

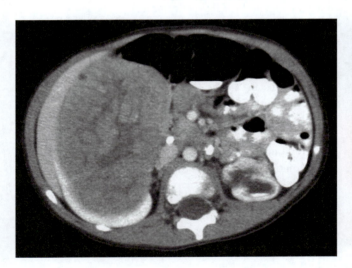

Fig. 92.1 A computed tomography scan of a large righted Wilms tumor

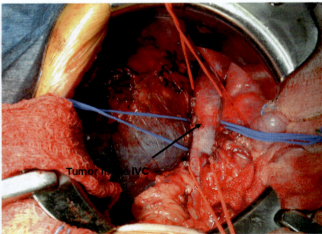

Fig. 92.2 An intraoperative picture of a Wilms tumor extending into the inferior vena cava. The inferior vena cava is isolated by vessel loops

preparation, does not use ionizing radiation and can usually help determine if the mass arises from the kidney. Color Doppler US imaging should be used routinely to assess the renal vein and inferior vena cava (IVC) for evidence of intravenous tumor extension (Fig. 92.2). It rarely extends down into the ureter. About 11% of patients with WT present with renal vein involvement, while 4% have IVC or atrial involvement. There have been reports of patient deaths due to embolism when unrecognized tumor thrombus has been dislodged during nephrectomy, highlighting the need to document this preoperatively. US is not sensitive enough to determine the full local extent of disease or for the identification of bilateral Wilms tumor or nephrogenic rests.

Computed tomography (CT) scan of the abdomen will confirm the renal origin of the mass and provide a better assessment of local extent of disease. Since common sites of metastatic spread of WT include the lungs and the liver, abdominal and pulmonary imaging should be included in the study.

Abdominal CT may also reveal or confirm the extent of renal and IVC tumor thrombus and is especially useful in demonstrating contralateral renal involvement. Early generations of CT scans missed perhaps as many as 10% of bilateral lesions and it was therefore always mandated that the surgeon explore the contralateral kidney prior to doing a nephrectomy for Wilms tumor. However, a recent review looking at the use of modern helical CT scan technology in patients with WT showed that only 0.25% of contralateral tumors failed to be identified and each was less than 1 cm in diameter. In fact, the newest surgical guidelines do not include mandatory formal exploration of the contralateral kidney at the time of the nephrectomy.

CT does not always allow us to differentiate WT from hyperplastic or sclerotic nephrogenic rests, benign lesions that can undergo malignant degeneration. Magnetic resonance imaging (MRI) can be helpful in this regard, but to date has not been shown to be superior to CT for baseline assessment. Likewise, though positron emission tomography (PET) appears to be useful in the work up of patients with cancer, including a few with WT, its role has yet to be defined.

With very few exceptions, a preoperative biopsy should never be done in a child with a renal tumor as this invariably results in tumor spillage and upstages the tumor to stage III. This may result in the child having to receive radiation therapy that might otherwise have been unnecessary.

Staging

The prognosis for children with Wilms tumor is affected by certain patient and tumor characteristics, the most important of which are histologic grade and tumor stage. Others include the age of the patient, the size of the tumor and whether the tumor demonstrates loss of heterozygosity.

Though WT is the most common renal tumor of childhood, the pediatric surgeon will occasionally encounter one of the rarer tumors, clear cell sarcoma of the kidney (CCSK), rhabdoid tumor (RTK), renal cell (adenocarcinoma) or mesoblastic nephroma. For a time, CCSK and RTK were thought to be histologic variants of WT but it is now clear that they are separate entities requiring distinct therapies. Mesoblastic nephroma is a benign hamartoma of the kidney. It is the most common renal neoplasm seen in the first 12 months of life, but since 20% of renal tumors in infants will turn out to be WT, the surgeon always assume that it could be a malignant tumor and rigorously adhere to surgical oncology standards.

The histology of a Wilms tumor is described as either *favorable* or *unfavorable*. Favorable tumors consist of blastemal, stromal and epithelial elements (Fig. 92.3). Unfavorable tumors are anaplastic and represent approximately 10% of all Wilms tumors (Fig. 92.4). Patients with favorable histology have a better overall survival for any given stage. Because

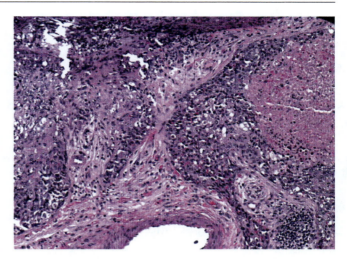

Fig. 92.3 A high power H and E stained micrograph of favorable histology Wilms tumor

anaplasia is a marker of tumor resistance and does not necessarily correlate with the biological aggressiveness of tumor, it is important that the pathologist note whether the anaplasia is focal or diffuse. For stage I tumors, any degree of anaplasia makes it unfavorable, whereas for stages II, III, or IV, only those tumors with diffuse anaplasia are considered unfavorable. Regardless of the histology, the completeness of surgical resection can determine the ultimate outcome.

The tumor stage is determined by the results of the imaging studies and both the surgical and pathologic findings at nephrectomy (Table 92.3). The staging system has been gradually revised as the features associated with prognosis have been defined. Patients are classified both by local stage, which pertains to the primary tumor, as well as disease stage. For example, a child with a small primary tumor confined to the kidney may have a local stage I tumor but could have distant metastases (stage IV) or a contralateral tumor (stage V). Likewise, the tumor may be "upstaged" by biopsy or spillage. Current therapy recommendations are based on a consideration of both the local stage and the disease stage.

Other factors that appear to affect prognosis are patient age and size of the primary tumor. For stage I tumors, children who are less than 2 years of age have a better overall survival than children who are older than two. And children with tumors that weigh less than 550 g have a better prognosis than those with larger tumors.

Loss of heterozygosity (LOH) refers to a chance loss of genetic material such that a defective allele inherited from one parent is no longer balanced by the functional one inherited from the other parent, leading to inactivation of tumor suppression genes in the tissue affected by the mutation. LOH on chromosomes 11p, 16q and 1p has been found in some children with WT. Retrospective studies suggest that children with LOH have poorer outcomes independent of stage or histology than those without LOH. This has been confirmed by at least one prospective study and as a result, ongoing Wilms tumor studies currently utilize LOH as a determinant of therapy.

Surgical Management

The standard surgical management of all patients with a unilateral renal tumor includes radical nephro-ureterectomy and retroperitoneal lymph node sampling. A transabdominal, transperitoneal incision is standard, as it provides adequate exposure for most tumors and access to the hilar vessels and retroperitoneal lymph nodes. For very large tumors or those that come off the superior pole and extend up to the diaphragm, a thoraco-abdominal incision that extends through the eighth or ninth intercostal space may be necessary. I place a bump under the child on the side of the tumor to improve the exposure. Immediately upon entering the

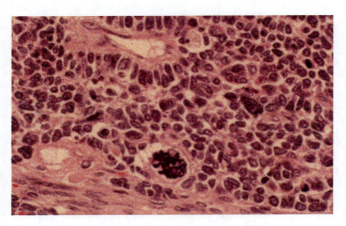

Fig. 92.4 A high power H and E stained micrograph of unfavorable histology (anaplastic)

abdomen, I perform a complete exploration of the abdomen to look for liver metastases, evidence of peritoneal seeding, signs of preoperative tumor rupture and presence of ascites. If preoperative imaging is satisfactory and does not suggest a bilateral process, routine exploration of the contralateral kidney is not necessary. On the other hand, if imaging studies are suggestive of a possible contralateral kidney lesion, the contralateral kidney should be formally explored both visually and by careful palpation to rule out bilateral involvement. This should be done *prior* to nephrectomy. Any areas suggestive of a contralateral tumor should be biopsied and sent for frozen section analysis. If positive for Wilms tumor, the nephrectomy should *not* be performed (see below).

Once the abdomen has been fully assessed, I begin to mobilize the kidney. The colon is mobilized to the midline and the bowel is reflected to expose the kidney. Wilms tumors can be very large and preliminary ligation of the renal artery and vein should not be pursued if technically difficult or dangerous. In these cases, after palpating the renal vein to rule out the presence of a tumor thrombus, I prefer to identify the ureter first and divide it as distally as possible. I then mobilize the kidney laterally, inferiorly and superiorly, coming to the hilum last so that the kidney is attached only by a vascular pedicle. Dissection needs to be gentle as these tumors are soft and the capsule can tear easily. If the capsule is violated or ruptured during mobilization of the tumor, tumor spillage is the result and needs to be documented as the patient will subsequently require postoperative radiation therapy. Obviously, this should be avoided if at all possible.

There are specific anatomic considerations depending on which side the tumor is located. On the right, the renal vein is short and easier to tear during dissection, and the adrenal vein is sometimes adherent to the tumor itself. To help expose the vein and IVC, it is useful to perform a Kocher maneuver. On

Table 92.3 National Wilms Tumor Study Group/Children Oncology Group Wilms tumor staging

Stage I
The tumor is limited to the kidney and has been completely resected
The tumor was not ruptured or biopsied prior to removal
No penetration of the renal capsule or involvement of renal sinus vessels

Stage II
The tumor extends beyond the capsule of the kidney but was completely resected with no evidence of tumor at or beyond the margins of resection
There is penetration of the renal capsule or
There is invasion of the renal sinus vessels

Stage III
Gross or microscopic residual tumor remains postoperatively including: inoperable tumor, positive surgical margins, tumor spillage surfaces, regional lymph-node metastases, positive peritoneal cytology or transected tumor thrombus
The tumor was ruptured or biopsied prior to removal

Stage IV
Hematogenous metastases or lymph-node metastases outside the abdomen (e.g., lung, liver, bone, brain)

Stage V
Bilateral renal involvement is present at diagnosis and each side may be considered to have its own stage

the left, the renal vein crosses over the aorta and the left gonadal and adrenal veins enter the renal vein directly. Mobilizing the spleen and pancreas superior and medial to the tumor will facilitate exposure for left-sided tumors. On either side, if the adrenal gland is adherent to the tumor it is best to remove it with the kidney rather than risk tumor spillage.

Once the renal vein is exposed, I carefully palpate the vein and IVC to rule out extension of tumor. If tumor extension is present, this should be removed en bloc with the kidney, prior to ligation of the vein. Note should be made of whether tumor penetrates the vessel wall or is attached to the intima. Patients with extension of tumor thrombus above the level of the hepatic veins should have a biopsy of the primary tumor followed by neo-adjuvant chemotherapy. This approach will often achieve significant shrinkage of the intravascular thrombus, facilitating subsequent surgical removal.

Laparoscopy

At present, there is no role for laparoscopy in the management of WT. A single case series that included eight cases has been published. Although the procedure was completed in four patients, the incision was the same size as that used for an open procedure. In most cases, the potential benefits of laparoscopy do not justify the combined risk of complications and spillage associated with trying to resect these typically large tumors. There may someday be a role for laparoscopy in patients with bilateral WT and small tumor that only require a partial nephrectomy.

Contiguous Organs

Wilms tumors typically displace adjacent organs, but frank invasion is rare. Tumors may be densely adherent to other structures but can usually be separated by careful dissection. En bloc resection, for example partial hepatectomy, is not generally warranted. A small section of diaphragm, psoas muscle or tip of the pancreas is acceptable and sometimes necessary. Extensive resection of multiple organs, such as spleen, pancreas and colon, is also not advised as this is associated with significant risk of complications. In these situations, a biopsy followed by chemotherapy will usually allow for a safer resection at a later date.

Lymph Node Documentation

The presence or absence of metastatic disease in hilar and regional lymph nodes is an extremely important factor in the accurate staging of a patient with WT. Children with positive lymph nodes are classified as stage III and they receive more intensive chemotherapy as well as abdominal radiation. It is therefore mandatory for the surgeon to routinely sample lymph nodes from the renal hilum and the pericaval or para-aortic areas. Tumor relapse diminish survival to 40%. Studies have highlighted two key factors that affect relapse: (1) failure to biopsy lymph nodes, which increases the local relapse rate greater than lymph node involvement itself (Relative risk 2.6 (1.1, 6.0)) and (2) tumor spillage (RR 2.86 (1.33–6.17)) even when correcting for histology, age and lymph node status. Failure to sample lymph nodes is a major technical error and has been noted to occur in 10–12% of operations for Wilms tumor. The implications of this omission are greatest for children under 2 years of age with stage I Wilms tumors that are less than 550 g. These children can be treated with surgery only with a survival of 98.7% and without the risks associated with receiving chemotherapy. However, they are only candidates for this approach if their lymph nodes are sampled and shown to be negative for tumor.

Tumor Spillage

The local stage of the tumor and the conduct of the operation play an important role in directing adjuvant therapy. *Spillage* refers to violation of the tumor capsule during operative removal and results in a stage III designation. Studies have shown a higher risk of recurrence in patients with tumor spillage irrespective of the cause or extent of the spill. Percutaneous or incisional biopsy prior to nephrectomy is also considered a spill, as is transection of the renal vein or ureter at the site of tumor extension. When tumor extends into the renal vein or inferior vena cava, it must be clearly stated in the operative report if the tumor thrombus was removed *en bloc,* if it was removed completely and if there was evidence of either adherence or invasion of the vein wall.

Rupture refers to either the spontaneous or post-traumatic disruption of the tumor preoperatively, allowing tumor cells to disseminate throughout the flank or peritoneal cavity. Bloody peritoneal fluid should be examined carefully for evidence of malignant cells. Tumor may also grow through the renal capsule and the overlying peritoneum, bringing the neoplastic tissue in free communication with the peritoneal cavity.

When is a Tumor Unresectable?

There are four reasons a tumor might be classified as initially unresectable. The first is a patient with extension of tumor thrombus above the level of the hepatic veins. Second, tumors that involve contiguous structures (not including the adrenal gland) whereby the only means of removing the kidney tumor requires removal of the other structure. A third is if in the surgeon's judgment a nephrectomy would result in significant morbidity or mortality, diffuse tumor spill or residual tumor. Fourth, children who have extensive pulmonary compromise from a massive tumor or widespread pulmonary disease, which makes them high-risk surgical candidates. Children with unresectable disease should receive chemotherapy prior to their definitive operation.

In most cases, pretreatment with chemotherapy can reduce tumor bulk and allow safer resection. The maximum response to chemotherapy typically occurs by week 6, which is when radiographic assessment should be performed. However, neo-adjuvant chemotherapy based solely on radiographic data does not result in improved survival and could result in the loss of important staging information. It is therefore recommended that most patients undergo initial operative exploration to assess resectability directly.

Special Situations

Nephroblastomatosis/Nephrogenic Rests

Nephroblastomatosis or nephrogenic rests (NR) are remnants of renal embryonic tissue that are considered precursor lesions to Wilms tumor and are defined as persistent metanephric tissue that persists after the 36th week of gestation (Fig. 92.5). They can be found in a perilobar, intralobar or panlobar location. When a rest is found in a kidney that contains a WT, it suggests that the child is at increased risk of developing a metachronous contralateral tumor.

A more difficult scenario is when a rest is found as a primary lesion. These children can go on to develop Wilms tumors and must be followed carefully.

It can be difficult to distinguish a nephrogenic rest from Wilms tumor. NR are classified based on histologic appearance (hyperplastic, regressing or sclerosing) and growth phase (incipient or dormant). Diffuse hyperplastic perilobar nephrogenic rests (DHPLNR) form a thick rind around the kidney and are generally easy to identify. Hyperplastic NR, on the other hand, are actively proliferating neoplasms that can produce masses as large as a typical Wilms tumor. These are very difficult to distinguish from a WT. Malignant degeneration of NR is the biggest challenge for the surgeon managing these patients. Unfortunately, incisional biopsies are of no value. It is critical to examine the interface between the lesion and the renal parenchyma. Another clue is that hyperplastic NR lack a pseudocapsule, while most Wilms tumors will have this feature.

The prevalence of NR is 41% in cases of unilateral WT, 90% in bilateral synchronous WT, and 94% in metachronous bilateral WT. Serial imaging is recommended in children with WT and nephroblastomatosis, as the hallmark of malignant transformation of benign nephroblastomatosis is renal enlargement. US is the most cost effective screening tool but T1-weighted MRI is the best way to confirm the diagnosis.

Intravascular Extension

Vascular extension into the renal vein, IVC and atrium presents special surgical challenges, especially when there is invasion or adherence to the intima of the vein. Preoperative chemotherapy decreases the size and extent of the tumor thrombus, facilitating

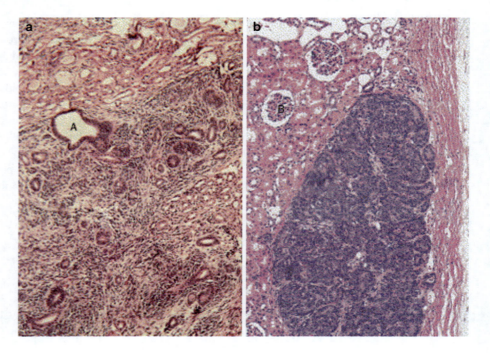

Fig. 92.5 Neprhogenic rests

subsequent excision. The tumor that extends into the renal vein and cava may simply extend as a floating attachment. Control of the renal vein and IVC above and below the thrombus with vessel loops is necessary. The tumor should not be transected. Stitches can then be placed on either side of the renal vein. This will help with vascular control and limit bleeding. The tumor and kidney should be completely mobilized prior to removing vascular thrombus; traction on the vascular pedicle allows the top of the thrombus to come down lower in the IVC making control of the vein above the thrombus somewhat easier. The renal vein is opened and the tumor pulled out of the vein. A Foley balloon technique can also be used to pull out the tumor. When the thrombus is fixed to the vascular intima, extraction is more difficult and the venotomy may need to be extended along the IVC. A similar technique to remove plaque for a carotid endarterectomy is helpful to lift the tumor off the vein wall. If after preoperative chemotherapy the tumor still extends above the hepatic veins, sternotomy while on cardiopulmonary bypass is needed to allow the intra-atrial or retrohepatic IVC thrombus to be excised.

Synchronous Bilateral Wilms Tumors

Current therapy for children with bilateral Wilms tumor (BWT) emphasizes sparing renal parenchyma. A review of National Wilms Tumor Study Group/Children's Oncology Group (NWTSG/COG) patients found that 9.1% of those with synchronous BWT developed renal failure. The cause of renal failure in 74% of the patients was bilateral nephrectomy for persistent or recurrent tumor in the remaining kidney. Current surgical guidelines emphasize avoiding total nephrectomy at initial surgery. Initial therapy for a child with BWT is chemotherapy. In contrast to the child with a unilateral tumor, a pathological diagnosis prior to chemotherapy is not mandated because the initial therapy would not be affected by the results of the biopsy. Extensive algorithms have been developed to help direct therapy for children with BWT. These can be found on the COG website (www.childrensoncologygroup.org). When faced with a patient with BWT, it is strongly advised that the surgeon review the published guidelines, which are regularly updated and, when in doubt, contact one of the surgical experts listed on the website for guidance.

After initial chemotherapy the patient is evaluated by repeat imaging at 6 weeks and then, if nephron-sparing surgery is still not deemed feasible, again at 12 weeks after further chemotherapy. If it appears that a partial nephrectomy is a viable option, a second-look procedure should be performed. It is also important to examine lymph nodes at this time. With regard to radiation therapy, each kidney is treated differently, depending on the local stage of each tumor and the completeness of resection on that side. The goal of surgery, whether at week 6 or 12, is to achieve complete resection of tumor with negative margins while preserving as much viable kidney as possible.

A good response by imaging is usually associated with a good response histologically but the converse is not always true. Tumors with complete necrosis and predominantly regressive changes can increase in size during therapy. Chemotherapy can also induce differentiation towards stroma- and epithelial-predominant tumors. These histologic subtypes may demonstrate a poor clinical response to therapy but have an excellent prognosis if the tumor is completely excised. For patients with unilateral tumors and <50% reduction in size, partial resection is not always feasible, making nephrectomy necessary. The surgeon should always attempt to achieve negative surgical margins. Enucleation of the tumor is reserved for children with favorable histology BWT if removing a margin of renal tissue would compromise the vascular supply to the kidney. Biopsy should be done for non-responding tumors and before considering enucleation, because if anaplasia is identified, enucleation is contraindicated. The finding of anaplasia (10% of BWT) also alters chemotherapy recommendations. An incisional biopsy is less likely to result in sampling error and is strongly preferred over needle biopsy. Children with BWT who require bilateral nephrectomies can be considered for renal transplantation after therapy is completed but are at risk of tumor reactivation.

Horseshoe Kidney

Resection of a WT in a child with a horseshoe kidney presents unique challenges. Preoperative imaging is critical and at operation identification and isolation of the renal vessels and ureters are critical. Exposure and mobilization of the kidney including the isthmus and ipsilateral ureter are carried out as if one is performing a unilateral resection. A partial nephrectomy is carried out on the side containing the tumor. Again, it is important that the lymph node are sampled for staging purposes. Nephron-sparing surgery should be considered for children known to be at increased risk for development of metachronous WT.

Lung Metastasis

Standard therapy in North America for patients with Wilms tumor lung metastases has included adjuvant chemotherapy and 1,200 cGy of external beam radiation (RT) to both lung fields. However, because RT is a major cause of long-term morbidity and because patients with pulmonary lesions detectable only by CT scan who are treated with a two-drug regimen have worse outcomes than those treated with three drugs *regardless* of whether they received pulmonary RT, the routine use of lung irradiation is being reexamined. Moreover, it has been shown that patients with complete resolution of pulmonary nodules on CT scan after 10 weeks of chemotherapy have a favorable prognosis, suggesting that there may be some patients for whom the added risk associated with RT is unnecessary. As a result, new therapies for children with pulmonary lesions are to be response-based. For example, if lung lesions are still present after 6 weeks of therapy, more intensive chemotherapy and RT will be the standard recommendation.

Regarding children with pulmonary metastases, there are three situations in which a surgeon may be asked to intervene. The first is at diagnosis, when resection of a single small lesion that may prove to be benign could mean the difference between a stage I designation, for which surgical resection alone is sufficient, and stage IV, for which a more toxic regimen is required. Since only two-thirds of children with lung lesions detected by CT scan at the time of diagnosis will prove to have metastatic tumor on biopsy, CT-only lesions should be biopsied for histopathologic confirmation. Another opportunity is when lesions shrink but do not go away completely after the first round of chemotherapy. It is sometimes valuable to assess the histology of the lesion prior to considering RT. Finally, if tumor remains after both chemotherapy and RT, the surgeon may be asked to attempt a curative resection of remaining lung lesions.

Summary Points

- Wilms tumor is the most common primary malignant renal tumor of childhood and the second most common pediatric solid abdominal tumor (after neuroblastoma).
- Treatment for Wilms tumor is multidisciplinary and requires the surgeon to have knowledge of current surgical, chemotherapeutic and radiation protocols.
- Overall survival for children with WT is 85%.
- The primary imaging modalities are ultrasound and computed tomography.
- Ultrasound with color Doppler should be used to assess tumor in the renal vein, inferior vena cava and right atrium.
- Radical nephro-ureterectomy is the treatment of choice for unilateral tumors and provides essential staging data.
- Wilms tumors are large but mobile, and rarely invade other organs.
- Tumor size does not correlate with spread or stage.
- Key prognostic factors are stage, histology, presence of loss of heterozygosity, age of child and tumor size.
- Tumor recurrence has a negative impact on survival, as do technical errors such as failure to sample lymph nodes and intra-operative spillage.

Editor's Comment

Radical nephro-ureterectomy for Wilms tumor is usually straightforward but can occasionally present challenges. In Europe, standard treatment guidelines include preoperative tumor shrinkage with neo-adjuvant chemotherapy and delayed nephrectomy, whereas the standard for unilateral tumors in the United States is up-front nephrectomy followed by adjuvant chemotherapy. The principal advantage of the former approach is the significant minimization of the risk of intra-operative rupture and subsequent relapse – the operation is certainly much easier after the tumor has been treated – but the downside is that all children are treated with an intensive three-drug chemotherapy regimen.

The European approach also creates a dilemma related to diagnostic confirmation – biopsy always results in tumor spillage while treating patients without tissue exposes children with benign lesions to the risks of chemotherapy and risks under treating those with anaplasia. Nevertheless, a neo-adjuvant approach is often used for tumors that have ruptured, for extremely large tumors that are metastatic or inoperable,

when intracaval tumor thrombus extends above the hepatic veins or into the right atrium and for bilateral tumors. Tumors that have ruptured can be biopsied percutaneously without upstaging the patient or can be treated without tissue diagnosis. When patients present with large tumors and lung lesions, I prefer to biopsy the lung lesions, which can usually be done thoracoscopically, rather than the primary tumor. This avoids tumor spillage in the abdomen and confirms that the lung lesions are genuinely metastatic. Chemotherapy will usually allow tumor thrombus to shrink back towards the primary, allowing control of the IVC above the tumor and removal at the time of the nephrectomy. Tumors that do not retract are either poor responders or adherent the wall of the vessel. In these situations, it is relatively straightforward to have a cardiac surgery colleague perform a sternotomy and place the child on cardio-pulmonary bypass. This allows for resection and reconstruction of the retrohepatic cava as well as atriotomy for removal of intracardiac tumor. Occasionally, the top of the thrombus can be pulled down below the liver by manual traction on a kidney that has been completely mobilized and only attached by the renal vein. In these cases we will have the cardiac team on standby.

Finally, while it is true that even very large Wilms tumors rarely invade local structures, a possible exception is the posterior aspect of the diaphragm, where the tumor can be quite adherent and which is a common location for recurrence. In these cases, it is probably best to excise this tissue with the tumor.

Diagnostic Studies

- Ultrasound with color Doppler
- Computed tomography of the abdomen and chest

Parental Preparation

- Major operation with a large incision
- Diagnosis is likely to be a childhood cancer
- Treatment is multidisciplinary
- Surgery is the first stage of treatment
- Need for central venous access for chemotherapy

Preoperative Preparation

☐ Informed consent.
☐ Type and cross.
☐ PT/PTT to rule out coagulopathy.
☐ Monitor for hypertension before and after surgery.
☐ Ensure that the pediatric oncology team is involved in the care of the patient early on.
☐ Review the surgical protocol for renal tumors either through the American Pediatric Surgical Association Website (www.eapsa.org) or the Children's Oncology Group web site (www.childrensoncologygroup.org).

Differential Diagnosis

- Wilms tumor
- Clear cell sarcoma
- Adenocarcinoma
- Rhabdoid tumor of kidney
- Mesoplastic nephroma
- Angiomyolipoma
- Cystic nephroma
- Metanephric tumor
- Ossifying renal tumor of infancy
- Diffuse hyperplastic perilobar nephroblastomatosis
- Nephrogenic rest
- Oncocytic renal neoplasms following neuroblastoma

Technical Points

- The surgical procedure for all unilateral renal tumors is a radical nephro-ureterectomy and lymph node sampling.
- Failure to sample lymph nodes is the major technical error noted in Wilms tumor surgery.
- Pre-operative and intra-operative biopsies prior to removing the kidney should avoided.
- Patients with extension of tumor thrombus above the level of the hepatic veins should be managed with preoperative chemotherapy.
- Wilms tumors displace other organs, and in the majority of cases the organs can dissected freely from the tumor. Radical *en bloc* resection, e.g., partial hepatectomy, is not warranted.
- Preoperative rupture and intra-operative spillage increases disease recurrence and must be noted at the time of surgery so that treatment can be intensified.

Suggested Reading

Dome JS, Cotton CA, Perlman EJ, et al. Treatment of anaplastic histology Wilms' tumor: results from the fifth National Wilms' Tumor Study. J Clin Oncol. 2006;24(15):2352–8.

Ehrlich PF, Ritchey ML, Hamilton TE, et al. Quality assessment for Wilms' tumor: a report from the National Wilms' Tumor Study-5. J Pediatr Surg. 2005;40(1):208–12.

Ehrlich PF, Hamilton TE, Grundy PE, et al. The value of surgery in directing therapy of Wilms tumor patients with pulmonary disease: a report from The National Wilms Tumor Study Group (NWTS -5). J Pediatr Surg. 2006;41(1):162–7.

Grundy PE, Breslow N, Li S, et al. Loss of heterozygosity for chromosomes 1p and 16q is an adverse prognostic factor in favorable-histology Wilms tumor: a report from the National Wilms Tumor Study Group. J Clin Oncol. 2005;23(29):7312–21.

Hamilton TE, Green DM, Perlman EJ, et al. Bilateral Wilms' tumor with anaplasia: lessons from the National Wilms' Tumor Study. J Pediatr Surg. 2006;41(10):1641–4.

Perlman EJ, Faria P, Soares A, Hoffer FA, et al. Hyperplastic perilobar nephroblastomatosis: Long term survival in 52 patients. Pediatr Blood Cancer. 2006;46:203–21.

Ritchey ML. Renal sparing surgery for Wilms tumor. J Urol. 2005; 174(4 Pt 1):1172–3.

Shamberger RC, Guthrie KA, Ritchey ML, et al. Surgery related factors and local reccurance of Wilms tumor in the National Wilms tumor study 4. Ann Surg. 1999;229(2):292–7.

Shamberger RC, Ritchey ML, Haase GM, et al. Intravascular extension of Wilms tumor. Ann Surg. 2001;234(1):116–21.

Shamberger RC, Haase G, Argani P. Bilateral Wilms' tumors with progressive or nonresponsive disease. J Pediatr Surg. 2006;41(4):652–7.

Chapter 93
Adrenal Tumors

Daniel von Allmen

When one thinks of adrenal tumors in children, neuroblastoma is usually the first consideration. However, there are several other neoplastic processes that can involve the adrenal gland in the pediatric population and run the gamut from aggressive malignancies with a very poor prognosis to benign processes with an excellent prognosis. They might be completely asymptomatic or express a broad variety of endocrine behaviors. Although heterogeneous by nature, they share the fact that surgery is the primary mode of therapy.

Adrenocortical Tumors

Adrenocortical carcinoma (ACC) and adrenocortical adenomas are very rare in children, accounting for less than 0.2% of all pediatric malignancies. ACC is more common in females than males and has a somewhat bimodal age distribution, with a peak less than 2 years of age and a second peak near the end of the first decade of life. For reasons that are somewhat unclear but most likely based on genetic predisposition, the incidence of adreoncortical tumors is ten times higher in Brazil than in the United States. By combining data on this uncommon tumor, investigators from the Children's Oncology Group and from Brazil are joining forces to improve our understanding of the disease.

A significant number of patients with adrenocortical tumors have a p53 mutation. More than half of patients in the United States with ACC have germline mutations in the p53 DNA-binding domains (exons 4–8) while a single mutation in exon 10 of the *TP53* gene is consistently observed in patients from Brazil. A genetic predisposition can be associated with specific syndromes: ACC is 100 times more frequent in patients with Li-Fraumeni syndrome, which is characterized by a p53 mutation, than in the normal population. Similarly, ACC has been associated with Beckwith-Wiedemann syndrome,

characterized by LOH for IGF-2, another recognized genetic risk factor.

Although ACC presents as an asymptomatic mass in about 10% of cases, it frequently presents with evidence of hormonal stimulation. Though true precocious puberty is rare, it is not uncommon for children with ACC to present with virilization, characterized by an increase in the size of the genitals, pubic hair, deepening voice, and hirsutism, or signs of cortisol excess, including acne, hypertension, moon face, centripetal fat, weight gain, and a buffalo hump.

The work up for a patient presenting with any of these findings includes imaging and laboratory studies. Ultrasound is usually the first imaging study because it is relatively inexpensive and usually rapidly obtained. The presence of a mass suggestive of an adrenal lesion then leads to more sophisticated imaging such as CT or MRI. The laboratory work up includes urine for 17-ketosteroids and the androgen dehydroepiandrosterone sulfate (DHEA-S). Plasma is sent for cortisol, DHEA-S, testosterone, renin activity, deoxycortisol, 17-hydroxyprogesterone, aldosterone, and adrostenedione.

Treatment

The treatment of any adrenal mass is primarily surgical. Adrenal masses identified in the face of abnormal clinical and laboratory findings require surgical resection. While small, well circumscribed lesions are sometimes amenable to the laparoscopic approach, larger lesions and those with evidence of invasion into surrounding structures mandate an open exploration with aggressive attempts at resection. In patients with larger tumors (stage II), the impact of a formal retroperitoneal lymph node dissection is being evaluated by the Children's Oncology Group. Tumor extending up the right adrenal vein and inferior vena cava is sometimes an indication for obtaining intrapericardial control of the inferior vena cava or cardiopulmonary bypass to allow for resection of the venous extension in continuity with the primary tumor (Fig. 93.1). Distinguishing between adenoma and carcinoma can be difficult but infiltration of surrounding tissues suggests

D. von Allmen (✉)
Department of Pediatric Surgery, University of North Carolina,
North Carolina Medical Hospital, Chapel Hill, NC 27599, USA
e-mail: vonallme@med.unc.edu

P. Mattei (ed.), *Fundamentals of Pediatric Surgery*,
DOI 10.1007/978-1-4419-6643-8_93, © Springer Science+Business Media, LLC 2011

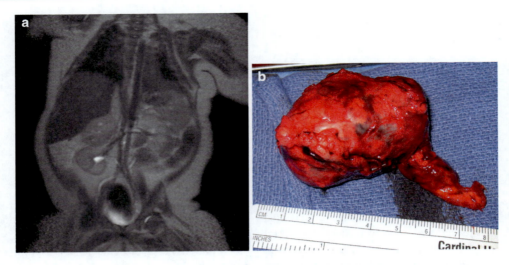

Fig. 93.1 Five month old with right adrenal tumor. (**a**) MRI sagittal view showing extension of tumor up the vena cava to the level of the diaphragm; (**b**) Resected tumor specimen with caval extension removed in continuity with adrenal mass

Table 93.1 Staging for adrenocortical tumors

I	Small tumors totally excised (<100 g and <200 cm³) with normal post-operative hormone levels
II	Completely resected large tumors (≥100 g and ≥200 cm³) with normal post-operative hormone levels
III	Unresectable, gross or microscopic residual disease
	Tumor spillage
	Patients with Stage I and II tumors who fail to normalize hormone levels after surgery
	Patients with retroperitoneal lymph node involvement
IV	Presence of distant metastasis

malignancy and, given the absence of effective chemotherapy, dictates aggressive attempts at resection. This includes partial gastrectomy or splenectomy for invasive or adherent left sided tumors and non-anatomic liver resections on the right.

Staging of adrenal tumors is post-surgical and is based on the size of the tumor and degree of resection (Table 93.1). Distinguishing between malignant carcinoma and benign adenoma in children can be very difficult. The histopathologic distinction is based on mitotic index, extent of tumor necrosis, presence of atypical mitoses, and nuclear grade (Table 93.2). The clinical behavior of the tumor also provides an indication of the aggressiveness of the tumor.

Unfortunately, there is little in the way of proven medical therapy for adrenocortical carcinoma. Mitotane is an adrenolytic insecticide that can be used in either low doses to inhibit steroid synthesis or in higher doses to destroy adrenocortical cells. The response rate to the drug is 20–30%, but there has been no change in overall mortality. Evaluation of the efficacy of neoadjuvant chemotherapy in stage III and IV patients is ongoing. Study patients are treated with cisplatin, etoposide, and doxorubicin both before and after definitive surgery, followed by an 8-month course of mitotane.

The overall survival for ACC is between 50 and 75%. There is a sharp distinction based on stage with a greater than

90% survival for patients with stage I disease and less than 10% survival for patients with stage IV disease. Younger patients (less than 4 years old) have a higher incidence of low stage disease and therefore a higher survival rate. Local recurrence occurs in 30 to 50% of stage II and III tumors and the outcome for stage III and IV disease remains very poor.

Pheochromocytoma

Pheochromocytomas arise from the chromaffin cells of the adrenal medulla. Paragangliomas are extra-adrenal manifestations of the same process and typically arise within the sympathetic ganglia. Both are characterized by synthesis of catecholamines including epinephrine, norepinephrine, and dopamine. Pheochromocytomas are rare tumors that usually present between the ages of 6 and 15 years and, unlike ACC, they are slightly more common in boys. Although pheochromocytomas are seen in association with hereditary syndromes including MEN-2A, MEN-2B, and NF-1, most tumors are sporadic and do not share the same chromosomal abnormalities as the familial variants. In patients with MEN-2, abnormalities of the RET proto-oncogene are common.

Eighty-five percent of pheochromocytomas occur in the adrenal gland while the remainder arise in other areas associated with sympathetic tissues such as the sympathetic ganglia near the renal hilum and the organ of Zuckerkandl. Thirty percent of patients have multiple tumors.

Most pediatric patients have signs and symptoms of sustained hypertension rather than the paroxysmal hypertension more commonly seen in adults. Central nervous system manifestations, including mental status changes, visual changes, and decreasing school performance have all been described. Headaches, palpitations, sweating, and anxiety

Table 93.2 Histologic grading, modified Weiss criteria for pediatric adrenocortical tumors

Diagnosis	Mitotic index	Confluent necrosis	Atypical mitosis	Nuclear pleomorphism
Adrenocortical adenoma	0–5	Absent	Absent	Mild–moderate
ACC-low grade	6–20	Present	Present	Marked
ACC – high grade	>20	–	–	–

Source: Bugg MF, et al. Am J Clin Path. 1994;101(5):625–29. © 1994 American Journal of Clinical Pathology; © 1994 American Society for Clinical Pathology

Mitotic index = mitotic figures/high power field

are also commonly reported. Other than hypertension, the physical exam findings are usually limited.

The diagnosis can be confirmed by measuring elevated catecholamines, metanephrines, vanillylmandelic acid (VMA), and homovanillic acid (HVA) in urine that is collected for 24 h. The radiologic workup includes CT or MRI of the abdomen, which typically reveals a smooth, well-circumscribed lesion less than 5 cm in diameter. A nuclear medicine ^{131}I-metaiodobenzylguanidine (MIBG) scan is helpful in identifying multiple lesions. The preoperative work up should include an echocardiogram to look for left ventricular hypertrophy due to chronic hypertension. In some patients, congestive heart failure can be the presenting sign.

Treatment

The primary treatment for pheochromocytoma is surgical resection. Classically, patients have been prepared for operation with alpha-blockade and volume loading to counteract the chronic vasoconstriction induced by catecholamine excess. During the operation, the anesthesiologist must be prepared for rapid changes in blood pressure such as spiking hypertension when the tumor is manipulated and rapid loss of alpha stimulation leading to hypotension when the adrenal vein is ligated. Adrenalectomy is usually curative and the tumors are often relatively small and well circumscribed, making them amenable to a laparoscopic approach. Bilateral tumors are sometimes amenable to partial adrenalectomies leaving residual functional adrenal gland on one or both sides. On the other hand, if bilateral adrenalectomy is necessary, life-long replacement with glucocorticoids and mineralocorticoids becomes necessary.

Obviously, associated paragangliomas should be completely resected. Less than 10% of tumors are malignant. Malignant tumors can be treated with ^{131}I-MIBG, octreotide, or tumor chemoembolization but the prognosis is poor with unresectable or metastatic disease.

Summary Points

- Adrenal tumors are a heterogeneous group and can be benign or malignant, but for most surgery is the primary mode of therapy.
- Adrenocortical carcinoma are very rare in children, accounting for less than 0.2% of all pediatric malignancies.
- A significant number of patients with adrenocortical tumors have a p53 mutation.
- Although adrenocortical carcinoma presents as an asymptomatic mass in about 10% of cases, it frequently presents with evidence of hormonal stimulation.
- The absence of effective chemotherapy for adrenocortical carcinoma dictates aggressive attempts at resection.
- Although pheochromocytomas are seen in association with hereditary syndromes including MEN-2A, MEN-2B, and NF-1, most tumors are sporadic.
- Most pediatric patients with pheochromocytoma have signs and symptoms of sustained rather than paroxysmal hypertension.
- The primary treatment for pheochromocytoma is surgical resection.

Editor's Comment

Many of the adrenal masses encountered in children can be resected laparoscopically, including pheochromocytomas, most ganglioneuromas, and even some neuroblastomas. The size of the mass might be a limiting factor depending on the experience of the surgeon. Tumors for which spillage is potentially disastrous, such as adrenocortical carcinomas, should probably not be approached using a minimally invasive approach. In most cases, a lateral, transabdominal approach can be used for both right and left adrenal lesions. The majority of the operation can be performed using blunt dissection, dividing small vessels with the harmonic scalpel or hook electrocautery. Control of the adrenal vein can be particularly hazardous, especially on the right where it is typically very short and enters directly into the IVC. It is easily torn by overly aggressive dissection but once identified can be clipped near its origin and divided.

Newborns with incidentally identified adrenal masses have neuroblastoma or adrenal hemorrhage. These are difficult to differentiate but the distinction is usually irrelevant, because either lesion, if small, can be safely observed. Resection is rarely necessary but sometimes demanded by anxious parents. Careful surveillance with serial ultrasound appears to be safe, but should probably be done as part of a clinical trial.

Adrenal ganglioneuromas are often found incidentally in teenagers who undergo CT or MRI for unrelated symptoms or as part of a trauma evaluation. The vast majority of these lesions are benign and could theoretically be safely observed indefinitely, however because a very small percentage of these will turn out to harbor a tiny neuroblastoma (ganglioneuroblastoma) resection is usually recommended. In fact, although most "incidentalomas" in children are benign, size and imaging characteristics do not necessarily predict the likelihood of malignancy. In practice then, a pediatric surgeon is asked to resect almost every adrenal mass identified in a child beyond the newborn period. Fortunately, these lesions can almost always be removed laparoscopically.

All but the smallest adrenocortical carcinomas should be resected using an open approach through a generous incision in order to make every effort to avoid breach of the capsule and even the slightest degree of tumor spillage. These tumors are generally unresponsive to chemotherapy and therefore complete resection offers the greatest (and sometimes only) chance for cure. Spillage upstages the tumor and can significantly diminish survival. The tumor capsule is often very delicate and tears easily. A meticulous and very gentle approach is imperative. Locally invasive tumors should be resected *en bloc,* including portions of adjacent spleen, liver, stomach or diaphragm if necessary to achieve negative margins. All patients should undergo an extensive ipsilateral retroperitoneal lymph node dissection for staging purposes. Unlike the case with Wilms tumor, adrenocortical carcinoma with tumor thrombus extension into the IVC or atrium almost never shrinks in response to neoadjuvant chemotherapy. If, even after complete mobilization of the primary tumor, the thrombus cannot be pulled down into the infrahepatic IVC to allow placement of a vascular clamp above it, cavotomy on cardiopulmonary bypass must be used.

Diagnostic Studies

For Adrenocortical Tumors

- CT or MRI
- Urine for 17-ketosteroids and DHEA-S
- Serum for cortisol, DHEA-S, testosterone, renin activity, deoxycortisol, 17-hydroxyprogesterone, aldosterone, adrostenedione

For Pheochromocytoma

- CT or MRI
- MIBG scan
- Twenty-four hour urine for catecholamines, metanephrines, VMA, and HVA

Parental Preparation

- There is a risk of bleeding and, for adrenocortical carcinoma, tumor spillage, and, for phechromocytoma, hypertensive crisis.

Preoperative Preparation

- ☐ Careful surgical planning with 3-dimensional radiographic imaging.
- ☐ Alpha and beta blockade for pheochromocytoma.
- ☐ For adrenocortical tumors that extend into the retrohepatic IVC or atrium, arrangements for cardiopulmonary bypass or cardiac surgery on standby.

Suggested Reading

Bugg MF, Ribeiro RC, Roberson PK, et al. Correlation of pathologic features with clinical outcome in pediatric adrenocortical neoplasia. Am J Clin Pathol. 1994;101:625–9.

Michalkiewicz E, Sandrini R, Figueiredo B, et al. Clinical and outcome characteristics of children with adrenocortical tumors. An analysis of 254 cases from the International Pediatric Adrenocortical Tumor Registry. J Clin Oncol. 2004;22:838–45.

Rescorla FJ. Malignant adrenal tumors. Semin Pediatr Surg. 2006;15: 48–56.

Sullivan J, Groshong T, Tobias JD. Presenting signs and symptoms of pheochromocytoma in pediatric-aged patients. Clin Pediatr (Phila). 2005;44(44):715.

Zancanella P, Pianovski MA, Oliveira BH, Ferman S, Piovezan GC, Lichtvan LL, et al. Mitotane associated with cisplatin, etoposide, and doxorubicin in advanced childhood adrenocortical carcinoma: mitotane monitoring and tumor regression. J Pediatr Hematol Oncol. 2006;28:513–24.

Chapter 94
Rhabdomyosarcoma

Ravi S. Radhakrishnan and Richard J. Andrassy

Rhabdomyosarcoma (Greek: rhabdos = rod, myos = muscle, sarkos = flesh) is a primary malignancy in children and adolescents that arises from embryonic mesenchyme with the potential to differentiate into skeletal muscle. Rhabdomyosarcoma accounts for over half of all soft tissue sarcomas in children and, with approximately 250–300 new cases per year in the United States, the third most common solid tumor in infants and children behind neuroblastoma and Wilms tumor. In adults, rhabdomyosarcomas arise mostly in the extremities, while in children they can occur in any anatomical location of the body, even in places where there is no skeletal muscle, such as the urinary bladder or biliary tree. In fact, the disease can arise at any site and in any tissue in the body except bone. The most common sites are the head and neck region and the genitourinary tract, with only 20% occurring in the extremities.

In 1950, Stobbe demonstrated improvement in outcome in head and neck sites when radiation therapy was added after incomplete resection. In 1961, Pinkel and Pinkren advocated adjuvant chemotherapy after complete surgical excision and postoperative radiation therapy, which was the beginning of the multimodal approach to solid tumors.

Although the trend has been toward far less mutilating surgery, the surgeon plays an even greater role in initial biopsy and staging, as well as primary re-excision, appropriate wide local resections, and second-look operations. The surgeon should be involved early in the multimodal approach to treatment.

Diagnosis

The diagnosis of rhabdomyosarcoma is usually made by direct open biopsy. There are no helpful markers or specific imaging studies. The pathologist is expected to identify the histologic subgroups to allow adequate staging and to direct therapy. Several grams of tissue are therefore usually needed. Biopsies of genitourinary primaries frequently are performed endoscopically. Needle biopsies that are performed to establish the diagnosis of prostatic tumors are difficult to interpret and must include several cores.

Trunk and extremity rhabdomyosarcoma should have excisional or incisional biopsy, with the incision placed so that it will not interfere with the incision required for subsequent wide local excision. For extremity tumors, this usually means a longitudinal incision. Wide local excision with clear margins is the ultimate goal. Regional lymph nodes are evaluated depending on location of the primary. Trunk and extremity lesions have a high incidence of lymph node involvement and sentinel lymph node mapping is advised. Patients also require a complete workup before definitive surgery. The preoperative evaluation includes imaging, blood work, and bone marrow biopsy.

Staging and Clinical Grouping

Pretreatment staging for RMS is performed to stratify the extent of the disease for different treatment regimens as well as to compare outcome. This classification is a modification of the TNM staging system and is based on primary tumor site, primary tumor size, clinical regional node status, and distant spread (Table 94.1). Pretreatment size is determined by external measurement or three-dimensional imaging, depending on the anatomic location. Staging is based on clinical criteria and should be done by the responsible surgeon based on preoperative imaging and physical findings. Intraoperative and pathologic results do not affect staging but do affect clinical grouping.

The clinical grouping system was developed by the intergroup Rhabdomyosarcoma Group (IRS) and is based on the pretreatment and operative outcome (Table 94.2). The underlying premise is that total tumor extirpation at the original site is the best hope for cure and thus it allows patients to be stratified according to their degree of resection. In the past,

R.S. Radhakrishnan (✉)
Department of Surgery, MD Anderson Cancer Center, Memorial
Hermann Hospital, 6431 Fannin Street, MSB 4.200, Houston,
TX 77030, USA
e-mail: ravi.radhakrishnan@uth.tmc.edu

P. Mattei (ed.), *Fundamentals of Pediatric Surgery*,
DOI 10.1007/978-1-4419-6643-8_94, © Springer Science+Business Media, LLC 2011

Table 94.1 Pretreatment staging classification

Stage	Sites	T	Size	N	M
1	Orbit, head and neck (excluding parameningeal), bladder/non-prostate	T1 or T2	a or b	N0 or Nx	M0
2	Bladder/prostate, extremity, cranial parameningeal, other (trunk, perineal, thoracic)	T1 or T2	a	N0 or Nx	M0
3	As in Stage 2	T1 or T2	a	N1	M0
			b	N0/N1/Nx	M0
4	All	T1 or T2	a or b	N0/N1/Nx	M1

Definitions:

Tumor

T1   Confined to anatomic site of origin

a: ≤5 cm diameter in size

b: >5 cm diameter in size

T2   Extension and/or fixation to surrounding tissue

a: ≤5 cm diameter in size

b: >5 cm diameter in size

Regional node

N0   regional nodes not clinically involved

N1   regional nodes clinically involved by neoplasm

Nx   clinical status of regional nodes unknown

Metastasis

M0   no distant metastasis

M1   distant metastasis present

Table 94.2 Clinical grouping of rhabdomyosarcoma

Group I	Tumor completely excised with microscopic negative margins
Group II	Tumor completely excised with microscopic positive margins
Group III	Tumor excised with gross residual tumor
Group IV	Distant metastases

this had led to aggressive and often mutilating procedures. This system does not take into account the biological nature or natural history of the tumor, nor does it account for the experience and the aggressiveness of the surgeon. Group I includes patients who have had complete resection of the primary tumor with microscopic negative margins. Group II patients have had a gross total resection of the tumor with microscopic positive margins or positive regional lymph nodes. Group III have gross residual disease. Group IV have metastatic disease.

With more frequent use of biopsy and neoadjuvant chemotherapy, there has been a "group shift" in clinical trials from Group I or II to Group III, where biopsy is generally followed by neoadjuvant chemotherapy. Group assignment is based on intra-operative findings and postoperative pathologic status and most include final pathologic verification of margins, residual tumor, node involvement, and, when applicable, cytological examination of pleural and peritoneal fluid. Both clinical grouping and pretreatment staging have been shown to correlate with outcome.

Based on the findings from previous IRS trials I through IV, risk groups have been established for treatment in IRS-V. The

IRS-V Study combines group, stage, and histology subtype to allocate patients to three different therapeutic protocols according to risk of recurrence. Low-risk patients were defined as those with Stage 1 and 2 disease and no nodal spread, or patients with orbital involvement with incomplete resection. High-risk patients were those with metastatic disease, with all other patients falling into the intermediate risk category. Low-risk patients have an estimated 3-year failure-free survival (FFS) rate of 88%, intermediate-risk patients 55–76%, and high-risk patients less than 30%. Multidisciplinary treatment is recommended as defined by histologic subtype and primary site, as well as the extent of disease at diagnosis and response to treatment. The goal is to achieve local control with preservation of form and function.

Treatment

The approach to the treatment of rhabdomyosarcoma has been multimodal for more than 30 years. The advances in understanding the biology and treatment of this disease can largely be attributed to the IRS studies I–V. And specific surgical treatment has progressively been less aggressive and less mutilating while maintaining the excellent survival statistics of earlier studies.

The surgical treatment of RMS is site-specific, however the general principles include complete wide excision of the primary tumor and surrounding uninvolved margins while preserving cosmesis and function.

Initial biopsy is generally incisional except for small lesions that can be safely excised. Some lesions will have a pseudocapsule, which might allow the lesion to be shelled out, giving the surgeon the false notion that the entire lesion has been removed. At many anatomic sites, there will be gross or microscopic residual and pretreatment re-excision is warranted if this can be done without disfigurement.

Biopsy of any lesion potentially involves the need for subsequent re-operation and wide excision. Longitudinal incisions are frequently better than horizontal incisions on areas such as an extremity. A biopsy to confirm malignancy requires that the biopsy tract be excised at the time of reoperation; if the biopsy site is inappropriately placed, this excision may require much larger incisions or resections than would otherwise be necessary.

Solid-tumor biopsies are traditionally divided into excisional biopsies, in which the entire tumor is included in the specimen, and incisional biopsies, in which only a portion of the tumor is included. In an excisional biopsy, margins should be carefully marked to allow re-resection should the biopsy reveal a positive margin. Ideally, excisional biopsies are planned to allow resections that will leave behind only negative margins. If such an excisional biopsy results in too large of a resection, then incisional biopsy is more appropriate.

If biopsy margins are not carefully marked on the specimen and in the operative field (usually by sutures or clips), the ability of the surgeon to subsequently obtain negative margins is severely compromised. Testicular masses should be approached through an inguinal rather than a scrotal incision so that proximal control of the cord can be obtained and a wide local excision performed without seeding the scrotum with tumor. The proximal spermatic cord should be examined for free margins with more proximal excision necessary if tumor is still present. Biopsy of the tumor through the scrotum often leads to the need for scrotal resection and an increased risk of local recurrence.

Secondary excision after initial biopsy and neoadjuvant therapy has a better outcome than does partial or incomplete excision. Despite the shift of more patients into clinical group III, chemotherapy followed by delayed or second-look surgery has allowed for better prognosis with less mutilating surgery. Biopsy of regional nodes, or sentinel lymph node mapping to evaluate nodes, is warranted in selected sites such as the extremity.

In some patients with extremity or trunk tumors, initial tumor resection is thought to be complete, but then histopathologic review reveals microscopic residual disease corresponding to clinical Group IIa. In many of these patients, primary re-excision (PRE) is possible, achieving wider disease-free margins. The benefits of PRE have been demonstrated in IRS-I and IRS-II, where 154 patients with extremity or trunk RMS were initially placed in clinical Group IIa, then 41 patients underwent successful PRE and were converted to clinical Group I prior to the onset of adjuvant therapy. These patients were compared with 113 patients who had microscopic residual disease and did not undergo PRE and with 73 patients who were free of disease after the initial resection (clinical Group I). Among these 41 patients, the 3-year Kaplan–Meier survival estimate was 91%, compared with 74% for Group IIa patients not undergoing PRE and 74% for patients who were initially Group I. This approach might also be applicable to tumors of other locations. Primary re-excision should be strongly considered when the initial resection was not a "cancer operation" (malignancy was not suspected at initial excision), even if the margins are apparently negative.

Second look operation (SLO) has been used for several pediatric tumors to evaluate therapeutic response and to remove any residual tumor after completing initial therapy. The use of SLO was evaluated in IRS-III and shown to be beneficial in clinical Group II patients. The performance of SLO changed the response status in a significant number of patients: 12% of presumed complete response (CR) patients were found to harbor residual tumor, while 74% of re-excision patients were recategorized as CR after operation. The survival rate of these recategorized patients was similar to that of patients confirmed to be CR at re-exploration.

The general surgical principles learned from IRS I to IRS IV and thus considered in IRS V include: (1) Patients with localized, completely resected disease (Group I) generally have the best prognosis and overall survival. Patients with metastases at diagnosis (Group IV) have the worst outlook, and those with Group II and III disease have an intermediate prognosis. Thus, it has been preferable to try to remove all visible tumor, if feasible without excessive morbidity. (2) When a lesion has been resected, primary re-resection is indicated if the primary operation was not a cancer operation or there are positive margins. Any question of margin status should warrant re-resection. In addition, Group I patients with embryonal rhabdomyosarcoma are not subjected to postoperative external-beam radiotherapy. (3) It is desirable to preserve organ function and thus spare such structures as the eye, vagina, and bladder, especially since patients with tumor at or near these sites generally have a good prognosis. Primary chemotherapy followed by radiation therapy is the recommended approach. Delayed excision of initially unresected tumor may improve prognosis by changing a partial response into a complete response after initial shrinkage of the tumor by chemotherapy, with or without radiation therapy. (4) There is a relationship between age at diagnosis and likelihood of regional lymph node involvement in boys with nonmetastatic paratesticular rhabdomyosarcoma. Survival in IRS IV was better for boys younger than 10 years of age, as the nodal relapse rate was lower than in those 10 years of age and older. We now recommend performing a modified ipsilateral retroperitoneal lymph-node dissection in older boys who have no clinical evidence of regional node involvement. If the nodes are uninvolved, cyclophosphamide and XRT are withheld, whereas if tumor is present in the nodes, cyclophosphamide and XRT are given in addition to vincristine and actinomycin D.

Other considerations for IRS V include a more aggressive approach to evaluating lymph nodes. In earlier IRS studies, lymph node involvement was thought to be rare at most sites, but the nodes were rarely evaluated. More recent studies have suggested that the incidence of involved lymph nodes in patients with extremity tumors may be higher than initially suspected. Sentinel lymph-node mapping, using a vital dye such as isosulfan blue (Lymphazurin) along with radio-labeled technetium sulfur colloid, can localize the regional node most likely to contain tumor cells. If the node is positive, then the nodal basin is irradiated. The utility of sentinel-lymph node mapping is being currently being evaluated in IRS V.

For patients whose tumors are initially deemed unresectable, a second-look procedure should be considered after initial chemotherapy. Imaging studies have not been consistently reliable in determining actual response to treatment. In IRS III, 75% of children with Group III tumors with evidence of partial or no response on imaging studies had either a pathologically complete response (CR) or were converted to such a response by resection of all remaining tumor. However, most (but not all) patients who have shown a CR on imaging studies are confirmed as having such a response by secondary surgery. Survival was better in those patients converted to CR. Secondary surgery is less beneficial in children with Stage IV disease. Second-look surgery is least useful for tumors in the head and neck but is appropriate for trunk and extremity tumors. A trend toward improved survival in patients converted to CR by means of second-look operations has been enduring.

Metastatic Disease

Metastatic disease most commonly involves the lung (58%), bone (33%), regional lymph nodes (33%), liver (22%), and brain (20%). Of patients enrolled in the IRS-III, 14% were clinical group IV at the time of diagnosis. Primary sites more likely to generate metastases include the extremities (23%), parameningeal (13%), retroperitoneal, trunk, gastrointestinal, and intrathoracic sites. Primary sites with a low incidence of metastases include the orbit (2%), non-parameningeal/non-orbital head and neck (5%) and genitourinary sites. Metastatic disease is the single most important predictor of clinical outcome, with a 3-year FFS of only 25%.

The lung is the most common site of metastatic disease. Patients with lung-only metastases appear to have a somewhat better prognosis than those with multiple sites or metastases to bone or liver and have a higher incidence of favorable sites and favorable histology. Since rhabdomyosarcomas are generally highly chemosensitive, resection of numerous metastases does not appear indicated. However, from our own experience, isolated single metastases to the lung have a better prognosis than multiple metastases. For this reason, we believe it is of value to biopsy a single metastasis to confirm histology. Persistent or recurrent disease after chemotherapy might warrant resection both for diagnosis and to decrease tumor burden. Overall, there has been little improvement in survival for patients with metastatic disease. The estimated overall survival and FFS at 3 years was 39 and 25%. Overall survival at 3 years was influenced by histology (47% for embryonal, 34% for all others) and increasing number of metastatic sites. By multi-variate analysis, the presence of two or fewer metastatic sites was the only significant predictor.

Postoperative Care

Prior to multimodal therapy, surgery alone for RMS resulted in survival rates of <20%. Local micrometastatic disease, nodal disease, or unrecognized/untreated distant disease frequently led to early recurrence and subsequent death due mainly to advanced metastatic disease. The development of adjuvant and later neoadjuvant chemotherapy has led to a marked increase in survival. The IRS studies have shown progressively better survival rates with less mutilating surgery and less chemotoxicity.

Agents with known activity in the treatment of RMS include vincristine (V), actinomycin D (A), doxorubicin (Dox), cyclophosphamide (C), ifosfamide (I), and etoposide (E). The gold standard for combination chemotherapy in the treatment of rhabdomyosarcoma has been VAC (vincristine, actinomycin D, cyclophosphamide). Consecutive large randomized trials have allowed for modifications of this combination tailored to specific subgroups according to clinical group and site of disease. Patients with metastatic disease have a poor prognosis despite aggressive therapy. Intensive, multi-agent combinations (carboplatin/epirubicin/vincristine) have been used in an attempt to improve survival and have resulted in a reported response rate of around 50%.

Complications of treatment for rhabdomyosarcoma are varied and extensive. These include chemotherapy toxicity and death, acute and long-term complications related to radiation therapy, and standard surgical complications of biopsy and resection. Long-term follow-up for delayed complications and second malignancies is warranted in all patients.

Outcomes

The overall trend has been an increase in survival for each subsequent IRS study. The survival rate depends on clinical group, stage, and primary site. The overall 5-year survival rate in IRS III Study was 71%: 90% for clinical group I, 80% for clinical group II, 70% for clinical group III, and 30% for clinical group IV. The survival rate by pretreatment staging classification was 80% for Stage I, 68% for Stage II, 49% for Stage III, 21% for Stage IV. Overall, FFS rates for the patients treated on IRS-IV did not differ from those seen for similar patients treated on IRS III.

Summary Points

- Rhabdomyosarcoma is the most common soft tissue sarcoma and the third most common solid tumor in children.
- Preoperative staging and subsequent clinical grouping help predict response to treatment and survival.
- Multimodal management (surgery, chemotherapy, radiation) of rhabdomyosarcoma has been shown to offer the best outcomes.
- Re-operation for complete resection of tumor has led to improved survival.

Editor's Comment

Despite its name, rhabdomyosarcoma does not necessarily arise from skeletal muscle. In fact, it commonly arises in tissue that contains no skeletal muscle. Unlike most other cancers, the approach to treatment and the prognosis of rhabdomyosarcomas vary greatly depending on the site of origin, with certain sites being considered favorable and others unfavorable. This characterization mostly correlates with the histologic subtype – tumors that arise in favorable sites are usually embryonal, while those from unfavorable sites are typically alveolar. So important is the site of origin that it is a primary factor in determining tumor stage. Rhabdomyosarcomas that arise within hollow organs such as the bladder, nasal cavity, or biliary tree are often described as botryoid ("cluster of grapes"), which is a type of embryonal and associated with the best prognosis. Age is also an important prognostic factor but mostly because it correlates with histology and site or origin: in general, children under 1 year of age and older than 10 have a worse prognosis. Like other small round blue cell tumors (lymphoma, Ewing's/PNET, neuroblastoma), rhabdomyosarcomas have a tendency to metastasize to the bone marrow, which is why bone marrow biopsy is always performed as part of the initial work up.

Tumors in favorable sites are treated with biopsy and neoadjuvant chemotherapy with little need for more than a limited surgical exploration to confirm the absence of residual tumor. Complete resection with a margin is rarely needed. Unfavorable tumors, on the other hand, require elaborate attempts at local control with either aggressive surgery or, if surgical resection is not feasible or safe, external beam radiation. Multiple operative attempts to render the patient free of tumor might be reasonable in certain situations. For certain sites, such as an extremity or the trunk, sentinel lymph node biopsy is often requested. The technique is straightforward and should include both lymphoscintigraphy and injection of blue dye. Often two lymph nodes are identified, sometimes in different nodal regions (popliteal and inguinal), both of which need to be excised.

At second- or third-look operations for resection, the previous scar and all tissue planes violated at the previous operation must be excised with a margin, which can result in a significant soft tissue defect. Entering the previous site potentially increases the risk of recurrence but can be difficult to avoid even with preoperative high-resolution three-dimensional imaging. An ideal margin is 1–2 cm; but if the tumor is adjacent to vital structures or bone, a negative tissue fascia plane is acceptable.

Botryoid tumors arising from the vagina should be biopsied and treated with chemotherapy. Mutilating surgery is almost never indicated and the prognosis is usually excellent. Biliary rhabdomyosarcoma also carries a relatively good prognosis, especially if it is of the botryoid variety. Biopsy can be performed through a common duct exploration or through the cystic duct after cholecystectomy. At planned re-operation, we have used choledochoscopy to confirm the absence of residual tumor after chemotherapy. Depending on the stage and extent of disease, some of these patients will also require liver resection or the addition of radiation therapy. Extremity tumors often occur in adolescents, are usually alveolar, and carry a guarded prognosis. Although therapy to control the primary tumor must be aggressive, limb-salvage should be considered if at all possible.

Differential Diagnosis

- Leukemia
- Lymphoma
- Ewing sarcoma/PNET
- Liposarcoma
- Neuroblastoma
- Osteosarcoma
- Wilms tumor

Diagnostic Studies

- History/physical (ht. wt.)
- Laboratory
  - CBC w/differential
  - Electrolytes, creatinine, LFTs, LDH
  - Urinalysis
- Imaging
  - Chest X-ray
  - MRI or CT of primary
  - CT Chest
  - Bone scan
- Bone marrow biopsy/aspirate
- CSF cytology (for parameningeal)

Parental Preparation

- Prognosis is site specific and based on histology, stage, and grouping.
- Possibility of needing further operations.
- If the tumor is unresectable, it is best to biopsy, treat with chemotherapy and then try to resect the tumor at a second operation.

Preoperative Preparation

☐ Informed consent
☐ Radio-labeled technetium sulfur colloid lymphos-cintigraphy for sentinel lymph node biopsy
☐ Type and crossmatch

Technical Points

- Longitudinal incision for biopsies to facilitate inclusion in re-operations.
- Wide excision of primary lesion to remove microscopic residual tumor.
- Orient and mark margins of excision in specimen and in tumor site to allow for re-excision if necessary.

Suggested Reading

Andrassy RJ. Soft tissue sarcomas. In: Carachi R, Azmy A, Grosfeld JL, editors. The surgery of childhood tumors. Chapter 14. Berlin: Springer; 2008.

Breneman JC et al. Prognostic factors and clinical outcomes in children and adolescents with metastatic rhabdomyosarcoma – a report from the Intergroup Rhabdomyosarcoma Study IV. J Clin Oncol. 2003;21:78.

Crist WM et al. Intergroup rhabdomyosarcoma study IV: results for patients with nonmetastatic disease. J Clin Oncol. 2001;19:3091.

Li FP, Fraumeni Jr JF. Rhabdomyosarcoma in children: epidemiologic study and identification of a familial cancer syndrome. J Natl Cancer Inst. 1969;43:1365–73.

Miller SD, Andrassy RJ. Complications in pediatric surgical oncology. J Am Coll Surg. 2003;197:832–7.

Neville HL, Andrassy RJ, Lobe TE, Bagwell CE, Anderson JR, Womer RB, et al. Preoperative staging, prognostic factors, and outcome for extremity rhabdomyosarcoma: a preliminary report from the Intergroup Rhabdomyosarcoma Study IV (1991–1997). J Pediatr Surg. 2000;35:317.

Chapter 95
Sacrococcygeal Teratoma

Helene Flageole

Sacrococcygeal teratoma (SCT) is the most frequently encountered tumor in the fetus and newborn. It is also the most common extra-gonadal germ cell tumor. While the majority present at birth or prenatally because of a large sacral mass, a small but significant number of patients will present later on with symptoms of urinary or intestinal obstruction because they have a completely intra-pelvic tumor.

The incidence of SCT is approximately 1 in 30,000 live births and they are three times more prevalent in females. Most are benign at birth, however the incidence of malignant transformation increases rapidly thereafter: by 4 months of age 40% or so are malignant, and after 1 year virtually all of them are. The most common malignant elements are yolk sac tumor and embryonal carcinoma, hence the value in monitoring alpha-fetoprotein and β-HCG.

Twenty percent of infants born with SCT have associated congenital anomalies. Some cases have been reported with cardiac defects or GI malformations such as trachea-esophageal fistula, imperforate anus, or anal stenosis. Others have spina bifida, myelomeningocele, and genito-urinary anomalies. Many patients have functional or structural abnormalities of adjacent organs (hip dislocation, hydronephrosis) due to the mass effect created by a large teratoma.

SCTs are classified according to the relative extent of intra- and extra-pelvic involvement (Fig. 95.1). Type 1, the most common, is primarily external, with minimal pre-sacral involvement. Type 2, the next most common, has both external and internal components. Type 3 is primarily internal but is still somewhat visible externally, while Type 4 tumors are entirely internal and not visible externally.

Prenantal Diagnosis

SCTs are increasingly being diagnosed prenatally. Some can be seen at the first antenatal ultrasound, which is typically performed around 18 weeks, while many others will be found on studies done between 20 and 32 weeks for larger than expected uterine size. Findings consist of an external mass originating from the sacral area with solid and cystic components, as well as occasional foci of calcification (Fig. 95.2). Myelomeningoceles are occasionally confused for an SCT.

The prognosis for prenatal SCT is much more guarded than that of postnatal SCT because of the higher proportion of highly vascular tumors, which tend to cause high-output cardiac failure and fetal hydrops. The overall mortality for prenatally diagnosed SCT exceeds 50%. Tumors with a large solid component are more vascular and are associated with a much higher risk of hydrops fetalis and placentomegaly, presumed to be due to a hyperdynamic state induced by the low resistance vessels in the teratoma. There is also a higher risk of maternal mirror syndrome, in which the mother develops severe preeclampsia and edema, the severity of which "mirrors" that of the fetus. Unless there is an intervention, the outcome for fetuses that develop hydrops is uniformly fatal. Therefore, when an SCT is identified in utero, serial ultrasound and close monitoring for signs of hydrops are imperative. Expectant patients also need to be watched closely for signs of preterm labor, which is quite frequent because of the associated polyhydramnios. The aim is to prevent dystocia, tumor rupture, and bleeding, which is associated with premature labor and uncontrolled delivery.

The optimal treatment for the fetus with SCT and hydrops is urgent cesarean section, but this can only be performed safely if lung maturity is achieved. Recently, some fetuses that were too early in gestation to be delivered have successfully undergone debulking of the SCT in utero. Advanced cardiac failure and maternal mirror syndrome are contraindications to fetal intervention.

Fetuses with predominantly avascular cystic lesions have a much better prognosis. In some cases with very large cystic components, aspiration of fluid at the onset of labor has made

H. Flageole (✉)
Department of Surgery, McMaster Children's Hospital,
1200 Main Street, Hamilton, ON L8N325, Canada
e-mail: flageol@mcmaster.ca

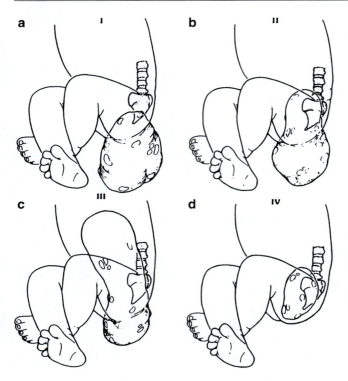

Fig. 95.1 Altman classification of sacrococcygeal teratoma. Type I (45%) are almost entirely external, with only a small internal component. Type II (35%) have external and internal components of approximately equal size. Type III (10%) are mostly internal, with only a small external component. Type IV (10%) are entirely internal with no tumor visible externally. (From Grosfeld JL, Billmire DF. Teratomas in infancy and childhood. Curr Probl Cancer. 1985;9(9):1–53. Reprinted with permission from Elsevier)

a vaginal delivery possible. As a general guideline, SCTs that are larger than 5 cm in diameter or have a significant solid component should be delivered by caesarean section, while smaller, cystic ones can proceed vaginally (Fig. 95.3).

Postnatal Diagnosis

If not identified antenatally, 90% of SCT will be noted at delivery. The diagnosis is usually rather evident just by inspection (Fig. 95.2). A careful rectal examination must be conducted to assess for the presence of an intra-pelvic component. Tumor markers (AFP, β-HCG) should be measured as well.

Imaging in the form of plain pelvic films will identify sacral defects and tumor calcifications. Computed tomography can also give valuable information such as the extent of pelvic involvement, the presence of urinary obstruction, and evidence of distant metastases. When the diagnosis is uncertain or if spinal involvement is suspected, MRI is more useful.

Those SCT that are not visible at birth because they are completely intra-pelvic (10%), will invariably present later in life, typically between the ages of 4 months and 4 years. The presenting symptoms are variable and include anal stenosis, constipation or bladder compression. Due to the high incidence of malignancy in tumors identified late, a full metastatic workup, including tumor markers and CT scan of chest and abdomen, should also be performed.

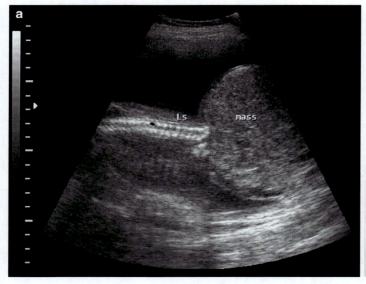
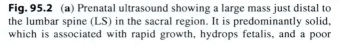
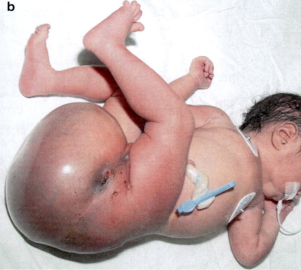

Fig. 95.2 (**a**) Prenatal ultrasound showing a large mass just distal to the lumbar spine (LS) in the sacral region. It is predominantly solid, which is associated with rapid growth, hydrops fetalis, and a poor prognosis. (**b**) An otherwise healthy-appearing newborn with a large sacrococcygeal teratoma. Note the severe anterior displacement of the anus

Curarino's Triad

First described in 1981, this triad consists of anal stenosis, sacral bony defect, and a presacral mass. The presacral mass is most often a teratoma but it can also be a meningocele, a dermoid or an enteric cyst. A significant number of these patients (up to 20%) will also have a tethered spinal cord.

Most patients will present with constipation and there is a positive family history in 50%. For teratoma or dermoid cysts,

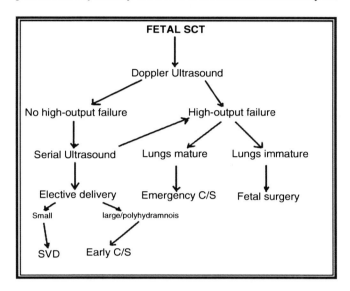

Fig. 95.3 Algorithm for the treatment of sacrococcygeal teratoma

a posterior surgical approach will be adequate to address both the presacral mass and the anal stenosis. Rarely, a combined abdominal approach will be required. When the presacral mass is a meningocele, it is repaired first. The anorectal malformation is addressed at a later date to prevent to risk of meningitis that is associated with a combined approach.

Treatment

Complete surgical excision is the treatment of choice for SCT. This is best accomplished early in the newborn period as a semi-elective procedure, once the baby is properly resuscitated and necessary investigations have been conducted. The type of tumor dictates the surgical approach. For types 1 and 2, a posterior approach is usually adequate (Fig. 95.4).

The goals of surgical resection of an SCT are: (1) complete tumor excision, (2) removal of the coccyx, (3) reconstruction of the pelvic floor and anorectal sphincter, and (4) an acceptable cosmetic appearance. Failure to remove the coccyx is associated with a high rate of recurrence.

After inserting a urinary catheter, the patient is placed in the prone jack-knife position. A V-shape incision is made at the superior margin of the tumor. It is important to identify the course of the anus by placing a Hegar dilator in the anal canal. After raising skin flaps, the muscles are dissected from the tumor. It very important to try to preserve these attenuated fibers.

The teratoma is then mobilized close to its capsule. The superior margin of dissection is where the surgeon will encounter the coccyx, which must be excised, preferably in continuity with the tumor. This is also where the main blood supply to the tumor, from the middle sacral artery or branches of the hypogastric arteries, will be identified. After division of these vessels, the tumor is then separated from the rectum.

Attention is then directed to reconstruction of the anorectal muscles, followed by skin closure. I usually leave a closed suction drain under the skin flaps and keep the patient in the prone position for several days postoperatively.

Challenging Cases

There are situations where the standard method of resection is not applicable and modifications must be made to improve the likelihood of success.

Premature infants with large vascular tumors represent a very high surgical risk. In such cases, one can attempt to initially control the middle sacral and hypogastric arteries through a transabdominal approach or even by laparoscopy. There are also reports describing the use of intra-abdominal devascularization followed by staged resection, extracorporeal membrane oxygenation (ECMO), or hypothermic hypoperfusion.

Postoperative Care

The most serious complication of SCT resection is hemorrhage. In the early postoperative period, there is a risk of urinary retention and wound infection or dehiscence. Other potential complications include urinary or fecal incontinence and an unsatisfactory cosmetic appearance.

After excision, there is a risk of local or distant recurrence. For mature teratoma, the risk of recurrence is approximately 10% and for those with immature elements up to 5% recur. Of those that recur, approximately half are malignant. Recurrent tumors should be resected, if at all possible, along with the coccyx if remains after the initial operation. Malignant yolk sac tumor (endodermal sinus tumor) is usually highly sensitive to chemotherapy, which accounts for a high salvage rate even in the case of malignant degeneration.

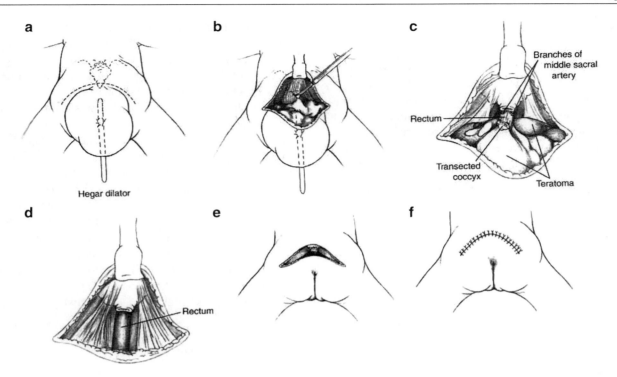

Fig. 95.4 Posterior approach to resection of a sacrococcygeal teratoma. (a) Prone positioning of the infant. It is helpful to place a Hegar dilator partially into the rectum to facilitate its identification during the tumor resection. (b) A "frown" or inverted V posterior incision facilitates access to the tumor and the coccyx, which is being deviated. (c) Middle sacral vessels after division of the coccyx. Once these vessels are ligated and divided, the tumor can be dissected from the rectum and separated from the gluteal and levator muscles. (d) Tumor has been removed and underlying rectum and pelvic muscles can be visualized. (e) Anatomic reconstruction of the anorectal muscles is performed. (f) Final closure of the incision. (From Grosfeld JL, ed. Pediatric surgery. 6th ed. Philadelphia, PA: Mosby; 2006, p. 561. Reprinted with permission from Elsevier)

Because of the risk of local or distant recurrence, it is important to closely follow patients with SCT for at least 4 years. Our practice has been to monitor patients at 3-month intervals for the first 3 years, and 6-month intervals for the next 2 years. Monitoring consists of a physical examination, including a careful rectal examination, and serum AFP levels. Any abnormal finding on examination or elevation of serum markers is pursued with CT or MRI of the abdomen and pelvis and a CT of the chest.

Summary Points

- SCT is the most frequently encountered tumor in the fetus and newborn and is also the most common extra-gonadal germ cell tumor.
- The incidence of SCT is 1 in 30,000 and they are three times more prevalent in females.
- Most SCTs are benign but the incidence of malignancy increases rapidly with age.
- Malignancy is most commonly in the form of yolk sac tumor (endodermal sinus tumor).
- Most are now detected by prenatal ultrasound.
- Factors associated with a poor prognosis include: prenatal detection, more solid than cystic, and fetal hydrops.
- Twenty percent of infants with SCT have associated congenital anomalies.

Editor's Comment

The vast majority of SCTs are now detected by antenatal ultrasound. Thanks to the efforts and experience of fetal treatment centers over the past 10–15 years, treatment algorithms are continually being refined. Predominantly cystic teratomas can usually be safely observed to term, but aspiration of fluid is sometimes indicated for very large cysts that threaten to cause premature labor. Tumors that are predominantly solid are usually well-vascularized, tend to grow rapidly, and are associated with hydrops and fetal demise. If lung maturity can be achieved, early delivery is indicated. If hydrops develops too early in gestation for delivery, in utero resection has been performed with some success. For cases associated with concomitant fetal anomalies, maternal mirror syndrome, or early severe hydrops, delivery is the only alternative.

Managing an infant with a large SCT at birth can be a challenge. The tumor can literally weigh as much or more than the baby and the blood flow to the tumor usually accounts for the majority of cardiac output. After rapid resuscitation and placement of monitoring access, operation should be undertaken rather urgently. Hemorrhage is a devastating complication and can be difficult to prevent and nearly impossible to control once it occurs. Some have attempted to wrap the tumor tightly with an elastic bandage until the operation can be undertaken, but the benefit of this maneuver is unknown. There are compelling reports of those who have attempted to control the blood supply of the tumor by ligating the middle sacral artery using a trans-abdominal approach before proceeding with a standard posterior resection.

Type IV (abdomino-pelvic) SCTs typically present late and therefore have a high rate of malignant degeneration. The diagnosis should be considered in toddlers who develop a change in bowel habits. The tumor can usually be detected by careful digital rectal examination and confirmed by CT or MRI of the pelvis. Tumor markers (AFP, HCG) must be sent and a thorough metastatic work up performed. Surgical resection with coccygectomy is the mainstay of therapy but this can be a difficult operation – too low for a trans-abdominal approach and too high for a perineal approach. A combined approach might be necessary, in which case the trans-abdominal operation should be performed first in order to control the blood supply and mobilize the pelvic and intra-abdominal portion of the tumor.

Although yolk sac tumors that arise within SCTs in young children are usually chemosensitive, malignant germ cell tumors that arise in the sacral region in otherwise healthy adolescents can be very difficult to treat. They are infiltrative and sometimes locally invasive, extremely difficult to resect in their entirety, and poorly responsive to chemotherapy or radiation. It is sometimes necessary to perform multiple operations in an attempt to eradicate all residual and recurrent tumor. It is unknown whether these tumors arise de novo or within an occult SCT, but either way they usually arise from or near the coccyx, making coccygectomy in all cases a reasonable recommendation.

Diagnostic Studies

- CT or MRI of the abdomen and pelvis
- AFP, quantitative β-HCG
- CT of the chest (metastatic work up)

Preoperative Preparation

- ☐ 3D imaging
- ☐ Type and crossmatch
- ☐ Bowel decompression
- ☐ Prophylactic antibiotics

Parental Preparation

- This is a major operation with significant risks of hemorrhage, injury to adjacent structures, and, for infants with high-output heart failure, death.
- After successful resection, children are monitored closely for 4–5 years for possible recurrence and malignancy.
- Long term, children are at risk for bowel and bladder dysfunction (constipation, incontinence).

Technical Points

- The goals of surgical resection are: complete tumor excision, removal of the coccyx, reconstruction of the pelvic floor and anorectal sphincter, and an acceptable cosmetic appearance.
- The posterior approach is standard and usually allows for complete resection of the tumor.
- The blood supply is from the middle sacral artery or branches of the hypogastric arteries.
- The anus and rectum are severely displaced by the tumor and a dilator placed in the anorectum during the operation helps to avoid inadvertent injury.

Suggested Reading

Bittmann S, Bittmann V. Surgical experience and cosmetic outcomes in children with sacrococcygeal teratoma. Curr Surg. 2006;63:51–4.

Cozzi F, Schiavetti A, Zani A, et al. The functional sequelae of sacrococcygeal teratoma: a longitudinal and cross-sectional follow-up study. J Pediatr Surg. 2008;43:658–61.

Derikx JP, De Backer A, van de Schoot L, et al. Long-term functional sequelae of sacrococcygeal teratoma: a national study in the Netherlands. J Pediatr Surg. 2007;42:1122–6.

Derikx JP, De Backer A, van de Schoot L, et al. Factors associated with recurrence and metastasis in sacrococcygeal teratoma. Br J Surg. 2006;93:1543–8.

Draper H, Chitayat D, Ein SH, Langer JC. Long-term functional results following resection of neonatal sacrococcygeal teratoma. Pediatr Surg Int. 2009;25(3):243–6.

Gabra HO, Jesudason EC, McDowell HP, et al. Sacrococcygeal teratoma – a 25 year experience in a UK regional center. J Pediatr Surg. 2006;41:1513–6.

Hedrick HL, Flake AW, Crombleholme TM, et al. Sacrococcygeal tera-
    toma: prenatal assessment, fetal intervention, and outcome. J Pediatr
    Surg. 2004;39:430–8.
Kaneyama K, Yamataka A, Kobayashi H, et al. Giant, highly vascular
    sacrococcygeal teratoma: report of its excision using the Ligasure
    vessel sealing system. J Pediatr Surg. 2004;39:1791–3.

Tran KM, Flake AW, Kalawadia NV, et al. Emergent excision of a prenatally
    diagnosed sacrococcygeal teratoma. Pediatr Anaesth. 2008;18:431–4.
Wakhlu A, Misra S, Tandon RK, et al. Sacrococcygeal teratoma. Pediatr
    Surg Int. 2002;18:384–7.

Chapter 96
Ovarian Tumors

Kirk W. Reichard

Ovarian pathology can present in a variety of ways including abdominal pain, abdominal mass, abnormal vaginal bleeding, precocious puberty, and on routine antenatal ultrasound. Because the ovary is composed of epithelial, sex cord-stromal and germ cell elements, there are many different neoplastic and non-neoplastic conditions that may develop. Fortunately, the majority of these lesions in children are benign, and a rational differential diagnosis and treatment plan can be developed based on the patient's age, presenting symptoms, and the appearance on initial diagnostic imaging.

Most girls with suspected ovarian pathology will undergo pelvic ultrasound examination as the initial diagnostic study. Cystic lesions can be readily identified and the fluid characterized as simple or complex, with debris and septa that suggest either hemorrhage or torsion. It is crucial that a Doppler flow study be performed in this case, to confirm the presence of pulsatile blood flow within the ovary. Ultrasound can also identify fat and calcifications that are found in teratomas. Large, poorly circumscribed, complex masses with areas of necrosis or hemorrhage are suspicious for malignancy.

Further diagnostic imaging is indicated for patients with complex cystic or solid lesions. Computed tomography provides better delineation of the soft tissue components of the mass, including fat and calcification, is valuable in detecting evidence of metastases in the liver or lymph nodes, and, as the initial modality in patients who present with abdominal pain, can help to rule out other pathology. However, it is worth remembering that small, simple ovarian cysts are normal in pre-adolescents and adolescents and in the absence of rupture, hemorrhage or excessively large size are an unlikely cause of pain. MRI is said to be superior to CT for the imaging of pelvic organs, as it is more specific in characterizing soft tissue and fluid components and can show evidence of torsion or PID. Nevertheless, in most institutions CT is more readily available and usually provides the information necessary to proceed with the proper course of therapy.

Many neoplastic and non-neoplastic ovarian masses are hormonally active. Functional cysts and sex cord-stromal tumors occasionally produce sufficient estrogen to cause precocious puberty and gonadotropin suppression in premenarchal girls. Germ cell tumors may also secrete certain tumor markers. Alpha fetoprotein is normally secreted by certain embryonic and fetal tissue and is markedly elevated in patients with yolk sac (endodermal sinus) tumor as well as embryonal carcinoma. However, levels of AFP are normally well over 10,000 ng/dL in newborns and do not fall to normal levels for 6–8 months (Table 96.1). AFP has a serum half-life of 5–7 days, and can be used to determine adequacy of treatment as well as an early harbinger of recurrence. The β-subunit of human chorionic gonatrotropin (βHCG) is secreted by various germ cell tumors, including choriocarcinoma and embryonal carcinoma. It has a short half-life and so its level falls much more quickly than AFP after complete resection of tumor. CA-125 is a valuable marker in epithelial tumors, but has limited use in children. Some hormonally inactive tumors produce high levels of LDH based purely on bulky disease.

Purely Cystic Lesions

Functional cysts are non-neoplastic cysts that arise in response to endogenous or exogenous gonadotropins and can often be found incidentally on imaging studies of the pelvis. These cysts usually resolve spontaneously and can be managed expectantly.

In the fetal and neonatal period, follicular cysts develop in response to maternal gonadotropins and occur more commonly in pregnancies complicated by diabetes, preeclampsia or Rh disease. Neoplastic cystic lesions are quite rare in this age group. Non-echogenic, simple cysts that are asymptomatic and measure less than 5 cm can safely be observed with serial pelvic ultrasound, with resolution expected within the first 3–6 months of life. Cysts that are 5 cm or larger are thought to be at increased risk for torsion. These cysts can be percutaneously aspirated or drained and

K.W. Reichard (✉)
Thomas Jefferson School of Medicine, Alfred I. DuPont Hospital for Children, 1600 Rockland Road, Wilmington, DE 19803, USA
e-mail: kreichar@nemours.org

P. Mattei (ed.), *Fundamentals of Pediatric Surgery*,
DOI 10.1007/978-1-4419-6643-8_96, © Springer Science+Business Media, LLC 2011

Table 96.1 Average normal serum AFP in infants

Age	n	Mean ± SD (ng/mL)
Premature	11	134,734 ± 41,444
Newborn	55	48,406 ± 34,718
Newborn-2 weeks	16	33,113 ± 32,503
2 Week to 1 month	43	9,452 ± 12,610
1 Month	12	2,654 ± 3,080
2 Months	40	323 ± 278
3 Months	5	88 ± 87
4 Months	31	74 ± 56
5 Months	6	46.5 ± 19
6 Months	9	12.5 ± 9.8
7 Months	5	9.7 ± 7.1
8 Months	3	8.5 ± 5.5

Source: Reprinted with permission from Wu JT, et al. Serum AFP levels in normal infants. Pediatr Res. 1981;15:50

unroofed laparoscopically or at laparotomy. Occasionally, large fetal cysts are aspirated in an attempt to prevent antenatal torsion. Complex cysts should be managed surgically with ovarian sparing techniques whenever possible, although many of these lesions will prove to be ovaries that have undergone antenatal torsion.

In perimenarchal and adolescent girls, functional cysts are very common. Follicular cysts develop before ovulation, and can continue to grow if ovulation does not occur. Corpus luteum cysts develop after ovulation and can spontaneously hemorrhage. As long as normal blood flow can be demonstrated on Doppler examination, simple and hemorrhagic cysts that measure less than 5 cm are typically observed, generally resolving in 8–12 weeks. Cysts that are symptomatic, larger than 5 cm, or complex but not obviously hemorrhagic should be managed with cyst excision, taking care to spare the ovary. Aspiration, simple unroofing or marsupialization are less likely to cause ovarian damage, but are associated with higher recurrence rates. The lining of the cyst must be removed. Occasionally, adnexal mullerian remnants can develop into large cysts that preoperatively may be indistinguishable from ovarian cysts.

Ovarian Torsion

Girls who present with the acute onset of severe pelvic pain must be evaluated promptly for ovarian torsion. These patients can present with associated nausea and vomiting but usually do not exhibit the other signs of appendicitis. Ultrasound with Doppler examination is the diagnostic modality of choice. Underlying pathology, such as a functional cyst or teratoma, is found in the majority of patients with ovarian torsion, although nearly a quarter occur in otherwise normal ovaries. Torsion is less common in the setting of a malignancy, but torsion by no means rules it out with certainty. Occasionally,

acute hemorrhage into a fuctional cyst may mimic the clinical findings of torsion, and should be treated similarly if ultrasound findings are unclear and normal blood flow cannot be confirmed by Doppler preoperatively. The traditional treatment for an ovary that appears completely necrotic after detorsion has been oophorectomy, but recently many have challenged this approach, calling instead for detorsion and, in some cases, oophoropexy. Nevertheless, if underlying neoplastic pathology is suspected, or if a large amount of necrotic tissue is present, oophorectomy is still the procedure of choice. Torsion of the contralateral ovary is rare, particularly if a pathologic lesion is found on the first side. Contralateral pexy of a normal ovary is not routinely recommended unless there is evidence for laxity of the ovarian suspensory ligaments.

Mixed and Solid Masses

Unlike purely cystic lesions, mixed or solid neoplasms of the ovary are more likely to be malignant. Nevertheless, most are still benign, particularly in younger girls. Malignant tumors more frequently present as an asymptomatic mass, or with chronic pain and abdominal swelling. They are thought to undergo torsion less often than benign lesions, but can present with acute pain from hemorrhage. Solid masses in the perinatal period are extraordinarily rare.

Germ cell tumors make up nearly two thirds of all ovarian masses in children and adolescents, although sex cord-stromal tumors are relatively more common in young girls. In older adolescents and young adults, epithelial tumors begin to become more prominent, although they are usually benign or of low malignant potential (e.g., mucinous and serous adenomas). Invasive adenocarcinoma is quite rare in the pediatric age group.

Staging of pediatric ovarian masses has traditionally followed the International Federation of Gynecology and Obstetrics (FIGO) system used in adults, which was developed mainly for patients with epithelial tumors (Table 96.2). More recently, the Childen's Oncology Group (COG) has developed a staging system for patients with germ cell tumors that is used in all current clinical protocols. Both staging systems depend upon a standardized operative technique, which should be followed in all patients with complex mixed or solid masses. Given the different biological behavior in pediatric tumors and the desire to preserve fertility in young girls and adolescents, the operative approach to staging in children has become more conservative than that traditionally prescribed for adults (Table 96.3).

A midline laparotomy is generally employed, although a transverse mid-hypogastric incision may be appropriate, especially in younger girls. Laparoscopic approaches have

Table 96.2 Children's oncology group ovarian germ cell tumor staging and risk-based therapy

Stage	Extent of disease	Treatment (COG, AGCT 0132)
I	Limited to ovary or ovariesPeritoneal washings negative for malignant cells	Surgery only (low risk)
	No clinical, radiographic or histologic evidence of disease beyond the ovaries	
	Tumor markers normal after appropriate postsurgical half-life decline	
	The presence of gliomatosis peritonei[a] does not upstage patient	
II	Microscopic residual or positive lymph nodes (≤2 cm as measured by a pathologist)Peritoneal washings negative for malignant cells	PEB ×3 (intermediate risk)
	Tumor markers positive or negative	
	The presence of gliomatosis peritonei[a] does not upstage patient	
III	Lymph with malignant metastatic nodule (>2 cm as measured by a pathologist)Gross residual or biopsy only	PEB ×3 (intermediate risk)
	Contiguous visceral involvement (omentum, intestines, bladder)	
	Peritoneal washings positive for malignant cells	
	Tumor markers positive or negative	
IV	Distant metastases, including liver	PEB ×4 (high Risk)

PEB = compressed-dose cisplatin, etoposide and bleomycin

[a]Peritoneal nodules composed entirely of mature glial tissue and having no malignant elements

Table 96.3 Operative staging recommendations

Laparotomy
Collect peritoneal fluid/peritoneal washings
Inspect and palpate normal ovary (only biopsy suspicious lesions)
Inspect for tumor extension
    Omentum – omentectomy if involved
    Peritoneal surfaces – biopsy suspicious lesions
    Other organs – resection only if no functional consequence
Search for enlarged lymph nodes – biopsy and debulk when possible
Tumor resection – unilateral oophorectomy, with salphingectomy if there is tubal involvement, preserving fertility if possible

been described, but because of the increased risk of spillage and subsequent upstaging of the tumor it should only be considered when the lesion is small or the risk for malignancy is low. Immediately upon entering the abdomen, any free peritoneal fluid should be aspirated and sent for cytology. If no fluid is apparent, saline washings should be obtained. The contralateral ovary is then carefully inspected. A normal appearing ovary should not be bivalved or randomly biopsied, but suspicious nodules should be excised for histopathologic analysis. Pelvic and retroperitoneal lymph nodes should be inspected visually and by palpation and any enlarged or suspicious nodes should be removed. It is unnecessary to perform omentectomy for germ cell tumors unless the omentum is adherent to the tumor or when there is obvious tumor extension or nodularity. Any peritoneal nodules should be biopsied. The remainder of the intra-abdominal viscera should be inspected for tumor spread, and suspicious areas biopsied. Attention should then be turned to the primary tumor. The vast majority of pediatric ovarian tumors are adequately treated with unilateral oophorectomy, preserving of the fallopian tube if it is free of gross disease. Bilateral tumors are quite uncommon,

and so bilateral oophorectomy and hysterectomy are rarely indicated, especially at the first operation.

Germ Cell Tumors

The majority of ovarian neoplasms in children and adolescents are germ cell tumors, and the ovary is one of the most common sites for a germ cell tumor to develop, second only to the sacrococcygeal region when all age groups are considered. The specific type of tumor depends upon the pathway and degree of differentiation that the neoplastic primordial germ cells take (Fig. 96.1). Undifferentiated cells produce germinomas. Extra-embryonic differentiation leads to choriocarcinoma and yolk sac (endodermal sinus) tumors. Embryonal carcinomas develop from partial embryonic differentiation, while more complete embryonic differentiation yields mature and immature teratomas.

Teratomas

Mixed cystic lesions are usually benign in children and adolescents, with teratomas by far the most common. Teratomas contain elements from all three embryonic tissue layers: ectoderm, mesoderm and endoderm. One or more may predominate, and not all need be present in the same tumor, but there must be embryonic tissue elements in an ectopic location. Fat and organized calcifications, such as teeth or bone, are typically seen on preoperative imaging. They are often predominantly comprised of cysts, which may contain simple fluid or a significant amount of protein and cellular debris. Benign

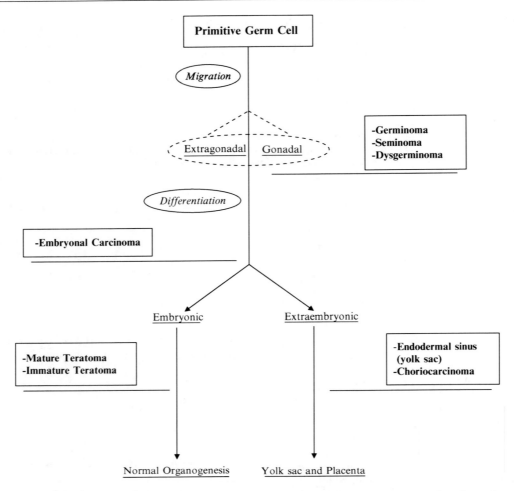

Fig. 96.1 Schematic diagram of the differentiation of the primordial germ cell and points where mutations or altered growth patterns lead to the various germ cell tumors encountered in clinical practice

teratomas are further classified as mature (more common) or immature, based upon the degree of cellular differentiation and presence of immature neural (glial) elements. The level of maturity is graded on a scale of 1–4, in ascending order of immaturity and likelihood of malignant potential. Patients with lesions that are grade 2 and above are typically treated with adjuvant chemotherapy. Patients with both mature and immature teratomas may be found to have plaques of glial tissue studding the peritoneal surfaces at laparotomy. These should be biopsied, but are not considered malignant, do not affect staging, and do not need to be completely removed.

Germ cell tumors, usually endodermal sinus or yolk sac, can rarely be seen arising within a teratoma and should be suspected in patients with significantly elevated preoperative AFP level. It should be noted, however, that the embryonic tissue in benign teratomas can produce modest elevations in AFP. Although quite unusual, any tissue type found in a teratoma can undergo malignant degeneration, giving rise to adenocarcinomas, sarcomas, or Wilms tumor, among others. The postoperative therapy for these malignant

tumors is guided by the histology and stage of the malignant component.

The operative approach should include the elements of the staging procedure described above. Teratomas must be resected intact. It is inappropriate to drain the fluid intraoperatively, as one might for a simple cyst. Although controversial, complete resection of the tumor with the affected ovary is the standard approach for unilateral disease. Enucleation of a mature teratoma with ovarian preservation leads to a marginally higher recurrence rate, but this approach is advocated by some authors for smaller, well-circumscribed tumors. Enucleation should clearly be attempted in patients with bilateral disease and those who have already had one ovary removed.

Patients with mature teratomas sometimes develop recurrence, including occasional reports of germ cell tumor, whether treated with oophorectomy or cystectomy. Therefore it is recommended that they undergo post-op monitoring with serum AFP and ultrasounds, obtained at 6–12-month intervals for 3–5 years.

Malignant Germ Cell Tumors

Germ cell tumors are the most common malignant ovarian neoplasm in childhood. Among this group, yolk sac tumor, also known as endodermal sinus tumor, prevails in most series. It is an aggressively malignant tumor and, in the vast majority of cases, is characterized by markedly elevated AFP levels.

Germinomas are somewhat less common in girls, but when combined with seminoma (which is the same cell type in males) and dysgerminoma (their extra-gonadal counterpart), they are the most common histological type in children overall. These tumors frequently present in association with other cell-types, so called mixed germ cell tumors. Germinomas can become quite large before presentation and although these tumors are generally not hormonally active, they usually produce high levels of lactate dehydrogenase (LDH).

Embryonal and choriocarcinoma are relatively less common germ cell malignancies. Both can produce isosexual precocious puberty or menstrual disturbances due to secretion of βHCG. Choriocarcinoma is particularly aggressive and can occur in various forms during pregnancy.

The general treatment approach is similar in all malignant germ cell tumors. Complete evaluation of tumor extent as outlined above is the first goal, as accurate staging guides subsequent therapy. To preserve fertility, unilateral oophorectomy or salphingo-oophorectomy is preferred whenever feasible. However, if tumor is identified in the contralateral ovary, bilateral oophorectomy is required. More extensive disease should be debulked, but neoadjuvant therapy followed by delayed resection is a reasonable course for advanced local disease.

The treatment of malignant germ cell tumors has been revolutionized by the advent of platinum-based chemotherapy, which is now the mainstay. The current COG protocol calls for surgery alone with careful surveillance for patients with stage I (low risk) ovarian tumors. Patients with stage II and III (intermediate risk) tumors receive compressed-dose cisplatin, etoposide and bleomycin (PEB) therapy. Patients with advanced disease may respond to standard PEB regimens. High-dose therapy combined with stem cell transplantation is utilized for unresponsive or recurrent disease.

Sex Cord-Stromal Tumors

Sex cord-stromal tumors arise from pre-committed mesenchymal cells destined to become granulose-theca cells in the ovary and sertoli-leydig cells in the testes. As a group, they are the second most common category of ovarian neoplasm in children and are nearly equal in incidence with germ cell tumors in younger girls. Patients with these hormonally active tumors typically present with precocious puberty. In younger girls, granulosa-theca cell tumors are more prevalent and cause true precocious puberty, whereas sertoli-leydig cell tumors predominate in older girls and generally produce virilization due to the secretion of testosterone.

Surgical staging guidelines are the same as for the germ cell tumors. Most patients with sex cord-stromal tumors present with stage 1 disease and carry a favorable prognosis, responding well to unilateral oophorectomy alone. More advanced lesions tend to be quite aggressive and require multimodal therapy, including radiation therapy in patients with granulosa-theca cell lesions.

Epithelial Tumors

Tumors that arise from the surface epithelial cells are the least common ovarian neoplasm in children and adolescents, but become the predominant tumor type in adult women. Most of these are benign mucinous or serous tumors that respond well to local surgical therapy. Malignant epithelial neoplasms differ from their adult counterpart in several ways, including a higher incidence of the mucinous cell type and higher incidence of tumors with borderline or low malignant potential, which make up a third of malignancies in adolescents.

Epithelial tumors are hormonally inactive and can present with very large tumors and bulky disease. They may also present with pain from torsion or hemorrhage. Most of these neoplasms elaborate CA-125, which, though not as specific as the other ovarian tumor markers, can be used as a diagnostic tool and as a measure of response to therapy.

After a proper staging laparotomy, ovarian epithelial malignancies are staged according to the FIGO staging system. Loco-regional spread is more common in these tumors and has a much greater impact on extent of surgery. Tumors isolated to one or both ovaries without capsular invasion can be treated with unilateral or bilateral salphingo-oophorectomy. Patients with more locally advanced disease require total abdominal hysterectomy and bilateral salpingo-oophorectomy. Cytoreduction is a key component to therapy. Adjuvant platinum-based chemotherapy is employed in nearly all cases. Borderline or low malignant potential tumors are usually treated with surgery alone, sparing fertility in many cases. Recurrences generally respond well to further surgery resection.

Ovarian tumors present in a variety of clinical scenarios, and represent a wide-ranging differential diagnosis (Table 96.4). The age of the patient, presenting symptoms

Table 96.4 Differential diagnosis and management strategy

Purely cystic	If symptomatic, complex or large: Laparoscopic/open drainage with resection of lining, and preservation of ovarian function (consider pexy)
Functional cysts	
Follicular (neonatal and peri-menarchal)	
Corpus lutean (peri-menarchal)	If asymptomatic and less than 5 cm: nonoperative management with serial US to confirm resolution
Mullerian remnants (e.g., para-tubal)	
Torsion	Urgent exploration and detorsion
Acute onset of pain (With abnormal ovary on ultrasound)	Inspect contralateral side
May have underlying pathology (Functional cyst, teratoma, malignancy)	Resection if
	Underlying pathology suspected (think about staging)
Hemorrhagic cysts (may be difficult to differentiate by ultrasound)	Large amount of necrotic tissue
	Pexy
	Ipsilateral if preserving
	Contralateral only of ligaments are lax
Complex/solid	Obtain CT or MRI to look for intra-abdominal spread
Germ cell neoplasms	Send tumor markers (AFP, βHCG, LDH, CA 125)
Teratomas (mature, immature)	Laparoscopy/mini-laparotomy ONLY for benign lesions
Malignant GCTs (endodermal sinus, germinoma, embryonal, and choriocarcinoma)	Malignant or uncertain lesions require formal staging laparotomy
Sex cord/stromal tumors	Large, bulky, and unresectable lesions can be biopsied initially, followed by neoadjuvant chemotherapy
Epithelial neoplasms	
Benign (cystadenomas)	
Malignant (mucinous or serous adenocarcinomas)	
Borderline/low malignant potential	

and appearance on imaging can help refine the diagnostic possibilities and therapeutic strategies. Functional cysts can generally be monitored unless they are large, symptomatic or have debris or septations on imaging. Teratomas are the most common benign ovarian neoplasm in children and can usually be managed with conservative resection that preserves fertility. Malignant lesions are derived from a variety of cell types and exhibit heterogeneous behavior. A careful preoperative evaluation and thorough intraoperative staging are the cornerstone of successful treatment, the ultimate goal of which is not only cure, but preservation of fertility.

Summary Points

- The ovary is composed of epithelial, sex cord-stromal and germ cell elements, each of which can produce neoplasms.
- Alpha fetoprotein is normally secreted by embryonic and is elevated in patients with yolk sac (endodermal sinus) tumor and embryonal carcinoma.
- Beta-HCG is secreted by choriocarcinoma and embryonal carcinoma.
- Non-echogenic simple cysts in newborns that are asymptomatic and less than 5 cm can be safely observed with serial pelvic ultrasound, with resolution expected within the first 3–6 months of life.
- In the setting of torsion, if underlying neoplastic pathology is suspected or if a large amount of necrotic tissue is present, oophorectomy is the procedure of choice.
- Germ cell tumors make up nearly two thirds of ovarian masses in children, although sex cord-stromal tumors are relatively more common in young girls.
- Given the different tumor biology and the desire to preserve fertility in young girls, the operative approach to staging in children is more conservative than it is for adults.
- Embryonal and choriocarcinoma can produce isosexual precocious puberty or menstrual disturbances due to secretion of βHCG.
- Tumors that arise from the surface epithelial cells are the least common ovarian neoplasm in children but are the predominant tumor type in adults.

Editor's Comment

Most of the diagnostic and treatment paradigms that we apply in the care of children with ovarian tumors are still based on the now somewhat dated concepts that were developed for women with epithelial ovarian cancer. Although there some similarities, the biology of germ cell tumors is typically different than that of epithelial cancers and therefore they should probably be approached differently. The unique psychosocial needs of adolescents and the importance of preserving sexual function and fertility are also factors to consider when determining the correct surgical approach. Nevertheless, based on the results of more recent clinical trials and the experience of many pediatric surgical oncologists, these protocols are gradually being updated and appropriately individualized.

As a rule, every ovarian mass in a young girl should be assumed to be malignant until proven otherwise. This even applies to large ovarian cysts (larger than 8 cm or growing rapidly) and mature teratomas, which though benign can contain immature (glial) elements that can seed the peritoneum (gliomatosis peritonei) or harbor a malignancy. In addition, a benign neoplasm (mucinous cystadenoma) can look just like a simple benign cyst but is associated with a risk of recurrence if incompletely excised or if its contents are spilled. Consequently, when treating a young patient with an ovarian mass: (1) surgical intervention should be undertaken without excessive delay, (2) serum tumor markers (AFP, βHCG) should be sent as part of the preoperative work up in all cases, and (3) the surgical approach must not put the patient at risk for spillage and subsequent up-staging of the tumor. This sometimes makes it difficult to consider a minimally invasive approach, which greatly increases the risk of spillage. As a general rule, laparoscopy should be used only in cases in which spillage is thought to be unlikely (small mature teratoma) or harmless (thin-walled simple cyst). When in doubt, it is recommended that a Pfannenstiel or lower midline incision be used and that precautions be taken to avoid even microscopic spillage. Tumors should be removed en bloc and with meticulous technique. To avoid a big incision when dealing with a large cyst, many surgeons will drain the cyst prior to performing the resection. This is technically considered spillage regardless of what precautions are taken. Some have resorted to creative maneuvers such as using cyanoacrylate adhesive to attach sterile plastic sheeting to the capsule of the tumor and thus create a barrier that is presumably impervious to spillage. Nevertheless, there is on-going debate as to the best way to balance the need to avoid harm (tumor spread) and the desire to minimize scarring.

Despite a lack of supportive data, traditional gynecology oncology guidelines often recommend ipsilateral salpingo-oophorectomy in all patients with an ovarian tumor. For most tumor types seen in girls, however, this is probably excessive. The approach recommended for young women with an ovarian mass is to preserve the fallopian tube unless it is directly involved with tumor and, when possible, to preserve part of the capsule of the ovary, which is where the ova reside. When the nature of the mass is not known, one can remove the entire mass using an ovary-sparing technique and send it for frozen-section analysis before deciding whether the ovary needs to be removed. When there is obvious metastatic disease, spillage is less of an issue and cyst drainage or incisional biopsy are acceptable. Although some surgical oncologists cringe at the concept of "tumor debulking," ovarian cancer is one of the few tumors for which reducing the gross volume of tumor is palliative and, in some cases, might also improve survival. Inspection and selective biopsy of suspicious iliac and para-aortic lymph nodes should be performed as part of the staging process but formal lymph node dissection is unlikely to be therapeutic and is associated with significant complications.

Diagnostic Studies

- Imaging
  - Pelvic ultrasound
  - Abdominal-pelvic CT scan
  - MRI (rarely)
- Laboratory
  - AFP
  - βHCG
  - Estrogens/testosterone (with precocious puberty or masculinization)

Parental Preparation

- We will try to preserve the fallopian tube and a portion of the ovary if it can be done safely.
- We might not be able to perform a proper operation through minimally invasive surgery because of the risk of spillage and the risk of tumor spread.
- Frequent follow up with blood tests for tumor markers and serial imaging will be necessary after proper surgical intervention has been performed.

Preoperative Preparation

- ☐ Thorough imaging studies
- ☐ AFP, βHCG levels

Technical Points

- A lower midline or transverse incision is usually best, unless the risk of malignancy or spillage is considered to be minimal.
- Torsed ovaries can be detorsed and preserved if there is no evidence of tumor.
- The fallopian tube and a portion of the ovary can be preserved in some cases.
- Proper staging is selective and includes aspiration of ascites and careful inspection of the contralateral ovary, omentum, peritoneum, and lymph node basins with biopsy of suspicious lesions only.
- It is paramount to avoid spillage of any cyst or tumor that could even remotely be malignant, even if this means using a larger incision than one would like.

Suggested Reading

Morowitz M, Huff D, von Allmen D. Epithelial ovarian tumors in children: a retrospective analysis. J Pediatr Surg. 2003;38(3): 331–5.

Pomeranz AJ, Sabnis S. Misdiagnoses of ovarian masses in children and adolescents. Pediatr Emerg Care. 2004;20(3):172–4.

Schultz KA, Ness KK, Nagarajan R, Steiner ME. Adnexal masses in infancy and childhood. Clin Obstet Gynecol. 2006;49(3): 464–79.

Templeman CL, Fallat ME. In: Grosfeld JL, O'Neill JA, Coran AG, Fonkalsrud EW, editors. Ovarian tumors: Pediatric surgery. 6th edn. Philadelphia: Mosby Elsevier; 2006. p. 593–621.

Ulbright TM. Germ cell tumors of the gonads: a selective review emphasizing problems in differential diagnosis, newly appreciated, and controversial issues. Mod Pathol. 2005;18 Suppl 2: S61–79.

von Allmen D. Malignant lesions of the ovary in childhood. Semin Pediatr Surg. 2005;14(2):100–5.

Chapter 97
Pediatric Testicular Tumors

Ismael Zamilpa and Martin A. Koyle

Primary testicular tumors in pediatric patients represent a rare entity, especially in the prepubertal male. The incidence of testicular neoplasms in children is approximately one tenth of that in adults. Although clinical presentation is similar, differences exist in terms of histological distribution, the incidence of malignancy, and the likelihood of metastatic disease. These differences have led to unique management strategies in children. Initial therapy still involves excision of the primary lesion. As in most adult patients, the prognosis in children is excellent, with overall patient survival approximating 100%. To help better define management of these tumors, the Prepubertal Testis Tumor Registry was established by the American Academy of Pediatrics in 1980 and has compiled data regarding presentation, treatment, and outcomes.

The majority of pediatric patients with a testicular neoplasm will present before the age of two. A painless scrotal mass is the most common initial complaint. Boys referred for the evaluation of precocious puberty also must be carefully evaluated for a testicular tumor, which can be very difficult to appreciate on examination. A thorough history and physical examination is paramount. Special attention should be paid to the genitalia and, in particular, the contralateral gonad, as bilateral testicular tumors can rarely be present. Transillumination of the testis can provide an indication of cystic or solid components.

A scrotal ultrasound is recommended to evaluate the mass and adjacent testicular parenchyma. This is especially helpful for preoperative preparation if a testis-sparing approach is being considered. A scrotal ultrasound is also recommended if the testicle cannot be adequately palpated, for example in the patient with a large, tense hydrocele. Testicular tumors can appear as solid or cystic lesions on ultrasound. Cystic tumors are more likely to be benign.

Testicular microlithiasis has been reported in association with yolk sac tumors.

Prior to surgical exploration, serum tumor marker levels should be measured. Alpha fetoprotein (AFP) is the only tumor marker necessary in children. Cell types associated with elevations in LDH or β-HCG (choriocarcinoma, seminoma, embryonal) are not seen in the pre-pubertal age group. Pre-operative tumor marker levels and histopathology findings following surgery will dictate additional imaging. The combination of normal serum AFP and benign features on ultrasound help to identify potential candidates for a testis-sparing surgical approach. Children under 6 months of age or an elevated AFP should have a metastatic work up, including a CT scan of the abdomen and pelvis and plain radiograph or CT of the chest.

Histological Distribution

Primary testicular tumors in children are of germ cell or stromal origin. Germ cell tumors include yolk sac tumors, teratomas, and epidermoid cysts. Stromal tumors include Leydig cell tumors, Sertoli cell tumors, juvenile granulosa cell tumors, and mixed gonadal stromal tumors. In the prepubertal male, yolk sac tumors and teratomas account for the majority of neoplasms. This is in contrast to the situation in adults, where mixed germ cell tumors and pure seminomas predominate. In addition, the incidence of benign lesions is much higher in children than in adults.

Yolk sac tumors represent the most common malignant neoplasms in children, the majority of whom will have an elevated serum AFP at presentation. It is important to note that elevations in AFP will be seen in newborns up to and beyond 6 months of age, therefore it may not be useful in distinguishing a yolk sac neoplasm from other scrotal pathology early in life.

Teratomas are possibly the most common testicular tumor in children, but the incidence is likely significantly underreported because they are generally benign. These tumors are composed of tissues derived from all germ cell layers

I. Zamilpa (✉)
Department of Pediatric Urology, University of Washington, Seattle Children's Hospital, 4800 Sand Point Way NE, W-7727, Seattle, WA 98105, USA
e-mail: ismael.zamilpa@seattlechildrens.org

P. Mattei (ed.), *Fundamentals of Pediatric Surgery*,
DOI 10.1007/978-1-4419-6643-8_97, © Springer Science+Business Media, LLC 2011

(endoderm, mesoderm, ectoderm) in various stages of maturation. Mature and immature teratomas are invariably benign. Epidermoid cysts are benign testicular lesions described as epithelium-lined cysts filled with keratin. Although once thought of as monodermal teratomas, they are now considered non-teratomatous benign masses.

Stromal testicular tumors are extremely rare. *Leydig cell tumors* behave in a benign fashion in pre-pubertal males and are often associated with precocious puberty or gynecomastia. In children, *Sertoli cell tumors* are hormonally inactive. Sertoli cell tumors and mixed gonadal stromal tumors are potentially malignant and metastases have been described. *Juvenile granulosa cell tumors* usually present within the first 6 months of age. They are hormonally inactive lesions that are often seen in patients with ambiguous genitalia or abnormal sex chromosomes but are considered benign entities.

Treatment

Surgical therapy is the standard of care and often the only treatment necessary. Operations for testicular tumors, including both radical orchiectomy and testis-sparing surgery, should always be done through an inguinal incision. The incision is made medial and parallel to the ipsilateral inguinal ligament, between the lateral edge of the pubic symphysis and the anterior superior iliac spine. The external oblique fascia is incised along the direction of its fibers. It is necessary to incise the fascia beyond the external inguinal ring in order to deliver the testicle without difficulty. The ilio-inguinal nerve can be identified traveling along the anterior surface of the spermatic cord. The nerve must be dissected away from the cord structures, and carefully secured outside the operative field. The spermatic cord should be mobilized from surrounding tissues, and encircled with a quarter-inch penrose drain that can be used later as a gentle tourniquet. Cremasteric muscle fibers are divided with bovie cautery. Prior to delivering the testicle, the operative field is isolated with sterile surgical towels and, before aggressive manipulation of the gonad is undertaken, vascular control is a must. Cord vessels should be occluded as close as possible to the internal inguinal ring. Once vascular control is achieved, the testicle is delivered. During a radical orchiectomy, a high ligation of the cord is performed. The use of non-absorbable sutures facilitates intra-abdominal identification of the cord structures if a retroperitoneal lymph node dissection is performed. Once the specimen is removed, the external oblique fascia can be approximated with absorbable suture. Skin edges should be approximated using a subcuticular closure with fine absorbable monofilament.

The child older than 6 months with an elevated AFP is presumed to have a yolk sac tumor and is recommended to undergo radical orchiectomy. Those with a normal AFP level and an ultrasound that suggests the potential for testicular preservation should undergo inguinal exploration with vascular control of the cord and excisional biopsy with frozen section analysis. If pathologic analysis reveals a malignant lesion, then radical orchiectomy should be performed. The diagnosis of a benign lesion, such as teratoma, epidermoid tumor or Leydig cell tumor, should lead to closure of the tunica albuginea with absorbable suture and replacement of the testis in the scrotum.

Lesions that are encapsulated or well-circumscribed are more amenable to a parenchymal sparing approach than infiltrating lesions, which can be difficult to remove without sacrificing a large amount of normal tissue. If sufficient normal parenchyma remains after excisional biopsy, it should be preserved. On the other hand, the biopsy must include some normal parenchyma at the margins. This is especially important in the case of teratomas in children who are approaching puberty: since teratomas in adolescents and adults are considered malignant, the presence of post-pubertal changes within the normal parenchyma mandates that a radical orchiectomy be performed.

Diagnostic uncertainty after frozen section analysis presents a significant challenge, especially given the low likelihood of an aggressive tumor. We will have discussed this rare scenario in advance with the family and will involve them in the decision. We have never had to return to remove a missed malignant neoplasm later identified on permanent section. In terms of recurrence and sustained growth of remaining testicular parenchyma, the results of testis-sparing surgery have been encouraging.

The staging (Table 97.1) and management of testicular tumors in children generally parallels that in adults. In fact, the recommendation in cases of scrotal violation have included hemiscrotectomy or the excision of the scrotal scar at the time of retroperitoneal node dissection. Unfortunately, due to the lack of evidence supporting a less aggressive approach, no conclusive recommendations are available for the pediatric patient.

After removal of a yolk sac tumors, serum AFP levels should be followed serially. The half life of AFP is 5–7 days. Failure of serum AFP to normalize following surgery suggests the presence of residual or metastatic disease. The majority of patients with a yolk sac tumor will present with a

Table 97.1 Staging (Children's Oncology Group)

Stage 1	Local disease, complete resection, markers normalize
Stage 2	Transcrotal orchiectomy, microscopic disease in the scrotum or high cord (<5 cm from proximal end), <2 cm diameter retroperitoneal lymph node, persistently elevated markers
Stage 3	>2 cm Diameter retroperitoneal lymph node
Stage 4	Distant metastases

lesion localized to the testicle and need no further therapy. In cases of metastatic or recurrent disease, excellent results have been achieved with platinum-based chemotherapy. Chemotherapy and radiation are recommended for metastatic sertoli cell and mixed gonadal stromal tumors, however, given their rarity, no specific treatment guidelines are available for these lesions.

Retroperitoneal lymph node dissection (RPLND) is rarely necessary in children. Hematogenous spread (predominantly to the lung) is more common than lymphatic metastasis to the retroperitoneum. Complications following RPLND, especially small bowel obstruction, are more common in children than in adults. It is also difficult to perform adequate nerve-sparing in smaller patients. In general, modified template RPLND is recommended for persistent tumor marker elevation or residual retroperitoneal masses following chemotherapy. In the rare patient with a yolk sac tumor and normal preoperative AFP levels, recurrent disease can be very difficult to detect. These patients might benefit from empiric RPLND.

Surveillance

Follow up for patients with stage I yolk sac tumors should include: monthly serum AFP, chest radiograph every 2 months for 2 years, and CT scan of the abdomen and pelvis every 3 months for the second year. Given the potential for metastasis, surveillance is also needed in patients with Sertoli cell tumors and those with mixed gonadal stromal tumors, although this has not been strictly defined.

No specific follow up is needed for prepubertal teratomas, epidermoid cysts, juvenile granulosa cell tumors or Leydig cell tumors. Following a testis-sparing procedure, preservation of adequate testicular volume should be confirmed by physical examination and scrotal ultrasound. Following radical surgery, it is important to discuss the option of testicular prosthesis with the patient and his family. Parents must also be warned about the potential for hypogonadism and the need for hormone replacement as the child gets older.

Summary Points

- Testicular neoplasms in children are rare.
- Teratoma and yolk sac are the most common cell types seen in children.
- An elevated AFP in a child older than 6 months suggests a yolk sac tumor.
- Sertoli cell and mixed gonadal stromal tumors are potentially malignant.
- Elevated AFP levels should normalize following surgery for yolk sac tumors.
- Platinum-based chemotherapy is the cornerstone of treatment for metastatic disease and persistently elevated tumor markers.
- Retroperitoneal lymph node dissection is recommended for residual mass following chemotherapy, elevated tumor markers following chemotherapy, and yolk sac tumor with normal pre operative markers.

Editor's Comment

Because a testicular mass might be encountered unexpectedly during inguinal hernia repair, hydrocelectomy or orchidopexy, it is important to understand the basic principles of the care of a child with a testicular tumor. Failure to do so could result in tumor spread or necessitate a hemiscrotectomy or orchiectomy that otherwise might have been avoided. Most surgical protocols are based on traditional adult protocols and certainly need to be updated, but this has yet to occur, probably due to the small numbers and a lack of controlled studies. Nevertheless, with the current trend towards

testis-sparing surgery, it should no longer be assumed that every testicle with a tumor must automatically be removed.

As a general rule, a testicular mass should never be approached through a scrotal incision or percutaneous transscrotal biopsy. This should only be done through an inguinal incision, usually made somewhat larger than a typical inguinal hernia incision and always involving opening the external ring so that the testis can be delivered easily into the wound without risk of rupture. If a testicular mass is discovered incidentally intra-operatively, the testis should be delivered through the inguinal incision and carefully inspected. A call should be made immediately to either a local pediatric urologic oncologist or to one of the national experts designated by the Children's Oncology Group, for purposes of an intra-operative consultation. At this point, depending on the circumstances and availability of expertise, the decision might be to remove the testis, to control the spermatic cord with a tourniquet and perform a biopsy for frozen-section analysis, or to place the testis back in its anatomic position in anticipation of a more definitive operation in the near future. The same approach should be used with paratesticular tumors, which can also be malignant and are treated using a very similar approach.

A painless testicular mass is presumed to be malignant until proven otherwise. The next step should always include scrotal US and measurement of tumor markers (AFP, HCG). Boys with gynecomastia should also be examined very carefully for the rare hormonally active testicular tumor but routine scrotal US is probably unnecessary and certainly not cost-effective. Metastatic workup for testicular tumors includes a chest X-ray and abdominal CT scan, and for paratesticular rhabdomyosarcoma includes a bone marrow biopsy.

A small testicular teratoma or epidermoid cyst in a prepubescent child can usually be easily excised with a small margin of normal parenchyma. Testicle-sparing surgery might also be recommended for Leydig cell tumors. For most other lesions, an incisional or excision biopsy with frozen-section diagnosis can usually help with decision making regarding orchiectomy. If orchiectomy is recommended, this should include a radical orchiectomy with high ligation of the spermatic cord. If the tumor is truly a surprise, it is usually best to consult the parents, intra-operatively if necessary, before an orchiectomy is performed. While it is generally considered better to have removed a testis for what was felt to be a possible malignancy than to preserve one that ultimately harbors a cancer, the decision should not be made lightly, especially since it would be difficult to justify the loss of an otherwise normal testis for a small benign lesion that could easily have been simply enucleated. Difficulty also arises in the rare situation of a testicular hematoma that is thought to possibly represent a ruptured testicular tumor. This is an extremely rare occurrence, but intra-operative biopsy should be performed if this a pathologist is available.

Retroperitoneal lymph node dissection for staging purposes in boys with testicular cancer is rarely necessary anymore, having been supplanted for the most part by modern medical imaging. This is a good thing as the morbidity from an extensive dissection can be severe. It is also sometimes requested in boys who have persistent tumor marker elevation but normal imaging after orchiectomy. There is probably little therapeutic benefit to removing positive retroperitoneal lymph nodes. We are occasionally asked to biopsy a suspicious node after the completion of therapy because of concerns about recurrence. If feasible, this should be performed laparoscopically.

Differential Diagnosis

- Germ cell tumors
  - Yolk sac tumors
  - Teratomas
  - Epidermoid cysts
- Stromal tumors
  - Leydig cell tumors
  - Sertoli cell tumors
  - Juvenile granulosa cell tumors
  - Mixed gonadal stromal tumors
- Trauma (hematoma, testicular rupture)
- Hydrocele/hernia
- Testicular torsion

Preoperative Studies

- Scrotal ultrasound
- CT scan of abdomen/pelvis
- Chest X-ray
- Alpha fetoprotein (AFP)
- βHCG
- LDH

Preoperative Preparation

☐ Tumor markers
☐ Informed consent

Parental Preparation

- Orchiectomy may be necessary, even if diagnosis is uncertain.

Technical Points

- Examine contralateral gonad for bilateral disease.
- Perform scrotal exploration through an inguinal incision.
- Preserve ilioinguinal nerve and occlude cord vessels prior to delivery of the testicle.
- Excisional biopsy for teratomas must include the evaluation of adjacent parenchyma.
- Radical orchiectomy needed for yolk sac, sertoli, mixed gonadal stromal tumors.
- Normal parenchyma remaining after excision of a benign mass must be preserved.

Suggested Reading

Agarwal PK, Palmer JS. Testicular and paratesticular neoplasms in prepubertal males. J Urol. 2006;176:875–81.

Borer JG, Tan PE, Diamond DA. The spectrum of sertoli cell tumors in children. Urol Clin North Am. 2000;27(3):521–41.

Phol HG, Shukla AR, Metcalf PD, et al. Prepubertal testis tumors: actual prevalence rate of histological types. J Urol. 2004;172:2370–2.

Ritchey ML, Shamberger RC. Pediatric urologic oncology. In: Wein AJ, Kavoussi LR, Novick AC, Partin AW, Peters CA, editors. Campbell-Walsh urology. 9th ed. Philadelphia: Saunders Elsevier; 2007. p. 3870–906.

Ross JH. Testicular tumors. In: Docimo SG, Canning DA, Khoury AE, editors. The Kelalis-King-Bellman textbook of clinical pediatric urology. 5th ed. United Kingdom: Informa Healthcare; 2007. p. 1329–38.

Ross JH, Rybick L, Kay R. Clinical behavior and a contemporary management algorithm for prepubertal testis tumors: a summary of the prepubertal testis tumor registry. J Urol. 2002;168:1675–9.

Valla JS. Testis-sparing surgery for benign testicular tumors in children. J Urol. 2001;165:2280–3.

Walsh C, Rushton HG. Diagnosis and management of teratomas and epidermoid cysts. Urol Clin North Am. 2000;27(3):509–18.

Walsh TJ, Grady RW, Porter MP, et al. Incidence of testicular germ cell cancers in U.S. children: SEER program experience 1973 to 2000. Urology. 2006;68:402–5.

Wu HY, Snyder HM. Pediatric urologic oncology: bladder, prostate, testis. Urol Clin North Am. 2004;31:619–27.

Chapter 98
Soft Tissue Tumors

Roman M. Sydorak and Harry Applebaum

Soft tissue tumors are relatively common in children and run the gamut from frequently seen lipomas to some of the rarest tumors in medicine. All three embryonal layers contribute to this group of tumors, with benign lesions far outnumbering malignant ones. Some of the more interesting benign soft tissue tumors include lipoblastomas, desmoid tumors (fibromatosis), inflammatory myofibroblastic tumors (IMT), and neurofibromas. Malignant tumors (sarcomas) comprise 7% of tumors in children. Nearly half of these are rhabdomyosarcomas. The remainder are grouped together as non-rhabdomyosarcoma soft tissue sarcomas (NRSTS), which include neoplasms of smooth muscle (leiomyosarcoma), connective tissue (liposarcoma), vascular tissue (hemangiopericytoma), and the peripheral nervous system (peripheral nerve sheath tumors). Synovial sarcomas, fibrosarcomas, and malignant peripheral nerve sheath tumors predominate in pediatric patients. NRSTS are more common in adults than in children; therefore, much of the information regarding the natural history and treatment of these lesions has been based on the results of adult studies. However, pediatric NRSTS are often associated with a better outcome than their adult counterparts. This difference is most pronounced for infants and children younger than 4 years, in whom tumors tend to be locally aggressive but not metastatic. These patients have an excellent prognosis when treated with surgical excision only. Soft tissue sarcomas in older children and adolescents often behave similarly to those encountered in adult patients.

Most soft tissue tumors occur sporadically. Rarely, genetic syndromes, such as neurofibromatosis, familial adenomatous polyposis, or Li–Fraumeni syndrome, are encountered. Cytogenetic anomalies are common and are fairly specific for tumor type. These can be found in small round cell tumors (Ewing's sarcoma), leiomyosarcoma of the gastrointestinal tract, dermatofibrosarcoma protuberans, and synovial cell sarcoma. Environmental factors also influence the development of NRSTS. Some NRSTS, particularly malignant fibrous histiocytoma, can develop within tissue that has been irradiated; others, like Kaposi's sarcoma, have been linked to viral infections.

The multiple histological types of soft tissue tumors often lead to confusion. There are dozens of named tumors. In general, these tumors are named according to the soft tissue cell they resemble. The less differentiated the tumors, the more difficult it is to pinpoint the exact origin and the less descriptive the name. Immunohistochemical staining, fluorescence in situ hybridization (FISH), electron microscopy (EM) and reversed transcriptase polymerase chain reaction (RT-PCR) is being used more frequently to make a diagnosis.

There is no clear-cut way to stage these diverse tumors as there is with rhabdomyosarcoma. Histological grade is currently the best indicator of the biological behavior of the tumor. They are graded 1–3, with the criteria including degree of differentiation, cellularity, mitotic index, and degree of spontaneous necrosis. There is some correlation with prognosis. As yet, there is no well-accepted staging system that is applicable to all childhood NRSTS; the system from the American Joint Commission for Cancer that is used for adults has not been validated in pediatric studies. Benign lesions are usually not graded, though some (IMT) have a tendency to invade locally and, in rare cases, can metastasize.

A multimodality treatment team provides the optimal care for these children. The skills of primary care physicians, pediatric surgical specialists, radiation oncologists and pediatric hematologist/oncologists ensure that children receive treatment that will achieve optimal survival and quality of life. Treatment for some of the rarer types of soft tissue tumors continues to be studied and numerous trials are underway primarily through the Children's Oncology Group (COG).

Diagnosis

Patients with soft tissue tumors tend to present with a painless solid mass and typically have a delay in diagnosis. The tumors are usually slow growing and symptoms, if any, are the result

R.M. Sydorak (✉)
Department of Pediatric Surgery, Kaiser Permanente Los Angeles Medical Center, 4760 Sunset Boulevard, 3rd Floor, Los Angeles, CA 90027, USA
e-mail: roman.m.sydorak@kp.org

P. Mattei (ed.), *Fundamentals of Pediatric Surgery*,
DOI 10.1007/978-1-4419-6643-8_98, © Springer Science+Business Media, LLC 2011

of compression or invasion of normal structures, thus varying by tumor location. They can occur anywhere in the body, with the extremities being the most common anatomic site. Cosmetic disfigurement may be present. New onset of rapid growth may be suggestive of malignant degeneration of a previously benign lesion. The initial diagnosis can include muscle strain, hematoma, lipoma or other benign disease. Physical examination should note the exact size of the mass, anatomic location, depth, mobility and relation to surrounding neurovascular structures. Systemic symptoms (fever, chills, weight loss, night sweats) are rare. Regional lymph nodes should be examined for enlargement.

As most of these lesions are benign, the need for radiological evaluation is often unclear. Difficulty with examination, size greater than 5 cm, symptomatic or potential invasion of surrounding structures, anatomic location or concern given the findings on physical examination usually prompts radiological evaluation. Conventional radiographs and ultrasound with Doppler often represent the first-line examinations and are sometimes sufficient to assess a mass adequately.

Careful imaging of the primary tumor is essential. CT or MRI help to determine relationship to bone, nerves, and vascular structures as well as the degree of tumor extension or invasion. Malignancy is suggested by involvement of multiple tissue compartments, poorly defined margins, heterogeneity of the tumor and, of course, the presence of metastases. While some argue that MRI provides more soft tissue detail, we have not found much improvement in soft tissue quality for MRI over CT. In addition, an MRI often mandates the use of general anesthesia with intubation and monitoring, especially in young children. For certain tumors, a CT scan of the chest, abdomen and pelvis is an important part of the evaluation for metastatic disease. PET scanning might provide additional information including spread to regional lymph nodes, but this has yet to be studied in detail.

Preoperative Preparation

Tissue analysis is essential for the diagnosis. Often core-needle biopsy can be used. This can be performed using ultrasound- or CT-guidance. The accuracy is excellent, with a high sensitivity and specificity. Younger children are often unable to tolerate such a procedure and incisional or excisional biopsy under general anesthesia is usually required. We prefer to attempt excision for tumors that are less than 5 cm in diameter and have no evidence of invasion of neurovascular structures, and incisional biopsy for larger or invasive tumors. The incision should be oriented in such a way that it can be excised en bloc with the tumor at a subsequent operation. For extremity tumors, this usually means a longitudinal incision. Fine-needle aspiration is rarely useful as it does not provide enough tissue for determination of histological subtype or grade.

Surgical Technique

Surgery remains the cornerstone of treatment for all soft tissue tumors. The primary surgical principle is en bloc excision of the tumor. Dissection is carried out through normal tissue planes. Surgical resection should include skin, subcutaneous tissue and soft tissue adjacent to the tumor. Some of these tumors have a pseudocapsule that allows the tumor to shell out fairly easily, giving the surgeon a false sense that the tumor has been totally excised, even though microscopic or even gross residual tumor remains. Ideally, the tumor should be excised with a 1–2 cm margin of normal tissue or, at minimum, uninvolved fascia. Frozen section is done at the time of operation only for areas suspicious for residual disease. The margins should be carefully inked by the pathologist for subsequent assessment of clearance. Closer margins should prompt consideration for re-excision, except when they are in proximity to vital structures or bone.

If the tumor is small, not suspicious and easily removed, complete surgical resection of the tumor is performed and pathological diagnosis is made following the operation. When the initial operation was done without the knowledge that cancer is present, a re-excision of the affected region should always be considered, even in the absence of a mass on postoperative imaging. The incision and any previous biopsy site need to be excised en bloc with the specimen.

Sacrifice of neurovascular structures is not usually necessary unless there is frank involvement. Nerves and arteries can often be dissected free from the tumor. Intra-operative Doppler can help with identification of arteries and veins. When tumors abut critical neurovascular structures, complete resection can compromise the integrity of distal structures. Under these conditions, adequate resection is often not possible and such patients require adjuvant chemotherapy or radiation.

Resection of neurovascular structures may render an extremity functionally useless, often more so than with an amputation. Therefore, particularly in an extremity, thoughtful preservation of function and limb salvage remain the key principles of resection. Local control rates with limb-sparing surgery for extremity sarcomas, with judicious use of adjuvant radiation therapy, approach 95%, equivalent to what was once obtained with amputation. Accordingly, amputation should be reserved for cases of major artery or nerve involvement, extensive bone involvement such that removal of the entire bone is required, or recurrence after previous resection and adjuvant radiation therapy.

Regional lymph nodes are usually not removed except when the tumor is positioned close to a nodal group. Sentinel lymph node mapping is employed at some centers to identify regional nodes that are the most likely to be involved, although its benefit has not been clearly defined in sarcomas.

Thoracic tumors (desmoids tumors, Ewing's sarcoma/PNET) typically require whole or partial rib resection to achieve negative margins. Reconstruction with prosthetic material is sometimes indicated, particularly in anterior or lateral regions of the chest wall. Large retroperitoneal masses usually necessitate extensive mobilization of the bowel with a wide Kocher or Mattox maneuver. Extensive bone, spine, nerve, or head and neck involvement might warrant the assistance of an appropriate surgical subspecialist.

Postoperative Care

After removal, efforts are made to close the dead space to prevent the development of a gross defect, seroma or hematoma. This may include transposition of adjacent musculature or rotational flaps. Closed suction drains are not recommended. External compression bandages are utilized, with elevation of the extremity or involved body part.

When there is concern about the adequacy of the surgical margin, radiation therapy is indicated. Because local control with radiotherapy alone is not achievable, radiation is only used to supplement surgery. This is particularly important in high-grade tumors with tumor margins less than 1 cm, for incompletely resected tumors, and for tumors invading neurovascular structures. Doses vary, but the entire compartment is usually irradiated, sparing the skin to prevent fibrosis. The morbidity of high-dose radiation therapy is of concern in infants and young children, both in terms of general toxicity and suppression of growth in the irradiated area. By using a combination of surgery and radiation, local control of the primary tumor can be achieved in more than 80% of patients. While radiation can be administered as adjuvant or neoadjuvant therapy, we prefer to avoid having to operate in an irradiated field given that the radiation can distort tissue planes and cause delayed wound healing. The most common exception is for very large tumors (10 cm or greater) or when surgical excision would be particularly difficult or dangerous. In these rare cases, preoperative radiation may make for a more straightforward and less morbid resection.

The results of adjuvant chemotherapy for soft tissue tumors have been disappointing. Intervention has varied depending on the tumor type, patient age, tumor size, histological grade, and location, but there has been very little improvement in overall survival. Virtually all trials of adjuvant chemotherapy for NRSTS present results for patients in aggregate. This can obscure important differences in histological subtypes of tumors. Nevertheless, for patients deemed at high risk for metastatic spread or in the presence of metastases, systemic chemotherapy is generally administered. Two drugs have been reliably shown to have some activity against a broad range of NRSTS as single agents: doxorubicin and ifosfamide. However, single agent therapy is rarely used and chemotherapeutic drug combinations are more common (Table 98.1). Certain tumors, including synovial cell sarcoma and the extraosseous Ewing's tumors, appear to be more chemosensitive than rhabdomyosarcoma and most other NRSTS. Some of the more aggressive benign tumors are sometimes treated with chemotherapy, and there several trials looking at the response of IMT and desmoids tumors to treatment with anti-inflammatory drugs and COX-2 inhibitors. Finally, a number of studies are exploring the utility of high dose chemotherapy followed by stem cell rescue in the treatment of some of the more aggressive soft tissue tumors.

Children with unresected NRSTS have a poor outcome. Only about one-third of patients treated with multimodality therapy remain disease free. The prognosis for children with metastatic soft tissue sarcomas is especially poor. Despite aggressive therapy that includes surgery, chemotherapy, radiation, and resection of metastases, fewer than one-third of these children survive.

Postoperative evaluation is designed to detect early recurrence. Follow-up is modified according to the risk of developing a recurrence and is therefore based on the type of tumor, histological grade, size, and location. In general, extremity tumors are followed by CXR and CT/MRI at 6-month intervals for at least 5 years. Most recurrences will occur within the first 2 years, after which the interval for the imaging studies is sometimes extended.

As many as a third of patients will develop recurrent disease. Half of all recurrences are local and reresection is often possible. Excision of metastatic disease, especially in the lung, appears to be of some value in prolonging survival. The best results are for isolated pulmonary metastases. Formal segmentectomy, lobectomy and mediastinal lymph node dissection are probably futile and therefore unnecessary.

The prognosis and biology of NRSTS tumors vary greatly depending on the age of the patient, the primary site, tumor size, tumor invasiveness, histological grade, depth of invasion, and extent of disease at diagnosis. Because of the need to minimize long-term related morbidity while maximizing disease-free survival, the ideal therapy for each patient is a carefully and individually determined plan utilizing prognostic factors before initiating therapy. Multimodality treatment approaches have significantly improved the quality of life and survival of patients with soft tissue tumors.

Table 98.1 Benefits of adjuvant therapy for common soft tissue tumors

Cell origin (soft tissue tumor)	Chemotherapy	Radiation
Fibroblastic/myofibroblastic		
Fibrosarcoma	A/C/I/Vinc	Yes
Dermatofibrosarcoma protuberans	Imatinib	No
Fibrous histiocytoma	None	No
Myofibroma/fibromatosis	Interferon	No
IMT	±	No
Desmoid tumor	NSAID/Vinb/M/T	Yes
Adipose tissue		
Lipoblastoma	None	No
Liposarcoma	None	Yes
Smooth muscle		
Leiomyosarcoma	None	No
Vascular		
Hemangioendothelioma	None	Yes
Kaposi's sarcoma	None	Yes
Hemangiopericytoma	None	Yes
Angiosarcoma	D	Yes
Peripheral nerve tumors		
Malignant peripheral nerve sheath tumor (MPNST)	None	Yes
Neurofibromatosis	None	No
Schwannoma	None	No
Tumors of uncertain origin		
Alveolar soft part sarcoma	±	Yes
Granular cell tumor	None	No
Myxoma	None	No
Synovial sarcoma	C/Da/I/Vinc	Yes
Rhabdoid tumor	A/C/Da/D/Vinc	±
Extraosseous bone tumors		
Chondrosarcoma	±	±
Extraosseous Ewing's sarcoma	C/D/Da/Vinc	±
PNET	C/D/Da/Vinc	±

A Actinomycin-D; *C* cyclophosphamide; *D* doxorubicin; *Da* dacarbazine; *I* ifosfamide; *M* methotrextate; *NSAID* non-steroidal anti-inflammatory drugs; *T* tamoxifen; *Vinb* vinblastine; *Vinc* vincristine

Summary Points

- Soft tissue tumors are common; benign lesions far outnumber malignant ones.
- Successful outcome is based on adequate surgical resection.
- Preoperative evaluation usually includes CT or MRI and incisional biopsy.
- Complete surgical excision based on intraoperative frozen section and consultation with a pathologist is critical.
- Postoperative treatment might include chemotherapy and radiation for incompletely excised tumors or metastatic disease.
- Long-term follow-up includes physical examination and medical imaging.

Editor's Comment

The variety of benign and malignant soft tissue tumors that are seen in children is considerable. They can arise from almost any tissue type and in any part of the body. Some malignant soft tissue tumors respond well to therapy and have a very good prognosis, while some that are technically benign can be locally invasive and extremely difficult to eradicate. They are overall quite rare and because they are easily confused with garden variety benign tumors (lipoma) or dismissed as traumatic lesions, the diagnosis is often a surprise. This also increases the chances that they are treated improperly at first, leading to unnecessary or disfiguring surgery.

Any soft tissue mass in a child should be considered potentially malignant until proven otherwise. In practical terms, this means that one should adhere to certain surgical principles so as to avoid spillage of the tumor and the eventual need to remove more tissue than would otherwise have been necessary. Tumors that are small and easily excised with a margin of normal tissue without creating large soft tissue defects or causing injury to neurovascular structures or normal organs may be excised up front. Larger tumors should be biopsied first. The incision and the tissue planes traversed should be planned carefully so that if a subsequent wide excision becomes necessary, one can incorporate the scar. For extremity lesions, this usually means a longitudinal incision. If the biopsy confirms the presence of a benign lesion, surgical extirpation is usually the only treatment modality available. Some can be simply enucleated while others require an aggressive attempt to remove all gross tumor. Desmoid and IMT are known to sometimes respond to anti-inflammatory drugs or COX-2 inhibitors but surgical resection is still considered the standard approach. For most malignant tumors, neoadjuvant chemotherapy can be used to shrink the tumor and render it resectable or at least minimize the amount of surrounding normal tissue that needs to be excised to achieve tumor-free margins. For most soft tissue sarcomas, the prognosis is the same whether the tumor is resected up front or after chemotherapy, as long as the entire mass is ultimately excised with a margin.

When a tumor needs to be re-excised after a biopsy or ill-advised attempt at resection, the resection plane must stay clear of all previous surgical planes. This entails making an elliptical incision around the previous scar and then staying outside of the postoperative seroma by at least 1–2 cm. Preoperative planning with high-resolution three-dimensional imaging is critical to achieving this goal. If the previous operative site is entered, the risk of subsequent recurrence is much higher. It is especially problematic when the previous operation was associated with significant bleeding or a hematoma, in which case previously uninvolved compartments must now be considered contaminated.

Though likely someday to be supplanted by PET scanning, sentinel lymph node biopsy is being used at some centers to assess the likelihood of metastasis and to guide therapy, especially for some of the more aggressive sarcomas (rhabdomyosarcoma, synovial cell sarcoma). The approach is similar to that used for melanoma, although the customary injection of radiotracer and lymphazurin dye under the skin raises concerns about whether lymphatic drainage from the deeper tissues will be the same. Formal lymph node dissection is rarely indicated. Resection of metastases is also rarely indicated except for the unusual situation in which there are a small number of isolated lung nodules.

Because of the many variations in approach to soft tissue tumors, it is best to consult with a pediatric oncologist before any planned operative procedure. One should always be thinking about the next step in order to avoid making an avoidable error. There are also nationally recognized experts in the COG who can answer questions and give advice regarding the optimal approach to the surgical management of these complex disorders.

Differential Diagnosis

- Hematoma
- Benign soft tissue lesions
- Rhabdomyosarcoma

Diagnostic Studies

- CT
- MRI

Parental Preparation

- An extensive operation might be necessary to remove the entire tumor with an adequate margin of normal tissue.
- Despite aggressive surgery, recurrence is possible and reresection is sometimes necessary.
- Unresectable and metastatic malignant soft tissue tumors have a poor prognosis.

Preoperative Preparation

- ☐ Review of pathology
- ☐ Consultation with pediatric oncologist
- ☐ Detailed three-dimensional imaging
- ☐ Informed consent

Technical Points

- Small tumors should be completely excised with a 1–2 cm margin.
- Larger tumors (>5 cm) should be biopsied and subsequent therapy recommendations based on pathology results.
- Avoid sacrificing major nerves and arteries to maintain function unless recurrent disease is present.
- Intra-operative Doppler can be a useful adjunct during the operation to avoid injury to major vascular structures.
- The entire previous scar including skin and subcutaneous tissues should be excised at the definitive resection.

Suggested Reading

Andrassy RJ. Advances in the management of sarcomas in children. Am J Surg. 2002;184:484–91.

Childhood Soft Tissue Sarcoma Treatment. National Cancer Institute. 2010. http://www.cancer.gov/cancertopics/pdq/treatment/child-soft-tissue-sarcoma/patient. Accessed 8 Feb 2010.

Park K, van Rijn R, McHugh K. The role of radiology in paediatric soft tissue sarcomas. Cancer Imaging. 2008;8:102–15.

Womer RB, Pressey JG. Rhabdomyosarcoma and soft tissue sarcoma in childhood. Curr Opin Oncol. 2000;12:337–44.

Chapter 99
Liver Tumors

Rebecka L. Meyers

An abnormal growth in a child's liver might be a malignant tumor, a benign tumor, or one of a wide assortment of congenital and acquired lesions (Table 99.1). For many of these other masses, the key to the diagnosis lies in identifying the underlying medical condition. One might expect to see a bacterial hepatic abscess in a child with chronic granulomatous disease, a fatty deposit in the liver of a child with hyperlipidemia, or perhaps an inspissated bile lake in a child with biliary atresia. Congenital liver cysts are rare and represent a spectrum that includes large simple cysts, intrahepatic choledochal cyst, and ciliated hepatic foregut cyst. Hydatid cyst will usually have a distinctive radiographic appearance. A small congenital liver cyst may be safely observed. If large and symptomatic (Fig. 99.1), excision might be indicated to relieve pain, prevent rupture, and guard against reported possibility of malignant transformation.

Primary liver tumors account for about 1% of all pediatric tumors. Age at presentation is often the key to the differential diagnosis. In newborns the most common tumor is infantile hepatic hemangioma. Hepatoblastoma is most commonly diagnosed between 4 months and 4 years of age. Benign tumors in toddlers are mesenchymal hamartoma and focal nodular hyperplasia. Hepatocellular carcinoma and hepatic adenoma are seen in older children. Other tumors are more rare (Table 99.2). Although the most common benign tumors often show classic distinguishing features on CT, imaging is not usually a reliable way to differentiate benign from malignant tumors.

Benign Liver Tumors

The three most common benign liver tumors have characteristic radiographic features (Table 99.3). Mesenchymal hamartomas have a characteristic multicystic appearance and the complex cysts are separated by thick vascular septae. Focal nodular hyperplasia (FNH) is usually a well demarcated and hyperenhancing lesion with a characteristic central stellate scar. An infantile hemangioma typically demonstrates bright peripheral enhancement.

Infantile Hepatic Hemangioma

Hemangioma is the most common benign tumor of the liver in infancy. Many of these lesions are discovered incidentally and are localized and small enough to be of no clinical significance. Symptoms sometimes seen with larger lesions include abdominal distention, hepatomegaly, congestive heart failure, vomiting, anemia, thrombocytopenia and consumptive coagulopathy, jaundice secondary to biliary obstruction, and associated cutaneous or visceral hemangiomas. Sometimes a large rapidly growing lesion can be life-threatening with intractable high-output cardiac failure due to intrahepatic arteriovenous shunting, Kasabach–Merritt syndrome, intraperitoneal hemorrhage, and respiratory distress as a result of pulmonary congestion and massive hepatomegaly. Kasabach–Merritt refers to a localized intravascular coagulopathy associated with platelet trapping within the tumor and is to be differentiated from the more global form of disseminated intravascular coagulopathy that might develop in severe cases.

The diagnosis of infantile hepatic hemangioma is usually straightforward and based on the combination of clinical symptoms and radiographic appearance on ultrasound and CT scan. Contrast-enhanced CT scan shows an area of diminished density, and after bolus injection of intravenous contrast there is contrast enhancement from the periphery toward the center of the lesion, and, after a short delay, there essentially is complete isodense filling of the lesion and liver. Angiography might be necessary in infants with refractory symptoms in whom either hepatic artery ligation or embolization is considered.

If a definitive diagnosis of simple infantile hepatic hemangioma can be made radiographically, management can be non-invasive because spontaneous regression occurs in most cases, especially in infants with focal tumors. The terminology is

R.L. Meyers (✉)
Primary Children's Medical Center, 100 North Medical Drive, Suite 2600, Salt Lake City, UT 84113, USA
e-mail: rebecka.meyers@hsc.utah.edu

P. Mattei (ed.), *Fundamentals of Pediatric Surgery*,
DOI 10.1007/978-1-4419-6643-8_99, © Springer Science+Business Media, LLC 2011

Table 99.1 Differential diagnosis of pediatric liver masses

Malignant tumors	Benign tumors	Other masses
Hepatoblastoma (HB)	Mesenchymal hamartoma	Vascular malformations
Hepatocellular carcinoma (HCC)	Focal nodular hyperplasia (FNH)	Hemangioma
Sarcoma	Infantile hemangioma	Hemangioendothelioma
Biliary rhabdomyosarcoma	Hepatic adenoma	Artiovenous malformation
Angiosarcoma	Nodular regenerative hyperplasia	Congenital/acquired cysts
Rhabdoid	Teratoma	Simple
Undifferentiated	Inflammatory myofibroblastic tumor (IMT)	Polycystic liver disease
Metastatic		Choledochal cyst
Wilms' tumor		Inspissated bile lake
Neuroblastoma		Biliary atresia
Desmoplastic SRCT		Parasitic cysts
Lymphoma		Amoebic
Germ cell tumor		Abscess
Colorectal		Bacterial
Carcinoid tumor		Fungal
Hemophagocytic lymphohistiocytosis (HLH)		Chronic granulomatous disease (CGD)
		Hematoma
		Fatty liver

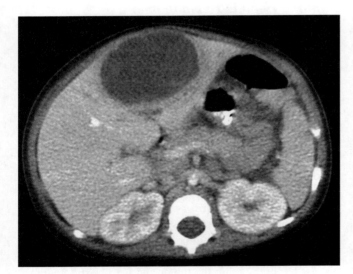

Fig. 99.1 Acquired hepatic cyst: amoebic abscess

confusing, however, with different authors often using the terms hepatic hemangioma, infantile hepatic hemangioma, and hepatic hemangioendothelioma interchangeably. True "hemangioendotheliomas" are usually a variant of kaposiform hemangioendothelioma and, unlike the more benign infantile hemangiomas, generally behaves in a biologically aggressive fashion and sometimes extends to involve extrahepatic structures such as the retroperitoneum, pancreas, or porta hepatis (Fig. 99.2). Historically, the initial medical intervention for symptomatic tumors has been corticosteroids. Many other medical treatment options exist, although no single treatment has been shown to be universally helpful. Congestive heart failure is treated with digitalis and diuretics. Anemia and coagulopathy are treated with corrective blood product replacement therapy. Platelets should be given judiciously because increased

platelet consumption accelerates the release of platelet derived grown factor (PDGF) which can promote tumor growth. Both success and complete failure have been reported variously with many other treatments including epsilon-aminocaproic acid, tranexamic acid, low-molecular-weight heparin, vincristine, cyclophosphamide, interferon 2-alpha, AGM-1470, and newer generation antiangiogenic drugs such as bevisuzimab and sorafanib. Multidrug chemotherapy regimens are sometimes required in aggressive forms of kaposiform hemangioendothelioma. Recent studies have shown that the large tumors can produce antibodies to TSH and screening to rule out secondary hypothyroidism is recommended. Reports demonstrate resolution of the hypothyroidism after liver transplantation in cases that fail medical management.

In infants who fail medical management, symptomatic solitary tumors can be treated by excision or embolization. Although potentially hazardous, hepatic arterial embolization can be life saving because it reduces arteriovenous shunting. There have been reports of orthotopic liver transplantation for cases in which the lesion is extensive and no other options exist. A treatment algorithm has been published by the vascular tumors study group at Boston Children's Hospital and stratifies treatment based upon whether or not the tumor is solitary, multifocal, or diffuse (Fig. 99.3).

Mesenchymal Hamartoma

Although mesenchymal hamartoma of the liver is the second most common benign liver tumor in children, its biology and pathogenesis are poorly understood. Historically, mesenchymal hamartoma has been described in the literature by various

Table 99.2 Age at presentation, primary liver tumors of childhood

Age group	Malignant	Benign
Infant/toddler	Hepatoblastoma 43%	Hemangioma/vascular 14%
	Rhabdoid tumor 1%	Mesenchymal hamartoma 6%
	Malignant germ cell 1%	Teratoma 1%
School age/adolescent	Hepatocellular (and transitional cell tumors) 23%	Focal nodular hyperplasia 3%
	Sarcomas 7%	Hepatic adenoma 1%

Modified from Von Schweinitz D. Management of liver tumors in childhood. Semin Pediatr Surg. 2006;15:17–24.

Table 99.3 Imaging characteristics that help to distinguish benign hepatic tumors

Mesenchymal hamartoma	*Complex multicystic* mass with solid septae
Focal nodular hyperplasia (FNH)	Hyperenhancing lesion with *central scar*
Infantile hepatic hemangioma	Very bright *peripheral contrast enhancement* with a central area of water attenuation
Hepatic adenoma	Enhancing lesion with *variable internal enhancement* and/or associated hemorrhage

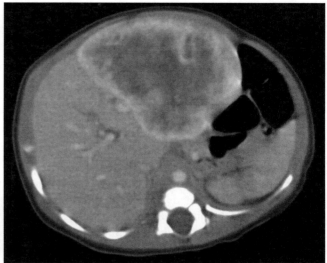

Fig. 99.3 Focal infantile hepatic hemangioma (most common benign liver tumor of infancy)

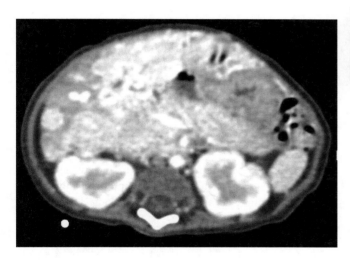

Fig. 99.2 Kaposiform hemangioendothelioma: Infant with invasive vascular tumor involving liver, retroperitoneum, pancreas, and base of mesentery who presented with heart failure, thrombocytopenia, and compression of portal triad

names including pseudocystic mesenchymal tumor, hepatic and giant cell lymphangioma, cystic hamartoma, bile cell fibroadenoma, hamartoma, and cavernous lymphangiomatoid tumor. Children with mesenchymal hamartoma typically present with abdominal swelling before 2 years of age. Before the widespread use of sophisticated diagnostic imaging, many of these tumors became very large, eventually presenting with mass effect such as vena cava compression, feeding difficulties, and respiratory distress. With the widespread use of ultrasound and CT these tumors are now usually detected early as a palpable mass in an otherwise asymptomatic child. The alpha-fetoprotein (AFP) level is variably elevated in this tumor confounding the differentiation from hepatoblastoma.

Mesenchymal hamartoma is more common in the right lobe of the liver. On ultrasonography one sees multiple echogenic cysts, but if the cysts are small the entire tumor might appear as an echogenic mass. The CT typically shows a well-circumscribed, multilocular, multicystic mass that contains low-density cysts separated by solid septae and stroma. The stroma and septae can be vascular and occasionally show contrast enhancement similar to that seen in infantile hemangioma. When the cysts are small and the lesion appears solid, biopsy might be required to eliminate the diagnosis of malignant neoplasm. The tumor tends to increase in size during the first several months of life and subsequently either stabilizes, continues to grow, or undergoes spontaneous regression. Traditionally, the surgical treatment has been complete tumor excision, either nonanatomically with a rim of normal tissue or as an anatomic hepatic lobectomy. If the tumor is unresectable, the surgical options include enucleation and marsupialization. Management continues to evolve, however, and because of many reports of spontaneous regression, there is a growing debate in the literature regarding the use of nonoperative management in the asymptomatic patient. Caution is warranted due to anecdotal reports of rare malignant transformation to undifferentiated (embryonal) sarcoma.

Focal Nodular Hyperplasia

The diagnosis of FNH can be made at any age. In children, it is usually seen between 2 and 5 years of age. It is a benign epithelial tumor that has been referred to by various names in the literature including benign hepatoma, solitary hyperplastic nodule, focal cirrhosis, cholangiohepatoma, and even mixed adenoma. Focal nodular hyperplasia is a well-circumscribed, lobulated lesion whose typical architecture on gross examination consists of bile ducts and a central stellate scar containing blood vessels that supply the hyperplastic process. Usually, there is no real capsule, but often the fibrous tissue surrounds the lesions, which can be single or multiple and vary in size from a few millimeters to more than 20 cm in diameter. Microscopically, the proliferating cells are practically identical to the surrounding hepatocytes.

Like other benign liver tumors, small lesions are usually incidentally found. Larger lesions eventually produce mass symptoms, usually abdominal pain. The diagnosis of focal nodular hyperplasia is suggested by the appearance on ultrasound or CT with intravenous contrast of a well-demarcated, hyperechoic, and homogenous lesion. Although approximately 50% of tumors will have normal accumulation of ^{99m}Tc sulfur colloid on liver scintigraphy, this finding is not specific as some of these children will turn out to have hepatoblastoma or hepatocellular carcinoma. In fact, although a radiographic "central stellate scar" is a characteristic finding, the radiographic appearance of FNH can be quite variable (Fig. 99.4). If biopsy does not definitively confirm the diagnosis, excision is usually necessary.

Complete surgical resection of biopsy-proven focal nodular hyperplasia is not mandatory in asymptomatic patients. Because spontaneous regression has not been reported, symptomatic patients will require either surgical excision or ablative therapy with ligation or embolization of the feeding hepatic arterial supply.

Hepatic Adenoma

Most common in young women, especially in response to birth control hormonal therapy, these tumors can rupture and bleed and therefore surgical excision is recommended. Differentiating them from FNH remains a challenge. Contemporary management might include percutaneous radiofrequency ablation.

Hepatic Teratoma

True hepatic teratoma is extremely rare. Twenty-four cases have been reported in the literature, 18 in children less than 3 years old, but about half are malignant. The characteristic histological finding is the predominance of hepatic tissue in the resected specimen.

Malignant Liver Tumors

In infants and toddlers, most malignant tumors are hepatoblastomas (HBL) and present with an asymptomatic right upper quadrant or epigastric abdominal mass. Some have fatigue,

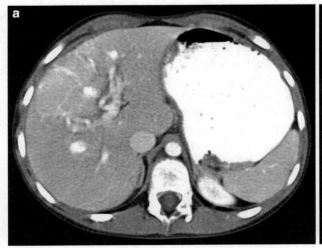
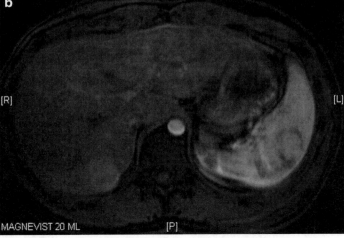

Fig. 99.4 Focal nodular hyperplasia (FNH): Though typically a hyperenhancing lesion with a central scar, these are examples of atypical appearing lesions: (**a**) hypervascular with unusual nest of dilated vessels encasing the tumor; and (**b**) isodense with liver on MRI T1, and T2; seen here (posterior right lobe) only after gadolinium contrast enhancement

fever, pain, anorexia, and weight loss. Rarely, they present with abdominal pain and hemorrhage after post-traumatic or spontaneous rupture of the tumor. Nonspecific symptoms of inanition or respiratory failure appear insidiously as the disease enters its advanced stages. As the cancer grows, the pain in the abdomen progresses to shoulder or back pain and becomes more pronounced. The child might also develop progressive anorexia and vomiting and appear thin and sickly. Tumor growth compresses the normal hepatic architecture causing: ascites, due to occlusion of the portal or hepatic veins; GI bleeding or splenomegaly, due to portal vein occlusion; or jaundice, scleral icterus, and pruritus, due to obstruction of the biliary tree. Symptoms are more common in older children, in whom the most common primary malignant liver tumor is hepatocellular carcinoma (HCC), primarily because it commonly presents at an advanced stage.

Although the exact cause of liver cancer is unknown, there are a number of conditions that are associated with an increased risk for developing hepatoblastoma or hepatocellular carcinoma. An embryonal tumor in the classic sense of incomplete differentiation, 90% of HBL cases are manifest by the age of 4, several have been present at birth, and there is a hypothesized association with prematurity. The incidence of HBL is 0.7–1 case per 1 million population per year in children in Western countries and has been increasing by about 3% per year. The Hepatoblastoma Origins and Pediatric Epidemiology (HOPE) study (www.cancer.umn.edu/research/programs) is a national study being conducted by researchers at the University of Minnesota who are trying to understand the epidemiology and increasing incidence of HBL. There is an increased risk of HBL in children with Beckwith–Wiedemann, hemihypertrophy, and familial adenomatous polyposis. Additional screening for cases in FAP kindreds is recommended by testing for germline mutations in the APC tumor suppressor gene. Additional biologic markers might include Trisomy 2, 8, and 20 and translocation of the NOTCH2 gene on chromosome 1.

The hallmark of increased risk for HCC in adults is underlying cirrhosis. Curiously, however, relatively fewer children with HCC have underlying cirrhosis compared to a majority (about 70%) of adults. Cirrhosis in children is usually due to biliary atresia, familial cholestatic syndromes, hepatitis B or C, or neonatal hepatitis. Other risk factors for HCC in childhood include type 1 glycogen storage disease, tyrosinemia, hemochromatosis, Fanconi's anemia, alpha-1 antitrypsin deficiency, autoimmune hepatitis, and primary sclerosing cholangitis. The fibrolamellar variant of HCC is rarely associated with cirrhosis, rarely produces alpha-fetoprotein, and tends to affect children more commonly than adults. Rarely, fibrolamellar HCC has been reported to arise in a background of focal nodular hyperplasia. Some patients with HCC have genetic alterations in tumor suppressor genes, which could explain the uncontrolled cell growth.

Diagnosis

Routine laboratory investigation should include complete blood count, liver panel (albumin, transaminases, glutamyl transferase, alkaline phosphatase, total and conjugated bilirubin), lactate dehydrogenase (LDH), tumor markers (AFP, βHCG, ferritin, CEA, catecholamines), and viral titers (hepatitis A, B and C, EBV).

The most important tumor marker is the serum AFP, which is elevated in 90% if children with HBL and 50% of children with HCC; however an increased AFP is not pathognomonic of a malignant liver tumor. Multicenter trials in Europe, Germany and North America have all concluded that hepatoblastomas that fail to express AFP at diagnosis (AFP level <100) are biologically more aggressive and carry a worse prognosis. Rarely, a well-differentiated, fetal-type, favorable prognosis HBL will not express AFP. Moreover, AFP levels must be interpreted with caution because AFP is normally elevated in neonates up to 6 months of age and is sometimes slightly elevated with other tumors, as well as after hepatic damage or during regeneration of liver parenchyma. There are many reports of both infantile hemangioendothelioma and mesenchymal hamartoma in children with very high AFP levels.

Other tumor markers that can be useful include: βHCG, elevated in germ cell tumors; ferritin, elevated in HCC and metastatic neuroblastoma; CEA, elevated in HCC and metastatic colorectal carcinoma; LDH elevated in many malignant tumors; catecholamines, elevated in metastatic neuroblastoma; Hepatitis C, in HCC; and EBV viral titers, in lymphoproliferative disorders.

Imaging

Hepatoblastoma appears as a large multinodular expansile mass, usually unifocal, but occasionally multifocal. The tumor is generally well demarcated from the normal liver but not encapsulated, and can invade hepatic veins, disseminate to the lungs, or penetrate the liver capsule to reach contiguous tissues. An initial ultrasound will identify the liver as the organ of origin; additional testing, usually a contrast-enhanced abdominal CT or MRI will more precisely define the vascular anatomy of the tumor.

In children with HBL, an abdominal CT, CT angiogram, or MRI outlines the anatomic extent of the tumor, clarifies the relationship of the tumor to the central venous structures, and evaluates for multicentric tumor nodules. The radiographic appearance of the tumor at diagnosis is used to assign the tumor a PRETEXT group (pretreatment extent of tumor). Devised by the International Society of Pediatric Oncology Liver Tumor Study Group (SIOPEL) in the early 1990s,

PRETEXT has been used by the European study group for risk stratification for many years. Although it has a slight tendency to overstage patients, PRETEXT shows good inter-observer agreement and is useful for monitoring the effect of neoadjuvant chemotherapy. The Children's Oncology Group (COG) will adopt the PRETEXT nomenclature to define surgical resectability in its new protocol starting to enroll patients in 2009. American pediatric surgical oncologists will need to become familiar with this system as it has become the international language of pediatric malignant liver tumors.

Building upon the Couinaud eight-segment anatomic structure of the liver (Fig. 99.5), PRETEXT divides the liver into four "sections." In the most recent version, the extent of tumor involvement at diagnosis is termed "PRETEXT," while the extent of tumor involvement after neoadjuvant chemotherapy is referred to as "POSTEXT" (Fig. 99.6). Extrahepatic growth is indicated by adding one or more of the following: V, vena cava or all three hepatic veins involved; P, main portal or both portal branches involved; C, involvement of the caudate lobe; E, extrahepatic contiguous growth (diaphragm, stomach, etc.), and M, distant metastases (mostly lungs, otherwise specify). Tumors are classified into one of four categories depending on the number of liver sections that are free of tumor (Fig. 99.7): I, three adjacent sections free of tumor; II, two adjacent sections free of tumor (or one section in each hemi-liver); III, one section free of tumor (or two sections in one hemi-liver and one nonadjacent section in the other); and IV, no tumor-free sections.

Chest CT is an essential part of the initial radiographic evaluation to rule out metastatic pulmonary disease. About 20% of children with HBL and 50% of those with HCC have lung metastasis at diagnosis (Fig. 99.8).

Treatment

If radiographic imaging is suspicious for malignancy, either a core needle biopsy, laparoscopic or open wedge biopsy, or definitive surgical resection can be performed (Fig. 99.9). The SIOPEL standard is biopsy followed by neoadjuvant chemotherapy for all PRETEXT groups. In an attempt to reduce chemotherapy toxicity, the Children's Oncology Group (COG) advocates definitive resection of PRETEXT I and II tumors at diagnosis, while PRETEXT III and IV are treated with biopsy and neoadjuvant chemotherapy. Postoperative chemotherapy is given to all patients except a small subset of HBL patients with a favorable histologic type known as "pure fetal" histology.

Definitive diagnosis of hepatoblastoma is made by biopsy or resection. Of the five histologic subtypes – fetal, embryonal, mixed epithelial, mesenchymal /macrotrabecular, and small cell undifferentiated – fetal carries the most favorable prognosis, small cell undifferentiated the worst. Even if unresectable at diagnosis, most hepatoblastomas are unifocal and chemosensitive, especially to the platinum-derived drugs. Since the routine addition of cisplatin in the late 1980s,

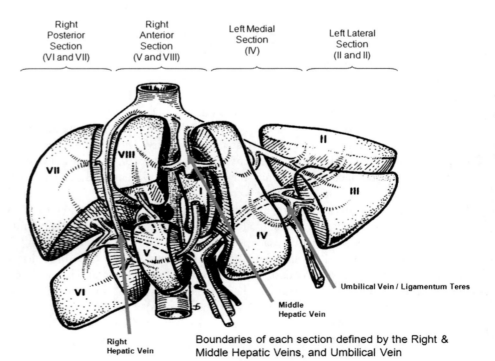

Fig. 99.5 PRETEXT is an extension of the Couinaud eight-segment anatomic division of the liver. PRETEXT defines four hepatic "sections"

Fig. 99.6 PRETEXT: *Pre*treatment *Ext*ent of disease. Anatomic extent of tumor to define resectability

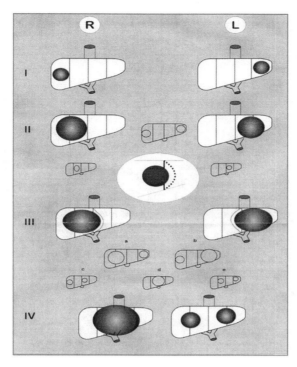

I ... 3 contiguous sections tumor free
II ... 2 contiguous sections tumor free
III ... 1 contiguous sections tumor free
IV ...no contiguous sections tumor free

In addition, any group may have:
V ...ingrowth vena cava, all 3 hepatic veins
P ...ingrowth portal vein, portal bifurcation
E ...extrahepatic
C ...caudate
M ...metastasis

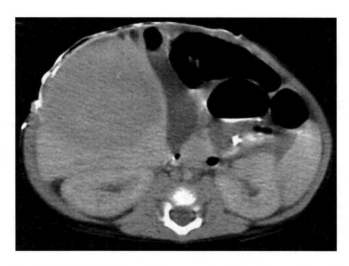

Fig. 99.7 PRETEXT II: a single tumor involving right anterior and posterior sections

overall survival in hepatoblastoma has increased from 30 to 70%. Twenty years later, cisplatin remains the backbone of the various different chemotherapy regimen in all four major multicenter study groups.

Cure from hepatoblastoma is not considered possible without a complete gross resection of the primary tumor at some point during the treatment regimen. There are two principal strategies (Fig. 99.9). The COG advocates for tumor resection at diagnosis whenever prudent and possible, arguing that toxicity is reduced by avoidance of unnecessary neoadjuvant

chemotherapy, that some tumors become resistant to prolonged courses of chemotherapy, and the highest survival rates have historically been observed in patients with initially resected tumors (although these tumors also tend to be the smaller and more favorable). Surgical guidelines advocate definitive surgical resection at diagnosis for localized, unifocal PRETEXT I and II tumors followed by chemotherapy. When the tumor is large, multicentric, or shows radiographic evidence of portal or hepatic venous invasion, or pulmonary metastatic lesions, the chance of curative resection might be improved by neoadjuvant chemotherapy and delayed primary resection.

Alternatively, the SIOPEL study group discourages resection of any tumor at diagnosis favoring neoadjuvant chemotherapy in all patients with the argument that the chemotherapy renders most tumors smaller, better demarcated, and more likely to be completely resected. This approach argues that the increased toxicity of neoadjuvant chemotherapy will be offset by the benefit of improved respectability.

The role of pulmonary metastasectomy has yet to be clearly defined, although it appears that surgical resection of lung deposits might be more likely to cure patients with disease that is present at diagnosis and persists after neoadjuvant therapy, rather than in patients with pulmonary relapse.

Data from the most recent COG study show 3-year event-free survival of 90% for Stage I–II (resected at diagnosis), 50% for Stage III (delayed primary resection), and only 20% for Stage IV (metastatic at diagnosis). In the most recent SIOPEL study, overall survival in the high-risk group increased to 73%, perhaps as a result of increased use of liver

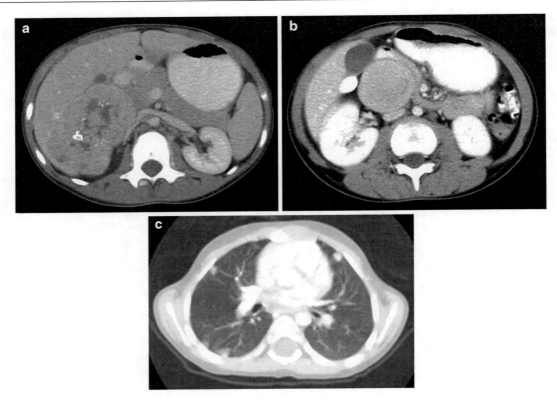

Fig. 99.8 Hepatocellular carcinoma (HCC): (**a**) primary tumor is PRETEXT II (involves right anterior and posterior sections); (**b**) large metastatic retroperitoneal lymph node obstructing duodenum; and (**c**) multiple metastatic lung nodules bilaterally

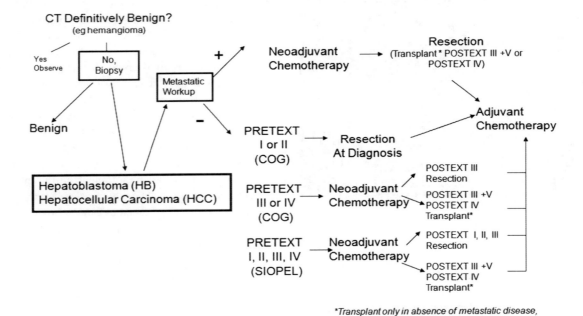

Fig. 99.9 Pediatric malignant liver tumor … *simplified treatment algorithm* (From SIOPEL 4 protocol book with permission from Piotr Czauderna)

transplantation in patients with extensive tumors. While "extreme" non-anatomic resection of such tumors might avoid the need for transplantation in some children, hazardous attempts at incomplete tumor resection in children with major venous involvement or with extensive multifocal tumors should be discouraged. Extensive hepatic surgery in children should be carried out in centers that have a facility for liver transplant, where surgical expertise, as well as willingness to embark on more radical surgery with a transplantation "safety net" is likely to be greater.

Hepatocellular Carcinoma

Unlike hepatoblastoma, hepatocellular carcinoma is relatively chemoresistant and therefore carries a poor prognosis and a 15% cure rate. Complete surgical resection or transplantation of localized disease is often the only hope. Tumors are commonly multifocal and carry a high risk of local relapse even after definitive resection with negative margins. In contrast to reports in the adult literature, the fibrolamellar histologic variant of HCC in children has been reported not to have a favorable prognosis or respond any differently to current treatment than typical childhood HCC. Children with initially respectable tumors had a good prognosis irrespective of histologic subtype, whereas outcome was uniformly poor for children who presented with advanced stage disease. Metastatic relapse is more common after transplantation for HCC, and therefore liver transplantation is restricted to patients whose tumor has always been clearly localized to the liver. The Milan criteria for liver transplant in adults with HCC (fewer than three nodules, largest nodule less than 5 cm) do not seem to apply to children. The transplant criteria used in SIOPEL 5, a study of non-cirrhotic HCC in patients under 30 years of age, are: (a) non-resectable unifocal tumors, independent of the upper size limit; (b) non-resectable multifocal tumors, fewer than five in number, largest less than 5 cm; and (c) presence of metastases, even if they clear after neoadjuvant chemotherapy, extrahepatic disease, hilar lymph nodes, and macroscopic vascular invasion are absolute contraindications.

New treatment modalities including metronomic chemotherapy and adjuvant anti-angiogenic therapy are the target of investigation based upon some early promising results. Most promising has been the recent adult experience with the anti-angiogenic agent sorafenib, which appears to improve survival in prospective trials in adults with unresectable HCC.

Hepatic Sarcomas

Primary hepatic sarcomas are rare. Outcome depends primarily on tumor histology, sensitivity to chemotherapy and/or radiotherapy, and the ability to achieve complete tumor resection.

Biliary Rhabdomyosarcoma

The classic presentation of biliary rhabdomyoscarcoma is in young children (average 3½ years) with jaundice and abdominal pain, often associated with distension, vomiting and fever. Histology is exclusively either embryonal or botryoid, both of which are associated with a favorable prognosis. Gross total resection is rare, but the tumor is often both chemo- and radiation-sensitive and long-term survival is seen in 60–70% of patients. Surgical intervention has two goals: to establish an accurate diagnosis and to determine the local-regional extent of disease. Although chemotherapy is generally effective at relief of the associated biliary obstruction, it is sometimes often too late. Patients remain at high risk of death from biliary sepsis during the first 2 months of their disease and empiric broad spectrum antibiotic coverage is of paramount importance in febrile patients.

Angiosarcoma

We have experienced rare cases that support the sporadic case reports in the literature of malignant transformation of infantile hemangioma to angiosarcoma. Histologic verification of malignancy can be difficult and this rare entity must be suspected if an infantile hemangioma shows unusual progression. Relatively chemoresistant, prognosis is generally poor.

Rhabdoid Tumor

Malignant rhabdoid tumor of the liver is a rare and aggressive tumor of toddlers and school age children which sometimes presents with spontaneous rupture. These rare tumors are often chemoresistant and fatal, although a recent case report suggests the potential for cure with multimodal therapy including ifosfamide, vincristine, and actinomycin D.

Undifferentiated Sarcomas

Undifferentiated (embryonal) sarcoma of the liver is a rare childhood hepatic tumor, and has historically been considered an aggressive neoplasm with an unfavorable prognosis. Survival has improved with multimodal approaches, designed for patients with soft tissue sarcomas at other sites, including conservative surgery at diagnosis, multiagent chemotherapy, and second-look operation in cases of residual disease.

Using these techniques, several small series have reported survival in up to 70% of children.

Metastatic Liver Tumors

Unlike the large body of literature concerning liver resection for metastatic colorectal tumors in adults, there is little published data that addresses the treatment of metastatic tumors in the liver from abdominal solid tumors in childhood. A recent series from a large metropolitan children's cancer center reported only 15 such patients over a 17-year period including: neuroblastoma (7), Wilms' tumor (3), osteogenic sarcoma (2), gastric epithelial (1), and desmoplastic small round cell tumor (2). Eleven of the fifteen died of progressive disease and four had a local recurrence. These results lead us to conclude that the overall prognosis in these patients remains poor and the decision to perform hepatic metastasectomy should be made with caution. The treatment approach should not, however, be uniformly nihilistic, because not all liver lesions in children with abdominal solid tumors turn out to be metastatic disease. Both nodular regenerative hyperplasia and focal nodular hyperplasia have been reported to mimic hepatic metastasis in children. Definitive diagnosis requires biopsy or resection.

Summary Points

- Age at presentation often the key to differential diagnosis:
  - Hepatoblastoma 0–4 year olds
  - Hepatocellular carcinoma 10–16 year olds
- Present with an asymptomatic epigastric or RUQ abdominal mass
- PRETEXT (Pretreatment Extent of Disease) can be used to stratify risk and predict surgical resectability
- Hepatoblastoma (HBL)
  - Alpha fetoprotein (AFP) elevated in 90%, when AFP not elevated = poor prognosis
  - Usually chemosensitive with a good prognosis if resectable
  - COG recommends resection of PRETEXT I and II at diagnosis
  - SIOPEL recommends biopsy and neoadjuvant chemotherapy in all patients
  - Multifocal PRETEXT III and PRETEXT IV might require liver transplant
- Hepatocellular Carcinoma (HCC)
  - AFP often not elevated
  - Cirrhosis less common than in adults
  - Usually chemoresistant with a relatively poor prognosis
  - Often very advanced at diagnosis
  - Milan Criteria for liver transplant might not apply to children
  - Encouraging early results in adult HCC with antiangiogenic agent, Sorafenib

Editor's Comment

Hepatoblastoma occurs with some frequency in children but in many cases is potentially curable. Given the importance of complete surgical excision and the intricacies of modern pediatric oncologic care, these children are best cared for at a center where surgical and oncological expertise are available and where transplantation capability is at hand. It is clear that survivability is nearly impossible without complete resection of the primary tumor with an adequate margin, and that salvage rates after a failed resection attempt or with recurrence after resection are not very good, even with transplantation. Therefore, it is extremely important to approach these patients with a careful plan of attack and with early involvement of the pediatric transplant surgeons.

The surgical approach is relatively straightforward: (1) If the tumor is relatively easily resectable *with an adequate margin* up front, then it is resected. (2) If the tumor is not safely resectable with a margin up front, the tumor is biopsied and the patient treated with neoadjuvant chemotherapy. After two and after four cycles of chemotherapy, the patient is reassessed for resectability and if it at any point it is considered resectable, then it should be resected. If it is still not resectable, even after four cycles, the option of transplantation should be discussed. (3) If it is clear that the tumor will not be resectable even after neoadjuvant chemotherapy, then liver transplantation as the primary surgical therapy should be considered. Application of the PRETEXT system is proving to be very helpful in making these sometimes difficult clinical decisions.

The decision about resection is made more difficult when it is thought that a non-traditional type of resection is necessary (extended trisegmentectomy, central hepatic resection, reconstruction of the vena cava), in which case it is an option at some centers to have a liver transplant surgeon perform the resection. At some institutions this can cause problems related to intramural politics, but this obviously should never be allowed to compromise the care of patient. Likewise, it is important to involve the transplant surgeons early whenever there is the possibility of difficult or dangerous resection as intra-operative challenges have been known to arise during hepatic resection for malignancy in children and an urgent last-minute phone call for help is usually a poor back-up strategy.

Intra-operative assessment of margins can be difficult when the lesion is deep or small. Preoperative imaging therefore needs to be of excellent quality, studied in detail ahead of time, and available for review in the operating room. This usually involves computer-enhanced three-dimensional CT- or MR-angiography to map out every large vessel within and around the liver. If the anatomic landscape is still confusing, intra-operative ultrasound can be extremely useful in these cases and should be readily available. An adequate parenchymal margin is generally considered to be at least 1 cm, though whether it is worth sacrificing a large vascular or biliary structure to achieve this is unclear. This is something that should be anticipated on the basis of the preoperative imaging and discussed with the oncologists in detail ahead of time.

The differential diagnosis of liver masses in children is broad but modern imaging, especially the combination of US and MRI, can usually allow the diagnosis to be made with a fair degree of accuracy. Most benign liver lesions can be observed and all should be followed with serial imaging, however parental anxiety can be extreme in these cases. It is rarely necessary to resect liver metastases but like some adult tumors there is sometimes a role for resection or ablation of certain types of tumors that have metastasized to the liver. Radiofrequency and cryoablation techniques are rarely used in children and can be dangerous especially in infants and small children, but smaller probes are being developed and collaboration with adult surgical oncologists should allow their safe application in appropriate cases.

Preoperative Preparation

☐ Detailed three-dimensional imaging (CTA or MRA)
☐ Type and crossmatch
☐ Informed consent

Suggested Reading

Awan S, Davenport M, Portmann B, et al. Angiosarcoma of the liver in children. J Pediatr Surg. 1996;31:1729–32.

Barnhart D, Hirschl R, Garver K, et al. Conservative management of mesenchymal hamartoma of the liver. J Pediatr Surg. 1997;32:1495–8.

Christison-Lagay ER, Burrows PE, Alomari A, et al. Hepatic hemangiomas: subtype classification and development of a clinical practice algorithm and registry. J Pediatr Surg. 2007;42:62–8.

Daller J, Bueno J, Guitierrez J, et al. Hepatic hemangioendothelioma: clinical experience and management strategy. J Pediatr Surg. 1999;34:98–106.

Isaacs Jr H. Fetal and neonatal hepatic tumors. J Pediatr Surg. 2007;42:1797–803.

Katzenstein HM, Krailo MD, Malogolowkin MH, et al. Fibrolamellar hapatocellular carcinoma in children and adolescents. Cancer. 2003;97:2006–12.

Meyers RL, Scaife ER. Benign liver and biliary tract masses in infants and toddlers. Semin Pediatr Surg. 2000;9:145–6.

Meyers RL, Katzenstein HM, Malogolowkin MH. Predictive value of staging systems in hepatoblastoma. J Clin Oncol. 2007a;25:737–8.

Meyers RL, Katzensten HM, Krailo M, et al. Surgical resection of pulmonary metastatic lesions in hepatoblastoma. J Pediatr Surg. 2007b;42:2050–6.

Meyers RL, Rowland JR, Krailo M, et al. Pretreatment prognostic factors in hepatoblastoma: a report of the Children's Oncology Group. Pediatr Blood Cancer. 2009;53:1016–22.

Reymond D, Plaschkes J, Ridolfi-Luthy A, et al. Focal nodular hyperplasia of the liver in children: review of follow-up and outcome. J Pediatr Surg. 1995;30:1590–3.

Roebuck DJ, Aronson D, Claypuyt P, et al. 2005 PRETEXT: a revised staging system for primary malignant tumors of childhood developed by the SIOPEL group. Pediatr Radiol. 2007;37:1096–100.

Rogers TN, Woodley H, Ramsden W, et al. Solitary liver cysts in children: not always so simple. J Pediatr Surg. 2007;42:333–9.

Spunt SL, Lobe TE, Pappo A, et al. Aggressive surgery is unwarranted for biliary tract rhabdomyosarcoma. J Pediatr Surg. 2000;35:309–16.

Stringer MD, Alizai NK. Mesenchymal hamartoma of the liver: a systematic review. J Pediatr Surg. 2005;40:1681–90.

Von Schweinitz D. Management of liver tumors in childhood. Semin Pediatr Surg. 2006;15:17–24.

Wang JD, Chang TK, Chen HC, et al. Pediatric liver tumors: initial presentation, image finding and outcome. Pediatr Int. 2007;49: 491–6.

Weitz J, Klimstra DS, Cymes K, et al. Management of primary liver sarcomas. Cancer. 2007;109:1391–6.

Chapter 100
Musculoskeletal Surgical Oncology

Jenny M. Frances and John P. Dormans

Musculoskeletal surgical oncology encompass a wide array of benign and malignant soft tissue and skeletal tumors, as well as lesions that can mimic a tumor. Among malignant tumors, only 900 soft tissue and 700 skeletal sarcomas are diagnosed yearly in children and adolescents in the United States, yet they consist of more than 50 different histological subtypes (Table 100.1).

The clinical presentation of a patient with a musculoskeletal tumor is highly variable and can include a recent onset of acute pain, a dull constant pain worsening over the previous few weeks, a painless mass, or an incidental radiographic finding. The key to successful treatment of musculoskeletal tumors is a prompt and accurate diagnosis. A delay in diagnosis is a pitfall that can limit treatment options and worsen outcomes. Survival and limb salvage rates decline when the diagnosis of a malignant sarcoma is missed or delayed. Yet, an overly aggressive work up for a benign lesion can lead to unnecessary tests and procedures, including unwarranted surgery. Familiarity with the basic principles of musculoskeletal oncology allows integration of clinical, radiographic and pathology data to optimize the probability of obtaining the correct diagnosis early. Knowing how to avoid all the things that can go wrong in the diagnostic process can have a profound and positive effect on patient outcome.

Diagnosis

When taking a musculoskeletal history, both the patient and the parents are important sources of information. The occurrence, duration, intensity, quality, and pattern of pain can help in formulating diagnosis and treatment plans. Useful tools in quantifying pain include a pain scale (1–10), recording the percentage of waking hours the pain is present, and determining what if anything makes the pain better or worse. Night pain is a red flag that should prompt further investigation. Pain that is worse at night and improves markedly with NSAIDs is a classic presentation for an osteoid osteoma. Pain with weight bearing can be a sign of a large benign or malignant bone lesion at risk for fracture, the presence of which should be ruled out with a radiograph. Some tumors, such as Ewing sarcoma or eosinophilic granuloma, can mimic infection and present with fevers, chills, and increased white blood cell count and c-reactive protein. When obtaining the history regarding a mass, ask how long it has been present and if it is growing, if the consistency of the mass has changed over time, and if there has been a fluctuation in size. Lesions that change in size can be indicative of a vascular lesion or a ganglion cyst. A family history of lumps and bumps, deformities, or short height can indicate familial diseases, such as multiple hereditary exostosis or neurofibromatosis.

The musculoskeletal exam must include a visual and physical exam of the entire body. It is important to look for café-au-lait skin lesions, the presence of more than three of which is suggestive of neurofibromatosis or McCune-Albright disease. Palpation of a mass characterizes the lesion and helps formulate the differential diagnosis. Is the mass soft and mobile like a lipoma, or hard and non-mobile, adherent to local tissue? Is the mass fluctuant and does it transilluminate like a ganglion cyst? Note whether the mass is superficial or deep. Deep soft tissue masses larger than 5 cm are considered sarcomas until proven otherwise. Is the mass tender? Are there any other masses? Observing the child walk barefoot helps to evaluate for the presence of a gait abnormality, suggesting the possibility of a spine or lower extremity lesion. The neuromuscular exam might reveal a deficit related to involved muscles or nerves, and thus indicate the location and regional effects of a lesion.

The more the musculoskeletal exam routine can be built into a game with younger children, the easier it will be to perform. For most of the exam, the child can be sitting comfortably on a parent's lap. Examining and testing normal, non painful body parts prior to the tender areas allow you not only to gain the confidence of younger patients, but also collect this information prior to a potential refusal of further participation.

J.M. Frances (✉)
Department of Orthopedic Surgery, New York University Hospital for Joint Diseases, New York, NY, USA
e-mail: jennymfrances@aol.com

P. Mattei (ed.), *Fundamentals of Pediatric Surgery*,
DOI 10.1007/978-1-4419-6643-8_100, © Springer Science+Business Media, LLC 2011

Table 100.1 Differential diagnosis of benign and malignant pediatric musculoskeletal tumors, classified by tissue of origin

Origin	Benign	Malignant
Bone	Osteoid osteoma	Osteosarcoma
	Osteoblastoma	
Cartilage	Osteochondroma	Chondrosarcoma
	Chondroblastoma	
	Chondromyxoid fibroma	
	Enchondroma	
	Periosteal chondroma	
Fibrous tissue	Nonossifying fibroma	Malignant fibrous histiocy-toma (MFH) of bone
	Fibrous dysplasia	
	Osteofibrouse dysplasia	
	Desmoplastic fibroma	
Miscellaneous	Unicameral bone cysts	Ewing sarcoma
	Aneurysmal bone cysts	Leukemia
	Giant cell tumor	Lymphoma of bone
	Langerhans cell histocytosis	
Metastatic tumors		Neuroblastoma retinoblastoma
		Hepatoblastoma
Bone lesions that can mimic tumors	Osteomyelitis	
	Tuberculosis	
	Avulsion fractures	
Vascular tumors	Hemangioma	
	Vascular malformations	
Nerve origin	Neurolemmoma	Malignant peripheral nerve sheath tumor (MPNST)
	Neurofibroma	
Fibrous origin	Fibromatosis	Fibrosarcoma
Muscular origin		Rhabdomyosarcoma
Miscellaneous	Ganglion	Synovial sarcoma
	Synovial cyst	Primitive neuroectodermal tumors (PNET)
		Soft tissue Ewing sarcoma
Soft tissue lesions that can mimic tumors	Abscess	
	Hematoma	
	Heterotopic ossification	
	Granuloma annulare	

The diagnostic work up will vary depending on what the suspected lesion is, as each has a characteristic presentation and potential for metastasis. However, the work up should start with a plain radiograph. Most skeletal lesions – although certainly not all – can be picked up by X-ray. Some soft tissue lesions have characteristic calcifications that can be seen on X-ray. In a child who complains of pain, most often the first step after history and physical should include anterior-posterior and lateral radiographs. Too many unfortunate stories circulate about children who have complained of pain for months, having been treated with multiple rounds of physical therapy prior to finally being sent for an X-ray that shows an osteogenic sarcoma. Perhaps more common nowadays is the opposite approach of always obtaining a CT or MRI without a specific diagnosis in mind, which is not advisable and can have unpredictable adverse effects.

When evaluating a radiograph of a bone lesion and trying to narrow down the differential diagnosis, it is useful to ask the following five questions: (1) What is the age of the patient? (2) Where is the lesion? (3) What is the lesion doing to the bone? (4) What is the bone doing to the lesion? and (5) What is the periosteal response? The first two questions regarding age and location are important as various bone lesions appear in classic locations in certain age groups (Fig. 100.1). Chondroblastoma, for instance, often presents as a discrete, lytic, round lesion located in the epiphysis of a skeletally immature patient. In the skeletally mature patient, a lesion that extends into the epiphysis might be a giant cell tumor.

The local effect of the lesion and the host bone's ability to contain the lesion can also provide clues as to the diagnosis. As such, the radiographic features between malignant and benign bone lesions differ markedly. Osteogenic sarcomas often present as locally aggressive, permeative metaphyseal lesions, with destruction of normal bone anatomy and marked reaction by surrounding bone (Fig. 100.2). Benign lesions, on the other hand, are typically more discrete, with narrow

Fig. 100.1 Differential diagnosis of bone tumors according to common locations. (Reprinted from Copley L, Dormans JP. Benign pediatric bone tumors. Pediatr Clin North Am. 1996;43:949, with permission from Elsevier)

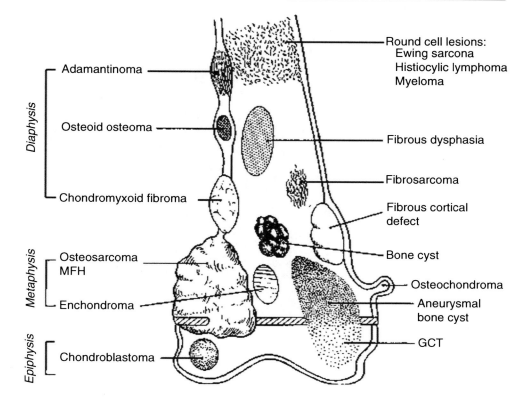

Fig. 100.2 (**a, b**) Anterior posterior and lateral radiographs of osteogenic sarcoma distal femur. (**c**) Coronal view of the ostegenic sarcoma showing the soft tissue extension and extent of intramedullary involvement. (**d**) Axial MRI showing close proximity, but not involvement, of the neurovascular structures to the tumor

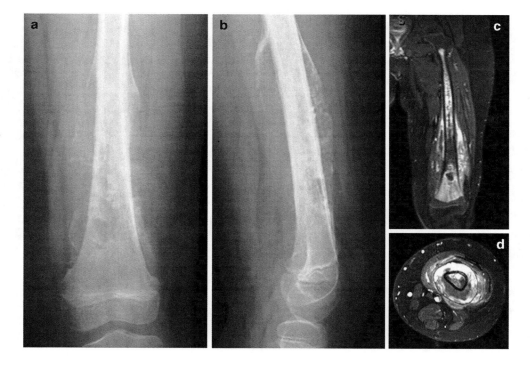

zones of transition between tumor and host bone and present in certain classic patterns (Figs. 100.3 and 100.4). Finally, the periosteal response to a well-contained, slowly growing benign lesion is a mature and solid cortical thickening, while the response to an aggressive lesion such as Ewing sarcoma is more likely to be interrupted and poorly consolidated, having the classic appearance of "hair on end," "sunburst," or "onion skin" calcification patterns.

Fig. 100.3 Benign bone tumors. (**a**) Pedunculated osteochondroma medial distal femur. (**b**) Non-ossifying fibroma of the distal tibia. (**c**) Large unicameral bone cyst of the proximal humerus. Note the proximity of the lesion to the growth plate

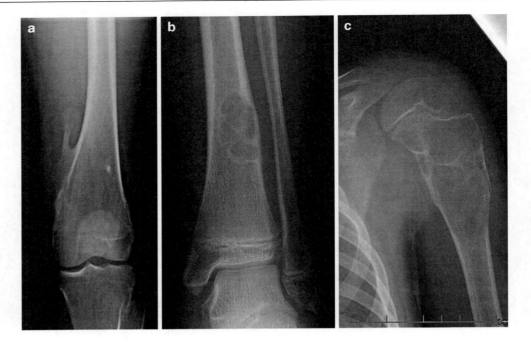

Fig. 100.4 Benign aggressive bone tumor. (**a**) AP radiograph of an aneurysmal bone cyst of the proximal fibula. Note the expansile bone cyst with multiple loculations. (**b**) MRI of the same bone lesion demonstrates a multiloculated cyst with fluid-fluid levels typically seen with aneurysmal bone cysts

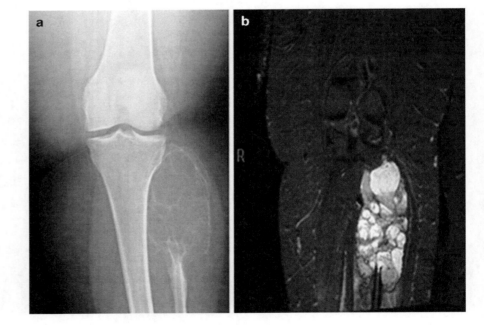

Benign Bone Tumors

Many asymptomatic benign bone tumors can be observed. This is particularly true of lesions that have a natural history of improving without intervention, such as unicameral bone cysts. Enlisting the help of an experienced musculoskeletal radiologist can corroborate the diagnosis and in doing so

prevent unnecessary biopsies of benign "no-touch" lesions. If the lesion is painful or the size and location of a benign lesion is such that there is risk for fracture, curettage and bone grafting might be indicated and is the treatment of choice for symptomatic benign lesions such as non-ossifying fibromas, some unicameral bone cysts, and fibrous dysplasia.

Locally aggressive benign lesions, such as chondroblastoma, giant cell tumors, chondromyxoid fibroma, and aneurysmal bone cysts (ABC) (Fig. 100.4), should be treated with an extended curettage using a burr, an adjuvant such as phenol or cautery, and bone grafting. When treating ABCs, in particular those that are large and aggressive, it is useful to remember that telangiectatic osteosarcoma is part of the differential diagnosis and to communicate this to the pathologist. The specific surgical treatment of some benign bone tumors depends on the lesion and location: patients with osteoid osteomas whose symptoms are not controlled by NSAIDs can be treated with radiofrequency ablation or surgical excision if the lesion is located in an area where radiation is not feasible.

Bone Sarcomas

The preoperative work up for suspected bone sarcomas includes a staging work up and a biopsy. Anterior-posterior and lateral radiographs are often diagnostic, at least in establishing the presence of a malignant process, but further studies are almost always needed. An MRI shows the extent of bone involvement and soft tissue extension and is very useful in planning the approach for biopsy or excision (Fig. 100.2). The relationship of the tumor to neurovascular structures also helps determine the feasibility of a limb-sparing approach. A bone scan is performed to look for skip lesions, multifocal disease, and metastases. Depending on the most likely diagnosis, a CT scan of the lungs is sometimes indicated to rule out the presence of lung metastases. Reported 5-year survival rates after resection of metastatic lung nodules in patients with osteosarcoma have been around 20% and even higher (up to 40%) if there are a small number of nodules and unilateral lung involvement.

The biopsy should preferably be performed by a surgeon with experience in dealing with bone tumors and who will be able to follow the patient through to the definitive stages of therapy. As the biopsy tract is always eventually excised, it is important to plan the incision such that it can be part of a future limb-sparing incision. In cases where the biopsy must be performed by someone other than the tumor surgeon, it is a good idea to consult with that surgeon to assure that the biopsy incision is in the same location as the incision of the final procedure. All biopsy incisions should be parallel to the long axis of the limb or body part, except some of those that are made around the pelvis or shoulder girdle, which should follow the incisional lines of an internal hemipelvectomy or scapulectomy (Fig. 100.5). The biopsy tract should approach through one muscle plane, rather than in between two muscles, and contamination of neurovascular structures should be avoided. This allows better preservation of tissues during the final procedure and is a prerequisite for allowing a limb-sparing operation. Careful hemostasis and meticulous closure is important. While prepping the lower extremity for biopsy, it is important to support the leg well, so to avoid a pathological fracture. Contamination of adjacent structures by hematoma a pathological fracture can either force an

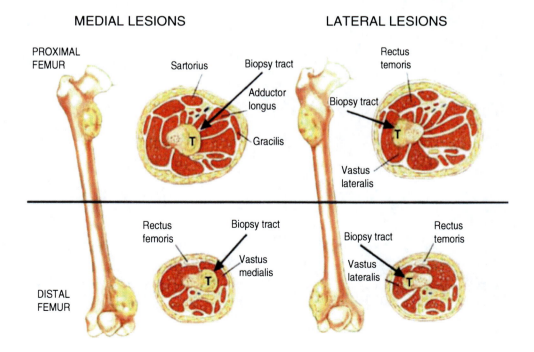

Fig. 100.5 Biopsy tract, proximal and distal femur. A distinction is made between lateral and medial lesions. (Adapted from Bickels et al. Biopsy of musculoskeletal tumors. Clin Orthop. 1999;368:212–9, with permission from Lippincott Williams & Wilkins)

amputation or potentially increase the local recurrence rate if limb-sparing surgery is performed.

An intra-operative incisional biopsy with hand-carried frozen section ensures that adequate tissue is obtained to make a diagnosis and has an accuracy of more than 90%. Personally carrying the specimen to the pathologist and conveying the clinical information leading up to the differential diagnosis eliminates errors and miscommunication. Working with an experienced musculoskeletal pathologist is key to obtaining a correct diagnosis. Based on the results of the frozen section analysis, central venous access and bone marrow biopsy is often done during the same general anesthetic (Fig. 100.6). Ultimately, cytogenetic tests that identify characteristic marker proteins and translocations for certain sarcomas aid greatly in establishing an accurate diagnosis.

Most patients with a bone sarcoma receive neoadjuvant chemotherapy prior to final resection. Though the response to chemotherapy varies, it usually shrinks the tumor, which in most cases allows for a more limited resection and preservation of limb function. It also targets the microscopic disease that is thought to be present in most patients and which can lead to metastases and local recurrence. After chemotherapy, preoperative planning must include new radiographs and another MRI.

Prior to the routine use of chemotherapy in the 1970s, survival rates for patients with osteogenic sarcoma were around 20% and the majority of patients were treated with amputation. With neoadjuvant chemotherapy, survival rates in the pediatric population today approach 70%, limb-sparing surgery can safely be done in 80% of cases, and local recurrence rates are down to 5–7%.

Surgical Technique

The most important goal of definitive surgery for a bone sarcoma is wide resection of the tumor with negative margins. All other goals are secondary. The art of the surgery includes the ability to obtain safe local control while preserving function whenever feasible. A wide resection of the tumor entails removing the tumor with the pseudocapsule (tumor), reactive tissue (satellite lesions), and a margin of normal tissue. What constitutes a "negative margin" depends on the tissue involved: for muscle and cancellous bone, 2–3 cm is considered adequate, while a single fascial layer or a physis is most likely a sufficient barrier to tumor progression in most cases. The local recurrence rate after wide resection is 2–4%. Intralesional excision (going into the pseudocapsule and tumor) and marginal excision (through the reactive zone with potential satellite lesions) can and probably do leave tumor cells behind and are therefore not appropriate when removing skeletal sarcomas.

The extent of resection is planned on the basis of the preoperative MRI. The entire tumor is excised, taking great care during the dissection to never violate the margin of the tumor or contaminate the field (Fig. 100.6). After resection, an intraoperative frozen section is done to evaluate for adequate mar-

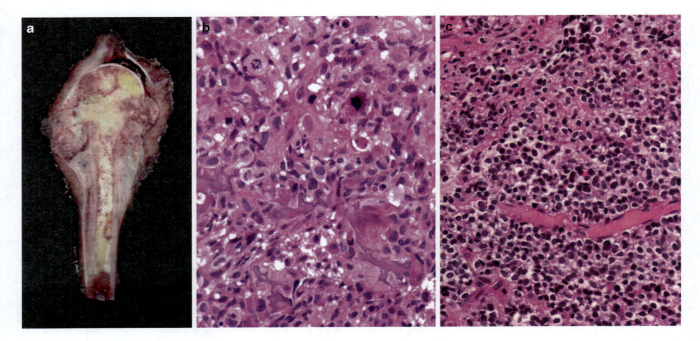

Fig. 100.6 (a) Gross anatomy of a resected osteosarcoma proximal humerus. Pathology evaluation demonstrated 50% viable tumor after neoadjuvant chemotherapy. (b) Histopathology of osteogenic sarcoma demonstrating pleomorphic spindle cells and osteoid production. (c) Ewing sarcoma histopathology demonstrating sheets of mono-morphic blue cells

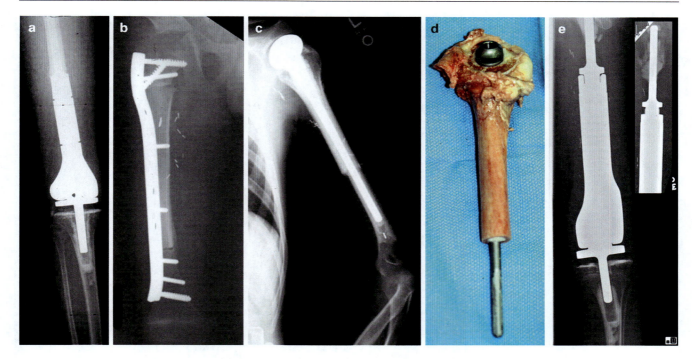

Fig. 100.7 Limb-sparing reconstructive options. (**a**) An endoprosthetic reconstruction. (**b**) An allograft intercalary reconstruction after resection of a diaphyseal Ewing sarcoma. (**c, d**) An allograft prosthetic composite (APC) reconstruction for a proximal humerus osteosarcoma enables improved soft tissue reconstruction. (**e**) An expandable growing endoprosthesis, with the inserted picture showing lengthening mechanism, can be used for skeletally immature patients with substantial growth left

gins, though it might take several days before the pathologist can give a final answer regarding margins, ultimate diagnosis, and the extent of tumor necrosis. Chemotherapy-induced tumor necrosis of more than 90% portends a better prognosis.

Reconstruction after resection can be done with allograft, metallic prosthesis, allograft-prosthesis composite, or free vascularized fibula grafts (Fig. 100.7). If possible, attempts to save the physis will allow for future growth of the limb. When the physis cannot be saved in a child with the potential for further growth, the use of a modular or extendable prosthesis should be considered. These children often undergo multiple procedures over several years to allow lengthening of the reconstructed limb. The risk of complications for these procedures is high and much time is invested in the limb. In the very young child, amputation is sometimes preferable. It entails a single operation and avoids the multiple return trips to the operating room, as well as the interruptions in life, potential complications, and periods of rehabilitation associated with each subsequent procedure.

One more option worth mentioning is rotationoplasty (Fig. 100.8), in which the tumor is resected *en bloc* and the distal tibia and foot are rotated 180° and reattached to the proximal femur. This provides a more functional limb than an above the knee amputation and is indicated for active patients who can accept the unusual cosmetic appearance of the rotationoplasty. Quality of life studies have not been able to show a significant quantitative difference between patients who undergo limb-sparing surgery or amputation, although it is likely that there are qualitative differences that have yet to be fully defined.

Postoperative Care

Prophylactic antibiotics are usually continued until drains are removed. Physical therapy, with attention to range of motion, is started early in the postoperative period. As long as the wound is healing appropriately, chemotherapy can usually be restarted after about 7–10 days. Follow-up radiographs are obtained regularly. Chest CT and bone scans to evaluate for metastases or recurrence are done with regular intervals per established protocols.

Careful monitoring for early postoperative complications such as infection and wound dehiscence is important, as these are somewhat more common due to exposure to chemotherapy and poor nutritional status. Postoperative joint contractures are also a concern, although early aggressive rehabilitation helps maintain range of motion. Long-term complications are not

Fig. 100.8 Rotationoplasty: (**a**) Scout view from a CT scan showing the rotationaplasty reconstruction on the left. After resection the tumor of the distal femur, the distal tibia is rotated 180° and attached to the proximal femur. (**b**) Clinical picture of a patient having undergone a rotationoplasty. Note how the ankle now essentially works as a knee within the prosthesis

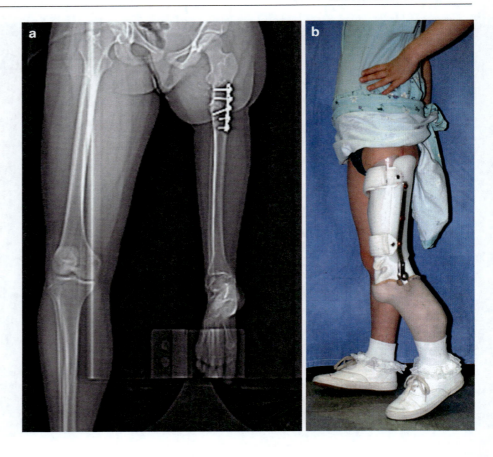

uncommon. They include endoprosthetic loosening, hardware failure, adjacent joint wear, allograft nonunion, allograft resorption, and late infection. The incidence of long-term complications depends on the initial tumor location, the type of reconstruction performed, and the patient's activity level. Children treated with amputation are at risk for terminal limb bone overgrowth.

Soft Tissue Sarcomas

Any deep (subfascial) mass larger than 5 cm is considered a sarcoma until proven otherwise. The preoperative work up for suspected soft tissue sarcomas is similar to that of bone sarcomas and includes an MRI, bone scan, chest CT, and incisional biopsy. Soft tissue sarcomas are usually treated with wide surgical resection. After resection of the primary tumor, plastic surgery expertise is sometimes needed for local reconstruction and wound closure.

Chemotherapy is more effective for certain soft tissue tumors, such as rhabdomyosarcoma or infantile fibrosarcoma. Although the specific indications for chemotherapy are complex and controversial, it is more likely to be offered to patients with chemo-sensitive tumors that are likely to

recur, and when there is evidence of metastatic disease. It is usually not indicated for sarcomas smaller than 5 cm and for superficial tumors that can be completely resected and are associated with a low expected risk of recurrence.

Some soft tissue tumors have a tendency to metastasize to lymph nodes, which makes a huge difference in the treatment strategy, especially with regard to chemotherapy. After careful physical examination, biopsy of clinically suspicious local and regional lymph nodes is indicated. For certain specific tumors (rhabdomyosarcoma, synovial cell sarcoma), sentinel lymph node biopsy should be used for staging purposes. Radiotherapy is occasionally indicated for local control of the primary tumor, particularly in cases where clear margins are not obtainable.

Unplanned Resections

What do you do if you find an unexpected malignancy when excising what you thought was a lipoma or some other benign lesion? The best advice is to avoid this situation by always obtaining an MRI prior to proceeding to the operating room. The information provided by MRI is easier to interpret in the absence of postoperative change and scarring and generally accurate in differentiating benign and malignant soft tissue tumors. Nevertheless, if for some reason you find yourself in this predicament, the most important thing is to recognize that the lesion is not a benign lesion and to *change* the operative plan. For any suspicious lesion, it is best to use a longitudinal incision, in case it turns out to be malignant. Start with obtaining a frozen section prior to attempting excision. If an immediate diagnosis is not available, convert the surgery from an excision to an incisional biopsy. Obtain tissue for diagnosis, achieve Hemostasis, and perform a water-tight closure over a drain placed in line with the longitudinal incision. Complete the indicated radiographic work up (MRI, bone scan, chest CT) while waiting for the final pathology results. About 60% of patients who undergo an unplanned sarcoma excision will have residual tumor present. This is why a second procedure to re-excise the tumor bed is recommended in cases where a presumed benign lesion turns out to be a sarcoma after final pathology.

The field of musculoskeletal oncology comprises a complex group of pathological processes. The specific treatment depends on the type of bone lesion, the location and in benign cases symptomatology. As these diseases are rare and expertise in this field greatly enhances the chances of optimal care, these cases should be referred to a musculoskeletal center. At the very least, a verbal consultation prior to proceeding with an incisional biopsy can help avoid a situation in which the ultimate treatment plan is compromised by mistakes in early diagnostic care. Increasing general awareness of the basic principles of surgical musculoskeletal oncology helps us to provide the best care possible for this patient group.

Summary Points

- Early diagnosis is key – avoid delays in work up.
- A radiograph is a good start and will help identify most bone sarcomas.
- Always consider the diagnosis of tumor in a child who complains of pain.
- Pain that wakes the child at night is a red flag for a bone sarcoma.
- An experienced musculoskeletal radiologist is crucial in helping differentiate benign lesions that should be left alone form those that warrant further workup.
- Although a biopsy is crucial for diagnosis, it should be performed by the treating institution.
- Poor technique in biopsy and lack of a good musculoskeletal bone pathologist can delay treatment or lead to unnecessary amputations for both benign and malignant lesions.
- Survival rates for Ewing and osteogenic sarcomas are approaching 60–70% with chemotherapy.
- Soft tissue tumors located deep to fascia or larger than 5 cm are presumed malignant until proven otherwise.

Editor's Comment

Nearly every child with a soft tissue mass or bone tumor associates it with a particular traumatic event. But it is helpful to recall a pediatric orthopedic surgery adage: "Every child falls every day." It is therefore important not to dismiss a deep tissue or bony lump as something merely related to an injury. Any large hematoma, especially one elicited by seemingly minor trauma, could be due to rupture of a soft tissue sarcoma. A follow-up US or MRI should be performed within 3–4 weeks to be sure that it is resolving as expected for a simple hematoma. Likewise, an osseous fracture that occurs with minor trauma should be considered a pathologic fracture until proven otherwise. It is still surprisingly common for a child with a sarcoma to finally have the diagnosis confirmed many weeks or months after initial presentation with a lump that was attributed to an injury. One should have a low threshold for obtaining an X-ray (for a bony lesion) or ultrasound (for a soft tissue mass) and always insist on a follow-up visit within 2–4 weeks.

Although it is rare to confuse it with a lipoma, a soft tissue sarcoma can often appear quite innocuous. Unless the diagnosis is certain, all soft tissue masses should be evaluated by US or MRI prior to attempting a resection or biopsy. Though an operation is not necessarily the wrong thing to do, the manner in which it is performed can make all the difference to a child whose mass later turns out to be malignant. This includes longitudinal incisions on the extremities, limiting the dissection to single muscle compartment, avoiding unnecessary dissection in adjacent planes, maintaining meticulous hemostasis to avoid a postoperative hematoma, which can increase the spread of the tumor, and staying clear of neurovascular structures. One must always think ahead to the next operation that might need to be performed. When re-excising a mass that has been operated on before, it is important to excise all tissue that has been touched by the other surgeon *en bloc* with a margin of normal tissue and without violating the previous planes of dissection or entering the seroma or hematoma that might still be present. These resections can lead to formidable residual wounds, especially in the chest or abdomen, that often require the expertise of a plastic surgeon for reconstruction.

Sentinel lymph node biopsy is useful for certain musculoskeletal tumors and should be part of the armamentarium of the pediatric surgical oncologist. The technique is rather straightforward but does require reliable Nuclear Medicine imaging resources and a Geiger counter for use in the OR. Whether a formal lymph node dissection should be performed in the event of a positive sentinel node is more controversial and should be based on the specific histology of the tumor and the clinical situation.

Osteogenic sarcoma is one of the few neoplasms for which surgical resection of metastatic lung lesions can improve survival. Patients with fewer than about ten lung nodules on chest CT should be considered for resection of all palpable nodules. This can be done through staged bilateral thoracotomies or median sternotomy. Thoracoscopy does not allow one to be thorough since tactile assessment of the lungs is not possible. Thoracotomy is standard and some feel that sternotomy fails to allow adequate access to all portions of the lung, especially the left lower lobe. We have had extensive experience with sternotomy, however, and have been pleased with the exposure. Additional benefits include less postoperative pain, the need for only one operation, and more rapid physical rehabilitation. The principal shortcoming is the scar, which most children prefer to avoid. Regardless of the approach, each lung needs to be excluded from ventilation while it is being inspected in order to increase the sensitivity of the examination. It is unlikely to be of any benefit to remove more than ten nodules but the exact upper limit is not known.

Diagnostic Studies

– Anterior-posterior and lateral radiographs
– MRI with contrast, including joint above and below
– Total body bone scan
– Chest CT
– Laboratory studies: CBC, ESR, CRP, Bun, Creatinine

Parental Preparation

– It can often help to talk to families that have undergone the procedure and treatment.
– Open and candid communication, sharing whatever information is known at the time and avoiding speculation helps reassure the family that the child is receiving optimal care.

Technical Points

• Extremity tumor biopsies should always be done with a longitudinal incision.
• If not referring the biopsy to a tumor surgeon, always consult prior to biopsy to ensure proper location of biopsy incision.
• The first objective of limb-sparing surgery is local control with tumor-free margins.
• Secondary objectives include maximizing function and cosmesis.
• Eighty percent of patients can undergo limb-sparing surgery with allograft, metallic endoprosthesis or composites for reconstruction.
• If encountering unexpected tissue when excising what was thought to be a benign lesion, abort and perform an incisional biopsy and frozen section instead.

Suggested Reading

Bui MM, Smith P, Agresta SV, Cheong D, Letson GD. Practical issues of intraoperative frozen section diagnosis of bone and soft tissue lesions. Cancer Control. 2008;15(1):7–12.

Copley L, Dormans JP. Benign pediatric bone tumors. Pediatr Clin North Am. 1996;43:949.

Dormans JP, Flynn JM. Pathologic fractures associated with tumors and unique conditions of the musculoskeletal system. In: Beaty JH, Kasser JR, editors. Rockwood and Wilkins fractures in children. 5th ed. Philadelphia: Lippincott Williams & Wilkins; 2001.

Greenspan A, Jundt G, Remagen W. Differential diagnosis in orthopedic oncology. Philadelphia: Lippincott-Raven; 2006.

Himelstein BP, Dormans JP. Malignant bone tumors of childhood. Pediatr Clin North Am. 1996;43:967–84.

Hosalkar HS, Dormans JP. Limb sparing surgery for pediatric musculoskeletal tumors. Pediatr Blood Cancer. 2004;42:295–310.

Hosalkar HS, Dormans JP. Surgical management of pelvic sarcomas in children. Pediatr Blood Cancer. 2005;44:305–17.

Malawer MM, Sugarbaker PH. Musculoskeletal cancer surgery treatment of sarcomas and allied diseases. Norwell: Kluwer Academic; 2001.

Peabody TD, Simon MA. Making the diagnosis: keys to a successful biopsy in children with bone and soft-tissue tumors. Orthop Clin North Am. 1996;27(3):453–9.

Schwartz HS. Orthopaedic knowledge update; musculoskeletal tumors 2. Rosemont: American Academy of Orthopaedic Surgeons; 2007.

Springfield DS, Gebhardt MC. Bone and soft tissue tumors. In: Morrisey RT, Weinstein SL, editors. Lovell and Winter's pediatric orthopaedics. 5th ed. Philadelphia: Williams & Wilkins; 2001. p. 507–62.

Chapter 101
Subcutaneous Endoscopy

Sanjeev Dutta

In many respects, we pediatric surgeons of the twenty-first century stand on the shoulders of giants. The outstanding scientific and innovative contributions of prior generations of surgeons enable us to definitively cure previously daunting pediatric surgical disorders. There is, however, "collateral damage" incurred by our operations. The most obvious example is the visible scarring that is left behind, but there is also the psychological impact of hospitalization, the exposure to painful procedures, and the impact of surgical illness on families. These factors are far less understood than the treatment of the diseases, perhaps because they are seen as unavoidable and necessary consequences of the operation.

Advances have been made toward addressing the visible scarring caused by common pediatric general surgical operations including those on the face, neck, chest wall, and abdomen. These techniques, sometimes referred to as "stealth" surgery, are achieved by combining minimal access surgery with novel surgical techniques in a way that completely hides the scars. Three of these techniques are: (1) trans-scalp endoscopy, for removal of forehead lesions, (2) transaxillary subcutaneous endoscopy, for removal of lesions of the neck and chest, and (3) single-port access/transumbilical laparoscopy, for abdominal procedures. In each, the goal is to perform a complex operation without leaving visible evidence and thus spare the child from the potential psychological and cosmetic impact of scars.

Diagnosis

The workup of the patient that is being considered for a stealth operation depends on the region of the body involved. In cases where subcutaneous endoscopy is utilized, such as the forehead, neck, or chest wall, a working space under the skin must be created. Obliteration of this space, such as from

significant burns, previous neck surgery or irradiation, will preclude use of this technique. The presence of active infection is also a contraindication. Finally, subcutaneous endoscopy should not be performed in children with skin that is excessively thin or easily injured, such as those with epidermolysis bullosa.

In general, stealth procedures should be limited to nonmalignant conditions that are well circumscribed, with the exception of thyroidectomy for follicular neoplasms, for which a transaxillary endoscopic technique is well-described. Very large lesions at any location can be more difficult to resect because of the difficulty in getting to the contralateral side, however goiters of up to 10 cm diameter have been removed, and I have removed a 15 cm diameter lipoma on the back of an adolescent.

Forehead and Brow Lesions

Dermoid cysts are the most common benign lesions removed from the forehead and brow by pediatric surgeons, but one may also encounter pilomatrixomas, lipomas, or osteomas. Midline dermoids found between the brows, called nasoglabellar cysts, can have intracranial extension and thus warrant three-dimensional imaging prior to resection. Dermoids can cause bony erosion, so parents should be alerted to a subtle crater effect after removal. As with the neck and chest wall, scalp or forehead scarring that prevents development of a subgaleal or subperiosteal plane contraindicates an endoscopic approach, but under such conditions the cosmetic benefits of the approach are minimal anyway.

Neck Lesions

Benign lesions of the neck that can be addressed using subcutaneous endoscopy include thyroglossal duct cysts, lymph nodes, torticollis, dermoid cysts, branchial cleft cysts, parathyroid adenoma, and goiter. The preoperative workup is the

S. Dutta (✉)
Department of Surgery, Lucile Packard Children's Hospital, Stanford University, 780 Welch Road, Suite 206, Stanford, CA 94305, USA
e-mail: sdutta1@stanford.edu

P. Mattei (ed.), *Fundamentals of Pediatric Surgery*,
DOI 10.1007/978-1-4419-6643-8_101, © Springer Science+Business Media, LLC 2011

same as for open procedures. It is not advantageous to remove lesions with significant skin involvement using subcutaneous endoscopy since a noticeable cutaneous defect will be created. However, lesions for which limited (<3 mm) skin excision is required can still result in a nearly invisible scar. The dermal portion is excised last to prevent loss of carbon dioxide insufflation.

Resection of the thyroid is limited to benign lesions and small follicular neoplasms. Lobectomy, isthmectomy, and total (or near-total) thyroidectomy have been described, but children will most commonly undergo total gland removal. Early experience should consist of glands less than 5 cm in diameter.

For hyperparathyroidism, single adenomatous parathyroids are most commonly removed, however a 3½ gland parathyroidectomy for hyperplasia has been described. Preoperative sestamibi scan and intra-operative ultrasound localization confirm a solitary adenoma and help determine the appropriate axilla to access. Intra-operative rapid parathyroid hormone assay is also helpful.

Abdominal Conditions

Single site laparoscopic access through an incision hidden in the umbilicus is emerging as a reasonable option for "scarless" abdominal surgery, specifically for appendectomy, cholecystectomy, and total splenectomy, however virtually all abdominal procedures can be performed in this way.

While a history of open abdominal operation is not an absolute contraindication to laparoscopy, previous large incisions traversing the umbilicus portend difficulty with the umbilical approach due to dense adhesions. Finally, large solid organ resections that require an intact specimen for histopathology cannot be performed through a transumbilical incision since the fascial defect is too small for intact specimen removal.

Surgical Technique

Trans-Scalp Subcutaneous Endoscopy

The procedure is performed under general anesthesia and cefazolin is administered preoperatively. The patient is positioned supine with the head placed at the foot of the bed and elevated on foam padding so that the neck is slightly flexed. The surgeon and assistant are positioned at the foot of the bed and a monitor is placed adjacent to the head of the bed. Betadine scrub is used to prepare the skin of the forehead and scalp, and baby shampoo is used to clean the hair. The hair is not shaved or clipped, but directed away from the planned incision site using a sterile comb and Bacitracin ointment.

An endoscopic brow lift set is used, including a rigid endoscope introducer with attached retractor (Fig. 101.1), a 3-mm 30° laparoscope, a periosteal elevator, curved endoscopic scissors/dissector and a vascular-tip suction device. The curved shaft of these dissection instruments aids in navigating the curve of the skull in the forehead region. One can also use standard 20-cm long, 3-mm laparoscopic instruments.

Local anaesthetic (0.25% bupivacaine with 1:200,000 epinephrine) is injected at a site 2 cm posterior to the hairline that vertically corresponds to the location of the lesion. The injection is carried through to the subperiosteal or subgaleal planes and a path is hydrodissected toward the lesion. A single 2.5-cm V-shaped skin incision (apex posterior) is made with a #11 blade at the site of the injection. A V-shaped incision is better camouflaged by typical hair growth than a

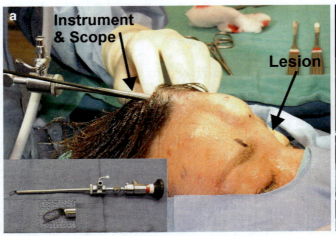
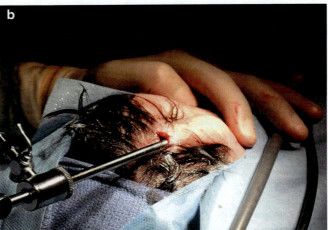

Fig. 101.1 (**a**) Telescope and instrument placement for trans-scalp endoscopic removal of a midline nasoglabellar cyst. The telescope is inserted through a browlift introducer/retractor (*inset*). (**b**) Trans-scalp endoscopic removal of a lateral brow dermoid cyst

transverse incision. For dermoid cysts, the incision is carried through to the subperiosteal plane and subperiosteal elevators are used to complete dissection of the path toward the lesion.

Endoscopic surgery on the forehead requires familiarity with the neural structures in the region, specifically the temporal branch of the facial nerve, the supratrochlear nerve, and the superficial branch of the supraorbital nerve. The temporal nerve supplies motor function to the frontalis muscle and the orbicularis oculi, and is at risk during excision of lateral brow masses. The main trunk of this nerve runs within the superficial temporal fascia while the terminal branches are in a subcutaneous plane and so are at even greater risk. Injury to this nerve during endoscopic surgery is avoided by maintaining a subperiosteal plane of dissection until the lesion is reached. Aggressive retraction should be avoided to prevent neuropraxia. The supratrochlear and supraorbital nerves run lateral to the midline in the subperiosteal plane. When dissecting toward a nasoglabellar cyst, the dissection should remain in the midline and extend in a subperiosteal plane, then advance into the subgaleal plane approximately 2 cm above the supraorbital rim. The supraorbital nerve emerges from the supraorbital foramen, which can occur up to 2 cm above the supraorbital rim. An incision overlying the lesion would be perpendicular to the course of the nerves, increasing chances of transection. The endoscopic dissection runs parallel to the nerves, hence conferring less risk of injury.

After inserting the introducer/retractor, the endoscope is advanced into the dissection path, giving excellent visualization. A trocar or insufflation are not necessary. Fingertip palpation on the skin is helpful to localize the lesion. All instruments are placed alongside the telescope, through the single scalp incision. Two instruments can be placed through the incision to allow two-handed dissection. If necessary, a separate, tiny, lateral scalp stab incision with its own tunnel can be used to introduce another instrument to allow some triangulation around the pathology. Once near the lesion, dissection involves separating the lesion from the surrounding tissues. A periosteal elevator is effective for lesions that are firmly attached to periosteum and bone.

The lesion is removed through the endoscope tract when free of all surrounding tissues. The dissection is generally bloodless, however a 3-mm hook endocautery can be used if necessary. Rupture of dermoids might occur during dissection but this is not a problem so long as the contents and capsule are removed completely. Once removed, the dissection path is irrigated copiously with saline, the fluid is completely expressed, hemostasis is ensured and any hairs introduced into the tract are removed under direct visualization. The skin incision is closed with a running absorbable intradermal suture. No attempt is made to re-approximate the galea.

Transaxillary Subcutaneous Endoscopy

The patient is positioned supine with the ipsilateral arm (or sometimes both arms) abducted 90° and secured on a padded arm board (Fig. 101.2). The neck is hyperextended with a shoulder roll in place. The neck, anterior chest, axillae, and shoulders are prepared with betadine solution. Prior to commencing the procedure, landmarks including the sternal notch, the sternocleidomastoid muscle, and the clavicle are clearly marked on the overlying skin.

For lateralized lesions, a 5-mm incision is made in the ipsilateral mid-axilla parallel to the lateral border of the pectoralis

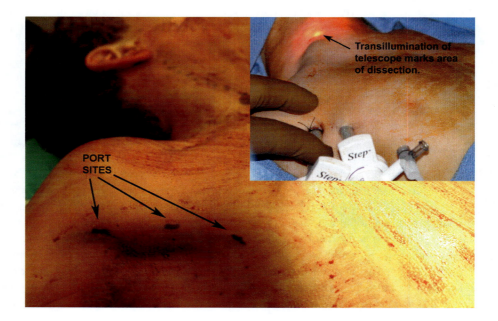

Fig. 101.2 Patient positioning and port placement (*inset*) for transaxillary subcutaneous endoscopy. (Reprinted with permission from Dutta S, Slater B, Butler M, Albanese CT. "Stealth surgery": Transaxillary subcutaneous endoscopic excision of benign neck lesions J Pediatr Surg. 2008;43(11):2070–4.)

major muscle, and the subcutaneous plane is dissected free with a hemostat in the direction of the lesion for about 3 cm. It is easy to accidentally dissect into the subfascial plane and this should be avoided. A 5-mm sheath trocar over a Veress needle is introduced followed by a 5-mm port, which is secured to the skin using a 3-0 silk suture. The skin forms a secure air-tight seal around the port.

The subcutaneous space is insufflated with 10 mmHg CO_2 at a flow rate of 3 L/min and a 5-mm 30° telescope is inserted and used as a dissection tool to carefully expand the subcutaneous space. With the initial workspace created, additional 3-mm ports are placed 2.5 cm to either side of the first port, again at the lateral border of the pectoralis (Fig. 101.2). A 3-mm monopolar hook cautery is used to take down connective tissue attachments and further expand the workspace. This space is largely avascular, and the dissection straightforward. Finger palpation on the skin is helpful to guide dissection, which is carried over the pectoralis fascia and the clavicle, through the platysma and toward the lesion. Care is taken not to cauterize near skin to avoid any cutaneous burns. It is critical to create a wide, cavernous work space to avoid subcutaneous tunneling, which can be problematic for navigation and exchange of instruments. Once an adequate workspace is created, the insufflation pressure is reduced to 7 mmHg.

For lateralized lesions and midline dermoids, standard 3-mm 20-cm long laparoscopic instruments are used to carry out the dissection through the ipsilateral axilla. The pathology is localized by finger palpation, and by directing the dermal transillumination of the telescope toward the lesion. Landmarks that help to guide dissection include the pectoralis fascia, the clavicle, the two heads of sternocleidomastoid muscle, and the sternal notch. Once the lesion is visualized, dissection is similar to that for standard laparoscopy. Hook cautery is the primary dissection tool but care must be taken not to cauterize the dermis, which can result in a full thickness burn. For adolescents in whom a generous workspace is created, 5 mm wristed instruments placed through 5-mm ports can be used. These instruments amplify dexterity by providing two additional degrees of freedom and enable circumferential dissection of lesions. Surgical robotics have been applied in the same way.

For thyroglossal duct cyst excision, where it is necessary to follow a midline tract and resect the hyoid bone, a presternal transverse 5 mm incision at the level of the nipples is used for the camera port site and a port is placed in each axilla to optimize triangulation of instruments around the cyst (Fig. 101.3). The patient is positioned in the frog-leg or lithotomy position at the foot of the bed with the operating surgeon positioned at the feet or between the legs. A subcutaneous tract anterior to the sternum is created and a 5-mm port and telescope are inserted. Axillary incisions are created bilaterally for introduction of one 3-mm port through each axilla. The cyst is dissected circumferentially and the tract

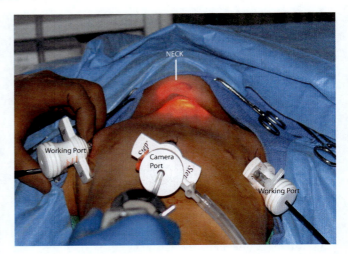

Fig. 101.3 Patient positioning and port placement for the anterior approach to thyroid resection and for thyroglossal duct cyst excision. A presternal port placed at nipple level is used for the telescope, and ports in each axilla allow introduction of dissection tools that triangulate around the target pathology. (Reprinted with permission from Dutta S, Slater B, Butler M, Albanese CT. "Stealth surgery": Transaxillary subcutaneous endoscopic excision of benign neck lesions J Pediatr Surg. 2008;43(11):2070–4.)

carefully followed to the hyoid bone, which is divided on either side of the thyroglossal duct with hook scissors. An absorbable endoscopic loop is then used to ligate the base of the tract beyond the hyoid.

For total thyroidectomy, two approaches are possible: anterior or bilateral. In the anterior approach (Fig. 101.3), a presternal port allows introduction of a telescope and one working port is placed in each axilla. Dissection is accomplished with an ultrasonic or radiofrequency dissector, or with hook cautery. A subcutaneous transverse platysmal flap is created in the midline to expose the strap muscles. These are divided in the midline and retracted laterally. The gland is then approached from an inferolateral direction, taking the inferior thyroid vein and working superiorly toward the middle thyroid vein and inferior thyroid artery. The parathyroids and recurrent laryngeal nerves are visualized and preserved. The superior thyroid vessels are divided, and the ligament of Berry is detached to free the gland.

In the purely bilateral approach, three trocars are placed in each axilla and each lobe is dissected from the ipsilateral axilla. A single axilla can be used for a hemithyroidectomy. A midline port is not used and the strap muscles are not divided in the midline. The clavicular head of the sternocleidomastoid muscle is partially divided after incising the supraclavicular platysma, and the deep cervical fascia is entered posterior to the sternal head to approach the gland from a lateral direction. Alternatively, a plane can be created anterior to the sternocleidomastoid, going between the sternal head and the sternohyoid and sternothyroid muscles. In both approaches, the strap muscles are retracted anteriorly, and the middle thyroid vein and inferior thyroid artery are divided. The gland is raised medial to lateral, preserving the parathyroids and recurrent laryngeal nerve. The inferior thyroid vein is divided, exposing the ligament of Berry, which is then detached to free the gland from the trachea. Finally, the superior thyroid vessels are divided. The contralateral lobe is mobilized in a similar fashion through the contralateral axilla.

The parathyroids can also be approached either anteriorly or laterally. Inferior adenomas are readily identified with the lateral approach, and typically found just medial to the middle thyroid vein, which is divided to gain exposure (Fig. 101.4). Once exposed, the adenoma and its vascular pedicle can be dissected free by staying right on the gland with a hook cautery.

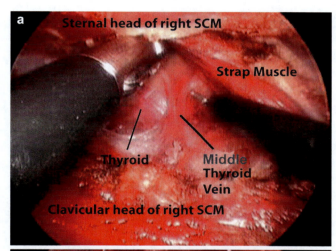

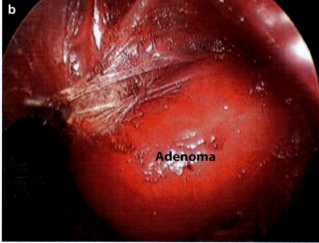

Fig. 101.4 Subcutaneous endoscopic view of the lateral approach to parathyroid adenoma excision with exposure of (**a**) the middle thyroid vein and (**b**) the adenoma after division of the vein. (Reprinted with permission from Dutta S, Slater B, Butler M, Albanese CT. "Stealth surgery": Transaxillary subcutaneous endoscopic excision of benign neck lesions J Pediatr Surg. 2008;43(11):2070–4.)

After excision of each lesion, the instruments and ports are withdrawn and all carbon dioxide insufflation is removed by massaging the skin toward the trocar sites. Local anesthetic (1:1 mixture of 0.25% bupivacaine and 1% lidocaine) is then injected around the sites and the skin is reapproximated with intradermal 5-0 absorbable sutures.

Single-Port Access Abdominal Surgery

All procedures are performed under general anesthetic and orotracheal intubation. Prophylactic antibiotics are administered and appendectomy patients have urinary catheters placed for the duration of the case. Operating room setup is the same as for standard laparoscopy. Wristed 5-mm instruments (Fig. 101.5) are used to perform dissection, including a hook cautery, Maryland dissector, standard grasper, and a thermal ligation device. These hand-held laparoscopic instruments have 7° of freedom that includes a pitch and yaw wrist action, which allows for triangulation around the pathology despite a near-parallel co-location of the instrument shafts at the abdominal wall. The instruments are crossed to achieve this triangulation (Fig. 101.6).

Single-port access (SPA) surgery is becoming the accepted nomenclature for this approach. While the name implies that a single port device is used (a single device that incorporates multiple conduits for telescope and instrument placement), in actuality, the key element is the use of a single small incision through which multiple instruments are placed. Although there are commercially available single-port devices that provide a convenient conduit for instruments, they are not critical for achieving the intended goal. One can create a similar effect simply by placing multiple ports side by side in the small incision.

SPA operations are currently the only clinical application of stealth surgery for abdominal conditions. Other scarless procedures such as natural orifice transluminal endoscopic surgery (NOTES) are still experimental and their application in children seems not only conceptually unappealing (transvaginal access is unlikely to be considered) but also currently associated with an unacceptable risk of leak and infection, especially with transgastric or transrectal access.

Transumbilical port access is the key. Dissection techniques are essentially the same as for standard laparoscopy, but require experience to become comfortable with the novel configuration and functionality of the wristed instruments. The single access site is created by making a vertical incision through the umbilical skin in the midline, extending to the very edge of the umbilical ring, and if necessary a millimeter or two beyond in either direction. For cholecystectomy and gastro-esophageal procedures, the incision is oriented transversely. The incision is carried through the center of the

Fig. 101.5 External appearance of a single-port appendectomy. Ports are placed through a single incision at the umbilicus (*inset*). (Reprinted from Dutta S. Early experience with single incision laparoscopic surgery (SILS): eliminating the scar from abdominal operations. J Pediatr Surg. 2009;44(9):1741–5, with permission from Elsevier)

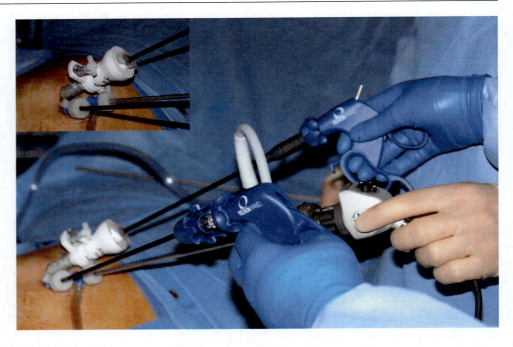

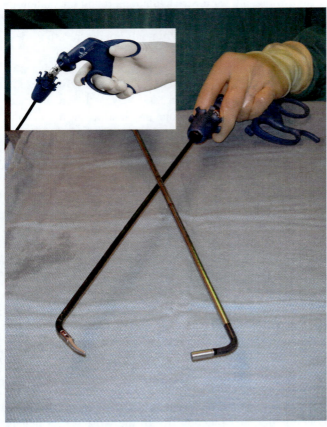

Fig. 101.6 Crossing the instrument shafts in this manner allows intra-abdominal triangulation around the target pathology. The wrist action of the instrument tip is actuated by flexing the handle where it meets the shaft (*inset*: tip movement mirrors hand movement). (Reprinted from Dutta S. Early experience with single incision laparoscopic surgery (SILS): eliminating the scar from abdominal operations. J Pediatr Surg. 2009;44(9):1741–5, with permission from Elsevier)

umbilical stalk, and each half of the stalk is detached from the underlying fascia. A wide prefascial plane surrounding the incision is created with blunt and cautery dissection. At full retraction, the skin incision typically measured 2–2.5 cm. A Veress needle is passed through the midline at the congenital umbilical fascial defect and CO_2 is injected to 15 mmHg. Three trocars are placed through this single incision in a triangular configuration, including two 5-mm "apple core" trocars and one 12 mm sheath-type trocar (Fig. 101.5).

For appendectomy, the mesoappendix is divided with cautery or an endostapler with a vascular cartridge. The appendix is transected at its base using a vascular cartridge endostapler or endoloops and the specimen removed using an endo-bag.

For cholecystectomy, cephalad retraction of the gallbladder fundus and liver is achieved by transabdominal passage of a heavy-gauge polypropylene suture high in the right upper quadrant, taking a generous bite of the gallbladder fundus under telescopic visualization. The triangle of Calot is dissected with the wristed instrumentation to identify the cystic duct. Small branches of the cystic artery on the gallbladder wall are divided using hook cautery, obviating the need to divide more proximally with clips. The cystic duct is then divided between clips. The remainder of the gallbladder is dissected from the liver bed and the specimen removed in the standard fashion.

For splenectomy, two instruments are used for retraction and dissection. The 12-mm port should be large enough to accommodate a roticulating endostapler. Inferior attachments and vessels are divided with the thermal ligation device, followed by the short gastric vessels. The hilum is divided with one or more firings of a roticulating endostapler using a vascular cartridge, with the stapler sharply angulated

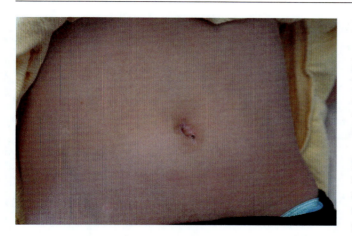

Fig. 101.7 Cosmetic outcome 1 week after single-port splenectomy. The single incision at the umbilicus will be imperceptible. (Reprinted from Dutta S. Early Experience with single incision laparoscopic surgery (SILS): eliminating the scar from abdominal operations. J Pediatr Surg. 2009;44(9):1741–5, with permission from Elsevier)

cephalad. The remaining avascular attachments are then divided and the spleen placed in an endoscopic bag. For spleens larger than 10 cm in maximum dimension, the 12-mm port is upsized to a 15-mm port and a large bag is used to retrieve the spleen. In all cases, the bag is brought through a larger fascial defect that is created by joining the 12 mm defect with one of the 5 mm defects, and the spleen is morcellated with a sponge clamp.

The fascial incisions are closed using absorbable suture. The umbilical stalk is tacked down to the fascia using 5-0 absorbable suture, and the umbilical skin is reapproximated using the same suture in a simple interrupted fashion. Cosmetic results are consistently outstanding (Fig. 101.7). Bupivicaine is injected as a field block around the umbilicus.

Postoperative Care

For subcutaneous endoscopy, patients are discharged home the same day and acetaminophen is usually an adequate analgesic. Patients who have undergone single-port operations are managed postoperatively as they are after equivalent laparoscopic procedures.

The long-term effects of scarring from general surgical procedures remain to be studied, as does the impact of scarless surgery. There is an abundance of evidence in the psychology and surgical (mainly burn and cleft lip) literature to suggest that visible scarring in children can result in reduced self-esteem, impaired socialization skills, and lower self-ratings of problem-solving ability. Furthermore, other children judge children with facial deformities more negatively than those without facial deformities. In one particular study in which children were asked their impressions of images of other children with facial scars, participants aged 8–16 years rated individuals with facial deformities as less popular, friendly, and smart, and were less likely to choose these individuals as friends. Surgeons are being encouraged to more closely monitor the effects of scarring and other side effects of their treatments in the follow-up of their patients.

Scarring is an unfortunate consequence of many of the operations that pediatric general surgeons perform, one that can have a significant impact on the psychological well-being of the child. Early minimal access surgery, namely laparoscopy and thoracoscopy, was an evolution toward addressing the issues surrounding scarring, in addition to improving pain and recovery time. Stealth surgery takes this paradigm one step further by allowing the surgeon to perform complex operations without leaving visible evidence.

Summary Points

- Visible scarring can have a life-long impact on the psychological development of the child.
- Lesions of the forehead, neck, and chest wall can be removed scarlessly by utilizing a subcutaneous endoscopic approach that exploits hidden areas of the body as entry points, such as the scalp and axilla.
- Most abdominal operations can be performed without visible scarring using a single port access technique that hides the incision in the umbilicus.
- Pediatric general surgeons can readily apply these techniques by combining traditional MAS techniques with some novel maneuvers and new enabling technologies.

Editor's Comment

Though not yet widely available, subcutaneous endoscopic procedures and single-port surgery are the next steps along the continuum of progress in the field of minimal access surgery. Eventually, camera lenses and instruments will have multiple joints or will be entirely flexible to allow most procedures to be performed through a single umbilical port. Until then, progress will need to be incremental and driven forward by mavericks in the field. Though each of us undoubtedly applauds this progress, we should also be mindful of the fact that patients, especially children, are not experimental subjects. In addition, cutting-edge procedures should not be attempted unless we have a reasonable expectation that the risks are as low or lower than what would be expected for the standard of care.

Standard minimally invasive procedures in the abdomen can be modified to improve cosmesis: using the minimum number of ports necessary; creating a true intra-umbilical incision rather than the standard periumbilical incision; placing an instrument next to the umbilical camera port incision rather than placing a second port; placing all port site incisions as far lateral on the abdomen as possible and avoiding the upper abdomen and the midline whenever possible; placing instruments that do not require replacement during the operation, such as a liver retractor, through the abdominal wall without using a port; and using U-stitches to retract or suspend certain structures (gall bladder, falciform ligament, stomach) instead of placing an extra port merely for a retractor.

Subcutaneous endoscopic procedures are useful for neck lesions, including the thyroid and parathyroid, but are technically demanding. In addition to the standard axillary incisions, peri-areolar incisions are also well positioned and cosmetically acceptable. The subcutaneous working space should be created with gentle blunt dissection whenever possible and only the minimum pressure of CO_2 insufflation needed to maintain the space should be used. Excessive pressure can create widespread subcutaneous emphysema. Finally, one should be aware that there is a risk of burning the skin if the tip of the laparoscope comes into contact with the dermis for more than a few seconds, just as can occur externally when the scope touches the skin or the surgical drapes.

Differential Diagnosis

Forehead

- Dermoid cyst
- Lipoma
- Nasoglabellar cyst
- Osteoma
- Pilomatrixoma

Neck (Lateral)

- Lymph node
- Branchial cleft cyst
- Torticollis

Neck (Midline)

- Dermoid cyst
- Lymph node
- Parathyroid adenoma
- Thyroglossal duct cyst
- Thyroid follicular neoplasm

Chest Wall

- Dermoid cyst
- Gynecomastia
- Lipoma
- Pilomatrixoma

Diagnostic Studies

Head, Neck, and Chest Wall

- Clinical exam alone
- Ultrasound
- Computed tomography scan
- Magnetic resonance imaging
- Sestamibi (for parathyroid adenoma)
- Fine needle aspiration (thyroid nodules)

Abdominal

- Per usual practice

Parental Preparation

- Potential for mild "crater" effect after removal of forehead dermoid cysts that exhibit bony erosion.
- Possibility of neuropraxia after brow dermoid excision, secondary to retraction.
- Possibility of hematoma, seroma, or ecchymosis formation after subcutaneous endoscopy (usually self resolving).
- With single-port surgery, there is always the possibility that we will need to convert to a standard laparoscopic or open operation.

Preoperative Preparation

☐ Appropriate imaging.

☐ Appropriate instrumentation.

☐ Preoperative localization of parathyroid adenoma (sestamibi scan).

☐ For nasoglabellar cyst, rule out intracranial extension with computed tomography.

☐ For subcutaneous endoscopy, confirm location of lesion and mark overlying skin and relevant landmarks prior to insufflating subcutaneous space.

Technical Points

Trans-scalp Subcutaneous Endoscopy

- Avoid aggressive retraction to avoid neuropraxia
- Become familiar with forehead neural anatomy

Transaxillary Subcutaneous Endoscopy

- Create broad, cavernous subcutaneous workspace before dissecting the lesion
- Liberal use of finger palpation to identify landmarks and target lesion
- Follow cutaneous transillumination of telescope to guide dissection
- Ensure hemostasis to prevent postoperative hematoma or ecchymosis

Single-port Access Surgery

- Start with appendectomy before progressing to more complex procedures such as cholecystectomy
- Splenectomy should be attempted only after considerable experience with SPA
- Insert ports to different depths to avoid port backend collisions
- Use different length instruments through each port to avoid instrument backend and camera collisions

Suggested Reading

Dutta S, Albanese CT. Endoscopic excision of benign forehead masses: a novel approach for pediatric general surgeons. J Pediatr Surg. 2006;41(11):1874–8.

Dutta S, Albanese CT. Transaxillary subcutaneous endoscopic release of the sternocleidomastoid muscle for treatment of persistent torticollis. J Pediatr Surg. 2008;43(3):447–50.

Dutta S, Slater B, Butler M, Albanese CT. Stealth surgery: subcutaneous endoscopic excision of benign neck lesions. J Ped Surg. 2008;43(11):2070–4.

Dutta S. Single port access transumbilical surgery: eliminating the scar of abdominal operations in children. Submitted for Publication.

Miyano G, Lobe TE, Wright SK. Bilateral transaxillary endoscopic total thyroidectomy. J Pediatr Surg. 2008;43(2):299–303.

Chapter 102
Benign Skin Lesions

Michael D. Rollins and Sheryll L. Vanderhooft

Virtually every child has a number of benign growths on the skin. Parents of children who ask their pediatrician to look at a growth are usually concerned that the lesion may be cancerous or precancerous. Many papules and nodules that arise in children have very characteristic clinical features that allow a diagnosis to be made without the aid of histological or radiographic evaluation. However, some lesions may be very non-specific in appearance and require a biopsy to make a diagnosis. In some situations, obtaining an imaging study is desirable before a biopsy is performed. For example, lesions along the midline of the face, scalp, and back frequently have connections to the brain or spinal cord, and care must be taken to avoid biopsy of any midline lesion until such a communication is ruled out, usually by CT or MRI.

More than 75% of soft tissue tumors that present between birth and 12 months of age are benign. There are several features of a cutaneous neoplasm that heighten the concern about malignancy. These include onset during the neonatal period, rapid or progressive growth, skin ulceration, fixation to or location deep to the fascia, and a firm mass greater than 3 cm in diameter. In the absence of any of these findings, there is a greater than 99% chance that the lesion will prove to be benign.

Cutaneous Lesions

Verrucae

Human papillomaviruses (HPV) infect epithelial tissues of skin and mucous membranes and clinically manifest as warts (verrucae). Infection occurs by skin-to-skin contact, with maceration or sites of trauma predisposing patients to inoculation. The incubation period of these viruses ranges from 2 to 6 months. The virus induces epidermal proliferation, causing rough surfaced papules and plaques, often with superficial thrombosed capillaries. The natural history of warts is spontaneous resolution once the host immune response occurs. However, this may take several years. On average, 75% of warts in children will spontaneously resolve within 3 years, even if no treatment is attempted.

In children old enough to comply with therapy, reasonable first line therapies for common, plantar, and palmar warts include: salicylic acid, liquid nitrogen cryotherapy, or cantharidin blistering. For patients with facial lesions, topical agents such as 5-FU, tretinoin, or imiquimod may be useful. Topical or intralesional immunotherapy for recalcitrant lesions may be effective with less scarring. This type of treatment is often best accomplished in conjunction with a dermatologist. When selecting a method of treatment, the extent and location of the lesions, age of the child, and willingness of the child to participate in treatment should be considered. The least painful methods should be used initially, reserving more destructive therapies for recalcitrant lesions and lesions in which cosmesis is less important.

Calcinosis Cutis

Cutaneous calcification arises secondary to trauma or in association with metabolic diseases (parathyroid neoplasms, hypervitaminosis D, renal disease) and connective tissue diseases (CREST syndrome, dermatomyositis). It may be a focal process or more widespread. Calcinosis cutis presents as hard nodules with chalky material within them. The clinical differential diagnosis includes osteoma cutis and the treatment of choice is surgical removal.

M.D. Rollins (✉)
Department of Surgery, Division of Pediatric Surgery, Primary Children's Medical Center, University of Utah School of Medicine, 100 North Mario Capecchi Drive, Suite 2600, Salt Lake City, UT 84113-1100, USA
e-mail: Michael.Rollins@hsc.utah.edu

P. Mattei (ed.), *Fundamentals of Pediatric Surgery*,
DOI 10.1007/978-1-4419-6643-8_102, © Springer Science+Business Media, LLC 2011

Keloid

Keloids are benign fibrous growths present in scar tissue that form due to an exaggerated connective tissue response to dermal injury. Keloids differ from hypertrophic scars in that they extend beyond the margin of the original scar. These lesions may be asymptomatic or frequently they are pruritic, tender, or cause sharp, shooting pains. Keloids do not spontaneously resolve and may continue to enlarge. Management consists of potent topical steroid massage, intralesional steroid injections, or topical silicone gel. Intralesional corticosteroids are first-line therapy for keloids with up to 70% of patients responding, although recurrence rates are high. Triamcinolone (5–40 mg/mL) is injected into the bulk of the keloid using just enough to make the keloid blanch. Injections may be repeated at monthly intervals using increasing concentrations of triamcinolone. Do not exceed 40 mg of the drug per visit due to the risk of atrophy and hypopigmentation. Surgical revision of a keloid may be considered, but recurrences are common.

Pyogenic Granulomas

Pyogenic granulomas are solitary polypoid lesions that often occur after a history of trauma or local irritation. They are associated with capillary proliferation and are commonly found on the skin as red, raised, occasionally bleeding lesions. The lesion typically develops over a few days to weeks and treatment may be indicated for cosmesis or if the lesion bleeds easily with minor trauma. Treatment strategies include topical silver nitrate, liquid nitrogen, or ligature of the polyp neck. Most commonly these are shaved off and the base cauterized. Rarely is more extensive surgical excision required.

Dermatofibroma

Dermatofibromas are benign neoplasms of dermal connective tissue that may vary tremendously in appearance. They sometimes occur as the result of trauma or an insect bite but are often idiopathic. Some dermatofibromas present as small, firm, reddish-brown, sclerotic papules, less than 1 cm in size, that exhibit dimpling of the overlying skin when they are squeezed. Others present as dome-shaped pink, red, or reddish-brown tumors. Dermatofibromas are freely movable over the subcutaneous fat. They may grow slowly and then remain stable for years. They are found most commonly on the anterior surface of the lower extremities. No treatment is required unless the lesion is symptomatic, has recently changed in size or color, or is bleeding. If the lesion protrudes above the skin surface it may be subject to repetitive trauma, in which case excision could be considered. Excision of a progressively enlarging lesion is indicated due to the rare development of dermatofibrosarcoma protuberans.

Neurofibroma

Neurofibromas are benign neoplasms of nerve tissue that may appear as solitary lesions in otherwise healthy individuals or as multiple lesions in association with neurofibromatosis. They appear initially in early childhood or adolescence as firm, polypoid, irregular nodules which gradually increase in size. In patients with neurofibromatosis, lesions may increase in number. Neurofibromas occur anywhere on the cutaneous surface, but palms and soles tend to be spared. When moderate digital pressure is applied to the surface of a small neurofibroma, it may invaginate into the dermis, which is referred to as "buttonholing." Although most neurofibromas are intradermal lesions, large plexiform lesions may occur in the subcutaneous layer. Surgical excision is performed on tumors that are disfiguring, interfere with function, or are subject to irritation, trauma or infection. It is important to evaluate any patient with a neurofibroma for the characteristic skin findings of neurofibromatosis type 1, which includes the presence of six or more café-au-lait macules, two or more neurofibromas of any type or one plexiform neurofibroma, and freckling in the axillary or inguinal regions. If these classic skin lesions are identified, the patient should be referred to a medical geneticist.

Subcutaneous Lesions

Lipoma

Lipomas and lipoblastomas arise from subcutaneous fat. They are soft, mobile and nontender subcutaneous nodules with a lobular and rubbery texture. They may be difficult to differentiate from deep hemangiomas or lymphangiomas. They may arise anywhere on the body, but most commonly they are found on the neck, shoulders, back, and abdomen. Lipomas are benign and generally asymptomatic and may be left untreated unless they become uncomfortable, are growing, or are cosmetically unacceptable. Radiographic imaging may be considered for lesions located in the deeper soft tissue of the extremities, the neck, or the paraspinous region. Complete surgical excision is typically curative. It is usually possible to differentiate lipomas from the surrounding fat intraoperatively because they have a firmer consistency. Lipoblastoma should be considered in the differential diagnosis of a rapidly enlarging subcutaneous mass in children under 3 years of age. Although lipoblastoma is a benign lesion, it may recur up to 25% of the time and long-term follow up is recommended.

Granuloma Annulare

Although granuloma annulare is an idiopathic inflammatory process involving the dermal collagen and not a neoplasm, the firmness of the lesions often raises the concern about malignancy. The cutaneous type presents most commonly in children and young adults as localized firm aggregates of flesh-colored or reddish-brown papules that coalesce into annular plaques, often with central clearing. There is a subcutaneous variant that presents in healthy young children as a firm, painless, nonmobile, lobular mass usually on the lower extremity, which often raises the concern about malignancy. Spontaneous resolution occurs within several years in the majority of patients. Reassurance, therefore, is an important aspect of management, and expectant observation is a reasonable approach. Symptomatic lesions may be treated with topical or intralesional steroids with varying success. Occasionally, an incisional biopsy is required to confirm the diagnosis in the subcutaneous type although clinical presentation along with MRI findings may be sufficient to support observation.

Infantile Myofibromatosis

Infantile myofibromatosis is a neoplasm derived from myofibroblasts and is the most common fibrous tumor of infancy. The tumors are rubbery, firm, rounded dermal and subcutaneous nodules that may be present at birth or appear in early infancy. They may be reddish-brown or purple and range from 1 to 7 cm in diameter. The condition occurs in two forms: *solitary* (more common) and *multicentric*. The solitary form more commonly affects the trunk, head and neck. It is more common in males and is characterized by one tumor involving the skin and/or soft tissue that regresses spontaneously within 1–2 years with less than 10% recurrence. The multicentric form is more common in females and is characterized by several tumors involving the skin, soft tissue, viscera, and/or bone. It also follows a benign course in most circumstances with spontaneous resolution in a few years. However, the condition may be fatal in infants with extensive visceral involvement, especially the lung. Biopsy of the cutaneous tumors is essential to exclude soft

tissue sarcoma, fibrosarcoma and rhabdomyosarcoma. Although these tumors have a high rate of spontaneous regression, visceral myofibromas that affect function should be surgically excised. Recurrence is unusual but should be managed by re-excision. All children with myofibromas should be evaluated for bone and visceral involvement with imaging studies.

Cysts

Epidermoid Cyst

Epidermoid cysts, also called epidermal inclusion cysts, are the most common type of cutaneous cysts. They arise from occluded pilosebaceous units or from traumatic implantation of epidermal cells into the dermis. They are often erroneously referred to as "sebaceous cysts." The cyst wall consists of normal epidermis that produces keratin and they grow slowly as keratin accumulates within them. They present as elevated, round, flesh-colored or somewhat yellow papules or nodules, often with a discernible overlying punctum, and are freely movable. When they rupture, the keratin that is released has a cheesy consistency, often with a sour odor. Although epidermoid cysts typically appear after puberty, they are not unusual in young children. They arise most commonly on the face, scalp, neck, back and scrotum. Another relatively common location in toddlers is within the umbilical scar. Removal of the entire epidermal lining of the cyst is necessary to prevent recurrence. If the cyst ruptures when it is being removed, care must be taken to irrigate all of the keratin out of the wound to prevent formation of a foreign body granuloma. Epidermoid cysts may become infected, which can make excision more difficult and the final cosmetic result less acceptable. It is best to treat these with antibiotics with or without drainage and delay excision until all signs of the acute infection have resolved.

Dermoid Cyst

Dermoid cysts arise primarily along lines of embryonic fusion. They are most commonly located along the lateral third of the eyebrow, forehead and scalp. Dermoids are usually round, soft, and fixed to deep tissue or bone. They usually present as a painless mass 1–2 cm in diameter but can grow larger if left untreated. They contain keratin and some may also contain hair, bone, tooth, or nerve tissue. Dermoids in the head often cause an indentation in the outer table of the skull, which may be apparent on skull radiograph. Cysts arising near the medial canthus of the eye, along the nose, or along suture lines of the skull may have an intracranial extension, and therefore radiographic imaging with CT or MRI is recommended before attempting surgical removal. Definitive treatment is surgical excision. Incisions on the scalp should follow lines of tension. An incision just above and parallel to the eyebrow should be used for improved cosmesis in dermoids located at the lateral eyebrow.

Pilomatrixoma (Calcifying Epithelioma of Malherbe)

Pilomatrixomas are benign tumors of hair follicle origin. They present as slow-growing solitary papules or nodules with a rock-hard consistency in the subcutaneous fat just below the dermis. The overlying skin may have a yellow, red, or blue hue. These nodules occur almost exclusively in children and young adults with more than half located on the head and neck. The tumors are usually asymptomatic but may become inflamed and tender. The clinical differential diagnosis includes epidermoid cyst, other cystic lesions, and calcinosis or osteoma cutis. Surgical excision is the treatment of choice for these tumors and should include the small area of overlying dermis. Recurrence rates are low.

Ingrown Toenails

Ingrown toenails most commonly affect the great toe and occur when the lateral nail plate pierces the lateral nail fold and enters the dermis. Predisposing factors include poorly fitting shoes, excessive trimming of the lateral nail plate, and trauma. Treatment of ingrown toenails depends on the severity of the lesion. Patients should be educated about proper nail trimming, which includes allowing the lateral nail plate to grow beyond the lateral nail fold and trimming the nail horizontally. Mild to moderate lesions may be treated by soaking the affected foot in warm water three times per day and pushing the lateral nail fold away from the nail plate. A small cotton wedge may be placed under the lateral nail plate to relieve pressure. For more severe lesions in which there is significant pain, erythema, or pustular discharge, treatment involves removing the lateral portion of the nail. This may be accomplished using a digital nerve block or under general anesthesia. A straight hemostat is inserted under the nail to separate it from the nail bed and the lateral nail fold is excised. A curette should be used to remove granulation tissue. Following excision, dilute hydrogen peroxide should be used to clean the site two to three times per day followed by application of bacitracin ointment. The intraoperative application

of 10% NaOH to the adjacent germinal matrix to accomplish a chemical matrixectomy prior to curettage may reduce recurrence rates.

Foreign Bodies

Children are often referred for various nodular and cystic lesions that are usually removed in order to relieve parental anxiety and obtain a definitive diagnosis. One should keep in mind that lesions that are tender or show signs of inflammation may represent a local reaction to a foreign body. The history is frequently suggestive but plain radiographs or ultrasonography should be performed for documentation and to help guide surgical intervention. Removal of soft tissue foreign bodies may occasionally be performed in the emergency department with sedation and local anesthetic but is usually best accomplished in the operating room. Intraoperative fluoroscopy or ultrasonography may be helpful for localization and to ensure that all fragments have been removed. Depending on the nature of the wound, the skin may either be left open to granulate or loosely closed. Postoperative radiographic documentation of complete removal of the foreign body is imperative, as a retained foreign body can cause significant discomfort, recurrent infection and the need for multiple procedures.

Lymph Nodes

Enlarged lymph nodes may cause great concern to parents and primary care providers. These are most commonly secondary to infectious or otherwise nonspecific processes although malignancy must be considered. The interview should help the surgeon distinguish infectious from noninfectious causes. Questions should focus on how long the node has been present, if there has been any change in size, and if it is causing any symptoms. Presence of constitutional symptoms including fevers, chills, night sweats, and weight loss (more than 10% body weight) should be sought. In addition, orthopnea or the recent onset of dyspnea suggests a mediastinal component. Other pertinent aspects of the history are recent foreign travel and exposure to cats.

Certain characteristics on physical exam may suggest a benign versus a malignant process, although it is impossible to determine based on exam alone. Physical exam should focus not only on the involved lymph node but on identification of a local infectious process near the enlarged lymph node, an exam of all major nodal basins and an abdominal exam to evaluate for hepatosplenomegaly or an abdominal mass. Lymphadenopathy present in only one region suggests local causes. An obvious infection near the anatomically drained area may be present but often there is no clinical evidence of an inoculation site. Generalized lymphadenopathy is the enlargement of more than two noncontiguous lymph node regions and is generally the result of systemic disease. A node that is smaller than 1 cm and asymptomatic may safely be observed. If the node is tender, has overlying skin changes, or is fluctuant, it is likely infectious and a trial of antibiotics or drainage should be considered. Asymptomatic lymph nodes greater than 2 cm, symptomatic lymph nodes greater than 1 cm, nodes that are getting progressively larger, are firm or fixed or are located in the supraclavicular region are worrisome and should be biopsied or excised. Prior to excision, a complete blood count, erythrocyte sedimentation rate, chest X-ray, cat-scratch (*Bartonella henselae*) titers, Epstein–Barr virus titer or Monospot test should be obtained. In certain situations, a PPD or HIV test may be indicated.

When excision of a lymph node is required, one must be careful not to injure adjacent structures, especially peripheral nerves. The incision should be made along the lines of tension in the skin. Mobilization of the lymph node should be almost exclusively by blunt dissection in a plane immediately adjacent to the capsule of the node and the vascular pedicle cauterized or ligated only when clearly visualized and separated from adjacent structures. If the lymph node is part of a matted group of nodes then an incisional biopsy large enough for diagnosis is all that is required. If there is a suspicion for lymphoma, the specimen should be sent fresh to pathology. Cultures should be performed if an infectious process is suspected.

Cervical Lymphadenitis

Cervical lymphadenitis is common in childhood and is usually caused by a viral upper respiratory illness. Cervical lymphadenitis caused by viral or bacterial infection may be acute or subacute and may present with unilateral or bilateral involvement. Lymph node enlargement caused by a viral upper respiratory illness are typically small, rubbery, mobile and discrete without erythema. They may be minimally tender. Although the clinical course is self-limited, the enlarged lymph nodes may persist for several weeks.

Chronic Cervical Lymphadenitis

Children occasionally have enlarged nodes that do not appear to be acutely infected. The nodes may be less erythematous or have no erythema and are less tender than those in acute

bacterial adenitis. In the absence of a history or physical exam that suggests a malignant process, the child should be evaluated for tuberculosis, atypical mycobacterial infection, and cat-scratch disease. Most children should receive a 2 week course of an oral antistaphylococcal antibiotic with repeat examinations by the same physician to assess response to therapy. An oral antibiotic effective against methicillin-resistant staphylococcus may be a reasonable choice depending on the prevalence of the organism in the hospital or region. A single dominant lymph node present for longer than 6–8 weeks, which has not responded to appropriate antibiotic therapy, should probably be completely excised, cultured, and submitted for histologic exam to rule out neoplasm.

Mycobacterial Lymphadenitis

Atypical mycobacteria are now the most common causative agents of mycobacterial lymphadenitis. These are characterized as acid-fast bacilli using light microscopy. Atypical (or nontuberculous) mycobacterial adenitis is generally considered a local infectious process in immunocompetent hosts. It is not contagious and the portal of entry in an otherwise healthy child is thought to be the oropharynx. The common clinical presentation is in a child between 1 and 5 years of age with focal, unilateral involvement of the jugulodigastric, preauricular, or submandibular nodal group. The involved nodal group is usually minimally tender, firm, and rubbery to palpation, is well circumscribed and may be adherent to underlying structures. The involved lymph nodes may enlarge over weeks to months without prominent systemic symptoms. Skin testing with tuberculin PPD may yield an intermediate reaction due to cross-reactivity. The treatment of choice is complete surgical excision with primary wound closure. Some would advocate a prolonged course of clarithromycin in addition to surgical excision. If complete excision is not possible, curettage is the next best option although recurrence of the infection and the development of a chronic draining sinus are possible sequelae. There is some evidence that observation alone may be effective after the diagnosis is confirmed by fine needle aspiration, though resolution of the lymphadenitis may take up to 12 months.

Cat-scratch Disease

Cat-scratch disease is a common cause of lymphadenitis in children. The causative organism is *Bartonella henselae*. Most cases can be directly related to contact with a cat, and the usual site of inoculation is a limb. The disease begins as a superficial infection or pustule forming in 3–5 days and is followed by regional adenopathy in 1–2 weeks, although adenopathy may occur as long as 60 days following the event. Although the diagnosis can often be made by history alone, commercially available tests to detect antibodies against *B. henselae* or PCR may confirm the diagnosis. Although early systemic symptoms of fever, malaise, myalgia, and anorexia are common, the disease usually follows a benign, self-limiting course with resolution of lymphadenopathy in 6–8 weeks even without specific treatment. Excisional biopsy may be warranted if a draining sinus tract develops or if the diagnosis is uncertain.

Peripheral Lymphadenopathy

Normal lymph nodes in most regions are usually less than 1 cm in their longest diameter. Exceptions are the epitrochlear region (less than 0.5 cm in diameter) and the inguinal region (less than 1.5 cm in diameter). Although the concern for malignancy in unexplained peripheral lymphadenopathy is high, one large series found the prevalence of neoplasia to be 13% with 52% of peripheral lymph node biopsies demonstrating reactive hyperplasia of undetermined etiology. However, *supraclavicular* lymphadenopathy is associated with a high rate of malignancy. Right-sided nodes are associated with cancer of the mediastinal lymph nodes whereas left-sided nodes suggest intra-abdominal malignancy, most often lymphoma. *Axillary* lymphadenopathy is commonly the result of infections or trauma to the arm, thoracic wall, or breast. *Inguinal* lymphadenopathy in children is usually not associated with a specific etiology unless the nodes are very large (>3 cm). Palpable *epitrochlear* nodes are often pathologic in children. The differential diagnosis includes infections of the forearm or hand, leukemia, lymphoma, and atypical mycobacterial infections.

Vascular Lesions

Hemangioma

Infantile hemangiomas are the most common tumor of infancy, occurring in 10–12% of infants. They are vascular tumors that grow by endothelial proliferation and generally occur within the first few weeks of life. They are classified as superficial (epidermal and dermal involvement), deep (subcutaneous), and mixed depending on the depth of soft tissue involvement. They are usually well-circumscribed lesions that may be flesh-colored, bright red or blue. Growth is characterized by two phases: proliferative (birth to 12 months)

and involutive (1–10 years). Hemangiomas typically double in size during the first 2 months of life, with the average hemangioma achieving 80% of its final size by 5 months.

Complications may occur due to extensive size, involvement of vital structures, bleeding, ulceration, secondary infection, platelet trapping (Kasabach–Merritt syndrome), and associated abnormalities. Kasabach–Merritt phenomenon occurs with the more invasive kaposiform hemangioendothelioma or tufted angioma. Worrisome lesions include lumbosacral lesions, large facial lesions, periocular lesions, lesions in the beard distribution on the face, and occasionally multiple lesions. Lumbosacral lesions can be associated with genitourinary anomalies and spinal dysraphism. Large facial hemangiomas can occur as part of the PHACES syndrome (posterior fossa malformations, hemangiomas, arterial anomaly, coarctation of the aorta and cardiac defects, eye abnormalities and occasionally sternal defects). Eyelid and periocular hemangiomas represent ophthalmologic emergencies because of potential visual impairment from pressure on the globe or visual obstruction. Lesions that are prone to ulceration include those on the lip, axillae, neck, and buttock. Hemangiomas occurring in the beard distribution of the face can be associated with airway involvement with hemangioma. Multiple papular small hemangiomas can be seen in association with visceral hemangiomas involving the liver, gastrointestinal tract, lungs, brain, and other organs. High-output cardiac failure can develop with large liver hemangiomas. Lesions that pose significant cosmetic concerns, such as those involving the lip, nasal tip, and ear, may require early medical intervention in an attempt to halt growth and prevent permanent deformation.

Most hemangiomas can simply be observed. Regression is complete in half of children by age 5, in 70% of children by age 7, and in the remainder by age 10. In the involuted phase, nearly normal skin is restored in approximately 50% of children. Yellow pulsed-dye laser treatment may halt progression of growth of early hemangiomas and should be considered for all facial hemangiomas. Steroids (intralesional or systemic) are recommended for large hemangiomas, those that cannot safely be excised, and those that compromise vital structures and function. Vincristine may be considered for steroid-unresponsive hemangiomas. Surgical excision is recommended for lesions that have not completely involuted, skin ulceration, recurrent bleeding, or if the location of the lesion poses significant health concerns.

Vascular Malformations

Vascular malformations are localized or diffuse lesions that result from errors of embryonic development and may affect any segment of the vascular system, including arterial, venous, capillary, and lymphatic vessels. Most vascular malformations are sporadic with an overall prevalence of 1.2–1.5%. Lesions are categorized as slow-flow or fast-flow anomalies.

Lymphatic malformations are slow-flow vascular anomalies best characterized as microcystic, macrocystic, or mixed. They most commonly appear as ballotable masses with normal overlying skin, although a blue hue may be present with large underlying cysts. Lymphatic malformations are generally evident at birth or before age two. Radiologic documentation is best performed by MRI although ultrasound may be useful to characterize the flow within the malformation and confirm the presence of macrocysts. Malformations are commonly located in the axilla/chest, cervicofacial region, mediastinum, retroperitoneum, buttock, extremities, and anogenital areas. The two main complications of lymphatic malformations are intralesional bleeding and infection. Analgesia, rest, and time are sufficient therapy for intralesional bleeding. Infection may result in cellulitis requiring prolonged intravenous antibiotics.

The two strategies available for treating lymphatic anomalies are sclerotherapy and surgical resection. Macrocystic lesions are more amenable to treatment with sclerotherapy. Commonly used agents include hypertonic saline, sodium tetradecyl sulfate, absolute ethanol, and doxycycline. OK-432, a treated strain of *Streptococcus pyogenes*, is an investigational agent which has had excellent reported success. Side effects of sclerosants include local necrosis, blistering, and local neuropathy. Complete clinical resolution has been reported in 60–100%. In some cases, especially lesions that are predominantly microcystic, surgical resection might be the only way to cure lymphatic malformations, but this can be difficult due to extent of the lesion and incorporation of vital structures. Staged resections may be necessary for large lesions. Recurrence is common after resection and reported in 40% of lesions following incomplete resection and 17% after macroscopically complete excision.

Venous malformations are the most common of all vascular anomalies and are frequently misdiagnosed as hemangiomas. The typical appearance is a blue, soft, and compressible mass. They demonstrate proportional growth with the growth of the child. Most venous malformations are solitary, but multiple cutaneous or visceral lesions can occur. Phlebothrombosis is common and can be painful. If large and located on the extremity, they may cause limb length discrepancies, painful hemarthrosis, and degenerative arthritis. These anomalies are best imaged by MRI.

Treatment options include sclerotherapy and surgical resection. For small cutaneous malformations, injection with 1% sodium tetradecyl sulfate is often successful. However, recanalization can occur leading to recurrence. Excision of a venous malformation is usually successful for small, well-localized lesions. Sclerotherapy may be useful 24–72 h prior to resection in order to shrink the lesion.

Nonmelanocytic Nevi

Epidermal Nevi

Epidermal nevi present as yellowish-brown, velvety, granular, or warty plaques. They may occur as single or multiple lesions and typically have a linear or whorled configuration, following the lines of Blaschko. Epidermal nevi may be present at birth, but they most often appear during early childhood and evolve until puberty. They may arise anywhere on the cutaneous surface and may also involve the oral mucosa and ocular conjunctiva. Most epidermal nevi measure several centimeters or less in length but can extend along an entire limb or traverse the chest, abdomen, or back. Malignant degeneration (e.g., basal cell or squamous cell carcinoma) of epidermal nevi is rare. Epidermal nevi may be generalized and associated with abnormalities of the skeletal, ocular, genitourinary, central nervous, and cardiovascular systems, commonly referred to as the epidermal nevus syndrome.

Treatment of these lesions is unnecessary unless the nevus results in cosmetic disfigurement. Topical therapies can help smooth the epidermal nevi but need to be used long term to maintain the effect. Full-thickness surgical excision is curative for a completely developed epidermal nevus, however, excision of a lesion that has not completely evolved may lead to recurrence. Surgical excision therefore should be delayed if possible until puberty.

Nevus Sebaceus of Jadassohn

Nevus sebaceus is a collection of normal sebaceous glands. It presents at birth as a solitary well-circumscribed round or oval hairless yellowish orange plaque, often with a lobular texture. The predominant sites of involvement are the scalp, face and neck. Nevus sebaceus grows in proportion to the child's growth but is usually less than 2–3 cm in diameter. With the onset of puberty, the sebaceous glands within the nevus become functional, which causes thickening of the plaque. Secondary neoplasias arise in 10–15% of these lesions, typically in adulthood, and are most commonly benign tumors of epidermal appendage origin. Malignant degeneration (basal cell carcinoma, squamous cell carcinoma) is uncommon and estimated to be less than 1%. Changes of the nevus sebaceus that should prompt consideration of a biopsy include friability, focal nodularity, or rapid enlargement. Periodic evaluation for changes during infancy, early childhood, and into adulthood is recommended. Management includes biopsy of any changing area or full-thickness excision if the lesion is bothersome. Prophylactic excision before puberty is no longer routinely recommended.

Becker's Nevus

Becker's nevi are epidermal nevi that present initially as a hyperpigmented patch, predominantly in males during childhood or adolescence. The lesion commonly develops hypertrichosis limited to the area of pigmentation. It is usually a large lesion, 10–20 cm in diameter and frequently located over the back, shoulder, or upper arm. Becker's nevus is characterized by increased androgen receptor sensitivity, which explains why it is seen predominantly in males. It is a benign lesion and therefore surgical excision is not necessary. Treatment of the pigmentation and hypertrichosis may be attempted with lasers. Shaving, depilatories, and electrolysis also can address the issue of hair overgrowth.

Postoperative Care

After surgery, routine follow up is essential to assess wound healing and discuss pathology results. Lesions not excised on the first visit should be evaluated on serial office visits by the same examiner. Enlarged lymph nodes may require repeat examination every 2–3 weeks for up to 8 weeks, whereas nevi may need to be followed for up to a year. The surgeon should be thoughtful and sensitive when dealing with these minor skin lesions as parental anxiety is often high.

Summary Points

- Most skin lesions in infants and children are benign.
- Approximately 75% of warts will spontaneously resolve within 3 years.
- Evaluate any patient with a neurofibroma for skin findings of NF type I.
- Most hemangiomas can simply be observed but parental reassurance is necessary.
- Lesions that pose significant cosmetic concerns such as those involving the face may require early medical intervention.
- Nevi that have an atypical appearance or have changed abruptly require complete excision.
- Prophylactic excision of nevus sebaceus is no longer recommended.

Editor's Comment

The back is a common place for subcutaneous lesions such as lipomas, lymphangiomas, and fibromas to arise in infants and children. Typically off the midline and below the level of the scapula, these tend to be large, flat lesions with indistinct borders and a high risk of recurrence after surgical excision. Ultrasound or MRI can be useful to determine the true extent and to help with surgical planning. It is also helpful to delay excision until the child is more than a year of age when the dissection planes within the fat are somewhat easier to delineate. These will sometimes turn out to be due to nodular fasciitis, an inflammatory lesion that causes the fascia of the paraspinous muscles to thicken and fibrose. Excision usually leaves the muscle without investing fascia, which is functionally not an issue. In the end, these lesions are all benign and mostly of cosmetic concern, therefore the least invasive operation with the best cosmetic result should be the goal.

Other uncommon but challenging skin lesions occasionally seen in a typical pediatric surgical outpatient practice include tick bites and myiasis. Tick bites create a lot of anxiety in some parts of the country because of concerns about Lyme disease, but surgeons are sometimes asked to assess a child who has had a tick removed in such a way that the mouth parts have been left embedded in the skin. This can cause an intense foreign body reaction or even a local vasculitis. If the lesion persists after a 2-week period of observation, surgical excision is sometimes necessary. Cutaneous myiasis is due to growth within the skin of the larva of the botfly, which is indigenous to parts of Central and South America. The dermal lesion is typically red, raised, and itchy with a small central hole (breathing pore) through which a serosanguinous discharge (feces) is intermittently seen. Patients will sometimes also describe the feeling that something is wriggling within the lesion. The larva will eventually come out on its own and the course is benign, but few patients or parents in the US will tolerate such "therapy." Home remedies abound, including the application of petrolatum to suffocate the larva, but surgical extraction under general anesthesia is often the best option.

For dermoid cysts that are located within a slight concavity of the skull, it is important to remove the underlying periosteum to prevent recurrence. It is tempting to attempt retrieval of a foreign body in the foot in the office or Emergency Department, but this is often a frustrating exercise that can push the foreign body deeper. The foot has many intersecting subcutaneous fibrous septae that are difficult to navigate, can allow the foreign body to hide, and can make the practitioner appear to be incompetent in the eyes of the parents. Unless the foreign body is directly visible, it is always best to perform the extraction in the operating room, under general anesthesia, and, if the foreign body is radiopaque, under fluoroscopic or ultrasound guidance. When dealing with any foreign body extraction, it is important to warn the parents about the possibility of a retained foreign body and carefully document that the foreign body has been extracted, usually with a follow-up radiograph. Always insist on a follow-up visit so that you can be sure that the wound has healed well with no evidence of infection or foreign body. These situations are often highly charged, both emotionally and legally.

Diagnostic Studies

- CT/MRI lesions arising near the medial canthus of the eye, along the nose, or along suture lines of the skull to rule out intracranial extension
- Ultrasound or MRI may be useful to characterize lesions and evaluate extent/depth of the lesion
- MRI of brain/spine to rule out CNS involvement pre operatively in giant congenital melanocytic nevi involving posterior midline
- Ultrasound or plain radiograph to document foreign body

Parental Preparation

- Reassurance is needed for lesions not excised on first visit.
- Discussion of risks: wound infection, seroma, hematoma, scarring.

Technical Points

- The entire lining of an epidermoid cyst must be removed to prevent recurrence.
- Excise worrisome lesions initially with a narrow margin.

Suggested Reading

Chang LC, Haggstrom AN, Drolet BA, et al. Growth characteristics of infantile hemangiomas: implications for management. Pediatrics. 2008;122(2):360–7.

Christison-Lagay ER, Fishman SJ. Vascular anomalies. Surg Clin North Am. 2006;86(2):393–425.

Coffin CM, Dehner LP. Soft tissue tumors in first year of life: a report of 190 cases. Pediatr Pathol. 1990;10(4):509–26.

Coffin CM, Dehner LP. Fibroblastic-myofibroblastic tumors in children and adolescents: a clinicopathologic study of 108 examples in 103 patients. Pediatr Pathol. 1991;11(4):569–88.

Fraser L, Moore P, Kubba H. Atypical mycobacterial infection of the head and neck in children: a 5-year retrospective review. Otolaryngol Head Neck Surg. 2008;138(3):311–4.

Lyon VB. Lumps and bumps in children-when to worry: recent trends in recognition and pathology of hemangiomas of infancy and Spitz nevi. Curr Opin Pediatr. 2004;16(4):392–5.

Oguz A, Karadeniz C, Temel EA, et al. Evaluation of peripheral lymphadenopathy in children. Pediatr Hematol Oncol. 2006;23(7):549–61.

Price HN, Zaenglein AL. Diagnosis and management of benign lumps and bumps in childhood. Curr Opin Pediatr. 2007;19(4):420–4.

Santibanez-Gallerani A, Marshall D, Duarte AM, et al. Should nevus sebaceus of Jadassohn in children be excised? A study of 757 cases, and literature review. J Craniofac Surg. 2003;14(5):658–60.

Soldes OS, Younger JG, Hirschl RB. Predictors of malignancy in childhood peripheral lymphadenopathy. J Pediatr Surg. 1999;34(10):1447–52.

Chapter 103
Atypical Nevi and Malignant Melanoma

Kenneth W. Gow

Pigmented lesions of childhood are a frequent indication for referral to a pediatric surgeon. The majority of lesions are benign. However, in the rare instance of melanoma, some believe that pediatric outcomes are worse than those in adults. This poses the challenge of choosing which lesions can be observed and which should be biopsied. Adding to this difficulty is that some lesions possess both benign and malignant features. It is therefore important for a surgeon to become familiar with those disorders for which there is established therapy and those whose management is less well-defined.

Ordinary melanocytes are cells derived from the neural crest and reside in the basal layer of the epidermis. They are evenly dispersed as single units and produce melanin, providing the natural pigmentation of the skin. The production of melanin is an intricate process in which melanosomes travel along melanocyte dendrites and are transferred to surrounding keratinocytes. This allows transport of melanin to protect cells in the skin from ultraviolet light injury.

Nevus cells are anomalous melanocytes that cluster as nests within the lower epidermis or dermis and do not have dendritic processes. Melanocytic nevi (moles) are benign proliferations of nevus cells, of which many variants are encountered, each with specific clinical, histologic, and molecular characteristics. They are initially formed by melanocytes that have been transformed from highly dendritic single cells normally interspersed among basal keratinocytes to round cells that grow in nests along the dermoepidermal junction.

Melanoma is thought to arise when melanocytes or melanocytic nevi are exposed to ultraviolet radiation, which leads to damage of the DNA and subsequent malignant changes and uncontrolled growth. While considered the most serious type of skin cancer, it is also quite rare in children. Nonetheless, due to its varied presentations and poor prognosis, diagnosis and management continue to be a significant challenge.

K.W. Gow (✉)
Department of Surgery, Children's Hospital and Regional Medical Center, University of Washington, 4800 Sand Point Way NE, MIS W-7729, PO Box 5371, Seattle, WA 98105, USA
e-mail: Kenneth.Gow@seattlechildrens.org

Diagnosis

In most cases, the pediatric surgeon will not be the first person to have seen the child with a questionable skin lesion. Very often children will be referred from the primary medical provider and a biopsy might already have been performed. But even if you are not the first to work up a particular lesion, you should obtain a complete history, with attention to moles, changes (ABCDE – asymmetry, border irregularity, color, diameter >6 mm, evolution), family history of skin malignancies, sun exposure, and, especially, a history of sunburn. While none of these criteria are absolute, any unusual features will increase the possibility of a malignancy.

Melanoma differs in children in that it can arise from certain conditions that are known to be associated with development of melanoma: (1) transplacental melanoma (transmitted from the mother with melanoma), (2) giant congenital melanocytic nevi, (3) xeroderma pigmentosum (defect in repair of DNA after damage induced by ultraviolet light), (4) immunosuppression (from hematologic or infectious disease or following organ or hematopoietic stem cell transplantation), and (5) dysplastic nevi syndrome.

The physical examination should include a thorough evaluation of the entire skin surface with special attention to other suspicious lesions. Areas that are often overlooked are the scalp, nail beds, palms, soles and all lymph node basins (cervical, axillary, and groin). Photography is helpful if lesions are being followed over time. Mucous membranes and the digits and interdigital spaces are important regions to scrutinize.

Due to the rare nature of melanoma in children, it is often not recognized or considered seriously in the differential diagnosis, leading frequently to a potentially detrimental delay in diagnosis and treatment. Confounding this further is the fact that benign lesions can have alarming melanoma-like features, whereas melanomas can present atypically: nodular, pedunculated, amelanotic lesions, or simulating a pyogenic granuloma. These confusing parameters make it difficult for parents and caregivers to sort out what needs further attention.

Children with numerous moles tend to develop nevi with a particular clinical appearance, or a "signature nevus."

A large number of acquired nevi and the presence of clinically atypical nevi each represent a marker of increased risk of melanoma. Since most cutaneous melanomas are not associated with a prior nevus, there is no benefit from prophylactic removal of nevi. However, a nevus that has different characteristics from other nevi in the same patient should be viewed with caution. As mentioned, baseline photographs can prove helpful for serial examination purposes.

If a biopsy has already been performed, it is imperative to obtain the slides and review them with an experienced dermatopathologist. If local expertise is not readily available, have the slides sent out to experts at other centers for a second opinion. This is critical but it can be challenging, even for very experienced histopathologists. Recently it has been suggested that 40% of lesions initially diagnosed as melanoma were subsequently classified as benign after review. If you have received the slides and have confirmed the diagnosis of melanoma, particular attention should be paid to important features that will guide decisions for further therapy: Breslow thickness, presence or absence of ulceration, mitotic rate, Clark level, and the status of the margins.

If no biopsy has been performed and the lesion has worrisome features, then you should consider biopsy to inform further management. If the lesion is less than 1.5 cm, an excisional biopsy should be performed. Remember that when orienting the incision it is important to anticipate what type of incision might need to be made if wide excision becomes necessary. It is usually best to make the incision parallel to the long axis on the extremities and along traditional planes on the trunk. It is important to have about a 5 mm margin of normal skin around the lesion (Fig. 103.1). For lesions that are larger than 1.5 cm, an incisional or punch biopsy is usually preferable. A shave biopsy is strongly discouraged as it will only provide the uppermost aspect of the lesion, and will

therefore be useless in determining the depth of the lesion, making staging a challenge.

Histopathologic features that appear to be the most useful for distinguishing melanomas from benign nevi include: size >7 mm, ulceration, high mitotic activity, mitoses in the lower third of the lesion, asymmetry, poorly demarcated lateral borders, lack of maturation, dusty melanin, and marked nuclear polymorphism.

The diagnosis and management of malanoma can be quite challenging and, while our role as surgeons cannot be understated, it is important to work as part of a qualified multidisciplinary team. This should include an experienced dermatopathologist, a pediatric oncologist, and an adult oncologist with experience treating patients with melanoma. Finally, it is sometimes necessary to consult a radiation oncologist or plastic surgeon, especially if soft tissue coverage is a potential issue after wide excision. While not every patient will require the entire team, you should certainly become conversant with specialists in your facility or region to facilitate management.

Congenital nevi are classically defined as melanocytic nevi present at birth or within the first few months of life, however some congenital nevi present between 3 months and 2 years. Acquired nevi appear after the first 6 months of life and the number increases during childhood and adolescence, usually reaching a peak in the third decade and then slowly regressing with age. Nevi can be located at various depths of the skin, with deeper lesions being more elevated and less pigmented. They tend to be symmetrical and less than 8 mm in diameter with a homogeneous surface, even pigmentation, round or oval shape, regular outline, and sharply demarcated border.

Both environmental and genetic factors play a role in the development of acquired melanocytic nevi. Sun exposure is the main environmental influence, especially when intense and intermittent. Sunscreen use might limit the development of such nevi. From a genetic standpoint, individuals with lightly pigmented skin have more nevi than those with darker complexions. Freckling represents a heritable phenotypic feature that is also associated with more numerous nevi.

Congenital Nevi

About 1% of newborns have a congenital melanocytic nevi (CMN). Compared to acquired nevi, the melanocytes in CMN tend to extend deeper into the dermis and even the subcutaneous tissues, and track along appendages such as hair follicles. As such, they are classified based on the most apparent location: *junctional* (at the epidermodermal junction), *compound* (both the epidermodermal junction and dermis), or *dermal* (confined almost entirely to the dermis).

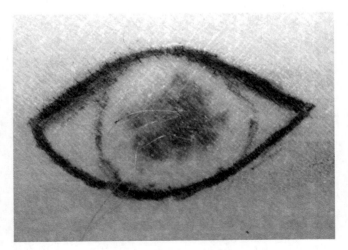

Fig. 103.1 A nevus should be measured circumferentially with 0.5 cm margins. This is an elliptical excision oriented along the extremity

Congenital nevi enlarge in proportion to the child's growth. The lesions are categorized on the basis of size into three groups: *small* are less than <1.5 cm in diameter, *medium* are between 1.5 and 20 cm, and *large* are larger than 20 cm, or, in a neonate, more than 9 cm on the head and more than 6 cm on the body. The color ranges from tan to black, and the borders are often geographic and irregular. As children grow, the nevi change from flat to a more irregular surface. There is ongoing debate as to the melanoma risk associated with CMN. In general, large CMN tend to be associated with systemic disease (central nervous system), whereas the effects of small and medium sized CMN are usually limited to the skin. The risk of development of cutaneous melanoma in small and medium CMN is thought to be only up to 1% over a lifetime and usually arise after puberty.

Small and medium CMN are managed individually, factoring in ease of monitoring, clinical history, parental concern, and cosmetic issues. Lesions that have worrisome features should be excised. Those that are difficult to excise completely can be treated using laser therapy. Nonetheless, in view of the overall good prognosis, prophylactic removal is generally not needed as long as monitoring is available and feasible.

The risk of developing melanoma within a large CMN is estimated to be between 5 and 10% over a lifetime, with about half occurring during the first 5 years of life. In some patients, the site of primary melanoma is the central nervous system or retroperitoneum. The patient with a "giant" (>40 cm) CMN in a posterior axial location with numerous satellite nevi has the greatest risk of developing melanoma. Of note, deep soft tissue malignancies other than melanoma, such as rhabdomyosarcoma and peripheral nerve sheath tumors, can also develop in association with large CMN.

Early and complete surgical removal of large CMN is recommended, although this can be challenging given the size, location, and frequent involvement of deeper structures. Excision therefore often requires staged excision with the use of tissue expanders and skin grafting. Further, even if achieved successfully, complete excision does not reliably eliminate the risk of melanoma, as primaries in the central nervous system and other sites can occur. When surgical excision is not feasible, cosmetic benefit can be obtained from curettage, dermabrasion, and ablative laser therapy. Regardless of the extent of resection, these patients must be followed closely and should undergo biopsy if any concerning changes occur. In addition, they must be screened with MRI of the brain, preferably during the first 6 months of life if the nevus overlies the posterior axis, and then followed with serial neurologic examination.

Speckled lentiginous nevi (SLN) or nevus spilus might represent a subtype of CMN. The tan patch background (café-au-lait macule-like) of an SLN is noted at birth with spots appearing over time. The risk of developing melanoma in SLN is thought to be similar to CMN of the same size. Accordingly, SLN should be followed clinically with periodic examinations and biopsy of suspicious areas. The development of melanoma has been rarely described in association with speckled lentiginous nevi, however, and typically only in adulthood.

Halo Nevi

The halo nevus is also known as Sutton's nevus or leukoderma acquisitum centrifugum. It is a melanocytic nevus surrounded by a round or oval halo of symmetric depigmentation, which usually present as multiple lesions on the back. They are sometimes associated with atopic dermatitis, Turner syndrome, or autoimmune disorders. This pigment loss often heralds spontaneous regression of the central nevus presumably through an immune response to nevus antigens. The process lasts weeks to years and occurs in four clinical stages: (1) pigmented nevus surrounded by a halo of depigmentation, (2) pink nevus surrounded by a halo of depigmentation, (3) circular area of depigmentation, with disappearance of the nevus, and (4) normal-appearing skin after repigmentation of the halo. Halo nevi have often been confused with melanoma because melanomas that undergone regression can appear pale. It is important to point out that halo nevi are entirely benign and of only cosmetic significance.

Atypical Nevi

Atypical nevi are also known as dysplastic nevi or Clark's melanocytic nevi. They are benign acquired nevi that share some clinical features of melanoma such as asymmetry, border irregularity, color variability, and a diameter greater than 6 mm. While previously referred to as dysplastic nevi, current recommendations are to avoid using this confusing term. Histologically, they are nevi with architectural disorder and with varying degrees of atypia (none, mild, moderate, or severe).

Atypical nevi usually begin to appear around puberty and continue to develop throughout life. In general, the density of atypical nevi is greater on areas of the body that receive intermittent sun exposure than in covered sites. They usually are variegated with often different colors (pink, tan, brown), and are usually flat with an elevated center (a "fried egg" appearance). The borders can be irregular and are characteristically ill defined. They are usually larger than common nevi (>5 mm) but in general terms, size is not associated with the degree of atypia; more telling is that they often occur in the setting of a high mole count.

A patient with multiple atypical nevi is at increased risk of developing melanoma. Such patients need periodic total body skin examinations (TBSE). Compared to the general population, patients with atypical nevi tend to develop melanoma at an earlier age. The relative risk varies from 2 to 8 times in those with no personal or family history of melanoma, to over 100 times in those with two or more family members with melanoma.

Some children are normal at birth but develop large numbers of morphologically common nevi in early childhood. These become more numerous and acquire atypical clinical features within a decade. New lesions continue to develop throughout life. Such children may have dysplastic nevus syndrome (DNS). Other names for DNS include familial atypical mole-malignant melanoma syndrome (FAMMM) and B-K mole syndrome (the initials of the family names of the first two kindreds studied). There is no consensus about the minimum essential criteria for diagnosis, but a reasonable range is 50–100 lesions. The nevi are usually large (>5 mm) and irregular with an ill-defined border. The color is variable with a mixture of pale and dark brown, and pink. Vital to note is that melanoma-prone family members with atypical nevi have a lifetime risk of developing melanoma of 100%. The benefits of the early introduction of protective measures such as reduction of exposure to solar UV, adequate clothing, regular TBSE, and regular use of sunscreen are thought to be of some benefit.

Blue Nevi

Blue nevi are benign proliferations of dendritic dermal melanocytes that produce melanin. The blue color of these cells is due to the preferential scattering of shorter wavelengths of light by dermal melanin (Tyndall effect). This is to be differentiated from Mongolian spots, which are bluish patches that usually appear in the sacral region. Clinically, blue nevi appear similar to nodular melanoma but they typically lack rapid growth. There is a form of malignant blue nevi, which usually arises in the scalp. Nonetheless, should such lesions remain stable, most can be managed expectantly. Patients with blue nevi that are difficult to follow due to color or location should be offered the option of surgical excision.

Spitz Nevi

Spitz nevus (also Reed nevus) was first seen in a cohort of children with melanocytic lesions that behaved in a benign manner but shared histological features with melanoma. Most Spitz nevi appear during childhood, most commonly on the face and lower extremities. They may arise de novo or in association with an existing melanocytic nevus. Lesions can be pink, tan, red, or brown, are usually solitary, dome-shaped, papules or nodules, and sometimes grow at a rapid rate. However, not all such lesions present with classic features, and thus the differentiation of a Spitz nevus from malignant melanoma can be difficult. Further, there are no ancillary studies such as immunohistochemical markers or molecular markers that will reliably distinguish between these two entities.

Spitz nevi tend to present in children younger than 10 years and most by the first two decades of life. There is general agreement that any presumed Spitz nevus with atypical features (size >10 mm, asymmetry, ulceration) should be excised. However, other aspects of the management are less clear, such as the need to achieve clear margins, or the need for staging procedures such as sentinel lymph node biopsy.

Occasionally, clearly distinguishing between an atypical Spitz tumor and melanoma is simply not possible. Such lesions will need to be carefully evaluated and discussed with local experts. However, there is enough uncertainty regarding the behavior of Spitz nevi that a standardized approach cannot be established at this time.

Melanoma

Melanoma is still considered a rare cancer of childhood, accounting for only 1–3% of all pediatric malignancies. Compared to adults, childhood cases are more common in females (61%) and non-Whites (6.5%). There has also been an increase in the incidence of melanoma in adolescents by 85% from 1973 to 1996. The incidence for teenagers was higher in the southern regions of the US, which suggests that sun exposure is a factor. Melanomas in children arise commonly on the head and neck (20%) and the remainder distribute equally on the trunk and extremities. From a histologic standpoint, when compared to adults, childhood melanomas appear to have a higher percentage of atypical clinical features (amelanotic and raised lesions), nodular histology, thicker lesions, and having a higher metastatic rate to lymph nodes. Despite such biologic differences, reports indicate that children have similar outcomes to adults and have an overall lower incidence of recurrence, thereby refuting the impression that melanoma is a more aggressive disease in children and adolescents. Currently, there is a paucity of large studies to guide our overall management of the child with melanoma.

Diagnosis and Staging

The staging in children is the same as that used for adults (Table 103.1). Despite early enthusiasm for the use of positron emission tomography to provide further information about

Table 103.1 TNM staging categories for cutaneous melanoma

T categories

Tis: Melanoma in situ

T1a: Melanoma ≤1.0 mm thick without ulceration and mitosis $<1/mm^2$

T1b: Melanoma ≤1.0 mm thick with ulceration or mitoses $≥1/mm^2$

T2a: Melanoma 1.01–2.0 mm thick without ulceration

T2b: Melanoma 1.01–2.0 mm thick with ulceration

T3a: Melanoma 2.01–4.0 mm thick without ulceration

T3b: Melanoma 2.01–4.0 mm thick with ulceration

T4a: Melanoma >4.0 mm without ulceration

T4b: Melanoma >4.0 mm with ulceration

N categories

N0: No spread to nearby lymph nodes

N1: Spread to 1 nearby lymph node; a: Micrometastasis; b: Macrometastasis

N2: Spread to 2 or 3 nearby lymph nodes; a: Micrometastasis; b: Macrometastasis; c: In transit metastases/satellites without metastatic nodes

N3: Spread to 4 or more lymph nodes, OR matted nodes, or in transit metastases/satellites with metastatic nodes

M categories

M0: No distant metastasis

M1a: Distant metastases to skin or subcutaneous tissue or distant nodal metastases and normal serum LDH

M1b: Lung metastases and Normal Serum LDH

M1c: All other visceral metastases and Normal Serum LDH OR Any distant metastasis and Elevated Serum LDH

Anatomic stage groupings for cutaneous melanoma

Stage 0	Tis, N0, M0
Stage IA	T1a, N0, M0
Stage IB	T1b or T2a, N0, M0
Stage IIA	T2b or T3a, N0, M0
Stage IIB	T3b or T4a, N0, M0
Stage IIC	T4b, N0, M0
Stage IIIA	T1-4a, N1a or N2a, M0
Stage IIIB	T1-4b, N1a or N2a, M0; T1-4a, N1b or N2b or N2c, M0
Stage IIIC	T1-4b, N1b or N2b or N2c, M0; Any T, N3, M0
Stage IV	Any T, Any N, M1

Source: Used with permission from the American Joint Committee on Cancer (AJCC®), Chicago, IL. The original source for this material is the AJCC Cancer Staging Handbook, Seventh Edition (2009), published by Springer Science and Business Media, LLC, www.springerlink.com

melanoma staging in adults, it has been associated with low rates of detection of metastatic disease and high false positive rates. This latter issue is perhaps even more relevant in children where inflammation is more common. Consequently, PET is not routinely indicated for early or late stage melanoma. Brain metastases are best assessed with MRI, lung and liver metastases by CT, and small lymph nodes by ultrasound. However, while certainly useful, ultrasound cannot replace sentinel lymph node biopsy since involved nodes are not necessarily enlarged.

Surgical Therapy

The visible lesion is often not the true extent of the microscopic disease. The guiding principle of surgical therapy for melanoma is wide excision with clear margins, which helps avoid local recurrence and improves overall outcome. The extent of resection has been reduced over the years from the 5 cm recommended several decades ago to the current standards that

Table 103.2 Surgical guidelines for melanoma

Tumor	Surgery
<1 mm	1 cm Excision margins, consider sentinel lymph node biopsy
1–2 mm	1–2 cm Excision margins, sentinel lymph node biopsy
>2 mm	2 cm Excision margins, sentinel lymph node biopsy
Any +ve nodes	Complete lymph node dissection

are based on the diameter of the lesion (Table 103.2). Briefly, for lesions 1 mm or less, a 1-cm margin is considered adequate; for lesions 1.1–2 mm, the margin should be 1–2 cm, and for lesions larger than 2 mm, the margin should be at least 2 cm. The depth of resection should include the superficial fascia. The excisional specimen must be oriented to allow the surgeon to potentially return to perform a wider excision to achieve a complete resection. Again, if the resection will create a defect that will be difficult to close, a flap or skin graft might be required (Fig. 103.2).

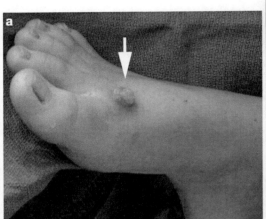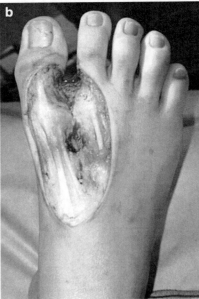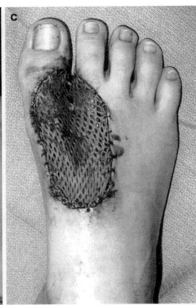

Fig. 103.2 (**a**) Pedunculated lesion in a teenage girl that was initially treated as a wart. A biopsy eventually revealed a deep melanoma. (**b**) A wide local excision with 2-cm margins was performed. (**c**) A full thickness skin graft was used to establish closure

Sentinel Lymph Node Biopsy

Introduced in 1992, sentinel lymph node biopsy has become the standard method to accurately stage patients with malignancies that have the potential to spread via the lymphatic route. Since its original application for melanoma and breast cancer, it has gained wide acceptance in many other adult cancers. Several small studies have demonstrated its usefulness for diagnosis and staging in childhood skin neoplasms.

Sentinel lymph node positivity has been found to be one of the most important prognostic indicators and the technique has been shown to accurately identify occult nodal metastases that would otherwise have grown to palpable size with a the traditional watch-and-wait approach. The surgical technique is generally straightforward. The patient is brought to the hospital on the morning of the operation to undergo lymphoscintigraphy, which identifies the location of the node of interest. This should be performed by an experienced nuclear radiologist and should be confirmed with a hand-held gamma probe prior to taking the patient to the operating room. To provide a second, confirmatory method of isolating the sentinel lymph node, the surgeon should inject isosulfan blue (Lymphazurin 1%) around the lesion after induction of general anesthesia and before sterilely preparing the skin. Performing frozen sections is not generally necessary or recommended. If on permanent sections the node is involved with metastatic melanoma, it is recommended that the patient return to the operating room for a complete lymph node dissection, as this has been shown to double survival when compared to delaying resection until the disease is clinically apparent. If available, RT-PCR (reverse transcriptase-polymerase chain reaction) should be used to assess for micrometastases, as it has been shown to be more sensitive than standard histopathology alone.

In children with melanoma, SLNB is positive in 22–60%, a higher rate than that seen in adults. The technique is especially well suited to the management of lesions arising from the head, neck or trunk, where the lymph node drainage patterns are less predictable (Fig. 103.3).

Surgery is considered key not only for diagnosis and staging, but also for the eradication of the disease. Further, though the issue is still somewhat controversial, we advocate completion lymphadenectomy in patients with positive sentinel lymph nodes as it appears to achieve better outcomes. Nevertheless, the risks of complete node dissection, such as wound infection and lymphedema, cannot be overlooked and probably have more lasting implications in this age group.

Adjuvant Therapy

Systemic therapy for metastatic melanoma is under investigation. Unfortunately, pediatric patients are not included in most trials of adjuvant therapy for melanoma; therefore treatment plans for children must be extrapolated from adult studies.

Melanoma appears to be radiosensitive but this is only used in high-risk patients. It has further been shown that hypofractionation (larger doses of radiation given in fewer treatment sessions over a shorter period of time) achieve the best results. In addition, intensity-modulated radiation

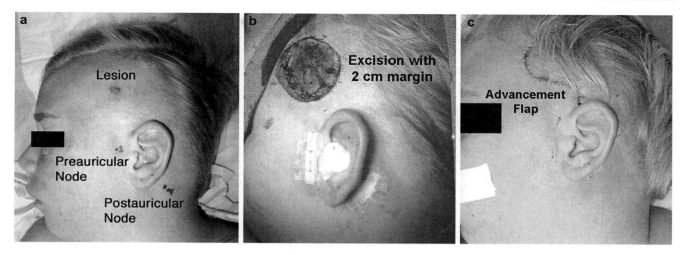

Fig. 103.3 (**a**) Sentinel lymph node mapping is essential in the head and neck region as the lymph node drainage pattern can be unpredictable. In this patient, a scalp primary had both preauricular and postauricular sites mapped by lymphoscintigraphy. (**b**) Wide local excision with 2-cm margins was performed. (**c**) An advancement flap was used to close the defect

therapy has been used and appears to reduce the dose to adjacent normal structures.

Immune therapy has been studied in two forms: melanoma vaccines and immunomodulating drugs. Despite initial excitement, the results of recent trials with vaccines have been disappointing. Further, drugs that stimulate autologous immune modulation, such as interleukin-2 and interferon α-2b, have been used in some patients to achieve durable complete remission. However, the current protocols are long (about 1 year) and associated with significant side effects (anorexia, leukopenia, depression, fatigue). Initial limited experience in children has shown feasibility with acceptable toxicity and promising long-term survival data.

Prognosis

Due to the infrequency of the disease, it has been difficult to establish reliable outcome data for melanoma of childhood. Recent data indicate that there are approximately 18 deaths due to melanoma in individuals less than 20 years of age in the United States every year. The mortality rates are highest in the oldest age group (age 15–19 years), 8–18 times higher than the younger age groups. Numbers currently cited indicate survival of pediatric melanoma as 89 and 79% at 5 and 20 years post diagnosis, respectively. The majority of deaths are attributable directly to melanoma (72%). Outcomes may be related to the site of disease with survival for melanoma on the head and neck and extremities generally better than if it presents on the trunk. Further, though more common in females, when adjusting for age and site outcomes in girls are somewhat better. A recent case-matched series between adult and pediatric melanoma has shown that children often have a thicker melanoma at the time of presentation, which is an important determinant of outcome. However, while stage is considered a prognostic indicator in children, other indicators that have been shown to be useful in adults have not been found to be predictive. Recent studies further show that children with a positive sentinel lymph node can still expect long-term survival with a low incidence of recurrence.

Summary Points

- Malignant melanoma is rare in children but outcomes are worse than those in adults.
- Melanoma is thought to arise when melanocytes are exposed to ultraviolet radiation.
- Characteristic changes ("ABCDE") that increase the likelihood of melanoma include: asymmetry, border irregularity, color, diameter >6 mm, evolution.
- Most cutaneous melanomas are not associated with a prior nevus.
- Up to 40% of lesions initially diagnosed as melanoma are subsequently classified as benign after review.
- The risk of developing melanoma within a large congenital melanocytic nevus is estimated to be between 5 and 10% over a lifetime, with about half occurring during the first 5 years of life.
- Survival of pediatric melanoma is approximately 90% at 5 years and 80% at 20 years.

Editor's Comment

Parents are often very anxious about their children's moles. In some centers, it is one of the more common requests for surgical intervention. However, except for giant melanocytic nevi and syndromes associated with atypical nevi, melanoma only rarely arises from a long-standing congenital nevus, regardless of its features. It is much more of a concern in a nevus that arises de novo or in moles that have changed dramatically or become symptomatic. Nevertheless, when there is no other way to reassure them, it is practically impossible to deny a request for biopsy when parents are anxious about the possibility of cancer.

The diagnosis of malignant melanoma is surprisingly difficult to confirm with certainty and there is often disagreement among dermatopathologists in different parts of the country upon review of the same lesion. Until a genetic signature or biochemical identification becomes available, there will continue to be the need to solicit multiple expert opinions and make the best recommendation with the available information. It is probably best in most cases to err on the side of being more aggressive given the consequences of under-treating a true malignant melanoma, but this is difficult when wide excision becomes necessary on a functionally or cosmetically important part of the body. At least the recommended margin of the wide excision has been decreased to no more than 2 cm (compared to the 5-cm margin that had been mandated until recently).

Giant melanocytic nevi pose a problem in that the risk of developing melanoma is not insignificant but reconstruction can be a challenge. Depending on the part of the body involved, options include skin grafting, tissue expanders, rotation flaps, and, rarely, myocutaneous free flaps. In some sites, staged excision is possible, which allows growth and relaxation of surrounding skin between operations. Each elliptical excision should be within the borders of the nevus such that the scar can be excised at the next operation and the surrounding normal skin remains untouched until the final stage.

Sentinel lymph node biopsy is an important adjunct that should be available at any children's medical center that provides care for children with melanoma. It is not technically challenging but it does require the availability of expertise in Nuclear Medicine and some special equipment (Geiger counter). On the morning of the scheduled procedure, lymphoscintigraphy is performed to identify the sentinel node. The radioactivity remains trapped in the node for several hours. To provide a visual aide in identifying the node at operation, blue dye is injected at the same cutaneous site as the radiotracer, usually just before the area is sterilely prepared for surgery. AT surgery, the node is identified using the Geiger counter and an appropriate incision is made to allow excision of the node. Measuring high radioactivity in the excised node and minimal residual in the operative field confirms that the correct node was excised. Complications are rare but include seroma, lymphedema, and false negative results.

Differential Diagnosis

- Melanoma
- Atypical nevus
- Congenital melanocytic nevus
- Halo nevus
- Blue nevus
- Spitz nevus
- Speckled lentiginous nevus
- Pygenic granuloma

Diagnostic Studies

- Total body examination
- Serial examination with photography
- Sentinel lymph node biopsy

Preoperative Preparation

☐ Careful consideration of anatomy and need for subsequent wide excision

Parental Preparation

- The diagnosis of melanoma can be very difficult to confirm or exclude, sometimes requiring multiple opinions from around the country.
- We might start with an incisional biopsy or an excisional biopsy with a 5-mm margin, but wide excision might eventually become necessary.

Technical Points

- The visible lesion is often not the true extent of the microscopic disease.
- The guiding principle of surgical therapy for melanoma is wide excision with clear margins.
- For lesions 1 mm or less, a 1-cm margin is considered adequate; for lesions 1.1–2 mm, the margin should be 1–2 cm, and for lesions larger than 2 mm, the margin should be at least 2 cm.
- The depth of resection should include the superficial fascia.
- Histopathologic features that can help distinguish melanomas from benign nevi include: size >7 mm, ulceration, high mitotic activity, mitoses in the lower third of the lesion, asymmetry, poorly demarcated lateral borders, lack of maturation, dusty melanin, and marked nuclear polymorphism.
- Sentinel lymph node positivity is one of the most important prognostic indicators.
- Some advocate completion lymphadenectomy in patients with positive sentinel lymph nodes as it might achieve better outcomes.

Suggested Reading

Brady M, Weinberg H, Kraus D, Lewis J, Coit D, LaQuaglia M, et al. Lymphatic mapping in the management of melanoma in children. Pediatr Dermatol. 1998;15(6):421–5.

Ceballos PI, Ruiz-Maldonado R, Mihm Jr MC. Melanoma in children. N Engl J Med. 1995;332(10):656–62.

Hamre MR, Chuba P, Bakhshi S, Thomas R, Severson RK. Cutaneous melanoma in childhood and adolescence. Pediatr Hematol Oncol. 2002;19:309–17.

Lewis KG. Trends in pediatric melanoma mortality in the United States, 1968 through 2004. Dermatol Surg. 2008;34(2):152–9.

Pappo AS. Melanoma in children and adolescents. Eur J Cancer. 2003;39(18):2651–61.

Rao BN, Hayes FA, Pratt CB, Fleming ID, Kumar AP, Lobe T, et al. Malignant melanoma in children: its management and prognosis. J Pediatr Surg. 1990;25(2):198–203.

Rhodes AR. Pigmented birthmarks and precursor melanocytic lesions of cutaneous melanoma identifiable in childhood. Pediatr Clin North Am. 1983;30(3):435–63.

Roaten JB, Partrick DA, Pearlman N, Gonzalez RJ, Gonzalez R, McCarter MD. Sentinel lymph node biopsy for melanoma and other melanocytic tumors in adolescents. J Pediatr Surg. 2005;40(1):232–5.

Schaffer JV. Pigmented lesions in children: when to worry. Curr Opin Pediatr. 2007;19(4):430–40.

Spitz S. Melanomas of childhood. 1948. CA Cancer J Clin. 1991;41(1):40–51.

Chapter 104
Necrotizing Soft Tissue Infections

Eric R. Scaife

Surgical consultation for soft tissue infections is a common if not banal part of our practice. It is tempting to react with a sense of annoyance at having to trudge over to see yet another case of inguinal lymphadenitis or a leg cellulitis in the emergency department. However, every once in a while, the referring physician's description over the phone carries some vague sense of trepidation that this infection is somehow different and indeed the case becomes legendary to the practitioners who care for the child. How do we decide when a case is a simple soft tissue infection and how do we pull the trigger on surgical aggression that can result in loss of limb or disfiguring removal of tissue? Is it intuition or are there surgical signs that help us appropriately to accelerate our care?

Necrotizing infections are characterized by destruction of the soft tissues, systemic toxicity, and a high mortality. A variety of names have been applied to these aggressive infections. Necrotizing fasciitis, hospital gangrene, Meleney cellulitis, synergistic cellulitis, and the popular lay term "flesh-eating bacteria" have all been used to describe a process in which there is extensive tissue destruction, thrombosis of arterioles, and bacteria spreading along fascial planes. Necrotizing fasciitis is classically defined as Type I or Type II. Type I is a polymicrobial infection and Type II is monomicrobial, usually secondary to a Group A streptococcal infection.

The disease is more common in adults but it is certainly not unheard of in children. Most busy children's centers can expect to see a true necrotizing soft tissue infection once or twice per year while consultation for cellulitis or a soft tissue abscess occurs several times per week. Adults often have predisposing factors, such as peripheral vascular disease or diabetes, which foster the development of a severe soft tissue infections. With the exception of those who are immunocompromised, children usually have no predisposing factors. Surgical wounds, trauma, vaccination wounds, varicella lesions, necrotizing enterocolitis, and omphalitis encompass some of the scenarios in which we see pediatric necrotizing

soft tissue infections. Primary necrotizing fasciitis implies that no portal of entry can be identified. The mortality of these serious infections is estimated to range from 20 to 40%.

We have seen aggressive Group A streptococcal infections complicate routine inguinal hernia surgery in infants. The infant develops a rapidly spreading erythema around the inguinal incision. The erythema is accompanied by induration and the child is febrile, irritable, and tachycardic. Tragically we cared for a boy who lost his leg and shortly thereafter his life when he developed Group A streptoccal myositis days after a baseball pitch struck him in the thigh. Complications of varicella lesions are vanishing as the vaccination program has matured, but necrotizing cellulitis at the site of one of these otherwise relatively innocuous lesions was not unheard of in the past. In infants, omphalitis is a feared soft tissue infection with a recognized mortality that can also result in significant soft tissue loss in the abdominal wall. In premature infants, necrotizing enterocolitis can occasionally seed the abdominal wall with a dangerous and aggressive Type I polymicrobial infection.

Diagnosis

The primary focus of the diagnostic workup is to determine whether the infection requires aggressive surgical intervention. The physical examination can offer clues as to whether an infection is simple cellulitis or something more menacing. Pain that is out of proportion to the physical exam implies ischemia and severe inflammation within the deeper tissues. Erythema is ubiquitous for cellulitis but a rapidly spreading pattern or one associated with induration and edema is very concerning. It is common for these skin changes to be outlined with a marking pen. One of our burn surgeons likes to say that if an infection has been outlined with a pen then the next advancing line should be drawn with a knife. Tissue necrosis can be seen with patchy infarction of the skin and gas-forming bacteria can cause crepitance when the gas begins to infiltrate along fascial planes. A late sign that is particularly worrisome is spreading erythema that evolves

E.R. Scaife (✉)
Department of Pediatric Surgery, University of Utah, 100 N. Mario Capecchi Drive, Street 2600, Salt Lake City, UT 84113-1103, USA
e-mail: eric.scaife@hsc.utah.edu

P. Mattei (ed.), *Fundamentals of Pediatric Surgery*,
DOI 10.1007/978-1-4419-6643-8_104, © Springer Science+Business Media, LLC 2011

into bullae, often filled with a violaceous fluid. In some patients, the disease is deep with few superficial signs. If the infection causes myonecrosis, the patient may develop a compartment syndrome and severe pain with passive or active range of motion of the muscle group.

As the infection progresses, local signs begin to include systemic signs of sepsis. Fever is seen in both common and alarming infections but unrelenting tachycardia is a feature of an overwhelming process. Local tissue destruction, release of bacterial toxins, and an uncoupled systemic inflammatory response combine to create a physiologic storm. White blood cells are mobilized and consumed. The cell count is left-shifted with a significant bandemia and one can find either leukocytosis or leucopenia. Rhabdomyolysis can be extensive and the resultant myoglobinuria can cause renal failure. Liver cells lyse and release aminotransferases. Hypotension can be profound and will lead to death if the infection cannot be controlled.

In ambiguous cases, a biopsy with a frozen section can help to confirm or exclude the diagnosis. The biopsy is diagnostic of a necrotizing infection if there is necrosis of the superficial fascia. Leukocytic infiltration with polymorphic neutrophils predominating in the fascia, subcutaneous tissue and dermis are also consistent with the diagnosis. Finally, fascial arteriolar and venous thrombosis and visible bacteria in the specimen on frozen section are also signs of a necrotizing infection.

The differential diagnosis usually includes typical cellulitis. Unless accompanied by an abscess, cellulitis responds to antibiotics within 24–48 h whereas a necrotizing infection is unresponsive to medical treatment and the patient will show signs of rapid deterioration. Erysipelas, pyoderma gangrenosum, and purpura fulminans are other skin conditions that can be confused with a necrotizing infection.

The imaging studies used to evaluate necrotizing soft tissue infections include CT and MRI. A non-contrast CT is the better of the two. It is expedient, and capable of outlining the extent of the process, especially if there is gas in the tissue. The MRI can be overly sensitive and is perhaps only really helpful if you are trying to rule out necrotizing fasciitis when the diagnosis has been raised but the clinical suspicion is low. If the clinical suspicion is high, neither study should keep you out of the operating room.

Preoperative Preparation

When the decision is made to go to the operating room perhaps the most important part of the preparation is discussing the consequences of a necrotizing infection with the parents and the patient, if mature enough to understand the gravity of the situation. Surgery to radically remove the infected tissue can result in severe disfigurement or amputation. Death is a real possibility in severe infections and it is shocking to escalate from what was thought to be a simple boil to the possibility of loss of limb or life.

These patients should be treated like unstable trauma patients. Laboratory studies and intravenous and arterial access are obtained preoperatively. They need blood and fresh frozen plasma. The patients are anemic due to hemolysis and coagulopathic due to disseminated intravascular coagulation. Intravenous vasopressors should be available to help control systemic vascular resistance as hypotension progresses.

Treatment

A necrotizing soft tissue infection can only be effectively treated with surgical removal of the infected tissue. The affected tissue is overwhelmed with bacteria, which spread along the avascular planes of the fascia. The arterioles thrombose and the infection effectively isolates itself from the immune system and systemic antibiotics. Prompt and radical excision of the infection is the only hope for turning the tide against the infection. The obviously affected tissue is removed down to the fascia and the border of the resection is defined by reaching tissue that bleeds. The muscle under the fascia must also be interrogated. If the muscle and fascia are grey, bleed poorly or show pathetic contraction to stimulation with electrocautery, then that tissue must be removed as well. In order to control the infection one must be able to get beyond the infected tissue and into healthy tissue. This means that one must be prepared to amputate or disarticulate a limb in order to get ahead of the infection. Infections that involve the trunk or retroperitoneum can be more difficult to treat because it is more difficult to establish a perimeter around the infection. It is common to have to return to the operating room for multiple debridements but one should be aggressive with the initial operation in order to optimize the chance for survival.

Surgical excision is accompanied by appropriate antibiotic coverage. Necrotizing fasciitis can be caused by a number of organisms including Group A *streptococcus*, *Staphylococcus aureus*, *Clostridium septicum*, *Clostridium perfringes*, *Escherichia coli*, *Enterococcus faecalis*, and *Bacteroides fragilis*. Antibiotic therapy should initially be broad in spectrum to cover a Type I infection. Antibiotics like imipenum or meropenum currently fill this role, but the addition of clindamycin or vancomycin should be part of the initial therapy.

Type II infections are most commonly caused by Group A streptococcus, however necrotizing fasciitis caused by community acquired methicillin-resistant *S. aureus* (MRSA) is an emerging clinical syndrome. Clindamycin is an important drug directed against Group A streptococci. It helps to facilitate phagocytosis of Streptococcus pyogenes by inhibiting the production of the virulence factor, M-protein. It also suppresses toxin production and has a long postantibiotic effect. Intravenous administration of high dose gammaglobulin has been advocated to neutralize the exotoxins but the efficacy of this strategy has yet to be clearly established. Empiric therapy should be started immediately. If severe MRSA infections are encountered in your population, then therapy must also include agents active against this infection. In surgery, a Gram stain, culture, and antibiotic sensitivities should be sent to focus the medical treatment.

After radical surgery, the patient will be supported in the intensive care unit. The care at this point deals with the multisystem effects of this process. The child will likely be on a ventilator and require vigorous fluid resuscitation. It is common to require vasopressors to increase the systemic vascular resistance. If myonecrosis has been a part of the infection then one must guard against the effects of rhabdomyolysis. If after 12–24 h the child's sepsis shows no signs of abrogation, then you should consider returning to the operating room to explore for advancing infection and tissue that requires further debrided.

Hyperbaric oxygen therapy has been used for necrotizing soft tissue infections but no clear benefit has been identified. The rationale for hyperbaric oxygen therapy is that by increasing the oxygen tension in an ischemic environment one might be able to improve host immune defenses and wound healing. Most of the studies looking at hyperbaric therapy have struggled to provide adequate controls and therefore outcomes are compared to historical controls without convincing evidence that patient care is improved with hyperbaric therapy. In addition, there are logistical problems with hyperbaric therapy. These patients are critically ill and it might be unsafe to place them in the unregulated environment of the hyperbaric chamber and pediatric institutions are not likely to have ready access to a hyperbaric chamber.

After the infection has been excised, the surgeon is often left with a huge wound to manage. Typically, I will apply a vacuum-assisted wound dressing, which is usually simple for the nursing staff to manage. It helps to remove debris and bacteria from the site and it is quite effective in encouraging the wound base to granulate. After the sepsis has cleared and the wound is clean and covered with granulation tissue, it is time to consider closure or coverage. If skin flaps can be raised, the wound should be closed primarily, but split-thickness skin grafts or rotational flaps are often required. If there is absence of the abdominal wall, a biologic acellular matrix may be needed to reconstruct the wound.

Postoperative Care

After the storm of a necrotizing infection has passed, the patient and family are left with the results of sometimes significant tissue destruction. This might mean dealing with unsightly scars or the deformity of an amputation. It might also involve joint limitation from scars that wrap and tether limbs and fingers. Tragically, it can mean suffering the grief of losing a child. This is a disease that can steal away a family's hopes and dreams. There are support groups and web-based memorials for families affected by necrotizing fasciitis and certainly we should call upon our own resources, including physical therapy, rehabilitation medicine, plastic surgery, social work, or the clergy to help our patients with the recovery process. As surgeons, it is our hope that when we encounter such an infection that we can respond with the appropriate judgment and degree of surgical aggression to limit the losses.

Summary Points

- Necrotizing soft tissue infections are rare but real occurrences in children and a surgeon must have an appropriate index of suspicion to identify these dangerous infections.
- Local signs that are worrisome for a necrotizing infection include: rapidly spreading erythema, tissue induration, tissue infarction, and violaceous bullae.
- Systemic signs include tachycardia, mental status changes, rhabdomyolysis, low urine output, and hypotension.
- Radical surgical excision of the infected tissue, broad spectrum antibiotics, and intensive supportive care are the pillars of treatment.

Editor's Comment

A necrotizing infection in a child can test the judgment and skills of a pediatric surgeon like few other clinical problems can. The decision to rush a child off to the operating room for disfiguring or potentially debilitating surgery must often be

made quickly and on the basis of the clinical picture alone. And, of course, time is of the essence – a delay of even a few hours can literally mean the difference between life and death. One does not have the luxury of waiting for imaging studies or delaying surgery until the next morning. To make matters worse, there are no pathognomonic signs, except those that occur when it is too late to make a difference. The decision to operate is made on the basis of the unforgettable appearance of a child who demonstrates: (1) panic, irritability, or lethargy; (2) extreme discomfort (analogous to the exquisite pain characteristic of peritonitis); (3) unusual skin changes (violaceous hue, bullae, crepitance, severe and well-demarcated edema, exquisite tenderness); and (4) hemodynamic changes consistent with systemic sepsis, all out of proportion to that expected for a simple soft-tissue cellulitis or abscess. When in doubt, it is far better to perform an operation that later proves to have been unnecessary than to miss an opportunity to limit the extent of spread of a necrotizing infection.

Although fasciitis is the archetypical form of the disease, a necrotizing infection can involve tissue other than fascia, including muscle, tendons, or subcutaneous tissues (necrotizing cellulitis). The surgical approach is always the same – aggressive debridement of all necrotic tissue down to structures that bleed and are therefore likely to be viable. As there are no reliable bedside indicators of disease progression, a planned second-look operation in 12–24 h should be strongly considered in all cases. Omphalitis can develop into a particularly devastating type of necrotizing infection because the full-thickness of the abdominal wall is often involved and might need to be debrided, exposing the abdominal contents and requiring extraordinary measures to achieve adequate coverage. A type of Fournier's gangrene can also occur after inguinal hernia repair or circumcision, requiring extensive debridement of the perineum.

Reconstruction after the successful treatment of these devastating infections and their surgical aftermath can be quite challenging. Vacuum dressings and elaborate tissue transfer techniques have proven valuable, while hyperbaric oxygen therapy and the application of topical growth factors have not. In most cases, partial-thickness skin grafts applied directly to fascia or muscle in young children provide an acceptable functional and cosmetic solution. For more devastating lesions, collaboration with a pediatric plastic surgery team is often necessary.

Preoperative Preparation

- ☐ IV hydration
- ☐ Type & cross for both packed red blood cells and fresh frozen plasma
- ☐ Consider need for central venous and arterial access
- ☐ Plan for admission to the intensive care unit

Parental Preparation

- – Significant skin and soft tissue loss are possible
- – Possible disfigurement
- – Possible amputation
- – Serious threat of mortality

Diagnostic Studies

- – Surgical exploration with frozen section biopsy
- – CT/MRI
- – Wound culture

Technical Points

- Excise all of the affected tissue until you reach tissue that bleeds normally.
- If the underlying muscle is affected, it too must be resected.
- If the patient does not improve within the first 12–24 h, then return to the OR for additional debridement is necessary.
- Vacuum dressing for post operative wound care.

Suggested Reading

Angoules AG, Kontakis G, Drakoulakis E, Vrentzos G, Granick MS, Giannoudis PV. Necrotising fasciitis of upper and lower limb: a systematic review. Injury. 2007;38 Suppl 5:S19–26.

Bisno AL, Stevens DL. Streptococcal infections of skin and soft tissues. N Engl J Med. 1996;334(4):240–5.

Fustes-Morales A, Gutierrez-Castrellon P, Duran-Mckinster C, Orozco-Covarrubias L, Tamayo-Sanchez L, Ruiz-Maldonado R. Necrotizing fasciitis: report of 39 pediatric cases. Arch Dermatol. 2002;138(7):893–9.

Martin JM, Green M. Group A streptococcus. Semin Pediatr Infect Dis. 2006;17(3):140–8.

Miller LG, Perdreau-Remington F, Rieg G, et al. Necrotizing fasciitis caused by community-associated methicillin-resistant Staphylococcus aureus in Los Angeles. N Engl J Med. 2005;352(14):1445–53.

Sakata S, Das Gupta R, Leditschke JF, Kimble RM. Extensive necrotising fasciitis in a 4-day-old neonate: a successful outcome from modern dressings, intensive care and early surgical intervention. Pediatr Surg Int. 2008;25(1):117–9.

Chapter 105
Hemangiomas and Vascular Malformations

David W. Low

Pediatric vascular anomalies can be generally classified into two broad categories: hemangiomas and everything else. More specifically, clinicians must understand the difference between hemangiomas (and a handful of other biologically active, proliferative vascular anomalies) and biologically inactive, non-proliferative vascular malformations.

It is important to make a distinction between the two, as the treatment options and timing of intervention sometimes differ drastically. Parents today have ready access to the internet and support groups, and it is not unusual to have parents who are well-informed, or sometimes misinformed, by non-peer-reviewed online information. There might also be medicolegal implications if parents sense they have been given a misdiagnosis or an inappropriate recommendation that has resulted in a permanent deformity.

Hemangiomas are the most common benign neoplasm of infancy, occurring in 10% of full term babies and as many as 25% of premature babies weighing less than a kilogram. Many clinicians still erroneously call all vascular birthmarks hemangiomas, and since all hemangiomas regress spontaneously and usually require no surgical intervention, parents are usually advised to wait patiently for 5 years for the hemangioma to "disappear." Unfortunately, 30% of hemangiomas leave significant deformities that cannot be entirely corrected by surgery, and vascular malformations have no ability to regress, leaving a population of children and parents with inappropriate therapy and overly optimistic expectations. Vascular malformations include abnormally formed capillaries, arteries, veins, lymphatics, or combinations of different vessels that occur in utero, are present at birth (although not always clinically evident), and persist throughout life.

Spectrum of Lesions

The typical hemangioma presents in the first few weeks of life as a small strawberry-colored skin lesion that begins to grow out of proportion to the growth of the infant (Fig. 105.1). The proliferative phase may continue for 6–12 months until the angiogenic factors that stimulate endothelial growth begin to turn off. The first signs of regression include a pale grayish-white color change and a decrease in tissue turgor as the vessels begin to involute. The average hemangioma takes about 5 years to fully regress.

A small subset of rapidly involuting congenital hemangioma (RICH) are present at birth and undergo rapid involution during the first year of life (Fig. 105.2). Conversely, non-involuting congenital hemangiomas (NICH) never seem to involute, are bluish in pigmentation with a fine telangiectatic pattern and are warm to the touch, resembling arteriovenous malformations (Fig. 105.3). Subcutaneous hemangiomas appear blue but are nevertheless composed of proliferating capillary endothelial cells rather than larger vessels; they are still often erroneously referred to as "cavernous" hemangiomas. Some hemangiomas have both dermal and subcutaneous components and therefore present with a combination of protruding strawberry and subcutaneous blue bulky soft tissue (Fig. 105. 4).

Although they can occur in any location, 60% of all true hemangiomas are located on the head and neck. Visceral hemangiomas (hepatic and splenic) can also occur. Babies with six or more cutaneous hemangiomas warrant an abdominal ultrasound to rule out this potentially life-threatening condition, which can also be associated with failure to thrive and high-output cardiac failure. In addition, hemangiomas are sometimes part of a syndrome or association. The PHACES association includes *p*osterior cranial fossa abnormalities such as Dandy-Walker cysts, a large facial *h*emangioma, *a*rterial anomalies, *c*ardiac defects or *c*oarcation of the aorta, *e*ye abnormalities, and *s*ternal cleft. Children with PELVIS syndrome have a large *p*erineal or sacral hemangioma associated with *e*xternal genitalia abnormalities, *l*ipomyelomeningocele with a tethered spinal cord, *v*esicorenal abnormalities, *i*mperforate anus and perineal *s*kin tag.

D.W. Low (✉)
Department of Surgery, Division of Plastic Surgery, University of Pennsylvania School of Medicine, Children's Hospital of Philadelphia, Philadelphia, PA 19104, USA
e-mail: david.low@uphs.upenn.edu

P. Mattei (ed.), *Fundamentals of Pediatric Surgery*,
DOI 10.1007/978-1-4419-6643-8_105, © Springer Science+Business Media, LLC 2011

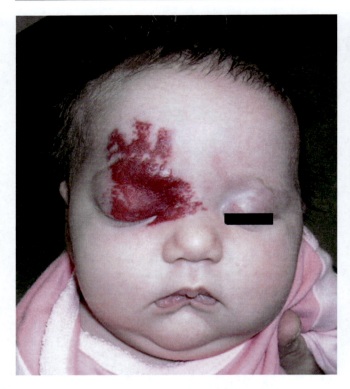

Fig. 105.1 Periorbital hemangioma in the proliferative phase

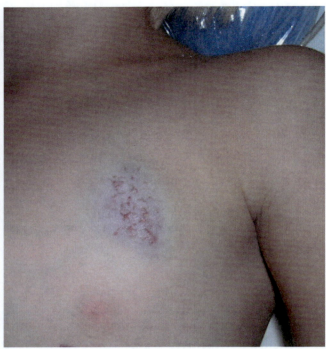

Fig. 105.3 Non-involuting congenital hemangioma of the chest

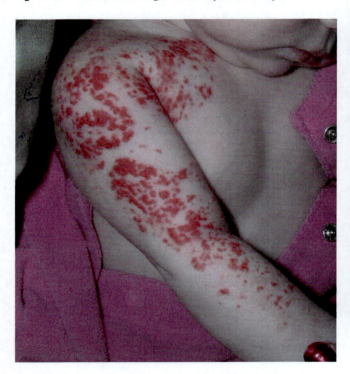

Fig. 105.2 Rapidly involuting congenital hemangioma of the arm

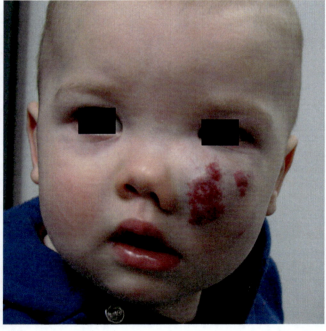

Fig. 105.4 Hemangioma with both subcutaneous and dermal components

Other proliferative vascular anomalies that occur in infancy include *Kaposiform hemangioendothelioma* (Fig. 105.5) and *angioblastoma* (tufted angioma). Both can cause platelet-trapping and life-threatening thrombocytopenia (Kasabach-Merritt syndrome) and often require a tissue biopsy to make the diagnosis. *Angiosarcomas* are extremely rare malignant tumors that occur mostly in the elderly, but have been reported in children.

Pyogenic granuloma, more accurately termed *lobular capillary hemangioma*, occur at any age, might be caused by

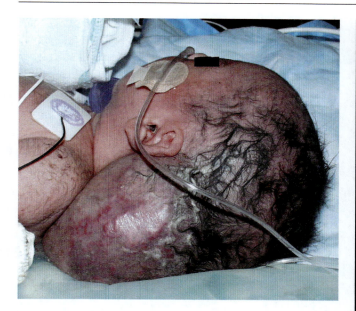

Fig. 105.5 Kapsiform hemangioendothelioma

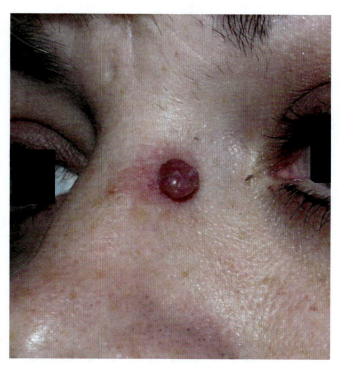

Fig. 105.6 Pyogenic granuloma

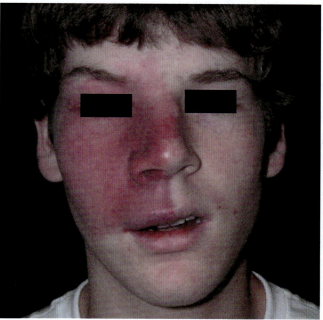

Fig. 105.7 Capillary vascular malformation (port wine stain)

Capillary vascular malformations (port wine stains) are usually present at birth as patches of pink or purple skin, often in a dermatomal distribution (Fig. 105.7). If the ophthalmic dermatome (V1) of the trigeminal nerve is involved, there can be simultaneous ocular or CNS involvement (*Sturge-Weber syndrome*), which can cause glaucoma and seizures.

Macular stains (stork bite) resemble port wine stains in the central forehead and posterior occipital/neck region and have the inexplicable ability to lighten significantly during the first year of life.

Venous malformations appear as clusters of subcutaneous veins that engorge when the affected area is dependent and then empty and soften when the area is elevated (Fig. 105.8). Rapid enlargement can occur but is more likely due to vascular rupture and hematoma formation rather than actual growth of the abnormal vessels. Pain and swelling can also be associated with thrombosis of the dilated veins due to sluggish or stagnant flow. They can occur anywhere on the body and sometimes involve underlying subcutaneous tissue, muscle, or viscera. Some can even be transmural: a venous malformation of the cheek might extend from the dermis, through the muscles, and into the submucosal layer. Venous malformations of the head occasionally communicate intracranially with the sagittal sinus.

The *blue rubber bleb nevus syndrome* (Fig. 105.9) is a genetically transmitted form of venous malformation that occur in multiple sites all over the body, including the gastrointestinal tract, leading to bleeding and anemia or bowel obstruction due to intussusception. Venous malformations first

minor skin trauma with inappropriate angiogenesis, and are characterized by small vascular lobules. They have a fragile epidermal cover and can bleed profusely (Fig. 105.6).

Vascular malformations, unlike hemangiomas, are present at birth (although not always clinically evident) and grow proportionately with the child. They are not vascular tumors, do not expand rapidly unless there is intralesional bleeding or lymph accumulation and they do not regress spontaneously.

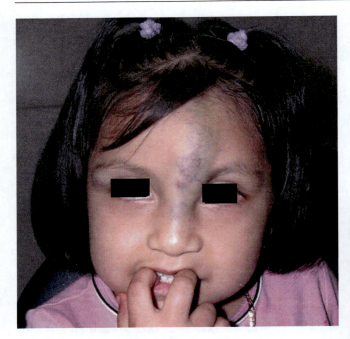

Fig. 105.8 Venous vascular malformation of the forehead and nose

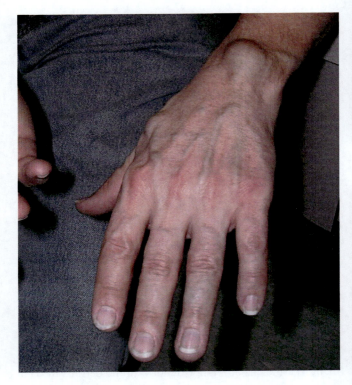

Fig. 105.9 Blue rubber bleb nevus syndrome (acquired venous malformations)

appear in infancy but the appearance of new malformations continues into adulthood.

Glomus tumors or glomangiomas look like small clusters of bluish-purple dermal or subcutaneous vessels and are composed of glomus cells, which normally regulate cutaneous

circulation (Fig. 105.10). They are often tender to touch and can be exquisitely tender when located beneath a fingernail in the nail bed.

Lymphatic malformations sometimes manifest at birth as obvious soft tissue masses with severe soft tissue hypertrophy (Fig. 105.11). They are composed of thousands of tiny lymphatic cysts or several large macrocysts (in the cervicofacial region these historically have been called cystic hygromas). Dermal or mucosal involvement results in visible lymphatic vesicles. Blood can leak into the dermal lymphatics, resulting

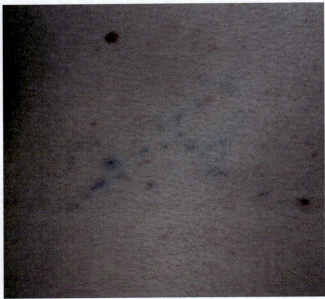

Fig. 105.10 Glomus tumor of the trunk

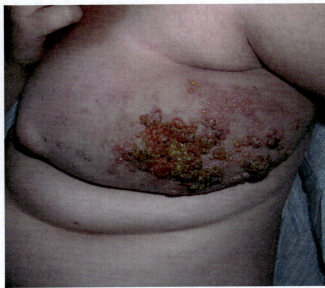

Fig. 105.11 Lymphatic malformation of the breast with cutaneous vesicles

in crusty cutaneous lesions (*angiokeratomas*) that might appear to bleed profusely but the discharge is predominantly lymph stained with blood pigmentation. Some large cystic lymphatic malformations appear to have the capacity to regress, which is probably due to repeated episodes of infection or inflammation that gradually cause fibrosis of some of the abnormal lymphatic spaces.

An *arteriovenous malformations* (AVM) presents as warm, pulsatile masses that occur anywhere on the body (Fig. 105.12). The AVM may include a patchy cutaneous capillary vascular malformation and hypertrophy of the involved area (Parkes-Weber syndrome). High turbulent flow within the lesion often causes a bruit or thrill to be appreciated on examination. There is sometimes a noticeable increase in size during puberty, presumably due to hormonal stimulation and additional vascular shunting.

Spider angiomas are common dermal vascular malformations with a central feeding vessel and a radiating pattern of tiny telangiectasias (Fig. 105.13). When compressed, the lesions blanch, then readily refill from the center to the periphery when pressure is released.

Klippel-Trenaunay syndrome describes a patchy capillary vascular malformation overlying a low-pressure, low-flow venolymphatic malformation, usually with local tissue hypertrophy (Fig. 105.14). In the lower extremity, a markedly dilated lateral vein is sometimes noted and represents a remnant from fetal development. The skin sometimes exhibit multiple angiokeratomas scattered diffusely over the areas of port wine stain.

Proteus syndrome is an overgrowth condition that affects the entire body to varying degrees, creating vascular malformations, lipomas, epidermal nevi, and thickened, wrinkled

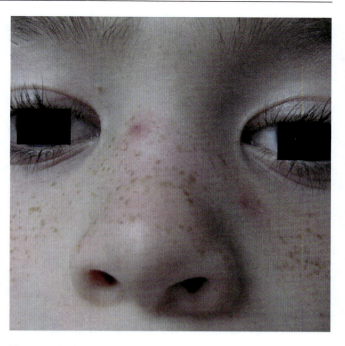

Fig. 105.13 Spider angiomas commonly seen on the face

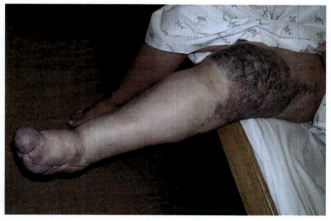

Fig. 105.14 Klippel-Trenaunay syndrome with extreme hypertrophy of the leg

plantar surfaces. John Merrick, the Elephant Man, is thought to have had Proteus syndrome, not neurofibromatosis.

Maffucci's syndrome includes enchondromas of the hands, vascular malformations in unrelated areas, rare angiosarcomas, and a 15–20% lifetime risk of developing chondrosarcoma.

Diagnosis

In the majority of cases, history and physical examination will allow an accurate diagnosis and further testing is unnecessary. In some patients, serial clinical examinations

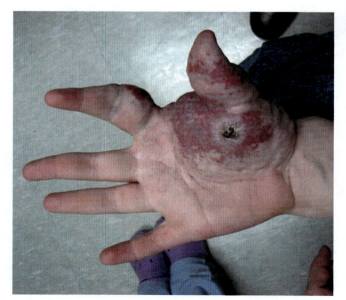

Fig. 105.12 Arteriovenous malformation of the hand

will make the diagnosis, based upon the growth or lack of growth of the vascular anomaly. For example, a flat patch of vascular pigmentation initially thought to be a capillary vascular malformation (port wine stain) might become strawberry red and raised and increase its area of involvement, which is indicative of a hemangioma.

An MRI with contrast will usually distinguish the true etiology of most vascular anomalies and is indicated for atypical hemangiomas when the diagnosis is in doubt, for lesions involving the head and neck (to assess the extent of periorbital, parotid and airway involvement or posterior cranial fossa abnormalities), and for those overlying the spine to rule out lipomyelomeningocele with spinal cord tethering. An ultrasound to exclude hepatic or splenic involvement is indicated in patients who have more than six cutaneous hemangiomas, while an echocardiogram is sometimes needed to rule out cardiac abnormalities if the lesion is thought to be part of a syndrome.

Although an MRI can usually demonstrate the extent of vascular malformations, particularly if they have muscular or visceral involvement, it is only necessary if it will change therapy: the best treatment for Klippel-Trenaunay syndrome with obvious involvement of the leg is conservative compression therapy, and so an MRI is not needed to make the diagnosis or to recommend therapy. On the other hand, if one is planning to attempt sclerotherapy or venous ligation and removal of abnormal veins, an MRV might be useful to not only document the course of the anomalous veins but also to ensure the presence of normal draining veins.

For a suspected AVM, an MR-angiogram is a better initial screening test, reserving an angiogram for those cases that require additional diagnostic and potentially therapeutic arteriography. An ultrasound-guided needle can facilitate injection of lymphatic and venous malformations for sclerotherapy. Although urinary levels of basic fibroblast growth factor (bFGF) are elevated during the proliferative phase of a hemangioma, the test is rarely necessary as the diagnosis is usually obvious. Thyroid function tests are indicated in patients with hepatic hemangioma, as the active form of thyroid hormone can be inactivated by increased levels of type 3 iodothyronine deiodinase, resulting in hypothyroidism.

Treatment of Hemangioma

Pediatricians advise the vast majority of parents whose infants have hemangiomas to be patient and wait for eventual cessation of growth and gradual involution. Half of all hemangiomas will finish involuting by 5 years of age and 70% will have involuted by age seven. Approximately 70% of all hemangiomas will involute satisfactorily without requiring any further intervention; however at least 30% will leave a residual deformity in the form of redundant skin, dermal scarring, bulky fibrofatty tissue or facial disfigurement.

Hemangiomas of the lips, nose and cheeks commonly leave behind redundant and distorted tissue that will require surgical attention and result in some kind of surgical scar.

With the advent of the internet, parents are increasingly eager to take an active role in the management of their child's hemangioma. Rather than watch them become progressively more deformed, they desperately hope to abort the natural history of the hemangioma. They seek early laser therapy or surgical excision and some will shop around until they find a surgeon who will take an aggressive approach. A balanced approach is necessary and the surgeon must always weigh the risks and benefits of a surgical scar and operative complications against the possibility that natural involution will leave a better final result. My personal philosophy is that because surgery leaves a scar 100% of the time, before proceeding with surgery one should be reasonably confident that natural involution will leave a worse deformity. Also, the decision to operate before complete involution increases the risk of bleeding, and decreased visibility may increase the risk of damage to nerves and other key anatomic structures.

Life-threatening subglottic hemangiomas and vision-threatening periorbital hemangiomas cannot be managed conservatively. The initial treatment of choice is oral corticosteroid therapy, most often given in the form of prednisolone 2–4 mg/kg/day mixed with the infant's formula because of its unpalatable taste. An H2-blocker (ranitidine 3 mg/kg/day) is given throughout the course of therapy to decrease gastrointestinal side effects. Various tapering schedules exist, but a slow gradual taper is preferable to cycling on and off alternate months. Side effects include increased irritability, change in appetite, temporary and reversible growth suppression, hypertension, and Cushingoid appearance. Small hemangiomas have also been treated with intralesional injection and topical clobetasol propionate (Temovate) cream, but the rate, distribution and amount of steroid delivered is much less predictable.

In 2008, the potential benefit of oral beta blocker (propranolol) therapy to suppress and shrink hemangiomas was first reported. There has since been increasing enthusiasm for the use of beta blockers as potential first-line therapy for problematic hemangiomas to avoid the side effects of prolonged steroid therapy. Initial treatment sometimes includes several days of inpatient observation and cardiology consultation for side effects such as hypoglycemia, hypotension, and bradycardia. The dose can then be adjusted on an outpatient basis. Time will tell if beta blocker therapy replaces steroids as first line therapy for problematic hemangiomas.

Laser photocoagulation with a pulsed yellow dye laser is sometimes useful for small, flat hemangiomas, but because the light can only penetrate about 1 mm into the dermis it is generally not useful for bulky or subcutaneous lesions. Most parents will describe a couple weeks of regression after laser therapy followed by some rebound growth, therefore repeated treatments are often necessary to suppress the hemangioma until permanent involution occurs. The laser is also useful for painful or ulcerated hemangiomas. Although somewhat unpredictable, in many cases laser therapy appears to be able to suppress pain within 24–48 h, possibly by photocoagulation of the sensitive nerve endings in the lesion, and accelerate healing, perhaps by suppressing inappropriate vascular proliferation.

In most situations, surgical excision or debulking is similar to excision of a nevus or cyst. Hemangiomas that leave redundant skin or excess fibrofatty scar tissue will often benefit from elliptical excision, trading the hemangioma for a linear scar. The timing of excision is a judgment call which will be influenced by the degree of deformity, the size of the hemangioma, the amount of residual vascularity, the location (less cosmetically important hemangiomas tend to carry less urgency), the anxiety level of the parents, and the experience of the surgeon. Large hemangiomas might require staged excision, particularly if debulking surgery is elected prior to complete involution, increasing the potential for significant operative bleeding. Large hemangiomas in the lip or nasal regions benefit from early debulking to facilitate feeding and social acceptance, with the understanding that a secondary surgical revision will be necessary in the future.

Nasal tip hemangiomas commonly splay apart paired tip cartilages and leave behind excess skin and bulky fatty tissue after the vessels have involuted. Correction commonly requires judicious trimming of nasal skin and hemangioma, and suturing the tip cartilages together. Lip hemangiomas are usually asymmetric, and surgical debulking or removal of a hemangioma essentially creates a cleft lip deformity. Techniques for cleft lip repair, often with minor adjustments to individualize the procedure for a given patient, provide a strategy for addressing these very challenging deformities (Fig. 105.15).

Subcutaneous hemangiomas that leave excess fibrofatty tissue will occasionally be amenable to debulking by liposuction if enough time is allowed for complete vascular involution.

Scalp hemangiomas will often cause dermal scarring and damage the hair follicles, leaving a patch of alopecia. Excision (alopecia reduction) is the treatment of choice, rather than punch or micro hair grafting.

Cheek hemangiomas can leave problematic deformities in an area that is normally very smooth. Surgical scars in the middle of the cheek are often equally noticeable, and therefore one must be fairly certain that natural regression will leave a worse result than a surgical scar before proceeding with excision. Options for surgical intervention include: standard elliptical excision, excision with a purse-string closure, carbon dioxide laser skin resurfacing, or pulsed dye laser and sclerotherapy for residual vessels. Excision of redundant skin and subcutaneous tissue caused by a parotid hemangioma must be undertaken very carefully to avoid injury to branches of the facial nerve.

Ear hemangiomas can cause significant skin and subcutaneous excess, but the subcutaneous component often

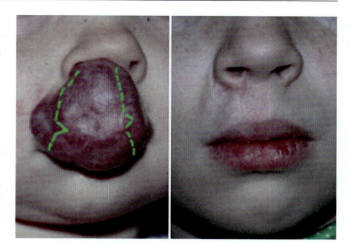

Fig. 105.15 Upper lip hemangioma before and after debulking

involutes dramatically. To avoid a soft tissue deficiency, it is often safer to postpone debulking until the ear hemangioma has almost completely involuted.

Treatment of Vascular Malformations

The treatment of *capillary vascular malformations* (port wine stains) most commonly involves the use of a pulsed yellow dye laser. The wavelength can vary with the type of laser, but currently the third and fourth generation pulsed yellow dye lasers carry a 585 or 595 nm wavelength, which is absorbed by oxyhemoglobin. The handpieces most often deliver circular pulses of variable width and power density. A cryogen cooling spray to accompany each laser pulse decreases the pain of the laser pulse and protects the skin from thermal injury. Protective goggles for all personnel and protective goggles or corneal shields for the patient are essential. Depending upon the age of the patient and the location of the lesion, topical anesthetic cream or general anesthesia might be necessary. Clinicians must inform parents that despite multiple laser treatments (average 6–8) it is highly unlikely that the birthmark will ever completely fade. Furthermore, the laser typically leaves extremely dark bruises for 2–3 weeks and, if the power density is too high or the pulses are delivered too close together, scarring can occur. Because it can take 2–3 months to see the full benefit of each treatment, laser treatments are separated by at least 2 months. The laser is not equally effective on all areas of the face and it is less effective as one moves distally on the extremities towards the hands and feet. Parents and patients should be made aware that results are sometimes disappointing. Additionally, despite successful laser treatment, some will darken with age as residual vessels further dilate. In this situation, laser treatment can be resumed and might offer additional benefit.

Facial capillary vascular malformations, particularly those on the lips, can also cause significant hypertrophy, which often necessitates surgical debulking. Again, plastic surgical techniques for cleft lip repair or reconstruction can be applied to obtain cosmetically acceptable results after major debulking (Fig. 105.16).

The treatment of *venous malformations* might include laser therapy, sclerotherapy, surgical excision or combinations of all three. Venous malformations of the head and neck are often best approached by sclerotherapy, as the malformation is usually transmural, visible just beneath the epidermis and through the oral mucosa. In such situations, surgical debulking may be accompanied by excessive bleeding that is difficult to control, inability to adequately resect the involved area or excessive scarring and post-surgical deformity. A series of sclerotherapy sessions using alcohol or sodium tetradecyl sulfate under fluoroscopic or ultrasound guidance is often the best treatment option. The laser or milder sclerosing agents can be used for superficial dermal components. The potassium-titanyl-phosphate or KTP laser, a 532-nm green light laser, delivers a continuous beam of laser energy rather than pulses of light, and is useful for intraoral coagulation. The laser light travels down a fiberoptic cable which can be inserted directly into the malformation for intralesional photocoagulation. However the technique is highly operator dependent, the amount of laser energy delivered is difficult to judge, and the thermal effects can be difficult to limit, making it less precise than sclerotherapy.

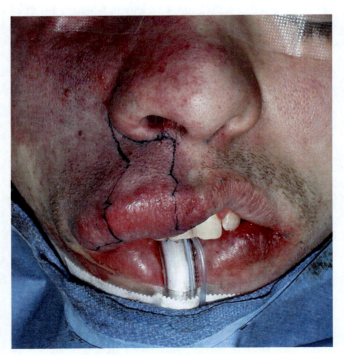

Fig. 105.16 Debulking strategy for a hypertrophied upper lip associated with a capillary vascular malformation

Venous malformations of the tongue can be directly excised or significantly debulked with very limited blood loss by clamping the base of the tongue with cushioned vascular clamps. The incised edge can be oversewn prior to release of the clamps. Because of the anticipated postoperative tongue edema, patients will require in-hospital observation for airway monitoring or overnight intubation.

Lower extremity venous malformations can be treated only if the malformation does not serve as the main vascular runoff for the involved leg. Sclerosis of a major venous malformation or varicosity using ultrasound guidance is commonly performed by interventional radiologists. To prevent the passage of sclerosant or clot into the circulation, it is occasionally necessary to ligate vessels that communicate with a major normal draining vein prior to an attempt at sclerotherapy.

Lymphatic malformations are among the most frustrating of the vascular malformations to treat surgically. Hours of painstaking dissection often result in minimal benefit, facial nerve injuries or postoperative edema that takes a very long time to subside. The best results are with macrocystic lymphatic malformations that are amenable to repeated sclerotherapy, often obviating direct surgical debulking. Sclerosing agents have included alcohol, doxycycline, and Picibanil (OK432, still awaiting FDA approval). Microcystic lymphatic malformations do not always respond to sclerotherapy and therefore require direct surgical debulking, especially for cervicofacial malformations and those in other areas that cannot be managed conservatively with compression garments. Sometimes a combination of surgical debulking and postoperative compression will help to maintain a reasonable decrease in size. The carbon dioxide laser can be used to vaporize cutaneous lymphatic vesicles, offering limited palliative improvement for draining dermal lymphatics.

Arteriovenous malformations can either be followed conservatively with periodic palliative selective embolization, or excised in their entirety. Simple ligation of the major feeding vessels without removal of the malformation is contraindicated, as the AVM will readily recruit flow from other regional arteries making future management even more difficult. Preoperative embolization a day prior to surgery might significantly decrease intraoperative blood loss and also provide the surgeon with a vascular roadmap. Ideally, the malformation should be completely excised to remove all vascular shunting. The subsequent defect sometimes requires sophisticated flap reconstruction to optimize the postoperative outcome.

Complications

Surgical excision of a vascular lesion always carries a risk of bleeding, therefore the surgeon must decide which cases require a type and crossmatch or preoperative embolization. If the risk of bleeding is significant, most parents will prefer a directed donor unit in spite of evidence that banked blood statistically is safer. Particularly with hemangiomas, the surgeon should be confident that the surgical scar will be better than the deformity left by natural involution. Hemangiomas that are debulked prior to complete involution can have greater intra-operative bleeding, increased risk of nerve damage due to poor visualization and distorted anatomy, and poor healing with dehiscence of the incision since sutures are often placed into skin edges compromised by vascular tissue. When the breast is involved in girls, early debulking is contraindicated as injury to the breast bud will affect normal breast development.

The use of any laser can cause scars, ocular injury, and operating room fires. The pulsed dye laser for port wine stains can cause a flash burn if it causes upper lip and nasal hairs to singe in an oxygenated environment.

Summary Points

Proliferative (biologically active) Vascular Anomalies

- Hemangioma
- Pyogenic granuloma (lobular capillary hemangioma)
- Kaposiform hemangioendothelioma
- Tufted angioma (angioblastoma)

Non-proliferative (biologically inactive) Vascular Malformations

- Capillary (port wine stain)
- Venous
- Lymphatic/venolymphatic
- Arterial/arteriovenous
- Glomus cell
- Spider angioma

Hemangioma Syndromes

- PHACES (*p*osterior cranial fossa abnormalities, facial *h*emangioma, *a*rterial anomalies, *c*ardiac defects or *c*oarcation of the aorta, *e*ye abnormalities)
- PELVIS (*p*erineal hemangioma, *e*xternal genital abnormalities, *l*ipomyelomeningocele, *v*esicorenal abnormalities, *i*mperforate anus, perineal *s*kin tag)

Vascular Malformation Syndromes

- Sturge-Weber (V1 capillary malformation with eye or CNS involvement)
- Klippel-Trenaunay (capillary malformation with underlying venolymphatic malformation, hypertrophy)
- Parkes-Weber (capillary malformation with underlying AVM)
- Blue rubber bleb nevus (venous malformation, GI involvement, hereditary)

Editor's Comment

"Birthmarks" cause a great deal of anxiety, and sometimes genuine anguish, for parents and grandparents. Vascular lesions should always be taken seriously. Parents need to be made aware of all available options and actively involved in the decision-making process. All too often, especially with hemangiomas, their concerns are casually dismissed because the lesion is considered merely cosmetic or likely to resolve spontaneously. The care of children with vascular malformations has also greatly improved with the increased use of interventional radiographic techniques such as embolization and sclerotherapy, as well as the emergence of the multi-disciplinary "vascular malformation clinic" that makes available the expertise of devoted specialists and state-of-the-art treatments.

Large dermal lesions pose a challenge because the aesthetic results of surgical therapy might be no better than if the lesion were left untreated. These patients are probably best treated by an experienced pediatric plastic surgeon or vascular malformation clinic. Subcutaneous lesions cause a significant amount of angst for parents because of concerns about a potential malignancy. Unless imaging studies confirm with a high degree of certainty that the mass represents a hemangioma and is therefore likely to resolve spontaneously, most of these should patients should be offered excision. If there is any possibility of involvement of deeper structures, an ultrasound or MRI should be done to avoid surprises in the operating room. It is probably unnecessary to leave a drain except when very large tissue flaps are created. It is usually possible to ignore a postoperative seroma, unless it is symptomatic or infected, in which case it can be drained painlessly with a needle placed directly into the incision, which is insensate. Recurrence of vascular malformations is generally rare; however notable exceptions include lymphatic malformations and intramuscular venous malformations, for which embolization or sclerotherapy should be considered.

Large facial hemangiomas, especially those that threaten the airway or compromise vision, pose a significant dilemma. Even if they resolve spontaneously, the fibrofatty residual can be cosmetically unappealing. Recent reports of success with the use of propranolol are exciting. This has the potential to revolutionize the treatment of these challenging lesions. Patients should be carefully monitored for potentially serious adverse effects as well as unforeseeable consequences, ideally as part of a controlled clinical trial.

Differential Diagnosis

Hemangioma

- Dermoid cyst
- Glioma
- Lipoma
- Lipoblastoma
- Other vascular anomalies

Diagnostic Studies

- MRI with contrast provides the most information
- MRA in the case of suspected arteriovenous malformations
- MRV in the case of venous and venolymphatic malformations prior to sclerotherapy
- Ultrasound to rule out visceral involvement, cardiac, and great vessel anomalies
- Diagnostic arteriograms or venograms may be indicated at the discretion of the interventional radiologist

Parental Preparation

- Laser therapy for capillary vascular malformation (Port wine stain) will cause significant bruising for 2 weeks, multiple laser treatments will be necessary for best results, and the laser is expected to lighten but not remove the lesion.
- Complete surgical excision of vascular malformations in many cases is not possible, and there is often a significant risk of injury to adjacent structures, surgical scarring and possible recurrence of the primary lesion.

Preoperative Preparation

- Preoperative hemoglobin and type and screen if moderate blood loss possible, Type and crossmatch if significant blood loss possible
- Preoperative arteriogram or MRA
- Consider embolization 24 h preop for large AVMs
- Informed consent

Technical Points

- Intra-operative blood loss can be decreased by application of a tourniquet when an extremity is involved, injection of lidocaine with epinephrine around the area to be excised when a tourniquet cannot be utilized, digital pressure surrounding the lesion to be excised or debulked, temporary application of cushioned vascular clamps on tongue and lip lesions, and preoperative embolization in the case of arteriovenous malformations.
- For small lesions that can be excised in their entirety, blood loss can be minimized by operating in normal tissue, avoiding incisions into the vascular lesion itself.
- The bayonet bipolar cautery can be extremely useful as a hemostatic dissector. In some cases residual parts of a hemangioma or vascular malformation can be simply cauterized between the tips of the bipolar forceps without having to excise them. This can be especially useful with larger malformations and hemangiomas where the surgeon is doing a debulking rather than a complete excision.
- Surgical drains should be placed for large excisions, especially with venous venolymphatic excisions, to prevent problematic hematomas and seromas.

Suggested Reading

Boon LM, MacDonald DM, Mulliken JB. Complications of systemic corticosteroid therapy for problematic hemangioma. Plast Reconstr Surg. 1999;104(6):1616–23.

Bradley JP, Zide BM, Berenstein A, et al. Large arteriovenous malformations of the face: aesthetic results with recurrence control. Plast Reconstr Surg. 1999;103(2):351–61.

Lawley LP, Siegfried E, Todd JL. Propranolol treatment for hemangioma of infancy: risks and recommendations. Pediatr Dermatol. 2009;26(5):610–4.

Low DW. Hemangiomas and vascular malformations. Semin Pediatr Surg. 1994;3(2):40–61.

Mulliken JB, Young AE. Vascular birthmarks: hemangiomas and malformations. Philadelphia: Saunders; 1988.

Zide BM, Glat PM, Stile FL, et al. Vascular lip enlargement: Part I. Hemangiomas – tenets of therapy. Plast Reconstr Surg. 1997a;100(7):1664–73.

Zide BM, Glat PM, Stile FL, et al. Vascular lip enlargement: Part II. Port-wine macrocheilia – tenets of therapy based on normative values. Plast Reconstr Surg. 1997b;100(7):1674–81.

Chapter 106
Disorders of the Breast

Mary L. Brandt

Lesions of the breast in the pediatric population are relatively common and nearly always benign. The problems seen by a pediatric surgeon fall into four major categories: developmental, inflammatory/infectious, traumatic, and neoplastic. Many pediatric breast lesions do not require surgical intervention. When surgery is indicated, the overriding principles of pediatric breast surgery include: preservation of developing tissue, periareolar access whenever possible, and adequate resection based on pathology.

Developmental Disorders

Breast development begins during the sixth week of embryonic development. At this stage, epidermal cells migrate into the mesenchyme of the ventral surface of the embryo, creating a ridge of tissue. These mammary ridges or "milk lines" extend the length of the embryo, from groin to axilla. During the tenth week of development, atrophy occurs superior and inferior to the pectoral region.

The mammary ridge differentiates into breast tissue as the main lactiferous ducts and mammary glands begin to develop from the epidermal portion of the ridge. The adipose and connective tissue develops from the mesenchyme, which is of mesodermal origin. The areola develops at approximately 5 months' gestation, and the nipple appears shortly after birth.

Failure of the milk line to atrophy may lead to the development of supernumerary breast tissue. *Polythelia*, or extra nipples, is common, occurring in 0.6–2.2% of the population. This occurs as commonly in men as it does in women. Although usually sporadic, familial polythelia has been reported. Although polythelia is often thought of as cosmetic,

malignant degeneration has been reported, leading some authors to suggest resection of all pigmented lesions located in the milk line. *Polymastia*, or supernumerary breast tissue, is less common than polythelia and occurs most commonly in the axilla or near the inframammary crease (Fig. 106.1). Supernumerary breast tissue can occur outside of the milk line, although this is exceedingly rare. Breast tissue has been reported on the back, shoulder, buttocks and even the face. Failure of formation of the glandular structure of the breast leads to a condition called pseudomamma. In patients with pseudomamma, the breast tissue is composed exclusively of adipose and connective tissue.

Bilateral *breast hypoplasia* is usually normal, although distressing to an adolescent girl. Rarely, bilateral hypoplasia may be a sign of ovarian failure, gonadal dysgenesis (Turner syndrome), androgen excess (congenital adrenal hyperplasia), androgen-producing tumor, or hypothyroidism. Radiation therapy to the prepubertal chest can also result in breast hypoplasia. True *amastia*, or absence of the breast is rare, and is associated in up to 40% of patients with other conditions, such as congenital ectodermal defects. The *tuberous breast anomaly* is a specific form of breast hypoplasia in which the base of the breast is small, and the breast tissue essentially herniates into a large areolar complex. Reconstructive surgery is usually required to obtain a normal appearance.

Asymmetry is common in breast development and is often more pronounced during puberty. Up to 25% of adult women have significantly asymmetric breasts. The presence of scoliosis or a rib cage deformity can create the illusion of asymmetry when none exists. Unilateral breast hypoplasia or absence is sometimes iatrogenic, due to neonatal surgery (central lines, chest tubes or thoracotomy, Fig. 106.2) or associated with Becker's nevus or Poland syndrome. Becker's nevus is an androgen-sensitive lesion which becomes apparent during puberty. Patients with Poland's syndrome have absence or hypoplasia of the pectoralis muscle, ipsilateral hand deformity, abnormal or missing ipsilateral ribs and absent or hypoplastic breast tissue. Plastic surgery reconstruction of the breast and chest wall is often required.

M.L. Brandt (✉)
Department of Pediatric Surgery, Baylor College of Medicine, Texas Children's Hospital, 6621 Fannin Street, Houston, TX 77030, USA
e-mail: brandt@bcm.edu

P. Mattei (ed.), *Fundamentals of Pediatric Surgery*,
DOI 10.1007/978-1-4419-6643-8_106, © Springer Science+Business Media, LLC 2011

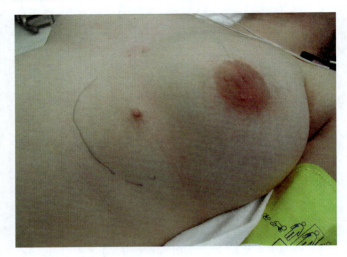

Fig. 106.1 Supernumerary breast (polymastia)

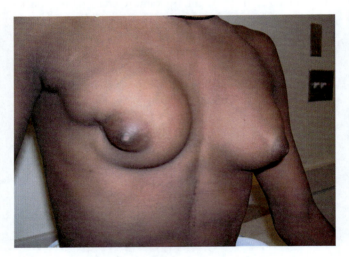

Fig. 106.2 Abnormal breast growth in an adolescent resulting from neonatal tube thoracostomy

Thelarche

In most girls, appearance of breast tissue, or thelarche marks the beginning of puberty. In African American girls, pubic hair is often apparent before thelarche. Thelarche occurs at a mean age of 8.9 years for African-American girls and 9.9 years for Caucasians. Neonates, both male and female will often have palpable breast tissue because of the response to maternal estrogen. This occurs in up to 70% of infants and might be worsened with manipulation. It typically resolves within 12 months in boys but can take up to 2 years to regress in girls. Girls who are obese experience thelarche earlier than girls of normal weight.

Breast development is graded using the Tanner Stages (Table 106.1). During thelarche, asymmetry is common, with one breast bud developing first. Parents and physicians may become alarmed at what appears to be a mass. Biopsy is

Table 106.1 Tanner stages of breast development

Stage 1	(Preadolescence) elevation of the breast papilla only
Stage 2	Elevation of the breast and papilla as a small mound enlargement of the areola diameter
Stage 3	Further enlargement of the breast and areola with no separation of their contours
Stage 4	Further enlargement with projection of the areola and papilla to form a secondary mound above the level of the breast
Stage 5	(Mature stage): projection of the papilla only, resulting from recession of the areola to the general contour of the breast

Source: Templeman. Obstet Gynecol Clin North Am. 2000;27(1):19–34

contraindicated as this may harm the breast bud and lead to significant breast deformity.

Premature thelarche is defined as breast development before age eight, in the absence of other signs of puberty. This occurs in up to 2% of girls, and typically presents between 1 and 3 years of age. Premature thelarche may rarely be due to exposure to exogenous estrogen or to underlying disorders, such as McCune-Albright syndrome. Up to 14% of girls with premature thelarche go on to develop precocious puberty. It is therefore important to continue to follow these girls closely for secondary sexual characteristics or a change in growth velocity. In idiopathic premature thelarche, regression of the breast tissue occurs in most patients, but can take up to 6 years. Premature thelarche does not affect subsequent puberty, breast development or change the risk of developing other breast disorders.

Gynecomastia

The most common hormonally induced breast lesion in boys is gynecomastia. Gynecomastia occurs when there is excessive estrogen or decreased testosterone production. Hormonal fluctuations during puberty leads to physiologic gynecomastia in up to 65% of pubertal boys. Boys who are obese are more likely to develop physiologic gynecomastia, probably because of increased estrone, produced by aromatization of adrostenedione in fatty tissue. In a small percentage of boys, there is an underlying cause for the gynecomastia. Increased estrogen can result from tumors that secrete estrogen or human chorionic gonadotropin, liver dysfunction, hyperthyroidism or inadvertent administration of exogenous estrogen. Decreased testosterone can occur from primary gonadal dysfunction, such as Klinefelter's syndrome, androgen insensitivity, or defects in testosterone biosynthesis. There are numerous drugs associated with gynecomastia (Table 106.2). A pathologic cause should be suspected when puberty is early (tumors) or late (gonadal dysfunction), when breast tissue appeared before puberty, when there is rapid breast growth, or if there is nipple discharge. If the breast tissue is

Table 106.2 Drugs that may cause gynecomastia

Anabolic steroids
Cimetidine
Ranitidine
Isoniazid
Metronidazole
Marijuana
Methotrexate
Alkylating agents
Cyclophosphamide
Furosemide
Spironolactone
ACE inhibitors
Nifedipine
Verapamil
Tricyclic antidepressants
Phenothiazines
Clonidine
SSRIs
Theophylline
Cyclosporine

Source: Reprinted with permission from Pediatr Rev. 28:e57–68, Copyright © 2007 by the AAP

greater than 4 cm in diameter it is also more concerning for an underlying disorder.

Physiologic gynecomastia resolves in 75% of boys within 2 years. Boys who are obese take longer for the gynecomastia to resolve. Recent work has implicated elevated leptin levels as a possible etiology of persistent gynecomastia in boys. Although many adolescent boys present requesting surgery, the most appropriate therapy is reassurance. Surgery should be reserved for boys who have had no decrease in breast size over the period of a year or if there is excessive fibrosis of the breast tissue. Surgery is indicated in these boys because of a known, albeit small risk of malignant degeneration. Boys with Klinefelter's syndrome are at particular risk for carcinoma, and resection of the breast tissue should be considered a prophylactic mastectomy in these boys. There have been other cases of otherwise normal adolescents with gynecomastia who developed ductal carcinoma in situ or frank carcinoma of the breast. In addition to the clear medical indication for surgery, severe gynecomastia is a psychologically debilitating condition for a young man in puberty. Even small changes in breast size can have significant impact on quality of life and normal psychosocial development.

Juvenile (Virginal) Hypertrophy

Juvenile hypertrophy of the breast is a condition of extreme and often rapid growth of one or both breasts. In this condition, the breasts may become enormous, occasionally weighing as much as 50 lb each. This is a morbid condition as these girls have tremendous back and neck pain, psychological problems, and limitation of daily activities as a result of the breast hypertrophy. Interestingly, bulimia may also be a co-morbid condition, as some girls resort to disordered eating to normalize their appearance. The etiology of juvenile hypertrophy is not known, although elevated sensitivity of the breast tissue to steroid secretion during puberty has been suggested. It is slightly more common in African-American girls. Treatment begins with confirming the diagnosis by ruling out neoplastic lesions such as a giant fibroadenoma or lymphoma. Ultrasound can usually distinguish these, but a core needle biopsy is sometimes necessary. Breast reduction is indicated and should be performed at the end of puberty to avoid additional surgery to achieve breast symmetry. Occasionally, the asymmetry is so significant and the symptoms so pronounced that earlier reduction may be necessary. In these cases, a second reduction may be necessary after puberty is completed. The use of drugs such as medroxyprogesterone or tamoxifen to avoid recurrence has been suggested for severe cases.

Infections

Mastitis

Mastitis, or infection of the breast tissue, occurs most commonly in newborns and in lactating women. In the newborn, *mastitis neonatorum* can lead to injury to the breast bud and systemic sepsis. *Staphylococcus aureus* is the most common organism causing neonatal mastitis. Because of the increasing prevalence of methicillin-resistant *Staphylococcus aureus*, antibiotics to cover MRSA should empirically be given. Warm soaks to the breast can help decrease the discomfort and speed healing.

Abscess

Abscesses of the breast develop as a consequence of mastitis or from external inoculation of the breast by trauma, sexual trauma, hair pulling, or piercing. Approximately 50% of infants with mastitis develop a breast abscess. Antibiotics are an important part of therapy, but the cornerstone of treatment is drainage of the abscess. A small abscess in an otherwise stable infant can be initially treated by aspiration alone. For larger or recurrent abscesses or if the infant is ill, a formal incision and drainage is indicated. A periareolar incision is used for cosmetic reasons. In neonates and small children, a 14-gauge needle can be passed from one areola border to the other (through the abscess) and used to pass a vessel loop through the center of the abscess. The vessel loop can then be tied in a loop to serve as a drain.

Trauma

Blunt trauma to the breast is not common. It most often occurs from shoulder restraints during a motor vehicle accident. Other causes of injury can be from non-accidental injury (blow with a fist or blunt object), injury from an animal (such as a horse kick) or during an athletic event. Complete subcutaneous rupture of the breast has been reported. More commonly, girls develop bleeding into the breast tissue, which can be impressive and quite painful. Significant crush injury of the breast may also result in fat necrosis. Surgery for trauma to the breast is rarely indicated, although there are rare exceptions in which evacuation of a painful or expanding hematoma is indicated. Significant force can result in a serious injury to the breast bud in a pre-pubertal girl and can result in asymmetry of the breasts. Particularly in sports such as gymnastics, protection of the developing breast with a padded bra is recommended. Iatrogenic trauma to the breast is a particular problem for pre-pubertal girls, especially neonates. Chest tubes, central lines and thoracic surgery can all lead to injury to the breast bud with abnormal or absent breast growth (Fig. 106.2).

Burns

Burns to the breast are a particularly challenging injury. The type and depth of burn have significant impact on subsequent breast development in the prepubertal child. Since progenitor cells for breast tissue are located at the base of the nipple areola complex (NAC), if the NAC is not involved by the burn, breast development will most likely be unaffected. Scald injuries rarely result in loss of breast development. For deeper burns, the usual algorithm of rapid excision and grafting may not be the best choice as this can result in injury to the progenitor cells. A conservative debridement, avoiding a margin of 2–3 cm around the areola, is recommended. If the progenitor cells are not damaged, the breast will develop but can be entrapped by superficial scar. Surgery to release what is in effect a contracture is often indicated. If the developing breast tissue is destroyed by the injury, subsequent reconstruction can be accomplished by autologous flap or implants.

Breast Masses

Infantile Breast Masses

True breast masses in the infant are rare (Table 106.3). Vascular and lymphatic malformations are among the most common lesions (Fig. 106.3). It is very important to understand the classification of vascular lesions, as defined by Mulliken; an accurate diagnosis will dictate management and prognosis. The decisions to treat any vascular lesion is based on how fast they are growing (and therefore the risk of injuring the breast bud with this growth), the risk of resection, and the probability of involution. Although hemangiomas of the breast will usually spontaneously involute with time, other vascular and lymphatic lesions will not. In rare instances of rapid growth, hemangiomas of the breast can be treated with topical, intralesional or systemic steroids if the rapid growth is at risk to injure the breast bud. Hemangiomas typically experience a 4–6-month period of vascular growth before involution but involution can take several years to complete. Unlike hemangiomas, vascular malformations, including lymphangiomas, do not involute. Imaging with ultrasound and, if necessary, MRI may help plan the appropriate approach if these appear to be surgically resectable.

Table 106.3 Etiology of breast masses in children

	Neonatal	Pre-pubertal	Pubertal
Common	Gynecomastia Hemangioma Vascular malformation Lymphangioma	Breast bud from thelarche or premature thelarche	Fibroadenoma Fibrocystic changes Retroareolar cyst (cyst of montgomery)
Less common		Simple cyst	Fat necrosis Simple (blue-domed) cyst
Rare		Juvenile papillomatosis Intraductal papilloma Giant cell fibroblastoma Carcinoma	Papilloma Phyllodes tumor Neurofibroma Carcinoma Rhabdomyosarcoma, non-Hodgkins lymphoma Malignant fibrous histiocytoma Metastatic disease

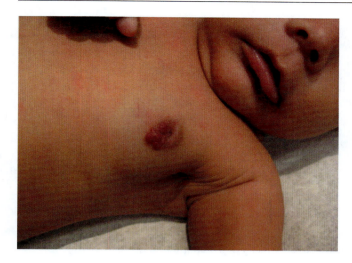

Fig. 106.3 Hemangioma of the breast in a neonate

If surgery does not seem the best option, endovascular or percutaneous sclerotherapy may be useful in managing the lesion.

Pre-Pubertal Breast Masses

Breast masses in prepubertal children are uncommon and are virtually all benign. The most common breast "mass" in prepubertal children is actually a physiologic *breast bud*. It is common for one breast to begin to develop before the other; this asymmetry is often a cause for concern for families and referring doctors. It is very important to recognize this as physiologic and reassure the families. Biopsy is contraindicated, as it can result in breast deformity by injuring the breast bud.

Juvenile papillomatosis is a rare lesion has been reported in children as young as 7 months of age, although it is more common in girls older than 10. It is important to know that juvenile papillomatosis is a marker for increased risk of breast cancer, both for the child and in other family members. Up to 15% of patients with juvenile papillomatosis will have carcinoma present in the lesion, usually a secretory carcinoma. Juvenile papillomatosis usually presents as a palpable mass, similar to a fibroadenoma on exam. The treatment is excision. This well demarcated mass, when divided, has a "Swiss cheese" appearance, with multiple cysts present in the lesion. Single intraductal papillomas have been reported in children as young as 4 years of age.

Other rare masses in prepubertal children include the *giant cell fibroblastoma*. This is a very rare soft tissue neoplasm that can occur in association with dermatofibrosarcoma protuberans. This lesion should be excised with clear margins, as local recurrence has been reported. Although *phyllodes tumor* occurs most commonly in teenagers, it has

been reported in girls as young as 11 years of age. *Carcinoma* of the breast is almost unheard of in prepubertal children, but case reports have been published of a lipid-secreting carcinoma in a 10 year old and a secretory carcinoma in three preschool children.

Pubertal Breast Masses

Fibroadenoma is the most common solid lesion women up to the age of 30. Most series of surgically resected breast lesions in adolescent girls report that 75–90% of lesions removed are fibroadenomas. These are usually isolated lesions that are well circumscribed, ovoid, mobile and rubbery in consistency. The natural course is usually rapid growth over 6–12 months with subsequent stabilization. *Giant fibroadenoma* is defined as any fibroadenoma larger than 5 cm in diameter. Physical examination usually suffices but ultrasonography provides additional information. Up to 25% of girls have multiple fibroadenomas, which are often more easily identified on ultrasound. Mammography is not indicated, as the dense tissue of the adolescent breast and extremely low risk of malignancy leads to unnecessary radiation exposure. Because fibroadenoma can resolve spontaneously, the initial plan should be observation. If there is growth or if the lesion is larger than 5 cm, removal is indicated. If there is no change, there are two options that can be offered the family: the lesion can be observed, with or without needle biopsy, or resected. For many families, this is preferable because it obviates the need for sequential examination and helps reduce the anxiety associated with waiting.

Phyllodes tumors, previously (and inaccurately) termed *cystosarcoma phyllodes* are rare fibroepithelial tumors that more commonly occur in mature women (average age 42 years). Patients most commonly present with a firm, large tumor, very similar to a giant fibroadenoma. If there is any suspicion of a phyllodes tumor, a needle biopsy is indicated before surgery to help with the surgical planning. These tumors are most often considered benign, but it is difficult to predict their biologic behavior. Approximately 20% of patients with phyllodes tumors (benign and malignant) experience a local recurrence. In addition, metastases have been reported in patients with apparently benign phyllodes tumors. For this reason, a wide local resection with clear margins is recommended for all phyllodes tumors. This can usually be accomplished with breast conserving surgery, but in some instances, a mastectomy is indicated.

Fibrocystic changes in the breast are physiologic but may be misinterpreted as a mass. Adolescents may present with nodular or cystic changes, increasing around the time of menstruation. There is no treatment necessary. Pain associated with these changes can be treated with firm support and oral analgesics. For some women, avoiding caffeine will improve breast pain. In severe cases, oral contraceptives may be of help.

Simple cysts, often described as blue-domed cysts, may occur in teenagers. These are single, large cysts of unknown etiology. Aspiration of the cyst usually leads to resolution and recurrence is unusual. Retroareolar cysts, or cysts of Montgomery, present either as a mass, sometimes associated with drainage from the areolar ducts, or as an acute infection. These cystic lesions are the result of hyperactive, and then obstructed, glands of Montgomery. On imaging, these lesions are single or multiple cysts which are invariably less than 2 cm in diameter. The natural history of these lesions is spontaneous resolution. Treatment of cysts of Montgomery is symptomatic with non-steroidal anti-inflammatory drugs for pain relief, warm soaks and antibiotics if infection is present. Resolution can take up to 2 years.

Intraductal papillomas are rare in teenagers, as these usually occur in women between the fourth and sixth decades of life. Multiple papillomas are slightly more common in younger patients and are often not associated with nipple discharge. Up to 25% of patients will have bilateral papillomas. A solitary papilloma is not considered a pre-malignant lesion, but patients with multiple papillomas are at increased risk for breast cancer. The treatment, if the lesion can be isolated to a single duct, is excision of the duct. Microdochectomy is effective and leads to better cosmesis in younger patients.

Fat necrosis, which occurs after traumatic injury to the breast, is unusual in teenagers but can present as a mass. The etiology is thought to be ischemia in the fatty tissue of the breast after following trauma, biopsy, or other surgery. It is often preceded by a hematoma or large ecchymosis. Unlike other masses, fat necrosis is usually tender on examination. Surgery may occasionally be indicated for pain control.

Malignant Tumors

Malignant tumors of the breast are exceedingly rare in children. The SEER (NCI) database reports only 75 children total in the United States as of 2008 with malignant breast disease, about half with phyllodes tumors and half with carcinoma. The youngest patient in this series was 11 and 84% of the children in this series were older than 15. The most common cell type in children with carcinoma of the breast is secretory adenocarcinoma. Ductal carcinoma is extremely rare in pediatric patients. The risk of carcinoma of the breast is increased 37-fold in children who have undergone mantle radiation for Hodgkin's lymphoma or other neoplasms. Higher doses of radiation and age less than 12 years at the time of treatment correlate with a higher risk. The algorithm used for most adult breast cancers, including the use of sentinel lymph node biopsy,

is recommended for children with malignant lesions of the breast. Other primary malignant tumors of the breast reported in children include rhabdomyosarcoma, non-Hodgkins lymphoma and malignant fibrous histiocytoma. Metastatic lesions of the breast have been reported in children from primary rhabdomyosarcomas and lymphomas.

Nipple Discharge

Discharge from the nipple can be caused by a variety of underlying problems. Milky discharge or galactorrhea may result from pregnancy or prolactinoma. Galactorrhea can also be caused by self-manipulation, drugs or hypothyroidism. The diagnosis of galactorrhea is made by the presence of fat globules in the discharge on microscopic staining. Serous or greenish discharge from the nipple is most often from a benign breast cyst. The differential of bloody discharge is age dependent.

Newborn infants often have galactorrhea as a result of the perinatal hormonal stimulation. This drainage, occasionally referred to as "witch's milk" by family members, will resolve spontaneously. Caregivers should be instructed not to squeeze the breast as this can prolong the time to resolution and increase the risk of mastitis. Newborn infants may develop bloody discharge in association with infantile gynecomastia. In boys, there are reports of subcutaneous mastectomy in the newborn period to control bleeding from the breast.

Breast discharge in the prepubertal child is most commonly from *ductal ectasia*, which is a congenital defect that results in dilation of the lactiferous ducts, with collection of secretions. This can occur from age 2–10 and usually presents with a bloody discharge (Fig. 106.4). The bleeding is felt to be secondary to superinfection of these stagnant secretions. Approximately 50% of children will have cultures positive for gram positive cocci (usually *Staph aureus*). Treatment is with empiric antibiotics to cover *Staph aureus*,

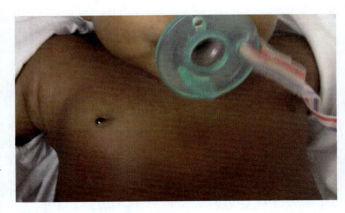

Fig. 106.4 Bloody discharge from ductal ectastia

with a change in antibiotics based on culture results. Both juvenile papillomatosis and papillomas have been reported in prepubertal children as a cause of bloody nipple discharge but are very rare.

The most common cause of bloody nipple discharge in pubertal children is a papilloma. Bloody discharge has been reported to occur in patients with an infarcted fibroadenoma and phyllodes tumors as well. Galactorrhea can occur in teenagers as a result of pregnancy, hypothyroidism, neurogenic lactation, pituitary tumors, or drugs. Hypothyroidism is reported in some series as the most frequent cause of

non-puerperal galactorrhea in adolescents. Neurogenic galactorrhea can occur after thoracotomy, burns, trauma, Herpes zoster or chronic nipple stimulation. Many drugs can cause galactorrhea, the most common of which are antipsychotics, antidepressants and histamine blockers. The nipple may be abraded during running or bicycling leading to chronic skin changes and bleeding. These injuries are more common in colder weather, when the nipple is more likely to be erect. Prevention is the best cure for this disorder. A dressing or a lubricant should be used over the nipples to prevent the abrasion. For girls, a well-fitted bra is important as well.

Summary Points

- The vast majority of breast lesions in children are benign.
- Breast disorders can be classified into four categories: developmental, infectious/inflammatory, traumatic, and neoplastic.
- Progenitor cells and developing breast tissue should be protected.
- Malignancy is more common in girls who have been exposed to radiation of the chest.
- Malignancy is rare but, if suspected, should first be confirmed with a core needle biopsy.
- Mammography is of limited (if any) use in children.
- Large abscesses should be drained, with a periareolar incision whenever possible.

Editor's Comment

"Breast mass" in a toddler is a common indication for referral to a pediatric surgeon. These cause tremendous anxiety for parents but almost always represent breast buds and should never be biopsied. There are women who have severe breast deformities or amastia due to a simple biopsy of a breast bud as a child. Reassurance and serial examinations should be the rule, with ultrasound performed for enlargement of the mass or extreme parental anxiety. Most breast masses in teenagers will turn out to be fibroadenomas, which can be multiple. Unless they are growing, larger than 4 cm in diameter, or causing pain, they should be followed. Many will resolve spontaneously after a few months or years of observation. Sometimes there is increased pressure to perform a biopsy because of an ultrasound report, usually dictated by an adult radiologist, that states that the lesion is "suspicious" and "must be biopsied." Repeat ultrasound performed by an experienced pediatric radiologist can sometimes provide the reassurance needed to avoid unnecessary surgery. Unless it occurs near the axilla, fibroadenomas should always be removed through a periareolar incision and, because they can usually be separated cleanly from the surrounding breast tissue with blunt dissection, the specimen should include little, if any, normal breast tissue. In addition, except in girls with a history of breast irradiation (Hodgkin's disease), resection of a breast mass with a margin is rarely necessary.

Fine needle aspiration is useful when dealing with a cyst but is rarely indicated in children. Most pediatric centers lack the expertise in performing the procedure and interpreting the results of cytologic analysis. Likewise, needle-localization biopsy is almost never indicated as this is usually performed in a woman with a nonpalpable lesion detected by screening mammography, which is never indicated in a child. Many adolescents complain of breast pain, for which there is often no effective treatment. When there is pain, many parents think they feel a mass when in fact there is only normal developing breast tissue, which can be very firm and tender to palpation, or simply fibrocystic change, which is not treated surgically.

Mastitis is treated with antibiotics, but an abscess should be aspirated or surgically drained, depending on its size. There is probably a greater risk of injury to the breast anlagen by uncontrolled infection than by incision and drainage performed carefully through a tiny incision at the areolar border. Abscess cavities should never be packed with gauze. Ectopic breast tissue most commonly occurs in the axilla and can be painful. The tissue is usually intimately adherent to the overlying dermis and an acceptable cosmetic result can be difficult to obtain. Gynecomastia can be psychologically distressing but usually resolves after the height of puberty. Many surgeons will refuse to operate (and insurance companies refuse to pay) until the patient has reached 18 years of age and can demonstrate that the breast tissue has failed to begin to diminish in size. The goal of mastectomy in these cases should be to remove only the breast tissue, although removing some fat is often necessary, especially in patients who are also obese. It is often difficult to know how much tissue should be removed from behind the nipple – removing too much can cause necrosis or nipple inversion, and leaving too much can result in recurrence, especially if the child is still young. It is usually best to leave a small amount and to warn the patient that recurrence could occur, albeit rarely.

The inframammary incision can be very useful and cosmetically superior to other thoracotomy incisions; however, when the incision is made while the patient is supine and under general anesthesia it will almost invariably end up being too high (on the breast). If there is any chance that an inframammary incision will need to be made, this site should be marked indelibly prior to the operation, preferably with the patient in an upright position.

Differential Diagnosis

- Fibrocystic change
- Fibroadenoma
- Papillomatosis
- Phyllodes tumor
- Mastitis/breast abscess
- Simple cyst
- Fat necrosis (trauma)
- Sarcoma (rare)
- Carcinoma (very rare)

Parental Preparation

- Despite all precautions, future breast development might be affected by an intervention performed at a young age.
- Breast cancer is exceedingly rare in children and adolescents.
- Most masses are benign fibroadenomas, which may resolve spontaneously and generally cause few problems.
- Some degree of breast asymmetry is normal and somewhat common.

Diagnostic Studies

- Ultrasound
- Fine needle aspiration (rarely indicated)
- CT/MRI (rarely indicated)

Preoperative Preparation

☐ Informed consent

Technical Points

- Breast incisions should be periareolar, unless malignancy has been confirmed.
- As most lesions are benign, removing a wide margin of normal breast tissue is usually unnecessary.
- Simple cysts can be aspirated.
- Microdochectomy is the best treatment for intraductal papilloma.
- Breast buds (and retro-areolar tissue) should never be excised or biopsied, except in the exceedingly rare case of a proven malignancy.

Suggested Reading

Barrio AV, Clark BD, Goldberg JI, et al. Clinicopathologic features and long-term outcomes of 293 phyllodes tumors of the breast. Ann Surg Oncol. 2007;14(10):2961–70.

De Silva N, Brandt M. Disorders of the breast in children and adolescents: Part 1: Disorders of growth and infections of the breast. J Pediatr Adolesc Gynecol. 2006a;19:345–9.

De Silva N, Brandt M. Disorders of the breast in children and adolescents: Part 2: Breast masses. J Pediatr Adolesc Gynecol. 2006b;19:415–8.

Greydanus DE, Matytsina L, Gains M. Breast disorders in children and adolescents. Prim Care. 2006;33(2):455–502.

Kapila K, Pathan SK, Al-Mosawy FA, et al. Fine needle aspiration cytology of breast masses in children and adolescents: experience with 1404 aspirates. Acta Cytol. 2008;52(6):681–6.

Lin HM, Teitell MA. Second malignancy after treatment of pediatric Hodgkin disease. J Pediatr Hematol Oncol. 2005;27(1):28–36.

Marler JJ, Mulliken JB. Current management of hemangiomas and vascular malformations. Clin Plast Surg. 2005;32(1):99–116.

Sadove AM, van Aalst JA. Congenital and acquired pediatric breast anomalies: a review of 20 years' experience. Plast Reconstr Surg. 2005;115(4):1039–50.

Templeman C, Hertweck SP. Breast disorders in the pediatric and adolescent patient. Obstet Gynecol Clin North Am. 2000;27(1):19–34.

Chapter 107
Kidney Transplantation

Peter L. Abt and H. Jorge Baluarte

The incidence of end stage renal disease in children is relatively low and only about 5% of kidney transplants in the United States are placed in children. In 2005, the United States Renal Data System reported 1,207 children 0–19 years of age with ESRD. In 2006, 893 renal transplants were performed in children, 312 from living donors and 581 from deceased donors. Deceased donors tend to be young and middle-aged adults, with essentially no use of extended-criteria organs. The mean age at transplant is around 11 years: 5% younger than 2, 15% between the ages of 2 and 5, 34% between 6 and 12, and roughly 46% older than 12. Sixty percent are male, 61% are white, 17% are black, and 16% are Hispanic.

The etiology of ESRD in children varies significantly with age. As a general rule, congenital structural lesions cause more renal failure in young children while glomerulonephritis is more common in older children. In fact, congenital, hereditary, and cystic diseases account for more than half of cases in children under six, whereas glomerulonephritis and focal segmental glomerulosclerosis account for more than a third of cases in those aged 10–19 years.

Early diagnosis is important because it is sometimes possible to slow the progression of chronic kidney disease, to treat comorbid conditions earlier, and to improve outcomes and quality of life long before renal replacement therapy becomes necessary. Though the diagnosis of renal disease is based on pathologic criteria and evidence of kidney damage, glomerular filtration rate (GFR) is considered an accurate reflection of the level of residual renal function regardless of the etiology or pathological diagnosis. Patients also need to be monitored for a multitude of other problems, including electrolyte abnormalities (hyponatremia, hyperkalemia, hypocalcemia) and metabolic derangements (metabolic acidosis, hyperuricemia, hyperperphosphatemia). Nutritional deficiencies can have an important impact on their growth and development. Anemia is the result of reduced erythropoietin synthesis, the presence of erythropoiesis inhibitors, blood loss, or hemolysis. Infants are especially vulnerable to developmental delays and are prone to seizures, dyskinesia and other central nervous system abnormalities. Growth failure, a major obstacle to full rehabilitation, often results from protein and calorie malnutrition, metabolic acidosis, growth hormone resistance, anemia and renal osteodystrophy. In addition, uremia is associated with nausea and loss of appetite. Many children with chronic renal insufficiency will require supplemental calories or enteral feeds delivered by a feeding tube. Children who fail to grow will sometimes respond to recombinant human growth hormone.

Bone disease and disorders of calcium and phosphorus metabolism frequently develop in children with chronic renal insufficiency, often resulting in secondary hyperparathyroidism. Decreased renal function reduces phosphate excretion and increases phosphate retention. An elevated serum phosphate level in turn suppresses calcitriol production, which is already low due to reduced renal mass. The result is reduced calcium absorption from the gastrointestinal tract and hypocalcemia. Hypocalcemia, reduced calcitriol synthesis and hyperphosphatemia act in concert to stimulate the production of parathormone, resulting in secondary hyperparathyroidism. Treatment includes dietary modifications that reduce phosphate intake and the administration of phosphate binders and vitamin D supplements.

Therapeutic Options

For the child with ESRD, renal replacement options include transplantation or dialysis. Renal transplantation is accepted as the therapy of choice for children with ESRD. This is based upon the belief that successful transplantation not only ameliorates uremic symptoms but also allows for significant improvement in skeletal growth, sexual maturation, cognitive performance, and psychosocial functioning. The child with a functional allograft has a quality of life that is far superior to that which is currently achievable with dialysis.

P.L. Abt (✉)
Department of Surgery, University of Pennsylvania, Children's Hospital of Philadelphia, Hospital of the University of Pennsylvania, Philadelphia, PA 19104, USA
e-mail: Peter.L.Abt@uphs.upenn.edu

P. Mattei (ed.), *Fundamentals of Pediatric Surgery*,
DOI 10.1007/978-1-4419-6643-8_107, © Springer Science+Business Media, LLC 2011

Transplantation also offers a distinct survival advantage over dialysis: the mortality rate for children on dialysis is three times higher than for those who have received a transplant.

Transplantation offers such an advantage over dialysis that every child who requires renal replacement therapy should be considered a potential transplant candidate. Dialysis may be required before transplantation to optimize nutritional and metabolic conditions, to allow small children to achieve an appropriate size, or to keep a patient stable until a suitable donor is available. Most centers strive for a recipient weight of at least 8–10 kg, which minimizes the risk of vascular thrombosis and allows the child to accommodate an adult-sized kidney. The target weight of 10 kg might not be achieved until 12–24 months of age.

Transplantation without prior dialysis (preemptive transplantation) accounts for 25% of pediatric renal transplants and offers several advantages. Most kidneys placed preemptively come from living donors, which have improved survival. Children with ESRD often have significant growth failure and development delay and a preemptive transplant might help to avoid these complications. It also helps to avoid the complications associated with placement of vascular access catheters and fistulas or grafts that are needed for hemodialysis and the abdominal complications associated with peritoneal dialysis. Potential candidates for preemptive transplantation need careful psychological assessment because there might be an increased tendency for noncompliance in this group of recipients. Nevertheless, there appears to be no impairment in graft outcome in pediatric recipients who have undergone preemptive transplantation when compared with those who have had dialysis before transplantation.

Absolute contraindications to transplant include: active untreated malignancy or a period of less than 12 months after treatment for a malignancy, active infection, current positive T-cell crossmatch, irreversible debilitating brain injury, active substance abuse, and severe multi-organ failure. Relative contraindications include: ABO incompatibility with the donor, human immunodeficiency virus (HIV) infection, long-standing history of medical noncompliance, severe psychomotor delay, psychiatric illness, inadequate social support, and active autoimmune disease such as systemic lupus erythematosus.

Due to advances in immunosuppressive therapy, earlier referral to transplant centers, better surgical techniques, and improved postoperative management, graft survival has improved substantially, with current 1-year patient survival approaching 98%.

Preoperative Planning

The pretransplant evaluation involves a multidisciplinary team that includes a pediatric nephrologist, transplant surgeon, psychiatrist or psychologist, transplant coordinator, dialysis nurse, dietitian, social worker, financial counselor, and pharmacist, assisted by consultation from a pediatric dentist, urologist, cardiologist, and anesthesiologist. Support from a social worker is essential as most families are ill-equipped to deal with the tremendous financial and psychological challenges of a chronically ill child.

The evaluation begins with a history and physical exam and a broad panel of laboratory studies. Potential recipients are screened for previous or active infection with cytomegalovirus (CMV), Epstein Bar virus (EBV), BK virus, hepatitis B and C, and HIV. It is important that children be immunized prior to transplantation as they may not be able to mount an adequate response while immunosuppressed. Live attenuated vaccines should be given prior to transplant and avoided following the initiation of immunosuppression.

Besides a routine chest X-ray, a selective approach to imaging is appropriate. Preoperative vascular studies are occasionally necessary in children who have had femoral dialysis catheters to document patency of the iliac vein and inferior vena cava and in those with congenital abnormalities associated with abnormal vascular anatomy. To avoid complications following transplant, it is essential that the lower urinary tract be adequately studied in children whose ESRD is due to urinary tract and bladder dysfunction associated with posterior urethral valves, neurogenic bladder, vesicoureteral reflux, outflow obstruction, prune belly syndrome or bladder extrophy. A voiding cystoureterogram (VCUG) and an estimation of bladder capacity should be performed. In some children with complex urogenital abnormalities, transplantation may be only one part of a series of operations planned to restore form and function and it is important that there exists a close working relationship between the transplant surgeon, urologist, and nephrologist.

In general, referral for transplantation should take place when the GFR is approximately 30 mL/min/1.73 m². A timely referral for transplantation is important as it allows time to address medical comorbidities, properly plan for the transplant and educate the patient and family. Early referral also forces children who never had to adhere to a strict medical regimen transition to the demanding regimen required after transplantation. This is extremely important as noncompliance causes 30–70% of long-term graft loss in children.

The timing of transplantation, especially whether preemptive transplantation should be considered, and the type of donor, living or cadaveric, are important issues that need to be discussed with the recipient and family. Receiving a kidney from a living donor offers two distinct advantages: it eliminates the potentially long wait for an organ from a deceased donor and the long-term graft survival is significantly better. Unadjusted 5-year graft survival data from the Scientific Registry of Transplant Recipients comparing living-donor graft recipients to deceased-donor graft recipients demonstrate markedly better graft survival for children who receive a living donor organ regardless of age: 89 vs. 75% for ages 1–5 years; 85 vs. 72% for ages 6–10; and 74 vs. 63% for ages 11–17.

Native nephroureterectomy is necessary in some patients and can be performed before transplant or at the time of transplant. The timing depends on the underlying cause of renal disease, coexisting medical conditions, availability of an allograft and the age of child. It should usually be performed in patients with malignant hypertension, vesicoureteral reflux, recurrent pyelonephritis, a genetic predisposition for renal malignancy (WT-1 mutations, such as Denys-Drash syndrome), large polycystic kidneys that compromise pulmonary function or cause early satiety, and nephrotic syndrome, which is associated with a hypercoagulable state and an increased risk of vascular thrombose within the transplanted kidney.

Operative Approach

Prior to transplantation, it is important to optimize the child's health status, which includes correcting acidosis, volume deficits and anemia, controlling hypertension, and ensuring that there are no active infections.

The operative approach to renal transplantation in children is guided by the size of the child and previous surgical therapy. In general, adult-sized kidneys are placed in children, as organs from pediatric donor have higher rates of vascular thrombosis and subsequent graft loss. A standard lower quadrant retroperitoneal approach with implantation of the renal graft into the external or common iliac vasculature can usually be performed in children who weigh 30 kg or more. For children who weigh less than 20 kg, a midline anterior abdominal approach to the distal abdominal aorta and inferior vena cava provides larger targets for implanting the donor artery and vein (Fig. 107.1). In addition, the peritoneal cavity offers more space for the kidney, which is usually too large for a retroperitoneal approach in a small child. Mobilization of the aorta and distal vena cava might require selective ligation of the lumber vessels. For children who are between 20 and 30 kg, the approach should be individualized based on a careful assessment of the child's body habitus.

The intra-operative management of the recipient's volume status is important, especially in small children, and requires close cooperation between the surgeon and the anesthesiologist. An adult graft can contain 250 mL of blood, or about 50% of the cardiac output in a small child. The recipient should be loaded with volume so that the central venous pressure is 10–15 mmHg before the kidney is reperfused. To maintain adequate perfusion, we use volume expansion with crystalloid and albumin to keep the mean arterial pressure no

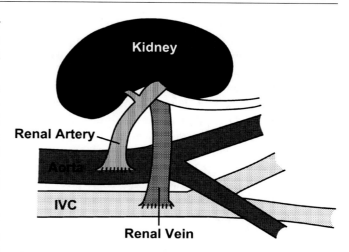

Fig. 107.1 Intraperitoneal placement of the renal allograft

lower than 60–70 mmHg. Occasionally, pressor support with dopamine is necessary. Acidosis and hyperkalemia develop readily in small children, particularly during aortic clamping, and should be aggressively corrected. Prior to reperfusion of the organ, intravenous mannitol and lasix are given. If at all possible, blood transfusion should be avoided in order to limit the patient's exposure to additional human leukocyte antigens. Most children will require another transplant in their lifetime and antigen sensitization can make future donor crossmatching much more difficult.

Once the kidney is reperfused, urinary drainage is established. A stent is usually not necessary for the routine ureteroneocystostomy but we use a stent for technically challenging situations, such as when the bladder mucosa is thin and friable. Certain circumstances mandate ureteroureterostomy or pyeloureterostomy, for which stenting is recommended. The anastomosis should be constructed with absorbable suture to avoid creating a nidus for stone formation. Occasionally two ureters are present in the donor kidney. These can either be implanted into the bladder with two separate anastomoses or joined together distally before being sewn into the bladder as a single anastomosis. The foley catheter usually is left in place for 3–5 days.

Postoperative Management

In the post-operative period daily laboratory studies and strict measurement of fluid balance are routine. In general, all intravenous lines and catheters are removed as soon as possible to reduce the risk of infection. Prophylactic antibiotics are given for 48 h and gastrointestinal prophylaxis with a proton pump inhibitor or histamine antagonist for stress gastritis in the setting of systemic corticosteroids is routine. Patients are initiated on prophylactic therapy for opportunistic infections: co-trimoxazol for *pneumocystis carinii* (dapsone or atovaquone in those with sulfa allergies) for 12 months, nystatin or clotrimazole troches for fungus for 6 months, and antiviral prophylaxis for CMV and herpes simplex virus for 6 months.

Fluid management is of upmost importance in the postoperative period. The new kidney produces copious urine, as a result of a reperfusion diuresis. Hourly urine replacement mL-per-mL with 0.45 saline and 22 mEq/L of sodium bicarbonate is routine for the first 24 h, which is then tapered or stopped over the next 24–72 h. The diuresis can be brisk, and a small child can easily become hypotensive if the urine output is not replaced. Infants sometimes need to be intubated for 24–48 h depending on their volume status and the safety of their airway.

Developments in immunosuppression account for much of the current success of transplantation (Table 107.1). Most drug regimens follow a similar approach, but immunosuppression can vary among transplant centers and among individual patients. Immunosuppression can be broadly viewed as having two phases. The perioperative period starts at the time of transplant and lasts through the first several months. It is during this time that the greatest risk of acute rejection exists. In general, immunosuppression medications are kept at higher doses. Over time, accommodation between the recipient and donor organ occurs and immunosuppression is usually able to be decreased somewhat.

At the time of transplant, many centers follow a course of induction therapy, weakening the immune system with either a polyclonal or monoclonal antibody. Depending on the antibody, these might be given as a one-time dose, or require repeated administration during the perioperative period. At most centers, a three-drug regimen of chronic immunosuppression is initiated following surgery, with the backbone consisting of a calcineurin inhibitor (either cyclosporine or tacrolimus), an antimetabolite (usually mycophenolate mofetil), and a corticosteroid taper. The calcineurin inhibitors are dosed based on serum levels. As chronic therapy, all three drugs are continued and, if immunologic acceptance of the kidney is observed, the calcineurin inhibitor dose is lowered based on trough levels. There is a growing movement to limit or even avoid recipients' exposure to corticosteroids in order to prevent some of the well-known complications of these medications (weight gain, acne, bone loss). Sirolimus, a TOR (target of rapamycin) inhibitor, is being used by some centers as a substitute for or in conjunction with lower doses of calcineurin inhibitors in order to prevent the long-term renal dysfunction attributed to calcineurin inhibitors.

Acute oliguria or anuria is a concerning sign and should initiate a rapid investigation and aggressive intervention, particularly in a patient who previously had good urine production. Common etiologies include obstruction of a Foley catheter from a blood clot in the bladder, hypovolemia, acute tubular necrosis (ischemia-reperfusion injury), ureteral leak, and compression of the kidney from a hematoma. Graft thrombosis and hyperacute rejection are other concerning causes of a sudden decrease in urine production. The initial evaluation includes: checking the patency of the urinary catheter, assessing volume status, and checking a hemoglobin level. If the cause is still unclear, duplex ultrasound of the graft or a nuclear medicine renal flow and excretion study should be performed next. A percutaneous renal biopsy might be warranted to detect rejection or acute tubular necrosis in patients who do not show improvement with other measures and who do not have a defined cause of graft dysfunction.

Delayed graft function is generally defined as the need for dialysis within the first week of transplant. Acute tubular necrosis is the most common cause of delayed graft function. It rarely occurs in the setting of living donor transplant where ischemia times are short, but occurs in 25% of deceased donor transplants. Acute tubular necrosis can take days or months to resolve. Little can be done to hasten renal recovery other than to support the kidney by avoiding hypoperfusion, maintain electrolyte balance, ensure an adequate hemoglobin, preserve volume status, and monitor the levels of calcineurin inhibitor, which are nephrotoxic. While waiting for renal function to resume, it is necessary to have a low suspicion for rejection and to biopsy the kidney judiciously to exclude rejection as an etiology of poor graft function.

Table 107.1 Commonly prescribed immunosuppressant medications

Class	Drug names	Mechanism
Antibodies	Anti-thymocyte globulin	Polyclonal antibody to human lymphocytes
	Muromonab	Monoclonal antibody to CD3 on T cells
	Basiliximab, Daclizumab	Bind and block IL-2 receptor on T cells
	Alemtuzumab	Binds CD52 on lymphocytes
Antimetabolites	Azathioprine	Interferes with nucleic acid synthesis
	Mycophenolate mofetil	Interferes with nucleic acid synthesis – more specific to lymphocytes
Corticosteroids	Prednisone, methylprednisolone	Inhibit production of T-cell lymphokines among other mechanisms
Calcineurin inhibitors	Cyclosporine	Binds to cyclophilin, inhibits IL-2 synthesis
	Tacrolimus	Binds to FK-binding protein, inhibits IL-2 synthesis
TOR inhibitors	Sirolimus	Inhibits T cell activation

Rejection is an anti-allograft response mounted by the recipient's T cells and is the major impediment to successful engraftment. This activation of T cells is initiated upon recognition of antigen-presenting cells, which stimulates a redistribution of cell-surface proteins, leading to a clustering of the T-cell receptor (TCR) and the CD3 complex with the CD4/CD8 antigens. The end result is the transcription and expression of genes essential to T-cell growth such as IL-2 and receptors for IL-2. The net consequence of cytokine production is the emergence of antigen-specific and graft-destructive T cells.

Any rise in serum creatinine concentration should be considered a result of acute rejection until proven otherwise. The traditional signs of acute rejection, fever and graft tenderness, are rarely seen in the current era of calcineurin inhibitors and prophylactic T-cell antibody therapy. Late diagnosis and treatment of rejection are associated with a higher incidence of resistant rejection and graft loss. Standard treatment of an episode of acute rejection is intravenous methylprednisolone (10 mg/kg/day to a maximum of 1 g/dose) for 3–5 days. Maintenance corticosteroid doses are then resumed at the pre-rejection levels or increased and tapered to baseline levels over a few days. Complete reversal of acute rejection, as judged by a return of the serum creatinine concentration to baseline, is achieved in about half of children and 40–45% achieve partial reversal. Steroid-resistant rejection episodes are treated with one of the currently available anti-T-cell antibodies. Conversion from cyclosporine to tacrolimus, or the addition of mycophenolate mofetil, might reverse or stabilize a rejection episode.

According to the 2007 Annual report of North American Pediatric Renal Transplant Cooperative Study (NAPRTCS), the probability of acute rejection at 12 months has decreased substantially. While historically over half of cadaveric organ recipients experienced an episode of acute rejection in the first few weeks post-transplant, the majority of patients now experience no episodes of acute rejection. Between 2003 and 2006, the probability of acute rejection for living organ recipients and deceased organ recipients was 13.7 and 17.9%.

Chronic rejection is the most common cause of graft loss and, according to the NAPRTCS 2007 annual report, it occurs in 35% of recipients. A more inclusive term of chronic allograft nephropathy is used at the present time because, in addition to the critical role of acute rejection, many other factors play a part in chronic rejection. The pathogenesis of chronic allograft nephropathy involves complex interacting immunologic factors like antigen-specific cellular and humoral immune mechanisms and nonimmune factors such as hypertension, hyperlipidemia, and long-term toxicity from calcineurin inhibitors.

Some complications do not become apparent for weeks or even months after transplant. Lymphoceles occur in those patients who have had a retroperitoneal approach to transplant and can cause compression of the renal vasculature or the iliac vein. While asymptomatic lymphoceles do not require therapy, symptomatic ones present with a palpable mass in the area of the transplant, ipsilateral leg swelling, or reduced renal function. Symptomatic lymphoceles can be drained percutaneously or into the peritoneal cavity using a laparoscopic approach. Late ureteral anastomotic strictures are usually due to ischemia. Treatment is initially nonoperative, by placing a percutaneous transrenal or retrograde stent. In general, a stricture that recurs or does not respond to a period of stenting requires surgical revision.

Recurrent disease accounts for 5% of graft loss of primary transplants and 10% of repeat transplants in pediatric recipients. Focal segmental glomerulosclerosis (FSGS) is the most common cause of graft loss from recurrent disease. This can occur immediately and is usually characterized by massive proteinuria and nephrotic syndrome. Though the etiology of the proteinuria remains uncertain, the existence of a circulating permeability factor has been implicated in view of the rapidity of the recurrence. Early post-transplant recognition of recurrent FSGS is important because plasmapheresis can decrease serum levels of the permeability factor and reduce graft loss. Other primary nephropathies and metabolic disorders like membranoproliferative glomerulonephritis, IgA nephritis, HSP nephritis, anti-GBM disease, atypical or inherited forms of hemolytic uremic syndrome, primary hyperoxaluria and cystinosis can affect function and cause graft loss.

Infections are the main cause of morbidity and mortality, accounting for 34% of all post-transplant deaths. Pneumonia and urinary tract infections are the most common bacterial infections. *Pneumocystis carinii* pneumonia (PCP), characterized clinically by dyspnea and hypoxemia, occurs in about 3% of renal allograft recipients. The risk is highest in the first month and trimethoprim-sulfamethoxazole (TMP/SMZ) prophylaxis should be provided for all patients and continued for 1 year.

Many young children have not been exposed to the herpes viruses (CMV, HSV, *varicella zoster* and EBV), and because they lack protective immunity, they are at increased risk for serious primary infections. The incidence of these infections is higher in children treated with antibody induction therapy and after treatment for acute rejection.

BK virus, a polyoma virus, is ubiquitous in the community and analysis of data from the US and Europe confirms a high level of seroconversion by late childhood. It is an important cause of allograft dysfunction, with up to 45% of infected grafts demonstrating BK interstitial infiltration. The intensity of post-transplant immunosuppression is believed to be directly related to BKV allograft nephropathy. The management of BK replication is not well studied and includes monitoring of viruria as a marker of viremia, reduction of immunosuppression, and consideration of empiric anti-viral therapy.

Hypertension is common immediately after renal transplantation and at 1 month posttransplant, 70% of patients require antihypertensive medication. The causes are multifactorial and primarily related to corticosteroid and calcineurin inhibitor therapy. Lipid abnormalities frequently occur after transplantation despite normal allograft function. Corticosteroids, calcineurin inhibitors, and sirolimus can induce hyperlipidemia. Patients should be screened during the first 6 months after transplantation and then annually. If dietary measures are not effective, therapy with statins can be started.

An increased incidence of cancer is a well-recognized complication of organ transplantation in children. These tumors are the result of a complex interplay of numerous factors including immunosuppressive drugs, the immunocompromised state per se, oncogenic viruses, and the possible synergistic effect of sunlight, infections, and hormonal factors. The pattern of malignancies in pediatric transplant recipients differs significantly from that in adults. Posttransplant lymphoproliferative disease is the most common, while skin carcinomas (squamous cell and basal cell carcinomas) are the second most common neoplasm. The mainstay of management of post-transplant lymphoproliferative disease is the drastic reduction or cessation of immunosuppressive treatment to allow recovery of the recipient's cytotoxic T-cell-directed EBV surveillance mechanism.

Rehabilitation and Quality of Life

Organ transplantation usually results in dramatic improvement of all aspects of physical, emotional, and social functioning. Cognitive skills improve after successful renal transplantation, suggesting stabilization of neuropsychologic functioning. Successful reentry into school after transplantation requires coordinated preparation of the child, family or caregivers, classmates and school personnel. Medication side effects, social and emotional difficulties, academic difficulties, use of school resources and caregiver attitudes all play a role and should be addressed. Within a year of successful transplantation, more than 90% of children attend school. Fewer than 10% are not involved in any vocational or education programs. By the 3-year follow-up nearly 90% of children are in appropriate school or job placement. Surveys of 10-year survivors of pediatric kidney transplants report that most patients consider their health to be good, engage in appropriate social, educational, and sexual activities, and experience a very good or excellent quality of life.

Summary Points

- Renal dysfunction in children can lead to multiple metabolic and nutritional deficiencies.
- Renal transplant offers a distinct survival advantage over dialysis.
- All children with end stage renal disease should be considered potential transplant candidates.
- Image the lower urinary tract if there is a history of urinary tract problems and prior to surgery.
- Living-donor renal transplant is preferable to an organ from a deceased donor.
- Intra-operative and postoperative volume management is important, especially in small children.
- Sudden cessation of urine production is an emergency that requires urgent investigation.
- Immunosuppression is required during the lifespan of the kidney transplant.
- Long-term outcomes are excellent, but life-long follow-up with a transplant physician is required to manage complications of immunosuppression.

Editor's Comment

Renal transplantation in children has become somewhat routine and the results have steadily improved over the past several years. Nevertheless, the degree to which receiving a kidney transplant changes the life of the child and his or her family should never be underestimated. These are very complex patients who are at risk for various general surgery problems including appendicitis, small bowel obstruction due to adhesions, lymphoceles, mesenteric or retroperitoneal lymphadenopathy, failure to thrive requiring gastrostomy placement, and the need for peritoneal dialysis catheters after

a failed intra-abdominal graft has been removed. Operative intervention for the treatment of any of these conditions can usually be performed laparoscopically, whether the graft is located in the retroperitoneum or peritoneal cavity, but one should anticipate significant adhesions. These adhesions can usually be lysed fairly easily using minimal access techniques.

Appendicitis is not uncommon in this population but can be approached in the usual fashion. Trocars should be placed carefully so as to avoid injury to the graft, preferably utilizing old scars. After placement of the camera port, the laparoscope itself can be used to lyse nearby adhesions to create some working space. Once two more ports are placed, a standard laparoscopic appendectomy can be performed. Obviously, antibiotics are necessary and spillage of luminal contents should be minimized. As with any patient who has undergone an intra-abdominal surgical procedure, small bowel obstruction due to adhesions can occur and will sometimes need to be relieved surgically. These patients are at risk for a rare form of adhesive bowel obstruction, sclerosing encapsulating peritonitis, which usually requires an extensive lysis of very dense adhesions. Although thought to be due to contamination of the peritoneal cavity during previous peritoneal dialysis treatments, perhaps by chlorhexidine, the sclerosing process is apparently sometimes accelerated by the initiation of immunosuppressants. Lymphoceles can cause pain or ureteral obstruction. The optimal treatment is the creation of a window between the lymphocele and the peritoneum, which can usually be fashioned using a laparoscopic approach. After renal transplantation, children are at risk for malignancy, the most common of which is lymphoproliferative disorder. The diagnosis is sometimes suspected on the basis of enlarged mesenteric or retroperitoneal lymph nodes. In most cases, these can safely be sampled laparoscopically. Gastrostomy button placement can also easily be performed laparoscopically – it is less invasive than open Stamm gastrostomy and is probably safer than the percutaneous approach in a child with multiple adhesions (fewer colon and liver injuries). Some patients who have had a failed intra-abdominal graft removed subsequently require insertion of a peritoneal dialysis catheter. This is made difficult by the loss of peritoneal domain due to extensive adhesions. We have had success using laparoscopic lysis of adhesions to create space and to aid in the placement of the catheter.

When treating children with ESRD, optimal surgical practice includes adherence to several general surgical principles: avoid blood transfusion (can cause blood antigen sensitization); be mindful of the location of the graft and the course of the ureter; exercise proper hygiene and use antibiotics judiciously to prevent infection; monitor blood loss and fluid status carefully; and avoid the administration of nephrotoxic drugs.

Diagnostic Studies

Preoperative

- Chest X-ray
- Voiding cystoureterogram

Postoperative

- Duplex sonography
- Nuclear renal scan

Parental Preparation

- Major operation, potential for long recovery
- Potential complications include graft thrombosis, rejection, urine leak, lymphocele
- Possibility of delayed graft function with potential need for post-transplant dialysis
- Lifelong need for immunosuppressive medications with potential complications
- Possibility of needing additional kidney transplant in the future
- Potential for disease recurrence in the transplanted kidney

Preoperative Preparation

- □ Optimize volume status
- □ Correct hyperkalemia
- □ No active infections
- □ Type and crossmatch
- □ Informed consent

Technical Points

- Flank incision via a retroperitoneal approach in children 20–30 kg and larger
- Midline incision is used to access the distal aorta and vena cava in children 20–30 kg or less
- Intraoperative heparin prior to clamping the recipient vasculature
- Minimize renal warm ischemic time
- A routine neoureterocystostomy does not require stenting
- The neoureterocystostomy should be created with absorbable suture

Suggested Reading

Baluarte HJ, Palmer JA, Petro J. Complications after renal transplantation. In: Kaplan BS, Meyers K, editors. The requisites series: pediatric nephrology and urology. Philadelphia: Elsevier Mosby; 2005a. p. 291–6.

Baluarte HJ, Palmer JA, Petro J. Evaluation for pediatric renal transplantation. In: Kaplan BS, Meyers K, editors. The requisites series: pediatric nephrology and urology. Philadelphia: Elsevier Mosby; 2005b. p. 284–90.

Baluarte HJ, Palmer JA, Petro J. Management of the pediatric renal transplant recipient. In: Kaplan BS, Meyers K, editors. The requisites series: pediatric and urology. Philadelphia: Elsevier Mosby; 2005c. p. 297–306.

Bartosh SM. Recipient characteristics. In: Fine RN, Webber SA, Olthoff KM, Kelly DA, Harmon WE, editors. Pediatric solid organ transplantation. 2nd ed. Malden: Blackwell Publishing; 2007. p. 146–52.

Fine RN. Renal transplantation in children: current practices. In: Ginss LC, Cosimi AB, Morris PJ, editors. Transplantation. Malden: Blackwell Science; 1999. p. 312–23.

Neu AM, Fivush BA. Outcomes and risk factors. In: Fine RN, Webber SA, Olthoff KM, Kelly DA, Harmon WE, editors. Pediatric solid organ transplantation. 2nd ed. Malden: Blackwell Publishing; 2007. p. 185–90.

North American Pediatric Renal Trials and Collaborative Studies. Annual Report. http://spitfire.emmes.com/study/ped/ (2007).

Papalois VE, Najarian JS. Historical notes. In: Fine RN, Webber SA, Olthoff KM, Kelly DA, Harmon WE, editors. Pediatric solid organ transplantation. 2nd ed. Malden: Blackwell Publishing; 2007. p. 139–45.

Patel UD, Thomas SE. Evaluation of the candidate. In: Fine RN, Webber SA, Olthoff KM, Kelly DA, Harmon WE, editors. Pediatric solid organ transplantation. 2nd ed. Malden: Blackwell Publishing; 2007. p. 153–60.

Scientific Registry of Transplant Recipients. Annual Report. http://www.ustransplant.org/ (2007).

Smith JM, McDonald RA. Post-transplant management. In: Fine RN, Webber SA, Olthoff KM, Kelly DA, Harmon WE, editors. Pediatric solid organ transplantation. 2nd ed. Malden: Blackwell Publishing; 2007. p. 174–84.

United States Renal Data System. Annual Report. http://www.usrds.org/ (2007).

Vukcevic Z, Ellis D, Bellinger M, Shapiro R. Donor evaluation, surgical technique and perioperative management. In: Fine RN, Webber SA, Olthoff KM, Kelly DA, Harmon WE, editors. Pediatric solid organ transplantation. 2nd ed. Malden: Blackwell Publishing; 2007. p. 161–6.

Wood EG, Hand M, Briscoe DM, et al. Risk factors for mortality in infants and young children on dialysis. Am J Kidney Dis. 2001; 37:573–9.

Chapter 108
Liver Transplantation

Maria H. Alonso

Few subspecialties have undergone the dramatic improvements in survival that have occurred in pediatric liver transplantation. In the early 1980s, survival rates of 30% limited the enthusiasm for this costly and work-intense operation. The introduction of more effective immunosuppression along with refinements in the operative and postoperative management of infants and children has improved survival rates to greater than 90%. When compared to the universally fatal outcome these patients would experience without transplantation, it is not surprising that liver transplantation has been embraced as the preferred therapy.

Indications

Children with extrahepatic biliary atresia constitute at least 50% of the pediatric liver transplant population. Successful biliary drainage achieving an anicteric state following the Kasai portoenterostomy is the most important factor affecting preservation of liver function and long-term survival. Primary transplantation without portoenterostomy is not recommended in patients with biliary atresia unless the initial presentation is at more than 120 days of age and the liver biopsy shows advanced cirrhosis. We believe that the Kasai portoenterostomy should be the primary surgical intervention for all other infants with extrahepatic biliary atresia. Patients with progressive disease following a Kasai procedure should be offered early orthotopic liver transplantation (OLT). The sequential use of these two procedures optimizes overall survival and organ use. Alagille syndrome (angiohepatic dysplasia) is an autosomal dominant genetic disorder manifest as bile duct paucity leading to progressive cholestasis, pruritus, xanthomas, malnutrition, and growth failure. Liver failure occurs late, if at all. Occasionally,

severe growth retardation, hypercholesterolemia, and pruritus can compromise the patient's overall well-being to the point where transplantation is valuable. Experience using external biliary diversion or internal ileal bypass accompanied by ursodeoxycholic acid therapy has demonstrated a significant decrease in both pruritus and complications of hypercholesterolemia. Both of these procedures can ameliorate or decrease the rate of ongoing parenchymal destruction and cirrhosis, obviating the need for liver transplantation.

Patients with fulminant hepatic failure without recognized antecedent liver disease present diagnostic and prognostic difficulties. Rapid clinical deterioration frequently makes establishment of a definitive diagnosis impossible before there is an urgent need for transplantation. Acute viral hepatitis of undefined type makes up the largest group, followed by drug toxicity and toxin exposure. Previously unrecognized metabolic disease must also be considered. Recently, an immune-based defect has been recognized as a cause of fulminant liver failure. This population needs to be identified as these children sometimes require a combination of bone marrow and liver transplantation to achieve long-term survival. When acceptable clinical and metabolic stability make liver biopsy safe, diagnostic information allowing directed treatment of the primary liver disease is helpful. The presence of ongoing coagulopathy often dictates the need for an open approach to biopsy.

Transplantation for hepatoblastoma is recommended for individuals who, after the administration of several cycles of chemotherapy, have a neoplasm confined to the liver that is un-resectable by conventional means. Children who had prior isolated metastasis that disappeared while undergoing preoperative chemotherapy can be considered in selected instances. Factors associated with a favorable prognosis include: (1) absence of prior surgical resection attempts; (2) unifocal rather than multifocal involvement; (3) absence of vascular invasion; and (4) fetal, as opposed to anaplastic or embryonal, histology. In addition to these staging factors, a favorable response to pretransplant chemotherapy suggests a more favorable long-term prognosis. Historically, recurrent disease has accounted for 50% of postoperative mortality; however, in our experience,

M.H. Alonso (✉)
Division of Pediatric and Thoracic Surgery, Cincinnati Children's Hospital Medical Center, 3333 Burnet Avenue, ML 2023, Cincinnati, OH 45229, USA
e-mail: alonm0@cchmc.org

P. Mattei (ed.), *Fundamentals of Pediatric Surgery*,
DOI 10.1007/978-1-4419-6643-8_108, © Springer Science+Business Media, LLC 2011

transplantation for unresectable hepatoblastoma followed by post-operative chemotherapy has lead to an overall survival of 88%. The role of transplantation has evolved such that in the upcoming Children's Oncology Group treatment study for the management of children with hepatoblastoma, early referral for transplant evaluation is recommended for those children who present with large lesions that appear un-resectable by conventional surgery.

Vascular tumors represent a group of patients with diffuse pathology who can benefit from transplantation. Children with intractable and progressive congestive heart failure, even when caused by non-neoplastic arteriovenous malformations or hemangioendothelioma, offer a unique opportunity for complete removal of the vascular malformation and correction of congestive heart failure. In our experience, transplantation in these instances offers significantly better long-term survival compared to embolization or hepatic artery occlusion which can precipitate sudden and widespread hepatic necrosis. For large or complex lesions it is essential to exclude angiosarcoma by pre-transplant biopsy.

The primary aim of the evaluation process is to define which patients require or would benefit from OLT and when such therapy should be undertaken. Evaluation should be directed toward the identification of: (1) progressive deterioration of hepatocellular function, (2) portal hypertension and gastrointestinal bleeding, or (3) malnutrition and growth failure. Referral for transplantation should occur when progressive deterioration is noted and before the development of life-threatening complications.

Contraindications

Contraindications to transplantation include: (1) extrahepatic unresectable malignancy, (2) malignancy metastatic to the liver, (3) progressive terminal non-hepatic disease, (4) uncontrolled systemic sepsis, and (5) severe irreversible neurologic injury. Relative contraindications to transplantation that need to be individually evaluated include: (1) advanced or partially treated systemic infection, (2) advanced hepatic encephalopathy, (3) severe psychosocial difficulties, (4) portal venous thrombosis extending throughout the mesenteric venous system, and (5) serology positive for HIV.

Donor Considerations

The single factor limiting the availability of OLT is the supply of donor organs. Since 1991, the number of patients awaiting liver transplantation has increased 11-fold. Available donor resources have not kept pace. As a consequence of this donor shortage, the time to transplant (waiting time) for all pediatric age groups has increased significantly, with young children and infants most affected. This severely limited supply of available donor organs has driven the advancement of many innovative liver transplant surgical procedures. The development of reduced-size liver transplantation allowed significant expansion of the donor pool for infants and small children. This not only improved the availability of donor organs but also allowed access to donors with improved stability and organ function. Evolution of these operative techniques has allowed the development of both split liver transplantation and living-donor (LD) transplantation. In the hands of experienced transplant teams, these procedures all have equivalent success to whole-organ transplantation. Furthermore, access to these many donor options has reduced waiting list mortality to less than 5%. Infants and children requiring transplantation benefit greatly by having access to all of these transplant options to minimize waiting time.

Assessment of donor organ suitability is undertaken by evaluating clinical information, static biochemical tests, and dynamic tests of hepatocellular function. Clinical factors identify donors who are at the limits of age, have had prolonged intensive care hospitalization and possibly sepsis, and have vasomotor instability requiring excessive vasoconstricting inotropic agents. Static biochemical tests identify pre-existing functional abnormalities or organ trauma but do not serve as good benchmarks to differentiate between acceptable and poor donor allografts. Donor liver biopsy is helpful in questionable cases to identify pre-existing liver disease or donor liver steatosis.

Anatomic replacement of the native liver in the orthotopic position requires selection or surgical preparation of the donor liver to fill but not to exceed available space in the recipient. When using full-sized allografts, a donor weight range 15–20% above or below that of the recipient is usually appropriate, taking into consideration body habitus and factors that would increase recipient abdominal size, such as ascites and hepatosplenomegaly. Surgical preparation of reduced-size liver allografts is based on the anatomy of the hepatic vasculature and bile ducts. Prolonged cold ischemic preservation allows the safe application of the extensive hypothermic bench surgery necessary for reduction techniques. The three primary reduced-size allografts used are the right lobe, the left lobe, and the left lateral segment, all prepared by ex-vivo hepatic resection.

The use of living donors has increased as the safety and success of this procedure has been demonstrated. One of the critical elements of LD transplantation is the proper selection of a donor, usually a parent or relative. This procedure is performed on the assumption that donor safety can be assured and that the donor's liver function is normal. Donors should be 21–55 years of age, have an ABO-compatible blood type, and have no acute or chronic medical conditions.

Careful attention must be paid to proper living donor consent. Parental concerns to help their ill child make true informed consent a challenge. A dedicated "donor advocate" not directly associated with the transplant team should assist with this process. Independent medical assessment of the donor is also essential. UNOS has recently established clear criteria for this process. After a satisfactory medical and psychological examination by a physician not directly involved with the transplant program, computed tomography is used to measure the volume of the potential donor segment to assure that it will meet the metabolic needs but not exceed the space available in the recipient. If acceptable, arteriography or CT angiography is undertaken to assess the hepatic arterial anatomy, thereby excluding potential donors with multiple arteries to segments 2 and 3, and facilitating minimal hilar vascular dissection at the time of transplantation. Experience has shown that 90% of donors who are deemed unacceptable were excluded on the basis of history, physical examination, laboratory screening, and ABO type. Donor safety has been excellent in all pediatric LD series.

Split-liver grafting involves the preparation of two allografts from a single donor. Two techniques have been used to accomplish hepatic division in the donor with similar overall success. The *ex-situ split* procedure divides the right lobe allograft (segments 5–8) from the left lateral segment allograft (segments 2 and 3) after the whole donor organ has been procured. Because this division is undertaken under vascular hypothermic conditions without hepatic perfusion, the vascular integrity of segment 4 is difficult to assess and it is frequently discarded. Conventional techniques for implanting the respective allografts are then used.

The successful experience with in-situ division of the living donor organ left lateral segment is a basis for the *in-situ split* procedure. Here the left lateral segment is prepared identically to a living related donor. The viability of segment 4 can be examined at the time of the division and it is usually incorporated with the right lobe graft to increase the cellular mass of the allograft. Because this procedure adds considerably to the donor procurement time, and the necessary skill of the donor team, it is more demanding and occasionally difficult to successfully orchestrate. Despite these considerations however, this technique is the preferred method for split-liver donor preparation.

The benefits of split-liver transplantation are best achieved when ideal donors are selected. Strict restrictions on age, vasopressor administration, predonation hepatic function, and limited donor hospitalization have been used to select optimal candidates for this donor procedure. When these donors are selected, the results from both in-situ and ex-situ techniques (Fig. 108.1) are similar, with both techniques now having patient survival for both allografts of 90–93% and graft survival rates of 86–89%.

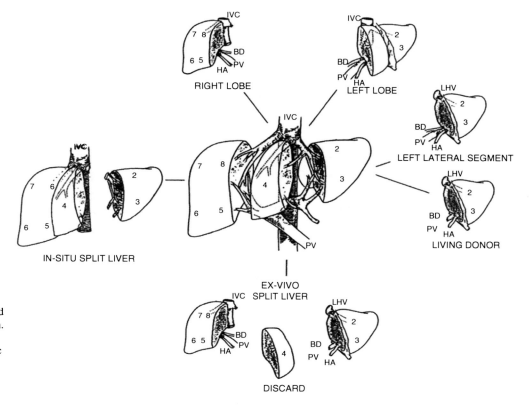

Fig. 108.1 Anatomic donor options available through surgical reduction. (Reprinted with permission from Ryckman FC, Alonso MH, Tiao GM. Solid organ transplantation in children. In: Ashcraft KW, Holcomb GW III, Murphy JP, editors. Pediatric surgery. Philadelphia: Elsevier Saunders; 2005. Copyright Elsevier 2005)

Surgical Technique

The transplant procedure is carried out through a bilateral subcostal incision with midline extension. Meticulous ligation of portosystemic collaterals and vascularized adhesions is necessary to avoid slow but relentless hemorrhage. Dissection of the hepatic hilum with division of the hepatic artery and portal vein above their bifurcation helps to achieve maximal recipient vessel length. The bile duct, when present, is divided high in the hilum to preserve the length and vasculature of the distal duct in case it is needed for primary reconstruction in older recipients. Preservation of the Roux-en-Y limb in biliary atresia patients who have undergone Kasai portoenterostomy simplifies later biliary reconstruction. Complete mobilization of the liver, with dissection of the suprahepatic vena cava to the diaphragm and the infrahepatic vena cava to the renal veins, completes the hepatectomy.

In children with serious vascular instability who cannot tolerate caval occlusion or who are receiving a LD organ, "piggy-back" implantation is necessary. In this procedure, the recipient vena cava is left intact and partial caval occlusion allows end-to-side implantation of a combined donor hepatic vein patch. Access to the infrarenal aorta to implant the celiac axis of the donor liver or iliac artery vascular conduits, provided by mobilizing the right colon and duodenum, is our preference for arterial reconstruction in complex allograft recipients.

Removal of the diseased liver is completed after vascular isolation is achieved. Retroperitoneal hemostasis is achieved before implanting the donor liver. In standard orthotopic transplantation, the suprahepatic vena cava is prepared by suture ligating any large phrenic orifices and creating one caval lumen from the confluence of the inferior vena cava and hepatic vein orifices. The donor liver is implanted using conventional vascular techniques and monofilament suture for the vascular anastomosis. When left lateral segment reduced-size grafts are used, the left hepatic vein orifice is anastomosed directly to the anterolateral surface of the infradiaphragmatic IVC using the combined right-middle hepatic vein orifices. The left lateral segment allograft is later fixed to the undersurface of the diaphragm to prevent torsion and venous obstruction of this anastomosis. Similar fixation is not necessary with right or left lobe allografts or with whole organ transplants.

Before completing the caval anastomosis, the preservation solution is flushed from the graft using 500–1,000 mL of hypothermic normokalemic intravenous solutions. When using full-sized grafts in older patients, we prefer to complete all venous anastomoses before reconstructing the hepatic artery. In reduced-size allografts and in small recipients where we prefer direct aortic vascular inflow reconstruction, the hepatic arterial anastomosis is completed before reconstructing the portal vein to improve visibility of the

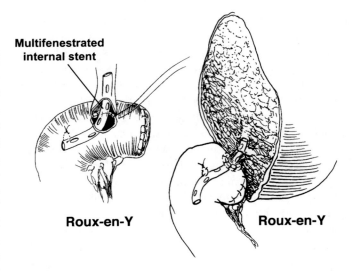

Fig. 108.2 Bile duct reconstruction using a Roux-en-Y with placement of an internal multi-fenestrated biliary stent into the common bile duct for a whole organ of left hepatic duct for a segment graft. (Reprinted with permission from Ryckman FC, Alonso MH, Tiao GM. Solid organ transplantation in children. In: Ashcraft KW, Holcomb GW III, Murphy JP, editors. Pediatric surgery. Philadelphia: Elsevier Saunders; 2005. Copyright Elsevier 2005)

infrarenal aorta without placing traction on the portal vein anastomosis. We often complete all anastomoses during vascular isolation before organ reperfusion, although some transplant teams reperfuse after venous reconstruction is complete.

Biliary reconstruction in patients with biliary atresia or in those weighing less than 25 kg is achieved through an end-to-side choledochojejunostomy using interrupted dissolving monofilament sutures. A multi-fenestrated silicone internal biliary stent is placed before completing the anastomosis (Fig. 108.2). In most cases, the prior Roux-en-Y can be used, with a 30–35 cm length being preferred. Primary bile duct reconstruction without stenting is used in older patients with whole organ allografts.

When closing the abdomen, increased intra-abdominal pressure should be avoided. In many cases, avoidance of fascial closure and the use of mobilized skin flaps and running monofilament skin closure are advisable. Musculofascial abdominal closure can be completed before patient discharge.

Postoperative Care

Most centers use an immunosuppressive protocol based on the administration of multiple complementary medications including corticosteroids and cyclosporine or tacrolimus. Additional antimetabolites (azathioprine, mycophenolate) are used when more treatment is needed. Prior protocols using polyclonal or monoclonal induction therapy have been abandoned in most cases due to the extent of the immunosuppressive potency. The

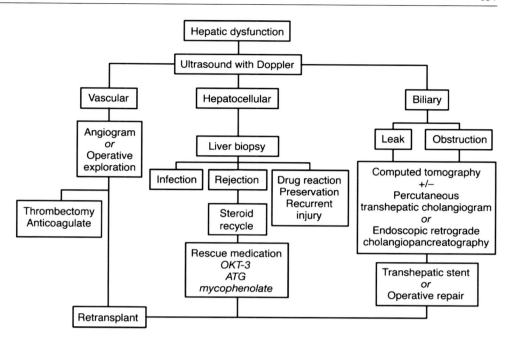

Fig. 108.3 Schematic flow diagram for management of postoperative liver allograft dysfunction. *ATG* antithymocyte globulin; *OKT-3* monoclonal antibody. (Reprinted with permission from Ryckman FC, Alonso MH, Tiao GM. Solid organ transplantation in children. In: Ashcraft KW, Holcomb GW III, Murphy JP, editors. Pediatric surgery. Philadelphia: Elsevier Saunders; 2005. Copyright Elsevier 2005)

recent introduction of humanized monoclonal antibodies to IL-2 (Basiliximab, Daclizumab) has stimulated interest in induction immunosuppression protocols, as these agents appear to have a low risk of opportunistic infections. The role that they will play in the future is not clear at present.

Most postoperative complications present as cholestasis, increasing hepatocellular enzyme levels, and on occasion fever, lethargy, and anorexia. This nonspecific symptom complex requires diagnostic evaluation before instituting treatment. Therapy directed at the specific causes of allograft dysfunction is essential (Fig. 108.3); empiric therapy of presumed complications is fraught with misdiagnoses, morbidity, and mortality.

Primary Nonfunction

Primary nonfunction (PNF) of the hepatic allograft implies the absence of metabolic and synthetic activity following transplantation. Complete nonfunction requires immediate retransplantation before irreversible coagulopathy and cerebral edema occur. More frequently, lesser degrees of allograft dysfunction occur and can be associated with several donor, recipient, and operative factors. The status of the donor liver contributes significantly to the potential for PNF. Ischemic injury secondary to anemia, hypotension, hypoxia, or direct tissue injury is often difficult to ascertain in the history of multiple trauma victims. Donor liver steatosis has also been recognized as a factor contributing to severe dysfunction or nonfunction in the donor liver. *Macrovesicular steatosis* on donor liver biopsy is somewhat more common in adult than pediatric donors and, when severe, is recognized grossly by

the enlarged yellow, greasy consistency of the donor liver. The risk of PNF increases as the degree of fatty infiltration increases. Microscopic findings are classified as mild if less than 30% of the hepatocytes have fatty infiltration, moderate if 30–60% are involved, and severe if more than 60% of the hepatocytes have fatty infiltration. Livers with severe fatty infiltration should be discarded, and donors with moderate involvement are used with some concern. Documentation of functional hepatic recovery is best undertaken by evaluating the ongoing hepatic output of clotting factors (V, VII) with improvement in coagulation parameters (PT, PTT) and the synthesis of bile. Protocol hepatic biopsies assist in the documentation of hepatic histologic and immunologic events, but they cannot accurately predict the likelihood of recovery.

Vascular Thrombosis

Hepatic artery thrombosis (HAT) occurs in children three to four times more frequently than in adult transplant series, most often within the first 30 days following transplantation. HAT presents with a variable clinical picture that might include fulminant allograft failure, biliary disruption or obstruction, or systemic sepsis. Doppler ultrasound imaging has been accurate in identifying arterial thrombosis and it is used as the primary screening modality to assess blood flow following transplantation or whenever complications arise. Acute HAT with allograft failure most often requires immediate retransplantation. Successful thrombectomy and allograft salvage is possible if reconstruction is undertaken before the onset of allograft necrosis. Biliary complications are particularly common following HAT. Ischemic biliary disruption with intraparenchymal biloma formation or anastomotic disruption presents with cholestasis associated with systemic sepsis. The development of systemic septicemia or multifocal abscesses in sites of ischemic necrosis secondary to gram-negative enteric bacteria, *Enterococcus*, anaerobic bacteria, or fungi can also be seen. Antibiotic therapy directed toward these organisms, along with surgical drainage, is indicated when specific abscess sites are identified. Percutaneous drainage and biliary stenting may control bile leakage and infection until retransplantation is undertaken.

Prevention of HAT requires meticulous microsurgical arterial reconstruction at the time of transplantation. Anatomic reconstruction is preferred in whole organ allografts; direct implantation of the celiac axis into the infrarenal aorta is recommended for all reduced-size liver allografts. All complex vascular reconstructions of the donor hepatic artery should be undertaken ex vivo whenever possible using microsurgical techniques before transplantation. When vascular grafts are required, they should also be directly implanted into the infrarenal aorta. No systemic anticoagulation was routinely used in our series, but aspirin (20–40 mg/day) is administered to all children for 100 days. Complex protocols administering both procoagulants and anticoagulants have also been very successful.

Portal vein thrombosis is uncommon in whole organ allografts unless prior portosystemic shunting has altered the flow within the splanchnic vascular bed or unless severe portal vein stenosis in the recipient has impaired flow to the allograft. Preexisting portal vein thrombosis in the recipient can be overcome by thrombectomy, portal vein replacement, or extra anatomic venous bypass. In biliary atresia recipients, pre-existing portal vein hypoplasia is best corrected by anastomosis to the confluence of the splenic and superior mesenteric veins in the recipient. When inadequate portal vein length is present on the donor organ, iliac vein interposition grafts are used. Early thrombosis following transplantation requires immediate anastomotic revision and thrombectomy. Discrepancies in venous size imposed by reduced-size allografts can be modified to allow anastomotic construction. Deficiencies of anticoagulant proteins, such as protein C and S, and antithrombin III deficiency in the recipient must also be excluded as a contributing cause for vascular thrombosis. Failure to recognize portal vein thrombosis can lead to either allograft demise or, on a more chronic basis, to significant portal hypertension with hemorrhagic sequelae or intractable ascites.

Biliary Complications

Complications related to biliary reconstruction occur in approximately 10% of pediatric liver transplant recipients. Their spectrum and treatment are determined by the status of the hepatic artery and the type of allograft used. Although whole and reduced-size allografts have an equivalent risk of biliary complications, the spectrum of complications differs. Primary bile duct reconstruction is the preferred biliary reconstruction in adults, but it is less commonly used in children. It has the advantage of preserving the sphincter of Oddi, decreasing the incidence of enteric reflux and subsequent cholangitis, and not requiring an intestinal anastomosis. Early experience using primary choledochocholedochostomy without a T-tube has been favorable. Late complications following any type of primary ductal reconstruction include anastomotic stricture, biliary sludge formation, and recurrent cholangitis. Endoscopic dilation and internal stenting of anastomotic strictures has been successful in early postoperative cases. Roux-en-Y choledochojejunostomy is the preferred treatment for recurrent stenosis or postoperative leak.

Roux-en-Y choledochojejunostomy is the reconstruction of choice in small children and is required in all patients with biliary atresia. Recurrent cholangitis, a theoretical risk, suggests anastomotic or intrahepatic biliary stricture formation or small bowel obstruction within the Roux limb or distal to the Roux-en-Y anastomosis. In the absence of these complications, cholangitis is uncommon. Reconstruction of the bile ducts in patients with reduced-size allografts is more complex. Division of the bile duct in close proximity to the cut-surface margin of the allograft, with careful preservation of the biliary duct collateral circulation, decreases but does not eliminate ductal stricture formation secondary to ductal ischemia. In our early experience, 14% of patients with left lobe reduced-size allografts developed a short segmental stricture requiring biliary anastomotic revision (Fig. 108.4). Operative revision of the biliary anastomosis and reimplantation of the bile ducts into the Roux-en-Y is necessary. Percutaneous transhepatic cholangiography is essential to define the intrahepatic ductal anatomy before operative revision, and temporary catheter decompression of the obstructed bile ducts allows treatment of cholangitis and elective reconstruction. Operative reconstruction is accompanied by transhepatic passage of exteriorized multifenestrated biliary ductal stents, which remain in place until reconstructive success is documented and late stenosis is unlikely. Dissection remote from the vasobiliary sheath in the donor has significantly decreased the incidence of this complication.

Biliary complications have been seen with an increased frequency following living donation in pediatric recipients. The left lateral segment 2 and 3 bile ducts are frequently separate at the plane of parenchymal division. The need for individual drainage of these small biliary ducts makes the development of late anastomotic stenosis more frequent. Individual segmental strictures do not always lead to jaundice in the recipient, but rather are identified by elevated serum gamma glutamyl transferase levels or through ultrasound surveillance. Re-operation after ductal dilatation

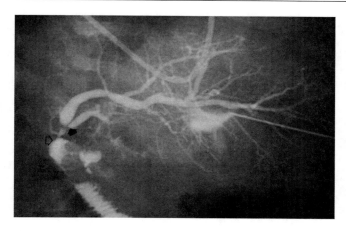

Fig. 108.4 Segmental bile duct stricture at the junction of the left lateral and left medial segmental bile ducts in a left lobe reduced size allograft. Solid arrow, bile duct stricture; open arrow, Roux-en-Y loop and bile duct anastomosis. (Reprinted from Ryckman FC, et al. Liver transplantation in children. In: Souchy FJ, editor. Liver disease in children, St. Louis: CV Mosby; 1994.)

allows for easier reconstruction due to the increased caliber of the segmental bile duct.

Acute Cellular Rejection

Allograft rejection is characterized by the histologic triad of endothelialitis, portal triad lymphocyte infiltration with bile duct injury, and hepatic parenchymal cell damage. Allograft biopsy is essential to establish the diagnosis before treatment. The rapidity of the rejection process and its response to therapy dictates the intensity and duration of antirejection treatment. Acute rejection occurs in approximately two thirds of patients following OLT. The primary treatment of rejection is a short course of high-dose steroids. Bolus doses administered over several days with a rapid taper to baseline therapy is successful in 75–80% of cases. When refractory or recurrent rejection occurs, antilymphocyte therapy using the monoclonal antibody directed against CD3 (OKT-3) or anti-thymocyte globulin (Thymoglobulin) is successful in 90% of cases.

Infection

Infectious complications have become the most common source of morbidity and mortality following transplantation. Multiple organism infection is common as are concurrent infections by different infectious agents. Bacterial infections occur in the immediate post-transplant period and are most often caused by gram-negative enteric organisms, *Enterococcus*, or *Staphylococcus* species. Intra-abdominal abscesses or infected collections of serum along the cut surface of the reduced-size allograft are best

addressed with extraperitoneal or laparotomy drainage; in our experience, percutaneous drainage has been less successful. Intrahepatic abscesses suggest hepatic artery stenosis or thrombosis and treatment is directed by the vascular status of the allograft and associated bile duct abnormalities. Sepsis originating at sites of invasive monitoring lines can be minimized by replacing or removing all intra-operative lines soon after transplantation. Antibacterial prophylactic antibiotics are discontinued as soon as possible to prevent the development of resistant organisms.

Fungal sepsis represents a significant potential problem in the early post-transplant period. Aggressive protocols for pretransplant prophylaxis are based on the concept that fungal infections originate from organisms colonizing the GI tract of the recipient. Selective bowel decontamination was successful in eliminating pathogenic gram-negative bacteria from the GI tract in 87% of adult patients and, in all cases, *Candida* was eliminated. However, these protocols have not been practical in pediatric patients because there is a long waiting time for pediatric organs and the palatability of the antibiotics used is poor. These regimens are commonly used in the preoperative preparation for combined liver/small intestinal transplantation. Fungal infection most often occurs in patients requiring multiple operative procedures and those who have had numerous antibiotic courses. Fungemia or urosepsis requires retinal and cardiac investigation and a search for renal fungal involvement; antifungal therapy should be undertaken promptly. Severe fungal infection is associated with greater than 80% mortality, making early treatment essential. All patients undergoing OLT should receive antifungal prophylaxis with fluconazole.

The majority of early and severe viral infections are caused by viruses of the Herpesviridae family, including Epstein–Barr virus (EBV), cytomegalovirus (CMV), and herpes simplex virus (HSV). CMV transmission dynamics are well studied and serve as a prototype for herpesvirus transmission in the transplant population. The likelihood that CMV infection will develop is influenced by the preoperative CMV status of the transplant donor and recipient. Seronegative recipients receiving seropositive donor organs are at greatest risk, with seropositive donor to recipient combinations at the next greatest risk. Use of various immune-based prophylactic protocols including IV IgG or hyper-immune anti-CMV IgG, coupled with acyclovir or ganciclovir/valganciclovir have all achieved success in decreasing the incidence of symptomatic CMV infection, although seroconversion in naive recipients of seropositive donor organs inevitably occurs.

EBV infection occurring in the perioperative period represents a significant risk to the pediatric transplant recipient. It has a varying presentation including a mononucleosis-like syndrome, hepatitis-simulating rejection, extranodal lymphoproliferative infiltration with bowel perforation, peritonsillar or lymph node enlargement, or encephalopathy.

In small children, its primary portal of entry is often the tonsils, making asymptomatic tonsillar hypertrophy a common initial presentation. EBV infection can occur as a primary infection or following reactivation of a past primary infection. When serologic evidence of active infection exists, an acute reduction in immunosuppression is indicated. It has become clear that continuous surveillance is necessary as the presentation is often nonspecific and the prognosis is related to early diagnosis. Screening by determination of EBV blood viral load by quantitative PCR appears to be the best current predictor of risk. Post-transplant lymphoproliferative disease (PTLD), a potentially fatal abnormal proliferation of B lymphocytes, can occur in any immunosuppressed individual. The importance of PTLD in pediatric liver transplantation is a result of the intensity of the immunosuppression required, its lifetime duration, and the absence of prior exposure to EBV infection in 60–80% of pediatric recipients. PTLD is the most common tumor in children following transplantation, representing 52% of all tumors compared to 15% in adults. About 80% of cases occur within the first 2 years following transplantation. The second pathogenic feature influencing PTLD appears to be EBV infection. Primary or reactivation infections usually precede the recognition of PTLD. A simultaneous increase in cytotoxic T-cell activity is the normal primary host mechanism preventing EBV dissemination. Loss of this natural protection as a result of the administration of T-cell inhibitory immunotherapy allows polyclonal B-cell proliferation to progress. Polyclonal proliferation of B-lymphocytes occurs following EBV viral replication and release. These EBV proliferating cells express specific viral antigens which represent possible targets for the immune system, thereby explaining the well described regression of PTLD after immunosuppressive tapering. With time, transformation of a small population of cells results in a malignant monoclonal aggressive B-cell lymphoma. Treatment of PTLD is stratified according to the immunologic cell typing and clinical presentation. Documented PTLD requires an immediate decrease or discontinuation of immunosuppression and institution of anti-EBV therapy. We prefer to use IV ganciclovir for initial antiviral therapy owing to the high incidence of concurrent CMV infection. Patients with polyclonal B-cell proliferation frequently show regression with this treatment. If tumor cells express B-cell marker CD20 at histology, the anti-CD20 monoclonal antibody Rituximab can be administered as weekly infusions of 375 mg/m².

Renal Insufficiency

The long-term success of liver transplantation has been related to effective immunosuppression with calcineurin-inhibitors (CNI) such as cyclosporine and tacrolimus. However, nephrotoxicity associated with their long-term use has become a major problem, affecting up to 70% of all non-renal recipients. Impaired glomerular filtration rate in pediatric recipients with stable graft function represents a serious problem. Up to 20% have a drop in GFR to below 50 mL/min/1.73m², and 5% progress to end-stage renal disease. Cyclosporin and tacrolimus both appear to be similar in risk. Efforts to reverse ongoing renal insufficiency using protocols that include instituting non-nephrotoxic agents, such as mycophenolate mofetil (MMF), while decreasing the CNI dose, have shown some success in improving GFR while protecting against unacceptable risks of acute rejection at the time of immunosuppressive drug conversion. Efforts to completely eliminate CNI administration have been complicated by acute or ductopenic rejection. Present efforts suggest that earlier staged reduction of the CNI prior to the development of severe GFR reduction will decrease but not eliminate this complication. Once established, chronic renal failure does not appear to resolve with CNI dose adjustment.

Retransplantation

The vast majority of retransplantation procedures in pediatric patients are done as a result of acute allograft demise caused by HAT or PNF. Acute rejection, chronic rejection, and biliary complications are less common causes. Many of these complications are associated with concurrent sepsis, which further complicates reoperation and compromises success. Survival following transplantation is directly related to prompt identification of appropriate patients and acquisition of a suitable organ. In our experience, when retransplantation is promptly undertaken for early graft failure, patient survival rate is 73%. However, when retransplantation is undertaken for chronic allograft failure, often complicated by multiple organ system insufficiency, survival is only 45%.

Outcomes

Although the potential complications following liver transplantation are frequent and severe, the overall results are rewarding. Improvements in organ preservation, operative management, immunosuppression, and treatment of postoperative complications have all contributed to excellent survival rates. Most successful transplant programs have reached overall 1-year survival rates of 90%, with greatly decreased risk thereafter. Similar if not better results have resulted from living donor transplantation, especially for small recipients. Infants younger than 1 year of age or weighing less than 10 kg have historically had survival rates of 65–88% overall, an improvement over initial reported rates of 50–60% during the early era of OLT development. Survival rates in infants now equal those seen in older children. Improved survival in these small recipients is consistent throughout all levels of medical urgency and results from a decrease in life-threatening and graft-threatening complications, such as HAT and PNF, in the reduced-size donor organ. Patients with fulminant hepatic failure have an overall survival rate that is significantly lower than other diagnostic groups, patients with metabolic disease having the highest survival rate. The most important factor determining survival is the severity of the patient's illness at the time of transplantation. When stratified for illness by PELD scores, Pediatric Risk of Mortality (PRISM) score, and the previous UNOS score, the PRISM score was the most accurate in predicting both survival and morbidity during the peri-operative period. Present efforts to use surgically altered allografts, such as RSOLT, LD-OLT, and split liver OLT, have experienced similar survival rates as those for whole organ recipients (Fig. 108.5).

The increased donor availability for small recipients achieved through the use of surgically reduced, split, or living donor organs has also brought about a significant decrease in waiting list mortality. In our center, mortality rate for patients awaiting transplantation decreased from 29 to 2%, and similar results have been reported by other pediatric centers. Efforts to enhance donor availability, allowing transplantation of children before they reach critical status is essential before major improvements in postoperative survival rates can occur.

The significant success now achieved following liver transplantation cannot overshadow the need for improved

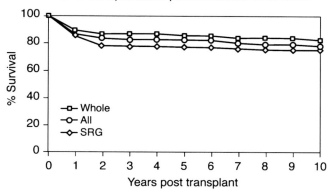

Fig. 108.5 Ten year patient and the allograft survival subdivided by whole and surgically reduced grafts, Cincinnati Children's Hospital Medical Center-Liver Care Center. (Reprinted with permission from Ryckman FC, Alonso MH, Tiao GM. Solid organ transplantation in children. In: Ashcraft KW, Holcomb GW III, Murphy JP, editors. Pediatric surgery. Philadelphia: Elsevier Saunders; 2005. Copyright Elsevier 2005)

management of post-transplant consequences of immunosuppression and pre-OLT chronic disease. The most significant factors contributing to long-term failure of the allograft or patient death in our program and others are consequences of immunosuppressive medications, such as late infection, PTLD, and chronic rejection of the allograft. Our ability to successfully address these challenges will determine the lifelong success of transplantation for our youngest recipients.

Summary Points

- Liver transplantation is a life saving intervention but carries long-term consequences.
- Biliary atresia is the most common indication for pediatric liver transplantation.
- Unresectable hepatoblastoma is an indication for liver transplantation.
- Technical advances have increased donor options for children reducing waiting list mortality.
- The transplant procedure remains technically challenging.
- Complications following transplant are extensive and varied.
- Life-long immunosuppression associated with attendant complications.

Editor's Comment

Pediatric liver transplantation programs currently achieve excellent results almost routinely. It is easy to forget that these are long and challenging operations with many potential complications, both technical and immunologic. Many of these children are quite ill and coagulopathic, making their preoperative assessment and preparation critically important aspects of their care. The task of "preopping" the patient often falls to a junior member of the surgical team, who might consider it a mundane chore; however, it is important to take this role seriously as poor preparation or a missed infection

can cause significant harm to the patient. Fortunately, when the liver has been placed and is functional, the patient often becomes immediately more stable and the coagulopathy resolves within the first 8–12 h.

Hepatoblastoma is a primary hepatic malignancy that affects young children and is only considered curable if the entire tumor is excised with negative margins. Some children with "unresectable" tumors are candidates for hepatectomy and liver replacement by transplantation. These patients should be referred for evaluation early in the course of their disease because, although primary hepatectomy and transplantation, even after neoadjuvant chemotherapy, is associated with a relatively high chance of cure, the results of salvage transplantation after a failed hepatic resection are not nearly as good. Likewise, if a hepatoblastoma appears to be resectable only by performing a non-anatomic or unorthodox resection, one should, depending on the experience and confidence of the general surgeon at his or her institution, consider referring the patient to an experienced transplant surgeon: their experience with performing split-liver transplants and living-related transplants is useful when having to excise a large tumor with a margin when this requires a creative biliary or vascular reconstruction.

There are other techniques more frequently used by transplant surgeons that can occasionally be useful for the general surgeon during hepatic resection or trauma. Aggressive liver tumor resection or extraction of an adherent Wilms tumor thrombus will sometimes require removal of a portion of the inferior vena cava in order to obtain a negative margin. Reconstruction of the vena cava can be challenging but can be accomplished with the use of a polytetrafluoroethylene graft material, usually as a patch that is cut to the appropriate size and shape. During a prolonged resection or repair of a large liver resection, especially if the vena cava is involved, it is sometimes necessary to employ the Pringle maneuver. To prevent bowel congestion due to prolonged portal vein obstruction and lower body edema during caval occlusion, shunt tubing can be inserted into mesenteric veins and the inferior vena cava, with the blood returning to a large systemic vein above the diaphragm. Finally, the techniques that have been developed to create a secure biliary-enteric can be applied in other hepatobiliary operations: meticulous mucosa-to-mucosa approximation with fine absorbable suture, placement of a stent when the bile duct is small, liberal use of roux-en-Y hepatico-jejunostomy, consistent use of closed suction drains.

Parental Preparation

- Extensive consultation with liver transplant team is vital.
- Perioperative and postoperative complications extensive.

Technical Points

- Recipient hepatectomy provides excellent technical experience.
- Understanding of donor procurement procedure is extremely beneficial as anatomy relevant to pediatric surgery tumor resections.

Suggested Reading

Broelsch CE, Whitington PF, Emond JC, et al. Liver transplantation in children from living related donors. Surgical techniques and results. Ann Surg. 1991;214(4):428–37.

Reyes JD, Carr B, Dvorchik I, et al. Liver transplantation and chemotherapy for hepatoblastoma and hepatocellular cancer in childhood and adolescence. J Pediatr. 2000;136(6):795–804.

Ryckman F, Fisher R, Pedersen S, et al. Improved survival in biliary atresia patients in the present era of liver transplantation. J Pediatr Surg. 1993;28(3):382–5.

SPLIT Research Group. Studies of Pediatric Liver Transplantation (SPLIT): year 2000 outcomes. Transplantation. 2001;72(3):463–76.

Chapter 109
Intestinal Transplantation

Thomas M. Fishbein

Intestinal transplantation is increasingly accepted as standard therapy for patients who develop intestinal and parenteral nutrition failure. While early attempts at intestinal transplantation more than 40 years ago met with limited success, progress has led to clinical success that parallels other solid-organ transplants. Intestinal transplants are now performed for children who suffer a failure of gut function from a variety of causes. In such cases, the state of nutritional failure is irreversible and no other therapy can guarantee long-term survival. In rare instances, gut function can be preserved, but anatomical defects, such as congenital malformation or mesenteric tumors require exenteration in order to preserve life. Thus, candidates fail parenteral nutrition, cannot adapt to life on parenteral nutrition, or require removal of the native gut in order to survive.

The principles of current intestinal transplant practice include appropriate patient and donor selection, organ procurement, the transplantation procedures, and early postoperative management. Currently, this practice is restricted to a small number of centers with considerable experience. However, the number of intestinal transplants performed in children has grown over the last decade and approval for reimbursement of these procedures, granted by the Centers for Medicare and Medicaid in 2001, heralded broader application of these procedures.

Candidates for intestinal transplantation are children who experience actual or impending irreversible loss of life-sustaining nutritional function of the gastrointestinal tract (Table 109.1). Three categories of disease account for most patients requiring intestinal transplants. (1) Short bowel syndrome (60%) resulting from neonatal and early childhood diseases requiring in most cases pediatric surgical intervention. Gastroschisis, omphalocele, necrotizing enterocolitis, volvulus, and extensive jejunoileal atresias account for the majority of such cases. More rarely, patients have short-gut syndrome due to vascular injury or other post-traumatic states. (2) Functional disorders of the intestine might also require transplantation. Epithelial disorders of enterocyte function, such as microvillus inclusion disease, tufting enteropathy, and autoimmune enteritis have all led to infantile diarrhea and preclude enteral feeding. In these cases, parenteral nutrition is required due to lack of absorptive function. Motility disorders, such as total intestinal aganglionosis (Hirschsprung disease), Berdon's syndrome (megacystis-microcolon hypoperistalsis syndrome), and other forms of visceral neuropathy or myopathy, also result in failure of intestinal function. (3) Tumors occurring in late adolescence, such as desmoids in the setting of Gardner syndrome, can also cause secondary complications leading to the need for intestinal transplantation. Usually, such tumors cause or threaten to cause ureteral or intestinal obstruction, fistula formation, central necrosis, and secondary superinfection. If such patients fail recognized medical therapies, radical exenteration and intestinal transplantation can be curative.

Patients undergoing intestinal transplantation have irreversible loss of gut nutritional function, and most such patients have failed parenteral nutritional therapy. While short-term parenteral nutrition is associated with excellent survival rates, long-term continuous therapy for intestinal failure is associated with significant risk of complications and death. The most common indication for intestinal transplantation is the evolution of parenteral nutrition-associated liver disease (PNALD). This can range from early mild cholestasis to cirrhosis and portal hypertension. The degree of liver disease is commonly underrepresented on liver biopsy. The mechanisms of liver disease associated with intestinal failure and parenteral nutrition delivery are incompletely understood, however it is usually a cholestatic process associated with early development of portal hypertension. Complications such as variceal bleeding due to esophageal or gastric varices are rare with this form of liver disease. Rather, when enteral tubes or stomas are present, varices frequently develop at mucocutaneous interfaces causing recurrent low-grade bleeding. This is a common sign of advanced PNALD.

T.M. Fishbein (✉)
Georgetown University Hospital, Transplant Institute, 3800 Reservoir Road, NW, 2 Main, Washington, DC 20007, USA
e-mail: thomas.m.fishbein@medstar.net

P. Mattei (ed.), *Fundamentals of Pediatric Surgery*,
DOI 10.1007/978-1-4419-6643-8_109, © Springer Science+Business Media, LLC 2011

Table 109.1 Diagnosis in 78 children undergoing intestinal transplantation by the author

Diagnosis	n	Percentage (%)
Gastroschisis	24	31
NEC	17	21
Motility disorder	15	19
Volvulus	9	12
Atresia	7	9
Epithelial disorder	6	8

Long-term parenteral nutrition is also associated with catheter-associated sepsis. Infections are more frequent among patients with intestinal motility disorders. Sepsis episodes associated with hemodynamic instability, respiratory failure, or frequent infections with pathogenic organisms suggest the need to consider transplantation. Loss of vascular access for parenteral nutrition delivery is another indication for intestinal transplantation. Children undergoing repeated line changes due to infectious or thrombotic complications can lose common routes of access for parenteral nutrition delivery.

Candidates for intestinal transplantation should have sufficient cardiopulmonary reserve to undergo transplantation and withstand an extensive ventilatory requirement. Patients with prior bronchopulmonary dysplasia, interstitial lung disease or oxygen requirement require close evaluation of their ability to tolerate the major volume shifts, massive transfusion, and prolonged ventilation that occur in the setting of a multiorgan transplant. Other relative contraindications include right-sided heart failure associated with severe congenital cardiac anomalies, limited outlook for neuropsychiatric or intellectual development, and concomitant diseases resulting in multisystem organ failure.

Candidates should have adequate renal reserve and endocrine pancreatic function. These factors can mitigate the type of transplant chosen, although they would likely not preclude transplantation. Patients with prior parenteral nutrition-associated pancreatitis, evolving liver disease, or renal insufficiency may require a multiorgan allograft.

Preoperative studies usually include small bowel and colonic contrast imaging, MRI or spiral CT to assess vascular access route patency, assessment of liver function and signs of portal hypertension, and urine creatinine clearance. Cardiopulmonary reserve is evaluated with two-dimensional echocardiogram and pulmonary function tests as indicated.

Parental preparation is an extremely important aspect of small intestinal transplantation. Intestinal transplantation is presented as life-saving therapy. The follow-up care is significant, and often requires frequent travel to a distant transplant program. Home administration of medications, enteral tube feeding, and frequent office visits are routine. Graft failure due to chronic dysfunction can occur years after transplantation. Parents should undergo a thorough psychosocial evaluation prior to the patient being listed for transplantation.

They should be informed of current survival and failure rates, the possibility of death while awaiting organ availability, and recognition of the potential for graft failure or death despite successful surgery.

Transplant Graft Types

Intestinal transplant evaluation must determine if a candidate should receive an isolated intestinal transplant or a multiorgan allograft. When only jejunoileum or jejunoileum and colon have been affected, an *isolated intestinal transplant* is usually indicated. When liver disease is pronounced, combined liver and intestine transplants are usually required. However, the liver can recover from cholestasis and even early fibrosis if parenteral nutrition is discontinued after successful intestinal transplantation. If other organs are required with the transplant, a decision between liver and intestine transplantation and multivisceral transplantation must be made. When gastric function is impaired significantly or a prior gastric resection has occurred, *multivisceral transplantation* is preferable. If the foregut of the candidate is intact, the stomach, duodenum, pancreas, and spleen can be salvaged and a combined *liver and small-bowel transplant* is preferable. We have obtained excellent results including colon for candidates who have no functional colon, but have a functioning rectum and sphincteric mechanism. An additional graft type is the *modified multivisceral transplant* in which the transplant recipient's liver is salvaged, but a stomach, pancreas, and jejunoileal allograft are transplanted. This en-bloc graft is drained through portal outflow into the native liver.

Isolated Intestinal Transplant

Isolated intestinal transplants refer to an allograft at the jejunoileum based on the superior mesenteric artery and vein. These can be performed with mesenteric vascular supply (inflow from the superior mesenteric artery and outflow through the superior mesenteric vein) or systemic drainage (inflow from the infrarenal aorta and outflow through the inferior vena cava). Enterectomy of the native small bowel and right colon is required in the case of dysmotility or an enterocyte disorder. This allows preservation of the superior mesenteric vessels for implantation of the graft. Proximal continuity is reestablished with a jejuno-jejunal anastomosis and a distal ileostomy is made. The mesenteric base must then be reconstructed to the retroperitoneum to avoid volvulus or internal herniation. The ileocolonic anastomosis can be performed with a proximal protective loop ileostomy or else a Santulli-type ileostomy can be made. If the right colon is transplanted with the allograft, a colo-colostomy is performed in conjunction with a proximal diverting loop.

Liver and Small-Bowel Transplant

This transplant includes a donor allograft of liver, duodenum, pancreas, and jejunoileum. The operations commences with a liver transplant incision and removal of the native liver. Preservation of the proximal foregut requires a portocaval shunt to be constructed providing venous outflow. Next, inflow needs to be obtained to the infrarenal aorta of the donor allograft. This brings blood supply to the donor superior mesenteric artery and celiac arteries, supplying the "en bloc" organ allograft. I prefer to transpose the pediatric donor's thoracic aorta as an interposition graft with anastomosis to the infrarenal aorta of the recipient. The end of this conduit is then anastomosed to the donor aorta just inferior to the superior mesenteric artery. Since the small baby aorta is deep in the retroperitoneum, the placement of this interposition grafts facilitates revascularization of the organs. Venous outflow is by piggy-back drainage of the suprahepatic vena cava of the donor liver to the cloaca of the recipient hepatic veins. Jejuno-jejunal continuity is then established distal to the graft ligament of Treitz by a recipient-to-donor anastomosis. Distal reconstruction is similar to that used for isolated intestinal transplantation.

Multivisceral Transplantation

In multivisceral transplantation, the entire gastrointestinal tract is eviscerated, leaving only the urogenital tract and retroperitoneum. The explant proceeds with mobilization of the recipient's liver off of the retrohepatic vena cava. A medial visceral rotation mobilizes the spleen, distal pancreas and stomach. The right colon, base of the mesentery, and duodenum are reflected medially from the right side, exposing the base of the SMA. Ligation of the SMA and celiac artery allows them to be transected. The hepatic veins can be clamped and the entire gastrointestinal tract removed after dividing the proximal stomach and left colon. Implantation of the allograft utilizes either direct reconstruction of celiac and superior mesenteric arteries or the use of supraceliac or infrarenal donor aortic conduit. Once the organs are reperfused, intestinal reconstruction is undertaken with a proximal gastrogastrostomy and a distal reconstruction. However, pyloroplasty or pyloromyotomy must be performed to provide gastric emptying, which is significantly impaired by transection of vagal innervation at organ procurement.

Postoperative Management

In all cases, we place a feeding tube to facilitate enteral medications and nutrition early after transplant. The ileostomy provides access for surveillance endoscopy and biopsy in the early phase. Patients are at early risk for bleeding, vascular thrombosis and ischemia, perforation, and anastomotic leak early after transplantation. Liberal use of second look laparotomy is encouraged. Peritonitis can result from translocation from the allograft after reperfusion and sometimes requires reoperation and peritoneal lavage. Peri-operative antibiotic use should provide prophylaxis against bacteria, fungi, and viruses (CMV, EBV). Peri-stomal hernia and internal hernias sometimes occur, as the mesenteric base is not naturally affixed to the retroperitoneum.

Nutrition

Semi-elemental enteral formula is begun after the first week due to intolerance to fat and intact protein early after transplantation because lymphatic reconstitution has yet to occur. Isosmolar feeding should be started due to the frequency of type 1 dumping syndrome. Formula is advanced and parenteral nutrition weaned over 2–8 weeks after transplantation. Isolated intestine recipients tend to tolerate feeding earlier, likely due to the presence of less severe organ dysfunction preceding transplantation. Early enteral feeding is transitioned to full enteral as tolerated over time.

Intestinal function after transplantation usually remains mildly abnormal, leading to the need for some dietary restriction. Foods containing insoluble cellulose or high in simple carbohydrates may cause type 1 dumping symptoms. Thus, the diet is modified by an individual clinician and patient according to tolerance. Patients with a longer colonic remnant or a transplanted colon seem to have improved function. The use of bulk forming agents, and strict adherence to a diet high in complex carbohydrates and protein and low in fat has an appreciable effect on graft function. Vitamin, mineral and micronutrient absorption is generally good and routine studies are not necessary. Several studies have shown linear childhood growth and development after transition to enteral feeding, but did not demonstrate "catch up" from the depressed growth curves seen in virtually all patients prior to transplantation.

Immunosuppression

Rejection has been the Achilles' heel of intestinal transplantation. Our understanding of the rejection process has evolved over time, and certain factors make it unique among solid organs currently transplanted. While T-cell priming usually occurs in recipient secondary lymphoid organs, it also occurs in the secondary lymphoid tissues of the intestinal donor allograft. This results in the arming of cytotoxic CD-8 cells against donor antigen, and the production of a predominantly IFN-gamma TH1 response from CD-4 cells. Additionally, factors predisposing to the development of inflammatory bowel disease, such as mutation of the NOD-2 gene, have recently been shown to dramatically increase the risk of severe rejection. These findings suggest that mechanisms of innate immunity of the bowel are critical to maintenance of homeostasis in the allograft.

Tacrolimus, a calcineurin inhibitor, remains the mainstay of prophylaxis against rejection. In our recent experience, the use of induction agents has decreased rejection rates from over 70% to less than 30%. Lymphocyte-depleting polyclonal anti-thymocyte antibodies or non-depleting agents such as monoclonal interleukin-2 antibodies have both been effective. Sirolimus has also been effective at decreasing the incidence and severity of rejection.

Follow-Up

Endoscopy with mucosal biopsy is performed at least weekly during the first few weeks after transplantation. This remains the gold standard to diagnose rejection, and the main pitfall remains distinguishing rejection from viral enteritis, which has a similar appearance. A combination of standardized grading criteria for rejection and evaluation of possible infections utilizing serum or plasma PCR to distinguish CMV, adenovirus, calcivirus or EBV infection has improved our ability do distinguish these disease states. Mild rejection can be treated with bolus steroids and increases in the calcineurin trough level. Rejection associated with mucosal ulceration requires the use of lymphocyte-depleting antibodies. Severe rejection is often associated with a septic state and early diagnosis is mandatory. This sometimes requires removal of the allograft. Alternatively, intestinal allograft enteritis is ideally treated with a combination of decreased calcineurin trough levels and an antiviral agent when one is efficacious against a particular pathogen. If graft function is good at 3 months after transplantation, the ileostomy can be reversed in those patients who have residual colon or in whom a colon has been transplanted.

Outcomes

Over the last decade there have been marked improvements in survival. According to data from the United Network of Organ Sharing, 1-year patient and graft survivals for recipients of intestinal and multiorgan transplants in North America in 2005 were 75 and 80%. Patient survival at 5 years for transplants performed between 1997 and 2000 remain modest at 54%. However, single centers where larger numbers of transplants are performed have achieved survival rates exceeding 90% at 1 year and should translate into better long-term survival. Factors associated with improved survival include: patients who come from home to receive transplants, younger age at transplant, first transplant, antibody-induction therapy, and the use of maintenance rapamycin. These findings collectively emphasize the importance of early referral of patients well enough to await transplantation at home and tolerate aggressive induction immunosuppression.

More than 80% of survivors attain freedom from parenteral support and resume regular activities. Few studies have considered quality of life among recipients of intestinal transplants. Those available suggest that the pre-transplant state is associated with significant psychosocial disability, increased narcotic dependence, and decreased quality of life, all of which improve after a successful transplant. Five years after transplant, children had similar responses on the Child Health Questionnaire as normal children, while their parents perceived mild decreases in physical and psychosocial functioning.

Summary Points

- Intestinal transplantation is increasingly accepted as standard therapy for patients with intestinal failure.
- Three categories of disease account for most patients requiring intestinal transplants: short bowel syndrome, functional disorders of the intestine, and tumors.
- The most common indication for intestinal transplantation is parenteral nutrition-associated liver disease (PNALD).
- Candidates for intestinal transplantation should have adequate cardiac, pulmonary, renal, and endocrine pancreatic function.

Editor's Comment

Not long ago, it was customary to close the abdomen of an infant with necrotic bowel, without performing a resection, and explain to the parents that there was no alternative but to let the child die. Today, it would be considered more appropriate to at least have discussed the option of intestinal transplantation with them before an irreversible decision had been made. Nevertheless, it is not yet an automatic decision or one to be taken lightly – the evaluation, pre-operative testing, wait for an organ to become available, the operation itself, the postoperative medical regimen, and the intensive follow-up care all combine to create a huge undertaking that is not a realistic option for every child or every family: it requires an enormous commitment, invariably causes tremendous emotional and financial strain, and disrupts nearly every aspect of home life. These patients and their families need to be supported in many ways while awaiting the transplant, with as much as possible of the work up preferably being performed close to home.

For some patients, small intestinal transplantation is the only alternative to long-term parenteral nutrition. This includes patients who have essentially no intestinal length and those with an irreversible motility or functional disorder of the gut. Children with short bowel can sometimes be treated effectively with a bowel lengthening operation, such as the STEP procedure, which in most cases is a reasonable consideration even if it is felt likely to only delay the eventual need for intestinal transplantation. Some of the visceral myopathy disorders that occur in adolescence will improve over time or are segmental, allowing palliation with some type of an enterostomy. Many children on long-term parenteral nutrition inevitably develop cirrhosis and thus will require liver transplantation in addition to small intestine transplantation. Finally, it is also important to do everything possible to preserve vascular access sites in patients with intestinal failure: using the smallest catheters compatible with therapy, not ligating veins, and taking all precautions to prevent central-line associated blood stream infections.

Differential Diagnosis

Intestinal failure

- Gastroschisis
- NEC
- Volvulus
- Atresia
- Bowel ischemia

Functional disorders

Epithelial disorders of enterocyte function

- Microvillus inclusion disease
- Tufting enteropathy
- Autoimmune enteritis

Motility disorders

- Total intestinal aganglionosis (Hirschsprung disease)
- Megacystis-microcolon hypoperistalsis syndrome (Berdon's syndrome)
- Visceral neuropathy/myopathy

Tumors

- Desmoid tumor
- Intestinal polyposis

Diagnostic Studies

- Contrast imaging of small bowel and colon
- MRI or spiral CT to assess vascular patency
- Liver function tests
- US to r/o portal hypertension, if necessary
- Liver biopsy, if necessary
- Creatinine clearance
- Two-dimensional echocardiogram
- Pulmonary function tests

Preoperative Preparation

- ☐ Psychiatric evaluation
- ☐ Assessment of organ function
- ☐ Type and crossmatching

Parental Preparation

- Intestinal transplantation is a life-saving treatment.
- The follow-up care is significant, often requiring frequent travel to the transplant program.
- Home administration of medications, enteral tube feeding, and frequent office visits are routine.
- Graft failure due to chronic dysfunction can occur years after transplantation.
- There is the possibility of death while awaiting organ availability.
- There is the potential for graft failure or death despite successful surgery.

Technical Points

- Depending on the status of the recipient's organs, intestinal grafts can be jejunoileal, liver/jejunoileal, or multivisceral (stomach, duodenum, pancreas, and/or colon).
- Jejunoileal transplantation can be performed with mesenteric or systemic vascular supply.
- In the case of a motility or enterocyte disorder, enterectomy of the native small bowel and right colon is required and allows preservation of the superior mesenteric vessels for implantation of the graft.
- The distal bowel is brought up as an ileostomy or Santulli-type construct.
- The mesentery needs to be fixed to the retroperitoneum to prevent volvulus and internal hernia.

Suggested Reading

Abu-Elmagd K, Fung J, Bueno J, et al. Logistics and technique for procurement of intestinal, pancreatic, and hepatic grafts from the same donor. Ann Surg. 2000;232:680–7.

Fishbein TM, Gondolesi GE, Kaufman SS. Intestinal transplantation for gut failure. Gastroenterology. 2003a;124:1615–28.

Fishbein TM, Kaufman SS, Florman S, et al. Isolated intestinal transplantation: proof of efficacy. Transplantation. 2003b;76: 636–40.

Reyes J, Mazariegos GV, Bond GM, et al. Pediatric intestinal transplantation: historical notes, principles and controversies. Pediatr Transplant. 2002;6:193–207.

Starzl TE, Todo S, Tzakis AG, et al. The many faces of multivisceral transplantation. Surg Gynecol Obstet. 1991;172:335–44.

Sudan D. Cost and quality of life after intestinal transplantation. Gastroenterology. 2006;130:S158–62.

Todo S, Tzakis AG, Abu-Elmagd K, et al. Intestinal transplantation in composite visceral grafts or alone. Ann Surg. 1992;216: 223–34.

Chapter 110
Gastrointestinal Bleeding

Katherine J. Deans

Gastrointestinal bleeding accounts for at least 3 of every 1,000 pediatric emergency room visits. Caring for children with gastrointestinal bleeding requires a thorough understanding of the possible etiologies and their respective symptoms. A detailed history and physical exam serve as the starting point for any work up of the child with gastrointestinal bleeding. The two most important factors are age and the nature of the bleeding episode. These two pertinent pieces of easily accessible information help to form the differential diagnosis, which serves as the basis for the diagnostic and therapeutic algorithm.

Gastrointestinal bleeding is usually classified based on the anatomic relationship between the suspected site of bleeding and the ligament of Treitz. Bleeding from sites proximal to the ligament of Treitz is considered upper gastrointestinal bleeding and bleeding from sites distal to the ligament of Treitz is considered lower gastrointestinal bleeding. Occult gastrointestinal bleeding refers to an initial presentation with a positive fecal occult blood test or iron deficiency anemia without visible evidence of blood loss. Patients with upper gastrointestinal bleeding typically present with melena, hematemesis, or blood clots mixed with emesis. Patients with lower gastrointestinal bleeding sometimes report bloody diarrhea, hematochezia, blood seen on toilet paper or blood streaks or clots mixed with stool. Patients with occult gastrointestinal bleeding sometimes present with non-specific signs and symptoms including fatigue, pallor, or anemia.

Certain types of gastrointestinal bleeding occur in children of any age; however, many etiologies are age-specific and warrant additional distinction (Tables 110.1 and 110.2).

Diagnosis

The first step in the evaluation of a gastrointestinal bleeding episode is to determine if the child is actually bleeding. In the neonate, maternal blood swallowed during birth or from cracked nipples during breast feeding can be mistaken for gastrointestinal bleeding, in which case an Apt test should be performed to determine whether the blood is maternal in origin. In addition, ingested foods or medicines containing red dye can look like blood in the stool, but is differentiated from gastrointestinal bleeding based on history and guaiac-based tests for occult blood. Also, children sometimes swallow their own blood from epistaxis or friable mucosa due to nose-picking, recent infection, or trauma. A careful history and thorough examination of the oropharynx, nasopharynx, and nares should allow you to safely eliminate these causes of bleeding.

The approach to any patient with gastrointestinal bleeding should begin with an assessment of hemodynamic stability and overall clinical condition (Table 110.3). After determining that the child is truly bleeding, one must characterize the severity of the bleeding and the patient's overall clinical condition to guide the urgency of diagnostic studies and therapeutic interventions. Small-volume or occult bleeding episodes without other clinical signs or symptoms such as altered vital signs, a fall in hemoglobin level, or worrisome findings on abdominal examination are usually not acutely life threatening. Conversely, any bleeding episode accompanied by abdominal tenderness or emesis indicate a potentially life-threatening pathologic process. Patients with substantial bleeding or who are ill-appearing should have reliable venous access established urgently. Circulating blood volume should be assessed and restored with crystalloid and blood products. Coagulopathy and platelet abnormalities should be corrected with additional blood products. Initial resuscitation should not rely on hematocrit measurements because, due to hemoconcentration, it is an unreliable index of severity of bleeding.

After resuscitation and stabilization is initiated, the site of bleeding must be established and a differential diagnosis should

K.J. Deans (✉)
Department of Surgery, Division of General Thoracic and Fetal Surgery, University of Pennsylvania, Children's Hospital of Philadelphia, 34th Street and Civic Center Boulevard, Wood Building, 5th Floor, Philadelphia, PA 19104, USA
e-mail: deansk@email.chop.edu

P. Mattei (ed.), *Fundamentals of Pediatric Surgery*,
DOI 10.1007/978-1-4419-6643-8_110, © Springer Science+Business Media, LLC 2011

Table 110.1 Age-based differential diagnosis of gastrointestinal bleeding

Age	Differential diagnosis	
	Upper gastrointestinal bleeding	Lower gastrointestinal bleeding
Newborn (<1 month)	Maternal or swallowed blood	Maternal or swallowed blood
	Allergic enterocolitis (milk or soy)	Allergic enterocolitis (milk or soy)
	Esophagitis	Anorectal fissure
	Gastritis	Necrotizing enterocolitis
	Gastroduodenal ulcers	Malrotation with midgut volvulus
	Mallory-Weiss tear	Hirschsprung disease
	Congenital malformation	Coagulopathy (Vitamin K deficiency)
	Intestinal duplication	Liver disease
	Coagulopathy (Vitamin K deficiency)	
	Liver disease	
Infancy (1 month–2 years)	Esophagitis	Anorectal fissure
	Gastritis	Allergic enterocolitis (milk or soy)
	Gastroduodenal ulcers	Intussusception
	Varices	Meckel's diverticulum
	Mallory–Weiss tear	Lymphonodular hyperplasia
	Hemangiomas	AVMs
	Dieulafoy's lesion	Infectious colitis
	Allergic enterocolitis (milk or soy)	Intestinal duplication
		Hemolytic uremic syndrome
		Henoch–Schonlein purpura
Preschool (2–5 years)	Esophagitis	Infectious diarrhea
	Gastritis	Juvenile polyps
	Gastroduodenal ulcers	Intussusception
	Varices	Meckel's diverticulum
	Mallory–Weiss tear	Lymphonodular hyperplasia
	Dieulafoy's lesion	AVMs
		Henoch–Schonlein purpura
		Hemolytic uremic syndrome
School age (>5 years)	Esophagitis	Infectious diarrhea
	Gastritis	Juvenile polyps
	Gastroduodenal ulcers	Inflammatory bowel disease
	Varices	AVMs
	Mallory–Weiss tear	
	Dieulafoy's lesion	

be generated based on the child's age and clinical presentation. A thorough history and physical exam (Table 110.4). will direct subsequent laboratory studies including a complete blood count, liver function tests, coagulation studies, serum electrolytes, BUN, creatinine, and a type and cross. Signs of cutaneous bruising, jaundice, ascites or prominent anterior abdominal wall veins suggest coagulopathy or liver disease as the underlying cause of gastrointestinal bleeding. Patients who present with a history of hematemesis, coffee-ground emesis, or melena are more likely to have an upper gastrointestinal source of bleeding, whereas patients who present with bright red blood per rectum, bloody diarrhea or hematochezia are more likely to have a lower gastrointestinal source of bleeding. Patients with occult gastrointestinal bleeding will need a combined workup to evaluate for both upper and lower gastrointestinal sources of bleeding.

In patients with suspected GI bleeding, a nasogastric tube lavage with room temperature or warmed fluid should be performed to assess the likelihood of an upper gastrointestinal source of bleeding and to remove particulate matter and clots from the stomach to facilitate upper endoscopy. A lavage that returns blood or coffee grounds indicates an upper gastrointestinal source of bleeding. An NG lavage that yields clear fluid does not rule out an upper gastrointestinal source because the pylorus is sometimes closed. Although there is a 20% false negative rate with a negative NG lavage, aspiration of non-bloody bilious fluid reflects an open pylorus and makes an upper gastrointestinal source of bleeding very unlikely.

For patients with suspected *upper gastrointestinal bleeding*, esophagogastroduodenoscopy is the diagnostic modality of choice, as it often allows identification and treatment of the bleeding source, and helps one predict the risk of rebleeding (Table 110.2). Endoscopy can be performed safely in children, but requires deep sedation or general anesthesia and the use of small endoscopes, which can limit interventional capabilities. It should be performed in children who present with severe bleeding, persistent low grade bleeding, or recurrent episodes of bleeding. Elective intubation should be considered in patients with ongoing hematemesis or altered respiratory or mental status to prevent aspiration and make EGD easier to perform. Also, the use of NG lavage and intravenous erythromycin (a motolin receptor agonist) prior to EGD might improve visualization and improve the diagnostic and therapeutic yield. When one is unable to determine the source of bleeding by EGD, angiography or a tagged red blood cell scan are useful diagnostic adjuncts. Angiography can allow detection of bleeding at a rate of 1–2 mL/min and tagged red cell scans can be used to detect bleeding at a rate as low as 0.1 mL/min. Barium studies are contraindicated because they make other studies (including EGD and angiography) more difficult to interpret.

The diagnostic workup for *lower gastrointestinal bleeding* depends on the patient's presentation and age (Table 110.2). Anorectal fissure can be confirmed on physical exam by

Table 110.2 Common presentation and workup of specific causes of gastrointestinal bleeding

Diagnoses	Suggestive history/physical findings	Age groups	Diagnostic test
Upper gastrointestinal bleeding			
Esophagitis, gastritis or gastroduodenal ulcers	Vomiting, GERD, epigastric pain, dysphagia, indwelling NGT or gastrostomy tube, critical illness, NSAIDs, alcohol, caustic ingestion	All age groups	EGD
Mallory–Weiss tear	Hematemesis after forceful vomiting	All age groups	EGD
Varices	Hematemesis with hepatomegaly, splenomegaly, jaundice or ascites	Infancy and older	EGD
Lower gastrointestinal bleeding			
Anorectal fissure	Painful defecation with streaks of red blood on stool	All age groups	Physical exam
Allergic colitis	Blood stained vomiting or diarrhea within 48 h of introducing formula	Neonates and infants	History
Necrotizing enterocolitis	Non-specific systemic signs of toxicity with abdominal distention, tenderness, vomiting, thrombocytopenia, or diarrhea with enteral feeding	Neonates (especially preterm)	KUB
Malrotation with midgut volvulus	Melena with abdominal distention and bilious emesis	Neonates	Upper GI series
Hirschsprung disease	Delayed meconium passage (>48 h) or progressive constipation with abdominal distention	Neonates	Contrast enema and suction rectal biopsy
Intussusception	Sudden onset, severe, colicky pain with vomiting and bloody mucoid stool; possible abdominal mass	Infants, preschool	Contrast enema or ultrasound
Meckel's diverticulum	Well child with large volume painless bleed	Infants, preschool	Meckel's scan
Lymphonodular hyperplasia	Painless bleeding after viral illness or allergic colitis	Infants, preschool	Colonoscopy
Juvenile polyp	Painless rectal bleeding with blood on top of the stool	Preschool, school age (up to 8 years old)	Colonoscopy
Infectious diarrhea	Bloody diarrhea with fever, pain, or tenesmus	Preschool, school age	History, stool cultures
Inflammatory bowel disease	Chronic bloody diarrhea with weight loss, anorexia, arthralgia or erythema nodusum	School age	Colonoscopy

Table 110.3 Clinical signs of severe gastrointestinal bleeding or pathology

Signs associated with significant blood loss	Signs associated with significant underlying pathology
Diaphoresis	Abdominal distention
Restlessness	Abdominal pain/tenderness
Pallor	Abdominal mass
Altered mental status	Fever
Delayed capillary refill	Emesis
Orthostatic blood pressure or heart rate	Altered mental status
Lethargy	
Ileus	
Hematocrit drop	

Table 110.4 Important components of history and physical exam

History	Physical exam
Blood in emesis, stool, or occult	Vital signs (orthostatic)
Time course of bleeding	Mental status (lethargy, restlessness)
Amount of bleeding	Skin color
Color and consistency of stool	Capillary refill
Location of blood in stool	Cutaneous bruising
History of previous GI bleed	Jaundice/scleral icterus
History of bleeding disorders/bruising	Oropharyngeal/nasopharyngeal mucosa
History of liver disease/varices	Abdominal distention/ascites
Medication/drug history	Abdominal tenderness/masses
Heart burn/dyspepsia symptoms	Abdominal wall veins
Abdominal pain	Nasal mucosa
Dysphagia/regurgitation	Rectal/peri-anal exam
Fever	
Weight loss/poor feeding	
Irritability	

spreading the perineal skin to evert the anal canal. Infants with recurrent fissures or patients with fissures occurring at older ages should be assessed for inflammatory bowel disease, sexual abuse, or rectal trauma secondary to a foreign body.

Milk- or soy-induced enterocolitis (allergic colitis) can be diagnosed presumptively by presenting three challenges with milk or soy formula and documentation of the resolution of symptoms upon elimination of the formula. Infants with milk protein allergy should be switched to a casein-hydrolysate formula. Gross bleeding should resolve within 3 weeks and occult bleeding by 12 weeks.

For neonates with concern for necrotizing enterocolitis (NEC) or intestinal obstruction, an abdominal radiograph might reveal an abnormal bowel gas pattern, a dilated solitary loop of bowel, or pneumatosis intestinalis. Neonates and infants with bilious emesis and melena need an urgent upper gastrointestinal series to rule out malrotation, unless they are ill-appearing or have a tense abdomen, in which case they should be prepared for urgent laparotomy. Infectious colitis (caused by organisms that produce a shiga-like toxin or are invasive) and pseudomembranous colitis (*Clostridium difficile*) are relatively common causes of lower gastrointestinal bleeding and are confirmed or ruled out with the appropriate stool culture or toxin assay.

For patients with suspected intussusception, an ultrasound or contrast enema should be performed. In patients with suspected Hirschsprung disease, a contrast enema is indicated and in many cases will demonstrate a segment of dilated colon proximal to the aganglionic segment. These patients should subsequently undergo a suction rectal biopsy to document aganglionosis. Rarely, a patient with Hirschsprung disease will present with large amounts of bleeding due to enterocolitis or megacolon and need immediate rectal decompression or urgent colostomy.

Children who present with painless rectal bleeding should be evaluated for Meckel's diverticulum. Bleeding is often profuse and usually intermittent but the children are typically otherwise asymptomatic. It is caused by a peptic ulcer within the diverticulum or in the adjacent ileal mucosa due to acid secreted by ectopic gastric mucosa that is sometimes present within the diverticulum. Patients with "painless rectal bleeding" suggestive of a Meckel's diverticulum should undergo a [99]technetium pertechnetate nuclear medicine ("Meckel's") scan. The tracer binds to gastric mucosa and is highly accurate, especially when enhanced by pretreatment with pentagastrin or an H_2-blocker, but it is not 100% accurate. Therefore, if the clinical suspicion is high, it might still be reasonable to recommend diagnostic laparoscopy despite a negative scan.

Colonoscopy is indicated for suspected lower gastrointestinal bleeding that cannot be explained on the basis on the patient's presentation and the studies outlined above. In patients for whom an upper gastrointestinal source of bleeding cannot be excluded, EGD should be performed in the same setting as colonoscopy. Other studies that can sometimes help to localize a lower gastrointestinal bleeding source include CT scan, ultrasound, tagged-RBC scan, angiography, capsule endoscopy, and CT enteroclysis.

Treatment

Most patients with upper gastrointestinal bleeding are hemodynamically stable. Bleeding mucosal lesions from gastritis or esophagitis are usually self-limited. Patients with suspected gastritis or esophagitis who are clinically well and have normal laboratory values may be placed on acid suppression therapy and followed as an outpatient. Patients presenting with significant hemorrhage from suspected gastroduodenal ulcers, gastritis or esophagitis should be placed on intravenous proton pump inhibitors and undergo EGD. An octreotide infusion might also be beneficial while awaiting EGD. Endoscopic therapies to stop bleeding include clipping, epinephrine injection, and contact thermal coagulation. Patients with continued bleeding from an identified source after EGD should be considered candidates for emergent surgical exploration with either oversewing or resection of the bleeding site. Angiography may also be considered for patients with continued bleeding prior to an operation. Once bleeding is controlled, all patients should be placed on acid suppression therapy with antacids, sulcrafate, H_2 blockers, or proton pump inhibitors to prevent rebleeding.

For patients with bleeding esophageal varices, an intravenous octreotide infusion should be started. Stable patients should undergo urgent EGD with sclerotherapy or banding of the varices. Unstable patients with bleeding varices should be admitted to the intensive care unit, intubated and fluid resuscitated. A Sengstaken–Blakemore tube may be used to tamponade the bleeding while preparations are made to perform EGD when the patient has been adequately resuscitated. The incidence of rebleeding from varices can be decreased by performing endoscopic sclerotherapy and banding, and using non-selective beta-blockers. In children, sclerotherapy can cause ulceration and is associated with a 15% incidence of esophageal stricture. Based on data in adults, banding might be more effective than sclerotherapy as it appears to result in improved survival, fewer episodes of rebleeding, and a lower complication rate. Patients with portal hypertension and intractable variceal bleeding may be considered for urgent transjugular intrahepatic portosystemic shunt, surgical portosystemic shunt, or liver transplantation.

Patients with lower gastrointestinal bleeding are usually stable and well-appearing. Children with lower gastrointestinal bleeding and abdominal pain should be evaluated for intestinal ischemia from midgut volvulus, intussusception, mesenteric thrombosis or an incarcerated hernia. These children should be aggressively resuscitated and prepared for emergency laparotomy. Patients with Meckel's diverticulum should undergo diverticulectomy or bowel resection, which can usually be performed using a laparoscopic-assisted or minilaparotomy approach. Patients with Hirschsprung disease require rectal decompression and subsequent surgical resection of the aganglionic segment and a pull-through procedure.

Stable patients with intussusception should undergo an air or water contrast enema to attempt reduction, with surgery reserved for radiographic failure. Patients with suspected intussusception and severe hemorrhage or shock should be resuscitated and brought immediately to the operating room. Colonoscopy can be used to treat polyps with snare polypectomy and cautery. Colonic ulcers, telangiectasias and hemangiomas can be treated during colonoscopy with epinephrine injection and either cautery or clipping. In patients with multiple polyps, polyposis syndromes (including Peutz Jeghers syndrome) should be considered and repeat colonoscopy should be performed every few years.

Neonates with NEC should be treated with ICU monitoring, bowel rest, and antibiotics, with surgical intervention reserved for disease progression or evidence of perforation. Milk or soy protein allergic colitis is treated by changing formulas. Children with anal fissures associated with constipation should be treated with stool softeners and lubricants and those associated with diarrhea should be treated by keeping the perineum clean and dry.

The approach to any patient presenting with gastrointestinal bleeding should begin with an assessment of hemodynamic stability and overall clinical status. Resuscitation is the first therapeutic step in any severe gastrointestinal bleeding episode. Subsequently, based on the patient's age, presentation, and the presumed source and severity of bleeding, appropriate and timely diagnostic and treatment algorithms should be instituted.

Summary Points

- The patient's age and clinical presentation are the most useful pieces of information in determining the likely cause of bleeding and for directing the diagnostic and treatment algorithm.
- The approach to any patient with gastrointestinal bleeding should begin with an assessment of hemodynamic stability and overall clinical status followed by resuscitation, diagnosis, and therapy.
- After resuscitation, the level of bleeding must be established and a list of potential diagnoses generated based on the child's age and clinical presentation.
- A nasogastric tube lavage helps to confirm or exclude an upper GI source of bleeding (proximal to the ligament of treitz) and to remove particulate matter and clots from the stomach to facilitate endoscopy.
- For patients with a suspected upper GI bleed, EGD helps identify the bleeding source, permits treatment of the identified bleeding lesions, and allows for stratification of the risk for rebleeding.
- For patients with a suspected lower GI bleed, the diagnostic workup depends on the suspected diagnosis based on the patient's age and presentation.
- Adjunct treatments for upper gastrointestinal bleeding may include intravenous proton pump inhibitors or octreotide.

Editor's Comment

As is the case in adults, determining the source of GI bleeding in children can be challenging and time consuming, but a systematic algorithm-based approach is usually best. In most institutions, the diagnostic and initial therapeutic steps are undertaken by pediatric gastroenterologists rather than surgeons, though a pediatric surgeon should be involved early in the care of these patients. This approach includes initial assessment/resuscitation (ABCs), careful history and physical examination, search for and correction of coagulation abnormalities, distinction between upper and lower GI sources of bleeding (NG lavage), and focused endoscopy and imaging studies. It is not uncommon for the clinicians who are treating these children to be anxious, disorganized, and quick to recommend surgery despite not yet having identified a source for the bleeding. The role of the surgeon is to maintain equanimity, keep the patient safe, and help guide a systematic diagnostic approach.

A true exploratory laparotomy in a child with GI bleeding should rarely be necessary. However, an operation will sometimes be necessary despite the source of bleeding having been only partially localized (right colon, stomach, mid-small bowel). Intra-operative techniques to localize the bleeding include: sequential isolation of short segments of the bowel using non-crushing bowel clamps, which might demonstrate a specific segment that fills with blood before your eyes; intra-operative endoscopy, in which the bowel is placed over the end of an endoscope passed through the mouth or anus by an assistant; serial enterotomies in the area of interest (stomach, duodenum, jejunum, ileum, colonic segment) with gross visualization of the mucosa; empiric resection of the bowel segment in question; and, only as a last resort, one or more temporary enterostomies to see, over the course of several hours or days postoperatively, which part of the bowel the bleeding is coming from. Though none of these techniques are easy to perform or particularly effective, I listed them here in decreasing order of preference. In general, it is best to avoid finding yourself in such a predicament by utilizing any and all localization techniques available to you *before* taking the patient to the operating room.

Given its limited effectiveness and relatively high complication rate, the Sengstaken–Blakemore tube should rarely, if ever, used in children with suspected variceal bleeding, except as an extreme measure to save a life or buy some time. It is more appropriate to use drugs, aggressive resuscitation with blood products, and emergent upper endoscopy by an experienced gastroenterologist or surgeon who is prepared to definitively treat the underlying varices.

Diagnostic Studies

Upper gastrointestinal bleed

– NGT lavage
– Esophagogastroduodenoscopy
– Angiography
– Tagged RBC scan

Lower gastrointestinal bleed

– Abdominal X-ray
– Upper gastrointestinal series
– Ultrasound
– Contrast enema
– Meckel's scan ([99]technetium pertechnetate)
– Colonoscopy
– Angiography
– Tagged RBC scan
– Computed tomography
– Video capsule endoscopy
– CT enteroclysis

Preoperative Preparation

☐ Airway, breathing, circulation
☐ Type and crossmatch for packed RBCs, plasma, and platelets
☐ Prophylactic antibiotics
☐ Informed consent

Parental Preparation

– Though it might seem like an unnecessary delay, it is important to take whatever time is needed to try to identify the source of bleeding in a systematic and meticulous fashion.

– No matter the cause or location, gastrointestinal bleeding is almost always intermittent and hard to pin down. (It is important to empathize with the family here as this can be disheartening and extremely frustrating.)
– The approach to the patient with GI bleeding usually involves a team including gastroenterologists, critical care doctors, radiologists, interventionalists, and surgeons.

Technical Points

• Regardless of the site or the cause, GI bleeding is almost always intermittent and elusive.
• Formulate a plan and work through it in a step-wise and systematic way.
• Your role as the surgeon, at least early on, is to maintain calm, guide the work up, and utilize good judgment when considering operative intervention.
• If your clinical suspicion is high, consider repeating a diagnostic study even if it was negative the first time.
• If you suspect bleeding from a Meckel's diverticulum and all other causes have been excluded, consider a diagnostic laparoscopy – but have a back-up plan if a Meckel's is not found.
• Be persistent about preoperative localization, but sometimes laparotomy is necessary despite not having identified a specific source.
• When you find yourself in an abdomen with no obvious source of bleeding, use a systematic approach that saves the most invasive option until it is unavoidable, anticipate having a gastroenterologist available to assist with intra-operative endoscopy, and, if at all possible, avoid the empiric removal of large segments of bowel unless there is a clear indication.

Suggested Reading

Arain Z, Rossi TM. Gastrointestinal bleeding in children: an overview of conditions requiring nonoperative management. Semin Pediatr Surg. 1999;8(4):172–80.

Boyle JT. Gastrointestinal bleeding in infants and children. Pediatr Rev. 2008;29(2):39–52.

Brown RL, Azizkhan RG. Gastrointestinal bleeding in infants and children: Meckel's diverticulum and intestinal duplication. Semin Pediatr Surg. 1999;8(4):202–9.

Fox VL. Gastrointestinal bleeding in infancy and childhood. Gastroenterol Clin North Am. 2000;29(1):37–66.

Kay MH, Wyllie R. Therapeutic endoscopy for nonvariceal gastrointestinal bleeding. J Pediatr Gastroenterol Nutr. 2007;45(2):157–71.

Lawrence WW, Wright JL. Causes of rectal bleeding in children. Pediatr Rev. 2001;22(11):394–5.

Chapter 111
Fetal Surgery

Foong-Yen Lim and Timothy M. Crombleholme

The extraordinary advances in molecular genetics and the ongoing technologic innovations in medical imaging now make it possible to prenatally diagnose virtually any condition with a high level of confidence. This has afforded the opportunity to consider prenatal treatment for an ever-expanding list of conditions and to avoid or minimize irreparable organ injury or death that can occur if treatment is delayed until after delivery. Fetal therapy has expanded the list of conditions that are considered for medical treatment including high-risk congenital pulmonary airway malformations (CPAM), fetal arrhythmias, congenital adrenal hyperplasia (CAH), and congenital diaphragmatic hernia (CDH). The indications for open fetal surgery have expanded with the development of interventions for myelomeningocele (MMC), sacrococcygeal teratoma (SCT), bladder outlet obstruction (BOO), and CPAM. Perhaps the most striking area of growth in fetal intervention has come in the field of fetoscopic techniques, which are used to treat conditions such as twin–twin transfusion syndrome (TTTS), twin reversed arterial perfusion (TRAP) sequence, and CDH.

Fetal intervention is only possible in the setting of precise prenatal imaging, a complete understanding of the maternal history, development of selection criteria for intervention, and the availability of techniques that are safe for both mother and fetus. In the past, fetal intervention was limited to conditions in which the life of a singleton fetus was threatened. In recent years, the indications for fetal intervention have been extended to non-life threatening conditions (MMC) and to multiple gestations. In fact, the most common indication for fetal surgery currently is TTTS. The sophistication of the average expectant mother has increased commensurately with the technical capabilities of fetal intervention. Expecting parents increasingly seek out expertise in fetal imaging, prenatal diagnosis and fetal intervention and are willing to travel if expertise is not locally available. The evolution of fetal intervention holds tremendous promise for altering the natural history of certain disorders in ways not possible after delivery. It also is fraught with potential risk for mothers who derive no direct benefit from these procedures. Critical appraisal of the potential maternal and fetal risks of fetal intervention must be carefully weighed by all parents considering these options.

Medical Fetal Therapy

Except for the use of steroids to enhance lung maturity in prematures, antenatal medical treatment options remain limited and include steroid administration for the treatment of CPAM, rapidly involuting congenital hemangiomas (RICH), and complete heart block in the setting of maternal systemic lupus erythematosus (SLE), and transplacental treatment of fetal tachyarrhythmias with antiarrhythmic medications.

Congenital pulmonary airway malformations can grow extremely rapidly between 20 and 26 weeks of gestation, which sometimes causes non-immune hydrops fetalis due to mediastinal shift, obstructed venous return, and compression of the heart. When dealing with non-cystic CPAM in the past, fetal surgery was the only treatment alternative for this uniformly fatal condition. Recently it has been reported that a course of maternal steroids (betamethasone 12.5 mg, intramuscularly × 2 doses) can arrest the growth of the solid component of the CPAM and allow the fetus to grow around the CPAM, however the response is variable and steroids do not completely eliminate the need for fetal surgery (Fig. 111.1).

Transplacental steroids can also induce regression of rapidly involuting congenital hemangiomas (RICH), which can cause high-output cardiac failure and hydrops. Fetal complete heart block in the setting of a structurally normal heart is usually due to transplacental passage of maternal SSA and SSB antibodies that crossreact with antigens expressed in the conduction system of the fetal heart. Maternal steroid administration can be used to treat the myocarditis, limit myocardial damage, and prevent further reduction in ventricular response rate. Maternal steroid administration for fetal

F.-Y. Lim (✉)
Department of Pediatric Surgery, Cincinnati Children's Hospital Medical Center, 3333 Burnet Avenue, MLC 11025, Cincinnati, OH 45229-3039, USA
e-mail: foong.yen.lim@cchmc.org

P. Mattei (ed.), *Fundamentals of Pediatric Surgery*,
DOI 10.1007/978-1-4419-6643-8_111, © Springer Science+Business Media, LLC 2011

Fig. 111.1 Management algorithm for prenatally diagnosed congenital pulmonary airway malformation (CPAM). *TA* thoraco-amniotic; *CVR* CPAM volume ratio (volume of CPAM/head circumference)

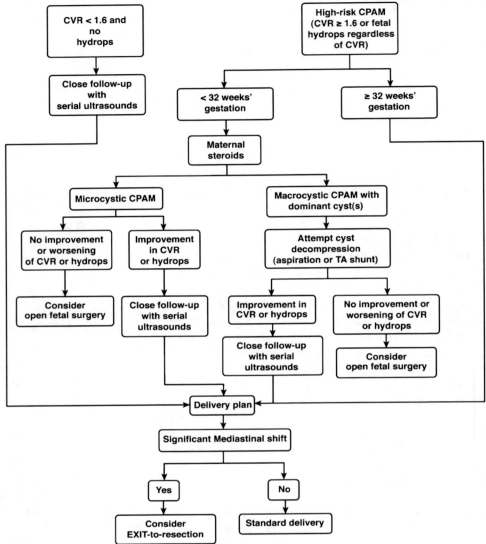

Management Algorithm for Prenatally Diagnosed Congenital Pulmonary Airway Malformation (CPAM)

TA = Thoraco-amniotic; CVR = CPAM volume ratio

complete heart block with or without the addition of beta-mimetic agents has been shown to improve survival.

In families known to be at risk for CAH, maternal steroid administration in the first trimester can prevent virilization in genotypic female fetuses. Ninety percent of cases of CAH are caused by 21 alpha-hydroxylase deficiency, which can be detected by measuring elevated 17-hydroxyprogesterone levels in the amniotic fluid. Virilization of the genitalia can only be prevented if maternal steroids are started prior to the ninth week of gestation. Treatment prior to 5 weeks might be necessary to prevent the virilizing effects on the fetal brain.

The most common fetal arrhythmia is supraventricular tachycardia (SVT) due to reentrant SVT or atrial flutter. Magnetocardiography provides a means of distinguishing different forms of SVT and allow the most appropriate transplacental administration of antiarrhythmic agent (sotalol, digoxin or flecainide). Inpatient continuous fetal monitoring is usually necessary in these cases to monitor response to treatment.

Fetal Surgery

Since the inception of fetal surgery, the development of fetal and maternal anesthetic technique has continued to evolve. For fetoscopic procedures, we prefer epidural anesthesia supplemented by local anesthetics and intravenous sedatives. This regimen is usually adequate even if a laparotomy is necessary (anterior placenta). For percutaneous shunting procedures, the combination of moderate sedation and local anesthetics with or without regional anesthesia is effective.

In the past, anesthesia for open fetal surgery and *ex utero* intrapartum therapy (EXIT) was established using a high concentration of volatile anesthetic agents to provide optimal uterine relaxation, which was necessary to preserve uterine-placental circulation; however this approach is frequently associated with maternal hypotension and direct fetal cardiac depression. To minimize these effects, it is more common now to start supplemented intravenous anesthesia (SIVA) after maternal epidural placement until uterine relaxation is required, at which point the concentration of desflurane is gradually increased and the SIVA infusion rate is decreased. Maternal blood pressure is maintained with judicious administration of intravenous fluids as well as phenylephrine and ephedrine. Tocolytics such as magnesium sulfate, indomethacin, nitroglycerine, and terbutaline are also sometimes useful. Standard maternal monitoring is performed using electrocardiography, pulse oximetry, blood pressure cuff (or arterial cannula) and foley catheter. When appropriate, fentanyl (5–20 μg/kg), atropine (20 mg/kg) and vecuronium (0.2 mg/kg) are injected intramuscularly into the fetus. Fetal monitoring during open procedure is achieved by pulse oximetry, fetal blood gases, and intraoperative fetal echocardiography. Perioperative antibiotics are administered as appropriate.

Fetoscopic Surgery

Fetoscopy is now the most commonly employed fetal surgical technique. The most common indication is TTTS, which affects 10–15% of monochorionic twin pregnancies and accounts for 17% of all prenatal mortality in twins. While the etiology is unknown, TTTS appears to be caused by vascular connections between the twins (chorioangiopagus), which causes polyhydramnios in the recipient twin and severe oligohydramnios and anemia in the donor twin. As the disease progresses, the recipient twin develops a hypertrophic cardiomyopathy and eventually cardiac failure. Selective fetoscopic laser photocoagulation (SFLP) of the vascular connections can arrest the progression of TTTS. Untreated TTTS is almost uniformly fatal, but with SFLP overall survival is 70–77%, with, up to 64% of pregnancies having both twins survive and 91% of pregnancies having at least one fetus survive. Other therapeutic options include amnioreduction, which is effective in 20–30% of patients, and ultrasound-guided radiofrequency ablation (RFA) of the umbilical cord, which should be considered as salvage therapy to

protect one twin from co-twin demise. When there is evidence of cardiomyopathy on fetal echocardiography, we have recently added nifedipine (20 mg orally every 6 h) as part of the treatment regimen. In addition, the need for additional tocolytics such as magnesium sulfate in these patients has diminished.

Twin reversed arterial perfusion (TRAP) sequence is another highly lethal anomaly in which vascular connections between a "pump" twin and an acardiac, acephalic twin result in polyhydramnios, preterm labor, heart failure, and fetal demise. Intrafetal RFA of the umbilical cord to the acardius results in 95% survival of the "pump" twin in cases in which adverse pregnancy outcome would be anticipated in 90% of cases.

In fetuses with congenital diaphragmatic hernia (CDH), tracheal occlusion has been shown in experimental models to increase airway pressure by blocking the normal egress of tracheal and lung fluid, which in turn increases fetal lung growth. In a prospective randomized trial of fetoscopic balloon tracheal occlusion, Harrison et al. found no difference in survival in left-sided CDH compared to postnatal therapy in cases with lung-to-head circumference ratio (LHR) <1.4, with the majority of patients having an LHR >0.9. The result was not surprising given the favorable outcome of fetuses with LHR >1.0. Deprest et al. have applied this fetoscopic technique to fetuses with LHR <1.0 and liver herniation, another indicator of poor prognosis. Balloon tracheal occlusion was then reversed prior to delivery. They reported a 57.1% survival, compared to an 11% survival with conventional postnatal care in European neonatal centers. This therapy is currently not available in the United States due to lack of an FDA-approved detachable balloon device. It is expected that such a device will become available soon and reversible fetoscopic tracheal occlusion will become an option for the most severely affected cases of CDH (Fig. 111.2).

Fetoscopic surgery has also been successfully applied in the treatment of amniotic band syndrome. Formed spontaneously or as a result of amniocentesis, amniotic bands encircle a limb and result in a tourniquet-like effect with subsequent limb amputation or death if the band involves the umbilical cord. Fetoscopic release of amniotic bands has prevented both limb amputation and death from cord accidents. Even after the bands are lysed, the involved limbs can still have sequelae, such as lymphedema or growth failure.

Congenital high airway obstruction syndrome (CHAOS) is a condition associated with non-immune hydrops in which complete intrinsic obstruction of the fetal airway prevents the egress of lung fluid from the tracheobronchial tree. Causes include tracheal or laryngeal atresia, web, or a cyst that completely occludes the airway. This life-threatening condition was previously thought to be rare. The prenatal

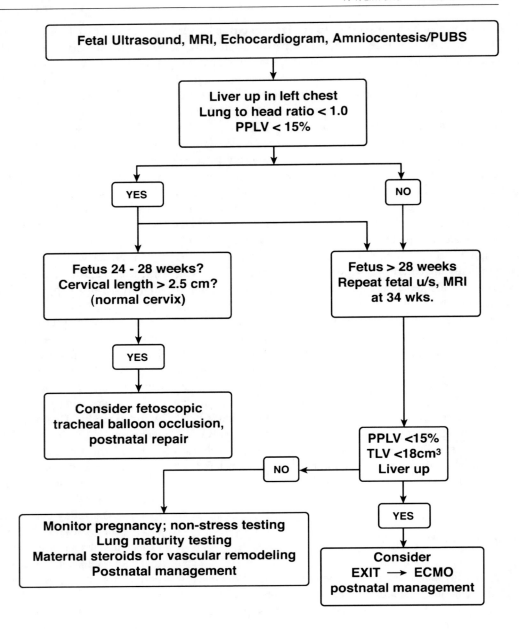

imaging findings of CHAOS include enlarged lungs with inverted diaphragms, cardiac hypoplasia, a dilated airway below the level of obstruction, and massive ascites. Without antenatal intervention or EXIT procedure, it is uniformly fatal. Up to one third of CHAOS cases will spontaneously perforate through the atresia into the larynx or esophagus with resolution of hydrops. Several patients have now undergone fetoscopic perforation of laryngeal or tracheal atresia to allow hydrops to resolve. An EXIT procedure is still necessary for delivery, but the resolution of hydrops results in a much healthier newborn.

Bladder outlet obstruction due to posterior urethral valves (PUV) results in bladder enlargement and oligohydramnios and, if untreated, severe renal dysplasia and death from pulmonary hypoplasia. This has been treated by vesicoamniotic (VA) shunting or open vesicostomy. Cases that present prior to 20 weeks gestation are candidates for fetoscopic/cystoscopic laser ablation of the PUV or transurethral catheterization with restoration of amniotic fluid volume, minimizing the risk of neonatal death from pulmonary hypoplasia. After 20 weeks gestation, the angulation between the bladder neck and the posterior urethra usually makes fetoscopic interventions too difficult, in which case open fetal vesicostomy or VA shunt should be considered (Fig. 111.3). It is unknown at this time if the fetoscopic approach will result in better renal outcome.

Compared to open fetal surgery, fetoscopic procedures and ultrasound-guided RFA seem to have a lower risk profile, but these procedures remain invasive and carry a risk to the mother and a substantial risk of preterm prelabor rupture of membrane (PPROM).

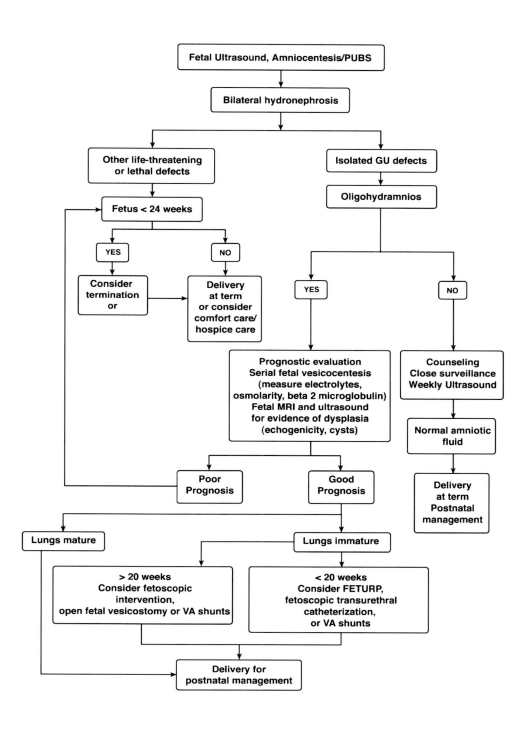

Fig. 111.3 Management algorithm for prenatally diagnosed lower urinary tract obstruction (LUTO). *VA* vesico-amniotic; *GU* genitourinary; *FETURP* fetoscopic transuterine release of posterior urethral valves; *PUBS* percutaneous umbilical blood sampling

Open Fetal Surgery

The indications for open fetal surgery remain relatively few. The maternal risks are higher than with fetoscopic intervention due not only to the large laparotomy incision required, but also large hysterotomy and aggressive tocolytic regimen required for management. With the notable exception of MMC, open fetal surgery is considered only when the life of the fetus is threatened. While the techniques used for specific diagnoses vary, the approach to anesthesia, entering the gravid uterus, fetal exposure, fetal and maternal monitoring and tocolytic management are largely the same. The maternal uterus is exposed through a low transverse abdominal incision. In posterior placentation, a midline fascial incision is used as the uterus will not need to be lifted out of the abdomen. In contrast, in the case of anterior placentation, the rectus muscles might need to be divided to allow tilting of the uterus out of the abdomen, facilitating a posterior hysterotomy. A large abdominal ring retractor is used to maintain exposure. Sterile intra-operative ultrasound is used to map the fetal position and to assist in marking the placental edge with electrocautery. The position and orientation of the hysterotomy is planned so as to stay 4–5 cm from and parallel to the closest placental edge. Under ultrasonographic guidance, a T-fastener is inserted into the amniotic cavity to lift up the uterine wall to allow safe placement of four traction sutures around the fastener to further elevate the membrane and myometrial wall from the fetus. A small hysterotomy is then made within the box created by the traction sutures using electrocautery. The T-fastener is removed and the hysterotomy incision is extended using an absorbable uterine stapler (US Surgical Corporation, Norwalk, CT), which is hemostatic and seals the membranes to the myometrium. To avoid cord compression or potential abruption, the amniotic volume is maintained with a continuous stream of warm lactated Ringer's solution delivered through a red rubber catheter attached to a Level I rapid infuser. The appropriate fetal part is then exposed, leaving the rest of the fetus within the uterus. An intravenous cannula is usually placed in the fetal extremity. A pulse oximeter is wrapped around the fetal palm or sole and secured with self-adhesive bandage material. Following repair of the specific defect, the fetus is returned to the uterus. The absorbable staples are left in place and a watertight, two-layer uterine closure is then performed using 0-polydioxanone sutures. Just prior to completing the first layer, amniotic fluid is restored with warm lactated Ringer's and antibiotics (nafcillin or clindamycin). Following uterine closure, the maternal laparotomy incision is closed in layers. The skin incision is closed in subcuticular fashion and covered by a transparent adhesive dressing or cyanoacrylate tissue adhesive to facilitate postoperative monitoring by a tocodynamometer and ultrasound examination.

Tocolysis begins as soon as the uterus is closed, starting with magnesium sulfate 6 g given over 1 h and followed by a continuous drip at 2 g/h or higher as indicated by uterine irritability. To supplement the magnesium sulfate, rectal indomethacin on a schedule of 50 mg every 4–6 h is also used for the first 48 h. The use of indomethacin requires close fetal monitoring by daily fetal echocardiography for evidence of ductal constriction and tricuspid regurgitation. Patient-controlled analgesia is an essential part of the tocolytic management as pain increases uterine irritability. We currently use a continuous epidural fentanyl and bupivacaine infusion and patient-controlled rescue doses.

Steroid-refractory CPAM or macrocystic lesions not responsive to decompression are an indication for open fetal surgery (Fig. 111.1). A fetal thoracoabdominal incision is used for exposure and care is taken to preserve even the tiniest of the compressed and hypoplastic portions of the lung. Survival after open surgery for hydropic CPAM is 60%; however, many losses occur when patients are referred late in the course of the disease with end-stage nonimmune hydrops. Those fetuses that are followed closely and show progression to hydrops despite steroid administration are better candidates for surgery when it is performed earlier in the course of the disease.

Sacrococcygeal teratoma (SCT) can grow rapidly, precipitating nonimmune hydrops, high output cardiac failure, polyhydramnios, preterm labor, and fetal demise. Almost uniformly fatal in the setting of hydrops, recently successful antenatal resections have been reported. The key to a successful outcome has been intervention early in the development of hydrops. The goal of fetal surgery in SCT is merely to interrupt the large vascular connections responsible for nonimmune hydrops. Care is taken to preserve the anorectal sphincter complex and a complete section of the SCT is not attempted. Completion of the resection of the pelvic component of the fetal SCT is performed postnatally. Only nine such cases have been attempted with six fetuses surviving to delivery. These infants must be followed for at least 3 years with serial alpha fetoprotein (AFP) levels, MRI, and physical examination in surveillance for recurrent SCT or malignant degeneration.

Like SCT, a large pericardial and mediastinal teratoma can result in nonimmune hydrops and must be followed closely. Open fetal resection of the teratoma by median stenotomy should be considered before end-stage nonimmune hydrops develops. Open fetal surgery has also been employed to treat other life-threatening conditions for which no other therapy exists or conventional approaches have failed, including fetal pacemaker placement for complete heart block and hydrops despite steroid and beta-mimetic therapy.

Perhaps the most significant recent change in the field of fetal surgery has been the application of these technique in non-life threatening conditions such as MMC. Although folic acid supplementation has reduced the incidence of MMC, it still occurs in up to 1 in 2,000 births. While no one would argue that MMC is not a devastating anomaly, it is not usually fatal in utero. Early reports suggest that fetal surgery to repair MMC can reverse the hindbrain herniation of the associated Chiari II malformation, slow the rate of progression of ventriculomegaly, and perhaps decrease the need for postnatal ventriculoperitoneal shunting. The Management of Myelomeningocele Study (MOMS Trial) is an NIH-sponsored prospective, randomized clinical trial comparing open fetal repair with conventional postnatal treatment. Endpoints include the need for postnatal shunting and neurodevelopmental outcome. Thus far, the MOMS Trial had recruited 130 of projected 200 patients over 5 years.

Bladder outlet obstruction due to PUV was the first structural anomaly treated by open fetal surgery. It was quickly supplanted by vesicoamniotic shunting due to the markedly less invasive nature of these shunts. While vesicoamniotic shunts can restore amniotic fluid and allow lung growth, they do not protect the kidney or the bladder from progressive injury. In fact, over 50% of successfully treated cases go on to develop renal failure. Often these children are poor transplant candidates due to a fibrotic, hypertrophied and poorly compliant bladder. Recently, open fetal surgery for vesicostomy creation in bladder outlet obstruction has again been employed as the most definitive means of decompressing the genitourinary tract and potentially protecting both the bladder and the kidney, especially when fetoscopic intervention fails (Fig. 111.3). Since severe oligohydramnios or anhydramnios is common, amnio-infusion is necessary prior to hysterotomy to avoid injury to the cord or the fetus. After the lower extremities of the fetus are exteriorized, a midline suprapubic incision is performed and the bladder is marsupialized to the abdominal wall with interrupted polydioxanone sutures. If both the maternal and fetal condition allow, flexible cystoscopy with release of the PUV can be attempted before the hysterotomy is closed and amniotic fluid restored.

No maternal deaths have been reported following open fetal surgery and subsequent fertility does not appear to be affected. Cesarean delivery is mandated after open fetal surgery and with subsequent pregnancies since the hysterotomy remains a weakened area and is at risk for rupture during active labor. Significant maternal bleeding, wound infection, chorioamniotic separation, and chorioamniitis are infrequent but occur more commonly than after fetoscopic interventions. Preterm labor and PPROM despite modern aggressive tocolytic regimens remain the greatest obstacle to successful outcome following fetal surgery. The median interval from fetal surgery to delivery is 5 weeks, with a range of several days to 15 weeks.

Ex Utero Intrapartum Therapy (EXIT)

Originally developed as a means of operating on placental support to remove surgical clips from the trachea of a baby with CDH at the time of delivery, the EXIT procedure has been used to treat airway obstruction due to large neck masses (cervical teratoma, lymphangioma), intrinsic airway obstruction (CHAOS), intrathoracic airway obstruction due to teratoma or CPAM, severe micrognathia, as well as a means of safe transitioning to ECMO support in CDH or severe congenital heart disease (CHD).

In all cases, the priority is to establish a secure airway while uteroplacental circulation and gas exchange is preserved (Fig. 111.4). The approach to entering the gravid uterus, fetal exposure, fetal and maternal monitoring, anesthetic, and tocolytic management are largely the same as that used in open fetal surgery. In some cases of cervical or mediastinal mass, partial or complete resection of the mass is necessary before the airway can be secured. Once the airway is secured, hand-ventilation is initiated and surfactant administered. Peripheral intravenous and umbilical catheterization is performed before the cord is clamped. Just before clamping of the cord and ending the EXIT procedure, volatile anesthetic is decreased or turned off entirely to prevent uterine atony. An intravenous oxytocin drip is used to enhance prompt return of uterine tone. The baby is then delivered, resuscitated and stabilized before being taken to the ICU or to a separate operating room for additional surgical intervention.

Currently, the indications for EXIT-to-ECMO are: (1) severe CDH with liver herniation, LHR<1.0, percent predicted lung volume (PPLV) lower than 15, and total lung volume less than 18 mL; (2) hypoplastic left heart syndrome associated with restrictive atrium; and (3) severe aortic stenosis associated with restrictive atrium. During EXIT-to-ECMO, after the airway is secured, ECMO cannulation is performed and support is started before the baby is delivered. This strategy avoids any period of severe hypoxia or acidosis during neonatal resuscitation, minimizes barotrauma, and allows safe transport of the baby to the ICU or to the cardiac catheterization suite for potential life-saving interventions.

Although the EXIT procedure is designed to optimize outcomes for a fetus, if not performed appropriately, there is a risk of maternal and fetal complications. The majority of these complications are due to inadequate uteroplacental gas exchange secondary to cord compression, placental abruption or loss of myometrial relaxation. Coordination between the surgical and anesthesiology teams is crucial to prevent uterine atony and maternal hemorrhage. There have been no maternal deaths and the average blood loss is comparable to cesarean section. Likewise, fertility is not affected but cesarean delivery for subsequent pregnancy is necessary to reduce the risk of uterine rupture if a low transverse hysterotomy is not

Fig. 111.4 Management
algorithm for EXIT procedure.
EXIT ex utero intrapartum
therapy

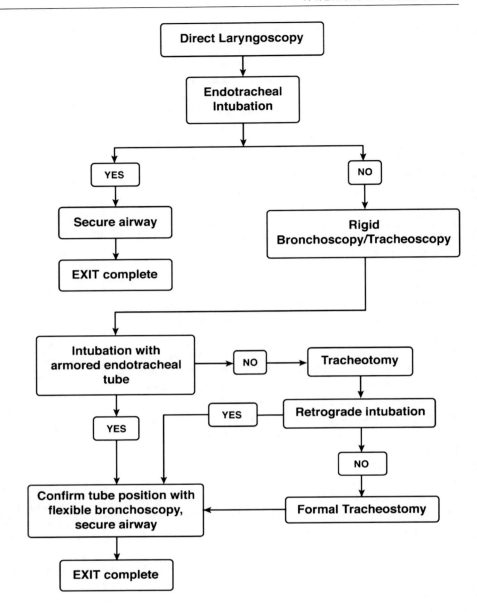

possible during the EXIT procedure. Careful orchestration among pediatric surgeons, obstetricians, neonatologists, anesthesiologists, cardiologists, sonographers, nurses, and technicians is vital to ensure maternal safety and a smooth transition of the baby to the postnatal environment. Everyone should be prepared for immediate delivery if the EXIT procedure must be abruptly terminated.

The evolution of fetal therapy holds tremendous promise to change the prenatal natural history and improve not only perinatal survival, but potential long-term outcomes as well. However, these efforts in developing innovative fetal treatment should not be mistaken for establishing fetal therapy as the standard treatment for any condition. Critical appraisal of the potential maternal and fetal risks of fetal intervention must be carefully weighed by parents and care givers. Nevertheless, collateral advances in multiple disciplines have occurred as a result of fetal interventions and the contribution of fetal surgery to advances in prenatal care and perinatal management have implications far beyond the narrow sphere of fetal therapy. With improved knowledge of perinatal disorders and extensive investigation in diminishing the potential risks of fetal intervention, the field of fetal therapy will continue to expand and provide new and exciting therapeutic options for the unborn patient.

Summary Points

- Fetal intervention requires precise high-quality prenatal imaging, a complete maternal history, strict selection criteria, and techniques that are safe for both mother and fetus.
- The most common indication for fetal surgery currently is twin–twin transfusion syndrome, which is usually treated by fetoscopy.
- Antenatal medical treatment options remain limited and include steroid administration for the treatment of congenital pulmonary airway malformations, rapidly involuting congenital hemangiomas, and complete heart block due to maternal lupus, and transplacental treatment of fetal tachyarrhythmias with antiarrhythmic medications.
- Fetoscopic surgery is currently used to treat: twin–twin transfusion syndrome, twin reversed arterial perfusion, amniotic band syndrome, congenital high airway obstruction syndrome due to tracheal atresia, bladder outlet obstruction due to posterior urethral valves, and, in experimental studies, congenital diaphragmatic hernia.
- Open fetal surgery is rarely indicated but is considered in conditions with a high mortality such as congenital lung lesions or sacrococcygeal teratoma with hydrops, and certain highly morbid conditions such as bladder outlet obstruction and myelomeningocele.
- Anesthetic and tocolytic techniques are currently quite effective but continually being refined.

Editor's Comment

Centers that specialize in fetal diagnosis and intervention are becoming increasingly common. Due to the efforts of experts in the field, the technology is advancing rapidly; though currently the indications for actual in utero fetal intervention remain few. Nevertheless, fetal diagnostic and surgical centers serve several important roles and, as such, have contributed greatly to the care of newborns with congenital anomalies: (1) genetic and obstetrical counseling, (2) state-of-the-art imaging and interventional diagnostics available in one location, (3) a source of reliable information for pregnant women and their families when a congenital anomaly has been identified antenatally, (4) the opportunity to pursue in utero intervention when indicated, (5) the ability to make plans for appropriate medical and surgical therapeutics for when the baby is born, and (6) the option of actually delivering the child in a children's hospital where care can be delivered without the delay associated with transfer (which at this time is available at only one center in the US).

Despite the fact that the results of fetal surgery for congenital diaphragmatic hernia have been disappointing in that the results have been no better than that achieved by the standard of care, the work has nonetheless contributed greatly to the understanding of this condition and effective fetal interventions appear to be finally within grasp. Operations for other conditions (congenital lung disease, sacrococcygeal teratoma, cervical masses) have proven somewhat more successful but only when the life of the fetus is in jeopardy.

Several technical problems encountered early on have been resolved, including achieving hemostasis of the hysterotomy incision, maintaining uterine volume and temperature during the procedure, balancing the needs of the mother and the fetus related to anesthetic issues, and avoiding injury to the placenta, which occupies a large proportion of the internal surface area of the uterus. Postoperative preterm labor remains a common and frustrating occurrence after fetal intervention. Nevertheless, it is inevitable, however, that someday soon fetal surgery will become more routine as the few remaining hurdles are removed.

Fetal operations, including procedures performed using the EXIT approach, involve a large team of dedicated specialists all working together to maintain the health and well-being of the fetus(es) and, most importantly, the mother. The planning and coordination of the team are clearly important to achieving this goal. During a typical fetal operation or EXIT procedure, the operating theater is filled with personnel, more than for any typical operation, each contributing something specifically important to the task at hand: pediatric surgeons, obstetricians, anesthesiologists, neonatologists, and nurses representing each of the specialties involved. Two operating rooms are usually required, one for the mother and another for the infant. The result is a tense but well-orchestrated process and usually a successful outcome. Eventually, it is likely that nearly every congenital anomaly will be detectable antenatally, in which case newer and better treatments will become available because of the ground-breaking work of the select few who are today's fetal surgeons.

Suggested Reading

Abe K, Hamada H, Chen YJ, et al. Successful management of supraventricular tachycardia in a fetus using fetal magnetocardiography. Fetal Diagn Ther. 2005;20:459–62.

Bianchi DW, Crombleholme TM, D'Alton ME, editors. Fetology: diagnosis and management of the fetal patient. New York: McGraw-Hill; 2000.

Biard JM, Johnson MP, Carr MC, et al. Long-term outcomes in children treated by prenatal vesicoamniotic shunting for lower urinary tract obstruction. Obstet Gynecol. 2005;106:503–8.

Breur JM, Visser GH, Kruize AA, et al. Treatment of fetal heart block with maternal steroid therapy: case report and review of the literature. Ultrasound Obstet Gynecol. 2004;24:467–72.

Deprest J, Jani J, Lewi L, et al. Fetoscopic surgery: encouraged by clinical experience and boosted by instrument innovation. Semin Fetal Neonatal Med. 2006;11:398–412.

Harrison MR, Evans MI, Adzick NS, editors. The unborn patient. 3rd ed. Philadelphia: WB Saunders; 2001.

Hedrick HL, Flake AW, Crombleholme TM, et al. Sacrococcygeal teratoma: prenatal assessment, fetal intervention, and outcome. J Pediatr Surg. 2004;39:430–8. http://www.fetalcarecenter.org.

Kohl T, Hering R, Bauriedel G, et al. Fetoscopic and ultrasound-guided decompression of the fetal trachea in a human fetus with Fraser syndrome and congenital high airway obstruction syndrome (CHAOS) from laryngeal atresia. Ultrasound Obstet Gynecol. 2006;27:84–8.

Lim FY, Crombleholme TM, Hedrick HL, et al. Congenital high airway obstruction syndrome: natural history and management. J Pediatr Surg. 2003;38:940–5.

Marwan A, Crombleholme TM. The EXIT procedure: principles, pitfalls, and progress. Semin Pediatr Surg. 2006;15(2):107–15.

Nimkarn S, New MI. Prenatal diagnosis and treatment of congenital adrenal hyperplasia. Pediatr Endocrinol Rev. 2006;4:99–105.

Peranteau WH, Wilson RD, Liechty KW, et al. Effect of maternal betamethasone administration on prenatal congenital cystic adenomatoid malformation growth and fetal survival. Fetal Diagn Ther. 2007;22:365–71.

Rossi AC, D'Addario V. Laser therapy and serial amnioreduction as treatment for twin-twin transfusion syndrome: a metaanalysis and review of literature. Am J Obstet Gynecol. 2008;198:147–52.

Sutton LN. Fetal surgery for neural tube defects. Best Pract Res Clin Obstet Gynaecol. 2008;22(1):175–88.

Chapter 112
Disorders of the Abdominal Aorta and Major Branches

Omaida C. Velazquez

Diseases of the subdiaphragmatic aorta in the pediatric population constitute a rare and highly heterogeneous group of disorders that present a tremendous challenge and require a multidisciplinary treatment approach. When viewed from the broad perspective of vascular surgical diagnosis and treatments, these conditions can be separated into two distinct entities: aneurysmal disease and stenotic/occlusive disease. Effective vascular reconstruction in these patients must take into account highly specialized issues related to the small size of the vessels being reconstructed, the limited availability of effective conduit for reconstruction, the optimal timing for operative repair, the anticipated life-long length of follow-up, and the principles of surgical technique that need to be incorporated to accommodate for anticipated growth. Equally important, the biology of the underlying specific diagnosis and the need for optimal medical therapy, family counseling, and social services must be understood, instituted, and carefully monitored by a team that, in our experience, has required the expertise of not only the pediatric and vascular surgeons, but also geneticists, nephrologists, rheumatologists, cardiologists, pediatric intensive care specialists, interventional radiologists, neurologists, gastroenterologists, neurosurgeons, plastics/microvascular surgeons, and transplantation surgeons.

Diagnosis

Aneurysms of the abdominal and its major named branches in the pediatric population are most commonly asymptomatic and usually noted incidentally by ultrasound, computed tomography, or magnetic resonance imaging being done for another, usually unrelated indication. When an aneurysm is detected in a child, it is essential that complete body imaging be done to determine whether this is an isolated pathology or part of a much more ominous systemic disease or connective tissue disorder. The head and neck region should be imaged with MRI and gadolinium-enhanced MR angiography. The prognosis for children with concurrent intracranial aneurysms is significantly worse than for those with an isolated abdominal aneurysm. In our experience, the presence of both aortic and intracranial aneurysms is highly lethal. Brain MRI/MRA might also reveal changes diagnostic of another rare disease, such as tuberous sclerosis. While MRA can also be used to image the chest, abdomen, pelvis, and extremities, CT angiography offers better blood vessel visualization for the trunk and extremities in small children. A classification for childhood arterial aneurysms has been proposed by Sarkar et al. (Table 112.1) and includes: arterial infection, giant cell aorto-arteritis, autoimmune vasculitis, Kawasaki disease, medial degeneration from genetic causes (Marfan and Ehlers–Danlos syndromes), other forms of medial degeneration, arterial dysplasia, idiopathic/congenital, and extravascular causes. Digital subtraction angiography is frequently not necessary for the diagnosis and complete imaging in these cases. The need for arterial puncture in DSA carries increased access-related complication risk in children. Thus, DSA should be reserved for cases where MRA and CTA imaging are inconclusive or when a therapeutic intervention like embolization is deemed necessary. Doppler ultrasound imaging is sometimes particularly useful, especially for serial follow-up of patient with an aneurysm involving the abdominal aorta, pelvis or an extremity. However, more detailed imaging by CTA or MRA is almost always required for planning a vascular reconstruction operation.

Unlike the aneurysmal diseases, the stenotic/occlusive diseases often present with symptoms, including, from most common to least common: hypertension, claudication, renal failure, congestive heart failure, limb-length mismatch, or intestinal ischemia. Less commonly, the diagnosis is made incidentally when diminished distal pulses are noted on physical examination or a bruit is heard on auscultation of the abdomen. The differential diagnosis includes: fibromuscular dysplasia (FMD),

O.C. Velazquez (✉)
Jackson Memorial Medical Center, University of Miami Hospital,
1611 NW 12th Avenue, Holtz Building, Room 3016 (R-310), Miami,
FL 33136, USA
e-mail: Ovelazquez@med.miami.edu

P. Mattei (ed.), *Fundamentals of Pediatric Surgery*,
DOI 10.1007/978-1-4419-6643-8_112, © Springer Science+Business Media, LLC 2011

Table 112.1 Classification of childhood arterial aneurysms

Class	Principal artery affected	Clinical characteristics and risk factors
Arterial infection	Aorta (particularly thoracic), iliac	Cardiovascular anomalies
		Umbilical catheterization
		Dyspnea
		Cough
		Chest pain
		Progression to rupture
		Death if untreated
Giant cell aortoarteritis	Aorta	Signs and symptoms vary from
		Absent to shock
	peripheral arteries (rare)	Untreated aortic lesions progress to rupture
Autoimmune vasculitis	Renal, hepatic and splenic arterial branches	Usually asymptomatic but may cause hematuria
		Perirenal hematomas, or
		Death with rupture
Kawasaki disease	Coronary (20–30%)	Often asymptomatic
	Axillobrachial	Myocardial infarction or tamponade (coronary)
	Iliofemoral	Limb ischemia (extremity)
	Hepatic	Obstructive jaundice (hepatic)
Medical degeneration, Marfan, and Ehlers–Danlos syndromes	Aorta	Aortic rupture or dissection common
		Arteriography and vascular reconstruction hazardous in type IV Ehlers–Danlos syndrome
Medical degeneration – other forms	Aorta	Associated with cardiac and aortic anomalies
	Peripheral arteries (rare)	Often present with aortic dissection or rupture
Arterial dysplasia	Renal	Usually asymptomatic
		Detected during arteriography for renovascular hypertension
Idiopathic, congenital	Iliofemoral, brachial, aorta	Often asymptomatic
		May cause limb ischemia
		Rupture not reported
Extravascular causes	Aorta, visceral, and extremity arteries	Aortic aneurysms often rupture
		Peripheral lesions asymptomatic
		Visceral lesions can cause GI bleeding

Source: modified from Sarkar R, Coran A, Cilley R, et al. Arterial aneurysms in children: clinicopathologic classification. J Vasc Surg. 1991;13:47–56, with permission from Elsevier

mid-aortic syndrome (MAS), neurofibromatosis, congenital abdominal coarctation, Williams syndrome, Takayasu's disease, and other vasculitides. FMD and MAS are the most commonly encountered entities among this mixed group of conditions. In these patients, the abdominal aorta and/or its major branches are stenotic or occluded. In our experience, the renal arteries are involved in 91% of cases, while the superior mesenteric artery and celiac artery are involved in 35%. For these conditions, DSA is the preferred diagnostic study, since CTA and MRA are often not fully diagnostic due to contrast-dilution and the very small diameter of the vessels. However, an attempt should be made to characterize the problem fully using state-of-the-art Doppler/ultrasound, CTA or MRA when possible, thus potentially avoiding the risks of DSA. In addition, MRA and CTA have the added benefit of showing inflammatory thickening of the wall of the aorta, an important finding that suggests an inflammatory or autoimmune etiology.

For children with either aneurysmal or stenotic/occlusive disease, echocardiogram and electrocardiography should be obtained since, depending on the specific underlying diagnosis, associated cardiovascular anomalies or left ventricular strain can occur. Renal function should be thoroughly assed in all these children. An elevated erythrocyte sedimentation rate or C-reactive protein levels raises suspicion for an active inflammatory process or vasculitis. Finally, in coordination with a rheumatologist, a full serologic panel should be ordered to screen for vasculitis and a thorough genetics evaluation should be requested in all these patients.

Preoperative Preparation

Hypertension should be medically managed in coordination with a nephrologist and with careful monitoring of renal function. In our experience, initial conservative blood pressure management of FMD or idiopathic MAS is feasible and safe in most cases. There are, however, some cases in which blood pressure control is unsatisfactory, renal function deteriorates, cardiac end-organ damage (ventricular hypertrophy) becomes evident by echocardiography, or disabling symptoms of claudication or intestinal ischemia develop. In these cases, prompt surgical reconstruction is indicated. On the other hand, if the hypertension can be adequately managed, it is possible to more carefully plan the vascular reconstructive procedure, which could potentially be delayed until after puberty to increase the availability of autogenous conduit material, allow for better size matching of the bypass to the native vessel, and optimize long-term patency.

A strong multidisciplinary effort to identify the exact diagnosis should be undertaken. Formal consultation with nephrology, rheumatology, and genetics is essential, while the surgeon might be asked to perform tissue or vessel biopsies to help make the diagnosis. If a vasculitis is confirmed, adequate medical treatment should be initiated, and operative reconstruction should be delayed, if possible, until the active inflammatory phase has subsided. The goals of medical therapy are to induce a remission and avoid recurrence or progression of the disease after reconstruction.

The choice for conduit when planning reconstruction needs to be determined in advance. Rather than a blind vein exploration in the operating room at the time of reconstruction, Doppler ultrasound vein mapping of the saphenous and jugular veins should be performed pre-operatively. Patients and their parents need to be aware of the expected additional incisions associated with harvesting autogenous vein conduits. Blood type-matched cryopreserved arterial allografts can be an effective alternative in a child too small for the use of an autogenous conduit (Fig. 112.1). We have used this type of conduit with success in three children presenting with aorto-iliac aneurysms. These conduits are readily available but need to be ordered ahead of the time.

Baseline pulse volume recordings (PVR), arterial Doppler ultrasounds and ankle-brachial indices of the lower extremities should be obtained prior to arterial reconstruction to allow for serial non-invasive physiologic follow-up of patients after reconstruction. Blood and coagulation products should be reserved in advance of the planned operative reconstructions. All potential risks, benefits and expected follow-up should be discussed with the parents in advance of the surgery and as part of the informed consent process.

Surgical Technique

A full midline laparotomy incision with left (and sometimes right) medial visceral rotation is the usual approach for these reconstructions. Though it is not usually necessary to mobilize the kidney and ureter, the descending and transverse colon, spleen, tail of pancreas and stomach are all mobilized medially to gain access to the aorta and named major branches. The left diaphragmatic crus is divided to expose the proximal abdominal aorta. Proximal and distal control is obtained of all vessels to be reconstructed. Heparin, 50–70 units/kg intravenous, is administered

3–5 min prior to clamping the vessels. Fully or partially interrupted suture lines are always used to allow for future circumferential growth of the vessel. Bypass grafts should purposely be created with built-in redundancy to allow for future longitudinal growth of the patient, however kinks must be avoided, as these can precipitate early graft thrombosis.

Aneurysmal disease is reconstructed end-to-end. Stenotic-occlusive disease is reconstructed end-to-side. Internal iliac artery aneurysms can be embolized or resected. All other aneurysms of the abdominal aorta and named branches require vascular reconstruction with restoration of flow.

For stenotic/occlusive disease, many options for treatment and reconstruction are available depending on the extent of disease. For treatment of renal artery stenosis, percutaneous transluminal angioplasty (PTA), vein or Dacron patch angioplasty, direct anastomoses/re-implantation, reversed saphenous vein grafting, partial or complete nephrectomy and nephrectomy with ex-vivo reconstruction and autotransplantation in the pelvis, are all acceptable treatment options. Choice of intervention should be carefully individualized to the specific extent of disease to optimize outcomes. Fibromuscular dysplasia can be treated with PTA, but repeated treatments are sometimes required and it is not advisable for branch lesions. In general, renal stents should be avoided in the pediatric population since their long-term durability is uncertain. If the aorta is not involved, reimplantation and patch angioplasty are good options for focal ostial lesions. When the aorta is involved, an aorto-aortic bypass with 10- to 14-mm Dacron and renal or visceral vein grafts (arising from the Dacron) may be required. Alternatively, the kidneys may be removed, reconstructed ex-vivo and re-implanted in the pelvis if the iliac artery inflow is not compromised by the disease, or if the aortic disease has already been bypassed. Autogenous vein bypass conduits should be re-enforced with 4 or 6 mm tubular Dacron mesh to decrease the known incidence of aneurysmal dilatation.

Complications

Bleeding, infection, thrombosis, reoperation, end-organ ischemia/failure and unforeseeable injuries to adjacent organs are all potential complications of these complex vascular reconstructions in the pediatric population. However, in our reported experience and that of others, the major complication rate ranges from zero to less than 0.5% and long-term outcomes appear to be excellent: more than 70% of reconstructions result in cure of hypertension and greater than 95% of grafts are patent at more than 5 years of follow-up. Chylous ascites and vein graft aneurysms were reported more frequently in earlier experiences, but have become relatively rare.

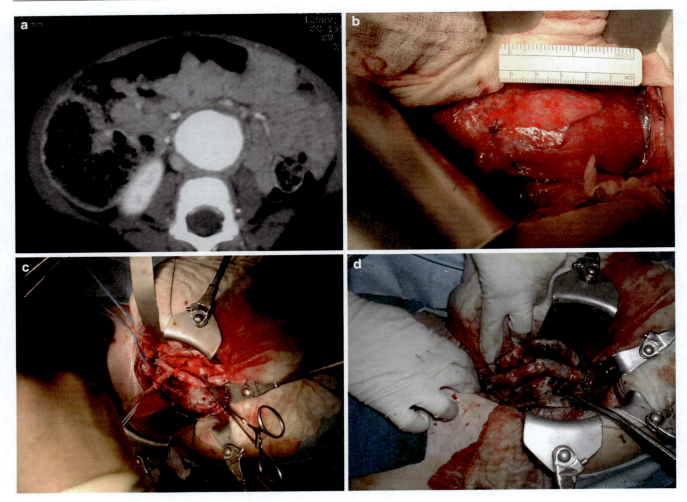

Fig. 112.1 (a) CTA abdomen in 14 month-old child with abdominal aortic aneurysm. (b–d) Intraoperative pictures of aneurysm repair with cryopreserved aorto-iliac arterial allograft. (b) Exposed infrarenal abdominal aortic aneurysm; (c) Proximal anastomosis is completed; (d) Completed reconstruction

Summary Points

- Management of pediatric aortic vascular disease requires a multidisciplinary approach.
- Autologous grafts greater than 3 mm in diameter and of sufficient length (greater saphenous vein, internal jugular vein, internal iliac artery) are preferred for vascular reconstruction to optimize patency.
- Vein grafts should be lined by Dacron tube external re-enforcement to decrease the risk of subsequent aneurismal dilatation.
- Aneurysmal disease carries high risk for rupture, thrombosis, or embolization and should be treated promptly with the intent to reconstruct using artificial graft material, cryopreserved human vessels, or autogenous conduit when available.
- Conservative management with medical treatments for blood pressure is feasible and safe for many patients with idiopathic mid-aortic stenosis.
- Indications for vascular reconstruction on stenotic/occlusive diseases include unsatisfactory medical control of hypertension, renal dysfunction with conservative therapy, evidence of cardiac end-organ damage, symptoms of severe claudication, limb-length discrepancy, or symptoms of intestinal ischemia.

Editor's Comment

There are few children's hospitals with staff surgeons who have the training and expertise to perform complex reconstructive operations of the aorta and its major branches in infants and children on their own. At some children's medical centers, the approach is multidisciplinary, with a team that consists of a vascular surgeon, a pediatric general surgeon, and an interventional radiologist. This approach combines the expertise of several skilled individuals who can work together to achieve excellent results in children with vascular problems that require major reconstruction.

Complex reconstructive vascular operations in children can certainly be challenging but are surprisingly well-tolerated. Patients with renovascular hypertension should have their blood pressure well-controlled, usually with beta-blocker therapy, prior to a planned procedure. At least one lower extremity should be sterilely prepared during any operation that could require the use of autologous vein graft material. Exposure is very important and usually entails a long midline or left thoracoabdominal incision. The spleen and left colon should be fully mobilized to expose the aorta and its major branches. If the right renal or iliac vessels need to be addresses, the right colon might need to be mobilized as well. Of course, proximal and distal vascular control is also very important. The thoracic aorta might need to be exposed by dividing the left crus to achieve proximal control. These exposures are generally more straightforward in children than they are in adults because of cleaner dissection planes, a paucity of fat and fibrosis, and pristine vessels free of atherosclerosis. The usual cardiac risks that are a major concern in adult vascular surgery are also rarely an issue in these children. Nevertheless, in these situations one can never afford to be cavalier.

Vascular anastomoses in children are performed with fine permanent monofilament sutures in the usual fashion, but one must always incorporate the possibility for growth at the anastomosis itself as well as in the length of the graft. Anastomoses should be performed at least partly with interrupted sutures although some surgeons prefer instead to incorporate a "growth stitch," which can gradually loosen over time as the child grows. Grafts should be created with some degree of redundancy to account for linear growth. Autologous venous grafts are ideal conduits but tend to become aneurysmal over time. A way to avoid these aneurysms is to reinforce the grafts with an outer covering of polytetrafluoroethylene graft. Depending on the caliber of the graft, 4- or 6-mm conduits are cut along their length and placed around the grafts after they have been sutured in place. Complications are rare and include bleeding, thrombosis, ischemia, and embolism. Long-term results have been excellent but close follow up and serial MR angiography are essential.

Differential Diagnosis

- Aneurysms
- Arterial infection
- Giant cell aortoarteritis
- Autoimmune vasculitis
- Kawasaki disease
- Medial degeneration from genetic causes – Marfan and Ehlers–Danlos syndromes
- Medial degeneration – other forms
- Arterial dysplasia
- Idiopathic/congenital
- Extravascular causes (trauma)
- Stenotic/occlusive disease
- Fibromuscular hyperplasia
- Neurofibromatosis
- Mid-aortic syndrome
- Arterial hypoplasia
- Congenital abdominal coarctation
- William's syndrome
- Takayasu's disease
- Other vasculitis
- Anastomosis stenosis

Diagnostic Studies

- Magnetic resonance imaging and angiography (MRI/MRA)
- Computer tomography (CTA)
- Doppler/ultrasonography (US)
- Digital subtraction angiography (DSA)
- Echocardiogram and electrocardiography

Parental Preparation

- Recommend genetic testing and counseling.
- Introduce family to social workers and case managers.
- Explain risks of operative reconstruction such as bleeding, infection, thrombosis, reoperation, end-organ ischemia/failure, and unforeseeable injuries to adjacent organs.
- Explain the nature of long-term follow up required (repeated imaging studies).
- Major operation, long recovery, large incisions.
- Possible need for post-operative anticoagulation.
- Likely need for ongoing medical treatments, including treatment for hypertension, in the first year post-operatively.

Preoperative Preparation

☐ Baseline pulse volume recordings (PVRs), arterial Doppler/ultrasound, and ankle-brachial indices (ABIs)

☐ Vein mapping studies defining any available autogenous conduit

☐ Type and Cross for blood, platelets, and coagulation products

☐ Complete body imaging

☐ Control of hypertension

☐ Informed consent

Technical Points

• Use a generous midline laparotomy incision with left (and sometimes right) medial visceral rotation; the kidney is not mobilized; the left diaphragmatic crus is divided to expose the proximal aorta; the colon, spleen, tail of pancreas, and stomach are all mobilized medially.

• Obtain proximal and distal control of all vessels to be reconstructed.

• Administer systemic heparin intravenously prior to clamping any vessels.

• Use interrupted suture lines to allow for future growth in diameter.

• Create grafts with built-in redundancy to allow for linear somatic growth.

Suggested Reading

English WP, Edwards MS, Pierce JD, et al. Multiple aneurysms in childhood. J Vasc Surg. 2004;39:254–9.

Kaye AJ, Slemp AE, Chang B, Mattei P, Fairman RM, Velazquez OC. Complex vascular reconstruction of abdominal aorta and its branches in the pediatric population. J Pediatr Surg. 2008;43(6): 1082–8.

O'Neil Jr JA, Berkowitz H, Fellows KJ, et al. Midaortic syndrome and hypertension in childhood. J Pediatr Surg. 1995;30:164–71.

Sarkar R, Coran AG, Cilley RE, et al. Arterial aneurysms in children: clinicopathologic classification. J Vasc Surg. 1991;13:47–56.

Sethna CB, Kaplan BS, Cahill AM, Velazquez OC, Meyers KE. Idiopathic mid-aortic syndrome in children. Pediatr Nephrol. 2008;23(7):1135–42.

Chapter 113
Ventricular Shunts for Hydrocephalus

Gregory G. Heuer and Phillip B. Storm

Hydrocephalus is the pathologic accumulation of cerebrospinal fluid within the ventricles of the brain. It is one of the most common conditions requiring the services of a pediatric neurosurgeon, occurring with an incidence of 1 in 2,000 births. The etiology is varied and includes obstructive causes, such as brain stem or posterior fossa tumors, intraventricular tumors, intracranial cysts, infection, encephalophele, genetic syndromes, or acute intracranial hemorrhage, as well as non-obstructive causes, which include congenital malformations, prematurity, some infections, and germinal matrix hemorrhage.

Untreated, hydrocephalus is usually fatal. Patients who present with hydrocephalus causing increased intracranial pressure require a procedure to divert the flow of CSF. Prior to the 1950s, most patients with hydrocephalus did not survive, as there were no effective long-term treatments. Surgeons used shunting devices as early as 1905 with little success. The modern shunt was developed in 1952 at The Children's Hospital of Philadelphia. This provided an effective surgical treatment for hydrocephalus and the management of this previously fatal condition changed dramatically.

Diagnosis

Hydrocephalus is a clinical diagnosis made when a patient has signs or symptoms of elevated intracranial pressure and evidence of ventricular enlargement on medical imaging. The presentation varies depending on the age of the patient and the etiology. Newborns and infants typically present with an enlarging head circumference, splayed cranial sutures, and a bulging anterior fontanelle. Because the fontanelle is still open and the sutures are not fused, infants can tolerate significant hydrocephalus without developing signs other than enlarging head size. Other signs in very young patients include irritability and somnolence, and, if a brain tumor is present, cranial nerve abnor-

malities. Elevated intracranial pressure can also cause newborns to have periods of apnea and bradycardia that are not a result of dysfunction of their cardiopulmonary system.

Although hydrocephalus typically presents in infancy, it can present in older children and adolescents, usually due to a tumor. Older children typically present with morning headaches, nausea, and vomiting. As the hydrocephalus worsens, the symptoms occur throughout the day and the headache intensifies. Because their sutures are closed they do not tolerate acute hydrocephalus as well as infants do. A late sign of hydrocephalus occurs when pressure is exerted on the superior colliculus of the midbrain causing an upgaze palsy ("setting sun sign"). The patient's eyes have a dramatic down-gaze and take on the appearance of a sun falling below the horizon (a component of Parinaud's syndrome).

Patients with a clinical picture suggestive of hydrocephalus should have neuroimaging to: (1) confirm the diagnosis of hydrocephalus; (2) ascertain the cause of the hydrocephalus; (3) identify any associated malformations (Dandy–Walker malformation); and (4) help develop a surgical plan for treatment. Hydrocephalus is often diagnosed and followed by ultrasound in infants while the anterior fontanelle is still open (Fig. 113.1). In older infants and children, CT is used to make the diagnosis. Some newly diagnosed patients require MR scan to identify structural abnormalities and tumors.

Patients who have had shunts placed previously for treatment of the hydrocephalus require additional imaging in the form of a shunt series, which consists of radiographs of the skull, neck, chest, and abdomen. The shunt series traces the entire course of the shunt tubing to confirm continuity of the system. These patients also should have a CT scan of the brain to compare the size of the ventricles.

Ventricular Shunt Devices

A standard ventricular shunt consists of three components (Fig. 113.2). The terms proximal and distal refer to the position of the shunt segment in relation to the valve. The proximal end is a silastic tube with a 2-cm section at the tip containing holes.

G.G. Heuer (✉)
Resident, Department of Neurosurgery, University of Pennsylvania, The Children's Hospital of Philadelphia, 877 N. 30th St. Philadelphia, PA 19130, USA
e-mail: gregory.heuer@uphs.upenn.edu

P. Mattei (ed.), *Fundamentals of Pediatric Surgery*,
DOI 10.1007/978-1-4419-6643-8_113, © Springer Science+Business Media, LLC 2011

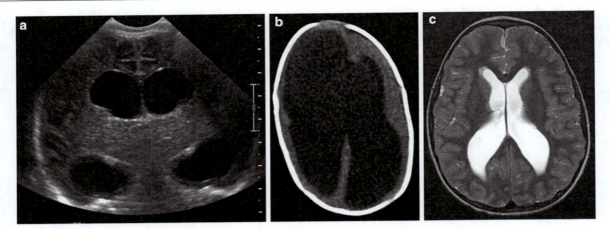

Fig. 113.1 Radiographic images demonstrating hydrocephalus. (**a**) Head ultrasound in a newborn demonstrating ventriculomegaly. (**b**) Head CT demonstrating ventriculomegaly. (**c**) Brain MRI demonstrating increased hydrocephalus associated with a posterior fossa tumor

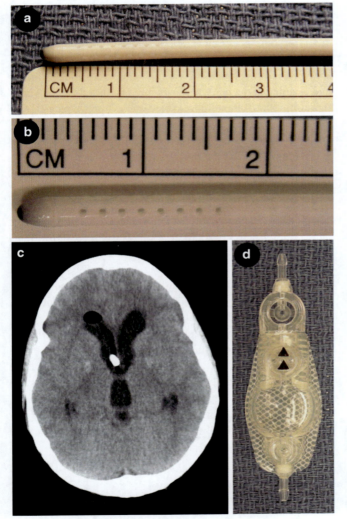

Fig. 113.2 Shunt system components. (**a**, **b**) Typical proximal ventricular shunt and 2-cm section at the tip containing side-holes. (**c**) Axial CT demonstrating the proximal catheter placed into the lateral ventricle. (**d**) Typical shunt valve (Medtronic, St Paul, Minn.)

The catheter is placed into the lateral ventricle through a frontal or occipital burr hole. The frontal burr hole is approximately 1–2 cm anterior to the coronal suture and approximately 3 cm off the midline, normally in the mid-pupillary line. The occipital burr hole is placed approximately 1 cm superior to the inion and about 4 cm lateral to the midline. Obviously some of these measurements will vary based on head size, but identifying bony landmarks is critical. Patients who have CSF systems that are not communicating sometimes require more than one proximal catheter into each CSF collection.

The second component of the shunt is the valve. There are a number of different types of valves. All function to regulate the flow of CSF and can have a pressure setting that is set or adjustable. Most shunt valve systems have a reservoir that allows for interrogation of the device and sampling of fluid.

The third component is the distal catheter, which extends from the valve to a body cavity where the CSF can be absorbed. The distal catheter typically is placed into the peritoneal cavity. If the peritoneal cavity is no longer an option because of a lack of adequate space, infection, or an inability to absorb CSF, the pleural cavity and the venous system are also options.

Treatment

Most patients presenting to an emergency department with a possible shunt failure are not in extremis and the neurosurgeon has time to obtain radiographic images and diagnose a proximal or distal malfunction, infection, or exclude a shunt problem entirely. Patients typically present with headache, nausea and vomiting, or a fever and should be evaluated with a head CT and a shunt series. The head CT should be compared to prior studies. If the ventricles are dilated, it is almost always diagnostic of a shunt malfunction. If the ventricles are stable, it is highly suggestive of a properly functioning shunt. However, because some patients have poorly compliant brains, they can have florid shunt failure despite an unchanged CT scan. The shunt series is evaluated for breaks in the tubing or for migration of the distal tubing. If there are no CT scans for comparison or the diagnosis cannot be made by the combination of history, physical examination, and imaging, the shunt must be interrogated.

A noninvasive way to interrogate the shunt is to depress the valve. If the valve remains collapsed or is very slow to refill in the setting of ventricles that are dilated, this is strongly suggestive of a proximal shunt malfunction. The exception is the patient with very small ventricles and little CSF. In these patients, a slowly refilling valve is consistent with a functioning shunt. If the valve pumps and refills briskly, the shunt is either working normally or there is a distal malfunction.

If the diagnosis is still in question or there is still a high suspicion for shunt malfunction, a 25-gauge butterfly needle is inserted through the skin into the reservoir. This not only allows measurement of the ICP but also allows analysis of CSF. A normal shunt tap will reveal a pressure less than 8 cm of water and the meniscus will vary with the heartbeat. Fluid is then easily aspirated and, in the case of a suspected infection, the CSF can be sent for cell count, gram stain, culture and sensitivity. In the setting of a distal obstruction, the fluid often overflows the top of the butterfly tubing and several milliliters of fluid are easily removed, often with immediate relief of symptoms. With a proximal obstruction, there is no fluid in the butterfly tubing or it does not vary with the heart rate, fluid usually cannot be removed, and the valve might collapse around the needle. And because fluid cannot be removed to ameliorate symptoms, a proximal obstruction should be considered urgent and, if the patient is symptomatic, a true emergency.

Once the diagnosis of shunt obstruction is made, stable patients are managed with dexamethasone (Decadron, 1 mg/kg/day divided every 6 h up to maximum daily dose of 16 mg), acetazolamide (Diamox, 30 mg/kg/day divided every 8 h up to a maximum daily dose of 1,500 mg) and ranitidine. We admit all of our hydrocephalus patients to the pediatric intensive care unit and plan surgical revision within 24 h.

Patients with newly diagnosed unshunted hydrocephalus or a proximal shunt obstruction presenting with obtundation, bradycardia, hypertension, or declining mental status require emergent intervention with intubation, hyperventilation, and mannitol or hypertonic saline. Newly diagnosed patients are usually treated with an externalized ventriculostomy placed in the emergency room, intensive care unit, or a shunt placed in the operating room. In extreme circumstances of proximal shunt obstruction we have inserted a 20-gauge spinal needle through the scalp, burr hole and brain along the trajectory of the obstructed catheter and let off CSF to temporally relieve the elevated pressure. The patient still needs a definitive procedure – ventriculostomy,

shunt placement, or revision – but they get immediate relief and a neurologic disaster is avoided.

Surgical Technique

Ventricular shunting is safe in patients of all ages and is useful for all types and causes of hydrocephalus. The peri-procedural mortality rate associated with shunt placement is less than 0.1%. The standard surgical technique is well established and routinely performed at all neurosurgical centers with relatively little variation.

Patients are placed supine on the operating room table and their heads are turned as far to one side as possible. Attempts are made to position the patient in such a manner as to make a straight path from the burr hole in the skull to the distal opening (Fig. 113.3). A role placed under the

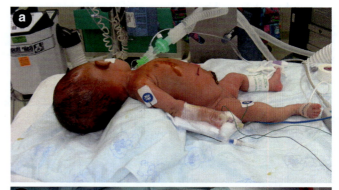
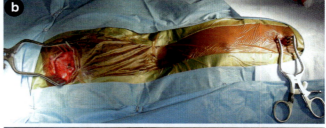
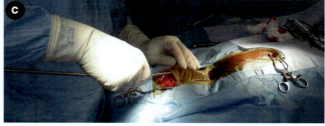

Fig. 113.3 Placement of a standard ventriculoperitoneal catheter. (**a**) Patient positioned supine on the operating room table. Note the placement of a roll under the shoulders which creates a straight line from the cranial incision to the abdominal incision. (**b**) Patient is prepared and draped, exposing the entire length of the path of the subcutaneous tunnel. A curvilinear incision is made in the skin and a burr hole is made in the skull just posterior to the ear. (**c**) Passage of the tunneling device in the subcutaneous space from the cranial incision to the abdominal incision

shoulder serves two purposes: it decreases the acuteness of the angle between the neck and the chest, reducing the risk of passing the tunneling device under the clavicle and into the chest, and it allows for proper placement of the occipital burr hole in patients who are obese or have necks that are have limited range of motion. The skin is sterilely prepared along the entire subcutaneous course of the shunt. A major problem with placement of shunt systems is infection. The rate of infection is significantly reduced by minimizing the handling of the shunt system and by completing the surgery quickly.

We favor an occipital approach because it allows the shunt to be passed from the cranial to the peritoneal incision without an intervening incision. In those cases where a frontal approach is used, a second incision behind the ear is required as a subcutaneous tunnel cannot be made from the burr hole to the site of the distal catheter. We use a frontal approach when the ventricles are small and cannot be accessed by an occipital approach. In these cases, intraoperative ultrasound or frameless stereotactic navigation can be invaluable. Fortunately, the vast majority of hydrocephalus patients have sufficiently dilated ventricles that an occipital approach is easily performed.

For new ventriculoperitoneal shunts the proximal and the distal ends are prepared by two surgeons working simultaneously. For the proximal end, a curvilinear incision is made in the skin and a burr hole is made in the skull. The dura is cauterized and opened sharply in a cruciate fashion with a #11 scalpel blade. After the dura is opened, its edges are cauterized along with the pial surface until meticulous hemostasis is achieved. Care is taken to minimize the opening to prevent the leakage of CSF around the catheter. A Kelly clamp is used to make a pocket for the reservoir. A metal tunneling device is passed under the skin in the subcutaneous tissue. The two challenges are not breaking through the skin when tunneling near the mastoid and the upper neck, and secondly not passing under the clavicle. Once the tunneling device is over the clavicle it passes easily to the small incision in the abdomen.

The peritoneum is prepared by making a linear incision in the abdomen. There are a myriad of acceptable locations, but we prefer a few centimeters below the costal margin. The underlying rectus fascial layer is exposed by bluntly dissecting through the subcutaneous fat. The fascia is sharply incised in a vertical fashion, the rectus muscle fibers are bluntly spread down to the peritoneum. The peritoneum is isolated between to hemostat clamps and sharply opened.

Once the tunneling device exits at the abdominal incision, a zero silk tie is secured on the end and the device is removed at the scalp end with the silk tie running along the subcutaneous tunnel that was just created. The distal end of the shunt is secured with the silk tie at the scalp and pulled back through the subcutaneous tissue. A blunt brain cannula is inserted through the brain into the ventricle until there is good egress of clear CSF. The brain cannula is removed and the proximal end of the shunt is passed into the ventricle through the track created by the cannula. Once flow of CSF from the distal catheter is confirmed, the catheter is placed into the peritoneal cavity under direct vision. The incisions are then closed in layers.

Postoperative Care

Patients are admitted to a monitored bed after shunt placement. They are observed for any signs of immediate shunt malfunction or complications (intracranial hemorrhage). A functioning shunt reduces ICP right away and patients normally have some immediate improvement in their signs and symptoms. Patients are routinely sent home on the first post-operative day. In the rare instance of suspected shunt failure in the immediate post-operative period, the shunt is evaluated with a head CT and one should consider accessing the valve with a 25-gauge needle to assess the proximal and distal portions of the shunt. We do not routinely order CT scans of the brain, only when we suspect a complication.

There are significant long-term complications of shunting devices, including sub-optimal shunting, mechanical failure, and infection. The 1-year failure rate varies but may be as high as 30 or 40%. This failure rate is significantly higher in premature and young infants because they often have numerous medical problems in addition to hydrocephalus. New designs may be able to overcome some types of mechanical failure and reduce infections. Some groups are retrospectively reporting that the use of programmable shunts and antibiotic impregnated catheters significantly decrease the rate of mechanical failures and infections; however, better controlled studies are needed to validate these claims and justify the increased costs.

Emerging Technology

In addition to ventricular shunts, other surgical techniques have been used for CSF diversion. One particularly useful technique for carefully selected patients is endoscopic third ventriculostomy. This technique involves placing an endoscope into the lateral ventricle and advancing it through the foramen of Monroe into the third ventricle. A hole is made in the floor of the third ventricle behind the posterior clinoid but in front of the basilar artery. The hole allows CSF to flow out of the ventricular system into the subarachnoid space, thus bypassing the obstruction.

At The Johns Hopkins Hospital, Walter Dandy successfully performed third ventriculostomies in several patients. In 1923, an urologist named William Mixter used a urethroscope to perform a third ventriculostomy in a patient with hydrocephalus. However, these early approaches were associated with a high complication and failure rates and therefore were not widely adopted. In recent years, more advanced surgical techniques and equipment have been developed that allow endoscopic third ventriculostomy (ETV) to be performed with an acceptable complication and success rates. Unfortunately, only patients with obstructive hydrocephalus below the level of the foramen of Monroe are candidates and they need to have the correct anatomy to ensure that the procedure can be performed safely. Also, this type of procedure is usually reserved for children older than 2 years of age, as very young patients have a high rate of ETV failure.

Hydrocephalus is a common and serious condition that the pediatric neurosurgeon encounters. It requires prompt evaluation and treatment. Special attention needs to be paid to the cause of the hydrocephalus in order to effectively treat and follow the hydrocephalic patient. Ventricular shunting is a safe and effective treatment for hydrocephalus. When performed at a center with considerable experience, this procedure can be accomplished with little morbidity. Future advances in the technology of shunt systems and in the development of ETV hold promise to further advance the treatment of pediatric hydrocephalus.

Summary Points

- Hydrocephalus is the pathologic accumulation of cerebrospinal fluid within the ventricles of the brain.
- It is one of the most common conditions requiring the services of a pediatric neurosurgeon.
- Because the fontanelle is still open and the sutures are not fused, infants can tolerate significant hydrocephalus without developing signs other than enlarging head size.
- Elevated intracranial pressure can also cause newborns to have periods of apnea and bradycardia.
- Older children typically present with morning headaches, nausea, and vomiting.
- A late sign of hydrocephalus is the "setting sun sign," an upgaze palsy that occurs when pressure is exerted on the superior colliculus of the midbrain.

Editor's Comment

Although gravity probably helps, the flow of CSF in a ventricular shunt relies on the gradient between the high pressure present in the ventricles of the brain and the lower pressure available in the peritoneal cavity, where the fluid can also be absorbed. When the peritoneum is not available due to adhesions or infection, other options include the pleural cavity and the right atrium (intravascular). Historically, other options have included the gallbladder or urinary bladder, however these procedures have largely been abandoned because of the risk of ascending infection and stone formation. Minimally invasive techniques can and should be used to place the distal catheter into the peritoneal cavity, the pleural space or the intravascular space whenever possible. This might include laparoscopy, thoracoscopy, or a modification of the Seldinger technique.

To avoid shunt malfunction or ascending infection (meningitis), precautions need to be taken when a patient with a ventricular shunt undergoes an operation for some other reason. Patients should receive prophylactic antibiotics for clean-contaminated or contaminated cases or if the shunt might come into contact with the skin. Obviously, incisions should be made carefully so as to avoid injury to the shunt. Although it apparently safe to create a pneumoperitoneum in the presence of a VP shunt that contains a one-way valve, to avoid infection and pneumocephalus it is probably safest to bring the distal end of the shunt out through a trocar site for the duration of the operation.

Some prefer to wrap the catheter in antibiotic-soaked gauze although this probably overkill. During inguinal herniorrhaphy, the catheter has been known to sometimes protrude through the inguinal hernia sac, where it can be injured or caught up in the ligation of the hernia sac. In the case of frank peritonitis, such as perforated appendicitis, the neurosurgeons will need to exteriorize the shunt and remove the distal catheter.

Patients with ventricular shunts occasionally develop complications that involve other surgical services. The intraperitoneal portion of the shunt can erode into the intestine and will sometimes even project through the anus after having eroded into the colon. This almost always creates more drama than danger and the treatment is nearly always simply the removal of the catheter (through the anus) and allowing the small opening in the bowel to heal itself. Cerebrospinal fluid draining into the peritoneum can sometimes create a pseudocyst which can be confused for an ovarian mass or other tumor. It can also result in a small bowel obstruction. The treatment is usually removal of the catheter and allowing the pseudocyst fluid to be resorbed. Only rarely does a lysis of adhesions or excision of the pseudocyst need to be performed. In infants with a patent processus, placement of a VP shunt will often lead to the formation of a large hydrocele or inguinal hernia. These should be repaired in the usual fashion before they become symptomatic or excessively large because this increases the recurrence rate. Patients with ventricular shunts that become infected usually present with classic signs and symptoms of meningitis, but young children with meningitis will sometimes present with what appears to be an acute abdominal process. Distinguishing the two can be difficult although three-dimensional abdominal imaging will usually help identify a source of pain in the abdomen such as appendicitis or pancreatitis. In these situations, cooperation between the general surgery and neurosurgery services is clearly important.

Diagnostic Studies

- CT
- MRI
- Shunt series
- Shunt interrogation
- CSF cell count and culture

Differential Diagnosis

Obstructive causes

- Brain stem or posterior fossa tumors
- Intraventricular tumors
- Intracranial cysts
- Infection
- Encephalophele
- Genetic syndromes
- Acute intracranial hemorrhage

Non-obstructive causes

- Congenital malformations
- Prematurity
- Infection
- Germinal matrix hemorrhage

Parental Preparation

- Standard therapy of hydrocephalus includes placement of a ventriculo-peritoneal shunt.
- VP shunts usually allow normal growth and function but, like any mechanical device, might require frequent revisions and modifications over time.
- Newer methods that include noninvasive endoscopic techniques are being developed.

Preoperative Preparation

- ☐ CT or MRI
- ☐ Treatment of underlying condition
- ☐ Prophylactic antibiotics

Technical Points

- A standard ventricular shunt consists of three components: proximal catheter, valve and distal catheter.
- The proximal end is placed through a burr hole placed in the skull and the distal end is placed in the peritoneal cavity where the CSF is absorbed.
- When the diagnosis of shunt obstruction is made, stable patients are managed with dexamethasone, acetazolamide, and ranitidine.
- All hydrocephalus patients who present with shunt obstruction are admitted to the pediatric intensive care unit and surgical revision is planned within 24 h.

Suggested Reading

Beni-Adani L, Biani N, Ben-Sirah L, Constantini S. The occurrence of obstructive vs absorptive hydrocephalus in newborns and infants: relevance to treatment choices. Childs Nerv Syst. 2006;22:1543–63.

Drake JM, Kestle JR, Milner R, et al. Randomized trial of cerebrospinal fluid shunt valve design in pediatric hydrocephalus. Neurosurgery. 1998;43:294–303.

Jallo GI, Kothbauer KF, Abbott IR. Endoscopic third ventriculostomy. Neurosurg Focus. 2005;19:E11.

Kestle JR, Hoffman HJ, Soloniuk D, Humphreys RP, Drake JM, Hendrick EB. A concerted effort to prevent shunt infection. Childs Nerv Syst. 1993;9:163–5.

Sciubba DM, Stuart RM, McGirt MJ, et al. Effect of antibiotic-impregnated shunt catheters in decreasing the incidence of shunt infection in the treatment of hydrocephalus. J Neurosurg. 2005;103:131–6.

Wiswell TE, Tuttle DJ, Northam RS, Simonds GR. Major congenital neurologic malformations. A 17-year survey. Am J Dis Child. 1990;144:61–7.

Chapter 114
Conjoined Twins

Gary E. Hartman

Conjoined twins are among the rarest developmental anomalies with incidence estimates ranging from 1 in 50,000 to 1 in 200,000 births. Most of the sets identified prenatally die either during pregnancy (25%) or within 24 h of birth (50%). While it is claimed that the incidence among stillborns is equal between boys and girls, girls predominate 3:1 among the live-born sets.

The twins are categorized by the location of the joining (thoraco-, omphalo-, cranio-) combined with the Greek term pagus ("that which is fixed") (Table 114.1). Twins joined at the chest and abdomen represent almost three quarters of the reported sets. There are two theories of the etiology of conjoined twins, the fission and the fusion theories. Historically it has been assumed that conjoined twins resulted from incomplete separation of a monozygotic twin embryo between the 13th and 15th day after fertilization. An alternative theory (fusion) is that two embryos fuse after initially being separate. There is no association with previous conjoining, maternal age or parity. While conjoined twins fit into the common classification categories with many similarities among them, it is best to consider each set a unique pair of individuals requiring careful anatomic evaluation and possessing separate moral and ethical identities.

Diagnosis

The diagnosis can be established by ultrasound as early as 12 weeks gestation by identifying constant relative positions of the fetuses, a single placenta with no separating membrane, or a single umbilical cord with more than three vessels. Follow-up scanning at 20 weeks provides reliable visceral detail and should include echocardiography.

While fetal echocardiography is quite accurate it tends to underestimate the degree of cardiac malformation and cannot reliably exclude myocardial fusion. Three-dimensional echocardiography provides greater detail. Since the chance of survival and separability are largely dependent on the extent of the cardiac anomalies, it is essential to obtain accurate cardiac imaging. In some instances, the imaging windows available are better prenatally than postnatally. If the pregnancy continues into the third trimester, a fetal MRI should be performed as it provides excellent soft tissue resolution and a larger field of view.

The frequency of associated anomalies and the site of fusion dictate the need for postnatal diagnostic studies. All sets should have plain X-rays of the chest and abdomen to identify associated anomalies such as diaphragmatic hernia, vertebral malformations, and cardiac lesions. Echocardiography and cranial ultrasound should also be performed in all cases. Additional studies are dictated by the location of the conjoining; the timing of these studies depends on their clinical condition. If the twins are stable, a few limited studies are obtained with the more complex imaging awaiting a period of transition and growth. If the twins' clinical condition is tenuous or discordant, suggesting that urgent separation might need to be considered, diagnostic studies should proceed with thoughtful multidisciplinary input.

In thoraco-omphalopagus twins the bowel gas pattern might appear to be separate on plain radiographs but more specific studies such as gastrointestinal contrast or CT with contrast should be obtained. Ultrasound of the liver, hepatic veins and abdominal viscera can provide valuable information about separability and can be accomplished with portable equipment if the infants are unstable. Computed tomography (Fig. 114.1) and MRI of head, chest and abdomen are obtained under general anesthesia and should be planned with sequences and timing of contrast injections optimized to provide as much dynamic information as possible while limiting the duration of the studies. Modern imaging software allows three-dimensional reconstruction that provides amazing detail and visualization of the proposed separation. The digital data from the cross-sectional

G.E. Hartman (✉)
Department of Pediatric Surgery, Stanford University School of Medicine, Lucile Packard Children's Hospital, 780 Welch Road, Suite 206, Stanford, CA 94305, USA
e-mail: ghartman@lpch.org

P. Mattei (ed.), *Fundamentals of Pediatric Surgery*,
DOI 10.1007/978-1-4419-6643-8_114, © Springer Science+Business Media, LLC 2011

Table 114.1 Types of conjoined twins

Category	Fusion	Percentage (%)
Thoracopagus	Chest/abdomen	20–40
Omphalopagus	Abdomen	18–33
Pygopagus	Sacrum/buttocks	18–28
Ischiopagus	Pelvis	6–11
Craniopagus	Cranium	2
Parapagus	Ventrolateral	New term

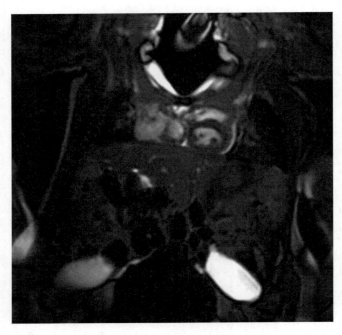

Fig. 114.1 Saggital CT of thoraco-omphalopagus conjoined twins

imaging can be used to make physical models of the twins and their viscera allowing further planning both for the separation and the reconstruction and calculations of the anticipated defect in the body wall resulting from the separation. In addition, the imaging allows flow estimations about twin–twin shunting at the cardiac and visceral levels. In cases of possible separation with structural cardiac anomalies, cardiac catheterization should follow the same indications as those of a singleton infant and might also reveal pulmonary hypertension or substantiate cross-circulation. Imaging of the biliary trees should be accurate from the MRI but in some cases should be supplemented by nuclear imaging.

Laboratory studies should include basic metabolic studies as well as oxygen saturations, arterial blood gases, and electrocardiograms. Twins with even small myocardial connections will usually have synchronous heart rates.

Twins joined at the pelvic and sacral regions (ischiopagus, pyopagus) often have complex vertebral, orthopedic, and genitourinary abnormalities; CT and MRI are required to identify the bony and visceral anomalies as well as possible fusion of the spinal cord. Multiplanar MRI is helpful in cataloging the pelvic viscera (uterus, bladders, fallopian tubes). Cross circulation is sometimes significant in these twins and, as in thoraco-omphalopagus, the contrast injection is done in one twin only and the scanning timed to obtain arterial and venous information. Delayed images are helpful in determining renal function. Complementary information is obtained by performing contrast studies of the genitourinary and gastrointestinal tracts. Cloacal anomalies and single rectum are common and accurate definition of the anatomy is critical to planning the surgical separation.

Twins joined at the head are classified as craniopagus or cephalopagus. Cephalopagus twins are usually also fused at the chest and have generally been thought to be nonviable, although a set of girls who are now 16 years old have chronicled their lives in short video clips on the internet. Craniopagus twins account for approximately 2% of all conjoining though they are more heavily reported in the lay press. Some cases have separate dura but most have significant connections of cerebral cortex and share at least a portion of the sagittal sinus.

Twins joined side to side are called parapagus and can have extensive connections with complex pelvic anatomy. They usually have a shared leg, a single symphysis pubis and one or two sacra. Unions that include the chest have complicated cardiac anomalies similar to the thoraco-omphalopagus twins and need extensive cardiac evaluation. The blood supply to the shared pelvis and lower extremity can be outlined with CT and MRI and rarely requires angiography.

Treatment

Multidisciplinary planning should begin prior to delivery. Counseling regarding viability and the possibility of separation should be accomplished with input from specialists with experience in the appropriate areas. Hospitalization is frequently indicated late in the pregnancy with a planned Cesarean section although obstetrical complications are frequent and often necessitate an urgent delivery. Stabilization in the neonatal ICU should include standard neonatal care with multidisciplinary evaluation and attention to privacy. While in the NICU, public and media exposure is usually well controlled but excessive or unnecessary examination by medical and hospital personnel is a risk and must be controlled. The optimal situation is stabilization of the infants such that they could be discharged home to return for further evaluation. The optimal time for elective separation is undetermined but has been suggested at between 4 months and 2 years. We have noted that even with separation at 4 months of age there are already significant musculoskeletal changes that require remodeling or physical therapy. On the other hand, larger size, more time for tissue expansion, and more "durability" of vessels and tissue are advantages of a delayed separation.

Emergency separation needs be considered when one twin is unstable or if both physiologically deteriorate due to their connection. If one twin dies, the other will succumb within 4–6 h from disseminated intravascular coagulation. In the absence of complete preparation for separation, emergency separation should only be considered when the death of one twin is imminent and the goal is salvage of the healthier twin. The specific management of each set of twins will depend on their physiologic status and specific constellation of conjoining and associated anomalies.

Thoraco-omphalopagus is the most common type of conjoining and with personal experience in the separation of five sets their treatment will be outlined here. Twins joined at the pelvis will require involvement of orthopedic, urologic, and neurosurgical colleagues and the operative plan will obviously be determined by the nature of their connections. Separation of craniopagus twins will not be discussed in detail.

The anesthetic and team coordination management of the twins begins with their diagnostic studies, as most will require general anesthesia. Experience with the twins' reaction to specific drugs, the degree of cross-circulation, and their recovery patterns are helpful in planning the separation procedure. We combine studies whenever possible, having obtained CT, MRI, and cardiac catheterization under a single anesthetic. Even with limiting of data acquisition this can take 6–8 h.

Tissue expansion is usually required to obtain adequate skin coverage of the large body wall defect created by the separation. We have used tissue expanders in twins as young as 2 months of age and have placed the expanders either on the connecting bridge itself or parallel to it. The expanders can be filled fairly rapidly, with weekly injections, usually either with topical anesthetic or a brief general anesthetic. Care must be taken to avoid excessive pressure, as the expanders are placed on both lateral surfaces of the twins. The timing of the insertion and expected expansion needs to be coordinated with the separation date.

Younger twins or those requiring a preoperative bowel preparation should be admitted the day prior to separation, though we have admitted older twins with separate gastrointestinal tracts on the day of surgery. Some centers insert all monitoring lines under a separate anesthetic on the day prior to separation. The induction, insertion of central and peripheral venous, arterial, and urinary catheters, temperature probes and positioning with careful padding of pressure points usually requires at least 2 h (Fig. 114.2).

The initial incision is centered at the midpoint of the connecting skin bridge and the tissue expanders on the "up" side of the twins are removed. The abdomen is easily entered at the umbilicus, which frequently has a small omphalocele membrane that is usually epithelialized by the date of separation. The abdominal portion of the body wall connection is opened and the peritoneal cavity of each twin is entered and

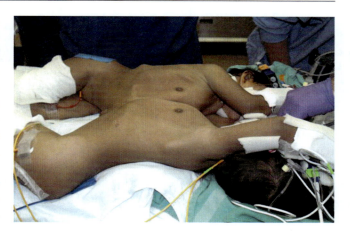

Fig. 114.2 Twins positioned with monitoring in place

the viscera inspected. The fused sternum on the "up" side is then carefully entered, which can be done without entering the common pericardium or separate pleural spaces. The pleurae of each twin can be bluntly dissected free of the sternal edges to expose the pericardium, which is entered again at the midpoint of the connection. The degree of any cardiac connection can now be assessed and preparation for potential cardiac bypass or pacing begun.

Opening of the abdomen and chest has thus allowed complete assessment of the visceral connections. Our strategy has then been to complete the separation of the abdominal viscera and the abdominal body wall of the "down" side prior to any cardiac procedures. Although cannulation for bypass is possible in the lateral position, this would allow for expeditious separation of the "down" sternum should either twin deteriorate.

The majority of thorac-omphalopagus twins have a fused liver, usually with separate biliary and vascular supply but with significant intraparenchymal vascular connections. On occasion, the livers are completely separate though touching. Bowel connections are separated with stapling devices and reconstruction deferred until separation is complete. Splitting of the diaphragm allows exposure to the contralateral surface of the liver connection, which can be encircled with umbilical tape or a penrose drain. We have had good results dividing the liver with a variety of devices including the harmonic scalpel, hydro-dissector, bipolar and monopolar coagulators, and direct suture ligation. At the completion of the separation, the raw surface can be sealed with the argon beam coagulator with little risk of a bile leak.

Attention is then turned to the cardiac separation. The cardiovascular strategy depends on the degree of connection, structural integrity of each heart, and the physiologic status of each twin. Sometimes the hearts are completely separate within a common pericardium, in which case the posterior body wall is separated and tissue expanders on the "down" side removed.

Myocardial connections can be small or large and are frequently atrial. A significant ventricular connection is usually identified preoperatively and precludes separation. The myocardial connections are test clamped to identify the physiologic consequences of their separation. While preparations for pacing or bypass are made ready prior to the division of the connection, they have not been necessary. Once the myocardial connection is severed and closed, the posterior body wall is completed and the twins rotated to the supine position.

In the absence of structural cardiac anomalies, one twin is moved to a separate operating room with his or her entire team so that reconstruction of the body wall can proceed simultaneously.

Structural cardiac malformations can be repaired or deferred depending on the magnitude of the corrective surgery, the need for cardiopulmonary bypass, and the physiologic status of the twin. Our most recent separation outlines the cardiac options and strategies. The twins shared a large atrial connection approximately 6 cm in cranio-caudal dimension. One twin had double-outlet right ventricle while the other had left main pulmonary artery stenosis with significant pulmonary hypertension. During test clamping of the atrial connection, both twins remained stable and separation was uneventful. The twin with pulmonary artery stenosis underwent patch angioplasty and definitive body wall reconstruction and closure. The twin with double-outlet right ventricle underwent definitive closure of the abdomen with skin closure of the chest. She was stabilized for 48 h and then underwent cardiac repair with reconstruction and closure of the chest. While bypass was available, the ability to avoid its use immediately after the liver separation appears to have contributed to the uneventful recovery of both twins.

Following separation, the abdominal and thoracic viscera are inspected and repaired (Fig. 114.3). Hemostasis is ensured and the abdomen is closed with minimal tension, which usually means placing a soft tissue patch in the upper fascial closure. Prosthetic material is used to provide a stable bridge between the sternal halves. We prefer sheets of material as opposed to struts and have had good experience with lactic acid polygylcolic acid copolymer products. The skin flaps are then generously mobilized and closed over drains placed in the mediastinal and subcutaneous spaces. If closure of both twins is completed at the same time, their return to the critical care area should be staggered.

Postoperative Care

A written plan for the postoperative care with individuals from each discipline identified and specific responsibilities spelled out in detail minimizes confusion postoperatively. Preprinted order sets that have been reviewed and agreed upon by all relevant disciplines are also helpful. Initial care is directed at optimization of respiratory and hemodynamic status. Careful fluid and ventilator management predominates in the first days but careful monitoring of liver function, fluid drainage, and the viability of skin flaps is also important. Early revision of any problems with the chest wall stabilization and skin flaps facilitates weaning from mechanical ventilation. Nutrition is critical and a period of tube feeding should be anticipated. As recovery progresses, a physical therapist should address the musculoskeletal issues imposed by the conjoining and the separation. Hospitalizations of 2–4 weeks should be anticipated for relatively uncomplicated recoveries and longer if any complications intervene. Long-term care is directed at any underlying structural anomalies that required correction and the body wall reconstruction.

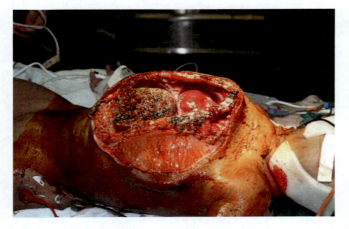

Fig. 114.3 One thoraco-omphalopagus twin after separation. The sternum is still split, revealing the heart and the cut edge of the divided liver bridge is visible below the diaphragm

Planning Process

Almost every series or case report about conjoined twins stresses the need for careful and intense planning for a successful outcome. A strategy that we have employed is regularly scheduled (weekly or every other week) meetings including a representative from every involved medical and surgical discipline, hospital operational departments, and nursing and hospital leadership (Table 114.2). A flow diagram of each step of the process with a responsible individual identified is helpful. This working group anticipates all outcome scenarios and develops strategies for each with information gathered along the way from diagnostic studies and the twins' responses to anesthesia and the environment. Mockups of the operating room with a specified location for

Table 114.2 Planning team – thoraco-omphalopagus

Anesthesia	Pediatric surgery
Cardiology	Cardiothoracic surgery
Radiology	Plastic surgery
Laboratory medicine	Critical care
Operating room director	Operating room nursing
Critical care nursing	Social services
Physical therapy	Admitting/registration
Medical records	Hospital administration
Security	Public relations/media

each individual and piece of equipment is done on paper and then tested in person with walk-throughs in the designated operating room (Fig. 114.4). All equipment should be turned on to test the electrical capacity of the room, which frequently needs supplementation with temporary power (up to 100 A or more).

On the day of separation attention to security and crowd control is facilitated by having a room general who has no clinical responsibilities but has the authority to remove anyone from the room. Accommodations for legitimate educational and clinical interest can be accomplished with a video feed to designated secure viewing areas. For particularly lengthy procedures, planning should include rest periods for staff and a designated individual to relay progress reports to the family.

Summary Points

- Conjoined twins are rare and are commonly associated with multiple congenital anomalies.
- The mortality rate is high, usually due to cardiac anomalies.
- Accurate prenatal imaging is important to obtain a realistic estimate of survival and separability.
- Manage the prenatal course as high risk with planned C-section.
- Multidisciplinary management and planning begin prenatally.
- Survival depends on the type of connection and associated anomalies.
- Emergency separation is associated with a 70% mortality.
- With careful planning and selection, elective separation can achieve survival of 70%.

Editor's Comment

Computer-enhanced three-dimensional imaging has allowed for much better pre-operative planning for these often extremely difficult and tedious operations, but the assembling of a team of experts and meticulous planning of each minute detail, including contingency plans for every conceivable snag, is still the most important aspect of the care of these unique individuals. Given the intense societal interest in these cases, it is also advisable to involve a team of bioethicists, hospital administrators, and public relations experts from the very beginning so that medical personnel can concentrate on providing excellent care without being distracted.

Technical Points

(Thoraco-Omphalopagus)

- Specify OR setup with specific location for each individual and piece of equipment.
- Walk-through with turn on and test of all equipment (may need more electrical supply).
- Select OR date and start time to ensure availability of all needed support and minimize disruption of OR and hospital operations.

- Limit entry to OR to authorized individuals with a clinical need.
- Provide audio–video feed to a designated viewing area.
- Identify two separate anesthesia and operating teams.
- Identify each individual's responsibilities and functions well in advance.
- Ensure adequate warming during prep and monitor insertions.
- Ensure adequate padding of all pressure points.
- Anticipate meticulous hemostasis from initial incision.
- Open "upper" portion of connection by entering at umbilicus and remove tissue expanders.
- Open abdomen and chest to assess degree of visceral fusion.
- Divide any intestinal connection reserving restoration of continuity until separation complete.
- Divide diaphragm and dissect posterior surface of fused liver.
- Divide liver using hydro-dissector, coagulation devices, or suture ligature and use argon beam.
- Divide posterior body wall to diaphragm.

Pre-Seperation Both in 1 O.R.

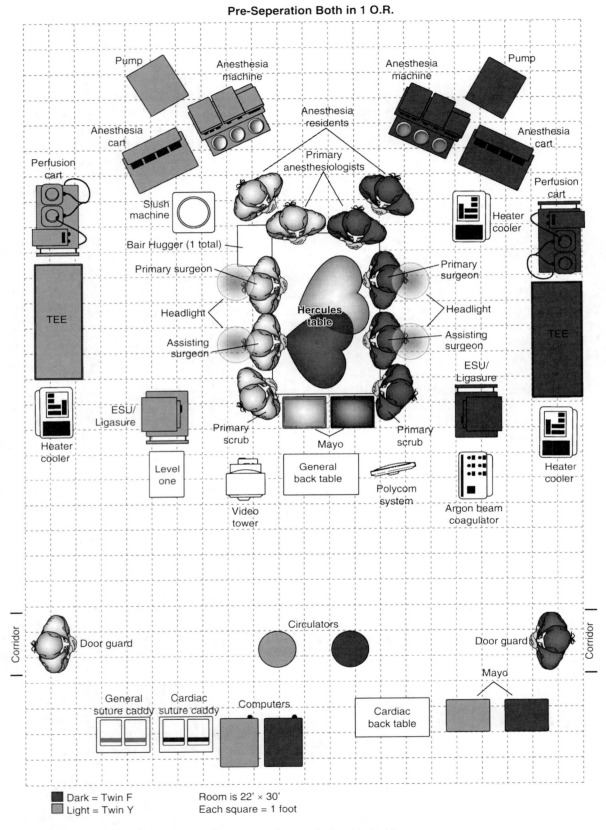

Fig. 114.4 Mockup of operating room with all personnel and equipment displayed in position

- Assess cardiac connection and position bypass/pacing personnel.
- Test clamp before dividing cardiac connection.
- Divide remainder of posterior body wall, removing any remaining tissue expanders.
- Rotate patients supine and cover with sterile occlusive dressings.
- Move one twin with team to adjacent OR.
- Re-prep and drape.
- Re-inspect abdomen and chest for hemostasis and complete any needed reconstruction of GI or biliary tracts
- Close abdomen without tension, which usually requires a soft-tissue patch.
- Mold rigid chest wall material to bridge sternal defect.
- Drain mediastinum and subcutaneous spaces.
- Mobilize and close skin flaps with minimal tension.
- Coordinate staggered transfer to critical care area.
- Predesignated postop care teams with predetermined order sets.

Parental Preparation

Prenatal

- Counseling regarding viability
- Obstetric management of high risk pregnancy
- Preparation for C-section
- Discuss parental preferences regarding privacy

Postnatal

- Outline diagnostic strategy/sequence of studies
- Review study results and possibility/risks of separation (multidisciplinary discussion)
- Identify social support needs
- Review all possible outcomes in detail including possibility of long-term disability
- Assist parents in dealing with media/interested individuals

Preoperative Preparation

- ☐ Flow diagram of all team members and responsibilities
- ☐ Confirm availability of all personnel and equipment
- ☐ Type and Crossmatch, CBC, coagulation and chemistry panels
- ☐ Blood bank has adequate supplies of products and factors
- ☐ Bowel prep with intravenous hydration, if necessary
- ☐ Informed consent (consider involvement of representative from Ethics Panel)

Diagnostic Studies

Prenatal

- Ultrasound
- Echocardiography
- MRI

Postnatal

- Plain radiograph
- Echocardiography
- Ultrasound
- MRI
- CT with 3D reconstruction
- GI contrast studies
- Voiding cystoureothrogram
- Cardiac catheterization

Suggested Reading

Hensel A and B. Conjoined Twins, Abby and Brittany Hensel Turn 16. www.youtube.com/watch?v=BkKWApOAG2g 2006.

MacKenzie TC, Crombleholme TM, Johnson MP, et al. The natural history of prenatally diagnosed conjoined twins. J Pediatr Surg. 2002;37:303–9.

O'Neill JA, Holcomb GW, Schnaufer L, et al. Surgical experience with thirteen conjoined twins. Ann Surg. 1988;208:299–310.

Pearn J. Bioethical issues in caring for conjoined twins and their parents. Lancet. 2001;357:1968–71.

Rode H, Fieggen AG, Brown RA, et al. Four decades of conjoined twins at Red Cross Children's Hospital – lessons learned. S Afr Med J. 2006;96:931–40.

Spencer R. Conjoined twins. In: Ashcraft KW, editor. Pediatric surgery. 3rd ed. Philadelphia, PA: W.B. Saunders; 2000. p. 1040–53.

Spitz L, Kiely EM. Conjoined twins. JAMA. 2003;289:1307–10.

Waisel DB. Moral permissibility as a guide for decision making about conjoined twins. Anesth Analg. 2005;101:41–3.

Index

A

Abdominal aortic disorders
  arterial aneurysms
    complications, 883
    diagnosis, 881–882
    preoperative preparation, 882–884
    surgical technique, 883
  complex reconstructive vascular operations, 885
  differential diagnosis, 885
  parental preparation, 885
  preoperative preparation, 886
  stenotic/occlusive diseases
    complications, 883
    diagnosis, 881–882
    differential diagnosis, 881–882
    preoperative preparation, 882–883
    surgical technique, 883
    symptoms, 881
    vascular reconstruction, 885
  vascular anastomoses, 885
Abdominal compartment syndrome (ACS), 78
Abdominal cysts
  adnexal, 365
  diagnosis, 367–368
  genitourinary abnormalities, 367
  liver, 366
  lymphangioma, 365–366
  mesenteric and omental, 366
  pancreatic, 366
  parental preparation, 371
  postoperative care, 369
  splenic, 366
  trauma/pseudocysts, 367
  treatment, 368–369
  tumors, 367
Abdominal pain. *See* Chronic abdominal pain
Abdominal trauma
  child abuse, 141
  diagnosis, 136
  differential diagnosis, 142
  impalements, 141
  intravenous access, 135
  isolated abdominal free fluid, 141
  parental preparation, 142
  penetrating injuries, 136
  physical findings, 135
  solid organ injuries
    bladder, 140
    colon, 141
    duodenum, 140
    hemorrhage/peritonitis, 137–138
    intestine, 140–141
    kidney, 139–140
    liver, 139
    non-operative management, 136–137
    operative intervention, 137–138
    organ injury scale, 137
    pancreas, 140
    rectum, 141
    spleen, 138–139
    treatment algorithm, 138
ABO incompatibility, neonatal hyperbilirubinemia, 562
ACC. *See* Adrenocortical carcinoma
Accreditation Council for Graduate Medical Education
    (ACGME), 42, 44
Achalasia
  diagnosis
    bird's beak deformity, 273, 274
    dysphagia, 273
    endoscopy, 273–274
    esophageal manometry, 274
    substernal chest pain, 273
  differential diagnosis, 278
  etiology, 273
  intra-operative perforations, 278
  parental preparation, 278
  postoperative care, 276–277
  preoperative preparation, 274, 278
  surgical technique
    four-trocar technique, 276
    laparoscopic Heller myotomy, 275–278
    patient positioning, 275
    trocars, 275
  treatment
    Heller myotomy, 274, 275
    nonoperative treatments, 274–275
    thoracoscopic approach, 275
Acute intermittent poryphyria, 434
Acute interstitial nephritis (AIN), 79
Acute kidney injury (AKI)
  abdominal compartment syndrome, 78
  acute interstitial nephritis, 79
  acute tubular necrosis phases, 73, 75
  cardiac surgery, 77
  categorization, 73–74
  definition, 73
  diagnosis, 74–75
  drug-related AKI, 77
  fractional excretion of sodium (FENa), 75
  hemolytic uremic syndromes, 78
  hepatorenal syndrome, 77
  HIV/AIDS, 79

Acute kidney injury (AKI) (*cont.*)
  malignancy, 78
  pathophysiology, 73–74
  prognosis, 79
  radiocontrast nephropathy, 79
  rhabdomyolysis, 78–79
  RIFLE criteria, 75–76
  thrombotic thrombocytopenic purpura, 78
  treatment, 75–77
  urinalysis, 75
Acute lung injury (ALI)
  clinical development, phases, 83–84
  definition, 84
Acute respiratory distress syndrome (ARDS)
  definition, 84
  inhaled nitric oxide (iNO), 88
  PEEP, 85
  permissive hypercapnea, 88
  permissive hypoxemia, 88
  prone positioning, 88
  surfactant therapy, 88
Acute tubular necrosis (ATN), 73
Adnexal cysts, 365
Adrenal tumors
  ACC
    clinical findings, 725
    staging, 726
    treatment, 725–726
  pheochromocytoma
    characterization, 726
    diagnosis, 727
    signs and symptoms, 726–727
    treatment, 727
Adrenocortical carcinoma (ACC)
  clinical findings, 725
  staging, 726
  treatment, 725–726
AFP. *See* Alpha fetoprotein
Aganglionosis, Hirschsprung disease, 479–480, 483
Air leak, pneumothorax
  catheterization, 307
  surgical therapy, 308
Airway pressure-release ventilation (APRV), 87
Airway/respiratory system, 3–5
AKI. *See* Acute kidney injury
Alpha fetoprotein (AFP)
  ovarian tumors, 741, 742
  testicular tumor, 749
American Pediatric Surgical Association (APSA), 43, 44
American Society of Anesthesiologists (ASA)
    physical status score, 3
Amnioinversion technique, omphalocele, 526–527
Amniotic band syndrome, 873
Amyand's hernia, 543
Anal fissure, 462–463
Anaphylactic shock, 49
Aneurysm. *See also* Arterial aneurysm
  classification, 882
  diagnosis, 881
Angioedema, chronic abdominal pain, 434
Angiosarcoma, liver, 769
Annular pancreas, 617–618
Ano-genital injuries, 171
Anorectal malformations
  anoplasty, 503–504
  classification, 499, 500
  colostomy, 501–503

diagnosis of, 502
    females, 500–503
    males, 499–500, 502
  differential diagnosis, 511
  distal colostogram, 504–505
  hydrocolpos, 502–503
  Malone procedure, 509–510
  parental preparation, 511
  posterior sagittal anorectoplasty
    females, 506–507
    males, 505–506
  posterior sagittal anorectovaginourethroplasty, 507–508
  postoperative care
    complications of, 508
    constipation, 509
    fecal incontinence, 509
    Hegar cervical dilators, 508
Anorectoplasty, posterior sagittal
  females, 506–507
  males, 505–506
Anorectovaginourethroplasty, 507–508
Antegrade continent enema (ACE) procedure
  anorectal malformation, 510
  constipation, 455–458
Aphallia, 659
Appendectomy
  appendicitis, 486–487
  intestinal rotational anomalies, 378
  meconium ileus, 398
Appendicitis
  Crohn's disease, 437–438
  diagnosis
    helical CT, 486
    laboratory evaluation of, 485–486
    physical examination, 485
    symptoms, 485
    ultrasound, 486
  differential diagnosis, 489
  etiology of, 485
  parental preparation, 489
  postoperative care, 488
  treatment
    appendectomy, 486–487
    fluid resuscitation, 486
    nonoperative therapy, 487–488
ARDS. *See* Acute respiratory distress syndrome
Arterial aneurysm
  complications, 883
  diagnosis, 881–882
  preoperative preparation, 882–884
  surgical technique, 883
Arteriovenous malformations (AVM)
  characterization, 823
  treatment, 826
Asthma, 4
Atlanto-occipital injuries, 153
Atresia
  biliary (*see* Biliary atresia)
  duodenal, 353–357
  esophageal (*see* Esophageal atresia)
  intestinal, 359–362
  long-gap esophageal (*see* Long-gap esophageal atresia)
  vagina
    Mayer–Rokitansky–Kuster–Houser syndrome, 701
    pedicle graft, 704
    surgical treatment, 701–703
    transverse obstructions, 702, 704

B

Bariatric surgery
  adjustable gastric band
    advantages of, 417, 418
    laparoscopic procedure for, 419
  biliopancreatic diversion, 416, 418
  complications, 420–421
  outcomes, 421
  parental preparation, 422
  patient selection, 415
  perioperative management, 418
  postoperative management, 419–420
  preoperative assessment
    nutritional and psychological evaluation, 416
    physical examination, 415–416
  Roux-en-Y gastric bypass
    laparoscopic procedure for,
      418–419
    mortality rate, 417
  vertical banded gastroplasty, 416–417
  vertical sleeve gastrectomy, 417
Bascom flap, pilonidal cyst, 470–471
Basilar skull fracture, 113
Becker's nevi, 802
Beckwith–Wiedemann syndrome, 524
Belly cleft. *See* Gastroschisis
Benign skin lesions
  cutaneous
    calcinosis cutis, 795
    dermatofibromas, 796
    keloids, 796
    neurofibromas, 796
    pyogenic granulomas, 796
    verrucae, 795
  cysts
    dermoid, 797–798
    epidermoid, 797
    pilomatrixomas, 798
  foreign bodies, 798
  ingrown toenails, 798
  lymph nodes
    cat-scratch disease, 799–800
    cervical lymphadenitis, 799
    incision, 799
    mycobacterial lymphadenitis, 799
    peripheral lymphadenopathy, 800
    physical exam, 798
  nonmelanocytic nevi
    Becker's nevi, 802
    epidermal, 801
    nevus sebaceus, 801
  parental preparation, 803
  postoperative care, 802
  subcutaneous
    granuloma annulare, 797
    infantile myofibromatosis, 797
    lipomas, 796–797
  vascular lesions
    hemangioma, 800
    vascular malformations, 800–801
Bezoar/foreign body, chronic abdominal pain, 431
β-human chorionic gonatotropin (βHCG), 741
Bianchi procedure, short bowel syndrome, 390
Bilateral renal agenesis (BRA), 642–643
Bilateral Wilms tumor (BWT), 721
Biliary atresia. *See also* Hyperbilirubinemia, neonatal
  anatomic classification, 567

  clinical classification, 567
  diagnosis
    hepatobiliary scintigraphy, 568
    neonatal cholestasis, 567–568
    percutaneous liver biopsy, 568
  differential diagnosis, 573
  parental preparation, 573
  postoperative care
    age at treatment, 570–571
    bile flow stimulation, 570
    bleeding, obstruction, and cholangitis, 570
    malnutrition, 570
    predictive markers, 571
  transplantation, 571
  treatment, 568–570
Biliary dyskinesia, diagnosis of, 580
Bird's beak deformity, 273, 274
Birth anomalies
  association, 18–19
  deformations, 18
  differential diagnosis of, 19
  disruption, 18
  dysplasia, 18
  malformation, 18
  sequence, 18
  syndrome, 18
Birth trauma, neonatal hyperbilirubinemia, 562
Bishop–Koop ileostomy, meconium ileus,
    397–398
Blast injuries, 165–166
Blue rubber bleb nevus syndrome, 821–822
Bochdalek hernia
  antenatal diagnosis, 535–536
  associated anomalies, 535
  etiology of, 535
  medical management
    cardiac monitoring, 536–537
    ECMO criteria, 537–538
    hypotension, 537
    mechanical ventilation, 537
    nitric oxide inhalation, 537
    principles of, 536
    pulmonary hypertension, 537
  minimally invasive method, 539–540
  outcomes, 539
  surgical management, 538–539
Botryoid tumors, 733
Bowel lengthening procedures, 390
Branchial cleft cysts
  antibiotics, 198
  first remnants, 198
  fistula, 197–198
  location, 197
  second remnants, 198
  surgical excision, 198
  third and fourth remnants, 198–199
Breast disorders
  development
    asymmetry, 829
    gynecomastia, 830–831
    hypoplasia, 829
    juvenile hypertrophy, 830–831
    polymastia, 829
    polythelia, 829
    Tanner stages, 830
    thelarche, 830
  differential diagnosis, 836

Breast disorders (*cont.*)
  infections
    abscess, 831–832
    mastitis, 831
  masses
    infantile, 832–833
    malignant tumors, 834
    prepubertal, 833
    pubertal, 833–834
  nipple discharge, 834–835
  parental preparation, 836
  trauma, 832
Bronchogenic cysts,
        199, 295, 327
Bronchopulmonary dysplasia (BPD), 10
Bronchopulmonary sequestration (BPS)
  arterial supply, 295
  extralobar, 294–295
  intralobar, 295
  surgical resection, 295
Bronchoscopy, 193
  anesthetic coordination
        and induction, 189
  complications, 191
  contraindications, 186
  differential diagnosis, 193
  endoscopic anatomy
    aryepiglottic folds, 188
    epiglottis and vallecula, 188
    stem bronchus, 189
    subglottis, 188
    tracheal rings, 188–189
  flexible bronchoscopy,
        189–190, 194
  foreign body removal, 191–193
  hazardous airway situations, 186
  indications
    child, 186
    infants, 185
    toddler, 185–186
  parental considerations, 191
  preoperative evaluation, 186–187
  preoperative preparation, 193
  radiographic evaluation, 187
  rigid bronchoscopy, 190–191
Budd–Chiari syndrome, 601
Burns
  antibiotic therapy, 132
  complications, 131
  depth characteristics, 124
  diagnosis, 123, 124, 132
  inhalation injury, 124–125
  Lund and Browder chart, 125
  parental preparation, 132
  postoperative care, 131
  preoperative preparation,
        130, 132
  prognosis, 131
  surgical technique, 130–131
  treatment
    airway, 124–125
    breathing, 126
    caloric intake, 129
    chemical burns, 129
    circulation, 126–127
    electrical burns, 130

    escharotomy, 128–129
    frostbite, 130
    laboratory studies, 127
    prophylactic systemic antibiotics, 127
    temperature regulation, 127
    wound care, 127–128

C
Capillary vascular malformations
  characterization, 821
  treatment, 825–826
Cardiogenic shock, 49
Castleman's disease, 215
Cat-scratch disease, 799–800
Caustic ingestions
  acids, 260–261
  age distribution, 260
  clinical features, 261
  differential diagnosis, 265
  esophageal anatomic narrowing, 261
  esophageal burn, 261
  injuries, classification, 261–262
  long-term complications, 263
  lye, 260
  physical form and pH, 260
  retrosternal pain, 261
  treatment
    acid suppression, 262–263
    antibiotics, 262
    colon interposition, 263
    corticosteroids, 262
    full-thickness injury, 263
    operative intervention, 263
CDH. *See* Congenital diaphragmatic hernia
Cervical lymphadenopathy
  acute cervical lymphadenitis, 213–214
  Castleman's disease, 215
  differential diagnosis, 218
  infections, 215
  Kawasaki disease, 215
  Kikuchi–Fujimoto disease, 215
  lymph nodes, 799
  malignancy, 214–215
  parental preparation, 219
  postoperative care, 217–218
  preoperative preparation
    fine needle aspiration, 216
    history, 215–216
    imaging studies, 216
    laboratory studies, 216
    operative intervention, 216
    physical examination, 216
  Rosai–Dorfman disease, 215
  sarcoidosis, 215
  subacute and chronic cervical lymphadenitis, 214
  surgical technique, 216–217
Cervical thymic cysts, 199
Chamberlain procedure, mediastinal masses, 325
Chemical burns, 129
Child abuse
  abdominal injuries, 170
  abdominal trauma, 141
  ano-genital injuries, 171
  burns, 170–171
  clinical evaluation, 172

diagnosis, 169
fractures, 170
head injuries, 169
inflicted bruises and bites, 171–172
Childen's oncology group (COG),
       742–743
Cholecystitis
    age and sex, 579
    complications, 584
    definition, 579
    diagnosis
        acute acalculous cholecystitis, 580
        differential diagnosis, 579
        physical examination, 580
        symptoms, 579
        ultrasonography, 580
    parental preparation, 585
    postoperative care, 583
    treatment
        endoscopic retrograde pancreatography, 582–583, 585
        fluid resuscitation, 580
        laparoscopic cholecystectomy, 580–582
        nonoperative therapies, 582
Choledochal cysts
    anatomic variations, 587, 588
    diagnosis, 587–588
    differential diagnosis, 591
    parental preparation, 591
    pathogenisis of, 587, 588
    postoperative care, 590
    surgical therapy
        for long-standing cyst, 589
        principle, 588
        type I and IV, 589–590
        type II and III, 590
        vitamin K supplement, intravenous, 588
Cholelithiasis. See Cholecystitis
Cholestasis, biliary atresia, 567–568.
           See also Intrahepatic cholestasis
Chronic abdominal pain
    acute intermittent poryphyria, 434
    anatomic/congenital GI disorders, 429–430
    bezoar/foreign body, 431
    diagnosis
        differential diagnosis, 427
        imaging methods, 428–429
        laboratory evaluation, 428
        physical examination, 427–428
        symptoms of, 426–427
    endometriosis, 433
    familial Mediterranean fever, 434
    functional abdominal pain
        etiology and pathogenesis, 425
        treatment for, 425–426
    gallbladder disease, 430–431
    hereditary angioedema, 434
    hypercalcemia, 433
    inflammatory bowel disease, 430
    intra-abdominal adhesions, 431
    intra-abdominal tumors, 432
    lead poisoning, 433
    organic etiology, 426
    ovarian cysts, 432
    pancreatic disease, 431
    parental preparation, 435
    pelvic inflammatory disease, 432

sickle cell disease, 433
surgical treatment, 429
tubo-ovarian abscess, 432–433
ureteropelvic junction obstruction, 432
vasculitis, 434
Chylothorax, 291, 292
    causes, 305, 306
    diagnosis, 305–306
    fluid composition, 306
    parental preparation, 311
    thoracic duct anatomy, 305, 306
    treatment
        nonoperative therapy, 306
        preoperative localization techniques, 307
        surgical objectives, 307
Circumcision
    Gomco clamp, 660
    techniques, 659
Clatworthy shunt, portal hypertension, 604
Cleft, belly. See Gastroschisis
Cloacal exstrophy
    embryology
        bladder exstrophy, 686
        cloaca division, 685
        malformations, 686
        mesodermal migration, 685
    hindgut refunctionalization, 685
    omphalocele-exstrophy-imperforate
            anus-spinal defects (OEIS), 685
    surgical treatment
        bladder exstrophy, 687
        differential diagnosis, 690
        evaluation, 686
        hindgut refunctionalization, 686–687
        osteotomies, 688
        parental preparation, 690
        patient care, 690
        patient stabilization, 686
        phallic reconstruction, 689
        postoperative appearance, 689
        pubic symphysis and
                scrotum separation, 689
        ultrasonography, 687
        vesico-intestinal fissure division, 687
COG. See Childen's oncology group
Colitis, Crohn's disease, 439–440
Collis–Nissen. See Fundoplasty
Colonic atresia, 361
Colostomy
    anorectal malformations, 501–503
    complications of, 448
    for fecal diversion, 446
    for high imperforate anus, 446
    indications, 443–445
    parental preparation, 449
    postoperative care, 447
    preoperative preparation, 445
    stoma closure, 447
Compartment syndrome, 165
Compression injuries, 154
Computerized physician order entry (CPOE), 42
Congenital adrenal hyperplasia (CAH),
       871–872
Congenital anomalies. See Birth anomalies
Congenital cystic adenomatoid malformation
       (CCAM), 293–294

Congenital diaphragmatic hernia (CDH), 871–872, 874
    anterior defect, 540
    parental preparation, 541
    posterolateral defect
        antenatal diagnosis, 535–536
        associated anomalies, 535
        etiology of, 535
        medical management, 536–538
        minimally invasive method, 539–540
        outcomes, 539
        surgical management, 538–539
Congenital heart disease, 5–6
Congenital high airway obstruction syndrome (CHAOS),
        873–874
Congenital lobar emphysema (CLE), 294
Congenital lung lesions
    bronchogenic cysts, 295
    bronchopulmonary sequestration (BPS), 294–295
    congenital cystic adenomatoid malformation, 293–294
    congenital lobar emphysema (CLE), 294
    differential diagnosis, 297
    indication, 293
    management, algorithm, 294
    parental preparation, 297
    preoperative preparation, 297
    surgical technique, 295–296
    thoracoscopic approach, 296
Congenital pulmonary airway malformations
        (CPAM), 871
Conjoined twins
    characterization, 893
    diagnosis
        classification, 894
        computed tomography, 893–894
        echocardiography, 893
        ultrasound, 893
    parental preparation, 899
    planning process, 896–898
    postoperative care, 896
    treatment
        abdominal and thoracic viscera, 896
        anesthesia, 895
        cardiac separation, 895–896
        thoraco-omphalopagus, 895
    types, 894
Constipation, 40
    complication rate of, 457
    definition, 453
    diagnostic evaluation
        contrast enema, 453–454
        newborns and infants, 454
        physical exam, 453
        school age children, 455
        toddlers, 454–455
    differential diagnosis, 458
    initial evaluation, 453
    parental preparation, 458
    surgical therapy
        irrigations of, 457
        Mitrofanoff and ACE procedure, 456
        Monti tube, 456–457
Cotton-Myer grading system, 179
C-reactive protein (CRP), 27
Critical airway
    costal cartilage harvest, 184
    cricotracheal resection, 182

diagnosis
    flexible laryngoscopy, 178
    history, 177
    physical examination, 178
    urgent intervention, 177
differential diagnosis, 184
laryngotracheal reconstruction, 181–182
operative airway evaluation
    airway sizing, 179
    bronchoscope, 179
    bronchoscopy table set up, 178–179
    Cotton–Myer grading system, 179
    laryngospasm, Philips laryngoscope blade, 179
parental preparation, 184
postoperative care, 183
preoperative preparation, 181, 184
tracheostomy (see Tracheostomy)
treatment, 180–181
Crohn's disease
    colitis, 439–440
    diagnosis, 438
    differential diagnosis, 442
    ileal disease, 437–438
    parental preparation, 442
    perirectal disease, 440–441
    postoperative care, 441
    surgical treatment, 438–439
Cross-trigonal (Cohen) technique, vesicoureteral reflux, 636
Cysts. See also Benign skin lesions; Branchial cleft cysts
    abdominal, 365–371
    cervical thymic cysts, 199
    choledochal, 587–591
    liver, 366
    neck masses
        differential diagnosis, 196
        embryologic development, 195
        pharyngeal clefts and pouches, 195
        thyroglossal duct cysts (see Thyroglossal duct cysts (TGDC))
    ovarian, chronic abdominal pain, 432
    pilonidal
        abscess drainage, 468
        differential diagnosis, 467–468
        etiology of, 467
        nonoperative management, 468–469
        postoperative care, 472
        prevalence in, 467
        sexual maturation affect in, 467
        surgical therapy, 469–472
    renal, 646–647
    splenic, 627–628

D
Depressed skull fracture, 112–113
Dermatofibromas, 796
Dermoid cysts, 797–798
Dialysis. See Peritoneal dialysis
Differentiated thyroid cancer, 205
Disorder of sex development (DSD)
    diagnosis, 694
    differential diagnosis, 694, 696
    gender assignment, 698–699
    gonadal dysgenesis (GD), 697
    46XX karyotype
        CYP21, 695
        genetic etiologies, 696

21-hydroxylase deficiency, 695
  lipoid adrenal hyperplasia, 696
  steroid biosynthetic pathway, 695
46XY karyotype, 697–698
laboratory evaluation, 693
nonpalpable testes, 694
ovotestictular, 698
parental preparation, 700
physical examination, 693
radiologic examination, 694
Double-volume exchange transfusion (DVET), 562–563, 565
DSD. *See* Disorder of sex development
Duodenal atresia
  diagnosis, 353
  incidence, 353
  laparoscopic repair, 355–356
  operative management, 354–355
  parental preparation, 357
  postoperative care, 356
  preoperative preparation, 353–354
Dysphagia, 273

E

ECMO. *See* Extracorporeal membrane oxygenation
Ectopic kidney, 647
Electrical burns, 130
Electrolyte disorders
  hyperkalemia, 62
  hypernatremia, 59–60
  hypokalemia, 60–62
  hyponatremia, 57–59
Empyema
  causes, 308
  diagnosis
    CT scan, 309–310
    ultrasonography, 308–309
    VATS, 310
  parental preparation, 311
Endocrine disorders, pancreas
  diagnosis, 619
  hyperinsulinism, 619
  localization, 620
  operative care, 619–620
  treatment, 619–621
  Zollinger–Ellison syndrome, 619
Endometriosis, chronic abdominal pain, 433
Endoscopic retrograde pancreatography (ERCP), 582–583, 585
Endotracheal tube immobilization, 125
Enteral nutrition
  advantages, 27
  caloric requirements, 27–28
  carbohydrates, 28
  complications, 31
  feed administration, 30–31
  feeding access, 28–29
  formulation, 29–30
  nutritional requirements, 27–28
  parental preparation, 32
  vitamins and trace minerals, 28
Enterocolitis, 867–868
  Hirschsprung disease, 480
  necrotizing, 381–385
Entero-enteric intussusception, 405. *See also* Intussusception

Epidermoid cysts, 797
Epidural anesthesia
  catheter placement, 24
  caudal approach, 23–24
  complications, 24, 25
  continuous epidural analgesia, 24
  dermatomal placement, 24
  epidural infusions, 24
  single injection technique, 24
Epidural hematoma (EDH), 113–115
Epiploceles, 545–546
Epispadias, 658–659
Erythrocyte enzyme deficiency, 627
Escharotomy, 128–129
Esophageal atresia, 231–232.
    See also Long-gap esophageal atresia
  complications
    anastomotic leaks, 227
    anastomotic stenosis, 228–229
    distal congenital stenosis, 228
    GER, 228
    recurrent TEF, 228
    tracheal narrowing, 227–228
    tracheomalacia, 228
  differential diagnosis, 232
  operative technique
    bronchoscopy, 224
    DeBakey forceps, 226
    extrapleural dissection, 225
    Foker technique, 225–226
    Replogle tube, 226
    suture-fistula technique, 225
    thoracotomy, 226
  parental preparation, 232
  postoperative care, 226–227
  preoperative preparation, 223–224
  prognostic classification, 229
Esophageal duplications, mediastinal masses, 327
Esophageal injuries
  anatomy/technical approach, 254–255
  caustic ingestions (*see* Caustic ingestions)
  complications, 259
  diagnosis
    antero-posterior and lateral radiographs, 253–254
    barium esophagogram, 254
    foreign body impactions, 253, 264–265
  differential diagnosis, 265
  endoscopy, 258–259
  esophageal replacement operations, 265
  Foley balloon catheter, 259
  foreign bodies
    blunt objects, 255
    button batteries, 257–258
    food impaction, 258
    large objects, 255–256
    magnets and lead, 258
    narcotic packets, 258
    sharp objects, 256–257
  full-thickness esophageal injury, 264–265
  immediate intervention, 261–262
  parental preparation, 265
  postoperative care, 258
  preoperative preparation, 265
  suture technique, 259
  symptoms, 253
  treatment, 255

Esophageal replacement, 251
    advantages and disadvantages, 248
    colon interposition, 247
    differential diagnosis, 251
    gastric transposition, 247–248
    gastric tube esophagoplasty, 248–250
    jejunal interposition, 250
    parental preparation, 251
    preoperative preparation, 252
Eventration, diaphragm
    congenital and acquired, 531
    diagnosis, 531, 532
    differential diagnosis, 533
    fundoplication, 533
    parental preparation, 533
    postoperative care, 532–533
    treatment of, 532
Evidence-based medicine (EBM), 41
Extracorporeal membrane oxygenation (ECMO)
    cannula selection, 91
    cannulation, 98
    complications, 96–97
    decannulation, 96
    diagnostic studies, 98
    goals on, 94–95
    indications, 91, 92
        cardiac failure, 92
        hypercarbia, 92
        hypoxia, 91–92
        metabolic acidosis, 92
    initial management, 94
    neonatal ECMO cannulation, 93–94
    parental preparation, 99
    pediatric and adult cannulation, 94
    preoperative preparation, 92–93, 99
    surgery, 96
    survival outcomes, 97
    VV vs. VA-ECMO, 93
    weaning process, 95–96
Extrahepatic portal vein obstruction (EPVO), 600
Ex-utero intrapartum therapy (EXIT), 873, 877–878

F
Facet fracture-dislocation, 153–154
Familial polyposis (FP), 495–496
Fast-track postoperative protocol
    ambulation, 39
    constipation, 40
    diet, 39
    discharge criteria, 40
    indications, 37–38
    intravenous fluid, 39
    nasogastric tubes, 38–39
    pain management, 39
    patient expectations, 38
    pediatric surgery, 38
    postoperative ileus, 37
Femoral hernia, 543–544
Fetal surgery
    antenatal medical treatment, 871
    congenital adrenal hyperplasia, 871–872
    congenital diaphragmatic hernia,
        871–872, 874
    congenital pulmonary airway malformations, 871
    ex utero intrapartum therapy, 873

fetal intervention, 871
fetoscopy
    amniotic band syndrome, 873
    congenital diaphragmatic hernia, 873
    congenital high airway obstruction syndrome, 873–874
    lower urinary tract obstruction (LUTO) management, 875
    twin–twin transfusion syndrome, 873
myelomeningocele, 875
open fetal surgery
    ex utero intrapartum therapy, 877–878
    myelomeningocele, 876–877
    sacrococcygeal teratoma, 876
    tocolysis, 876
supplemented intravenous anesthesia (SIVA), 873
[^{18}F]fluoro-L-DOPA, 612
Fibrinolytics, empyema treatment, 310
Fibromuscular dysplasia (FMD), 882
Fistula-in-ano, 462
Flexible bronchoscopy, 189–190, 194
Flexion-distraction injuries, 154–155
Floppy Nissen fundoplication (FNF).
            See Fundoplasty
Foley catheter, 107, 110
Fowler–Stephens orchidopexy, undescended testis, 675
Fractional excretion of sodium (FENa), 75
Frostbite, 130
Fundoplasty
    dumping, 337
    dysphagia, 338
    feeding, 336–337
    gas bloat, 337
    medications, 337
    post-prandial hypoglycemia, 337–338
    principles, 335–336
    recurrent GERD, 338
    retching, 338

G
Gallbladder disease, chronic abdominal pain,
        430–431
Gallstones. See Cholecystitis
Gas bloat syndrome, 337
Gastroesophageal reflux disease (GERD), 6
    diagnosis, 334
    fundoplasty (see Fundoplasty)
    gastric contents viscosity, 333–334
    nonoperative therapy, 334–335
    physiology of, 333
    postoperative management, 336–338
    surgical treatment, 335–336
    symptoms and signs, 333
Gastrointestinal bleeding
    classification, 865
    diagnosis
        clinical signs, 867
        colonoscopy, 868
        enterocolitis, 867–868
        esophagogastroduodenoscopy, 866
        hemodynamic stability assessment, 865
        nasogastric tube lavage, 866
        physical findings, 867
        rectal bleeding, 868
    differential diagnosis, 866
    parental preparation, 870
    treatment, 868–869

Gastroschisis
  diagnosis
    echocardiography, 516
    ultrasound, 515
    umbilical ring contracture, 516
  etiologies of, 515
  parental preparation, 521
  plastic sutureless repair, 520
  postoperative care, 519–520
  treatment
    intubation and ventilation, 516
    silo-assisted closure of, 517–518
    Smead–Jones knots for, 519
Gastrostomy, surgical enteral access
  indications for, 347
  jejunostomy tubes, 349
  laparoscopic guided method, 348–349
  open type, 348
  parental preparation, 352
  percutaneous endoscopy, 349
  postoperative care
    accidental tube dislodgement, 350
    of balloon leak or rupture, 349–350
    skin erosion, 350
    tissue granulation, 350
  tube removal, 351
Genetic inheritance mechanisms
  autosomal dominant diseases, 17
  autosomal recessive inheritance, 17
  chromosomal mosaicism, 18
  genomic imprinting, 18
  X-linked dominant disorders, 18
  X-linked recessive disorders, 17–18
Germ cell tumors
  malignant, 745
  primordial germ cell and point mutations, 744
  sex cord-stromal tumors, 745
  teratomas, 743–744
Glasgow Coma Scale, 106
Glomus tumors, 822–823
Glucose infusion rate (GIR), 615
Gomco clamp, circumcision, 660
Graves' disease, 204–205
Grynfelt-Lesshaft hernia, 544
G-tube/gastro-jejunostomy (GJ) tube, 29
Gynecomastia, 830–831

H
Haller index, pectus deformities, 313
Hand injuries, 166
  amputations, 164–165
  blast injuries, 165–166
  compartment syndrome, 165
  diagnosis, 161, 162
  differential diagnosis, 166
  flexor tendon lacerations, 164
  metacarpophalangeal dislocations, 163
  nerve injuries, 164
  parental preparation, 167
  phalangeal neck and condyle fractures, 161–162
  preoperative preparation, 166
  scaphoid fracture, 163
  Seymour fracture, 163
  vascular injuries, 164
Hashimoto's thyroiditis, 204

HB. See Hepatoblastoma
HCC. See Hepatocellular carcinoma
Head trauma
  diagnosis
    Glasgow Coma scale, 112
    medical therapy, 112
    neurologic exam, 111
    ventriculostomy, 111–112
  differential diagnosis, 116
  hematoma (see Hematoma)
  parental preparation, 116
  preoperative preparation, 116
  skull fracture (see Skull fracture)
Hegar cervical dilators, 508
Hemangiomas
  characterization, 819
  spectrum of lesions, 819–821
  treatment, 824–825
Hematoma
  cerebral contusion, 114
  epidural hematoma (EDH), 113–114
  intraparenchmal hemorrhage, 114
  subdural hematoma (SDH), 114
  traumatic brain injury, 114
Hemolytic uremic syndrome (HUS), 78
Hemoptysis, 118–119
Hepatic artery thrombosis (HAT). See Vascular thrombosis
Hepatic resection
  diagnosis
    laboratory assessment, 594
    physical examination, 593–594
    radiographic evaluation, 593
  differential diagnosis, 597
  fibrin sealant application, 597
  and hepatoblastoma, 593
  indications, 593
  parental preparation, 598
  postoperative care, 596
  preoperative preparation, 594–595
  surgical technique
    bilateral subcostal incision, 595
    parenchymal transection, 595–596
    resectability determination, 595
    trisegmentectomy, 596
Hepatic vein obstruction, 601
Hepatobiliary scintigraphy, biliary atresia, 568
Hepatoblastoma (HB), 764–765
Hepatoblastoma, hepatic resection, 593
Hepatocellular carcinoma (HCC), 769
Hepatorenal syndrome (HRS), 77
Hereditary spherocytosis (HS), 626
Hermaphroditism. See Ovotesticular DSD
Hernia. See also Congenital diaphragmatic hernia (CDH);
      Inguinal hernia
  Bochdalek, 535–540
  epigastric, 545–546
  femoral, 543–544
  inguinal, 543
  lumbar, 544
  Morgagni, 540
  and omphalocele, 527
  traumatic abdominal wall, 545
  umbilical cord, 547–548
HI. See Hyperinsulinism (HI)
High frequency oscillatory ventilation (HFOV),
      86–87, 91

Hirschsprung disease. *See also* Constipation
   diagnosis
      rectal biopsy, 476
      water-soluble contrast enema, 476
   enterocolitis, 480
   etiology of, 475
   incontinence, 480
   long-segment, 480–481
   near-total intestinal aganglionosis, 481
   obstructive symptoms
      aganglionosis and motility disorder, 479–480
      functional megacolon, 480
      internal sphincter achalasia, 480
      mechanical obstruction, 479
   other anomalies, 476
   parental preparation, 483
   postoperative care, 478–479
   treatment
      resuscitation, 476–477
      surgical management, 477–478
   variant, 481–482
Hodgkin's disease (HD), 205, 325, 326
Horseshoe kidney
   renal abnormalities, 647
   Wilms tumor (WT), 721
HPS. *See* Hypertrophic pyloric stenosis
Hydrocele
   contralateral exploration, 666–667
   diagnostic studies, 671
   embryology, 663
   laparoscopic repair, 667–669
   postoperative care, 669–670
   trans-illumination, 665
   treatment, 665
Hydrocephalus
   diagnosis, 887
   differential diagnosis, 892
   endoscopic third ventriculostomy, 891
   parental preparation, 892
   postoperative care, 890
   surgical technique, 889–890
   treatment, 888–889
   ventricular shunt devices, 887–888
Hydrocolpos, anorectal malformations, 502–503
Hyperbilirubinemia, neonatal. *See also* Biliary atresia
   ABO incompatibility, 562
   birth trauma, 562
   cause, 561
   clinical manifestation of, 561
   differential diagnosis, 565
   laboratory evaluation, 562
   parental preparation, 565
   physical exam, 562
   treatment
      double-volume exchange transfusion, 562–563
      phototherapy, 562
   UPDGT activity of, 562
   in utero bilirubin level, 561–562
Hypercalcemia, chronic abdominal pain, 433
Hyperinsulinism (HI)
   diagnosis
      diffuse and focal forms, 611–612
      histopathology, 613
      hypoglycemia, 612
      K_{ATP} channel, 611
      medical management, pediatric endocrinology, 612

      mutations, 611
      radiology tests, 612–613
      sulfonylurea receptor 1 (SUR1), 611
   differential diagnosis, 616
   parental preparation, 616
   postoperative care, 615
   surgical technique
      focal lesions, 614
      pancreatectomy, 614
      PET scan localization, 614–615
Hyperkalemia, 62
Hypernatremia
   definition, 59
   etiology and treatment, 59–60
   hypervolemia, 60
   hypovolemia, 60
Hyperparathyroidism
   postoperative care, 210
   primary, 208, 209
   secondary, 208
   surgical technique, 209–210
   tertiary, 209
Hypertrophic pyloric stenosis (HPS), 345
   diagnosis, 341
   incidence, 341
   parental preparation, 345
   postoperative care, 343–344
   preoperative preparation, 341–342
   surgical technique, 342–343
Hypokalemia
   cell movement, 61
   definition, 61
   etiology, 61
   increased non-renal losses, 61
   increased renal losses, 61
   treatment, 61–62
Hyponatremia
   etiology and treatment, 58
   euvolemia, 59
   hypervolemia, 59
   hypovolemia, 58
   pseudohyponatremia, 59
   symptoms, 57
Hypoplasia, 829
Hypospadias
   complications
      blood supply, 655
      hypospadias repair, 656
      meatal stenosis, 655
   surgical technique
      cover penis, 654
      deglove penis, 652
      repair, CHOP approach, 655
      straighten penis, 652–653
      Z-plasty closure, 656
Hypotension, 111
Hypovolemic shock, 49

I
Ileal disease, 437–438
Ileal pouch anal anastomosis (IPAA). *See* Ulcerative colitis (UC)
Ileocecal intussussception. *See* Intussusception
Ileocecectomy
   Crohn's disease, 438–439
   inflammatory bowel disease, 430

Ileo-colic intussusception, idiopathic, 403–405. *See also* Intussusception
Ileostomy
    Bishop–Koop technique, meconium ileus, 397–398
    colitis, 439
    complications of, 448
    ileal pouch anal anastomosis, 494
    indications
        end stoma, 444
        function and types, 443–444
        permanent stomas, 445
    loop ileostomy, 446
    parental preparation, 449
    postoperative care, 447
    preoperative preparation, 445
    primary incision, 445–446
    stoma closure, 447
Ilioinguinal and iliohypogastric block, 25
Immune thrombocytopenic purpura (ITP), 627
Indomethacin therapy, PDA, 284, 287
    contraindications, 284–285
    risk, 285
Inflammatory bowel disease, 430
Inguinal hernia
    contralateral exploration, 666–667
    diagnostic studies, 671
    differentiation, 664
    embryology, 663
    incarceration, 669
    laparoscopic repair, 667–669
    parental preparation, 671
    physical examination, 664
    postoperative care, 669–670
    surgical repair, 665–666
    treatment, 665–666
Inhalation injury, 124–125
Innocent heart murmurs, 5
Intestinal atresia
    apple-peel lesion management, 362
    colonic, 361
    diagnosis, 359
    differential diagnosis, 362
    duodenal, 360 (*see also* Duodenal atresia)
    incidence, 359
    jejunoileal, 360–361
    parental preparation, 362
    postoperative care, 361
    treatment, 360
Intestinal failure (IF). *See* Short bowel syndrome
Intestinal failure-associated liver disease (IFALD), 34, 35
Intestinal neuronal dysplasia (IND), 481–482
Intestinal rotational anomalies. *See* Rotational anomalies, intestine
Intestinal transplantation
    differential diagnosis, 861
    endoscopy, 860
    mucosal biopsy, 860
    parental preparation, 858, 861
    patients, 857
    postoperative management
        immunosuppression, 859–860
        nutrition, 859
    preoperative care, 858

principles, 857
    transplant graft type
        isolated intestinal transplant, 858–859
        liver and small-bowel transplant, 859
        multivisceral transplantation, 859
Intrahepatic cholestasis
    complications, 577
    differential diagnosis, 577
    disorders of, 575
    parental preparation, 577
    postoperative care, 576
    surgical technique, 575–576
Intraparehchmal hemorrhage, 114, 115
Intussusception
    diagnosis
        contrast studies, 402
        differential diagnosis, 403, 406
        physical examination, 401, 402
        plain abdominal radiographs, 401, 402
        ultrasound, 401–402
    incidence, 401
    parental preparation, 407
    treatment, 403
        entero-enteric intussusception, 405
        idiopathic ileo-colic intussusception, 403–405
    and Wilms tumor, 407
ITP. *See* Immune thrombocytopenic purpura

J
Jaundice. *See* Biliary atresia; Hyperbilirubinemia, neonatal
Jejunoileal atresia, 360–361
Juvenile hypertrophy, 830–831

K
Karydakis procedure, pilonidal cyst, 470
46XX Karyotype
    CYP21, 695
    genetic etiologies, 696
    21
    -hydroxylase deficiency, 695
        lipoid adrenal hyperplasia, 696
        steroid biosynthetic pathway, 695
Kawasaki disease, 215
Kidney transplantation
    diagnosis, 845
    operative approach, 841
    parental preparation, 845
    postoperative management
        acute oliguria, 842
        anti-allograft, 843
        delayed graft function, 842
        fluid management, 842
        focal segmental glomerulosclerosis (FSGS), 843
        hypertension, 844
        immunosuppression, 842
        infections, 843–844
        prophylactic therapy, 841
    preoperative planning, 840–841
    quality of life, 844
    rehabilitation, 844
    therapeutic options, 839–840
Kikuchi–Fujimoto disease, 215
Klippel–Trenaunay syndrome, 823

L

Ladd procedure, intestinal rotational anomalies,
    377–378
Laparoscopic Heller myotomy, 275–277
Laparoscopic splenectomy, 629
Laryngeal mask airway, 5
Laryngotracheal injury, 120
L-dihydroxyphenylalanine (L-DOPA), 612
Lead poisoning, chronic abdominal pain, 433
Linear skull fracture, 112
Liver cysts, 366
Liver dysfunction, short bowel syndrome,
    388–389
Liver transplantation
    contraindications, 848
    donor considerations, 848–849
    indications
        biliary atresia, 847
        evaluation, 848
        fulminant hepatic failure, 847
        hepatoblastoma, 847–848
        vascular tumors, 848
    outcomes, 854–855
    parental preparation, 856
    postoperative care
        acute cellular rejection, 853
        biliary complications, 852–853
        infection, 853–854
        primary nonfunction (PNF), 851
        renal insufficiency, 854
        vascular thrombosis, 851–852
    retransplantation, 854
    surgical technique, 850
Liver tumors
    angiosarcoma, 769
    benign
        focal nodular hyperplasia(FNH), 764
        hepatic adenoma, 764
        hepatic teratoma, 764
        infantile hepatic hemangioma, 761–763
        mesenchymal hamartoma, 762–763
    biliary rhabdomyoscarcoma, 769
    diagnosis, 765
    differential diagnosis, 762
    hepatic sarcomas, 769
    hepatocellular carcinoma, 769
    imaging
        abdominal CT, 765
        CT angiogram, 765–766
        pretreatment extent of tumor (PRETEXT),
            766–767
        treatment, 766
    malignant, 764–765
    metastatic colorectal tumors, 770
    preoperative preparation, 771
    rhabdoid tumor, 769
    treatment
        biopsy, 766
        gross resection, 767
        SIOPEL study, 767
        staging, 767–768
    undifferentiated/embryonal sarcoma, 769–770
Lobectomy
    chest tube, 301
    differential diagnosis, 302
    Ligasure device, 300–301

    lower lobes, 301
    postoperate care, 301
    upper lobes, 301
Long-gap esophageal atresia, 244
    complications, 241–242
    definition, 233
    diagnosis, 233–234
    differential diagnosis, 244
    esophageal reconstruction, 237–241
    esophageal replacement
        colon interposition, 242
        gastric transposition, 242–243
        gastric tube, 242–243
        infants, 243
        jejunum, 243
        mediastinal routes, 242
    gap measurement, 236–237
    gastrostomy, 235–236
    parental preparation, 244
    postoperative care, 240–241
    preoperative preparation, 244
    tracheoscopy, 234–236
Lumbar hernia, 544
Lund and Browder chart, 125
Lung biopsy
    children, 300
    diagnosis, 299–300
    differential diagnosis, 300
    indications, 299
    patient position, 300
    postoperate care, 300
    preoperative preparation, 300
    procedure, 300
Lymphangioma cysts, 365–366
Lymphatic malformations
    characterization, 822
    treatment, 826

M

Macular stains, 821
Maffucci's syndrome, 823
Malignant hyperthermia
    characterization, 10–11
    genetic susceptibility, 11
    treatment, 11
Malone procedure
    anorectal malformations, 509–510
    constipation, 455–457
Malrotation. *See* Rotational anomalies, intestine
Marsupialization, pilonidal cyst, 469–470
MAS. *See* Mid-aortic syndrome
Mayer–Rokitansky–Kuster–Houser syndrome, 701
MCDK. *See* Multicystic dysplastic kidney
Mechanical tamponade,
    portal hypertension, 603
Mechanical ventilation
    advanced modes, 86–87
    basic modes, 86
    non-invasive positive pressure, 87
Meckel's diverticulum
    diagnosis, 410–411
    differential diagnosis, 412
    embryologic origin of, 409
    heterotopic mucosa types, 409
    incidence, 409

parental preparation, 412
presentation of
    bowel obstruction, 409–410
    inflammation, 410
    painless gastrointestinal bleeding, 409
treatment, 411
Meconium ileus
complications of, 399
diagnosis, 395–396
differential diagnosis, 400
parental preparation, 400
postoperative care, 398–399
treatment
    gastrostomy, 398
    ileostomy, 397–398
    laparotomy, 397
    nonoperative therapy, 396–397
Mediastinal masses
biopsy techniques, 325–326
diagnosis
    biopsy, 324–325
    chest X-ray and MRI, 324
    physical examination, 324
    symptoms, 323–324
differential diagnosis, 329
mediastinum, 323
postoperative care, 328
preoperative preparation, 325, 328
treatment
    anterior compartment lesions, 326–327
    posterior mediastinal masses, 327
Melanoma
adjuvant therapy, 810–811
diagnosis
    atypical nevi, 807–808
    biopsy, 806
    congenital nevi, 806–807
    development, 805
    halo nevi, 807
    measurement, 806
    physical examination, 805
    Spitz nevi, 808
differential diagnosis, 812
parental preparation, 812
preoperative preparation, 812
prognosis, 811
sentinel lymph node biopsy, 810
staging, 808–809
surgical therapy, 809–810
Mesenteric cysts, 366
Metacarpophalangeal dislocations, 163
Metastatic colorectal tumors, 770
Methicillin resistant *Staphylococcus aureus* (MRSA),
    shock, 49
Micropenis, 659
Mid-aortic syndrome (MAS), 882
Mikulicz operation, meconium ileus, 398
Monti–Yang ileocecostomy, 455–457
Morgagni hernia, 540
Multicystic dysplastic kidney (MCDK)
diagnosis, 643–644
etiology, 643
lateral retroperitoneoscopic nephrectomy, 645–646
macroscopical analysis, 643
nonoperative treatment, 644
surgical therapy, 644–645

Musculoskeletal surgical oncology
benign, 776–777
bone sarcomas
    biopsy, 777
    neoadjuvant chemotherapy, 778
    postoperative care, 779–780
    preoperative technique, 777
    surgical technique, 778–779
diagnosis
    pain scale, 773
    radiographic technique,
        774–775
    visual and physical examination, 773
differential diagnosis, 774, 775
limb-sparing reconstruction, 779
osteosarcoma, resected, 778
parental preparation, 782
rotationoplasty, 780
soft tissue sarcomas, 780
unplanned resections, 780–781
Mycobacterial lymphadenitis, 799
Myectomy-myotomy, Hirschsprung disease, 481
Myelomeningocele (MMC), 875–877

N
Narcotics, 39
Nasogastric feeding tubes, 28
National Surgical Quality Improvement Program
    (NSQIP), 44
Neck injuries, 121
diagnosis and initial management
    airway assessment, 118
    hemorrhage, 117–118
    laryngotracheal injury, 118–119
    neurological injuries, 119
management, 120
neck, anatomy, 117, 118
operative technique
    laryngotracheal injury, 120
    pharyngo-esophageal injuries, 120
    vascular injury, 119
Necrotizing enterocolitis
colostomy, 446
diagnosis, 381
differential diagnosis, 385
ileostomy, 445
parental preparation, 386
postoperative care, 384
preoperative preparation,
    381–382
rectal bacterial microbiome, 382
surgical technique
    laparotomy, 383–384
    peritoneal drainage, 382–383
Necrotizing fasciitis
causes, 816
characterization, 815
classification, 815
diagnosis, 815–816
parental preparation, 818
postoperative care, 817
preoperative preparation, 816
treatment
    hyperbaric oxygen therapy, 817
    surgical removal, 816

Neisseria gonorrhoeae, 680
Neuroblastoma
    bone marrow/stem cell transplantation, 711
    chemotherapy, 711
    clinical presentation, 709–710
    diagnosis
        histopathology, 710
        risk stratification, 710–711
        staging, 710
    differential diagnosis, 713
    immunotherapy, 711
    parental preparation, 713
    radionuclides therapy, 711–712
    retinoid therapy, 711
    surgery, 711
    treatment, 711–712
Neurofibromas, 796
Neurogenic shock, 49
Nissen–Rosetti. *See* Fundoplasty
Non-Hodgkin's lymphoma (NHL), 205, 326
Non-invasive positive pressure mechanical ventilation (NIPPV),
        87–88
Nonpalpable testis, 673
Non-rhabdomyosarcoma soft tissue sarcomas (NRSTS), 755
North American pediatric renal transplant cooperative study
        (NAPRTCS), 843

O
Obesity
    bariatric surgery
        complications, 420–421
        laparoscopic procedure, 418–419
        outcomes, 421
        parental preparation, 422
        patient selection, 415
        perioperative management, 418
        postoperative management, 419–420
        preoperative assessment, 415–416
        surgical options, 416–418
Obstructive sleep apnea, 4
Omental cysts, 366
Omphalitis infection, umbilical disorders, 548
Omphalocele
    bladder extrophy, 528
    complications, 527–528
    diagnosis, 523–524
    differential diagnosis, 528
    etiology and incidence, 523
    operative treatment
        amnioinversion, 526–527
        delayed closure, 525–526
        primary closure, 524–525
    parental preparation, 529
    postnatal care, 524
Omphalocele-exstrophy-imperforate anus-spinal defects
        (OEIS), 685
Ovarian cysts, 432
Ovarian torsion, 742
Ovarian tumors
    alpha fetoprotein (AFP), 741, 742
    cystic lesions
        corpus luteum, 742
        neoplastic, 741–742
        non-neoplastic, 741
    differential diagnosis, 746

    epithelial cells, 745–746
    germ cell tumors
        malignant, 745
        primordial germ cell and point mutations, 744
        sex cord-stromal tumors, 745
        teratomas, 743–744
    imaging techniques, 741
    management strategy, 746
    mixed and solid masses
        laparotomy, 742–743
        malignant, 742
        staging, 742–743
    ovarian torsion, 742
    parental preparation, 747
    pathology, 741
Ovotesticular DSD, 698
Oxygen delivery, 50

P
Palpable testis, 673
Pancreas disorders
    anatomic abnormalities
        annular pancreas, 617–618
        pancreas divisum, 618–619
        pancreatic cysts, 618
    endocrine disorders
        diagnosis, 619
        hyperinsulinism, 619
        localization, 620
        operative care, 619–620
        treatment, 619–621
        Zollinger–Ellison syndrome, 619
    pancreatitis
        causes, 621
        etiological factors, 620
        imaging techniques, 621–622
        physical examination, 621
        symptoms, 621
        treatment, 622
    pseudocyst, 622
Pancreas divisum, 618–619
Pancreatectomy, 614–615
Pancreatic cysts, 366, 618
Pancreatic pseudocyst, 622
Pancreatitis
    causes, 621
    etiological factors, 620
    imaging techniques,
        621–622
    physical examination, 621
    symptoms, 621
    treatment, 622
Parathyroid disorders
    adenomas, 211
    hyperparathyroidism
        (*see* Hyperparathyroidism)
    parental preparation, 212
    preoperative preparation, 212
Parenteral nutrition
    administration routes, 33–34
    calories, 34
    carbohydrates, 34
    complications, 35
    electrolytes, 35
    fat, 34–35

home parenteral nutrition, 35
indications, 33
nutrient requirements, 34–35
protein, 34
Patent ductus arteriosus (PDA)
bleeding, 287
complications, 286
diagnosis, 284, 287
differential diagnosis, 287
ductal closure, phases, 283
fetal development, 283
incidence, 283
indomethacin, 284
morbidity, 283–284
parental preparation, 287
posterolateral thoracotomy, 287
preoperative preparation, 287
surgical closure, complications, 286–287
treatment strategies, 284–286
vascular structure, erroneous ligation, 287
Pectus carinatum
bracing technique, 319–320
etiology, 319
symptoms, 319
technical points, 321
Pectus excavatum
anatomic classifications, 313–314
cardiac effects, 314–315
cause, 313
characteristics, 313
deformity depth, 314
exercise program for, 314
incidence rate, 313
preoperative evaluation, 315–316
pulmonary effects, 315
surgical technique
and aerobic sports, 317
antibiotics, 317
complications of, 318
marking of, 316
open technique, 318–319
pectus bar removal, 319
pressure effects on, 316–317
stabilizer, 317
substernal tunnel correction, 316, 317
thoracoscopy, 316
technical points, 321
thoracic kyphosis, 314
Pediatric surgery
computerized physician order entry (CPOE), 42
evidence-based practice, 43
medication error, 41–42
surgical morbidity and mortality (M&M), 42–43
surgical outcomes research, 43–44
Pediatric trauma resuscitation, 103, 110
cardiac arrest, algorithm, 104
diagnostic procedures
CT scanning, 108–109
diagnostic peritoneal lavage, 109
plain radiographs, 108
ED thoracotomy, 109
parenteral preparation, 110
prehospital care
airway management, 103
chest X-ray, 103–104
c-spine immobilization, 104

primary survey
airway, 104–105
breathing, 105
circulation, 105–106
disability, 106–107
exposure, 107
secondary survey
chest X-ray, 107
digital rectal exam, 108
Foley catheter, 107
laboratory studies, 107–108
nasogastric tube, 107
re-evaluation, 108
tertiary survey, 109
Pelvic inflammatory disease (PID), chronic abdominal pain, 432
Penile anomalies
aphallia, 659
circumcision
Gomco clamp, 659
techniques, 659
congenital penile curvature, 657
epispadias, 658–659
hidden penis, 651
hypospadias
complications, 653, 655–657
surgical technique, 652–653
megameatus intact prepuce (MIP), 657
micropenis, 659
parental preparation, 662
phimosis, 657–658
preputial glanular adhesions, 657
urethral duplication, 659
Penile nerve block, 25
Percutaneously with endoscopic (PEG), 29
Perianal disease
anal fissure, 462–463
differential diagnosis, 465
fistula-in-ano, 462
pilonidal sinuses, 463
rectal prolapse, 461–462
Peripherally inserted central catheter (PICC), 33, 65
Peripheral lymphadenopathy, 800
Perirectal disease, 440–441
Peritoneal dialysis
parental preparation, 557
postoperative care, 555–556
catheter-care procedures, 555
exit-site infections, 556
intra-abdominal pressure, 555–556
peritonitis, 555
preoperative preparation, 553
surgical technique
laparoscopic method, 554–555
open method, 553–554
Petit hernia, 544
PFIC. See Progressive familial intrahepatic cholestasis
Phalangeal neck fractures, 161–162
Pharyngo-esophageal injuries, 120
Pheochromocytoma
characterization, 726
diagnosis, 728
signs and symptoms, 726–727
treatment, 727
Phimosis, 657–658
Phototherapy, jaundice, 562
Pigtail catheter, pneumothorax treatment, 307

Pilomatrixomas cysts, 798
Pilonidal cyst
    abscess drainage, 468
    differential diagnosis, 467–468
    etiology of, 467
    nonoperative management, 468–469
    postoperative care, 472
    prevalence in, 467
    sexual maturation affect in, 467
    surgical therapy
        cleft lift procedure, 470–471
        complex flaps, 471–472
        excision with primary closure, 470
        lateral advancement flap, 470
        marsupialization, 469–470
        wide excision, 469
Pilonidal sinuses, 463
Ping-pong ball fractures, 113
Pneumothorax
    initial evaluation, 307
    parental preparation, 311
    physical examination of, 307
    treatment
        catheterization, 307
        oxygen therapy, 307
        surgical therapy, 308
Polymastia, 829
Polyposis, familial, 495–496
Polythelia, 829
Portal hypertension
    causes of, 599, 600
    definition, 599
    diagnosis, 601
    endoscopic intervention for
        band ligation, 603
        liver transplantation, 609
        non-shunt procedures, 608
        portosystemic shunt operations, 603–607
        sclerotherapy, 603
        transjugular intrahepatic portosystemic shunt, 607–608
    intra-hepatic causes, 600
    mechanical tamponade, 603
    nonoperative treatment, 601–602
    parental preparation, 610
    pharmacologic intervention, 602
    post-hepatic causes, 601
    pre-hepatic obstruction, 600
Portoenterostomy, biliary atresia
    postoperative care, 570–571
    procedure, 568–570
Post-prandial hypoglycemia (PPHG), 337–338
Post-pyloric feeding tubes, 28
Prenatal diagnosis
    array-based comparative genomic hybridization (array CGH), 20–21
    birth anomalies (see Birth anomalies)
    chromosome analysis, 20
    fluorescence in situ hybridization (FISH), 20
    genetic inheritance mechanisms (see Genetic inheritance mechanisms)
Preoperative assessment
    airway/respiratory system, 3–5
    allergy, 12
    anemia, 7
    anesthesia risks, 3
    anterior mediastinal mass, 8–9
    cerebral palsy, 9

congenital heart disease, 5–6
    corticosteroids, 7
    developmental disorders, 9
    diabetes, 6–7
    fasting, 13
    gastroesophageal reflux disease, 6
    hemoglobin/hematocrit, 14
    herbal/homeopathic medications, 12
    hypotonia, 9
    malignancy, 8
    malignant hyperthermia, 10–11
    medications, 12
    NSAIDs and aspirin, 12
    obesity, 6
    pregnancy testing, 14
    prematurity, infants, 9–10
    sickle cell anemia, 8
    thyroid disease, 7
    trisomy 20, 11–12
    Von Willebrand disease, 8
Proctectomy, ulcerative colitis, 493–494
Progressive familial intrahepatic cholestasis (PFIC)
    complications, 577
    differential diagnosis, 577
    parental preparation, 577
    partial external biliary diversion (PEBD), 575–576
    postoperative care, 576
    types of, 575
Proteus syndrome, 823
Pseudocysts, 367
Pseudohermaphroditism. *See* 46XX Karyotype
Pseudohyponatremia, 59
Pyloromyotomy, hypertrophic pyloric stenosis, 344
    complications, 343
    parental preparation, 345
    postoperative course, 343
    principles, 342–343
    supraumbilical *vs.* laparoscopic method, 343–344
Pyogenic granulomas, 796

R
Radiocontrast nephropathy, 79
Rectal prolapse, 461–462
Rectus sheath block, 25
Regional anesthetic techniques
    advantages, 23, 25
    epidural anesthesia (*See* Epidural anesthesia)
    ilioinguinal and iliohypogastric block, 25
    penile nerve block, 25
    rectus sheath block, 25
    spinal anesthesia/analgesia, 24–25
Renal abnormalities
    anomalies of fusion, 647
    autosomic recessive (ARPKD), 648
    bilateral renal agenesis (BRA), 642–643
    diagnostic studies, 649
    ectopic kidney, 647
    MCDK
        diagnosis, 643–644
        etiology, 643
        lateral retroperitoneoscopic nephrectomy, 645–646
        macroscopical analysis, 643
        nonoperative treatment, 644
        surgical therapy, 644–645
    parental preparation, 649
    polycystic kidney, 646

renal cyst, 646–647
URA
  imaging techniques, 642
  ipsilateral adrenal gland, 642
  mutation, 641
  ultrasound, 641
  urogenital tract, 641
Renal cyst, 646–647
Resting energy expenditure (REE), 34
Reverse rotation. *See* Rotational anomalies, intestine
Rex shunt, portal hypertension, 605–607
Rhabdomyolysis, 78–79
Rhabdomyosarcoma
  clinical staging and grouping, 729–730
  diagnosis, 729
  differential diagnosis, 734
  metastatic disease, 732
  parental preparation, 734
  postoperative care, 732
  survival rate, 732
  treatment
    biopsy, 730–731
    imaging studies, 732
    primary re-excision (PRE), 731
    secondary excision, 731
    surgical principles, 731–732
Richter's hernia, 543
Rigid bronchoscopy, 190–191
Rosai–Dorfman disease, 215
Rotational anomalies, intestine
  diagnosis
    abdominal radiograph, 375
    bilious vomiting, 374
    ultrasound, 375–376
  differential diagnosis, 379
  embryology
    malrotation, 373–374
    nonrotation and reverse rotation, 374
    normal intestinal rotation, 373
  parental preparation, 380
  postoperative care, 378
  treatment
    aggressive intravenous hydration, 377
    appendectomy, 377, 378
    surgical method, 377–378
Roux-Y technique, gastrostomy, 349

S
Sacrococcygeal teratoma (SCT), 876
  parental preparation, 739
  postnatal diagnosis, Curarino's triad, 737
  postoperative care, 738
  prenantal diagnosis, 735–736
  preoperative preparation, 739
  treatment, 737–738
Santulli–Blanc operation, meconium ileus, 398
Sarcoidosis, 215
Scaphoid fracture, 163
Sclerotherapy, 200
Scrotal pain
  diagnosis
    cremasteric reflex, 680
    etiology, 679
    history, 679
    palpation, abdomen, 680

differential diagnosis, 682
manual detorsion, 681
neonate torsion, 681
parental preparation, 683
postoperative care, 681–682
surgical management, 681
urinalysis, 680
SCT. *See* Sacrococcygeal teratoma (SCT)
Septic shock, 49
Serial transverse enteroplasty (STEP), 390
Sex development disorders.
      See Disorder of sex development (DSD)
Seymour fracture, 163
Shock
  anaphylactic shock, 49
  cardiogenic shock, 49
  definition, 49
  diagnosis, 49–50
  goal-directed guidelines, 51
  hypovolemic shock, 49
  intensive care unit, 52
  neurogenic shock, 49
  physiologic principles, 50–51
  resuscitation, first hour, 51–52
  septic shock, 49
Short bowel syndrome
  causes of, 387
  diagnosis
    citrulline levels, 388
    feeding intolerance, 388
    intra-operative measurement, 387
    stool analysis, 387–388
  parental preparation, 393
  postoperative care
    essential fatty acid deficiency, 391
    infections of, 391–392
    persistent anemia, 391
  treatment strategies
    medications, 389
    nutrition, 388–389
    surgical technique, 390–391
Sickle cell anemia
  chronic abdominal pain, 433
  preoperative assessment, 8
  spleen disorders, 627
Silo-assisted closure, gastroschisis, 517–518
Single-port access abdominal, 789–791
Skull fracture
  basilar, 113
  complications, 113
  depressed, 112–113
  linear, 112
  surgical intervention, 113
Smead–Jones knots, gastroschisis, 519
Soave procedure, Hirschsprung disease, 477
Soft tissue tumors
  adjuvant therapy benefits, 758
  benign lesions, 755
  cytogenetic anomalies, 755
  diagnosis, 755–756
  differential diagnosis, 759
  histological types, 755
  parental preparation, 759
  postoperative care, 757
  preoperative preparation, 756
  surgical technique, 756–757

Somatostatin, portal hypertension, 602
Spider angiomas, 823
Spigelian hernia, 544
Spinal anesthesia/analgesia, 24–25
Spinal cord injury without radiological abnormality
    (SCIWORA), 151
Spine trauma
    atlanto-occipital injuries, 153
    clinical signs, 151
    complications, 155
    compression injuries, 154
    diagnosis, 152
    differential diagnosis, 156
    facet fracture-dislocation, 153–154
    flexion-distraction injuries, 154–155
    incidence, 151
    neurologic examination, 151–152
    parental preparation, 156
    preoperative preparation, 152–153, 156
    subaxial cervical spine injury, 153
    thoracic and lumbar spine, 154
    treatment, 153
Spleen disorders
    abscess, 627
    anatomy, 625
    cyst, 627–628
    cystectomy, 630
    differential diagnosis, 632
    erythrocyte enzyme deficiency, 627
    function, 625–626
    hereditary spherocytosis (HS), 626
    ITP, 627
    malignancy, 628
    parental preparation, 632
    partial splenectomy
        hemoglobin levels, 628
        immunoprophylaxis, 629
        laparoscopy, 629–630
        postoperative chemoprophylaxis, 629
        preoperative care, 628
    postoperative complications, 630
    preoperative preparation, 628
    sickle cell anemia, 627
    surgical technique, 629
    thalassemia, 626
Splenic abscess, 627
Splenic cystectomy, 629, 630
Splenic cysts, 366, 627–628
Spontaneous pneumothorax. *See* Pneumothorax
Stenotic/occlusive diseases
    complications, 883
    diagnosis, 881–882
    differential diagnosis, 881–882
    preoperative preparation, 882–884
    surgical technique, 883
    symptoms, 881
    vascular reconstruction, 884
Subaxial cervical spine injury, 153
Subcutaneous endoscopy
    diagnosis
        abdominal conditions, 786
        forehead and brow lesions, 785
        neck lesions, 785–786
    differential diagnosis, 792
    parental preparation, 792
    postoperative care, 791

preoperative preparation, 793
    surgical technique
        single-port access abdominal, 789–791
        transaxillary subcutaneous endoscopy,
            787–789
        trans-scalp subcutaneous endoscopy,
            786–787
Subdural hematoma (SDH), 114
Subjective global assessment (SGA), 27
Subtotal colectomy (SC), ulcerative colitis
    cyclosporine and toxic megacolon, 491
    infliximab, 491–492
    surgical technique, 492
Surgical morbidity and mortality (M&M), 42–45

T
Tension pneumothorax. *See* Pneumothorax
Teratomas, 743–744
Testicular tumor, pediatric
    characteristics, 749
    differential diagnosis, 752
    histological distribution
        epidermoid cysts, 750
        sertoli cell, 750
        teratomas, 749–750
        yolk sac tumors, 749
    parental preparation, 752
    staging, 750
    surveillance, 751
    treatment, 750–751
Testis. *See* Undescended testis
TGDC. *See* Thyroglossal duct cysts
Thalassemia, 626
Thelarche, 830
Thermal injuries
    burns (*see* Burns)
    etiology, 123
Thoracic trauma
    diagnosis, 145–146, 150
    initial management, 145
    parental preparation, 150
    treatment
        cardiac contusions, 146
        emergency department thoracotomy, 149
        esophageal perforation, 147
        penetrating thoracic trauma, 147–149
        pneumothorax and hemothorax, 148
        pulmonary contusions, 146
        ribs and thoracic cage injury, 147
        thoracic duct injury, 147
        tracheal and bronchial injuries, 146–147
        traumatic asphyxia, 146–147
Thoracoscopic biopsy and lobectomy, lung, 302
    biopsy (*see* Lung biopsy)
    French tube, 302
    hemithorax, 302
    lobectomy (*see* Lobectomy)
    parental preparation, 302
    pulmonary lobar lesions, 301
Thrombotic thrombocytopenic purpura (TTP), 78
Thyroglossal duct cysts (TGDC)
    acute infection, 196
    antibiotics, 197
    branchial cleft cysts (*see* Branchial cleft cysts)
    bronchogenic cysts, 199

carcinoma, 197
  cervical thymic cysts, 199
  epidermoid and dermoid cysts, 199
  external appearance, 196
  history and physical examination, 196
  incidence, 196
  lymphatic malformations, 199–200
  parental preparation, 201
  radioisotope scanning, 196–197
  recurrence risk, 197
  surgical excision, 197
Thyroid disorders, 212
  autoimmune inflammatory thyroid
    Graves' disease, 204–205
    Hashimoto's thyroiditis, 204
  carcinoma
    differentiated thyroid cancer, 205
    Hodgkins and non-Hodgkins lymphoma, 205
    medullary carcinoma, 205
    papillary and follicular thyroid carcinoma, 205
  differential diagnosis, 212
  functional thyroid disorders
    goiter, 203–204
    imaging studies, 203
    plasma T3 and T4 measurements, 203
    thyroid stimulating hormone (TSH), 203
  parental preparation, 212
  preoperative preparation, 212
  surgical therapy
    family history and physical exam, 206
    fine needle aspiration, 206–207
    near-total thyroidectomy, 207
    outcomes, 208
    pediatric thyroid nodules, 206
    radioablative therapy, 207–208
    subtotal thyroidectomy, 207
    surveillance, 208
    total thyroidectomy, 207
Tissue plasminogen activator (tPA), empyema, 310
Torsion, 681
Tracheoesophageal fistula
  complications, 227–229
  diagnosis and treatment, 231
  differential diagnosis, 232
  esophagram, 230
  Fogarty catheter and balloon, 230
  parental preparation, 232
  preoperative preparation, 232
  signs and symptoms, 230
Tracheostomy
  anatomical landmarks, 179
  cartilaginous structures, 179
  complications, 180
  endotracheal tube, 179–180
  polypropylene sutures, 179
Transaxillary subcutaneous endoscopy
  lateralized lesions, 787–788
  parathyroid adenoma excision, 789
  patient positioning, 787
  subcutaneous space, 788
  thyroglossal duct cyst excision, 788
Transjugular intrahepatic portosystemic shunt, portal hypertension, 607–608
Transplantation
  in biliary atresia, 571
  liver, endoscopic intervention for, 609

Trans-scalp subcutaneous endoscopy
  dissection, 787
  forehead, 787
  local anaesthesia, 786–787
  telescope and instrument placement, 786
Trauma, 705
  abdomen (*see* Abdominal trauma)
  burns (*see* Burns)
  child abuse (*see* Child abuse)
  hands (*see* Hand injuries)
  head (*see* Head trauma)
  neck injuries, 117–121
  pediatric trauma resuscitation
    (*see* Pediatric trauma resuscitation)
  spine (*see* Spine trauma)
  thoracic trauma (*see* Thoracic trauma)
  vascular injury, 157–160
Traumatic abdominal wall hernias (TAWH), 545
Traumatic brain injury, 114
Tubo-ovarian abscess (TOA), 432–433
Tumors, 367
  chronic abdominal pain, 432
  gastrointestinal tract, 410
  hepatic resection, 593–598
Twin–twin transfusion syndrome, 873

U
Ulcerative colitis (UC)
  ileal pouch anal anastomosis
    anti-inflammatory medications, 493
    catheterization, 493
    endorectal retraction, 493
    ileostomy, 494
    intravenous antibiotics, 492–493
    J-pouch construct, 493–495
    proctectomy, 493–494
    risks and uncertainties, 492
    steroid dependence, 492
  outcome, 495
  parental and family preparation, 497
  subtotal colectomy, 491–492
Umbilical disorders. *See also* Gastroschisis
  differential diagnosis, 552
  drainage defects of, 549
  granuloma, 547
  hernias, 547–548
  omphalitis, 548
  parental preparation, 552
  polyp, 547
  postoperative care, 551
  treatment, 550–551
  trunk-like umbilicus, 548
  umbilical-appendiceal fistula, 549–550
  urachal cyst, 548
Umbilicoplasty, 550–551
Undescended testis
  classification, 673
  diagnosis, 674
  differential diagnosis, 676
  parental preparation, 676
  postoperative care, 675
  treatment
    laparoscopic techniques, 675
    orchidopexy, 674
    surgical repair, 674

Unilateral renal agenesis (URA)
    imaging techniques, 642
    ipsilateral adrenal gland, 642
    mutation, 641
    ultrasound, 641
Ureteral advancement (Glenn–Anderson) technique, vesicoureteral
        reflux, 636
Ureteropelvic junction (UPJ) obstruction
    anastomosis, 637–638
    retroperitoneal approach, 637
Urinalysis, 75
Urine osmolality, 57–60, 75

V
Vagina
    anatomy, 702
    atresia
        Mayer–Rokitansky–Kuster-Houser syndrome, 701
        pedicle graft, 704
        surgical treatment, 701–703
        transverse obstructions, 702, 704
    diagnostic studies, 706
    embryology, 702
    foreign body, 705–706
    parental preparation, 706
    sexual abuse, 705
    trauma, 705
    tumors
        endodermal sinus, 703
        sarcoma botryoides, 702–703
        treatment, 703
VALI. See Ventilator-associated lung injury
Vascular access
    central venous catheter
        percutaneously inserted, 66, 69–70
        peripherally inserted, 65
        removal, 68
        tunneled, 66
    complications, 67
    difficult passage, 67
    implantable central venous access, 66
    parental preparation, 70
    peripheral intravenous access, 65
    trauma, 67–68
    umbilical vein, 65
    utrasound, 67
Vascular compression syndromes
    bleeding, 292
    complications, 291–292
    diagnosis, 289
    differential diagnosis, 292
    double aortic arch, 290
    innominate artery compression, 289
    ligamentum arteriosum, 290
    parental preparation, 292
    preoperative preparation, 292
    pulmonary artery slings, 289
    right-sided arch, 290
    treatment, 289–290
    vascular rings, 289
Vascular injury, 119
    diagnosis, 157–158
    outcomes, 158–159
    preoperative preparation, 160
    treatment, 158

Vascular malformations
    classification, 819
    complications, 827
    diagnosis, 823–824
    differential diagnosis, 828
    hemangiomas
        characterization, 819
        spectrum of lesions, 819–821
        treatment, 824–825
    parental preparation, 828
    preoperative care, 828
    spectrum of lesions
        arteriovenous malformations (AVM), 823
        blue rubber bleb nevus syndrome,
            821–822
        capillary, 821
        glomus tumors, 822–823
        Klippel–Trenaunay syndrome, 823
        lymphatic malformations, 822
        macular stains, 821
        Maffucci's syndrome, 823
        proliferative phase, 819
        proteus syndrome, 823
        spider angiomas, 823
        venous malformations, 821
    treatment, 825–827
Vascular thrombosis, 851–852
Vasculitis, 434
Vasopressin, portal hypertension, 602
Vasospasm, 158
Venous malformations
    characterization, 821
    treatment, 826
Ventilator-associated lung injury (VALI)
    goals, 84
    hypothetical regions, 84
    low tidal volume approach, 84
    oxygen toxicity, 85
    partial ventilatory support, 85
    PEEP, 84–85
    plateau airway pressures, 85
Ventricular shunt system.
            See Hydrocephalus
Vesicoureteral reflux
    diagnosis, 635
    differential diagnosis, 639
    hydronephrosis grading system, 636
    parental preparation, 639
    postoperative care, 638
    secondary reflux, 635
    surgical therapy
        cross-trigonal (Cohen) technique, 636
        cystoscopic injection, 637
        intervention, 636
        laparoscopy, 637
        ureteral advancement
            (Glenn–Anderson) technique, 636
    treatment, 636
    ureteropelvic junction (UPJ) obstruction
        anastomosis, 637–638
        retroperitoneal approach, 637
Video-assisted thoracic surgery (VATS)
    empyema, 310
    PDA, 285–286
    pneumothorax, 308
Von Willebrand disease (vWD), 8

W

WAGR syndrome, 715
Warren shunt, portal hypertension, 605
Werdnig–Hoffman syndrome, 531
Wilms tumor (WT)
    bilateral Wilms tumor (BWT), 721
    diagnosis
        computed tomography (CT),
            716–717
        ultrasound, 715–716
    differential diagnosis, 723
    horseshoe kidney, 721
    intravascular extension, 720–721
    lung metastasis, 721–722
    nephroblastomatosis/nephrogenic rests (NR), 720
    parental preparation, 723
    staging
        histology, 717, 718

        loss of heterozygosity (LOH),
            717–718
        pathologic findings, 717
    surgical management
        contiguous organs, 719
        laparoscopy, 719
        lymph node documentation, 719
        tumor spillage, 719
        tumor unresectable,
            719–720
Wilms tumor in,
        intussusception, 405
Witzel technique, gastrostomy, 349
WT. *See* Wilms tumor (WT)

Z

Zollinger–Ellison syndrome, 619